a LANGE medical book

CURRENT
Diagnosis & Treatment
in Orthopedics

third edition

Edited by

Harry B. Skinner, MD, PhD
Professor and Chair
Department of Orthopedic Surgery
College of Medicine
University of California, Irvine
Irvine, California

Lange Medical Books/McGraw-Hill
Medical Publishing Division

New York   Chicago   San Francisco   Lisbon   London   Madrid   Mexico City
Milan   New Delhi   San Juan   Seoul   Singapore   Sydney   Toronto

Current Diagnosis & Treatment in Orthopedics, Third Edition

ISBN: 0-07-138758-7 (Domestic)

1 2 3 4 5 6 7 8 9 0 DOC/DOC 0 9 8 7 6 5 4 3

Notice

Medicine is an ever-changing science. As new research and clinical experience broaden our knowledge, changes in treatment and drug therapy are required. The authors and the publisher of this work have checked with sources believed to be reliable in their efforts to provide information that is complete and generally in accord with the standards accepted at the time of publication. However, in view of the possibility of human error or changes in medical sciences, neither the authors nor the publisher nor any other party who has been involved in the preparation or publication of this work warrants that the information contained herein is in every respect accurate or complete, and they disclaim all responsibility for any errors or omissions or for the results obtained from use of the information contained in this work. Readers are encouraged to confirm the information contained herein with other sources. For example and in particular, readers are advised to check the product information sheet included in the package of each drug they plan to administer to be certain that the information contained in this work is accurate and that changes have not been made in the recommended dose or in the contraindications for administration. This recommendation is of particular importance in connection with new or infrequently used drugs.

This book was set in Adobe Garamond by Pine Tree Composition, Inc.
The editors were Shelley Reinhardt, Janene Matragrano, and Regina Y. Brown.
The production supervisor was Catherine Saggese.
The index was prepared by Katherine Pitcoff.
The book designer was Eve Siegel.
The cover designer was Mary McKeon.
R.R. Donnelley was the printer and binder.

ISSN: 1081-0056

This book is printed on acid-free paper.

INTERNATIONAL EDITION ISBN: 0-07-112413-6

Contents

5. Disorders, Diseases, & Injuries of the Spine 205

Serena S. Hu, MD, Clifford B. Tribus, MD, Bobby K-B Tay, MD, & Gregory D. Carlson, MD

6. Tumors in Orthopedics 286

R. Lor Randall, MD

7. Adult Reconstructive Surgery 370

Robert S. Namba, MD, Harry B. Skinner, MD, & Ranjan Gupta, MD

8. Orthopedic Infections 414

Scott C. Wilson, MD

9. Foot & Ankle Surgery 449

Jeffrey A. Mann, MD, Loretta B. Chou, MD, & Steven D. K. Ross, MD

Authors

Robert L. Barrack, MD
Professor of Orthopedic Surgery; Adjunct Professor
of Biomedical Engineering; Director, Adult
Reconstructive Surgery, Tulane University Medical
Center & Hospital, New Orleans, Louisiana
rbarrack@tulane.edu
Basic Science in Orthopedic Surgery

Michael S. Bednar, MD
Associate Professor, Department of Orthopedic Surgery
and Rehabilitation, Loyola University of Chicago,
Stritch School of Medicine, Maywood, Illinois
mbednar@lumc.edu
Hand Surgery

Vincent J. Caiozzo, PhD
Associate Professor, Department of Orthopedics,
College of Medicine, University of California, Irvine
vjcaiozz@uci.edu
Basic Science in Orthopedic Surgery

Gregory D. Carlson, MD
Assistant Clinical Professor, University of California,
Irvine; Orthopedic Spine Surgeon, Orthopedic
Specialty Institute, Orange, California
gcarlson@ocspine.com
Disorders, Diseases, & Injuries of the Spine

Loretta B. Chou, MD
Assistant Professor, Department of Orthopedic
Surgery, Stanford University School of Medicine,
Stanford, California
lchou@stanford.edu
Foot & Ankle Surgery

Stephen D. Cook, PhD
Lee C. Schlesinger Professor, Department of
Orthopedic Surgery; Director of Orthopedic
Research, Tulane University School of Medicine,
New Orleans, Louisiana
scook2@tulane.edu
Basic Science in Orthopedic Surgery

Edward Diao, MD
Professor, Department of Orthopedic Surgery;
Chief, Division of Hand, Upper Extremity, and
Microvascular Surgery, University of California,
San Francisco
diaoe@orthosurg.ucsf.edu
Musculoskeletal Trauma Surgery

Ranjan Gupta, MD
Assistant Professor, Department of Orthopedic
Surgery, Center for Biomedical Engineering,
University of California, Irvine
ranjang@uci.edu
*Basic Science in Orthopedic Surgery; Adult Reconstructive
Surgery*

Serena S. Hu, MD
Associate Professor, Department of Orthopedic
Surgery, University of California, San Francisco
hus@orthosurg.ucsf.edu
Disorders, Diseases, & Injuries of the Spine

Mary Ann E. Keenan, MD
Professor and Chief, Neuro-Orthopedics Program,
Department of Orthopedic Surgery, University of
Pennsylvania School of Medicine, Philadelphia
maryann.keenan@uphs.upenn.edu
Rehabilitation

Terry R. Light, MD
Dr. William M. Scholl Professor and Chairman,
Department of Orthopedic Surgery and
Rehabilitation, Loyola University of Chicago,
Stritch School of Medicine, Maywood, Illinois
tlight@lumc.edu
Hand Surgery

David W. Lowenberg, MD
Associate Professor of Clinical Orthopedic Surgery,
University of California, San Francisco; and Chief of
Fracture Service, California Pacific Medical Center,
San Francisco
dwlowenberg@yahoo.com
Musculoskeletal Trauma Surgery

Jeffrey A. Mann, MD
Private Practice, Oakland, California
jeffmann@msn.com
Foot & Ankle Surgery

Patrick J. McMahon, MD
Assistant Professor, Divisions of Sports Medicine, and
Shoulder and Elbow Surgery, Department of
Orthopedic Surgery, University of Pittsburgh School
of Medicine, Pittsburgh, Pennsylvania
Sports Medicine

Robert S. Namba, MD
Associate Clinical Professor of Orthopedic Surgery,
University of California, Irvine, College of
Medicine; Attending Surgeon, Southern California
Permanente Medical Group, Anaheim, California
robert.s.namba@kp.org
Adult Reconstructive Surgery

George T. Rab, MD
Ben Ali Shriners Professor of Pediatric Orthopedics,
Chair, Department of Orthopedic Surgery, Chief,
Division of Pediatric Orthopedics, University of
California, Davis, School of Medicine; Consulting
Physician, Shriners Hospitals for Children, North-
ern California
george.rab@ucdmc.ucdavis.edu
Pediatric Orthopedic Surgery

R. Lor Randall, MD, FACS
Assistant Professor, Department of Orthopedics,
University of Utah School of Medicine; Director,
Sarcoma Services and Chief, SARC Laboratory,
Huntsman Cancer Institute; Attending Physician,
University Hospital, Primary Children's Medical
Center, Shriner's Hospital Intermountain, LDS
Hospital, Salt Lake City, Utah
Tumors in Orthopedics

Steven D.K. Ross, MD
Clinical Professor, Department of Orthopedic Surgery,
University of California, Irvine College of Medicine,
Orange, California
sdross@uci.edu
Foot & Ankle Surgery

John R. Shank, MD
Fellow in Foot and Ankle Surgery, Harborview
Medical Center, Seattle, Washington
johnrshank@yahoo.com
Musculoskeletal Trauma Surgery

Harry B. Skinner, MD, PhD
Professor and Chair, Department of Orthopedic
Surgery, University of California, Irvine
hskinner@uci.edu
*Basic Science in Orthopedic Surgery; General Considera-
tions in Orthopedic Surgery; Musculoskeletal Trauma
Surgery; Sports Medicine; Adult Reconstructive Surgery*

Douglas G. Smith, MD
Associate Professor, Department of Orthopedic
Surgery, University of Washington School of
Medicine, Seattle; Director, The Prosthetics
Research Study, Seattle, Washington; Medical
Director of the Amputee Coalition of America,
Knoxville, Tennessee
dgsmith@u.washington.edu
Amputations

Wade R. Smith, MD
Assistant Professor of Orthopedic Surgery, University
of Colorado School of Medicine, Denver, Colorado;
Director of Orthopedic Surgery, Denver Health
Medical Center, Denver, Colorado
wsmith@dhha.org
Musculoskeletal Surgery

Bobby K-B Tay, MD
Assistant Professor in Residence, Department of
Orthopedic Surgery, University of California at
San Francisco
tayb@orthosurg.ucsf.edu
Disorders, Diseases, & Injuries of the Spine

Clifford B. Tribus, MD
Associate Professor, Division of Orthopedics,
University of Wisconsin School of Medicine,
Madison, Wisconsin
tribus@surgery.wisc.edu
Disorders, Diseases, & Injuries of the spine

Robert L. Waters, MD
Clinical Professor of Orthopedics, University of
Southern California School of Medicine; Medical
Director, Ranchos Los Amigos National
Rehabilitation Center, Downey, California
Rehabilitation

Scott C. Wilson, MD
Assistant Professor of Orthopedic Surgery, Tulane
University School of Medicine, New Orleans,
Louisiana
mshinn@tulane.edu
Orthopedic Infections

Preface

This *Current Diagnosis & Treatment in Orthopedics* is the third edition of the orthopedic surgery contribution to the Lange CURRENT series of books. It is intended to fulfill a need for a ready source of up-to-date information on disorders and diseases treated by orthopedic surgeons and related physicians. It follows the same format as other Lange CURRENTs with an emphasis on major diagnostic features of disease states, the natural history of the disease where appropriate, the work-up required for definitive diagnosis, and finally, definitive treatment. Because the book focuses on orthopedic conditions, treatment of the patient from a general medical viewpoint is de-emphasized except when it pertains to the orthopedic problem. Pathophysiology, epidemiology, and pathology are included when they assist in arriving at a definitive diagnosis or in understanding the treatment of the disease or condition.

References to the current literature were carefully chosen for the first and second editions and updated for the third edition so that the reader can investigate topics to greater depth than would be possible in a text of this size. Selected references to the older literature are also included when those articles are landmarks in the advancement of the understanding of orthopedic diseases and conditions.

INTENDED AUDIENCE

Students will find that the book encompasses virtually all aspects of orthopedics that they will encounter in classes and as sub-interns in major teaching institutions.

Residents or house officers can use the book as a ready reference, covering the majority of disorders and conditions in emergency and elective orthopedic surgery. Review of individual chapters will provide house officers rotating on subspecialty orthopedic services with an excellent basis for further, in-depth study.

For emergency room physicians, especially those with medical backgrounds, the text provides an excellent resource in managing orthopedic problems seen on an emergent basis.

Family practitioners and internists will find the book particularly helpful in the referral decision process and as a resource to explain disorders to patients.

Lastly, practicing orthopedic surgeons, particularly those in subspecialties, will find the book a helpful resource in reassuring them that their treatment in areas outside their subspecialty interests is current and up-to-date.

ORGANIZATION

The book is organized primarily by anatomic structure. Because of the natural subspecialization that has occurred in orthopedic surgery over the years, strict anatomic divisions are not always possible and in those cases subspecialties are emphasized. Thus, there is some overlap and some artificial division of subjects. The reader is encouraged to read entire chapters or, for more discrete topics, to go directly to the index for information. For example, the house officer rotating onto the foot and ankle service would find reading the foot and ankle chapter to be a prudent method of developing a baseline knowledge in foot surgery. A knee problem might be best approached by looking in the sports medicine chapter or in the adult reconstructive surgery chapter.

The first chapter serves as a basis for the rest of the book because it summarizes current basic information that is fundamental in understanding orthopedic surgery. Chapter 2 introduces aspects of interest in the perioperative care of the orthopedic patient. Management of orthopedic problems arising from trauma is covered in Chapter 3, while Chapter 4 deals with sports medicine with emphasis on the knee and the shoulder. Chapter 5 covers all aspects of spine surgery including degenerative spinal problems, spinal deformity, and spinal trauma.

Chapter 6 provides comprehensive coverage of tumors in orthopedic surgery, including benign and malignant soft tissue and hard tissue tumors. Adult joint reconstruction, including the disorders that lead to joint reconstruction, are covered in Chapter 7. In Chapter 8, infections with their special implications for orthopedic surgery are covered. Chapter 9 discusses foot and ankle surgery and Chapter 10, hand surgery. Chapter 11 covers diseases in orthopedics unique to children. The final two chapters deal with amputation and all aspects of rehabilitation fundamental to orthopedic surgeons in returning patients to full function.

OUTSTANDING FEATURES

- Careful selection of illustrations maximizes their benefits in pointing out orthopedic principles and concepts.
- The effect of changes in imaging technology on optimal diagnostic studies is emphasized.
- Bone and soft tissue tumor differential diagnosis are simplified by comprehensive tables that categorize tumors by age, location, and imaging characteristics.
- Concise, current, and comprehensive treatment of the basic science necessary for an understanding of the foundation of orthopedic surgery patient care is given.

NEW TO THIS EDITION

- Ethics, pain management, blood replacement, and treatment and prevention of deep venous thrombosis and pulmonary embolism now included in "General Considerations" chapter
- Up-to-date information on shoulder evaluation
- Advances in the understanding of back pain
- The latest on the molecular biology of neoplasm in the chapter on musculoskeletal tumors
- Help in diagnosing hip and knee problems based on the patient's age at presentation
- More on the new COX-2 inhibitors
- Surgical management of osteoporosis using techniques such as kyphoplasty and vertebroplasty
- More guidance on the operative care of shoulder arthritis
- Guidelines for predicting function, such as ambulatory capability after spinal cord injury
- Coverage of materials that have recently come onto the market for joint replacement, including the new polyethylenes and ceramics
- The latest on the increasingly important growth factors

   Taken as a whole, these new features, combined with a review and update of the entire text and references, make this edition a significant improvement over the last.

Harry B. Skinner, MD, PhD
Orange, California
May 2003

Basic Science in Orthopedic Surgery | 1

Ranjan Gupta, MD, Vincent Caiozzo, PhD, Stephen D. Cook, PhD, Robert L. Barrack, MD, & Harry B. Skinner, MD

BIOMECHANICS & BIOMATERIALS

Ranjan Gupta, MD, Vincent Caiozzo, PhD,
Stephen D. Cook, PhD, Robert L. Barrack, MD,
& Harry B. Skinner, MD

Orthopedic surgery is the branch of medicine concerned with restoring and preserving the normal function of the musculoskeletal system. As such, it focuses on bones, joints, tendons, ligaments, muscles, and specialized tissues such as the intervertebral disk. Over the last half century, surgeons and investigators in the field of orthopedics have increasingly recognized the importance that engineering principles play both in understanding the normal behavior of musculoskeletal tissues and in designing implant systems to model the function of these tissues. The goals of the first portion of this chapter are to describe the biologic organization of the musculoskeletal tissues, examine the mechanical properties of the tissues in light of their biologic composition, and explore the material and design concepts required to fabricate implant systems with mechanical and biologic properties that will provide adequate function and longevity. The subject of the second portion of the chapter is gait analysis.

BASIC CONCEPTS & DEFINITIONS

Most biologic tissues are either **porous materials** or **composite materials.** A material such as bone has mechanical properties that are influenced markedly by the degree of porosity, defined as the degree of the material's volume that consists of void. For instance, the compressive strength of osteoporotic bone, which has increased porosity, is markedly decreased in comparison with the compressive strength of normal bone. Like composite materials, **alloyed materials** consist of two or more different materials that are intimately bound. Although composite materials can be physically or mechanically separated, alloyed materials cannot.

Generally, composites are made up of a matrix material, which absorbs energy and protects fibers from brittle failure, and a fiber, which strengthens and stiff-ens the matrix. The performance of the two materials together is superior to that of either material alone in terms of mechanical properties (eg, strength and elastic modulus) and other properties (eg, corrosion resistance). The mechanical properties of various types of composite materials differ, based on the percentage of each substance in the material and on the principal orientation of the fiber. The substances in combination, however, are always stronger for their weight than is either substance alone. Microscopically, bone is a composite material consisting of hydroxyapatite crystals and an organic matrix that contains collagen (the fibers).

The mechanical characteristics of a material are commonly described in terms of stress and strain. **Stress** is the force that a material is subjected to per unit of original area, and **strain** is the amount of deformation the material experiences per unit of original length in response to stress. These characteristics can be adequately estimated from a **stress-strain curve** (Figure 1–1), which plots the effect of a uniaxial stress on a simple test specimen made from a given material. Changes in the geometric dimensions of the material (eg, changes in the material's area or length) have no effect on the stress-strain curve for that material.

Mechanical characteristics can also be estimated from a **load-elongation curve,** in which the slope of the initial linear portion depicts the **stiffness** of a given material. Although similar in appearance to the stress-strain curve, the load-elongation curve for a given material can be altered by changes in the material's diameter (cross-sectional area) or length. For instance, doubling the diameter of a test specimen while maintaining the original length will double the stiffness because the increased diameter doubles the **load to failure** (ie, it doubles the force that a material can withstand in a single application) without changing the total elongation. Conversely, doubling the length of the test specimen while maintaining the original diameter will decrease the stiffness by half because doubling the length in turn doubles the elongation without changing the load to failure.

Because of this difference between the stress-strain curve and load-elongation curve, any comparison of the characteristics of specimens requires that the same type of curve be used in the evaluation. If the load-elongation curve is used, the geometric dimensions of the

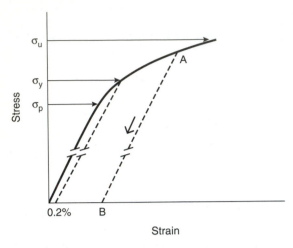

Figure 1–1. A generalized stress-strain diagram illustrating the mechanical properties of a material subjected to stress. The proportional limit (σ_p) of a material is the stress at which permanent or plastic deformation begins. Because the proportional limit is difficult to measure accurately for some materials, a 0.2% strain offset line parallel to the linear region of the curve is constructed. The stress corresponding to this line is defined as the yield stress (σ_y). If stress is removed after the initiation of plastic deformation (point A), only the elastic deformation denoted by the linear portion of the stress-strain curve is recovered. The ultimate tensile strength (σ_u) is the maximal stress that a material can withstand in a single application before it fails.

specimens must also be the same. In this chapter, subsequent discussions will pertain to the stress-strain curve, although differing terminology in the load-elongation curve will be noted parenthetically.

The initial linear or elastic portion of the stress-strain curve (see Figure 1–1) depicts the amount of stress a material can withstand before permanently deforming. The slope of this line is termed the **modulus of elasticity** (stiffness) of the material. A high modulus of elasticity indicates that the material is difficult to deform, whereas a low modulus indicates that the material is more pliable. The modulus of elasticity is an excellent basis on which different materials can be compared. When materials such as those used in implants are compared, however, it is important to remember that the modulus of elasticity is a property only of the material itself and not of the structure. Implant stiffness in bending—or, more correctly, flexural rigidity—is a function both of material elastic modulus and of design geometry.

The **proportional limit,** or σ_p, of a material is the stress at which permanent or plastic deformation be-

gins. The proportional limit, however, is difficult to measure accurately for some materials. Therefore, a 0.2% strain offset line parallel to the linear region of the curve is constructed, as shown in Figure 1–1. The stress corresponding to this line is defined as the **yield stress,** or σ_y. If stress is removed after the initiation of plastic deformation (point A in Figure 1–1), only the elastic deformation denoted by the linear portion of the stress-strain curve is recovered. The **ultimate tensile strength** (failure load), or σ_u, is the maximal stress that a material can withstand in a single application before it fails.

When subjected to repeated loading in a physiologic environment, a material may fail at stresses well below the ultimate tensile strength. The **fatigue curve,** or **S-N curve,** demonstrates the behavior of a metal during cyclic loading and is shown in Figure 1–2. Generally, as the number of cycles (**N**) increases, the amount of applied stress (**S**) that the metal can withstand before failure decreases. The **endurance limit** of a material is the maximal stress below which fatigue failure will never occur regardless of the number of cycles. Fatigue failure will occur if the combination of local peak stresses and number of loading cycles at that stress are excessive. Although most materials exhibit a lower stress at failure with cyclic loading, some do not, such as pyrolytic carbon, making it appropriate for high-cycle applications such as heart valves. Environmental conditions strongly influence fatigue behavior. The physiologic environment, which is corrosive, can significantly reduce the

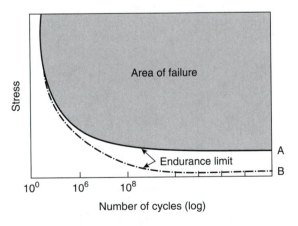

Figure 1–2. A generalized diagram comparing two fatigue curves, or S-N curves, for the same material. Curve A illustrates the material's endurance limit in a noncorrosive environment, and curve B illustrates its endurance limit in a corrosive environment. The body is an example of a corrosive environment for implant materials.

number of cycles to failure and the endurance limit of a material.

Materials can be evaluated in terms of ductility, toughness, viscoelasticity, friction, lubrication, and wear. These properties will be introduced here, and many of them will be explored in detail in subsequent sections.

Ductility is defined as the amount of deformation that a material undergoes before failure and is characterized in terms of total strain. A brittle material will fail with minimal strain caused by propagation because the yield stress is higher than the tensile stress. A ductile material, however, will fail only after markedly increased strain and decreased cross-sectional area. Polymethylmethacrylate (PMMA, a polymer) and ceramics are brittle materials, whereas metals exhibit relatively more ductility. Environmental conditions, especially changes in temperature, can alter the ductility of materials.

Toughness is defined as the energy imparted to a material to cause it to fracture and is measured by the total area under the stress-strain curve.

Because all biologic tissues are viscoelastic in nature, a thorough understanding of **viscoelasticity** is essential. A viscoelastic material is one that exhibits different properties when loaded at different strain rates. Thus, its mechanical properties are time-dependent. Bone, for example, absorbs more energy at fast loading rates, such as in high-speed motor vehicle accidents, than at slow loading rates, such as in recreational snow skiing.

Viscoelastic materials have three important properties: hysteresis, creep, and stress relaxation. When a viscoelastic material is subjected to cyclic loading, the stress-strain relationship during the loading process differs from that during the unloading process (Figure 1–3). This difference in stress-strain response is termed **hysteresis.** The deviation between loading and unloading processes is dependent on the degree of viscous behavior. The area between the two curves is a measure of the energy lost by internal friction during the loading process. **Creep,** which has also been called **cold flow** and is observed in polyethylene components, is defined as a deformation that occurs in a material under constant stress. Some deformation is permanent, persisting even when the stress is released. The constant strain associated with a decrease in stress over time is a result of **stress relaxation,** a phenomenon evident, for example, in the loosening of fracture fixation plates. The time necessary to attain creep, or stress relaxation equilibrium, is an inherent property of the material.

Friction refers to the resistance between two bodies when one slides over the other. Friction is greatest at slow rates and decreases with faster rates. This is because the surface asperities (peaks) tend to adhere to one another more strongly at slower rates. Mechanisms

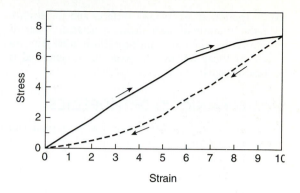

Figure 1–3. When a viscoelastic material is subjected to cyclic loading, the stress-strain curve during the loading process (solid lines) differs from that during the unloading process (dotted lines). This difference in stress-strain response is called **hysteresis.** The area between the two curves is a measure of the energy lost by internal friction during the loading process.

of **lubrication** reduce the friction between two surfaces. Several lubrication mechanisms are present in articular cartilage to overcome friction processes in normal joint motion. Similarly, mechanisms are present in polyethylene-metal articulations to overcome friction in joint replacements.

Wear occurs whenever friction is present and is defined as the removal of surface material by mechanical motion. Wear is always observed between two moving surfaces, but lubrication mechanisms act to reduce the detrimental effects of excessive wear. Three types of wear mechanisms are apparent in normal and prosthetic joint motion: abrasive, adhesive, and three-body wear. **Abrasive wear** is the generation of material particles from a softer surface when it moves against a rougher, harder surface. An example of the product of abrasive wear is sawdust, which results from the movement of sandpaper against a wood surface. The amount of wear depends on factors such as contact stress, hardness, and finish of the bearing surfaces.

Adhesive wear results when a thin film of material is transferred from one bearing surface to the other. In prosthetic joints, the transfer film can be either polyethylene or the passivated (corrosion-resistant) layer of metal. Regardless of the material, wear occurs in the surface that loses the transfer film. If the particles from the transfer film are shed from the other surface as well, they behave as a third body and also result in wear.

Three-body wear occurs when another particle is located between two bearing surfaces. Cement particles act as third bodies in prosthetic joints. Implant designers continue to search for compatible substances that reduce friction at articulating surfaces and thereby reduce the amount of wear debris generated. Wear of polyethylene is the dominant problem in total joint replacement today because the wear debris generated is biologically active and leads to osteolysis.

BIOMECHANICS IN ORTHOPEDICS

An analysis of the factors that influence normal and prosthetic joint function requires an understanding of free-body diagrams as well as the concepts of force, moment, and equilibrium.

Force, Moment, & Equilibrium

Forces and moments are vector quantities—that is, they are described by point of application, magnitude, and direction. A force represents the action of one body on another. The action may be applied directly (eg, via a push or a pull) or from a distance (eg, via gravity). A normal tensile or compressive force is applied perpendicular to a surface, whereas a shear force is applied parallel to a surface. A force that is applied eccentrically produces a moment.

The force generated by gravity on an object is the center of gravity. An object that is symmetric has its center of gravity in the geometrically centered position, whereas an object that is asymmetric has its center of gravity closer to its "heavier" end. The center of gravity for the human body is the resultant of the individual centers of gravity from each segment of the body. Therefore, as the body segments move, the center of gravity changes accordingly and may even lie outside the body in extreme positions, such as encountered in gymnastics. A moment is defined as the product of the quantity of force and the perpendicular distance between the line of action of the force and the center of rotation. A moment usually results in a rotation of the object about a fixed axis.

Newton's first law states that a body (or object) is in equilibrium if the sum of the forces and moments acting on the body are balanced; therefore, the sum of forces and moments for each direction must equal zero. The concept of equilibrium is important in understanding and determining force-body interactions, such as the increased joint reaction force occurring in an extended arm because of an external weight and such as the increased joint reaction force occurring in the hip at a specific moment during walking.

Free-Body Diagrams

A free-body diagram can be used to schematically represent all the forces and moments acting on a joint. The concepts of equilibrium can be extended to determine joint reaction or muscle forces for different conditions, as demonstrated in the following two examples.

Example 1: Determine the force on the abductor muscle of a person's hip joint (the abductor force, or F_{AB}) and the joint reaction force (the F_J) when the person is standing on one leg. The weight of the trunk, both arms, and one leg is ⅚ of the total weight (w) of the person. As illustrated in Figure 1–4, this weight will tend to rotate the body about the femoral head and is counteracted by the pull of the abductor muscles on the pelvis. The necessary equation to solve for the abductor force, F_{AB}, is as follows:

$$F_{AB} \times a = \frac{B}{nw} \times b$$

In solving the equation, assume that a = 5 cm and that b = 15 cm.

After this equation is solved, two of the three forces are known. The remaining force (the F_J) can be determined from a force triangle (see Figure 1–4), because according to Newton's first law, the sum of forces must equal zero.

Example 2: Determine the force on a person's deltoid muscle (the deltoid force, or F_D) and the force of the joint acting about the shoulder (the joint force, or F_J) when the person holds a metal weight (w) at arm's length (Figure 1–5). The weight of the arm is ignored because only the increase in forces about the shoulder caused by the metal weight is to be determined. F_D is determined by summing the moments about the joint center. The necessary equation is as follows:

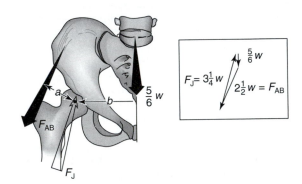

Figure 1–4. A free body diagram and force triangle illustrating the method for determining the force of the abductor muscle of a person's hip joint (F_{AB}) and the joint reaction force (F_J) when the person is standing on one leg and the total weight (w) of the person is known. See the discussion of example 1 in the text.

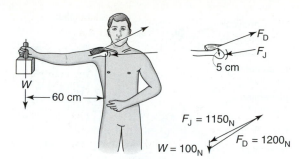

Figure 1–5. A free body diagram and force triangle illustrating the method for determining the force of a person's deltoid muscle (F_D) and the force of the joint acting about the shoulder (F_J) when the person holds a metal weight (w) at arm's length. See the discussion of example 2 in the text.

$$F_D \times a = w \times b$$

In solving the equation, assume that $a = 5$ cm and that $b = 60$ cm.

After this equation is solved, a joint reaction force of 1150 N is determined using a force triangle (see Figure 1–5).

Moments of Inertia

The orientation of the bone's or implant's cross-sectional area with respect to the applied principal load also greatly influences the biomechanical performance. Bending and torsion occur in long bones and are important considerations in the design of implants. In general, the farther that material mass is distributed from the axis of bending or torsion while still retaining structural integrity, the more resistant the structure will be to bending or torsion. The **area moment of inertia** is a mathematical expression for resistance to bending, and the **polar moment of inertia** is a mathematical expression for resistance to torsion. Both types of moment of inertia relate the cross-sectional geometry and orientation of the object with respect to the applied axial load. The larger the area moment of inertia or the polar moment of inertia is, the less likely the material will fail. Figure 1–6 summarizes the area moments of inertia for representative shapes important to orthopedic surgery. Creating an open slot in an object will significantly decrease the polar moment of inertia of the object.

Knowledge of moments of inertia is important for understanding mechanical behavior in relation to object geometry. For instance, the length of the long

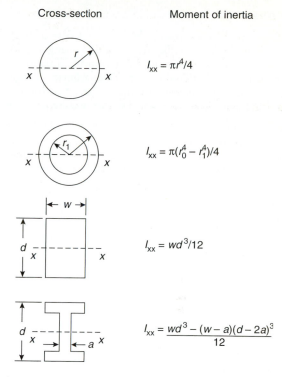

Figure 1–6. Summary of the area moments of inertia for representative shapes important to orthopedic surgery.

bones predisposes them to high bending moments. Their tubular shape helps them resist bending in all directions, however. This resistance to bending is attributable to the large area moment of inertia because the majority of bone tissue is distributed away from the neutral axis. The concept of moment of inertia is crucial in the design of implants that are exposed to excessive bending and torsional stresses.

BIOLOGIC TISSUES IN ORTHOPEDICS

The functions of the musculoskeletal system are to provide support for the body, to protect the vital organs, and to facilitate easy movement of joints. The bone, articular cartilage, tendon, ligament, and muscle all interact to fulfill these functions. The musculoskeletal tissues are integrally specialized to perform their duties and have excellent regenerative and reparative processes. They also adapt and undergo compositional changes in response to increased or decreased stress states. Specialized components of the musculoskeletal system, such as the intervertebral disk, are particularly suited for supporting large stress loads while resisting movement.

Bones

Bones are dynamic tissues that serve a variety of functions and have the ability to remodel to changes in internal and external stimuli. Bones provide support for the trunk and extremities, provide attachment to ligaments and tendons, protect vital organs, and act as a mineral and iron reservoir for the maintenance of homeostasis.

A. STRUCTURAL COMPOSITION

Bone is a composite consisting of two types of material. The first material is an organic extracellular matrix that contains collagen, accounts for about 30–35% of the dry weight of bone, and is responsible for providing flexibility and resilience to the bone. The second material consists primarily of calcium and phosphorous salts, especially hydroxyapatite $[Ca_{10}(PO_4)_6(OH)_2]$, accounts for about 65–70% of the dry weight of bone, and contributes to the hardness and rigidity of the bone. Microscopically, bone can be classified as either woven or lamellar.

Woven bone, which is also called **primary bone,** is characterized by a random arrangement of cells and collagen. Because of its relatively disoriented composition, woven bone demonstrates isotropic mechanical characteristics, with similar properties observed regardless of the direction of applied stress. Woven bone is associated with periods of rapid formation, such as the initial stages of fracture repair or biologic implant fixation. Woven bone, which has a low mineral content, remodels to lamellar bone.

Lamellar bone is a slower forming, mature bone that is characterized by an orderly cellular distribution and regular orientation of collagen fibers (Figure 1–7). The lamellae can be parallel to one another or concentrically organized around a vascular canal called a **Haversian system** or **osteon.** At the periphery of each osteon is a cement line, a narrow area containing ground substance primarily composed of glycosaminoglycans. Neither the canaliculi nor the collagen fibers cross the cement line. Biomechanically, the cement line is the weakest link in the microstructure of bone. The organized structure of lamellar bone makes it anisotropic, as seen in the fact that it is stronger during axial loading than it is during transverse, or shear, loading.

Bone can be classified macroscopically as cortical tissue and cancellous (trabecular) tissue. Both types are morphologically lamellar bone. Cortical tissue relies on osteons for cell communication. Because trabecular width is small, however, the canaliculi can communicate directly with blood vessels in the medullary canal. The basic differences between cortical tissue and cancellous tissue relate to porosity and apparent density. The porosity of cortical tissue typically ranges from 5% to

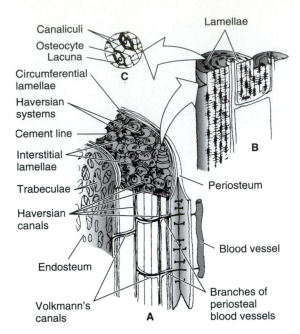

Figure 1–7. The structure of bone. **A:** A section of the diaphysis of a long bone, depicted without inner marrow. Each osteon is bounded by a cement line. **B:** Each osteon consists of lamellae, concentric rings composed of mineral matrix surrounding the Haversian canal. **C:** Along the boundaries of the lamellae are small cavities known as lacunae, each of which contains a single osteocyte. Radiating from the lacunae are tiny canals, or canaliculi, into which the cytoplasmic processes of the osteocytes extend. (Reproduced, with permission, from Nordin M, Frankel VH: Biomechanics of bone. In: Nordin M, Frankel VH, eds: *Basic Biomechanics of the Musculoskeletal System.* Lea & Febiger, 1989.)

30%, and that of cancellous tissue ranges from 30% to 90%. The apparent density of cortical tissue is about 1.8 g/cm, and that of cancellous tissue typically ranges from 0.1 to 1.0 g/cm. The distinction between cortical tissue and cancellous tissue is arbitrary, however, and in biomechanical terms the two tissues are often considered as one material with a specific range in porosity and density.

The organization of cortical and cancellous tissue in bone allows for adaptation to function. Cortical tissue always surrounds cancellous tissue, but the relative quantity of each type of tissue varies with the functional requirements of the bone. In long bones, the cortical tissue of the diaphysis is arranged as a hollow cylinder to best resist bending. The metaphyseal region of the long bones flares to increase the bone volume and surface area in a manner that minimizes the stress of joint contact. The cancellous tissue in this region provides an intricate network that distributes weight-bearing forces and joint reaction forces into the bulk of the bone tissue.

B. BIOMECHANICAL BEHAVIOR

The mechanical properties of cortical bone differ from those of cancellous bone. Cortical bone is stiffer than cancellous bone. Cortical bone will fracture in vivo when the strain exceeds 2%, but cancellous bone does not until the strain exceeds 75%. The larger capacity for energy storage (area under the stress-strain curve) of cancellous bone is a function of porosity. Despite different stiffness values for cortical and cancellous bone, the following axiom is valid for all bone tissue: the compressive strength of the tissue is proportional to the square of the apparent density, and the elastic modulus or material stiffness of the tissue is proportional to the cube of the apparent density. Therefore, any increase in porosity, as occurs with aging, will decrease the apparent density of bone, and this in turn will decrease the compressive strength and elastic modulus of bone.

Variations in the strength and stiffness of bone also result from specimen orientation (longitudinal versus transverse) and loading configuration (tensile, compressive, or shear). Generally, the strength and stiffness of bone are greatest in the direction of the common load application (longitudinally for long bones). With regard to orientation, cortical bone (Figure 1–8) is strongest in the longitudinal direction. With regard to loading configuration, cortical bone is strongest in compression and weakest in shear.

Tensile loading is the application of equal and opposite forces (loads) outward from the surface. Maximal stresses are in a plane perpendicular to the load application and result in elongation of the material. Microscopic studies show that the tensile failure in bones with Haversian systems is caused by debonding of the cement lines and pull-out of the osteons. Bones with a large percentage of cancellous tissue demonstrate trabecular fracture with tensile loading.

The converse of tensile loading is **compressive loading,** which is defined as the application of equal and opposite forces toward the surface. Under compres-

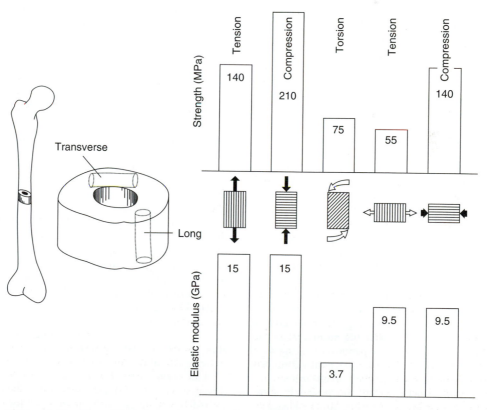

Figure 1–8. The effects of specimen orientation and loading configuration on the strength and elastic modulus of cortical bone from the diaphyseal region of a long bone.

sion, a material shortens and widens. Microscopic studies show that compressive failure occurs by oblique cracking of the osteons in cortical bone and of the trabeculae in cancellous bone. Vertebral fractures, especially associated with osteoporosis, are associated with compressive loading.

The application of either a tensile load or a compressive load produces a shear stress in the material. **Shear loading** is the application of a load parallel to a surface, and the deformation is angular. Clinical studies show that shear fractures are most common to regions with a large percentage of cancellous bone, such as the tibial plateau.

Bone is a viscoelastic material, and its mechanical behavior is therefore influenced by strain rate. Bones are approximately 50% stiffer at high strain rates than at low strain rates, and the load to failure nearly doubles at high strain rates. The result is a doubling of the stored energy at high strain rates. Clinical studies show that the loading rate influences the fracture pattern and the associated soft-tissue damage. Low strain rates, characterized by little stored energy, result in undisplaced fractures and no associated soft-tissue damage. High strain rates, however, are associated with massive damage to the bone and soft tissue owing to the marked increase in stored energy.

Bone fractures can be produced either from a single load that exceeds the ultimate tensile strength of the bone or from repeated loading that leads to fatigue failure. Because bone is self-repairing, fatigue fracture occurs only when the rate of microdamage resulting from repeated loading exceeds the intrinsic repair rate of the bone. Fatigue fractures are most common during strenuous activity when the muscles have become fatigued and are therefore unable to adequately store energy and absorb the stress imposed on the bone. When the muscles are fatigued, the bone is required to carry the increased stress.

C. REMODELING MECHANISMS

Bone has the ability to alter its size, shape, and structure in response to mechanical demands. According to Wolff's law regarding bone remodeling in response to stress, bone resorption occurs with decreased stress, bone hypertrophy occurs with increased stress, and the planes of increased stress follow the principal trabecular orientation. Thus, bone remodeling occurs under a variety of circumstances that alter the normal stress patterns. Clinically, altered stress patterns resulting from fixation devices or joint prostheses have caused concern about effects on the long-term bone architecture.

Bone mass and body weight are positively correlated, especially for weight-bearing bones. Therefore, immobilization or weightlessness (as experienced by astronauts) decreases the strength and stiffness of bone.

The subsequent loss in bone mass results from the alteration or absence of normal stress patterns. Bone mass, however, is regained with the return of normal stress patterns. The loss of bone mass in response to immobilization or weightlessness is a direct consequence of Wolff's law. Associated bone resorption in response to orthopedic implants can be deleterious to bone healing, however. Although bone plates provide support for fractured bone, the altered stress patterns associated with stiff metal plates cause resorption of bone adjacent to the fracture or underneath the plate. Therefore, removal of the plate may precipitate another fracture. Resorption of bone has also been reported in total hip and knee replacements. This is particularly common with larger diameter noncemented femoral stems, which have an increased moment of inertia and thus have less flexibility than do smaller diameter cemented stems.

The resorption of bone in response to a stiff implant, which alters the stress pattern the bone carries, is termed **stress shielding.** The degree of stress shielding is not dependent on the absolute flexibility of the prosthesis but, rather, on the amount of reduced flexibility in the implant in relation to the flexibility of the bone. Clinically, stress shielding could also be detrimental to the longevity of implant fixation. In an effort to reduce stress shielding designers of implants are using materials with a degree of flexural rigidity that approximates the flexibility of bone.

D. HEALING MECHANISMS

The fracture healing process involves five stages: impact, inflammation, soft callus formation, hard callus formation, and remodeling. Impact begins with the initiation of the fracture and continues until energy has completely dissipated. The inflammation stage is characterized by hematoma formation at the fracture site, bone necrosis at the ends of the fragments, and an inflammatory infiltrate. Granulation tissue gradually replaces the hematoma, fibroblasts produce collagen, and osteoclasts begin to remove necrotic bone. The subsidence of pain and swelling marks the initiation of the third, or soft callus, stage. This stage is characterized by increased vascularity and abundant new cartilage formation. The end of the soft callus stage is associated with fibrous or cartilaginous tissue uniting the fragments. During the fourth, or hard callus, stage, the callus converts to woven bone and appears clinically healed. The final stage of the healing process involves slow remodeling from woven to lamellar bone and reconstruction of the medullary canal.

Three types of fracture healing have been described. The first type, endochondral fracture healing, is characterized by an initial phase of cartilage formation, followed by the formation of new bone on the calcified cartilage template. The second type, membranous fracture healing, is characterized by bone formation from direct mesenchymal tissue without an intervening cartilaginous stage. Combinations of endochondral healing and membranous healing are typical of normal fracture healing. The former process is observed between fracture gaps, whereas the latter is observed subperiosteally. The third type of fracture healing, primary bone healing, is observed with rigid internal fixation and is characterized by the absence of visible callus formation. The fracture site is bridged by direct Haversian remodeling, and there are no discernible histologic stages of inflammation or soft and hard callus formation.

Articular Cartilage

Articular cartilage is primarily avascular and has an abnormally small cellular density. The chief functions of articular cartilage are to distribute joint loads over a large area and to allow relative movement of the joint surfaces with minimal friction and wear.

A. STRUCTURAL COMPOSITION

Articular cartilage is composed of chondrocytes and an organic matrix. The chondrocytes account for less than 10% of the tissue volume, and they manufacture, secrete, and maintain the organic component of the cellular matrix. The organic matrix is a dense network of type II collagen in a concentrated proteoglycan solution. Collagen accounts for 10–30% of the organic matrix; proteoglycan accounts for 3–10%; and water, inorganic salts, and matrix proteins account for the remaining 60–87%.

The basic collagen unit consists of tropocollagen molecules, which form covalent cross-links between collagen molecules to increase the tensile strength of the fibrils. The most important mechanical properties of the collagen fiber are tensile strength and stiffness. Fiber resistance to compression is relatively ineffective because the large ratio of length to diameter (slenderness ratio) predisposes the fibers to buckling. The anisotropic nature of cartilage is thought to be related to several factors, including variations in fiber arrangements within the planes parallel to the articular surface, the collagen fiber cross-link density, and the collagen-proteoglycan interactions.

The mechanical properties of the cartilage are attributed to the inhomogeneous distribution of collagen fibrils (Figure 1–9). The superficial tangential zone contains sheets of fine, densely packed collagen fibers that are randomly woven in planes parallel to the articular surface. The middle zone contains randomly oriented and homogeneously dispersed fibers that are widely spaced to account for increased matrix content. Finally, the deep zone contains larger, radially oriented collagen fiber bundles that eventually cross the tidemark, enter the calcified cartilage, and anchor the tissue to the underlying bone.

Proteoglycans are monomers that consist of a protein core with glycosaminoglycan units (either keratan sulfate or chondroitin sulfate units) covalently bound to the core. Proteoglycan aggregation promotes immobilization of the proteoglycans within the collagen network and adds structural rigidity to the matrix. There are numerous age-related changes in the structure and composition of the proteoglycan matrix, including the following: a decrease in proteoglycan content from approximately 7% at birth to half that by adulthood, an

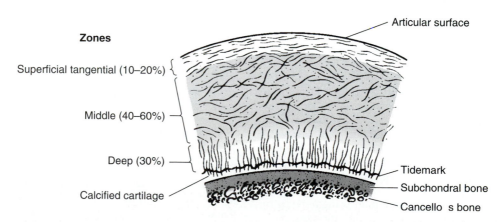

Figure 1–9. Orientation of the collagen fiber network in the three zones of the articular cartilage. (Modified and reproduced, with permission, from Mow VC et al: Biomechanics of articular cartilage. In: Nordin M, Frankel VH, eds: *Basic Biomechanics of the Musculoskeletal System.* Lea & Febiger, 1989.)

increase in protein content with maturity, a dramatic drop in the ratio of chondroitin sulfate to keratan sulfate with aging, and a decrease in water content as proteoglycan subunits become smaller with aging. The overall effect is that the cartilage stiffens. The development of osteoarthritis is associated with dramatic changes in cartilage metabolism. Initially, there is increased proteoglycan synthesis, and the water content of osteoarthritic cartilage is actually increased.

The water content of normal cartilage permits the diffusion of gases, nutrients, and waste products between the chondrocytes and the nutrient-rich synovial fluid. The water is primarily concentrated (80%) near the articular surface and decreases in a linear fashion with increasing depth, such that the deep zone is 65% water. The location and movement of water are important in controlling mechanical function and lubrication properties of the cartilage.

Important structural interactions occur between proteoglycans and collagen fibers in cartilage. A small percentage of the proteoglycans may serve as a bonding agent between the collagen fibrils that span distances too great for the maintenance or formation of crosslinks. These structural interactions are thought to provide strong mechanical interactions. In essence, the proteoglycans and collagen fibers interact to form a porous, composite, fiber-reinforced matrix, possessing all the essential mechanical characteristics of a solid that is swollen with water and able to resist the stresses and strains of joint lubrication.

B. BIOMECHANICAL BEHAVIOR

The biomechanical behavior of articular cartilage is best understood when the cartilage is considered as a viscoelastic and composite material consisting of a fluid phase and a solid phase. The compressive behavior of cartilage is primarily caused by the flow of interstitial fluid, whereas the shear behavior of cartilage is primarily caused by the motion of collagen fibers and proteoglycans. The creep behavior of cartilage is characterized by the exudation of interstitial fluid, which occurs with compressive loading. The applied surface load is balanced by the compressive stress developed within the collagen-proteoglycan matrix and the frictional drag generated by the flow of the interstitial fluid during exudation. Typically, human cartilage takes 4–16 h to reach creep equilibrium, and the amount of creep is inversely proportional to the square of the tissue thickness.

Similar to creep, stress relaxation is the response of the tissue to compressive forces on the articular surface. An initial compressive phase, characterized by increased stress, is associated with fluid exudation. In the subsequent relaxation phase, stress decay is associated with fluid redistribution within the porous collagen-proteo-

glycan matrix. The rate of stress relaxation is used to determine the permeability coefficient of the tissue, and the equilibrium stress is used to measure the intrinsic compressive modulus of the solid matrix. Microstructural changes in osteoarthritic cartilage reduce the compressive stiffness of cartilage.

Under uniaxial tension, articular cartilage demonstrates anisotropic and inhomogeneous properties. The tissue is stronger and stiffer parallel to the split lines and in superficial regions. Variations in the material characteristics are a result of the structural organization of the collagen-proteoglycan matrix in layering arrangements throughout the tissue. For example, the superficial tangential zone appears to provide a tough, wear-resistant, protective zone for the tissue. To examine the tissue's intrinsic response to tension, the biphasic viscoelastic effects of the tissue must be negated. This can be achieved by testing the tissue at low strain rates or by performing incremental testing and allowing for stress relaxation equilibrium to be achieved before continuing. The tissue tends to stiffen with increasing strain. Typically, specimens are pulled to the failure point at a displacement rate of 0.5 cm/min.

The shape of the stress-strain curve (Figure 1–10) can be described in morphologic changes of the collagen fibers: (1) the toe region designates collagen fiber pull-out, (2) the linear region designates stretching of the aligned collagen fibers, and (3) failure is the point at which all of the collagen fibers have ruptured. The tensile properties of the tissue are thus changed by an alteration of the molecular structure of collagen, an alter-

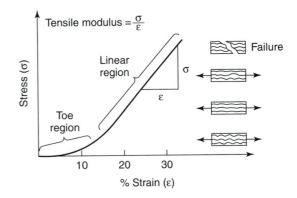

Figure 1–10. A stress-strain diagram for articular cartilage during tensile loading. The schematic representations on the right illustrate the orientation of the collagen fibrils in response to loading. (Reproduced, with permission, from Mow VC et al: Biomechanics of articular cartilage. In Nordin M, Frankel VH, eds: *Basic Biomechanics of the Musculoskeletal System.* Lea & Febiger, 1989.)

ation in the organization of the fibers within the collagenous network, or a change in collagen fiber cross-linking. For this reason, disruption of the collagen network may be a key factor in the initial development of osteoarthritis.

When the cartilage is tested in pure shear under infinitesimal strain conditions, no pressure gradients or volume changes are observed within the tissue as they are during tension or compression conditions. Thus, the viscoelastic shear properties of cartilage can be determined in a steady-state dynamic shear experiment. Cartilage shear stiffness is a function of collagen content or collagen-proteoglycan interaction. Increased collagen content reduces frictional dissipation of the load, and this in turn results in increased shear loading.

C. LUBRICATION MECHANISMS

Sophisticated lubrication processes are responsible for the minimal wear of normal cartilage under large and varied joint stresses. Four types of lubrication mechanisms are related to articular cartilage: boundary, fluid film, mixed, and self-lubrication. These mechanisms are inherent properties of the composition of the tissue with respect to water content and collagen-proteoglycan matrix orientation. Normal joints display all of the lubrication mechanisms just mentioned, whereas artificial joints are thought to primarily display elastohydrodynamic and boundary lubrication mechanisms.

The boundary mechanism protects the joint from surface-to-surface wear by means of an adsorbed lubricant. This mechanism, which depends chiefly on the chemical properties of the lubricant, is most important under severe loading conditions, when contact surfaces must sustain high loads.

The fluid film mechanism relies on a thin layer of lubricant that causes greater surface separation. The load on the joint surface is supported by the pressure on the film. Fluid film lubrication occurs with rigid (squeeze-film or hydrodynamic) bodies as well as with deformable (elastohydrodynamic) bodies. When two rigid surfaces are nonparallel and move tangentially with respect to each other, the pressure generated by the lubricant in the gap between the two surfaces is sufficient to raise one surface above the other. Moreover, when two rigid surfaces are parallel and move perpendicular to each other, the pressure generated by the lubricant is sufficient to keep the surfaces separated. This squeeze-film or hydrodynamic lubrication mechanism is able to carry high loads for short durations. When the squeeze-film mechanism generates a pressure great enough to deform the surface and thereby increase the amount of bearing surface area, elastohydrodynamic lubrication mechanisms will begin to make the necessary adjustments. Increased bearing surface area allows less lubricant to escape from between the surfaces, decreas-

ing the stress and increasing the duration associated with motion.

The mixed lubrication mechanism is a combination of the boundary and fluid film mechanisms. Boundary lubrication is essential in areas of asperity contact, and fluid film lubrication is present in areas of no contact. Therefore, most of the friction is generated in the boundary lubricated areas, whereas most of the load is carried by the fluid film.

Self-lubrication, or weeping, relies on the exudation of fluid in front of and beneath the surface of the rotating joint. Once the area of peak stress passes a given point, the cartilage reabsorbs the fluid and returns to its original dimensions. This lubrication mechanism results from the inhomogeneous character of the collagen and water distribution throughout the cartilage. When the pressure rises and strains are low, the tissue is most permeable and a large amount of water is exuded in front of the leading contact edge of the joint. As the joint advances, the load increases in the region of expelled fluid and the increased pressure and strains decrease the tissue permeability to fluid. This prevents the fluid on the articular surface from returning to the cartilage. As the contact surface moves past the point of contact, the pressure and strains are again low and the tissue permeability is increased, resulting in the return of fluid to the cartilage in preparation for the cycle to start again.

D. WEAR MECHANISMS

Wear is the removal of material from a surface and is caused by the mechanical action of two surfaces in contact. The principal types of wear experienced in articular cartilage are interface wear and fatigue wear.

Interface wear occurs when bearing surfaces come into direct contact with no lubricating film separating them. This type of wear may be found in an impaired or degenerated synovial joint. When ultrastructural surface defects in articular cartilage result in softer tissue with increased permeability, the fluid from the lubricant film may easily leak through the cartilage surface, thereby increasing the probability of direct contact between asperities. There are two forms of interface wear: adhesive wear, which occurs when surface fragments adhere to one another and are torn from the surface during sliding, and abrasive wear, which occurs when a soft material is scraped by a harder one.

Fatigue wear results from the accumulation of microscopic damage within the bearing material under repetitive stress. In the cartilage, three mechanisms are primarily responsible for fatigue wear. First, repetitive stress on the collagen-proteoglycan matrix can disrupt the collagen fibers, the proteoglycan molecules, or the interface between the two. In this case, cartilage fatigue is caused by the tensile failure of the collagen network, and proteoglycan changes could be considered part of the accumulated tissue damage. Second, repetitive and massive exudation and inhibition of interstitial fluid may cause a proteoglycan washout from the cartilage matrix near the articular surface. This results in decreased stiffness and increased tissue permeability. Third, during synovial joint impact loading, insufficient time for internal fluid redistribution to relieve high stress in the compacted region may result in tissue damage.

Numerous structural defects of the articular cartilage are caused or exacerbated by wear and damage. For example, fibrillations (splitting of the articular surface) are associated with wear and will eventually extend the full thickness of the cartilage. Destructive smooth-surface thinning is apparent when layers erode rather than split. In these and other types of surface damage of the cartilage, more than a single wear mechanism is likely to be responsible.

Several biomechanical hypotheses cover cartilage degradation. Factors associated with progressive failure of the tissue include the magnitude of imposed stress, the total number of sustained stress peaks, changes in the intrinsic molecular and microscopic structure of the collagen-proteoglycan matrix, and changes in the intrinsic mechanical property of the tissue. Failure-initiating mechanisms include a loosening of the collagen network, which allows for abnormal expansion of the proteoglycan matrix and swelling of the tissue, and a decrease in cartilage stiffness, which is accompanied by an increase in tissue permeability.

Biomechanically, conditions that cause excessive stress concentrations may result in increased tissue damage or wear. Joint surface incongruity, such as the incongruity of the hip joint in patients who had Perthes' disease during childhood, can result in abnormally small contact areas, which are associated with increased stress and increased tissue damage. Moreover, the presence of high contact pressures between the articular surfaces, such as that seen in patients with a shallow acetabulum (acetabular dysplasia), can reduce the probability of fluid film lubrication, allow for continued tissue damage, and also increase the risk of early degenerative arthritis.

Tendons & Ligaments

Tendons and ligaments are similar both structurally and biomechanically and differ only in function. Tendons attach muscle to bone; transmit loads from the muscle to the bone, which results in joint motion; and allow the muscle belly to remain an optimal distance from the joint on which it acts. Ligaments attach bone to bone, augment mechanical stability of the joint, guide joint motion, and prevent excessive joint displacement.

A. STRUCTURAL COMPOSITION

Both the tendons and the ligaments are parallel-fibered collagenous tissues that are sparsely vascularized. They contain relatively few fibroblasts (constituting approximately 20% of their volume) and an abundant extracellular matrix. The matrix consists of about 70% water and 30% collagen, ground substance, and elastin.

The fibroblasts secrete a precursor of collagen, procollagen, which is cleaved extracellularly to form type I collagen. Cross-links between collagen molecules provide strength to the tissue. The arrangement of the collagen fibers determines tissue function. In tendons, a parallel arrangement of the collagen fibers provides the tissues with the ability to sustain high uniaxial tensile loads. In ligaments, the nearly parallel fibers, which are intimately interlaced with one another, provide the ability to sustain loads in one predominant direction but allow for carrying small tensile loads in other directions.

Tendons and ligaments are surrounded by loose areolar connective tissue. The paratenon forms a protective sheath around the tissue and enhances gliding. At places where the tendons are subjected to large friction forces, a parietal synovial membrane is found just beneath the paratenon and additionally facilitates gliding. Each individual fiber bundle is bound by the endotenon. At the musculotendinous junction, the endotenon continues into the perimysium. At the tendoosseous junction, the collagen fibers of the endotenon continue into the bone as perforating fibers (Sharpey's fibers) and become continuous with the periosteum.

Tendons and connective tissues of the musculotendinous junction help determine the mechanical characteristics of whole muscle during contraction and passive extension. The muscle cells are extensively involuted and folded at the junction to provide maximal surface area for attachment, thereby allowing for greater fixation and transmission of forces. The sarcomeres directly adjacent to the junction of fast contracting muscles are shortened in length. This may represent an adaptation to decrease the force intensity within the junction. A complex intracellular and extracellular transmitting membrane consisting of a glycoprotein links the contractile intracellular proteins to the extracellular protein connective tissue.

The tendon insertions and ligament insertions to the bone are structurally similar. The collagen fibers from the tissue intermesh with fibrocartilage. The fibrocartilage gradually becomes mineralized, and this mineralized cartilage merges with cortical bone. These transition zones produce a gradual alteration in the mechanical properties of the tissue, resulting in a decreased stress concentration effect at the insertion of the tendon or ligament to the bone.

B. MECHANICAL BEHAVIOR

Tendons and ligaments are viscoelastic structures that have specific mechanical properties related to their function and composition. Tendons are strong enough to sustain high tensile forces resulting from muscle contraction during joint motion, but they are also sufficiently flexible to angulate around bone surfaces, to change the final direction of muscle pull. Ligaments are pliant and flexible enough to allow natural movements of the bones they connect; however, they are strong, are not extensible, and offer suitable resistance to applied forces and large joint movements. Because tendons and ligaments are viscoelastic structures, the injury they sustain is affected by the rate of loading as well as the amount of the stress load. The stress-strain and load-elongation curves for ligaments and tendons, like those for articular cartilage, have several regions that characterize the tissue behavior.

Figure 1–11 shows the load-elongation curve for progressive failure of the anterior cruciate ligament. Like the curve in Figure 1–10, the curve in Figure 1–11 has a toe region (correlating with the region labeled clinical test, when the anterior drawer test was administered) and a linear region preceding the failure region. In Figure 1–11, the curve in the toe region represents large elongations with small changes in load. This pattern is thought to reflect the straightening of the wavy, relaxed collagen fibers with increased loads. Within the linear region, the collagen fibers continue to become more parallel in orientation as physiologic loading proceeds. At the end of the linear region, small force reduc-

tions can be observed in the load-deformation curve. These dips are caused by the early sequential failure of a few maximally stretched fiber bundles. The final region represents major failure of fiber bundles in an unpredictable manner. Complete failure occurs rapidly, and the load-supporting ability of the tissue is substantially reduced.

The mechanical behavior characteristics of the anterior cruciate ligament differ somewhat from those of soft tissues that contain a high proportion of elastin fibers. These tissues can elongate up to 50% before stiffness markedly increases. After 50% elongation, however, the stiffness increases greatly with increased loading, and failure is abrupt with minimal further elongation. Load-elongation curves for several soft tissues are shown in Figure 1–12.

The viscoelastic behavior of ligaments is best exemplified in the bone-ligament-bone complex. Anterior cruciate ligaments in primate knee specimens were tested in tension to failure at both slow and fast loading rates to determine the viscoelastic nature of the bone-ligament-bone complex. At slow loading rates the bony insertion of the ligament was the weakest link, and an avulsion resulted. At fast loading rates, the ligament was the weakest link, and a midsubstance rupture generally was found. At slow rates, the load to failure was decreased by 20% and the stored energy was decreased by 30% in comparison with results with fast rates. The stiffness of the bone-ligament-bone complex was relatively unaffected by strain rate, however. Increased strain rates demonstrated a greater increase in strength for bone as compared with ligaments.

The mechanical properties of ligaments are closely related to the number and quality of the cross-links within the collagen fibers. Therefore, any process that affects collagen formation or maturation directly influences the properties of the ligaments. As aging continues, the number and the quality of cross-links increase, thereby increasing the tensile strength of the tissue. Moreover, the diameter of the collagen fibril increases with age. As aging progresses, however, collagen reaches a mechanical plateau, after which point tensile strength and stiffness decrease. There is also a decrease in the tissue collagen content, and this contributes to the continued decline in the mechanical properties of the tissue.

Tendons and ligaments remodel in response to mechanical demand. Physical training increases the tensile strength of the tendons and the ligament-bone interface, whereas immobilization decreases tensile strength. Even if the tissue maintains a relatively constant cross-sectional area during immobilization, the increased tissue metabolism results in proportionately more immature collagen and a decrease in the amount and quality of cross-links between molecules. Investigators who

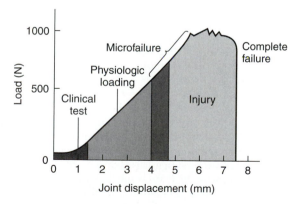

Figure 1–11. The load-elongation curve for progressive failure of the anterior cruciate ligament. (Reproduced, with permission, from Carlstedt CA, Nordin M: Biomechanics of tendons and ligaments. In: Nordin M, Frankel VH, eds: *Basic Biomechanics of the Musculoskeletal System.* Lea & Febiger, 1989.)

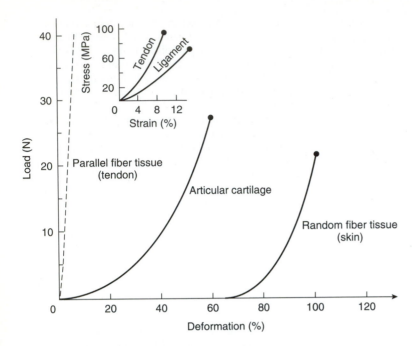

Figure 1–12. Load-elongation curves for several soft tissues. The range in mechanical properties of the tissues is attributable to collagen fiber orientation and interaction with the extracellular matrix.

studied ligaments that were immobilized for 8 weeks and control ligaments found that the previously immobilized ligaments required 12 months of reconditioning before they demonstrated strength and stiffness values comparable to those of the control ligaments.

Studies of nonsteroidal anti-inflammatory drugs (NSAIDs) such as indomethacin have demonstrated that treatment results in increases in the proportion of insoluble collagen and the total collagen content in tissue. It also leads to increased tensile strength, which is probably attributable to increased collagen molecule cross-links. Therefore, short-term NSAID therapy may increase the rate of biomechanical restoration of the tendons and ligaments.

C. Injury Mechanisms

Tendons and ligaments are subjected to less than one third of their ultimate stress during normal physiologic loading. The maximal physiologic strain ranges from 2 to 5%. Several factors lead to tissue injury, however. When tendons and ligaments are subjected to stresses that exceed the physiologic range, microfailure of collagen bundles occurs before the yield point of the tissue is reached. When the yield point is reached, the tissue undergoes gross failure and the joint simultaneously becomes displaced. The amount of force produced by the maximal contraction of the muscle results in a maximal tensile stress in the tendon. The extent of tendon injury is influenced by the amount of tendon cross-sectional area compared with that for muscle. The larger the

muscle cross-sectional area, the higher the magnitude of the force produced by the contraction and thus the greater the tensile load transmitted through the tendon.

Clinically, ligament injuries are characterized according to degree of severity. First-degree sprains are typified by minimal pain and demonstrate no detectable joint instability despite microfailure of collagen fibers. Second-degree sprains cause severe pain and demonstrate minimal joint instability. This instability is most likely masked by muscle activity, however. Therefore, testing must be performed with the patient under anesthesia for proper evaluation. Second-degree sprains are characterized by partial ligament rupture and progressive failure of the collagen fibers, with the result that ligament strength and stiffness decrease by 50%. Third-degree sprains cause severe pain during the course of the injury and minimal pain afterward. The joint is completely unstable. Most collagen fibers have ruptured, but a few may remain intact, giving the ligament the appearance of continuity even though it is incapable of supporting loads. Abnormally high stress on the articular cartilage results if pressure is exerted on a joint that is unstable owing to ligament or joint capsule rupture.

D. Healing Mechanisms

During tendon and ligament healing and repair, fibroblastic infiltration from the adjacent tissues is essential. The healing events are initiated by an inflammatory response, which is characterized by polymorphonuclear cell infiltration, capillary budding, and fluid exudation and which continues during the first 3 days following the injury. After 4 days, fibroplasia occurs and is accompanied by the significant accumulation of fibroblasts. Within 3 weeks, a mass of granulation tissue surrounds the damaged tissue. During the next week, collagen fibers become longitudinally oriented. During the next 3 months, the individual collagen fibers form bundles identical to the original bundles.

Sutured tendons heal with a progressive penetration of connective tissue from the outside. The deposited collagen fibers become progressively oriented until eventually they form tendon fibers like the original ones. This orientation of collagen fibers is essential because the tensile strength of repaired tendon is dependent on collagen content and orientation. If tendon is sutured during the first 7–10 days of healing, the strength of the suture maintains the fixation until adequate callus has been formed.

Tendon mobilization during healing is important to avoid adhesion of the tendon to adjacent tissue, particularly in cases involving the flexor tendons of the hand. Motion can be passive to prevent adhesion and at the same time to prevent putting excessive tensile stress on the suture line. The gliding properties of flexor tendons that have been mobilized are consistently superior to those of flexor tendons that have been immobilized during the healing process.

Direct apposition of the surfaces of a divided ligament provides the most favorable conditions for healing because it minimizes scar formation, accelerates repair, hastens collagenization, and comes closer to restoring normal ligamentous tissue. Care must be taken during the repair of ligaments to avoid subsequent common problems with healing, however. For instance, divided and immobilized ligaments heal with a fibrous tissue gap between the two ends, whereas sutured ligaments unite without a fibrous tissue gap. If excessive tension is placed on a suture, necrosis and failure to heal are observed. Unsutured ligaments can retract, shorten, and become atrophic, however, making repair difficult 2 weeks following the injury. In spite of this, many ligaments are not routinely repaired in orthopedic surgery.

The anterior cruciate ligament is often severely damaged in cases of midsubstance rupture and generally does not fare well following repair. The ligament is intra-articular, with synovial fluid tending to disrupt the repair. Instability of the knee also tends to place excessive stress on the repair unless the knee is immobilized, which leads to joint stiffness and muscle atrophy.

Skeletal Muscle

Skeletal muscles perform a wide variety of mechanical and biologic functions. From a mechanical perspective, it is obvious that skeletal muscles generate force and length changes. The generation of force and length change gives rise to the production of mechanical work and power. Less obvious is the fact that skeletal muscles are often subjected to so-called lengthening or eccentric contractions. During these types of contractions, muscles may act as so-called dynamic joint stabilizers and may store energy. From a biologic perspective, skeletal muscles are believed to secrete various growth factors such as insulin-like growth factor 1 (IGF-1), which is thought to play an important autocrine/paracrine role in regulating muscle fiber size. Additionally, it has been proposed that skeletal muscles play a key role in maintaining the health of motor neurons.

A. SKELETAL MUSCLE STRUCTURE

1. Macroscopic anatomy—Figure 1–13 provides both a macroscopic and microscopic perspective of the structure of skeletal muscle. From a macroscopic perspective, skeletal muscles are composed of tens of thousands of individual muscle fibers (muscle cells). Muscles that are involved in fine motor control usually contain a small number of muscle fibers compared with those muscles involved in activities requiring the generation of large forces and power outputs. Muscle fibers are usually found in so-called bundles that are also referred to as **fascicles.** Each fascicle typically contains about 10–30 muscle fibers that are encased in a connective tissue sheath known as the **endomysium.**

From an architectural perspective, muscles are often classified on the basis of the orientations of the muscle fibers' longitudinal axes relative to that of the entire muscle. For instance, **longitudinal** muscles are composed of muscle fibers whose longitudinal axis runs parallel to that of the whole muscle. Good examples of this type of architecture are the rectus abdominis and the sartorius muscles. In **fusiform** muscles, the fibers run parallel to the longitudinal axis throughout most of the muscle, but taper at the ends of the muscle. The soleus and brachioradialis muscles are typical of this architecture. Muscles can also exhibit a so-called **pennate** (unipennate, bipennate) architecture whereby the longitudinal axis of the individual muscle fibers runs diagonal to that of the whole muscle. A good example of a bipennate muscle is the gastrocnemius muscle. The muscle fibers of **angular** or **fan-shaped** muscles radiate from a narrow attachment at one end and fan out, resulting in a broad attachment at the other end as is seen in muscles like the pectoralis major.

Consistent with the theme of structure-function relationships, muscle architecture can be an important determinant of the mechanical properties of skeletal muscle. For instance, fusiform muscles typically have longer muscle fibers than bipennate muscles. Functionally, this means that a fusiform muscle should be able

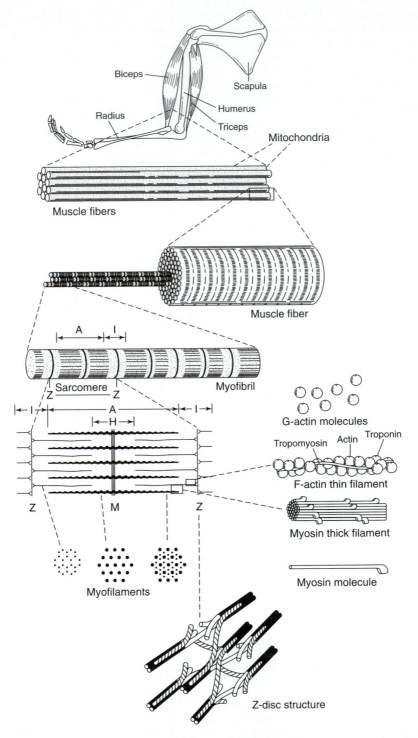

Figure 1–13. Overview of macroscopic and microscopic structure of skeletal muscle. (Reprinted, with permission, from McMahon TA. *Muscles, Reflexes, and Locomotion.* Princeton, NJ: Princeton University Press, 1984.)

to generate greater shortening velocities and muscle length excursions at the whole muscle level. In contrast, muscles with a pennate or bipennate architecture have shorter fibers, but the fibers are packed in such a manner that a larger number of muscle fibers are in parallel to one another, resulting in a larger physiologic cross-sectional area. Hence, the pennate muscle has a greater capacity for generating force.

2. Molecular anatomy of the myofibril—The structure of skeletal muscle at the molecular level is quite complex (see Figure 1–13). Each muscle fiber is made up of thousands of so-called **myofibrils** that are arranged in parallel to one another. Each myofibril has a cross-sectional area of approximately 1 μm^2. Hence, a muscle fiber with a cross-sectional area of approximately 1000 μm^2 would contain about 1000 myofibrils. Typically, the cross-sectional area of a muscle fiber can range from approximately 1000 to 7000 μm^2. Each myofibril consists of a repeating series of striations that are due to the arrangement of so-called **sarcomeres** in series. Each sarcomere is approximately 2–3 μm in length. Sarcomeres are often referred to as the contractile units of skeletal muscle.

In a general sense, sarcomeres consist of Z-lines, thin filaments, and thick filaments. The interdigitation of thick and thin filaments along with the presence of Z-lines is primarily responsible for the striation pattern of skeletal muscle. As shown in Figure 1–14, the Z-lines are dense thin structures that are found in the middle of the so-called I-band. In reality, each Z-line represents an anchor point to which thin filaments are attached. By definition, the collection of proteins between each Z-line is known as a sarcomere. Hence, the I-band represents a region where no overlap occurs of the thin filaments (by thick filaments), yielding a relatively light band. The A-band is composed of the thick filament and is strongly birefringent, producing a dark band on microscopic inspection. By definition, the length of the A-band is equivalent to the length of the thick filament. Normally, the thick and thin filaments partially overlap, and as a result a lighter region occurs in the middle of the A-band known as the H-zone.

Changes in sarcomere length and, as a result, muscle fiber length are due to the sliding of the thick and thin filaments relative to one another. In its most simplistic sense, this model states that contraction takes place not due to changes in the individual lengths of thick and thin filaments, but rather by the sliding of thin filaments past thick filaments. This model of contraction is known as the **sliding-filament hypothesis.** The changes in striation patterns during shortening contractions played a central role in developing the sliding filament hypothesis. In this context, Table 1–1 summarizes the changes in the striation pattern that occur during isometric, shortening (isotonic), and lengthening (eccentric) contractions.

3. Molecular anatomy of the sarcomere—As shown in Figure 1–14 and in Table 1–2, the overall structure of the sarcomere has become quite complex as more sophisticated techniques for studying skeletal muscle have evolved. On a basic level, the sarcomeric proteins and those associated with the sarcomere can be placed into four different categories: (1) contractile; (2) regulatory contractile; (3) structural; and (4) costameric.

As shown in Table 1–2, the primary contractile proteins are simply **actin** and **myosin.** These are referred to as contractile proteins, given their central role in the contractile process. Individual monomers of actin bind to one another to form so-called actin filaments. In contrast, the thick filament is composed primarily of myosin heavy-chain molecules packed in an antiparallel arrangement. A more detailed description of myosin is provided later. Regulatory contractile proteins are defined as those that turn the contractile apparatus on or off and those that can modulate the activity of the myosin heavy chain. In skeletal muscle, the regulatory contractile proteins involved in turning the contractile apparatus on or off are associated exclusively with the actin filament, and these proteins include **tropomyosin, troponin-T, troponin-I,** and **troponin-C.** Collectively, the thin filament is composed of the actin filament and these (ie, tropomyosin, troponin-T, troponin-I, and troponin-C) regulatory contractile proteins. Other regulatory contractile proteins are associated with the myosin heavy chain, and these are referred to collectively as **myosin light chains** (MLCs) because of their relatively low molecular weight. These MLCs may possibly be involved in regulating the kinetics of cross-bridge cycling.

Structural and costameric proteins play several essential roles. First, electron micrographs (see Figure 1–14) demonstrate that sarcomeres are organized in a very orderly fashion such that the Z-lines of adjoining sarcomeres appear to be in register with one another. As noted in Table 1–2, key intermediate filaments like **desmin** and **vimentin** are believed to play key roles in aligning the Z-line of one sarcomere with that of another. Other proteins like **synemin** are also thought to be involved in the alignment of sarcomeres. Structural proteins also play a key role in developing a mechanical linkage between sarcomeres and the extracellular matrix. These sites of connectivity between the sarcomere, cell membrane, and extracellular matrix have been referred to as **costameres** (see section 5. Molecular anatomy of the connection between the cytoskeleton and the extracellular matrix).

4. Molecular anatomy of myosin molecule—Although the term *myosin molecule* is often used, in reality the myosin molecule is a hexameric structure composed

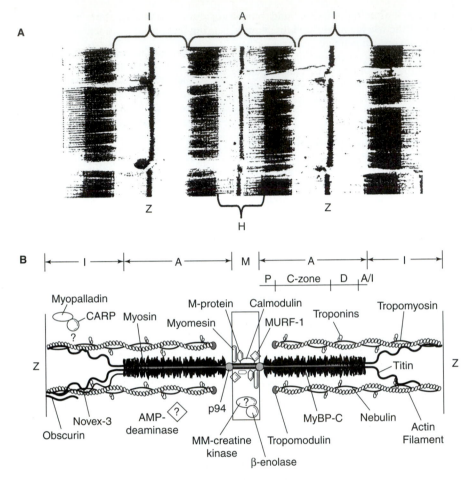

Figure 1–14. Striation pattern and various proteins associated with sarcomere. Electron micrograph of sarcomeres is shown in (**A**). A schematic illustration of the various structures and proteins of the sarcomere is shown in (**B**). p94 = muscle-specific calpain. MURF-1 = muscle ring finger-1, which is believed to be part of the ubiquitin-proteosome complex involved in protein degradation. MyBP-C = myosin-binding protein-C, otherwise known as C-protein. CARP = cardiac adriamycin-responsive protein. (**A** reproduced, with permission, from Aidley DJ: *The Physiology of Excitable Cells.* New York, NY: Cambridge University Press, 1998. **B** reproduced, with permission, from Clark KA et al: Striated muscle cytoarchitecture: an intricate web of form and function. Ann Rev Cell Dev Biol 2002;18:637.) Also, see Table 1–2.

of two myosin heavy chains, two so-called essential light chains (MLC$_1$ or MLC$_3$), and two regulatory light chains (MLC$_2$). The term *heavy* or *light* is used in reference to the molecular weights of each of these proteins. Each myosin heavy chain is composed of a rod region, lever arm (also known as S$_2$) and a globular head (also known as S$_1$). The rod region plays an important role in the packing of individual myosin heavy chains into thick filaments. The globular head contains the key

functional domains of this molecular motor. Within the globular head (Figure 1–15) are domains that contain (1) the actin-binding site, (2) the nucleotide (ATP)-binding site, and (3) the enzymatic (ATPase) properties responsible for converting chemical energy in the form of ATP into mechanical work and heat. The essential and regulatory light chains are bound to the so-called lever arm or s$_2$ region (see Figure 1–15). Each globular head has bound to it one essential and one reg-

Table 1–1. Effect of different types of contractions on the various bands, zones, lines, and length.

Type of Contraction	Z-line	I-band	A-band	H-zone	M-line	Sarcomere Length
Isometric	↔	↔	↔	↔	↔	↔
Shortening (isotonic)	↔	↓	↔	↓	↔	↓
Lengthening (eccentric)	↔	↑	↔	↑	↔	↑

↔ = no change in length; ↑ = increase in length; ↓ = decrease in length.

ulatory light chain. Mutations of some of these domains (eg, the actin-binding site) are thought to play roles in diseases such as familial hypertrophic cardiomyopathy. As noted earlier, the light chains are thought to play modulatory roles in regulating the kinetics of the crossbridge cycle.

The complexity of the myosin molecule is further complicated by the presence of isoforms for both the myosin heavy and light chains. Although it has long been recognized that muscles could be classified as **slow** or **fast twitch** (based on twitch properties), the importance of myosin heavy-chain isoforms has only been intensely studied during the past 20 years. In many smaller adult mammals (eg, mice, rats, rabbits), four myosin heavy-chains isoforms have been identified and classified as **slow Type I, fast Type IIA, fast Type IIX,** and **fast Type IIB** (in order of increasing ATPase activities and associated maximal shortening velocities). In adult humans, the slow Type I, fast Type IIA, and fast Type IIX myosin heavy-chain isoforms are expressed. This scheme of classifying myosin heavy-chains isoforms forms the basis for the nomenclature typically used to identify different muscle fiber types. Hence, a slow Type I muscle fiber would exclusively express the slow Type I myosin heavy-chain isoform.

It should be noted that there are isoforms for myosin heavy chains, myosin light chains, tropomyosin, troponin-T, troponin-I, and troponin-C. Hence, by mixing and matching these contractile and regulatory contractile proteins, the complexity that can arise in the design of sarcomeres becomes readily apparent.

The sequence of the crossbridge cycle is shown in (see Figure 1–15). First, myosin is detached from actin. Second, the head of the myosin heavy chain is attached to actin and releases Pi, leading to the power stroke (change in position of head between Figure 1–15B and 1–15C). Following completion of the power stroke, ADP is released, and subsequently ATP binds to the nucleotide-binding site (Figure 1–15D, E). The hydrolysis of ATP ultimately leads to the globular head of the myosin heavy chain returning to its original position. The magnitude of crossbridge cycling that occurs during a single contraction is enormous and can approach rates equivalent to 10^{17}–10^{18} crossbridge cycles per gram of muscle per second.

In thinking about the plasticity of the sarcomere and its constituent proteins, it should be noted that mechanical unloading and denervation lead to a decrease in the number of sarcomeres in parallel. From a functional perspective, this leads to a decrease in the capacity to produce force. In contrast, resistance training leads to an increase in the number of sarcomeres in parallel, and, as a consequence, increased capacity to produce force.

Factors such as mechanical unloading (eg, as accompanies cast immobilization) and altered thyroid hormone status will produce shifts in the contractile and regulatory contractile protein isoform profiles such that they will become faster. For instance, cast immobilization may lead to a transition from the slow Type I to the fast Type IIX myosin heavy-chain isoform. From a functional perspective, this will lead to an increase in maximal shortening velocity. Although it is commonly thought that strength training is an effective tool for increasing sprint speed, it should be noted that this will produce fast-to-slow transitions in myosin heavy-chain isoform expression.

5. Molecular anatomy of the connection between the cytoskeleton and the extracellular matrix— Costameres are important structures that link the cytoskeleton of skeletal muscle with the extracellular matrix (Figure 1–16). Currently, it is believed that the costameres serve at least three different functions: (1) aligning the sarcolemma with the cytoskeleton; (2) maintaining membrane integrity during different types of contractions, preventing injury to the sarcolemma; and (3) possibly playing a role in the lateral transmission of force. From a structural perspective, costameres are found aligned with the Z- and M-lines.

Table 1–2. Overview of proteins involved with the sarcomere and cytoskeletal-extracellular matrix interactions.

Classes and types of sarcomeric proteins	Molecular Wt (kDa)	Location	Function
Contractile proteins			
Myosin heavy chain	~200	Thick filament	Molecular motor; binds to actin; generates force and length change
Actin	~42	Thin filament	Binds myosin and translates force and/or length changes
Regulatory contractile proteins			
Tropomyosin	~37	Thin filament	Regulates interaction between actin and myosin; stabilizes thin filament
Troponin-T	~30	Thin filament	Couples troponin complex to actin?
Troponin-I	~22	Thin filament	Influences position of tropomyosin
Troponin-C	~18	Thin filament	Binds Ca^{+2}, influences position of tropomyosin
Myosin light chain-1	~22	Thick filament	Influences V_{max}?
Myosin light chain-2	~20	Thick filament	Influences tension–pCa^{+2} relationship
Myosin light chain-3	~18	Thick filament	Influences V_{max}
Structural proteins			
Associated with thin filament			
CapZ-α, CapZ-β	~36, ~32	Z-line	Caps free end of actin, regulates actin filament length; binds to α-actinin
Tropomodulin	~40	Thin filament	Caps pointed end of actin filament
Nebulin	~600–900	I-band	Anchors actin to Z-line; molecular ruler of actin filament length?
Associated with thick filament			
Myosin binding protein-C	~140	Thick Filament	Binds to lever arm and rod region of MHC; titin binding site
Myomesin	~185	M-line	Binds to myosin and titin; may play role in linking myosin and titin
MurF-1	~40	M-line	May play key role in degradation
Calpain-3; p94		M-line	Binds to titin
Titin	~3000–4000	Spans A–I bands	Molecular spring? Sarcomere template?
Associated with Z-line			
α-Actinin	~97	Z-line	Major protein of Z-line
LIM	~23	Z-line	Binds α-actinin, zyxin, β-spectrin
FATZ	~32	Z-line	Binds calcineurin to Z-line
Intermediate filaments			
Desmin	~53	Z-line	Longitudinal and lateral alignment of sarcomeres
Skelemin	~200	M-band	M-line integrity
Vimentin	~53	Z-line	Periodicity of Z-lines
Costameric proteins			
Ankyrin	17–440	Costamere	Localization
α-Dystrobrevin	~87	Costamere	Membrane stabilization; transmembrane signaling involved with NOS
α/β-Dystroglycan	~156, 43	Costamere	Prevents injury to sarcolemma
Dystrophin	427	Costamere	Stabilizes cytoskeleton and sarcolemma
α-Fodrin	85	Costamere	Attachment of cytoskeleton to ECM; signaling
Integrins	~90 and 150	Costamere	Stabilization of cytoskeleton
α-Sarcoglycan	~240	Costamere	Binds dystrophin and α-dystrobrevin; associated with NOS
α/β-Spectrin	~250	Costamere	Stabilization of sarcomere
Syntrophins	~57–60	Costamere	NOS?
Talin	~235	Costamere-MTJ	Role in stabilizing link between muscle fiber and tendon fibrils?
Vinculin	116 ~130	Costamere, MTJ	Role in stabilizing link between muscle fiber and tendon fibrils?

MHC = myosin heavy drain; LIM = cysteine-rich double zinc finger motifs that mediate protein binding; FATC = filamin, α-actinin and telethonin-associated Z-line protein; NOS = nitric oxide synthase; ECM = extracellular matrix.

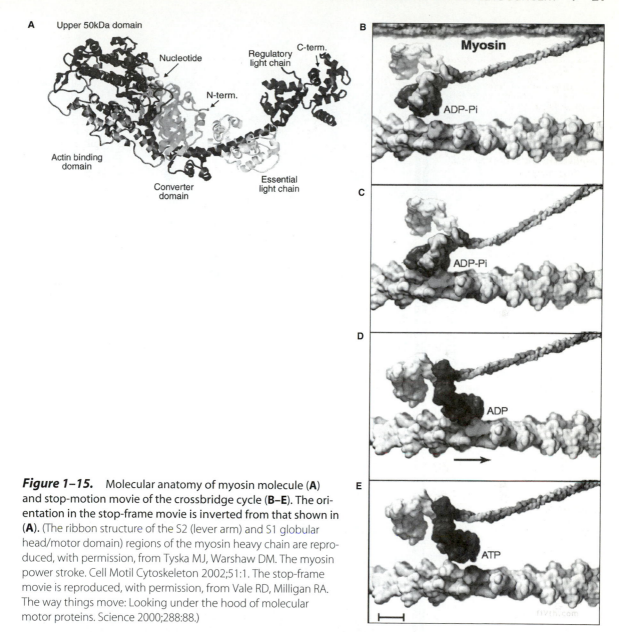

Figure 1–15. Molecular anatomy of myosin molecule (**A**) and stop-motion movie of the crossbridge cycle (**B–E**). The orientation in the stop-frame movie is inverted from that shown in (**A**). (The ribbon structure of the S2 (lever arm) and S1 globular head/motor domain) regions of the myosin heavy chain are reproduced, with permission, from Tyska MJ, Warshaw DM. The myosin power stroke. Cell Motil Cytoskeleton 2002;51:1. The stop-frame movie is reproduced, with permission, from Vale RD, Milligan RA. The way things move: Looking under the hood of molecular motor proteins. Science 2000;288:88.)

This linkage occurs as a result of so-called intermediate filaments. It should be noted that mutations in the costameric structure are thought to be involved in some of the muscular dystrophies. Additionally, these structures may play an important role in protecting muscle fibers from eccentrically induced muscle damage.

6. The on-and-off switch of the molecular motor: Excitation-contraction coupling—From a mechanical perspective, all of the sarcomeres must become activated in a synchronous fashion. An asynchronous activation of sarcomeres would lead to large heterogeneities in sarcomere length along the length of a muscle fiber with some sarcomeres actively shortening, whereas the nonactivated sarcomeres would be lengthened. The net result might be a contraction, whereby there is little overall shortening of the muscle fiber. The synchronous activation of all sarcomeres requires that there be an elaborate

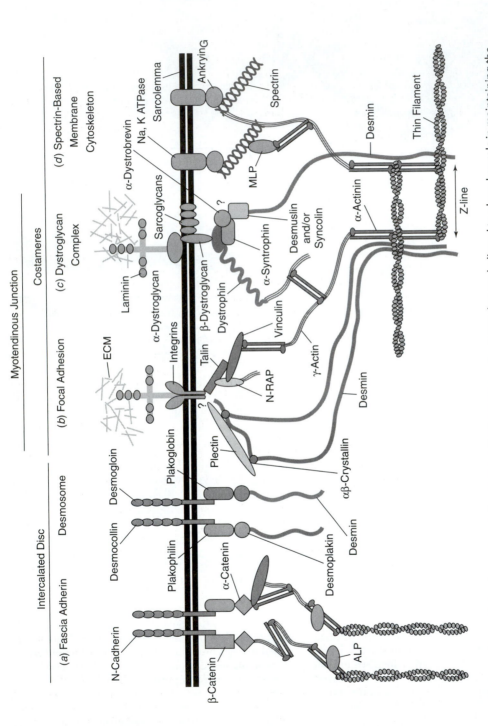

Figure 1–16. Molecular anatomy of costamere. Costameres are structures that are believed to play a key role in maintaining the mechanical integrity of the membrane during various types of contractions. They are localized at points of contact between the Z-line, M-line, and membrane (sarcolemma). They are also found at myotendonous junctions. The major proteins found localized at the costamere include ankyrin, cytokeratin, desmin, α-dystroglycan, β-dystroglyan, dystroglyan, dystrophin, α-fodrin, β-spectrin, alpha and beta subunits of the Na[+]/K[+] ATPase pump, sarcoglycan, sarcospan. The costamere forms a mechanical link between the sarcomeres within the muscle fiber and laminin located in the extracellular matrix. (Reproduced, with permission, from Clark KA et al: Striated muscle cytoarchitecture: an intricate web of form and function. Ann Rev Cell Dev Biol 2002;18:637.)

reticulum that functionally couples the depolarization of the sarcolemma (cell membrane) with activation of the sarcomere. The coupling between excitation and contraction involves extensive invaginations of the sarcolemma known as **transverse tubules** (T-tubules), which are associated with the **sarcoplasmic reticulum.** The sarcoplasmic reticulum is a network of membranes wrapped around the myofibrils, containing a large store of Ca^{2+}. When a skeletal muscle fiber is excited, the depolarization of the sarcolemma is propagated into the T-tubules. Excitation of the T-tubules then leads to the release of Ca^{2+} from the ends of the sarcoplasmic reticulum via so-called **Ca^{2+} release channels** (also known as ryanodine receptors). The Ca^{2+} quickly diffuses into the space occupied by the sarcomere, binding to troponin-C. This then causes tropomyosin to rotate about the longitudinal axis of the actin filament, uncovering the myosin binding sites of each actin molecule. The globular head of the myosin heavy chain will attach to this binding site and go through its power stroke, leading to the production of force or length change. Simply stated it is the binding of Ca^{2+} to troponin-C that turns on the contractile apparatus.

The contractile activity of the sarcomere is turned off by resequestering Ca^{2+} back into the sarcoplasmic reticulum via **Ca^{2+} ATPase pumps** located along the length of the sarcoplasmic reticulum. The dissociation of Ca^{2+} from troponin-C causes tropomyosin to rotate back into its original position, once again covering up or blocking the myosin-binding sites of each actin molecule. In this manner, the globular head of the myosin heavy chain is prevented from binding to actin, leading to decay in force production and causing the muscle to relax.

As mentioned earlier, there are a number of isoforms for the contractile and regulatory contractile proteins. Isoforms have also been identified for the Ca^{2+} release channels and Ca^{2+} ATPase pumps of the sarcoplasmic reticulum. These different isoforms play a key role in determining the rate of activation (ie, the release of Ca^{2+}) and relaxation (resequestration of Ca^{2+}). Mechanical unloading of skeletal muscle typically leads to an increased expression of the fast isoforms of the Ca^{2+} release channels, whereas reloading or strength training will produce the opposite effect.

B. SKELETAL MUSCLE FUNCTION

In a general sense, the mechanical activity of skeletal muscle is dependent on two factors: the pattern of stimulation and the extent of loading. The most basic unit of contractile response is known as a twitch. Simply stated, a twitch is the mechanical response of skeletal muscle to a single brief stimulus (Figure 1–17). This single stimulus leads to a single pulse of Ca^{2+} released

from the sarcoplasmic reticulum. This single pulse of Ca^{2+} is nonsaturating, meaning that it binds to only some of the troponin-C molecules. In turn, this causes only some of the tropomyosin molecules to rotate about the longitudinal axis of the actin filament, uncovering only some of the myosin-binding sites. From a mechanical perspective, this leads to a submaximal force transient called a **twitch** (Figure 1–17A). The Ca^{2+} is quickly resequestered by the sarcoplasmic reticulum, and force returns to resting levels.

The amount of Ca^{2+} released by the sarcoplasmic reticulum can be modulated by the pattern of stimulation. If a muscle is repetitively stimulated but with long durations between each stimulus, then the mechanical response will appear as a series of individual twitches, and the force produced will be submaximal. On the other hand, if the muscle is stimulated using a moderate frequency, then the mechanical response due to one stimulus will fuse with that of the second stimulus, leading to mechanical response known as **tetanus,** and the amplitude is dependent on the balance between Ca^{2+} release and resequestration. A greater frequency of stimulation will lead to a greater release of Ca^{2+} and production of force (Figure 1–17B). Tetanus has two types: one in which partial relaxation occurs between each stimulus (unfused) and another in which no discernible relaxation happens between stimuli (fused) (Figure 1–17B). During fused tetanus, all of the Ca^{2+}-binding sites of troponin-C are saturated, causing all of the myosin-binding sites to be exposed. This results in the greatest production of force.

As noted earlier, the loading of skeletal muscle also plays a key role in determining the mechanical response. For instance, if a muscle contracts against an immovable object, the muscle will not shorten, and hence muscle length will remain constant. This type of contraction is referred to as **an isometric contraction** (iso = same; metros = length), and it is under these loading conditions the muscle will produce maximal force. If a muscle contracts against a load that is submaximal (ie, less than the maximal force the muscle can generate), then the muscle will shorten. This type of contraction is often referred to as either a **shortening** or **an isotonic contraction.** Muscles not only work under these types of loading conditions, but work almost as often under conditions in which the muscle is activated and forcibly lengthened. These types of contractions are known as **lengthening** or **eccentric contractions.**

1. Conceptual framework of factors that determine muscle function—From an orthopedics perspective it would be beneficial to have a framework that would include the key factors that determine the mechanical function of skeletal muscle. Such a framework is laid

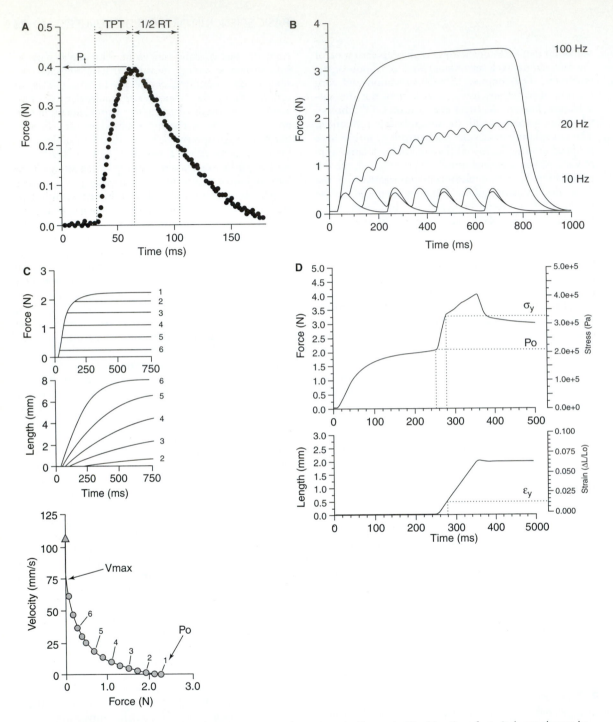

Figure 1–17. Various mechanical measurements that are typically made. The kinetics of a twitch are shown in (**A**). P_t = maximal twitch tension; TPT = time-to-peak tension; $1/2$ RT = one-half relaxation time. The importance of stimulation frequency in regulating the release of Ca^{2+} from the sarcoplasmic reticulum and ultimately force production is shown in (**B**). Methods used to determine the force-velocity relationship are shown in (**C**). V_{max} = maximal shortening velocity; P_o = maximal isometric tension. The mechanical response of a fully activated muscle to a strain of approximately 6% is shown in (**D**). σ = yield stress; ε = yield strain.

out in Figure 1–18 and revolves around the context of net mechanical work. In a general context, the net mechanical work produced by skeletal muscle during cyclic length changes (eg, cyclic sinusoidal length changes) is determined by those factors that determine the positive amount of work produced during the shortening phase and those factors that determine the amount of mechanical work done on relengthening the muscle (ie, negative work).

There are four determinants of the amount of positive work that can be produced during the shortening phase: (1) the length-tension relationship, (2) the rate of activation, (3) the force-velocity relationship in the shortening domain, and (4) the rate of relaxation. Two factors determine the amount of work done on the muscle during lengthening: (1) the force-velocity relationship in the lengthening domain and (2) the passive stiffness of the muscle. From an engineering perspective, each of these factors can be thought of as representing design constraints, one of which is static (the length-tension relationship) and others are dynamic. The term *static* in ref-

erence to the length-tension relationship implies that the basic dimensions of the sarcomere (and hence length-tension relationship) do not appear to be malleable. In contrast, the other factors can all be altered by factors influencing the mechanical loading of skeletal muscle (eg, immobilization), innervation (partial/complete denervation), and hormonal milieu (eg, thyroid, steroids).

2. Length-tension relationship—The amount of force a muscle can generate is dependent on muscle length; this length-tension relationship is shown in Figure 1–19. Typically, three regions of the length-tension relationship are described. The ascending limb extends from a sarcomere length of approximately 1.3–2.0 μm. In this region, the amount of isometric tension increases in direct proportion to the increase in sarcomere length. The plateau region extends from ~2.0 to 2.5 μm in mammalian fibers, and in this range there is an optimal overlap between the thick and thin filaments. Beyond a sarcomere length of 2.5 μm, the isometric force that can be produced decreases as a linear func-

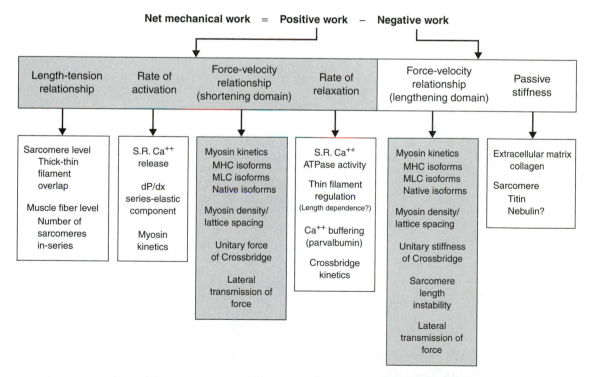

Figure 1–18. Various factors that limit the production of mechanical work and power. S.R. = sarcoplasmic reticulum. *dP/dx* = stiffness of series elastic component. MHC = myosin heavy chain. MLC = myosin light chain. (Modified, with permission, from Caiozzo VJ: Phenotypic plasticity of skeletal muscle: Mechanical consequences. Muscle Nerve 2002;26:740).

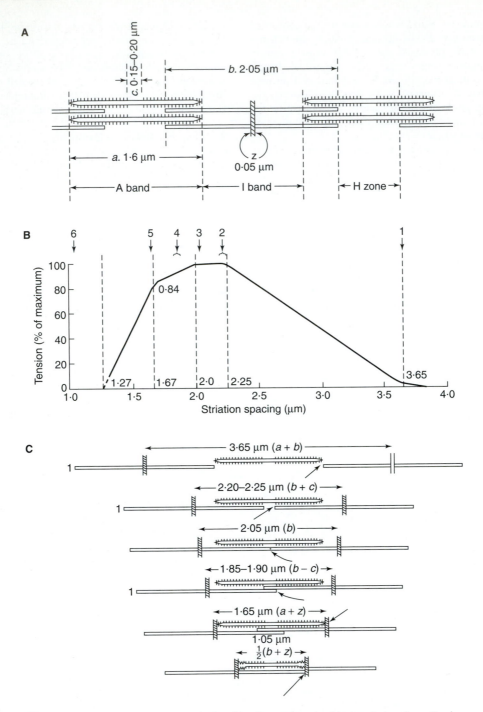

Figure 1–19. Length-tension relationship. (Reproduced, with permission, from Gordon AM et al: The variation in isometric tension with sarcomere length in vertebrate muscle fibres. J Physiol 1966;184:170.)

tion of increases in sarcomere length, reflecting a progressive decrease in overlap between the thick and thin filaments.

The length-tension relationship of the sarcomere is thought to represent a static design criteria, implying that it does not change with various types of interventions such as mechanical unloading. However, it is well known that muscles immobilized in a lengthened position will increase the number of sarcomeres in series, leading to the longitudinal growth of the fiber. In contrast, immobilization in a shortened position will reduce the number of sarcomeres in series, and result in a shorter muscle fiber. Hence, such manipulations have the potential for influencing the overall length-tension relationships of muscle fibers and whole muscles. Clearly, contractures may have a large effect on the number of sarcomeres in series and result in various clinical complications such as equinus contractures.

3. Force-velocity relationship in the shortening domain—When a muscle contracts against a light load, it will be able to shorten at a relatively high velocity. However, when a muscle contracts against a heavy load, it will shorten at a relatively slow velocity. The relationship between the force and shortening velocity is shown in Figure 1–17C and reveals that the force-velocity relationship in the shortening domain can be described by a rectangular hyperbola. Importantly, the shape and dimensions of this relationship are dependent on the types of contractile protein isoforms and how they are packaged. As noted earlier, **maximal shortening velocity** is primarily determined by the types of myosin heavy-chain isoforms present in the muscle fiber. For instance, a muscle fiber that expresses only the slow Type I myosin heavy chain will have a much slower V_{max} than one that expresses only the fast Type IIX or IIB myosin heavy-chain isoforms. V_{max} is not dependent on the cross-sectional area of the muscle fiber. The **maximal isometric tension** that a muscle can produce, often referred to as P_o, is largely independent of myosin heavy-chain isoforms but is heavily dependent on the number of sarcomeres in parallel (ie, cross-sectional area). Hence, in an individual who has marked atrophy, P_o would be expected to be significantly reduced but V_{max} would be unchanged. In this context, the force-velocity relationship can be referred to as a dynamic design criterion, meaning that changes in either cross-sectional area or myosin heavy-chain isoform expression can alter the shape and dimensions of this relationship. Importantly, this relationship represents a design criterion because the muscle can only operate on or below the force-velocity relationship.

The product of force × velocity is mechanical power. Hence, the force-velocity relationship also defines the maximal amount of mechanical power that can be produced under any given loading condition. This has important implications for a wide variety of movements.

4. Force-velocity relationship in the lengthening domain—When a muscle is maximally activated and then forcibly lengthened, the tension that can be generated is much greater than that observed under isometric conditions. However, at velocities beyond a relatively low lengthening velocity, tension will not rise any further. This is shown in Figure 1–20. Although muscles commonly perform lengthening contractions, our understanding of the factors that determine the shape of the force-velocity relationship in the lengthening domain is relatively poor. The shape and dimensions of the force-velocity relationship in the lengthening domain are much more complicated than these same dimensions in the shortening domain. In the shortening domain, the force-velocity relationship can be described by a planar curve with the axes of force and velocity. In the lengthening domain, the relationship is three-dimensional, being dependent on force, velocity, and time.

An example of the response of skeletal muscle to a lengthening contraction is shown in Figure 1–17D. Note that the muscle is stimulated, and force is allowed to move onto its isometric plateau. A constant-velocity stretch is then imposed on the muscle, and tension rises rapidly. However, at a strain of approximately 1–2% a sudden change occurs in the rise in tension such that the slope decreases dramatically. The initial force response is

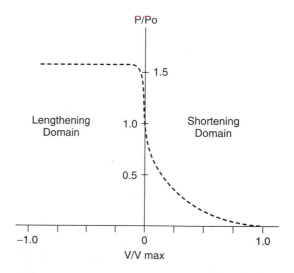

Figure 1–20. Force-velocity relationship in both the shortening and lengthening domains. (Reproduced, with permission, from Caiozzo VJ: Phenotypic plasticity of skeletal muscle: Mechanical consequences. Muscle Nerve 2002;26:740.)

often referred to as short-range stiffness. Note that both before and after the yield, force is constantly changing but the velocity of lengthening remains constant. This demonstrates the complexity of understanding the force-velocity relationship in the lengthening domain.

From a functional perspective, the force-velocity relationship in the lengthening domain is important because it determines the amount of work done on relengthening a muscle that is either fully or partially activated. Additionally, muscles are thought to act as dynamic joint stabilizers, so it might be hypothesized that stiffer muscles might better protect joints and ligaments (ie, anterior cruciate ligament) that are susceptible to injury. Recent studies have shown that mechanical unloading dramatically reduces both the stiffness and elastic modulus of skeletal muscle. The loss of elastic modulus occurs either due to a decrease in crossbridge density or to changes in the unitary stiffness of crossbridges.

5. Passive stiffness of skeletal muscle—The passive stiffness of skeletal muscle is influenced by both sarcomeric and extracellular matrix proteins. **Titin** is the largest known protein identified to date, and it attaches the thick filaments to the Z-line. Within the titin molecule is a unique region, the PEVK region, that functions like a molecular spring. It has been proposed that the passive tension of skeletal muscle fibers during stretch is, in part, due to the properties of titin. At the extracellular matrix level, the major protein component is **collagen.** It is currently believed that changes in the loading of skeletal muscle (via immobilization or resistance training) can alter the collagen content of skeletal muscle. The functional significance, however, has not been clearly delineated.

Aidley DJ: *The Physiology of Excitable Cells.* New York, NY: Cambridge University Press, 1998.

Caiozzo VJ: Phenotypic plasticity of skeletal muscle: Mechanical consequences. Muscle Nerve 2002;26:740. [PMID 12451599].

Clark KA et al: Striated muscle cytoarchitecture: An intricate web of form and function. Ann Rev Cell Dev Biol 2002;18:637. [PMID: 12142273]

Gordon AM et al: The variation in isometric tension with sarcomere length in vertebrate muscle fibres. J Physiol 1966;184:170.[PMID 5921536]

Tyska MJ, Warshaw DM. The myosin power stroke. Cell Motil Cytoskeleton 2002;51:1. [PMID 11810692]

Vale RD, Milligan RA. The way things move: Looking under the hood of molecular motor proteins. Science 2000;288:88. [PMID 10753125]

Intervertebral Disks

The intervertebral disks sustain and distribute loads and also prevent excessive motion of the spine. An individual's intervertebral disks account for 20–33% of his or her spinal column height. The disks are subjected to a large amount of stress during normal daily activity, and stress may double during increased activity, lifting, or trauma. Whether intervertebral disk failure occurs depends on loading rate and stress distribution.

A. STRUCTURAL COMPOSITION

Each intervertebral disk has a nucleus pulposus surrounded by a thick capsule called the annulus fibrosus (Figure 1–21). End-plates composed of hyaline cartilage separate the intervertebral disk from the vertebral body. The unique interplay of the nucleus pulposus, annulus fibrosus, and end-plates accounts for the ability of the disk to withstand compressive, rotational, and shear forces.

The nucleus pulposus lies in the center of the intervertebral disk, except in the lumbar spine, where it lies slightly posterior, at the junction of the middle and

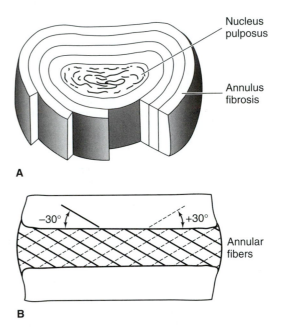

Figure 1–21. The intervertebral disk consists of a nucleus pulposus surrounded by the annulus fibrosus. In the first band of the annulus fibrosus, the collagen fibers are principally oriented at a 30-degree angle in one direction; in the second band, they are oriented at a 30-degree angle in the opposite direction; and the pattern continues (**A**), with the result that the annular fibers form an intricate crisscross arrangement (**B**). (Reproduced, with permission, from White AA, Panjabi MM: *Clinical Biomechanics of the Spine.* Lippincott, 1978.)

posterior thirds of the sagittal diameter. The nucleus pulposus is composed of a loose network of fine fibrous strands in a gelatinous matrix that contains water-binding glycosaminoglycans. The number of glycosaminoglycans decreases with age, thereby decreasing the hydration of the nucleus pulposus.

The annulus fibrosus is the ringlike outer portion of the disk and consists of fibrocartilage and fibrous tissue. The fibrocartilage is in a series of concentric laminated bands. In the first band, the collagen fibers are principally oriented at a 30-degree angle in one direction; in the second band, they are oriented at a 30-degree angle in the opposite direction; and the pattern continues (Figure 1–21A), with the result that the annular fibers form an intricate crisscross arrangement (Figure 1–21B). Centrally, the collagen fibers of the annulus fibrosus are attached to the cartilaginous end-plates. Peripherally, the fibers are attached to the bone of the vertebral body by Sharpey's fibers.

B. BIOMECHANICAL BEHAVIOR

The interaction between the nucleus pulposus and the annulus fibrosus accounts for the mechanical behavior of the intervertebral disk. The mechanical properties of the disk are viscoelastic and therefore depend on the loading rate and duration.

During compressive loading, the stress is transferred from the vertebral end plates to the intervertebral disk. With compression, pressure increases in the nucleus pulposus, and the fluid exerts hydrostatic pressure on the annulus fibrosus. As a result, the central portion of the vertebral end-plates are pushed away from one another, and the annular bands are pushed radially outward. The bulging annular bands develop tensile stress in all directions, the optimal orientation for maximal mechanical strength for the collagen fibers.

When the nucleus pulposus ages, its hydration decreases and its hydrostatic properties change. The load-transferring mechanism of the disk is greatly altered if sufficient hydrostatic pressure does not develop. In this situation, the annulus fibrosus transfers the stress to the periphery of the intervertebral disk; however, the fibers are subjected to compressive stress, which is not the optimal loading orientation for collagen fibers. This situation could lead to inadequate stress transfer from successive vertebral bodies, and this in turn could result in compression fractures of the vertebral bodies.

The nucleus pulposus has no effect during tensile loading of the intervertebral disk. Tensile loads are supported by tensile and shear stresses in the annulus fibrosus. The orientation of the collagen fibers of the annulus fibrosus provides no ability to resist shear stresses. Therefore, disk failure is greater with tensile loading than with compressive loading. Excessive shear stresses in the intervertebral disk may cause failure in pure rotational loading, when the nucleus pulposus has insufficient load to apply its hydrostatic effects to the annulus fibrosus.

Bao QB, Yuan HA: New technologies in spine: Nucleus replacement. Spine 2002;27:1245.

Bellucci G, Seedhom BB: Tensile fatigue behaviour of articular cartilage. Biorheology 2002;39:193.

Carlstedt CA et al: The influence of indomethacin on tendon healing: A biomechanical and biochemical study. Arch Orthop Trauma Surg 1986; 105:332.

Ding M et al: Mutual associations among microstructural, physical and mechanical properties of human cancellous bone. J Bone Joint Surg Br 2002;84:900.

Fung YCB: *Biomechanics: Mechanical Properties of Living Tissues.* Springer-Verlag, 1981.

Johnson LR: *Essential Medical Physiology.* Raven, 1992.

Kopperdahl DL et al: Quantitative computed tomography estimates of the mechanical properties of human vertebral trabecular bone. J Orthop Res 2002;20:801.

Kumaresan S et al: Contribution of disc degeneration to osteophyte formation in the cervical spine: A biomechanical investigation. J Orthop Res 2001;19:977.

Mow VC, Guo XE: Mechano-electrochemical properties of articular cartilage: Their inhomogeneities and anisotropies. Annu Rev Biomed Eng 2002;4:175.

Nordin M, Frankel VH, eds: *Basic Biomechanics of the Musculoskeletal System.* Lea & Febiger, 1989.

Rodger MM, Cavanagh PR: Glossary of biomechanical terms, concepts, and units. Phys Ther 1984;64:1886.

Silva MJ et al: Recent progress in flexor tendon healing. J Orthop Sci 2002;7:508.

Simunic DI et al: Biomechanical factors influencing nuclear disruption of the intervertebral disc. Spine 2001;26:1223.

Shinar H et al: Mapping the fiber orientation in articular cartilage at rest and under pressure studied by 2H double quantum filtered MRI. Magn Reson Med 2002;48:322.

Vanwanseele B et al: Knee cartilage of spinal cord-injured patients displays progressive thinning in the absence of normal joint loading and movement. Arthritis Rheum 2002; 46:2073.

Viidik A, Vuust J, eds: *Biology of Collagen.* Academic Press, 1980.

Wu JZ, Herzog W: Elastic anisotropy of articular cartilage is associated with the microstructures of collagen fibers and chondrocytes. J Biomech 2002;35:931.

IMPLANT MATERIALS IN ORTHOPEDICS

The body is a harsh chemical environment for foreign materials. An implanted material can have its mechanical and biologic properties significantly altered by body fluids. Degradation mechanisms, such as corrosion or leaching, can be accelerated by ion concentrations and pH changes in body fluids. The body's response to an implant can range from a benign to a chronic inflammatory reaction, with the degree of biologic response largely dependent on the implanted material. For optimal performance in physiologic environments, implant materials should have suitable mechanical strength, biocompatibility, and structural biostability. As the field of biomaterials science has developed, various classification schemes for implantable materials have been proposed, including schemes based on chemical composition and biologic response.

Implant materials can be classified as biotolerant, bioinert, and bioactive. **Biotolerant materials,** such as stainless steel and PMMA, are usually characterized by a thin fibrous tissue layer along the bone-implant interface. The fibrous tissue layer develops in part as a result of leaching processes that produce chemicals that irritate the surrounding tissues. Bioinert materials, such as cobalt-based alloys, titanium, and aluminum oxide, are characterized by direct bone contact, or osseointegration, at the interface under favorable mechanical conditions. Osseointegration is achieved because the material surface is chemically nonreactive to the surrounding tissues and body fluids. **Bioactive materials,** such as calcium phosphate ceramics, particularly hydroxyapatite, have a bone-implant interface characterized by direct chemical bonding of the implant with surrounding bone. This chemical bond is believed to be caused by the presence of free calcium and phosphate ion groups at the implant surface. The calcium phosphate materials can be used as implants or coatings. Other bioactive materials are the growth factors, which are finding application in stimulating desired responses from connective tissues.

Minimizing the local and systemic response to an implanted material through improved biocompatibility is only one engineering concern for reconstructive implant surgery. A prosthetic implant must appropriately transfer stress at the bone-implant surface to ensure long-term implant stability. Nonphysiologic stress transfer may cause pressure necrosis or resorption at the bone-implant interface. Necrotic and resorbed bone may lead to implant loosening and migration, thus compromising implant longevity. Polyethylene wear particles have been linked to osteolysis, also compromising implant longevity. Moreover, it is essential that materials have properties capable of sustaining the cyclic forces to which the implant will be subjected. For example, if the material properties are not adequate for load sharing, the implant may fail owing to fracture. If the geometry and material properties of the implant make it too rigid in comparison with the bone, then stress shielding of the bone is likely to occur, making bone resorption and implant loosening inevitable.

In addition to acceptable biocompatibility characteristics, biomaterials must demonstrate material properties suitable for their desired use. Materials used to manufacture total joint replacement systems must demonstrate a yield stress that is greater than the stress expected from

joint forces but must also have a flexural rigidity that will not result in unacceptable amounts of stress shielding of the bone. General stress-strain curves for the classes of materials allow for the comparison of material properties (Figure 1–22). For instance, ceramics are characterized by a high elastic modulus but are extremely brittle. In contrast with ceramics, metals have a lower elastic modulus but demonstrate increased ductility.

The most commonly used biomaterial combinations for orthopedic joint replacement are metals and metal alloys articulating with ultrahigh-molecular-weight polyethylene (UHMWPE). Stainless steel, an iron-based alloy, was used in Charnley's original hip prosthesis and is the material most commonly used for internal fixation plates, rods, and screws. Advances in materials science have produced stronger cobalt-based and titanium-based alloys. The wear resistance of cobalt-based alloys make them desirable for applications involving articulating surfaces. Titanium-based alloys, which have a modulus of elasticity closer to that of bone than the other metal alloys do, are currently being manufactured as femoral hip stems to reduce the effects of stress shielding.

Polymers and ceramics are also important classes of materials for orthopedic implant applications. Ultrahigh-molecular-weight polyethylene has a low coefficient of friction, making it ideal for an articulating surface. Polymethylmethacrylate has been used as a grouting agent in total joint arthroplasty to provide immediate fixation of total joint components to the skeleton. Porous-coated components require ingrowth of tis-

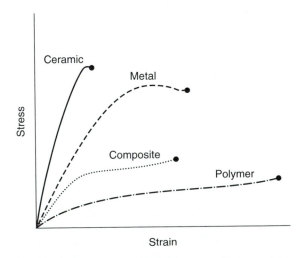

Figure 1–22. Representative stress-strain curves for the classes of materials used in orthopedic implants.

sue to the porous coating over a period of weeks or months to obtain stability. Aluminum oxide and zirconium oxide have gained popularity as materials for ceramic femoral heads because of their high wear resistance and low coefficient of friction. Finally, calcium phosphate ceramics, particularly hydroxyapatite, have been used in monolithic form as an augmentation material for metaphyseal bone defects and as a coating on metal devices for total joint arthroplasty.

Metals

The suitability of a metal component for maintaining longevity of a total joint replacement depends on the design of the implant and the biocompatibility, strength, wear, and corrosion characteristics of the metal. Materials scientists can improve on one or several of the characteristics of a metal alloy by varying the composition or by using different manufacturing processes.

An understanding of the terminology used to describe the strength and stiffness characteristics of a metal is essential in making informed decisions about the different metal alloys. The most important characteristics are elastic modulus, yield stress, ultimate tensile stress, and fatigue stress. As discussed at the beginning of this chapter, these properties can be determined from stress-strain curves and fatigue curves. The composition specifications and mechanical characteristics of all metals and their alloys used for orthopedic implants have been standardized by the American Society for Testing and Materials (ASTM).

The grain size, inclusion content, and surface porosity influence the strength characteristics of a metal. In general, the larger the grain size, the lower the tensile and fatigue strength at fracture. Excessive inclusions or a high surface porosity will weaken the metal by acting as stress risers and by providing areas for crevice corrosion. Manufacturing processes can be used to control these factors. For example, heating metal to a temperature near its melting point will increase the grain size, whereas forging processes will decrease the grain size.

Corrosion is a chemical reaction process that weakens the metal. Three types of corrosion are prevalent in implant materials: fatigue, galvanic, and crevice corrosion. Although all metals corrode in the physiologic environment, the severity of corrosion is determined by the chemical composition of the metal. Stainless steel corrodes more readily than either cobalt-based or titanium-based alloys. The chromium and molybdenum content of both stainless steel and cobalt-based alloys produces a corrosion-resistant surface layer. Titanium-based alloys have an adherent oxide passive film layer that provides their corrosion resistance.

The surfaces of all metallic implants are passivated (made passive to corrosion) with nitric acid to form an oxide surface layer that increases corrosion resistance. **Fatigue corrosion** may occur, however, if this passive film layer on the implant surface has been scratched or cracked and does not self-passivate in vivo. The ability to self-passivate may be hindered by wear processes or micromovement between modular components, a process called "fretting." Once corrosion begins, the implant weakens and will fail at a stress level below the endurance limit of the metal.

Galvanic corrosion occurs when an electric current is established between two metals that have different chemical or metallurgic compositions. Some differences arise from manufacturing processes and may be subtle, as in the difference between annealed bone plates and cold-worked screws made of stainless steel. Other differences that lead to galvanic corrosion arise from the close contact of two different metals in an implant, such as a titanium alloy femoral stem in contact with a cobalt alloy head. An evaluation of retrieved mixed metal femoral hip components consisting of a cobalt-chromium modular head on a titanium alloy stem demonstrated some degree of corrosion in the majority of the components. Further evaluation determined that corrosion occurred in all components that were implanted for longer than 40 months. The long-term clinical significance of the presence of corrosion caused by femoral component modularity is unknown. To avoid catastrophic galvanic corrosion, however, stainless steels should never be used with either cobalt-based or titanium-based alloys.

Crevice corrosion generally occurs when the fluid in contact with a metal becomes stagnant, resulting in a local oxygen depletion and a subsequent decrease in pH in relation to the rest of the implant. This form of corrosion is most prevalent underneath bone plates at the screw-plate junction. The mechanism of crevice corrosion, however, is apparent in point or structural defects in a metal. Corrosion of a defect results in progressive deepening of the defect, leading to the development of large stress concentrations and catastrophic failure of the implant.

A. IRON-BASED ALLOYS

There are four major groups of iron-based alloys or stainless steels, classified according to their microstructure. The group III (austenitic) stainless steels, which are labeled 316 and 316L, are used for orthopedic implants. The difference between 316 and 316L is that the latter contains a smaller percentage of carbon. Lowering the carbon content increases the corrosion resistance. Among the various elements contained in 316 and 316L stainless steels is molybdenum, which hardens the passive layer and increases pitting corrosion resistance.

Iron-based alloys have a wide range of mechanical properties (Table 1–3) that make them desirable for implant applications. Despite composition modifications, stainless steels are susceptible to corrosion inside the body, however. Therefore, they are most appropriate for temporary devices such as bone plates, bone screws, hip nails, and intramedullary nails.

Corrosion of stainless steels occurs for one of several reasons. The most common reason is incorrect metal composition, which increases the chance that galvanic corrosion processes will occur. Molybdenum is added to these metals to increase corrosion resistance; however, too much molybdenum can embrittle the alloy. Chromium carbide may form between the grain boundaries and result in grain boundary corrosion. This phenomenon is referred to as **sensitization.**

Another reason for corrosion is mismatch of implant components, especially when bone plates and screws are used, because even implants manufactured by the same company in different lots can be susceptible to corrosion processes caused by compositional differences. Crevice corrosion can occur at the junction of the screw with the bone plate and develops from local changes in pH and oxygen concentration that may result from slightly different manufacturing processes of the components.

Leaving plates and screws used to fix fractures in younger patients increases the risk of slow progressive corrosion over the years. Failure of the plate resulting from corrosion processes may also lead to bone fracture because stress shielding invariably occurs under the plate. Titanium alloy plates are gaining popularity because of their corrosion resistance and lower elastic modulus, properties that lower the degree of stress shielding.

B. Cobalt-Based Alloys

The mechanical properties that make cobalt-based alloys suitable for load-bearing implant applications are summarized in Table 1–3. Among the elements contained in these alloys is molybdenum, which is added to produce finer grains and thereby result in higher strength. The cobalt-based alloys are characterized by high fatigue resistance and high ultimate tensile strength levels, properties that make them appropriate for applications requiring a long service life and ability to resist fracture. The high wear resistance of these alloys also makes them desirable for load-bearing and articulating surface applications. Cobalt-chromium alloys are primarily used for components in total joint implants.

Despite the advantages of cobalt-based alloys, some cases have reported that surface porosities have acted as stress risers and led to premature fatigue failure. Hot isostatic pressing—a process that involves simultane-

Table 1–3. Minimum mechanical requirements for metal implant materials, as standardized by the American Society for Testing and Materials (ASTM).

Material Type	ASTM Number	Ultimate Elastic Modulus (GPa)	0.2% Offset Tensile Strength (MPa)	Yield Strength (MPa)	Elongation (%)	Reduction of Area (%)
Iron-based alloys						
Annealed stainless steel 316	F55-82	200	515	205	40	—
Annealed stainless steel 316L	F55-82	200	480	170	40	—
Cold-worked stainless steel 316 and 316L	F55-82	200	860	690	12	—
Cobalt-based alloys						
Cast Co-Cr-Mo alloy	F75-87	250	655	450	8	8
Wrought Co-Ni-Cr-Mo alloy	F562-84	240	793–1000	241–448	50	65
Titanium and titanium-based alloys						
Unalloyed titanium	F67-89	105	240–550	170–483	15–24	25–30
Cast Ti-6Al-4V alloy	F1108-88	110	860	858	8	14
Wrought Ti-6Al-4V ELI alloy	F136-84	110	860–896	795–827	10	25

ously applying both heat and pressure to consolidate powder into a solid form—has been adapted to significantly reduce surface porosity in cast metals. After this process is performed, the material must be heat-treated to attain maximal benefit. When performed properly, hot isostatic pressing increases the fatigue resistance, static strength characteristics, and corrosion resistance of cobalt-based alloys.

C. Titanium and Zirconium Alloys

Commercially pure titanium and titanium-based alloys are metals of low density (4.5 g/cm^3) and have chemical properties suitable for implant applications. Zirconium is in the same column in the periodic table. Both metals form an adherent oxide surface layer that makes them highly resistant to corrosion and chemically nonreactive to the surrounding tissues.

The mechanical properties of titanium and titanium-based alloys are summarized in Table 1–3. The elastic modulus value for titanium-based alloys is approximately 110 GPa, which is around half the value for iron-based or cobalt-based alloys but is still at least five times greater than the value for bone. Zirconium is alloyed with niobium (2.5%) and oxygen (0.11%) and has a modulus of 97.9(GPa). The higher the impurity content of the metal, the higher the strength and brittleness. Because of their low density, titanium and titanium-based alloys have superior specific strength (strength per density) over all other metals. Titanium has poor shear strength and wear resistance, however, making it unsuitable for applications involving articulating surfaces. It also exhibits notch sensitivity, which means that a small flaw or crack on the surface, such as might occur with mechanical damage, can cause a tremendous reduction in strength and increase the susceptibility to fracture.

New manufacturing techniques have been attempted to improve titanium-based alloys as bearing surfaces. Nitrogen ion implantation techniques were evaluated for their ability to increase the wear resistance and surface hardness of the alloys. The process of ion implantation accelerates elemental nitrogen ions toward the surface, where they become embedded. The presence of these ions causes distortions or strains within the crystal lattice of the metal and results in increased surface microhardness. The results have not been adequate to allow titanium or its alloys to be used as bearing surfaces. However, an oxidized zirconium alloy has produced a bearing surface that is showing promise. In vitro studies have shown that the increased surface hardness from the oxide layer significantly improves the wear resistance of the treated implant. The surface oxide layer is very thin (about 0.004 mm) but extremely adherent.

Polymers

Polymers have a wide range of properties attributable to variations in their chemical composition, structure, and manufacturing process, which make them suitable for several different implant applications. The choice of polymer for application is dictated by the effect of the physiologic environment on the stability of the material. Some polymers, such as PMMA, leach toxic substances into the surrounding tissues. Conversely, other polymers, such as silicone, absorb fluids from the body, and this absorption alters the mechanical properties. Despite the possible consequences of polymer implantation, the use of polymers as implant materials has been successful.

All polymers are composed of long chains of repeating units. These units may form linear, cross-linked, or branched chains. The individual chains may be organized in an orderly crystalline form having parallel or folded chains, or they may have an amorphous structure or a mixed structure. The molecular weight, chemical composition, degree of crystallinity, size and polarity of side groups, and degree of cross-linking determine the mechanical properties of the polymer. In general, as the molecular weight and crystallinity increase, the tensile strength and the resistance to cracking increase. The crystallinity is decreased by copolymerization, branching of chains, and large side groups.

A. Ultrahigh-Molecular-Weight Polyethylene

UHMWPE possesses an array of properties, including high abrasion resistance, low friction, high impact strength, excellent toughness, low density, ease of fabrication, biocompatibility, and biostability that makes it an attractive material for use in fabricating bearing surfaces for total joint replacements. UHMWPE is the material of choice for the liner of acetabular cups in total hip arthroplasties, the tibial insert, patellar components in total knee arthroplasties, and other load-bearing interfaces. The clinical performance of these components for nearly three decades has been excellent; however, there are concerns about the long-term wear of these devices. The concern is not only that the materials will wear out, but also that the wear debris generated will evoke an undesirable biologic reaction. It is known that particles in the submicron size undergo phagocytosis, resulting in a variety of biologic reactions. The reactions can include granulomatous lesions, osteolysis, and bone resorption. The phenomenon of wear of UHMWPE in total joint replacement is widely regarded as one of the most challenging problems in contemporary orthopedics.

A variety of factors influence the wear of polyethylene. These include the nature or quality of the starting material; the degree of crosslinking, strength, and toughness of the material; the manufacturing technique; the thickness of the polyethylene; the component sterilization conditions; and the storage environment and age of the component. The composition and physical properties of the starting materials used in the fabrication of UHMWPE components—in particular, molecular weight—have a profound effect on the materials performance. It is widely agreed that low-molecular-weight impurities and a high crystallinity are detrimental to the clinical performance. Increased crystallinity causes less resistance to crack initiation, crack propagation, and oxidation-enhanced wear.

UHMWPE is either machined from ram-extruded bar stock or compression molded directly from the starting powder. Ram extrusion is a two-step process in which the starting powder is first heated and pressurized in a polymerizing chamber followed by extrusion of bar stock. The second step, usually performed by the implant manufacturer is the machining of the component with a precision cutting lathe. By contrast, direct compression molding is a one-step process. A preshaped component and premeasured volume of starting powder are placed into a heated mold, and the component is then formed under pressure. Each manufacturing process has its own unique characteristics and problems. Some engineers believe that compression-molded components, although more expensive to produce, result in products with enhanced, in vivo wear performance.

In general, as the thickness of the UHMWPE components decreases, the stresses increases, and therefore, the wear also increases. This is because with an increase in thickness, the structural stiffness of the component increases, even when the value of the modulus of elasticity of the material remains unchanged. This effect has resulted in a recommendation for the minimal thickness of acetabular liners of about 5–6 mm and tibial inserts of 7–8 mm.

Several manufacturers have chosen gamma irradiation for sterilizing UHMWPE components at doses between 25,000 and 40,000 Gy. Gamma radiation causes both cross-linking and chain fission and is the major contributor to subsequent surface and subsurface oxidative degradation of the components. Other manufacturers have chosen surface sterilization techniques, such as ethylene oxide, or one of the several plasma techniques, which have no effect on the bulk properties of the polyethylene. There is considerable literature on the effect of a number of variables associated with sterilization, packaging, and aging of polyethylene on the in vivo and in vitro physical and mechanical properties. These include the method of sterilization, sterilization dosage, packaging atmosphere, and aging conditions. For example, irradiation and storage in an inert atmosphere reduces the oxidative degradation before implan-

tation. Because of this volume of work, no consensus has yet emerged on these effects. As noted, gamma sterilization, particularly in air, causes significant reduction of the various mechanical characteristics that have been shown to be related to the subsequent wear and performance of the material. These parameters include crystallinity, melting temperature, oxidation strength, tensile properties, and density.

Irradiation of polyethylene at much higher doses (50,000–150,000 Gy) followed by an annealing process has resulted in a cross-linked polyethylene with different properties. Early hip simulator wear studies indicate that this cross-linked polyethylene has very low wear rates and superior wear properties compared with conventional polyethylene. Early clinical trials seem to confirm these results.

B. POLYMETHYLMETHACRYLATE

Self-curing PMMA, commonly used as a grouting agent, is often called the weak link in total joint arthroplasty. Compared with cortical bone, bone cement has a lower elastic modulus and significantly inferior mechanical strength properties. The tensile strength of PMMA is similar to that of cancellous bone. The low modulus of elasticity allows for gradual transfer of stress from implant to bone. Mechanically, PMMA is weakest in shear loading and strongest in compression loading situations.

Implant design and cementing technique must compensate for weaknesses in tension, to avoid catastrophic failure of the cement. The poor fatigue strength of PMMA can be attributed primarily to porosity. Studies have shown that PMMA porosity is increased and fatigue strength is further decreased by mixing the cement with chilled monomer, rather than with monomer at room temperature. Therefore, if chilled monomer must be used, it is crucial to concurrently use porosity reduction techniques such as centrifugation and vacuum mixing. The fatigue strength of PMMA is also decreased by the presence of inclusions, such as bone chips and blood.

Aside from the inherent mechanical weakness of PMMA, the polymerization process causes local and systemic biologic effects. Locally, adjacent tissues can become necrotic owing to the extreme heat of polymerization, which can generate temperatures approaching 100 °C. Systemically, the leaching of monomer during the curing process may cause hypotension.

The fatigue properties of PMMA manufactured by different companies vary because of intrinsic compositional differences such as the size of the polymer beads, the addition of copolymers, and the presence of additives and radiopacifiers. In a study of the fatigue life of five commonly used bone cements (CMW, LVC, Palacos R, Simplex P, and Zimmer Regular), investigators prepared each cement in the manner suggested by its manufacturer. They found that Palacos R and Simplex P had equivalent fatigue strengths and that these two products had significantly greater fatigue strengths than the other three products. For each product, investigators compared the fatigue life of a regular sample with that of a sample that had undergone a process to reduce its porosity. In the case of each product, a reduction in the cement's porosity increased its fatigue life. Moreover, when investigators centrifuged two packages of Simplex P mixed with chilled monomer for 60 s, they found a fivefold increase in the fatigue properties of this cement.

Ceramics

Ceramics are wear-resistant and strong in compression, but they are extremely brittle and susceptible to cracking. Ceramic materials must be carefully chosen for specific implant applications because chemical composition affects the mechanical properties and biologic responses of each ceramic. For instance, in calcium phosphate ceramics, an alteration in the ratio of calcium to phosphorous can significantly alter the in vivo dissolution rate of the ceramic.

The mechanical properties of ceramics depend on grain size, porosity, density, and crystallinity. Strength is normally improved with increased density, increased crystallinity, and decreased porosity. The hardness and wettability of ceramics and the fact that ceramics can be polished to smooth surfaces make them ideal candidates for bearing surfaces. Nevertheless, for a ceramic implant to be reliable, its design must avoid sharp corners and notches, to overcome the predictable mechanical flaws of the material.

A. ALUMINUM OXIDE

The catastrophic effects of implant loosening associated with polyethylene wear debris led to interest in using other materials at the articulating surface. The use of aluminum oxide (Al_2O_3) was explored because it is a highly biocompatible material with high frictional resistance. In fact, the coefficient of friction for alumina-on-alumina articulations is approximately 2.3 times less than the coefficient for metal-on-polyethylene articulations. Studies have shown that alumina-on-alumina articulations demonstrate approximately 5000 times less wear than metal-on-polyethylene articulations do under experimental loading conditions.

In clinical practice, all-alumina acetabular components have not performed well, probably because of loosening due to the tremendous modulus mismatch between aluminum oxide and bone. Ceramic-on-polyethylene articulations have shown clinical promise, however. Aluminum oxide has excellent wear characteristics, and any ceramic wear debris that does accumulate at the interface may be less bioreactive than polyethylene or PMMA wear debris. Alumina-on-alumina articulations have demonstrated very low wear rates when clinically applied with a metal shell for attachment to acetabular bone. Although the alumina wear rates have been low, problems have occurred due to placement of the components, allowing impingement and abrasion of the neck of the femoral component.

Despite the excellent wear and friction characteristics of aluminum oxide, its fracture toughness and tensile strength are relatively low. It is also sensitive to microstructural flaws, which could result in wear and breakage. The elastic modulus of aluminum oxide is approximately 20 times greater than that of cortical bone. The modulus can be altered drastically with decreased crystallinity and increased porosity, however. Increased grain size decreases strength and a large grain size has been linked to reported cases of catastrophic wear. Careful regulation of manufacturing processes results in reliable aluminum oxide implants with small grain size, high density, high purity, adequate strength, and adequate component size.

B. ZIRCONIUM OXIDE

Recently, zirconium oxide (Zirconia) has become an attractive material for highly loaded joint replacement applications. Pure Zirconia undergoes room temperature transformation from the desired monoclinic structure to a mixture of tetragonal and cubic phases. Zirconium oxide can be maintained in a metastable state with the addition of a stabilizing oxide such as calcium or magnesium oxide. A stable, highly dense material having small grains can be obtained by mixing zirconium oxide with yttrium (Y_2O_3), however.

In comparison with aluminum oxide, zirconium oxide exhibits increased fracture toughness, increased bending strength, and decreased elastic modulus. Moreover, Zirconia-to-polyethylene articulations demonstrate 40–60% less wear than alumina-to-polyethylene articulations do in vitro. Because the mechanical and wear properties of zirconium oxide are superior to those of aluminum oxide, it is now possible to manufacture safer and smaller femoral heads for low-friction total hip arthroplasty. Again, careful regulation of manufacturing processes is required to prevent catastrophic failure as has been seen with these heads in Europe.

C. HYDROXYAPATITE

Calcium phosphate ceramics, classified as polycrystalline ceramics, have a material structure derived from individual crystals that have become fused at the grain boundaries during high-temperature sintering processes.

Tribasic calcium phosphate [$Ca_{10}(PO_4)_6(OH)_2$], which is commonly called **hydroxyapatite,** is a geologic mineral that closely resembles the natural mineral in vertebrate bone tissue. Tribasic calcium phosphate should not be confused with other calcium phosphate ceramics, especially tricalcium phosphate $[Ca_3(PO_4)_2]$, which is chemically similar to hydroxyapatite but is not a natural bone mineral.

Bulk hydroxyapatite is manufactured from a starting powder, and the manufacturing process consists of compression molding and subsequent sintering. Macroporous ceramics can be obtained by combining the starting mixture with hydrogen peroxide. Otherwise, a dense structure with a small percentage of micropores will result. Dense hydroxyapatite ceramics have a compressive strength greater than that of cortical bone; however, their tensile strength is approximately 2.5 times less than their compressive strength. Small reductions in density can significantly reduce tensile characteristics of the ceramic. Bulk hydroxyapatite can also be formed with a very uniform pore structure by the chemical conversion of calcium carbonate coral structures. This material can be used to augment bone graft in cancellous bone areas.

Although the static mechanical properties of bulk hydroxyapatite are good, the resistance to fatigue failure is low in physiologic conditions, as is common with sintered ceramics and particularly bioactive ceramics. Therefore, bulk hydroxyapatite is not suitable for applications requiring mechanical loading. Bulk hydroxyapatite has been used successfully in clinical practice as a bone graft substitute to fill metaphyseal defects associated with tibial plateau fractures. A composite prosthesis made by plasma spraying thin coatings of hydroxyapatite onto a metal substrate has recently been developed and is able to withstand the physiologic stresses imposed on it while providing an osteoconductive surface to achieve optimal bone apposition and ingrowth. Experimental results indicate that hydroxyapatite stimulates more extensive and uniform growth of bone into a porous-surfaced femoral stem or acetabular cup and probably aids bone growth across gaps between implants and surrounding bone.

Several formulations of an injectable hydroxyapatite have become available for minimally invasive surgery. These materials are similar to PMMA in that the setting process is a chemical reaction that yields the final product, in this case hydroxyapatite.

D. PYROLYTIC CARBON

Carbon occurs naturally in many forms, each having different structures, material properties, and uses. Coal is an example of carbon in its amorphous form with no crystalline structure. Graphite has an organized crystalline structure, in which carbon atoms are arranged in two-dimensional hexagonal sheets tightly joined by strong covalent bonds. Diamond is a third form of carbon having a three-dimensional cubic crystal structure with increased atomic bonds.

Pyrolytic carbon is a manufactured material formed by the pyrolysis, or heating of gaseous hydrocarbons. The resulting pyrolytic carbon is usually deposited on a graphite substrate in a turbostratic, two-dimensional crystalline structure with a high concentration of three-dimensional diamond cross-link bonding. In general, the physical properties of pyrolytic carbon fall between those of graphite and diamond. The form of pyrolytic carbon used as a surgical implant material has a very fine grain structure (approximately 50 Å), and isotropic physical and mechanical properties. Pyrolytic carbon is chemically inert and is resistant to wear and mechanical fatigue. It also has a high fracture strength, and low elasticity modulus (21–26 GPa), which falls within the range of moduli reported for cortical bone. Its biocompatibility is well documented and has been confirmed clinically in extensive use in cardiovascular implants for more than 30 years. Pyrolytic carbon has also proved to be extremely biocompatible in both osseous and soft tissues.

Pyrolytic carbon has been evaluated in cardiovascular, dental, soft-tissue, and orthopedic implants. It is the material of choice for the construction of mechanical artificial heart valves. The human heart beats on an average of 100,000 times per day or 35 million times per year. The carbon-on-carbon pivot systems in heart valves must resist stress and wear each time the heart beats. The history of successful function in heart valve components demonstrates the outstanding wear resistance of the carbon-on-carbon articulation, biocompatibility, and structural durability of the pyrolytic carbon material. Pyrolytic carbons have been evaluated clinically in orthopedics for replacement of the small bones and joints of the hands and feet. Nonconstrained pyrolytic carbon metacarpophalangeal joint replacements were evaluated between 1979 and 1987 in human clinical trials. A total of 151 pyrolytic carbon metacarpophalangeal joint replacements were implanted in 53 patients. Results at long-term follow-up ranging from 12 to 16 years demonstrated excellent performance of the implants with a 15-year survival rate of more than 70%. The long-term clinical outcome results of the metacarpophalangeal joint arthroplasties in humans demonstrated the biologic and biomechanical compatibility of pyrolytic carbons in a demanding orthopedic application.

Bucholz RW et al: Interporous hydroxyapatite as a bone graft substitute in tibial plateau fractures. Clin Orthop 1989;240:53.

Christel P et al: Mechanical properties and short-term in vivo evaluation of yttrium-oxide-partially-stabilized Zirconia. J Biomed Mater Res 1989;23:45.

Cook SD et al: Long-term follow-up of pyrolytic carbon metacarpophalangeal implants. J Bone Joint Surg (Am) 1999;81:635.

Clarke IC et al: Biomechanical stability and design. Ann NY Acad Sci 1988;523:292.

Collier JP et al: Results of implant retrieval from postmortem specimens in patients with well-functioning, long-term total hip replacement. Clin Orthop 1992;274:97.

Davies JP et al: Comparison and optimization of three centrifugation systems for reducing porosity of Simplex P bone cement. J Arthroplasty 1989;4:15.

Endo MM et al: Comparative wear and wear debris under three different counterface conditions of crosslinked and non-crosslinked ultra high molecular weight polyethylene. Biomed Mater Eng 2001;11:23. [PMID 11281576]

Food and Drug Administration, HHS: Medical devices; reclassification of polymethylmethacrylate (PMMA) bone cement. Final rule. Fed Regist 2002;67:46852. [PMID 12125716]

Friedman RJ et al: Current concepts in orthopaedic biomaterials and implant fixation. J Bone Joint Surg (Am) 1993;75:1086. [PMID 11132264]

Hamadouche M, Sedel L.: Ceramics in orthopaedics. J Bone Joint Surg (Br) 2000;82:1095.

Haraguchi K et al: Phase transformation of a Zirconia ceramic head after total hip arthroplasty. J Bone Joint Surg (Br) 2001;83:996. [PMID 11603539]

Lewis G, Carroll M: Rheological properties of acrylic bone cement during curing and the role of the size of the powder particles. J Biomed Mater Res 2002;63(2):191. [PMID 11870653]

Lim TH et al: Biomechanical evaluation of an injectable calcium phosphate cement for vertebroplasty. Spine 2002;27:1297. [PMID 12065977]

Ma L, Sines G: Fatigue behavior of a pyrolytic carbon. J Biomed Mater Res 2000 Jul;51(1):61. [PMID 10813746]

McKellop H et al: Development of an extremely wear-resistant ultra high molecular weight polyethylene for total hip replacements. J Orthop Res 1999 Mar;17(2):157. [PMID 10221831]

Morscher EW, Wirz D: Current state of cement fixation in THR. Acta Orthop Belg 2002;68:1. [PMID 11915452]

Murphy BP, Prendergast PJ. The relationship between stress, porosity, and nonlinear damage accumulation in acrylic bone cement. J Biomed Mater Res 2002;59:646. [PMID 11774326]

Oonishi H, Kadoya Y: Wear of high-dose gamma-irradiated polyethylene in total hip replacements. J Orthop Sci 2000;5(3):223. [PMID 10982661]

Ries MD et al: Polyethylene wear performance of oxidized zirconium and cobalt-chromium knee components under abrasive conditions. J Bone Joint Surg (Am) 2002;84 Suppl 2:129. [PMID 11712832]

Ries MD et al: Relationship between gravimetric wear and particle generation in hip simulators: Conventional compared with cross-linked polyethylene. J Bone Joint Surg (Am) 2001;83 Suppl 2 Pt 2:116.

Sharkey PF et al: The bearing surface in total hip arthroplasty: Evolution or revolution. Instr Course Lect 2000;49:41. [PMID 10829160]

Smith SL, Unsworth A: An in vitro wear study of alumina-alumina total hip prostheses. Proc Inst Mech Eng [H] 2001;215:443. [PMID 11726044]

Spector BM et al: Wear performance of ultra-high molecular weight polyethylene on oxidized zirconium total knee femoral components. J Bone Joint Surg (Am) 2001;83 Suppl 2 Pt 2:80. [PMID 11712839]

Vallo CI: Flexural strength distribution of a PMMA-based bone cement. J Biomed Mater Res 2002;63:226. [PMID 11870658]

GROWTH FACTORS
Biology

Growth factors hold great promise for the treatment of a variety of musculoskeletal conditions. The response of bone to structural damage is nearly unique in biology. The vast majority of tissues, when traumatized, heal with a fibrous scar, the cells and structure of which are not normal and are unable to fully assume the function of the tissue. In contrast, bone, the cornea, and the liver are capable of true cellular, morphologic, and functional regeneration. The initial phase of bone healing is characterized by an inflammatory response in consolidation of the hematoma within the fracture site. This is followed by the proliferation of periosteal, endosteal, and marrow stromal cells adjacent to the site, and recruitment of undifferentiated mesenchymal cells from nearby soft tissues. These cells and their progeny differentiate to become chondroblasts, chondrocytes, osteoblasts, and osteocytes. The cartilage formed is eventually replaced by bone, and the early woven bone is remodeled to a more mature lamellar structure.

Growth factors are polypeptides that serve as signaling agents for cells. These local proteins bind to specific receptors, occasionally with the assistance of extracellular binding proteins, to stimulate or inhibit functions inside the cell. The discovery of these substances revolutionized the field of cell biology by revealing the mechanisms of regulation of cell activities. Growth factors are present in plasma or tissues, and in concentrations measured in billionths of a gram; yet, they are the principal effectors of critical cellular functions, such as cell proliferation, matrix synthesis, and tissue differentiation. Cytokines are similar to growth factors as they are receptor-activating locally acting polypeptides. Although cytokines were originally characterized from cells of the hematopoietic and immune cell systems, the distinction is rather artificial as most authors currently consider growth factors to be a subset of cytokines.

Although the same growth factor is often found throughout the body, they have been named based on their function and tissue of origin. Several growth-promoting substances have been identified in bone matrix and at the site of fracture healing. These growth factors are believed to play a role in the healing process. Among these are the transforming growth factor beta (TGF-β), bone morphogenetic proteins (BMP), fibroblast growth factors (FGF), insulinlike growth factors (IGF), and platelet-derived growth factor (PDGF). These growth factors are produced by osteoblasts and incorporated into the extracellular matrix during bone formation. Small amounts of growth factors can also be trapped systemically from serum and incorporated into the matrix. The present hypothesis is that growth factors are located within the matrix until remodeling or trauma causes solubilization and release of the proteins.

A. Transforming Growth Factor Beta

The transforming growth factors beta (TGF-β) are a family of dimeric polypeptide growth factors and are coded by closely related genes. The family includes at least five molecules known as TGF-β 1–4, and by itself, is a member of a superfamily that includes BMPs, activins, and growth/differentiation factors (GDFs) among others that regulate morphogenesis in early development. The broad range of cellular activities regulated by TGF-βs include the proliferation and expression of differentiated phenotypes of many of the cell populations that make up the skeleton. Among these are the mesenchymal precursor cells for chondrocytes, osteoblasts, and osteoclasts. The presence of TGF-β in normal fracture healing suggests they play a role in the repair process. TGF-βs are secreted in an inactive form requiring acid pH or heat for activation. These dimeric, disulfide bonded molecules mediate their function through receptors that act as serine/threonine kinases. The receptors autophosphorylate after forming a complex with TGF-β, activate Smad intracellular pathways that translocate to the nucleus, and regulate gene transcription. Thus far, eight mammalian Smad proteins have been identified. After oligomerization, these proteins enter the nucleus to regulate transcription following assembly with transcriptional cofactors and comodulators.

B. Bone Morphogenetic Protein

Related to the TGF-β, the bone morphogenic proteins constitute a family of at least 15 growth factors originally identified for their ability to stimulate de novo bone formation. The BMPs are also referred to as osteogenic proteins (OPs); hence, there is some name confusion, because BMP-7 is also called OP-1. Bone morphogenic proteins are the only growth factors that can stimulate differentiation of mesenchymal stem cells into a chondroblastic (BMP-2) and osteoblastic (BMP-5, 6, and 7) direction. These BMP molecules are also quite effective osteoinductive agents. Noggin and chordin are extracellular binding proteins that alter binding of BMP molecules with their receptors. When implanted, most BMPs can stimulate a cascade of cellular events that closely mimics the process of endochondral ossification in normal fracture healing. Precursor cells are recruited and differentiated into chondrocytes that manufacture cartilage matrix. The cartilage is then gradually replaced by bone as osteoblasts populate the site. Eventually, bone marrow elements fill the newly formed intertrabecular spaces, and the bone remodels. Overexpression of BMP-4 in inflammatory cells is responsible for fibrodysplasia ossificans progressiva.

C. Fibroblast Growth Factors

Fibroblast growth factors are currently a group of eleven polypeptides that were originally discovered on the basis of their mitogenic effect on fibroblasts and have four known receptors. Acid fibroblast growth factor and basic fibroblast growth factor, also termed FGF-1 and FGF-2, respectively, have both been implicated in cartilage and bone regulation. Basic FGF is generally more potent than acid FGF. Fibroblast growth factors have a significant proliferative effect on osteoblasts but less effect on protein synthesis. FGFs probably enhance bone formation by increasing the number of cells capable of synthesizing bone collagen. FGFs are also angiogenic factors, which are important for neovascularization during bone healing. A defect in the FGF receptor 3 has been implicated as the cause for achondroplasia.

D. Insulinlike Growth Factor

The pivotal role of insulin growth factor in regulating endochondral ossification in skeletal growth suggests that this factor may also participate in endochondral ossification of bone healing. IGF regulates both bone matrix formation and cell replication. Of all the growth factors present in bone matrix, IGF-2 has the highest concentration; however, IGF-1 is four to seven times more potent than IGF-2. IGF-1, also known as somatomedin C, is produced in the liver and by skeletal tissue in response to stimulation with growth hormone. The cells that secrete IGFs also secrete any one of the six IGF-binding proteins that actually regulate the effectiveness of this growth factor.

Both IGF-1 and IGF-2 stimulate preosteoblastic cell replication by increasing the number of cells capable of synthesizing bone matrix. However, their mitogenic effect is less pronounced than those of other growth factors. IGFs also have independent effects on the differentiation of osteoblasts, increasing bone collagen production and inhibiting collagen degradation.

E. Platelet-Derived Growth Factor

Platelet-derived growth factor was discovered in serum as having a major mitogenic activity responsible for growth of cultured mesenchymal cells. It is a dimeric molecule that exists in two isoforms (A and B). When it is overproduced with some tumors, the proto-oncogene name is c-sis. PDGF is a potent regulator of bone cells and chondrocytes and has been shown to play a role in tendon healing.

F. Vascular Endothelial Growth Factor

This potent angiogenic agent is found in endothelial cells and is responsible for the formation of new vasculature. It has been found to be involved with the angiogenesis of calcified cartilage and distraction angiogenesis. Although not significantly involved in the formation of normal bone, VEGF has been shown to be involved with angiogenesis of malignancy. Clinical trials are being performed to evaluate the effectiveness of VEGF therapy into ischemic areas and the role of anti-VEGF therapy for treating malignancy.

Applications

Extensive efforts have been made to find methods by which growth factors can be used to stimulate local bone healing and bone formation in a variety of clinical models. The growth factors TGF-β, BMP, and basic FGF are the only growth factors that have been demonstrated to possess substantial capacity for in vivo bone stimulation. Growth factors are probably best able to exert a stimulatory effect when used in conditions associated with impaired healing. Research has begun to show increasing evidence that growth factors can be used in vivo to stimulate bone healing and bone formation. The growth factors BMP-2 and BMP-7, also known as **osteogenic protein-1 (OP-1),** are in the final stages of pivotal human trials. Issues of the best delivery system are currently being debated from the use of collagen gel/sponge carrier to ex vivo adenoviral-mediated delivery systems.

There are many challenges to the clinical application of growth factors. It is unlikely that cell-signaling molecules act independently of one another or are present in isolation from one another at their sites of action. Although therapeutic measures that employ single agents may be efficacious in some circumstances, it is likely that most clinical applications will require the development of combination or serial treatment regimens. In addition, because the specific actions of growth factors are context-dependent, it is critical to distinguish appropriate from inappropriate indications.

The therapeutic application of growth factors must also accommodate the fact that most factors have a widespread and variable distribution of target cells. A growth factor administered to elicit a desired response from one cell type may also influence other cell types, possibly in unintended or undesirable ways. Finally, in addition to demonstrating acceptable safety profiles and providing a physician-friendly delivery system in the current era of cost consciousness in health care, a growth factor treatment must demonstrate cost effectiveness along with clinical efficacy. Growth factors have many potential orthopedic applications. As challenges are met, it is plausible, if not probable, that growth factors will provide a means of treating patients with a variety of musculoskeletal disorders.

Musgrave DS et al: Gene therapy and tissue engineering in orthopaedic surgery. J Am Acad Orthop Surg 2002;10:6. [PMID 11809046]

Yoon ST, Boden SD: Osteoinductive molecules in orthopaedics: Basic science and preclinical studies. Clin Orthop 2002;395: 33. [PMID 11937864]

IMPLANT DESIGN & BIOLOGIC ATTACHMENT PROPERTIES

Total joint arthroplasty requires the type of implant materials and design that can support large functional loads. The implant must remain stable and rigid with respect to the bone while sustaining these loads. Adequate interface fixation requires interface micromotion of less than a hundred micrometers or gap spaces less than a fraction of a millimeter. Precise and uniform contact between the device and surrounding bone depends on the skill of the surgeon and the design of the instrumentation with which the site is prepared. The surface area of actual contact is probably small relative to the surface area of the implant. The contact points tend to induce areas of stress concentration rather than distribute the stress evenly. Bone maintains its structural integrity by responding to stress. In areas of stress concentration, bone resorption often occurs. Additionally, fibrous encapsulations of varying thicknesses are commonly found, and these further alter the ability of the implant to distribute stress uniformly. Implant loosening and migration may eventually occur and cause discomfort to the patient, in which case the implant may need to be removed.

Implant Fixation Mechanisms

Several types of implant fixation methods and surface texture designs have been investigated to obtain better surgical fit and stress distribution at the implant-bone interface. The methods include the use of a grouting agent, direct bone apposition to the implant surface, bone growth into porous-surfaced implants, and chemical bonding between bone and surface-active ceramic implant coatings.

A. GROUTING AGENTS

PMMA bone cement provides a mechanical interlock between the metal prosthesis and adjacent bone. Bone cement is not an adhesive; therefore, mechanical interlocking depends on the amount of interdigitation of the cement with trabecular bone and the quality of the fixation between the cement and the metal. The most favorable sign of cement fixation is immediate stability of the implant. Bone cement allows for load distribution over a larger area of bone, and this reduces stress concentrations that may result in pressure necrosis and remodeling. Despite the early clinical advantages of cement fixation, the long-term results have not been as encouraging. The poor fatigue properties of cement have led to fractures of the cement. These fractures result in altered stress patterns in the bone, eventually leading to bone remodeling and implant loosening. Particulate debris that results from cement fracture has been associated with osteolysis and aseptic loosening.

Improvements in the mechanical properties of cement and cementing techniques over the past two to three decades are leading to more promising results regarding the longevity of cemented prostheses. Femoral stems that were implanted with modern cement techniques have been shown to maintain stability and function beyond 10 years in 95–98% of the cases.

B. DIRECT BONE APPOSITION

Optimal osseointegration at the bone-implant interface is affected by the material properties and design of the implant. Implant design encompasses both the surface texture and geometry of the implant. The mechanical properties of the implant-bone interface have been investigated with various surface preparations, including smooth finishes, roughened or grit-blasted finishes, and grooved surfaces. Histologically, implants with smooth finishes have interfaces characterized by fibrous encapsulation, whereas implants with grit-blasted finishes have interfaces characterized by areas of direct bone apposition. Numerous studies have demonstrated that surface texture is a significant factor in obtaining adequate implant fixation with direct bone apposition methods.

Several materials with various polished and grit-blasted surfaces have been evaluated using transcortical models. The implant materials have included PMMA, commercially pure titanium, aluminum oxide, and low-temperature isotropic pyrolytic carbon. After the implant surface composition was varied by applying a coating of the low-temperature pyrolytic carbon to several implants, mechanical testing was performed. Comparison of the results demonstrated that the implant elastic modulus or surface composition did not significantly affect the interface attachment strength or histologic response. Surface texture significantly affected the interface mechanical properties, however. Implants with grit-blasted surfaces exhibited significantly higher interface attachment strengths than implants with polished surfaces did. Histologically, all implants with grit-blasted surfaces demonstrated areas of direct bone apposition, whereas all implants with polished surfaces demonstrated fibrous encapsulation (Figure 1–23), indicating that bone apposition required textured interface surface for attachment.

C. POROUS INGROWTH ATTACHMENT

The long-term problems associated with implant fixation with PMMA led to the development of methods intended for permanent biologic fixation, such as the

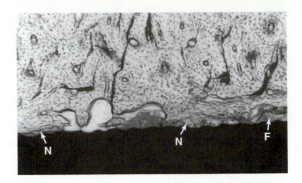

Figure 1–23. Histologic appearance of mechanically tested grit-blasted titanium alloy implants 10 weeks after implantation. Areas of direct bone apposition (N) and minimal fibrous tissue (F) were observed at the implant interface. The undecalcified histologic section was photographed using simultaneous transmitted and reflected illumination (basic fuchsin and toluidine blue stain; original magnification × 160).

porous coating of prostheses. It is generally accepted that an implant can achieve stabilization by tissue growth into the surface porous structure if (1) the material is bioinert, (2) there is direct apposition of the bone at the implant interface, (3) there is minimal or no movement at the implant site, and (4) the porous structure has appropriate pore size and morphology.

Porous coatings are effective as a means of biologic fixation because of their interface mechanical properties. The interface attachment strength of porous implants relying on bone ingrowth for fixation is at least an order of magnitude higher than that of nonporous implants relying on direct bone apposition for fixation.

To maintain optimal bone growth into a porous structure, the pores must be large enough to accommodate the development of bone tissue. Several groups of investigators have studied the degree and rate of bone ingrowth for different pore size ranges. Using porous ceramics, one group demonstrated that a pore size of 100 μm allowed bone ingrowth but that a pore size greater than 150 μm was necessary for osteon formation. Another group investigated the optimal pore size range for cobalt-based alloys by observing the rate of bone ingrowth and time necessary to attain maximal attachment strength. The results indicated that although a pore size range of 50–400 μm obtained the maximal attachment strength in the shortest time, osteon formation was not demonstrated histologically at this range. The mechanical results did not determine that osteon formation was a prerequisite to attain maximal attachment strength.

In addition to a minimal pore size, an effective porous coating must also have appropriate pore morphology. The available porous layer for bone growth must be large enough to accommodate a sufficient quantity of bone to maintain adequate fixation without compromising the mechanical properties necessary for a load-bearing prosthesis. A volume fraction porosity of 35–40% is accepted as optimal for effective biologic fixation of an implant with a strongly bonded porous layer. The volume fraction porosity is related to the interconnection pore size, particle interconnectivity, and particle size of the porous coating. Particle interconnectivity is important for ensuring adequate strength within the coating and between the coating and substrate. Too much particle interconnectivity can decrease the interconnection pore size and restrict the amount and type of ingrown tissue, however. A two-layer porous surface creates an interconnected and open porosity that is effective in creating a three-dimensional mechanical interlock of the ingrown bone.

Several different types of porous coatings have been evaluated, including the fiber mesh, void, beaded porous, and irregular plasma-sprayed types. The fiber mesh type of porous coating is composed of iron-based alloys, cobalt-based alloys, or commercially pure titanium wires that are cut and kinked to form the specific shape of the coating. The wires are then bonded to a solid metal substrate of the same metallic alloy through a sintering process in an inert gas environment or vacuum. The porosity obtained with this technique ranges from 40% to 50% with a mean pore size of 270 μm. A void type of porous coating has been obtained using a cobalt-based or titanium-based alloy. Magnesium microspheres are mixed with the base alloy by means of an investment casting technique. Under high temperatures, the magnesium evaporates, leaving pores on the surface of the alloy. This technique produces pores with different depths and connectivities. The most frequently studied porous coating is the beaded type. Cobalt-based alloy or titanium metal powder or macrobeads are either gravity compacted or applied with an organic binder onto a substrate. The beads are then sintered to the substrate at a submelting temperature for the base metal. The porosity ranges from 30% to 45% with pore diameters ranging from 100 to 400 μm. Production of another type of porous coating involves plasma-spraying titanium to either a titanium-based or cobalt-based alloy substrate. The plasma-spray technique is further discussed with regard to ceramic coatings (see following section).

The extent to which implants are covered with porous coating varies. On femoral stems, it ranges anywhere from complete coverage to coverage of the proximal third of the anterior and posterior pads. The extent of porous coating to achieve optimal stability has not been determined. Circumferential coverage is preferable, however, to prevent wear debris migration toward the distal portion of the prosthetic stem.

Clinically, the short-term results for porous-coated prostheses have been comparable to those for cemented prostheses. Histologically, retrieved human prostheses have demonstrated variable amounts of bone ingrowth, ranging from limited to extensive, with large amounts of fibrous tissue (Figure 1–24). Some retrieved prostheses have exhibited complete fibrous tissue infiltration into the porous surface. Components with limited bone ingrowth have shown fibrous tissue that was oriented in a fashion capable of load transmission. The bone ingrowth and extensive fibrous ingrowth are most likely effective mechanisms for early implant stabilization. A histologic analysis performed on six retrieved, noncemented, porous-coated femoral hip components demonstrated a significant increase in bone ingrowth from 19 to 53 months after implantation. The data showed that human bone remodels slowly and advances appositionally with limited endochondral ossification. Therefore, to achieve reproducible bone ingrowth, the porous coating must be adjacent to cortical bone.

D. CALCIUM PHOSPHATE CERAMIC COATINGS

Calcium phosphate coatings on metal surfaces were developed to overcome the mechanical problems of the ceramic as well as the biologic shortcomings of the metal. The new composite implants have the mechanical properties of the metal and the beneficial biologic properties of the bioactive ceramics. The bond between a metal substrate and a hydroxyapatite (HA) coating is critical to the success of a coated prosthesis. The processes and techniques of coating a prosthesis vary, and for this reason not all HA coatings perform equivalently.

A coating thickness of 50 μm is generally accepted as adequate for coverage. This coating thickness also represents a good compromise between the in vivo chemical dissolution that is associated with thin coatings and the potential fatigue failure under tensile loading that is associated with thick coatings. Various groups have studied the relationship of coating thickness and implant performance. One group reported chemical dissolution of an HA surface within the first few months of implantation when coating thicknesses of 15 μm or less were used. Another group found that HA coatings thicker than 100 μm not only demonstrated severe delamination at load levels below substrate yield strength but also demonstrated substrate fatigue at load levels below the endurance limit. In comparison, this group found that HA coatings that were 50 μm thick showed no delamination of the coating or substrate fatigue.

Studies have also been carried out to address concerns that HA coatings on porous-surfaced implants may occlude the pores or alter the morphology of the porous surface and thereby prohibit adequate bone

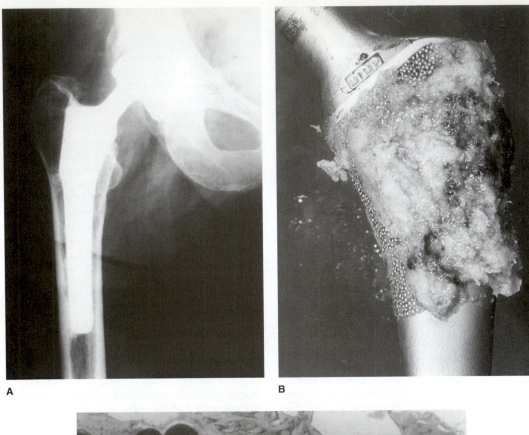

A

B

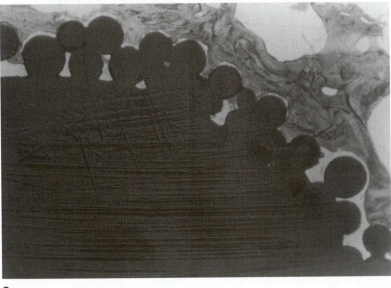

C

Figure 1–24. Four years after implantation, an uncemented porous-coated femoral stem was removed for revision because the patient suffered persistent thigh pain and limp. **A:** The radiograph taken prior to stem removal showed a relatively poor fit, without subsidence but with the presence of nonanatomic remodeling, as evidenced by the so-called pedestal sign. **B:** Gross specimen (posterior aspect) analysis suggested that the component was well fixed, as demonstrated by large amounts of bone. **C:** Histologic examination demonstrated extensive bone ingrowth (basic fuchsin and toluidine blue stain; original magnification × 24).

ingrowth. In these studies, investigators found that a coating thickness of 25–45 μm will not occlude the pores or alter the mechanical bone ingrowth properties of the porous surface.

Calcium phosphate coatings have been applied to substrates by means of a variety of methods, including dip coating, vacuum deposition, and plasma spraying. In dip coating, the substrate can either be dipped into a suspension of ceramic powder in a carrier or be dipped into a liquid form of glass ceramic. In vacuum deposition, ceramic material is removed from a source and deposited onto the target substrate.

Plasma-spraying methods are used by most manufacturers to apply calcium phosphate coatings to metal surfaces, particularly for load-bearing applications. A plasma or ionized gas is created by passing a gas or mixture of gases (usually argon or a mixture of nitrogen and hydrogen) through a high-energy, DC electric arc struck between two electrodes. Then the coating powder suspended in a carrier gas is introduced into this plasma stream, melted, and propelled onto the substrate target, usually at high velocities. The coating is applied in several layers, each approximately 5–10 μm thick. One modified method involves low-pressure plasma spraying in a vacuum chamber, which reportedly makes the coating more resistant to dissolution or bond strength degradation at the coating substrate interface.

Because of the high temperatures necessary for plasma spraying, the ceramic coating material may be chemically or structurally altered from the original ceramic. For this reason, all HA coatings are not identical and may vary among manufacturers in their composition, crystallinity, density, purity, and structure. These differences affect the bioactivity and bioresorbability of coatings and make it nearly impossible to predict their long-term in vivo behavior. To ensure the correct composition of HA coatings, manufacturers perform a variety of tests, including x-ray diffraction, infrared spectroscopy, scanning electron microscopy, and atomic absorption spectroscopy. Investigators concerned about the effects of plasma-sprayed HA coating on substrate surfaces have performed mechanical testing of HA-coated titanium and uncoated titanium and found no measurable differences in the fatigue properties of the metals for HA coatings less than 100 μm thick.

Several studies have shown that HA-coated implants are superior to uncoated implants in terms of interface attachment strength and bone apposition. Also, the properties of HA-coated implants with larger surface areas (macrotextured or porous surfaces) are superior to the properties of HA-coated implants with smaller surface areas (smooth surfaces).

Clinical experience with HA-coated orthopedic prostheses has been recent and limited. Therefore, only short-term studies based on clinical follow-ups and radiographic evaluations exist. In a prospective total hip replacement study, a prosthesis with HA-coated titanium components was evaluated. The HA coating covered the proximal 40% of the stem and covered over 50% of the outer sphere area of the threaded cup. During the first year following implant, there was a statistical correlation between signs of endosteal bone formation and scores in the Harris hip evaluation. At a minimum of 2 years after implantation, there were no signs of loosening or severe bone resorption in the femoral stem area. Similar excellent short-term results were reported for HA-coated, porous, cobalt-chromium primary and revision femoral hip stems. Other findings in early clinical studies of HA-coated porous implants have included decreased pain, decreased radiolucent lines around the implant, and improved bone remodeling.

When an HA-coated femoral stem and acetabular cup were retrieved from a 61-year-old woman 3 weeks after implantation and evaluated histologically, microradiographs showed cortical and trabecular thinning, indicative of osteoporosis. New bone was attached to approximately 10% of the HA surface on the stem and to approximately 20% of the HA surface on the cup. Bone spicules were connecting the bone chips and adjacent cancellous bone to the HA surface. The finding of bone formation on two surfaces supported the results of early animal studies that reported the osteoconductive effects of HA coatings. The bidirectional bone growth and osteoconductive properties of HA-coated prostheses (Figure 1–25) were further demonstrated after postmortem evaluation of an HA-coated implant and an uncoated implant, both retrieved from the same patient. Evaluation of the retrieved implants demonstrated 54% more bone in apposition to the HA-coated implant than in apposition to the uncoated implant on the contralateral side.

Not all studies in patients with HA-coated implants have reported positive findings. In fact, some recent studies have reported cell-mediated osteolysis, implant loosening, and other negative effects linked with the degradation or delamination of the HA coating, the generation and migration of HA particles, and the subsequent three-body wear of the implant that is caused by these particles.

Factors That Affect Biologic Attachment

Attachment at the bone-implant interface is affected by the material properties and design of the implant, surgical technique, initial implant stability, and direct contact with the surrounding bone. Initial implant stability and apposition with bone are not always achievable but are vital for implant longevity. Persistent micromotion

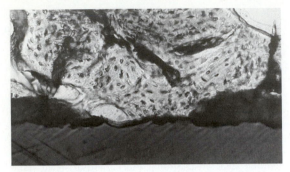

A

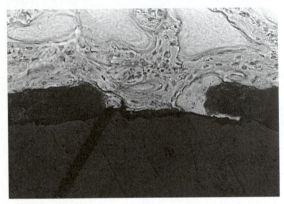

B

Figure 1–25. Histologic appearance of an HA-coated implant with a defect shown at two points in time: at 10 weeks after implantation (**A**) and at 32 weeks after implantation (**B**). Bone is observed in direct apposition to the HA coating and extending continuously from the edge of the HA material into the defect and along the metal substrate. The undecalcified histologic sections were photographed using simultaneous transmitted and reflected illumination (basic fuchsin and toluidine blue stain; original magnification × 160).

at the bone-implant interface causes bone resorption and necrosis, which can in turn result in fibrous tissue infiltration at the interface and in implant loosening. Moreover, any initial gap between the implant and surrounding bone may adversely alter the amount of osseointegration and the rate at which it occurs.

A. MOTION AT THE BONE-IMPLANT INTERFACE

Motion of an implant within the surgical site has a primary influence on biologic fixation and implant longevity. Initial implant stability is essential for the early tissue infiltrate within the porous structure to dif-

ferentiate into bone by either direct bone formation or appositional bone growth. When excessive early movement occurs at the bone-implant interface, bone formation within the pores is inhibited. The majority of research concerning motion at the interface has involved porous implants; however, the findings are applicable for press-fit implant systems.

Two studies of implants in a dog model have suggested that relative motion of greater than 150 μm at the bone-implant interface prevents bone formation. In one of the studies, a well-ordered fibrous tissue interface was maintained and provided adequate implant attachment. In the other study, bone ingrowth occurred when interface motion was 40 μm, but the calcified ingrown bone was not continuous with the surrounding bone. This finding further supports the idea that in order to obtain optimal bone growth into porous surfaces or bone apposition onto press-fit surfaces, it is necessary to have little or no initial micromotion at the interface.

In a recent study of HA coating in a continuous loaded implant model, investigators found that when interface motion led to the formation of a fibrous membrane, the HA coating was able to convert the membrane to bone.

B. SURGICAL FIT

The technical difficulties in cutting bone precisely to provide an exact fit around the implant often result in a poor surgical fit. Implant and instrumentation design may also make it difficult to achieve initial implant-bone interface apposition. When a femoral stem is press-fit into the femoral canal, only 10–20% of the prosthesis comes into direct contact with bone.

The effects of interface gaps and poor surgical fit of implants have been investigated by numerous groups. In studies of HA-coated prostheses, researchers found that the HA coating will not compensate for improper implant placement or poor surgical technique. The cell populations necessary for bone formation are identical across large interface gaps and in press-fit situations. In large gaps, the rate of gap filling and subsequent ingrowth will be delayed, and the quality of bone at the interface may also be reduced. Such studies indicate the potential benefits of robot controlled surgery, where much better initial apposition can be obtained.

Bach CM et al: No functional impairment after Robodoc total hip arthroplasty: Gait analysis in 25 patients. Acta Orthop Scand 2002;73:386. [PMID 12358109]

Bloebaum RD et al: Retrieval analysis of a hydroxyapatite-coated hip prosthesis. Clin Orthop 1991;267:97.

Bobyn JD et al: The optimum pore size for the fixation of porous-surfaced metal implants by the ingrowth of bone. Clin Orthop 1980;150:263.

Collier JP et al: Results of implant retrieval from postmortem specimens in patients with well-functioning, long-term hip replacement. Clin Orthop 1992;274:97.

Cook SD et al: Hydroxyapatite coating of porous implants improves bone ingrowth and interface attachment strength. J Biomed Mater Res 1992;26:989.

Cook SD et al: Quantitative analysis of tissue growth into human porous total hip components. J Arthroplasty 1988;3:249.

DeGroot K et al: Plasma sprayed coatings of hydroxylapatite. J Biomed Mater Res 1987;21:1375.

Fernandez-Pradas JM et al: Characterization of calcium phosphate coatings deposited by Nd-YAG laser ablation at 355 nm: Influence of thickness. Biomaterials 2002;23:1989. [PMID 11996040]

Freels DB et al: Animal model for evaluation of soft tissue ingrowth into various types of porous coating. Clin Orthop 2002;397:315. [PMID 11953623]

Geesink RG: Osteoconductive coatings for total joint arthroplasty. Clin Orthop 2002;395:53. [PMID 11937866]

Jinno T et al: Comparison of hydroxyapatite and hydroxyapatite tricalcium-phosphate coatings. J Arthroplasty 2002;17:902. [PMID 12375251]

Karabatsos B et al: Osseointegration of hydroxyapatite porous-coated femoral implants in a canine model. Clin Orthop 2001;392:442. [PMID 11716420]

LeGeros RZ: Properties of osteoconductive biomaterials: Calcium phosphates. Clin Orthop 2002;395:81. [PMID 11937868]

Manso M et al: Biological evaluation of aerosol-gel-derived hydroxyapatite coatings with human mesenchymal stem cells. Biomaterials 2002;23:3985. [PMID 12162331]

Noble PC et al: The anatomic basis of femoral component design. Clin Orthop 1988;235:148.

Paprosky WG, Burnett RS. Extensively porous-coated femoral stems in revision hip arthroplasty: Rationale and results. Am J Orthop. 2002;31:471. [PMID: 12216970]

Pilliar RM et al:: Observations on the effect of movement on bone ingrowth into porous-surfaced implants. Clin Orthop 1986;208:108.

Soballe K et al: Hydroxyapatite coating converts fibrous tissue to bone around loaded implants. J Bone Joint Surg Br 1993;75:270.

Thomas KA et al: The effect of surface macrotexture and hydroxylapatite coating on the mechanical strengths and histologic profiles of titanium implant materials. J Biomed Mater Res 1987;21:1395.

Thomsen MN et al: Robotically-milled bone cavities: A comparison with hand-broaching in different types of cementless hip stems. Acta Orthop Scand 2002;73:379. [PMID 12358108]

TISSUE RESPONSE TO IMPLANT MATERIALS

The effect of an implanted material on adjacent tissues depends on the amount and type of substance released into the tissues, the histologic response to the material, and the wear and corrosion properties of the material. The type of response to the implant determines the biologic classification of the material.

Biocompatibility

Biotolerant materials, such as stainless steel, PMMA, and UHMWPE, elicit the worst tissue response. When these materials are used, a fibrous tissue layer may form between the bone and the implant. This fibrous layer is generally observable as a radiolucent line on radiographs. Examination with light microscopy shows the presence of numerous macrophages near resorbing adjacent bone and the resulting fibrous tissue that contains macrophages and foreign body giant cells.

PMMA elicits adverse local and systemic effects from the moment of its introduction into the body. At the time of implantation, PMMA causes local tissue necrosis owing to the extreme heat of polymerization. During the polymerization process, monomer may leach into the surrounding tissues and cause hypotension. Over time, monomer may leach into the adjacent tissues and elicit a local inflammatory response, which results in bone resorption adjacent to the PMMA and the development of a fibrous membrane between the bone and the material. Finally, PMMA fragmentation particles elicit a chronic macrophage response at the implant-bone interface, and this can result in progressive osteoclasis and eventual aseptic loosening of the implant. Macrophages are stimulated by cell necrosis, bacteria, and foreign particulate matter. Particulate matter is the primary cause of aseptic loosening in cemented joint arthroplasties. In spite of this, bulk PMMA is well tolerated by the body, whereas particulate PMMA is not.

Bioinert materials, such as titanium and cobalt-chromium alloys, usually cause minimal tissue irritation. With stable implants of either titanium or cobalt-chromium alloys, appositional bone growth or osseointegration occurs. If titanium implants are used in articulating surface applications, however, they have poor wear resistance, and the excessive wear particles behave as biotolerant materials. These particles elicit a chronic macrophage response, which can lead to implant loosening.

Bioactive materials, such as calcium phosphate ceramics, offer the best biologic advantage of implant materials. The biocompatibility of the calcium phosphate ceramics is well documented. In response to these implanted ceramics, the body typically responds (1) without local or systemic toxicity, (2) without inflammatory or foreign body reaction, (3) without alteration of natural mineralization processes, (4) with functional integration of bone, and (5) with chemical bonding to bone via natural bone cementing mechanisms. The calcium phosphate ceramics are biocompatible with natural bone mineral and have a similar chemical composition, and these factors make them desirable bioactive materials.

Implant surfaces coated with HA have been characterized as being capable of forming direct, intimate bonds with the surrounding bone. The bonding area (approximately 50–200 nm) contains biologic apatite crystals that are highly oriented at the interface with a 10-nm periodicity similar to that of calcified tissue, as determined by electron diffraction studies. The bone apatite crystals are arranged against the implant surface in a palisade fashion, resembling the natural bonding between two bone fragments. The bonding area contains a ground substance that is heavily mineralized, although devoid of collagen fibrils, and has been likened to the natural bone cementing substance. The natural bone cementing substance is amorphous in structure, heavily mineralized, and rich in mucopolysaccharides. Because the bonding area contains a substance biologically similar to the natural bone cement substance, it is reasonable that the bond between the bone and the calcium phosphate ceramic is strong.

Problems Associated with Maintaining Implant Longevity

Implant loosening, which can result from bone loss that is caused either by stress shielding or by osteolysis, has been a problem associated with total joint arthroplasty since its inception. Periprosthetic osteolysis radiographically presents as diffuse femoral cortical thinning or as a focal cystic lesion. A focal lesion is associated with additional clinical complications.

Although the exact cause of osteolysis is unknown, it is thought to be a result of movement of the implant and generation of wear particles that migrate to the implant-bone interface, where they cause a tissue reaction. Recently, an in vitro mechanism was observed in which particulate debris stimulated bone resorption and eventually caused implant loosening. Macrophages that phagocytosed particulate debris were found to stimulate 15 times more osteoclastic bone resorption than control macrophages did.

The prevalence of osteolysis in stable cemented femoral components ranges from 3 to 8%. It appears, however, that osteolysis is observed earlier in patients with stable uncemented components and that the prevalence increases with time in vivo. The prevalence in uncemented systems ranges from 10 to 20% after 2–9 years in vivo.

In addition to osteolysis, another problem with total joint implants is the increase in metal ions released into the body. This problem is especially associated with uncemented porous-coated implants. Systemic and long-term effects caused by wear and corrosion are just being discovered. An understanding of the wear and corrosion mechanisms associated with decreasing implant longevity is vital for the development of improved implant designs and material manufacturing methods.

A. Surface Damage of Polyethylene Implants

Osteolysis, loosening, and other complications that reduce implant longevity have been attributed to polyethylene wear particles. Careful examination of retrieved polyethylene components has demonstrated a variety of modes by which surface damage occurs. These include scratching, burnishing, embedding of debris, pitting (the presence of shallow, irregular surface voids in the surface), surface deformation (permanent deformation on the articulating surface), abrasion (characterized by a tufted or shredded appearance of the polyethylene), and delamination (separation of large, thin surface sheets of polyethylene from implant components).

Fatigue has been suggested as the primary mechanism of polyethylene surface damage because the damage has been correlated with the length of time since implantation (number of cycles in the fatigue curve shown in Figure 1–2) and with patient weight (applied load or stress in Figure 1–2). Surface damage is noticeably less in acetabular components than in tibial components. The increased polyethylene damage in total knee arthroplasties can be attributed to reduced surface conformity and to compression-tension loading patterns. Nonconformity of articulating components in total knee arthroplasties results in contact stresses that approximate or exceed the strength of the polyethylene. Cruciate-retaining designs vary the location of contact over the entire articulating surface, thereby subjecting the implant components to alternating compression-tension contact stresses throughout the loading cycle. This cyclic process could contribute to the beginning and spread of cracks, which may lead to pitting, delamination, and other fatigue failure modes.

The elastic modulus and thickness of the polyethylene are significant predictors of contact stresses large enough to cause surface damage. An increased elastic modulus, as is found with carbon-reinforced polyethylene, raises contact stresses and can be expected to result in increased wear. This is important in component design because the elastic modulus of polyethylene near the surface may increase up to 100% over 10 years in vivo. A reduced level of polyethylene thickness, as is found in metal-backed acetabular and tibial components, can result in increased wear and creep, eventually leading to cracking and separation of the polyethylene from the metal. To avoid the high stresses that cause cracking, acetabular polyethylene thickness should be greater than 6 mm, and tibial polyethylene thickness should be greater than 8 mm. Another concern regarding metal-backed components is that loosening of the metal backing may cause the screws to break and migrate into the polyethylene insert, and this in turn can result in the generation of large amounts of metal and polyethylene wear debris.

B. Fatigue of Porous-Coated Implants

The primary failure mode of load-bearing orthopedic implants is fatigue. The majority of hip and knee systems have sintered porous coatings to maximize biologic fixation or cement impregnation. The fatigue properties of these porous-coated implants are influenced not only by the sintering treatment but also by a notch effect from the coating.

Sintering affects the fatigue properties of coated implants by altering the microstructure of their metal substrate. With titanium-based alloys, sintering requires that the material be heat-treated above the beta phase transition temperature, which reduces the fatigue properties of the material by about 40%. When post-sintering heat treatments are performed, the fatigue strength of the previously sintered titanium-based alloy increases by 25%. With cobalt-based alloys, sintering does not necessarily result in a reduction of fatigue strength. A dissolution of carbides and an increase in porosity occur, however, when cobalt-based alloys that have less than 0.3% carbon are exposed to sintering temperatures. Additionally, with improper cooling, the sintered cobalt-based alloys can develop continuous grain boundary precipitates.

Investigators have performed studies to determine the effects of sintering, postsintering heat treatments, and hot isostatic pressing techniques on the fatigue properties of nonporous and porous-coated cobalt-based alloys. They reported that sintered materials exhibited severe porosity and continuous grain boundary precipitates, which resulted in reduced fatigue and tensile strength. Hot isostatic pressing eliminated the porosity and grain boundary precipitation resulting from sintering, however. Moreover, hot isostatic pressing of the sintered materials increased the tensile and fatigue properties in implants with or without a porous coating.

Aside from manufacturing processes, which may alter the fatigue properties of the substrate, porous coatings have demonstrated a notch effect at the contact regions. These regions are susceptible to the initiation of cracks, which may continue to propagate along surface grain boundaries. This effect is most significant for the titanium-based alloys.

The fatigue properties that are caused by sintering and the notch effect of coating in load-bearing implants can be reduced by the following measures: (1) avoiding the use of porous coating in regions of maximal tensile stress, (2) using an additional heat treatment process on previously sintered titanium-based alloys, and (3) using

hot isostatic pressing on previously sintered cobalt-based alloys.

C. Ion Release and Surface Corrosion of Metal Implants

Any metal exposed to the physiologic environment will corrode. Corrosion is most evident in fracture fixation devices. Retrieval studies of stainless steel components have revealed evidence of pitting and crevice corrosion in about 75% of the components.

Apart from potential implant mechanical failure, the clinical significance of corrosion is determined by the type and quantity of metal ion that is released and by the local and systemic effects of ion release. The widespread use of porous coatings on metallic implants and the recent popularity of metal-on-metal bearing surfaces has raised additional concerns regarding metal ion release. Porous coatings increase the amount of surface area that is exposed to body fluids by a factor of 1.2 to 7.2. Depending on the type and morphology of the porous coating, the increased surface area could increase the corrosion and ion release rates by a factor of 1.2 to 5.2. Unlike the metallic surface of cemented implants, the metallic surface of porous implants is in direct contact with the endosteal bone surface and vasculature, creating an environment in which a cellular response to metallic ions is possible. The metal-on-metal bearing does not directly increase the corrosion area but does produce metal particulate debris that has a very large surface area to volume ratio. This debris then is available to corrode and put ions into the systemic circulation. Significantly increased levels of implant elements have been documented in serum and urine after implantation of these devices.

Released metal ions (Al, Co, Cr, Fe, Mn, Ni, Ti, and V ions) have one of four types of possible effects on the body: metabolic, bacteriologic, immunogenic, or oncogenic. With the possible exception of titanium, the metallic elements used to fabricate implants are either essential or toxic to processes of metabolism. Although it is known that excessive concentrations of essential elements can produce toxic effects, the ultimate fate of the released ions locally, systemically, or in remote organ systems remains to be determined.

Investigators recently studied the local and systemic effects of metal debris from 46 patients with total hip arthroplasties that required revision surgery. Among the implants studied were cemented and cementless titanium alloy and cobalt-chromium alloy stems, some of which were loose and some of which were well fixed. Examination of synovial fluid showed that metal ion concentrations were elevated in cases involving both cemented and cementless fixed and loose components. Examination of blood, however, showed that metal ion concentrations were elevated only in cases involving loose components. These findings suggest that metal ion release remains primarily a local problem until the implant becomes loose. They also suggest that early revision would decrease the systemic concentrations of metal ions.

Metal sensitivity induced by metal ion release is a common problem. Nickel, chromium, and cobalt are the ions most frequently responsible for metal sensitivity reactions. Some studies have shown that the released ions can form metal ion-protein complexes that behave as haptens by inducing an allergic response. Other studies have shown that metallic biomaterials elicit both B-cell-mediated and T-cell-mediated immune responses. When investigators studied porous-coated hip and knee devices retrieved from patients, they reported the finding of a cellular response in interfacial and interstitial tissues. Although none of the components had been removed because of infection and none had shown clinical or radiographic evidence of loosening, the investigators identified an inflammatory infiltrate with accompanying vascular proliferation in 22% of the components. The predominant cell types within the porous coatings were lymphocytes and histiocytes, although giant cells were also present. Several groups have reported that delayed hypersensitivity can produce an immunologic reaction in which T cells recognize a metal ion-protein complex, release a variety of lymphokines, and stimulate a mononuclear infiltration. Further research is necessary, however, to determine if an allergic or hypersensitivity response to metal ions is responsible for inflammatory infiltrates.

Metal ion release can be modified by applying a plasma-sprayed calcium phosphate coating to a porous metal. The ion release kinetics of the implant are altered in a variety of ways: (1) the ceramic can shield the metal; (2) nonuniform coatings can create a local exposure of the metal; (3) degradation of the coating with time can cause a variational release of ions; and (4) the metal surface can be structurally altered by the high temperatures used for the application process.

When investigators studied the in vitro corrosion behavior of cobalt-based alloys with and without HA coatings, they found that the use of HA coating decreased corrosion rates by an order of magnitude. They also found that the calcium in Ringer's solution deposited directly onto the HA coating.

Among the questions that remain unanswered concerning metal ion release are the following: What ion concentration for each metal results in adverse systemic effects? Once the systemic ion concentration becomes elevated, how long does it take before it decreases? Do metal ions preferentially attack certain tissues and organs and thereby cause adverse effects? Further research is needed to answer these crucial questions.

Anissian L et al: Cobalt ions influence proliferation and function of human osteoblast-like cells. Acta Orthop Scand 2002;73:369. [PMID 12143988]

Berzins A et al: Surface damage in machined ram-extruded and net-shape molded retrieved polyethylene tibial inserts of total knee replacements. J Bone Joint Surg (Am) 2002;84:1534. [PMID 12208909]

Brown SR et al: Long-term survival of McKee-Farrar total hip prostheses. Clin Orthop 2002;402:157. [PMID 12218479]

Collier JP et al: The biomechanical problems of polyethylene as a bearing surface. Clin Orthop 1990;261:107.

Cook SD et al: The effect of post-sintering heat treatments on the fatigue properties of porous coated Ti-6Al-4V alloy. J Biomed Mater Res 1988;22:287.

Edwards SA et al: Analysis of polyethylene thickness of tibial components in total knee replacement. J Bone Joint Surg (Am) 2002;84:369. [PMID 11886905]

Goldberg JR et al: A multicenter retrieval study of the taper interfaces of modular hip prostheses. Clin Orthop 2002;401:149. [PMID 12151892]

Cook SD et al: Inflammatory response in retrieved noncemented porous coated implants. Clin Orthop 1991;264:209.

Dorr LD et al: Histologic, biochemical, and ion analysis of tissue and fluids during total hip arthroplasty. Clin Orthop 1990; 261:82.

Freeman MA et al: Observations upon the interface between bone and polymethylmethacrylate cement. J Bone Joint Surg (Br) 1982;64:489.

Friberg L et al: Handbook on the Toxicology of Metals. Elsevier, 1986.

Georgette FS, Davidson JA: The effect of hot isostatic pressing on the fatigue and tensile strength of a cast, porous coated Co-Cr-Mo alloy. J Biomed Mater Res 1986;20:1229.

Hallab N et al: Metal sensitivity in patients with orthopaedic implants. J Bone Joint Surg (Am) 2001;83:428. [PMID 11263649]

Huang CH et al: Particle size and morphology of UHMWPE wear debris in failed total knee arthroplasties—A comparison between mobile bearing and fixed bearing knees. J Orthop Res 2002;20:1038. [PMID 12382971]

Maloney WJ et al: Endosteal erosion in association with stable uncemented femoral components. J Bone Joint Surg (Am) 1990;72:1025.

Merritt K, Brown SA: Distribution of cobalt chromium wear and corrosion products and biologic reactions. Clin Orthop 1996;329 Suppl:S233.

Merritt K, Rodrigo JJ: Immune response to synthetic materials. Sensitization of patients receiving orthopaedic implants. Clin Orthop 1996;326:71.

Murray DW, Rushton N: Macrophages stimulate bone resorption when they phagocytose particles. J Bone Joint Surg (Br) 1990;72:988.

Pilliar RM: Powder metal-made orthopedic implants with porous surface for fixation by tissue ingrowth. Clin Orthop 1983; 176:42.

Rao AR et al: Tibial interface wear in retrieved total knee components and correlations with modular insert motion. J Bone Joint Surg (Am) 2002;84:1849. [PMID 12377918]

Shrivastava R et al: Effects of chromium on the immune system. FEMS Immunol Med Microbiol 2002;34:1. [PMID 12208600]

Wright TM, Bartel DL: The problem of surface damage in poly-ethylene total knee components. Clin Orthop 1986;205;67.

■ GAIT ANALYSIS

Harry B. Skinner, MD, PhD

The science of studying human walking is called **gait analysis.** This science has evolved as a means of quantitating the individual components of gait. As measurement techniques have been refined to permit the determination of forces, moments, and movements of the human body, these techniques have been applied to functions other than walking. Thus, it has been possible to measure the functional demands of wheelchair motion and running, as well as activities as diverse as pitching a baseball. The study of gait analysis has been assisted by the development of devices that are able to measure gait in terms of (1) movement in space, (2) metabolic energy consumed during movement, (3) functional patterns of muscles during movement, and (4) forces applied to the ground during movement. Direct measurements of these factors have permitted the secondary determination of quantities concerning mechanical work, joint moments, and center of pressure, which in turn have been helpful in quantifying the function of prostheses and the effects of ataxia. The techniques of gait analysis have been applied to other facets of human function. Motion analysis, for example, has been applied to elucidate the kinesthetic changes in the spine occurring with fatigue in a study of repetitive lifting.

GAIT CYCLES, PHASES, & EVENTS

For uniformity in the reporting of gait measurements, investigators have adopted several definitions concerning gait cycle. One **gait cycle** is defined as the time from initial ground contact of one foot to subsequent ground contact of the same foot. This is then normalized to 100%, with the intervening phases, periods, and events (Figure 1–26) defined on this basis. Ground contact is chosen as the beginning of the cycle because it is easily defined. The duration of the gait cycle varies, depending on the height, weight, and age of the individual whose gait is being analyzed as well as on any pathologic process affecting the individual's movement. Normalization of the gait cycle into percentages facilitates comparison among individuals.

Two **gait phases** are recognized: the stance phase and the swing phase. The normal **stance phase,** when the extremity is on the ground, accounts for about 62% of the cycle, and the normal **swing phase** of that ex-

tremity accounts for the remainder. The proportions vary with speed. Each phase is divided into periods. The stance phase starts with double-limb support, is followed by single-limb support, and ends with a second period of double-limb support. Each period of double-limb support accounts for about 10% of the gait cycle. The swing phase is divided into early, mid, and late periods, with each period accounting for about 13% of the gait cycle. Swing phase for one limb corresponds to stance phase for the opposite limb.

The swing and stance phases are also divided into **gait events** (see Figure 1–26). Terms such as **heel strike** and **toe-off,** which have been used to describe the events in the gait cycle, were initially derived from the observation of normal gait. The nomenclature of gait analysis, however, is evolving to take into account the fact that these terms are inadequate in describing the gait of individuals who have joint contractures, joint instability, pain, spasticity, or other conditions that alter the gait so that the heel may never strike the floor or the heel and toe may strike simultaneously or depart simultaneously. In gait analysis, the various events are recognized by observation and can be correlated with measurements of the ground reaction force and motion variables. Observation is greatly enhanced through the use of slow-motion photography or video equipment.

GAIT MEASUREMENTS

The quantities that would be measured in a complete analysis of gait include three-dimensional translation, velocity, acceleration for all motion segments, forces exerted on the ground, electromyographic response of muscles during the gait cycle, and metabolic energy consumption. Obviously, a complete gait analysis would be an expensive and time-consuming procedure and perhaps not even possible within the endurance limits of some patients studied. A typical gait analysis is problem-oriented and focuses on information relevant to the disorder being addressed by the clinician.

Movement During Gait

A. STRIDE CHARACTERISTICS

The fundamental data needed for almost any gait analysis are basic measurements termed stride characteristics. These are necessary because they form a baseline for interpreting all of the other aspects of gait. The stride characteristic variables are velocity (speed), gait cycle, cadence, stride length, step length, single- and double-limb support time, and swing and stance time.

Velocity of gait is the measure of forward progression of an individual's center of gravity, which is generally located midline and anterior to the sacrum.

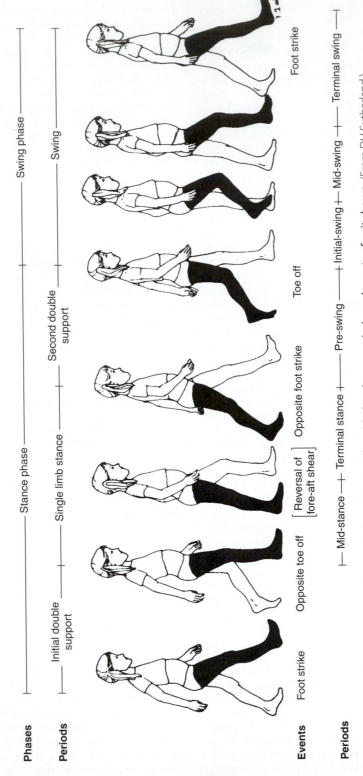

Phases

Stance phase ——— Swing phase

Periods

Initial double support ——— Single limb stance ——— Second double support ——— Swing

Events

Foot strike ——— Opposite toe off ——— [Reversal of fore-aft shear] ——— Opposite foot strike ——— Toe off ——— Foot strike

Periods

Mid-stance ——— Terminal stance ——— Pre-swing ——— Initial-swing ——— Mid-swing ——— Terminal swing

Figure 1–26. The typical normal gait cycle, with the phases, periods, and events of gait shown. (From DH Sutherland.)

Velocity is expressed as an average number of meters per minute, although it is obvious that the instantaneous velocity can vary somewhat.

Gait cycle is measured as the number of seconds from the initial ground contact of one foot until the subsequent ground contact of the same foot. **Cadence** is the number of steps per minute (the number of times both feet strike the ground per minute) and is different from the number of strides per minute (the number of times the same foot strikes the ground per minute).

Step length is measured as the distance (number of meters) covered from the time one foot strikes the ground until the opposite foot strikes. It differs from stride length, which is the distance (number of meters) covered from the time one foot strikes the ground to the next time the same foot strikes the ground. In normal individuals, the length of each step would be one-half of the stride length. But in people with pathologic processes that affect gait, the lengths of the two steps are different.

Single-limb and double-limb support times are periods of the gate cycle that can be measured in terms of seconds or in terms of percentage of the gait cycle (Table 1–4 and Figure 1–26). These periods in patients with a painful condition such as an ankle sprain generally differ from periods in normal individuals. Less obvious is the fact that the two double-limb support times (one following left foot strike and the other following right foot strike), which are usually of the same length in normal individuals, may be of two different lengths in patients with pathologic processes that affect gait. **Swing and stance times** can also be measured in terms of seconds or in terms of percentage of gait cycle.

Gait characteristics of normal men and women at free walking speed are shown in Table 1–4, and a sampling of these data for normal children at selected ages is presented in Table 1–5. Gait measurements are generally made at the **free walking speed** for each person because that speed is selected by the person to minimize energy consumption and is therefore considered the optimal gait velocity. Velocities that are slower or faster can be continuously maintained by individuals as long as the metabolic energy consumption remains in the aerobic range. These velocities are more costly in terms of energy expenditure, however.

Stride characteristics are sensitive indicators of diseases and disorders that affect gait. Many variables have a bearing on the stride measurements. Age, height, weight, and shoe wear are physiologic variables that will help define the basic parameters of velocity, cadence, and gait cycle. Abnormalities resulting from an anatomic change, such as joint replacement, degenerative disease of the lower extremities, or knee fusion, can be demonstrated as nonspecific and asymmetric variations in the stride characteristics. External variables such as those affecting the walking surface (eg, sand, concrete, and ice) can markedly alter stride measurements and must be considered in comparing data from different treatment groups or locations. Data are also sensitive to measurement technique. "Free" walking behavior in a laboratory may be different from that which takes place unobserved on a street and is definitely different from walking on a treadmill. Thus, to eliminate extraneous variables, care must be exercised not only in measuring stride characteristics but also in interpreting them.

Table 1–4. Gait characteristics of normal men and women at free walking speed.

Component (Unit of Measure)	Men (Mean ± 1SD)	Women (Mean ± 1SD)
Velocity (m/min)	91 ± 12	74 ± 9
Gait cycle (s)	1.06 ± 0.09	1.03 ± 0.08
Cadence (steps/min)	113 ± 9	117 ± 9
Step length (cm)[a]	78 ± 6	62 ± 5
Stride length (cm)	160	137
Single-limb support[a]		
Time (s)	0.44	0.39
As proportion of gait cycle (%)	40	38
Swing (s)[a]	0.41 ± 0.04	0.39 ± 0.03
Stance (s)[a]	0.65 ± 0.07	0.64 ± 0.06
Lateral motion of the head (cm)	5.9 ± 1.7	4.0 ± 1.1
Vertical motion of the head (cm)		
During right stance	4.8 ± 1.1	4.1 ± 0.9
During left stance	4.9 ± 1.1	4.1 ± 0.9
Hip flexion-extension used (degree)	48 ± 5	40 ± 4
Anteroposterior pelvic tilting (degree)	7.1 ± 2.4	5.5 ± 1.3
Transverse pelvic rotation (degree)	12 ± 4	10 ± 3

[a]Right equals left in normal individuals.

Data adapted, with permission, from Murray MP, Gore DR: Gait patients with hip pain or loss of hip joint motion. In: Black J, Dumbleton JH (editors). *Clinical Biomechanics: A Case History Approach*, Churchill Livingstone, 1981; and from Rancho Los Amigos Hospital data on normal values.

B. MOTION ANALYSIS

Motion analysis is necessary for the complete characterization of gait. Aside from simply recording motions, quantification of the dynamic range of motion of a joint or body segment is called kinematics Rather than measuring all limb segments, investigators generally focus on motion in certain limb segments and the

Table 1–5. Gait characteristics of normal children at free walking speeds for selected ages.

Component (Unit of Measure)	1 Year	2 Years	3 Years	4 Years	5 Years
Velocity (m/min)	38.2	43.1	51.3	64.8	68.6
Gait cycle (s)	0.68	0.78	0.77	0.77	0.83
Cadence (steps/min)	175.7	155.8	153.5	153.4	143.5
Step length (cm)[a]	21.6	27.5	32.9	42.3	47.9
Stride length (cm)	43.0	54.9	66.8	84.3	96.5
Single-limb support as proportion of gait cycle (%)[a]	32.1	33.5	34.8	36.5	37.6

[a]Right equals left in normal individuals.

Data adapted, with permission, from Sutherland DH et al: The development of mature gait. J Bone Joint Surg [Am] 1980;62:336; and from Sutherland DH et al: The development of mature walking. Clin Dev Med 1988;104:1.

trunk. Although major displacements of the lower extremities and upper extremities are occurring during gait, the center of mass of the body is only moving about 2–4 cm in a mediolateral direction and 2 cm in a superoinferior direction. Simultaneously, pelvic and trunk motion is occurring around the center of mass in a sinusoidal fashion. To conserve angular momentum, the upper extremity moves forward with the contralateral lower extremity.

Motion analysis has benefits and limitations. On the one hand, it provides more information to the clinician than does simple analysis of stride characteristics. For example, although stride analysis may show that the single-limb support time is reduced, motion analysis can clarify whether this is caused by decreased hip or knee motion, weakness of knee or ankle musculature, or some other condition and can also permit documentation of the benefit of intervention. On the other hand, motion analysis is labor-intensive and expensive from an equipment viewpoint. It also presents difficulties in accurately defining motion segments and sometimes in measuring relatively small movements. There are problems, for example, in placing the markers to determine mediolateral pelvic rotation or anteroposterior pelvic rotation and in measuring these movements, whereas measuring knee flexion and extension is much easier. Highly sophisticated motion analysis systems have been developed to maximize the accuracy and efficiency of these measurements, but there has been a concomitant increase in expense.

Energy Consumption During Gait

Energy expenditure results from muscle function and is possible as a direct result of the body's use of food. Steady-state aerobic metabolism is the optimal means of using oxygen to metabolize food, although less efficient anaerobic mechanisms are available. Measurements of oxygen consumption per unit of time can be converted to measurements of energy expenditure or power. An oxygen consumption measurement of 1 L/min is approximately equivalent to an energy consumption measurement of 5 kcal/min.

Energy expenditure per unit of body mass can be expressed per step, per unit of distance, or per unit of time. Most commonly, energy expenditure is measured in terms of **rate of oxygen uptake,** expressed as milliliters of oxygen per kilogram per minute (mL O_2/kg/min), and **net oxygen cost,** expressed as milliliters of oxygen per kilogram per meter (mL O_2/kg/m). Both the rate of oxygen uptake and the net oxygen cost depend on the velocity (v) of walking, expressed in terms of meters per minute (m/min). The approximate relations are as follows:

$$\text{Rate of oxygen uptake} = 0.001\, v^2 + 6.0$$

$$\text{Net oxygen cost} = \frac{6.0}{v} + 0.0011 v$$

The rate of oxygen uptake for normal adults is 11.9 ± 2.3 mL O_2/kg/min, and the net oxygen cost is 0.15 mL O_2/kg/m.

The rate of oxygen uptake increases with the square of the velocity (Figure 1–27). Body mass is obviously important in determining energetics, but location of the mass is even more important. An increase in weight around the center of mass (ie, the waist) is not nearly as energy-costly as an increase around the ankles. This is because the center of mass moves at a near constant velocity with relatively small motions. Conversely, the ankles must be accelerated and decelerated constantly during gait, with each acceleration and deceleration requiring energy. When net oxygen cost for normal in-

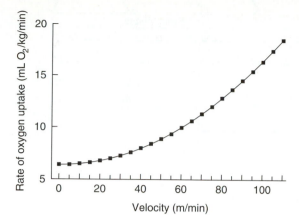

Figure 1–27. Rate of oxygen uptake as a function of velocity.

dividuals is expressed as a function of velocity, there is a minimum in the energy consumption curve at approximately 80 m/min, indicating that this is the most efficient velocity of ambulation (Figure 1–28).

Energy expenditure in gait assumes importance when gait efficiency decreases or when the most efficient gait velocity is markedly below normal. Attempts to increase velocity can increase energy costs to the point that sustained ambulation cannot be maintained. This can be seen, for example, in the case of traumatic transfemoral amputation. Although the amputee may ambulate with a net oxygen cost of about 0.28 mL O_2/kg/m, which is nearly 100% above normal (0.15 ± 0.02 mL O_2/kg/m), attempts to increase the speed could push the amputee into the anaerobic consump-

tion range and thereby limit the ambulation distance. A similar problem can be seen in the case of a paraplegic who has adequate muscle function to ambulate before gaining weight but finds that the net oxygen cost of increased weight makes wheelchair mobility more energy-efficient.

Muscle Function During Gait

Measurement of the function of muscles during gait is helpful in understanding and treating problems associated with cerebral palsy, stroke, poliomyelitis, and other diseases that alter the normal pattern of muscle function. The activity of muscles during gait is determined by **dynamic electromyography** through the use of either surface electrodes or fine wire electrodes inserted into muscles. Electrical activity generated from these muscles is monitored and recorded in an on-off fashion as a function of the gait cycle. Activity does not necessarily indicate agonistic (contracting) or antagonistic (lengthening) function, but this determination can be made with simultaneous motion analysis. At present, it is not possible to quantify the relationship between electromyographic activity and force.

Normal functioning of the muscles can be presented as a function of the gait cycle and is shown in Figure 1–29. Most muscle activity is generated at the beginning and end of the stance and swing phases of gait because it is necessary at these times to accelerate and decelerate the extremities.

Dynamic electromyography is particularly useful in disorders associated with spasticity, such as cerebral palsy and cerebral vascular accident. In these disorders, the results of functional muscle testing of the patient in the supine position can be markedly different from the results of testing in the upright ambulating position. For example, the tibialis anterior may function normally when the patient is supine, but dynamic electromyography may reveal a varus-deforming force of the hindfoot during ambulation.

Forces During Gait—Kinetics

Forces acting during ambulation arise from gravity, inertia, and ground reaction. At ambulation speeds, viscous drag can be ignored. The **gravitational force** (mass × gravity) must be considered because it will cause moments around centers of rotation for limb segments and body segments. The **inertial force** is proportional to the acceleration of the body segment and acts in the opposite direction because it resists acceleration. The **ground reaction force** is a measurement of the load applied to a device such as a force platform and has three components: vertical ground reaction force, fore-aft shear, and mediolateral shear.

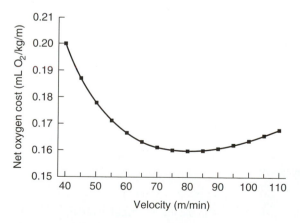

Figure 1–28. Net oxygen cost as a function of velocity.

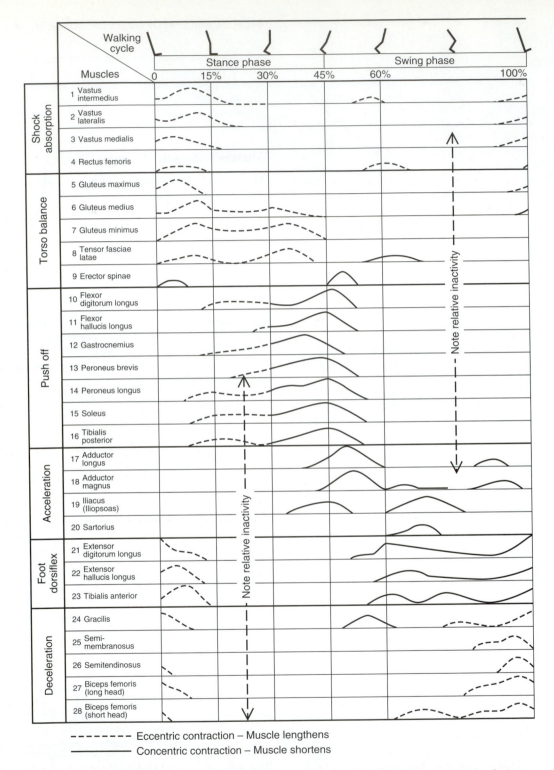

Figure 1–29. Tabulation of the on-off activity of the major muscles in the lower extremity during gait. Dashed lines show eccentric contraction (muscle lengthens); solid lines show concentric contraction (muscle shortens). (Reproduced, with permission, from Charles O Bechtel, Los Angeles, CA. American Academy of Orthopaedic Surgeons: *Atlas of Orthotics: Biomechanical Principles and Application.* Mosby, 1975.)

Typical curves for the three components of the ground reaction force are shown in Figure 1–30. The dip in the vertical force curve (Figure 1–30A) during the single-limb stance phase of gait occurs because the inertial forces reduce the ground reaction force below body weight. The fore-aft shear (Figure 1–30B) is negative after the heel strike because the foot is pushing the plate anterior. On toe-off, the converse is occurring so the shear force is in the opposite direction. Again, correlation of ground reaction forces to stride characteristics can be beneficial in interpreting gait data. Force platform data will show variations with walking speed, shoe wear, and compensatory mechanisms of gait, such as the avoidance of weight bearing on a painful extremity. The components of the ground reaction force in gait can be an indication of dynamic aspects of gait. The vertical ground reaction force tends to increase in magnitude and higher frequency content with increasing velocity and flatten with lower velocity and/or lower extremity pain. Examination of the frequency content especially in the medial-lateral shear component is an indicator of balance control, as in scoliosis. Static measurements provide center of pressure variations, also as a measure of balance control.

More sophisticated force measurement devices have been developed to permit measurement of pressure (force per unit area). These devices can yield both in-shoe pressures and pressures applied to the external surface of the shoe by a force platform. Thus discrimination of measures at the 1-cm^2 level is possible, allowing studies of feet of diabetic patients to discern differences shoe wear can have on the risk of skin breakdown.

Burnett RG et al: Comparison of mechanical work and metabolic energy consumption during normal gait. J Orthop Res 1983;1:63.

Chambers HG, Sutherland DH: A practical guide to gait analysis. J Am Acad Orthop Surg 2002;10:222. [PMID 12041944]

Perry J et al: Functional evaluation of the pes anserinus transfer by electromyography and gait analysis. J Bone Joint Surg (Am) 1980;62:973.

Sutherland DH et al: The development of mature gait. J Bone Joint Surg (Am) 1980;62:336.

ROLE OF GAIT ANALYSIS IN THE MANAGEMENT OF GAIT DISORDERS

Gait analysis has traditionally been a research tool and continues to find its primary use in the research arena. However, the impetus to document the benefit of medical intervention has resulted in a reliance on gait analysis to quantify gains made by surgery or other treatments. There continue to be proponents of gait analysis as a clinical diagnostic tool. New areas in which gait analysis is under investigation include Parkinson's dis-

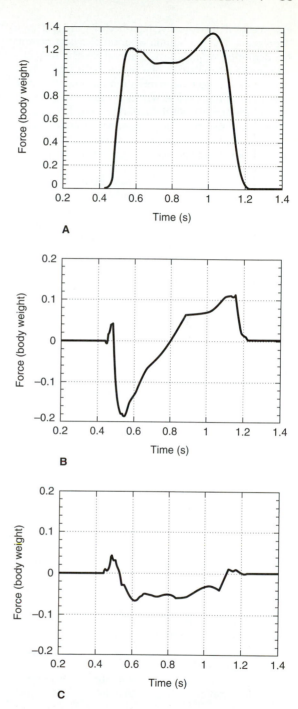

Figure 1–30. The typical ground reaction force for the left foot, shown with its three components. **A:** Vertical force. **B:** Fore-aft shear, which in this plot is negative for heel strike and positive for toe-off. **C:** Mediolateral shear, which in this plot is negative in the lateral direction. (Courtesy of S Rossi.)

ease, cervical myelopathy, high-heeled gait, and even depression. The publication of normative data permits the definition of pathologic gait and thereby defines a goal in the rehabilitation of a patient with a gait disorder. Analysis in gait laboratories can measure the initial deviation from normal as well as the improvements occurring through the rehabilitation process. Even as gait laboratories assume a more prominent role in evaluation of patients, however, the data generated from research laboratories have already affected clinical practice in a variety of ways.

New techniques of analysis have been developed as computer sophistication and availability have evolved. Gait is a process with inherent variability, which must be understood and accounted for in order to maximize its utility. Fractal analysis is one approach and may result in a better description of gait rhythm variations during maturation from childhood to adulthood. Understanding and predicting muscle activation patterns can be accomplished using artificial neural network models. These are particularly exciting as their use may lead to active control of prostheses. Part of the variability of gait arises from differences in body size. Scaling the gait data to body size can reduce intersubject variability and provide a tighter evaluation of abnormality. Identification of "abnormal" gait can be subtle in some cases in view of the variable and voluminous data generated. The common method of evaluation is principal component analysis, which quantifies the deviation of variables from normal. A more recent report evaluates variability based on an index that used the squared distance from the mean obtained from joint angle measurements of many subjects. These techniques promise to improve the usefulness of gait analysis in the evaluation and treatment of orthopedic patients.

Gait studies of patients with transfemoral and transtibial amputations have resulted in an objective evaluation of ambulatory potential after prosthetic replacement. Early studies demonstrated that amputations at more proximal levels resulted in greater loss of symmetry and increased energy expenditure (Table 1–6). These findings have stimulated renewed attempts to maintain amputations at the most distal level. Other studies showed that strengthening the muscles of the residual limb in patients with transtibial amputations resulted in velocities that were improved although still lower than normal. Recent electromyographic studies of gait in transfemoral amputees have demonstrated the importance of reattaching biarticular muscles that are transected at the amputation site to bone to maintain their function.

Techniques for gait analysis of amputees also provide the objective means of comparing various prosthetic components, such as the solid ankle cushion heel (SACH) foot, and the multiaxial and uniaxial feet.

Gait analysis has become a common tool in the treatment and evaluation of patients who have cerebral palsy or have suffered from a cerebrovascular accident or head injury. For disorders such as these, gait improvement can be expected for 6 months or more. Studies suggest that the natural history of gait in child and adolescent cerebral palsy is one of deterioration with aging, an important finding when evaluating long-term effects of intervention to improve gait. The use of electromyographic gait data can improve the results of muscle transfers in this group of patients. Knowledge of the activity period of a muscle (swing phase/stance phase) can allow prediction of the effect of transfer of that muscle. Thus, gait analysis has been applied to spastic equinovarus feet to determine the efficacy of transfers of tibialis anterior and tibialis posterior.

Clinicians can use gait analysis to provide objective clinical data whenever orthotics are prescribed. Gait analysis before and after the application of an orthosis can quantify the effects in an objective manner. In evaluating the results, clinicians should remember that an orthosis that eliminates motion of a joint may improve function by putting the joint in a better position without bringing the patient back to a normal state. With orthotic fitting, lack of motion at a joint such as the

Table 1–6. Results of free walking gait analysis in patients with transfemoral (TF) and transtibial (TT) amputations.

Cause and Level of Amputation	Velocity (m/min)	Cadence (steps/min)	Stride Length (m)	Gait Cycle (s)	Rate of Oxygen Uptake (mL/kg/min)	Net Oxygen Cost (mL/kg/m)
Traumatic TF amputation	55	86	1.26	1.42	12.7	0.28
Dysvascular TF amputation	36	72	1.00	1.66	12.6	0.35
Traumatic TT amputation	68	98	1.38	1.22	12.4	0.22
Dysvascular TT amputation	45	87	1.02	1.36	11.7	0.26

Data adapted, with permission, from Bagley AM, Skinner HB: Progress in gait analysis in amputees: A special review. Crit Rev Phys Rehabil Med 1991;3:101.

ankle will result in an increase in energy consumption and an alteration of gait symmetry. But without orthotic fitting, a poor joint position such as ankle equinus may make the gait even more inefficient and asymmetric. Similarly, AFOs thought to work through changes in spastic reflexes have been shown with gait studies to be less effective than hinged AFOs in CP children. Other studies have also shown that design of orthoses can be evaluated. In hemiplegic stroke patients, the use of a cane or the combination of a cane and an ankle-foot orthosis (AFO) has been found to significantly decrease energy consumption.

Gait analysis is also improving surgical decision making. A recent study allowed experienced clinicians to review videotape and clinical examination data before recommending a treatment plan. After reviewing complete gait data, the same clinicians changed recommendations in 52% of patients. A second study showed 39% of planned surgical procedures on children were deemed unnecessary after gait analysis. Evaluation of a patient's gait before and after a procedure can demonstrate the efficacy of the procedure and assist in postoperative care. A recent study demonstrated that the Van Nes rotational osteotomy allowed ambulation in children with proximal femoral focal deficiency at a more energy efficient rate than children with a Syme amputation. Gait analysis can allow objective comparisons of various procedures. This is primarily applicable, however, to those procedures in which the end point is an improvement of function. For example, walking efficiency as determined by velocity has been shown to be statistically the same for transfemoral amputation and for proximal tibial replacement for tumor, but below normal for both treatments for age. Such a comparison

Table 1–7. Results of free walking gait analysis in patients with total knee arthroplasty.

Study[a]	Patient Diagnosis	Time Since Surgery (yr)	Velocity (m/min)	Cadence (steps/min)	Stride Length (m)	Prosthesis Design
(1) Collopy et al (1977)	OA	1	57	100	1.2	Geometric
	RA	1	46	98	0.9	Geometric
(2) Simon et al (1983)	OA	3.3	63	100.6	1.2	Duopatellar
(3) Skinner et al (1983)	OA or RA	Preop	38.9	87.6	0.864	—
	OA or RA	5	46.5	91.5	1.01	Multiple
(4) Skinner et al (1983)	OA or RA	5.5	50.7	91	1.30	Polycentric
(5) Olsson and Barck (1986)	OA	9	62.4	107	1.14	Gunston-Hult
(6) Berman et al (1987)	Oa, with normal contralateral knee	1.5	49.6	—	1.07	Total condylar
	OA, with asymptomatic diseased contralateral knee	2.0	35.2	—	0.958	—
	OA in both knees	1.3	54.5	—	1.07	—
(7) Waters et al (1987)	RA	0.9	63	103	1.31	—
(8) Kroll et al (1989)	OA	1.1	64.1	109.7	1.18	—
(9) Steiner, Simon, and Pisciotta (1989)	OA or RA	1.0	69	114	1.18	Total condylar or unicompartmental

[a]References are as follows: (1) Collopy MC et al: Kinesiologic measurements of functional performance before and after geometric total knee replacement. Clin Orthop 1977;126:196. (2) Simon SR et al: Quantitative gait analysis after knee arthroplasty for monoarticular degenerative arthritis. J Bone Joint Surg [Am] 1983;65:605. (3) Skinner HB et al: Ambulatory function in total knee arthroplasty. South Med J 1983;76:1237. (4) Skinner HB et al: Correlation of gait analysis and clinical evaluation of polycentric total knee arthroplasty. Orthopedics 1983;6:576. (5) Olsson E, Barck A: Correlation between clinical examination and quantitative gait analysis in patients operated upon with the Gunston-Hult knee prosthesis. Scand J Rehab Med 1986;18:101. (6) Berman AT et al: Quantitative gait analysis after unilateral or bilateral total knee replacement. J Bone Joint Surg [Am] 1987;69:1340. (7) Waters RL et al: The energy cost of walking with arthritis of the hip and knee. Clin Orthop 1987;214:278. (8) Kroll MA et al: The relationship of stride characteristics to pain before and after total knee arthroplasty. Clin Orthop 1989;239:191. (9) Steiner ME, Simon SR, Pisciotta JC: Early changes in gait and maximum knee torque following knee arthroplasty. Clin Orthop 1989;238:174.
OA = osteoarthrosis; RA = rheumatoid arthritis.
Reproduced, with permission, from Skinner HB: Pathokinesiology and total joint arthroplasty. Clin Orthop 1993;288:78.

of therapy choices can aid in the surgical decision process or the informed consent process. Procedures such as joint replacement have pain as the primary indication for surgery, although improvement of function is also a desirable by-product.

The results of surgical procedures such as total knee arthroplasty and total hip arthroplasty depend on a whole host of variables, including the surgeons' experience and the patients' age, preexisting disease, cooperation, and motivation. Clinical evaluation of the results of these procedures is at best crude from a functional viewpoint. For example, evaluation criteria include walking distance and the ability to climb stairs sequentially. Although the application of sophisticated gait analysis techniques to total joint replacement is relatively new, normative data on total knee and total hip replacement surgery have appeared in the literature for some time. These data are shown in Tables 1–7, 1–8, and 1–9. To date, gait analysis has been unable to settle controversies that concern prosthesis design and are related to the efficacy of one type of cemented hip prosthesis versus another, the efficacy of cemented versus uncemented hip prostheses, and the efficacy of prostheses that sacrifice the posterior cruciate ligament of the knee versus those that preserve this ligament. As advances in prosthesis design and gait analysis continue, improvements in the management of patients with gait disorders will also continue.

Andriacchi TP et al: The influence of total knee replacement design on walking and stair climbing. J Bone Joint Surg (Am) 1982; 64:1328.

Bagley AM, Skinner HB: Progress in gait analysis in amputees: A special review. Crit Rev Phys Rehabil Med 1991;3:101.

DeLuca PA et al: Alterations in surgical decision making in patients with cerebral palsy based on three-dimensional gait analysis. J Pediatric Orthop 1997;17:608.

De Visser E et al: Gait and electromyographic analysis of patients recovering after limb-saving surgery. Clin Biomech 2000;15: 592. [PMID 10936431]

Fowler E et al: Energy expenditure during walking by children who have proximal femoral focal deficiency. J Bone Joint Surg (Am) 1996;78:1857.

Table 1–8. Results of free walking gait analysis in patients with total hip arthroplasty.

Study[a]	Patient Diagnosis	Time Since Surgery (yr)	Velocity (m/min)	Cadence (steps/min)	Stride Length (m)	Prosthesis Design
(1) Murray, Brewer, and Zuege (1972)	NA	—	50.0	—	0.98	McKee-Farrar
(2) Stauffer, Smidt, and Wadsworth (1974)	NA	0.5	37.1	80.4	—	Charnley
(3) Murray et al (1975)	OA or RA	2	65	106	1.23	McKee-Farrar
(4) Murray et al (1976)	OA or RA	0.5	62	102	—	Charnley
	OA or RA	0.5	57	102	—	Müller
	OA or RA	0.5	55	100	—	McKee-Farrar
(5) Murray et al (1979)	OA or RA	2	68	110	—	Charnley or Müller
(6) Brown et al (1980)	OA	1	55	101	1.12	—
(7) Olsson, Goldie, and Wykman (1986)	OA or RA	1	53.4*	97.2	1.08	Charnley
	NA	—	48.0*	93	1.00	H.P. Garches
(8) Mattsson, Brostrom, and Linnarsson (1990)	OA	1	80*	—	—	Charnley or H.P. Garches

[a]References are as follows: (1) Murray MP, Brewer BJ, Zuege RC: Kinesiologic measurements of functional performance before and after McKee-Farrar total hip replacement. J Bone Joint Surg [Am] 1972;54:237. (2) Stauffer RN, Smidt GL, Wadsworth JB: Clinical and biomechanical analysis of gait following Charnley total hip replacement. Clin Orthop 1974;99:70. (3) Murray MP et al: Kinesiology after McKee-Farrar total hip replacement: A two-year follow-up of one hundred cases. J Bone Joint Surg [Am] 1975;57:337. (4) Murray MP et al: Comparison of functional performance after McKee-Farrar, Charnley, and Müller total hip replacement: A six-month follow-up of one hundred sixty-five cases. Clin Orthop 1976;21:33. (5) Murray MP et al: Comparison of the functional performance of patients with Charnley and Müller total hip replacement. Acta Orthop Scand 1979;50:563. (6) Brown M et al: Walking efficiency before and after total hip replacement. Phys Ther 1980;60:1259. (7) Olsson E, Goldie I, Wykman A: Total hip replacement: A comparison between cemented (Charnley) and noncemented (H.P. Garches) fixation by clinical assessment and objective gait analysis. Scand J Rehab Med 1986;18:107. (8) Mattsson E, Brostrom LA, Linnarsson D: Walking efficiency after cemented and noncemented total hip arthroplasty. Clin Orthop 1990;254:170.
*Asterisk indicates velocity at fast walking speed; otherwise, velocity is at free walking speed.
NA = diagnostic data not available; OA = osteoarthritis; RA = rheumatoid arthritis.
Reproduced, with permission, from Skinner HB: Pathokinesiology and total joint arthroplasty. Clin Orthop 1993;288:78.

Table 1–9. Results of energy consumption analysis during gait in patients with total hip arthroplasty.

Study[a]	Patient Diagnosis	Time Since Surgery (yr)	Velocity (m/min)	Rate of Oxygen Uptake (mL/kg/min)	Net Oxygen Cost (mL/kg/m)
(1) Pugh (1973)	OA	—	—	10.0	0.15
(2) Brown et al (1980)	OA	1	55	11.86	0.22
(3) McBeath, Bahrke, and Balke (1980)	NA	2	64.5	12.13	0.186
(4) Mattsson, Brostrom, and Linnarsson (1990)	OA	1	80*	—	0.221

[a]References are as follows: (1) Pugh LG: The oxygen intake and energy cost of walking before and after unilateral hip replacement with some observations on the use of crutches. J Bone Joint Surg [Br] 1973;55:742. (2) Brown M et al: Walking efficiency before and after total hip replacement. Phys Ther 1980;60:1259. (3) McBeath AA, Bahrke MS, Balke B: Walking efficiency before and after total hip replacement as determined by oxygen consumption. J Bone Joint Surg [Am] 1980;62:807. (4) Mattsson E, Brostrom LA, Linnarsson D: Walking efficiency after cemented and noncemented total hip arthroplasty. Clin Orthop 1990;254:170.

*Asterisk indicates velocity at fast walking speed; otherwise, velocity is at free walking speed.

OA = osteoarthritis; NA = diagnostic data not available.

Reproduced, with permission, from Skinner HB: Pathokinesiology and total joint arthroplasty. Clin Orthop 1993;288:78.

Gefen A et al: Analysis of muscular fatigue and foot stability during high-heeled gait. Gait Posture 2002;15:56. [PMID 11809581]

Gore DR et al: Hip function after total versus surface replacement. Acta Orthop Scand 1985;56:386.

Huang G-F et al: Gait analysis and energy consumption of below-knee amputees wearing three different prosthetic feet. Gait Posture 2000;12:162. [PMID 10998614]

Hausdorff JM et al: When human walking becomes random walking: Fractal analysis and modeling of gait rhythm fluctuations. Physica 2001;302:138. [PMID 12033228]

Hesse S et al: Non-velocity-related effects of a rigid double-stopped ankle-foot orthosis on gait and lower limb muscle activity of hemiparetic subjects with an equinovarus deformity. Stroke 1999;30:1855.

Johnson DC et al: The evolution of gait in childhood and adolescent cerebral palsy. J Pediatric Orthop 1997;17:392.

Kay RM et al: The effect of preoperative gait analysis on orthopedic decision making. Clin Orthop and Rel Res 2000;372:217. [PMID 10738430]

Kay RM et al: Impact of postoperative gait analysis on orthopedic care. Clin Orthop Rel Res 2000;372:259. [PMID 10818985]

Nowak MD et al: Design enhancement of a solid ankle-foot orthosis: Real-time contact pressures evaluation. J Rehabil Res Dev 2000;37:273. [PMID 10917259]

O'Byrne JM et al: Split tibialis posterior tendon transfer in the treatment of spastic equinovarus foot. J Pediatric Orthop 1997;17:481.

Pierrynowski MR, Galea V: Enhancing the ability of gait analyses to differentiate between groups: scaling gait data to body size. Gait Posture 2001;13:193. [PMID 11323225]

Prentice SD et al: Artificial neural network model for the generation of muscle activation patterns for human locomotion. J Electromyogr Kinesiol 2001;11:19. [PMID 11166605]

Prodromos CC et al: A relationship between gait and clinical changes following high tibial osteotomy. J Bone Joint Surg (Am) 1985;67:1188.

Romkes J Brunner R: Comparison of a dynamic and a hinged ankle-foot orthosis by gait analysis in patients with hemiplegic cerebral palsy. Gait Posture 2002;15:18. [PMID 11809577]

Sanders JE et al: Effects of changes in cadence, prosthetic componentry, and time on the interface pressures and shear stresses of three trans-tibial amputees. Clin Biomech 2000;15:684. [PMID 10946102]

Schmalz T et al: Energy expenditure and biomechanical characteristics of lower limb amputee gait: The influence of prosthetic alignment and different prosthetic components. Gait Posture 2002;16:255. [PMID 12443950]

Tingley M et al: An index to quantify normality of gait in young children. Gait Posture 2002;16:149. [PMID 12297256]

Wilson H et al: Ankle-foot orthoses for pre-ambulatory children with spastic diplegia. J Pediatric Orthop. 1997;17:370.

REFERENCES

Cristal P et al, eds: *Biological and Biomechanical Performance of Biomaterials.* Elsevier, 1986.

Friberg L et al: *Handbook on the Toxicology of Metals.* Elsevier, 1986.

Fung YCB: *Biomechanics: Mechanical Properties of Living Tissues.* Springer-Verlag, 1981.

Gage JR et al: Instructional course lecture, The American Academy of Orthopaedic Surgeons. Gait Analysis: Principles and applications emphasis on its use in cerebral palsy. J Bone Joint Surg (Am) 1995;77:1607.

Perry J: *Gait Analysis: Normal and Pathological Function.* Slack, 1992.

Rose J, Gamble JG, eds: *Human Walking,* 2nd ed. Williams & Wilkins, 1994.

Zohman GL et al: Stride analysis after proximal tibial replacement. Clin Orthop 1997;339:180.

General Considerations in Orthopedic Surgery

Harry B. Skinner, MD

Orthopedic surgery encompasses the entire process of caring for the surgical patient from diagnostic evaluation to the preoperative evaluation and through the postoperative and rehabilitative period. Although the surgical procedure itself is the key step toward helping the patient, the preliminary and follow-up care can determine whether the surgery is successful.

DIAGNOSTIC WORK-UP

History and Physical Exam

Although it may seem obvious, the history and physical exam are still important in the evaluation of the patient. Every office visit is a history and physical exam, whether a new or a return visit. The completeness of the history and physical has assumed new importance in view of the complexities required for compliance with federal regulations. Regulations require that a chief complaint be specified and this must be clearly defined because it determines the direction for the rest of the history and physical. The history must address the key features of the problem to both elucidate the medical problem and to cover the subsidiary requirements for billing purposes. The social history and past medical history are similarly important because they change billing codes without necessarily affecting outcome or success of care. The physical again must cover the essentials necessary for diagnosis, and frequently the confirmation of the diagnosis is based on physical exam, but such things as skin condition and blood supply must be documented, despite the fact that this process is also part of the surgical evaluation. The next step is imaging and laboratory exams. The most important point here is to use the most cost-effective examination possible while keeping patient safety, satisfaction, and convenience in mind.

Imaging Studies

A. ROENTGENOGRAPHY

This is still the most cost-effective and most important initial diagnostic test in the orthopedist's armamentarium. Almost every patient should have a radiograph prior to going to a more sophisticated imaging study.

Certain situations are obvious; for example, a 68-year-old man with knee pain should have standing, flexed-knee posteroanterior (PA), lateral, and merchant plain film views taken. If those views show normal joint spaces, consideration of intra-articular pathology, such as a degenerative meniscus tear, can be worked up with magnetic resonance imaging (MRI). The normal views usually ordered are as follows:

1. **Neck pain**—No history of trauma, more than 4 weeks duration.

   Younger than 35 years: anteroposterior (AP) lateral, odontoid

   Older than 35 years: obliques

   History of trauma: flexion/extension laterals (obtain on first visit)

2. **Thoracic spine pain and tenderness**—

   Younger than 40 years, no reason to suspect malignancy: AP and lateral (if history of trauma, or possibility of osteoporosis on first visit, otherwise at 4 weeks).

   Consider cervical (C)-spine as a source of referred pain to thoracic (T)-spine if no tenderness in T-spine.

3. **Lumbar (L)-sacral (S)-spine**—

   Younger than 40 years, no reason to suspect malignancy after 4 weeks duration of the pain. With significant trauma, at first visit, or possible malignancy, ie, weight loss, malaise, fatigue: AP, lateral.

   Add obliques for chronic low back pain, ie, spondylolisthesis.

4. **Hips**—

   AP pelvis, lateral of affected hip.

   Consider L-S series if pain is in the buttock rather than in the groin.

5. **Knees**—

   Older than 40 or history of meniscectomy: Rosenberg, lateral, and sunrise films. Merchant views are similar to sunrise. The Rosenberg view is a 10-degree down shot of the PA of the knees while standing at 45 degrees of flexion.

For other knees AP, lateral, and sunrise.

In the child, up to age 16, consider a pelvis film with the complaint of knee pain and negative physical exam referable to the knee.

6. Femur, tibia, humerus, forearm—AP and lateral are indicated for trauma, palpable lesions, or suspected tumors.

7. Ankle—AP lateral and mortise.

8. Foot—AP, lateral, and oblique for routine evaluation.

9. Shoulder—AP, axillary, scapular Y, and outlet views.

10. Elbow—AP and lateral, (true lateral).

11. Hand/wrist—

Hand: PA and lateral.

Wrist: PA, lateral, and oblique

For suspected instability: clenched fist PA in radial and ulnar deviation.

Follow-up radiographs are obtained when a change in the radiographic findings would be expected. Remember that bone changes occur slowly, so radiographic changes take a comparable length of time. Radiographs are obtained in view of the clinical picture. For example, closed treatment of a distal radius fracture would not be expected to show changes due to healing for a minimum of 2 weeks. However, displacement of the fracture could occur sooner. Hence, radiographs to show displacement might be obtained at 1 week and 2 weeks. If no displacement is observed, the fracture position could be considered stable, and the next films might be obtained at 6 weeks—the earliest time healing might be observed. Similarly, closed treatment of an adult tibia fracture might be followed with radiographs at 2-week intervals, checking for displacement and healing, whereas a tibia fracture treated with an intramedullary rod, might be followed at monthly intervals to check for healing.

B. Magnetic Resonance Imaging

This imaging modality is very useful, but like electron beam computed tomography (CT) MRI is sometimes too revealing. This method should be reserved for clarifying a particular problem. Frequently in orthopedics, a bony lesion can be localized with a radiograph or bone scan, which then provides a focus for the MRI. MRI is useful for some bony lesions, such as osteonecrosis, tumors, fatigue fractures, and osteomyelitis. It is also helpful in some soft-tissue problems, such as knee meniscus tears and shoulder rotator cuff tears. It is important to realize that the MRI shouldn't be used when the diagnosis can be made with a less expensive test. For example, the use of the MRI in knee studies in patients older than 45 should always be preceded by plain films of the knee as noted earlier. An MRI of an arthritic knee adds little additional information because the meniscus and anterior cruciate ligament are likely to be damaged from the arthritic process already. On the other hand, the MRI can be very helpful in determining soft-tissue extension of tumors or infection.

The advent of new portable MRI units that perform limited studies with more resolution adds a new dimension to their use. These can provide data on the progression of disorders such as rheumatoid arthritis or osteomyelitis in a timely and cost-effective way. The possibility of osteomyelitis in the bones adjacent to ulcers on the foot is easily determined with this test because it shows the changes, typically edema, in the bone with osteomyelitis. A bone scan usually does not have the resolution to distinguish the inflammatory response in the soft tissue from the bony involvement. Osteomyelitis should be treated much differently from a soft-tissue ulcer, which does not affect the bone.

C. Computed Tomography

The CT scan is an extremely important imaging modality for examining bony lesions such as fractures. Frequently, plain films will provide some information about the fracture of interest, but the CT scan provides the three-dimensional information that can only otherwise be determined from the integration of the plain films in the surgeon's mind. The CT scan has added significantly to the management of such fractures as tibial plateaus, scapular fractures, ankle fractures, and cervical and lumbar spine fractures, as well as many others. Again, if little information can be gained that cannot be already discerned from the plain films, the CT scan only adds expense and patient inconvenience. The spiral CT has made imaging with this modality less expensive and much more rapid. The CT scan has also become the method of choice for determining whether a pulmonary embolus (PE) has occurred. Again, a CT for this indication is easier on the patient, more accurate, and is less invasive than angiography.

D. Technetium-99m Bone Scan

The bone scan finds many uses in orthopedic surgery. Keep in mind that the bone scan labels the osteoblast activity with the radioactive tracer, technetium-99; thus bone formation activity is recorded and little or no bone resorption activity is noted. Thus, any disorder that results in increased bone formation will result in a "hot" bone scan. This means that a disorder such as multiple myeloma may not show up on a bone scan because only osteoclastic activity is involved in the majority of lesions. This test is helpful in discerning loose total hip and total knee prostheses, however, even though the findings are nonspecific. It is very helpful in examining probable benign bone lesions because a cold bone scan largely rules out an aggressive process such as a malignancy. The bone scan is also helpful in diagnosing any disorder of unknown origin when there is pain localized to a particular region. A cold bone scan implies that the problem is a soft-tissue one, whereas a hot bone scan points to a region that may benefit from MRI.

Laboratory Exams

The two most important laboratory exams are for C-reactive protein and the erythrocyte sedimentation rate. These two tests indicate whether an inflammatory process, malignancy, or rheumatologic disorder are diagnostic considerations. If these tests are negative, systemic causes of a complaint can frequently be ruled out. In that situation a more localized disorder should be identified. The next most important test is the complete blood count. This test provides the general indication of the patient's health, revealing information about anemia, infectious processes, etc. The next most useful laboratory test for the orthopedic surgeon is the synovial fluid analysis. This test typically should include a culture and sensitivity. If there is any concern about infection, a cell count, differential, protein, and glucose measurement should be performed. Crystals should be looked for because they indicate chondrocalcinosis or gout. Elevated protein and reduced glucose levels suggest infection. The final factor that should be considered with any major surgery is the patient's nutritional status. This is evaluated with several tests including lymphocyte count and levels of pre-albumin, albumin, and serum iron transferrin.

Educating & Informing Patients & Their Families

Surgical procedures in orthopedics have varying degrees of difficulty and importance, ranging from a relatively simple clawtoe correction to the performance of a multilevel complex spinal fusion. After the decision to employ surgery as a therapeutic modality has been made, it is important to help the patient completely understand what to expect before, during, and after surgery. This process, called **informed consent** by the legal profession, has the more important purpose of ensuring the patient's cooperation and happiness.

To comply with the requirements of the legal profession and accrediting organizations, such as the Joint Commission on Accreditation of Healthcare Organizations (JCAHO), the surgeon must provide an explanation of the risks, prognosis, alternatives, and complications that might be encountered. The risks will be reviewed in some detail for the general risks encountered in typical orthopedic surgical procedures. The

risks and the complications that occur in surgery are intimately associated and thus will be dealt with together. The alternatives are sometimes straightforward. For example, a patient with an open fracture has a high risk of infection if not adequately treated with irrigation, debridement, and antibiotics. Thus, in such a situation, any reasonable and prudent person would consent to the procedure. The choice between alternatives can become significantly more subtle, however. For example, it is possible that a choice must be made between two different procedures or between a particular procedure and no procedure. In this situation, the surgeon must consider the psychosocial and physical attributes of the patient so as to assist him or her in making this decision. For example, consider men, both age 75 years, with severe degenerative disease in the right knee noted on radiograph. One individual is now at the point where he can't play golf, a situation that is reducing his physical exercise and a number of his social outlets. The other individual leads a relatively sedentary life-style, seldom walks more than a block, and obtains cardiorespiratory exercise by swimming, an activity in which his knee does not bother him. The surgeon should recommend knee replacement to one individual but not the other. At the same time, both individuals must be offered the alternatives, which include continued nonsteroidal anti-inflammatory medicine, bracing, sleeping medication, and analgesics.

Patients with an active life-style are becoming much more concerned about what will happen to them in the postoperative period, including how soon they can safely travel, when they can work, and when they can be fully able to take care of themselves. They are also concerned about what social services are available to help them if they cannot care for themselves fully. The surgeon must be prepared to address these questions and also advise patients with lower extremity or spinal problems about when they will be able to walk. In the same manner, after procedures on the hand or upper extremity, patients must be advised about when they will be able to use their hand. Advising the patient of these situations before surgery can prevent unexpected surprises in the postoperative period.

The patient should also be informed about the range of expectations for ambulation or use of the upper extremity because individuals vary in their response to surgery. For example, patients should be advised that after surgery on the hip or knee, they will need a walker for a few days, move to crutches, and typically be done with the crutches in the range of 2–4 weeks. They will use a cane before 6 weeks and be done with the cane before 3 months. Patients should be cautioned about travel after surgery, particularly with lower extremity injuries because of the risk of deep venous thrombosis. In such cases, discourage (for the first 6 weeks) plane trips longer than an hour and extended car trips made without stopping perhaps every 45 min. Anti-inflammatory medication (to reduce platelet adhesion) or anticoagulants should be recommended if such travel is unavoidable.

A. EXPLAINING THE PROCEDURES

An essential part of the patient's presurgical preparation and postsurgical cooperation is knowing what to expect at every step in the process. Nuances become important in the process of explaining the surgical procedures and their implications. For example, scheduling a bunion procedure 2 weeks prior to a patient's participation in her daughter's wedding could upset the patient if she fails to realize that she will be unable to wear the shoes she purchased for the event. Similarly, life-style considerations can affect the decision-making process in cases of medial gonarthrosis, in which the choice between a unicompartmental knee replacement and a high tibial osteotomy could be influenced by whether the patient plays tennis and holds a physically strenuous job or, alternatively, whether the patient is sedentary and works behind a desk most of the day.

B. REVIEWING THE RISKS AND POSSIBLE COMPLICATIONS

Reviewing the perioperative risks is important for all patients and optimally should be done well in advance and then repeated closer to the time of surgery. Some patients will require more detailed explanations, particularly if their relatives have undergone surgery in the past and had a problem with anesthesia or a complication such as a PE or infection. Based on the patient's responses to explanations, the health care team members will need to alter their approach to reach a balance between inadequately informing the patient and inducing unnecessary alarm that could make the patient refuse to undergo a procedure judged to be both beneficial and necessary.

Risk is a poorly understood concept in our culture. Some situations are considered to be higher in risk than they actually are. Some risks are understood better than others. It can help the patient to understand if these risks are put in perspective. The risks can be surprisingly high or low, but still disturbing to the patient. For example, many people have moved away from California to avoid an earthquake or refuse to fly commercial aircraft because of the risk, not realizing that the risk of death is 10–100 times higher while driving a car (Table 2–1). This lack of understanding of the risk can contribute to significant differences in the perception of liability associated with these activities. For example, the death benefit from a commercial airline accident might reach several million dollars per passenger, whereas death in an automobile accident might have no death

Table 2–1. Rates of death and complications associated with common activities.

Death or Complication	Percentage
Death (from MI after previous MI)	1
Major bleed (7 days, warfarin, INR 2.65)	0.02
GI ulcer/bleed perforation (naproxen 6 months)	1
Paralysis (from epidural)	0.02
Death (frequent flying professor/year)	0.001
Death (automobile/year)	0.016
Earthquake in California/per year	0.00018

benefit at all. Thus the *perception* of risk is very important and must be clarified in the patient's mind. Similarly, patients can understand and accept having a myocardial infarction after a major surgery because they can clearly see the strain on the heart from the surgery. However, they are not nearly as understanding of a lower extremity paralysis that can result from the epidural anesthetic for that surgery. The explanation of risks must be individualized for each patient. The patient with a previous myocardial infarction is clearly different from the healthy 20-year-old (see Table 2–1). Across-the-board rates of problems do not translate into direct risks for the individual patient.

Although all procedures carry some risks, the incidence and type of risks and complications will vary with the surgical procedure as well as with the patient's age and general health. Potential problems are listed and discussed here in alphabetical order.

1. Amputation—The potential problem of amputation is seldom of acute concern except in cases of significant trauma. The topic of amputation can frequently be discussed with the risk of infection because ischemia and infection can increase the risk of amputation.

2. Anesthesia—One of the major risks in orthopedic surgery is associated with anesthesia, not because complications of anesthesia are frequent but because they can be devastating. Death occurs at a rate of about 1 in 200,000 patients undergoing elective anesthesia. Other complications include but are not limited to the following: nerve damage and paraplegia from nerve blocks; headaches from dural leaks following use of spinal anesthetics; aspiration of stomach contents; and cardiac problems, including ischemia and arrhythmias. The surgeon should discuss these problems with the patient only in general terms, allowing the anesthesiologist to provide the most detailed explanations.

3. Arthritis—Virtually any procedure that will enter a joint, other than to replace it, has the potential to cause damage to that joint. In some instances, as in an intra-articular fracture, the surgery will likely lessen the risk of arthritis. Even in these instances, the patient should be told that the risk of damage is still real because the joint surface healing will not result in a normal cartilage surface.

4. Blood loss—Patients should be given a reasonably accurate estimate of blood loss as well as the opportunity to donate autologous blood prior to surgery. Designated donor blood is probably not safer but gives the patient who receives it a sense of security. To help minimize blood loss during surgery, the patient's use of nonsteroidal anti-inflammatory drugs (NSAIDs) should be discontinued about 2 weeks before surgery. Discontinuation of NSAIDs can significantly compromise comfort and incite rheumatoid flares in many patients who rely on these drugs. To minimize the risk, newer COX-II inhibitor NSAIDs may be used as a substitute during this period; no platelet disorders or bleeding time derangement occurs with these drugs, because they do not affect platelet function or inhibit thromboxane A_2.

5. Blood vessel damage—Arterial and venous damage take on greater significance as the size of the vessel increases and the arterial supply becomes more calcified with age and vascular disease. Patients generally understand this, but it must be emphasized where appropriate. Hip and knee replacement put unusual strains on the femoral and popliteal vessels, from positioning, and may damage calcified arteries.

6. Deep venous thrombosis/pulmonary embolism—Virtually all lower extremity and spine procedures in orthopedics involve some risk of deep vein thrombosis (DCT), and this should be explained to the patient. As many as 25% of patients who undergo a relatively high-risk procedure such as total hip arthroplasty will have venographically diagnosed DVT. The risk of PE is much less, however, and will be in the range of 0.3% for fatal emboli. This rate of fatal PE is about a 10-fold increase over the rate of fatal PE in the U.S. population in males older than 65 years of age. The risks associated with other procedures may be lower. In any case, the patient should be reassured that prevention procedures commensurate with risk will be undertaken.

7. Fracture—Many procedures in orthopedic surgery carry the risk of a bone fracture. Some procedures, such as uncemented hip replacement, present a higher risk for this complication, but virtually any orthopedic procedure could result in fracture of a bone. The patient must be informed of the risk in relation to the probability of the occurrence of such a problem.

8. Infection—The risk of infection in orthopedic surgery ranges from near zero in procedures such as arthroscopy to several percent in open fracture surgery. The problem of infection should be emphasized in proportion to risk. For example, if a diabetic patient is to undergo knee replacement, he or she should not only be assured that all steps will be taken to prevent infection (eg, administration of prophylactic antibiotics and use of ultrafiltration of air, or ultraviolet lights in the operating room) but should also be told of the various techniques that would be considered for use if infection occurred. These options include debridement, prosthesis removal, gastrocnemius flap, reinsertion, arthrodesis, and amputation. The common use of external fixation devices for fracture care is accompanied by the frequent problems associated with pin care. The patient and family should be informed about the problems caused by percutaneous devices to prevent the presumption that something has gone wrong. Skin problems are frequently associated with infection but may arise from other causes, such as adjacent scars compromising the blood supply to a surgical flap. Older patients and individuals who are smokers, have diabetes, or have wounds on the distal lower extremity are at increased risk. In such cases, the patient may be warned that delayed healing or necrosis of the skin edges may occur.

9. Loss of reduction—Although fracture care continues to improve, displacement of hardware or fracture fragments may necessitate a second procedure. The explanation of this risk should be individualized, based on the type of fracture. Loss of reduction may contribute to delayed union or nonunion of fractures. These problems may occur despite optimal care by the orthopedic surgeon. Poor vascular supply or smoking can be a factor leading to nonunion. The rate of nonunion is site-dependent but is only a few percent.

10. Nerve damage—Certain procedures are associated with nerve damage, although the damage is usually minor. For example, medial parapatellar incisions on the knee will cause some numbness from cutting the infrapatellar branch of the saphenous nerve. The patient should be informed in advance if some degree of minor nerve damage is anticipated in association with the particular surgical procedure being pursued and should also be informed of the risks of unexpected nerve damage that accompany all surgical procedures.

C. PROGNOSIS

The prognosis of the procedure is intimately related to the procedure. However, certain guidelines may be given. The expected time off work or time away from activities is important to the patient and depend on the patient's occupation, age, and available sick leave. The bank president with more control over his agenda will be able to return to work activities sooner than the day laborer. Driving is an important activity for many people, and limitations placed by a procedure can determine how much postoperative assistance a patient will need.

The patient should be given reasonable expectations about range of motion, strength, possible disability and when these should return to normal, if at all. Furthermore, walking or writing ability, ability to use a computer keyboard, and the time to expect to be able to do such activities may be appropriate for some patients. Again, these have to be individualized for each patient and determined for each home situation.

D. Keeping the Patient and Family Informed

Immediately before elective surgery, the surgeon can help comfort the patient and family by meeting them in the preoperative area and appearing relaxed, well rested, and positive about the outcome of the surgery. Giving the family a good estimate of the surgery time is important, but they should also be reassured that delays do not necessarily indicate the occurrence of complications that are detrimental to the patient. If the family members wish to be notified about delays, they should be encouraged to leave instructions about where they can be contacted. When surgery has been completed and the patient is no longer at risk of untoward accidents such as aspiration during extubation, a member of the surgical team should apprise the family of the outcome. At this time, it is appropriate to emphasize particular concerns to the family, such as the need to continue vigilance for infection in a diabetic patient who has undergone foot surgery.

Johnson BF et al: Relationship between changes in the deep venous system and the development of the postthrombotic syndrome after an acute episode of lower limb deep vein thrombosis. A one- to six-year follow-up. J Vasc Surg 1995;21:307.

Lillienfeld DE, Godbold JH: Geographic distribution of pulmonary embolism mortality rates in the United States, 1980 to 1984. Am Heart J 1992;124:1068.

Salvati E et al: Recent advances in venous thromboembolic prophylaxis during and after total hip replacement. J Bone Joint Surg Am 2000;82:252.

SURGICAL MANAGEMENT

Preoperative Care

A. The Team Approach

Inclusion of nurses, residents, anesthesiologists, and other members of the surgical team in the planning process can improve the efficiency and therefore affect the outcome of a surgical procedure. Good estimates of the length of the operative procedure and of the patient's anticipated blood loss and muscle relaxation requirements will minimize the risks from anesthesia and surgery. Reviewing the site of the operation and assessing the need for any special supplies and equipment, such as prostheses, lasers, or fracture tables, will also contribute to efficiency and optimal results. Special care must be exercised by all members of the operative team to prevent "wrong side" surgery. It has become a JCAHO standard to have the surgical team "mark" the surgical site.

B. Preparing and Positioning the Patient

Once the patient is in the operating room, every effort should be made to make him or her comfortable. A calm, efficient, and professional demeanor by everyone involved is necessary both before and after anesthesia has been induced. If the anesthesiologist indicates that placement of the antithromboembolic hose, intermittent pneumatic compression stockings, or tourniquets will improve efficiency, these can be put in place prior to induction. Placement of arterial lines, central lines, and Foley catheters should be done after the patient is anesthetized, if possible. Location of the operating table must be adjusted to ensure good lighting, optimize the efficiency of the surgeon and staff, and allow for maintenance of surgical sterile technique.

Positioning of the patient is the responsibility of both the surgeon and the anesthesiologist to facilitate the operation and to ensure the patient's safety. A perfectly executed operation can be marred by a nerve palsy that results from the failure to appropriately pad a remote area. If the patient is placed in the lateral decubitus position, the peroneal nerve at the knee and the brachial plexus of the downside shoulder girdle must be protected. During shoulder surgery, the surgeon must take care to avoid stretching the patient's brachial plexus or cervical nerve roots while attempting to maximize the operative field. Similarly, the patient's shoulder should not be abducted past 90 degrees, and joints with contractures should not be forced into unusual positions. These precautions are particularly necessary in treating rheumatoid patients or older osteoporotic patients. Injury to the extremities and loss of lines can be avoided by careful planning and synchronization when positioning patients into the lateral decubitus position or prone position.

C. Use of Antibiotics

Except in cases in which concern about infection requires unambiguous cultures to be obtained, prophylactic antibiotics should be started prior to skin incision. A first- or second-generation cephalosporin antibiotic is considered appropriate for orthopedic procedures.

D. USE OF A TOURNIQUET

A tourniquet can be extremely helpful in some procedures and is practically mandatory for others. The tourniquet stops the flow of blood to and from an extremity. To achieve this, the pneumatic tourniquet is inflated to a pressure that must be significantly higher than the arterial pressure because the pressure is dissipated in the soft tissue underneath the tourniquet.

1. Tourniquet size and placement—The tourniquet should be wide enough for the extremity while still permitting adequate exposure of the extremity. Particularly in cases involving surgery on muscles that cross the elbow or knee, the tourniquet should be placed as proximal as possible to ensure that the muscles have adequate stretch to permit full joint motion. When a tourniquet is used on a large extremity with a great deal of adipose tissue, care must be taken to ensure that the tourniquet does not slip distally, because this could result in wrinkles in the tourniquet and localized pressure on the skin. Slippage can be prevented by applying 5-cm (2-in.) adhesive tape to the skin in a longitudinal direction below the cast padding placed under the tourniquet.

2. Tourniquet time and pressure—The effects of tourniquets on tissues are a combination of time and pressure on individual structures. Neural and muscle tissue are most sensitive, with deleterious effects arising from direct pressure to structures and from distal ischemia.

Several considerations are involved in the selection of the level of tourniquet pressure. First, the level must be low enough to avoid pressure damage to sensitive neural structures but high enough so that the pressure around the arterial supply to the extremity is greater than systolic pressure (Figure 2–1). Second, if the patient's blood pressure is labile, a margin of safety is usually necessary. In a patient with a stable blood pressure, tourniquet pressures of 75 mm Hg above preinduction systolic pressure are typically adequate, although some surgeons use pressures as high as twice systolic. If the tourniquet is on an extremity with a great deal of adipose tissue, higher pressures are necessary to achieve adequate pressure at the artery to stop blood flow. Tourniquets should be calibrated and can be tested with an independent pressure measurement device or alternatively by palpation of the pulse and gradual elevation of pressure until the pulse disappears.

Complications will arise if tourniquets are used at high pressure for too long. The effects can sometimes be mitigated by using wider cuffs and curved cuffs, which allow for higher and more uniform pressure below the tourniquet. A rule of thumb is that tourniquet pressures should not be elevated for longer than

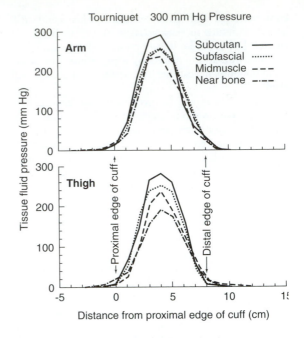

Figure 2–1. Distribution of tissue fluid pressure at four depths beneath pneumatic tourniquet with cuff pressure of 300 mm Hg applied on arms (**top**) and thighs (**bottom**). Values represent means for six limbs on each graph. (Reproduced, with permission, from Hargens AR et al: Local compression patterns beneath pneumatic tourniquets applied to arms and thighs of human cadavers. J Orthop Res 1987;5:247.)

2 h, and less time is preferable. In a canine study of the muscle tissue distal to the tourniquet, investigators found that 90-min tourniquet times with 5 min between reinflation minimized the ischemic damage. This finding points to the need for efficiency in performing surgical procedures under tourniquet. After tourniquet release, reflex hyperemia and edema are frequently encountered, making closure more difficult. Exsanguination with an Esmarch bandage prior to tourniquet inflation will facilitate emptying of large veins of the thigh and arm. Careful exsanguination may help prevent DVT, especially when reinflation of the tourniquet is planned.

Barwell J et al: J Bone Joint Surg Br 1997;79:265.

Classen DC et al: The timing of prophylactic administration of antibiotics and the risk of surgical wound infection. N Engl J Med 1992;326:281.

Hargens AR et al: Local compression patterns beneath pneumatic tourniquets applied to arms and thighs of human cadavers. J Orthop Res 1987;5:247.

Idusuyi OB, Morrey BF: Peroneal nerve palsy after total knee arthroplasty. Assessment of predisposing and prognostic factors. J Bone Joint Surg Am 1996;78:177.

Orkin FK, Cooperman LH: Complications in Anesthesiology. Lippincott, 1983.

Pedowitz RA et al: The use of lower tourniquet inflation pressures in extremity surgery facilitated by curved and wide tourniquets and an integrated cuff inflation system. Clin Orthop 1993;287:237.

Sapega AA et al: Optimizing tourniquet application and release times in extremity surgery. J Bone Joint Surg Am 1985;67:303.

Wiss DA, Stetson WB: Tibial nonunion: Treatment alternatives. J Am Acad Orthop Surg 1996;4:249.

Operative Care

The surgical team should make every effort to work efficiently during the period between the administration of anesthesia and the conclusion of the final steps of preoperative preparation, which may take from 10 to 30 min or longer. It is in the best interests of the patient to minimize the time between onset of anesthesia and the beginning of surgery.

A. INCISION SITES AND APPROACHES

Although the surgical wound "heals side-to-side, not end-to-end," the incorrect placement or the excessive length of a surgical incision for a given procedure only serves to increase surgical trauma to the patient, slow the healing process, and lengthen the rehabilitation period. If there is any doubt about the surgical incision site, roentgenographic examination should be considered. Use of an image intensifier should be considered in obese patients or in patients with previous surgery and retained hardware.

The incision should be made perpendicular to the skin, generally in a longitudinal manner and with a sharp knife. In tumor biopsies, longitudinal incisions are always made. The approach by the surgeon through the subcutaneous fatty layer is variable and depends on the location on the body. In most areas, sharp dissection with a knife through the subcutaneous tissue to the fascial layer is indicated. In the upper extremity and in areas where cutaneous nerves can be troublesome if injured, blunt dissection is used because cutaneous nerves travel in the fatty tissue. Many surgeons prefer blunt dissection with scissors used to spread tissue perpendicular to the wound. Hemostasis is obtained layer by layer. Usually, subcutaneous fat is not dissected from the skin, because this might devascularize it.

Surgeons must be extremely careful with the skin, making sure to avoid crushing it when forceps are used. The skin should never be clamped, nor should it be excessively stretched. A larger incision is much better for the skin than extreme tension is. Care of the soft tissues includes keeping them moist, avoiding excessive retraction, and being especially careful of neurovascular bundles. Nerves suffer damage from both traction and compression. Nerve palsies and paresthesias can spoil an otherwise well-performed operation in the eyes of both the surgeon and the patient. Care of the cartilage includes keeping it moist because drying has a deleterious effect.

Surgical approaches that go through internerve planes, such as between the deltoid and the pectoralis major, should be used to avoid denervation of muscles. The splitting of muscles in the surgical approach should also be avoided because splitting is generally more traumatic and more likely to denervate the muscle. This rule does not always apply in tumor surgery, because it is important to keep tumor cells in a single compartment.

B. ORTHOPEDIC INSTRUMENTS AND DRAINS

It is mandatory that tools be sharp at all times because the sharpness enables the surgeon to avoid the excessive pressure that creates problems in the depths of the wound. When an osteotome or elevator is needed, the concurrent use of a hammer is preferred because achieving exact control is possible by the strength and number of hammer taps, whereas control is difficult to achieve by pushing on an osteotome. With drill points and power saws, the sharpness of the instruments should be maintained to reduce necrosis secondary to heating and to facilitate the operation. Unless using a drill guide, the surgeon should start drilling bone in a perpendicular direction even though the final direction may be at some angle to the direction of the bone. This will prevent slipping off the desired bone entry point. Holes in long bones are stress concentration sites. Care should be taken to minimize the likelihood and degree of stress concentration by rounding holes and using drill holes to terminate saw cuts (Figure 2–2). When holes have been made in bone, especially in the lower extremity, the patient should be advised against torsional loading.

Obtaining hemostasis in bone can be troublesome, and the use of microcrystalline collagen is preferred to bone wax because of the foreign body response. Postoperative bleeding is common from bony surfaces. Despite the traditional use of drains by surgeons, evidence is accumulating that at least for some operations, such as total hip or total knee replacement, wound drainage may not be necessary and may lead to increased blood loss. If drains are used, they should be secured to prevent accidental removal and should be large enough to prevent clogging by clot formation. Drains are generally removed within 48 h of surgery unless they are used to eliminate dead space.

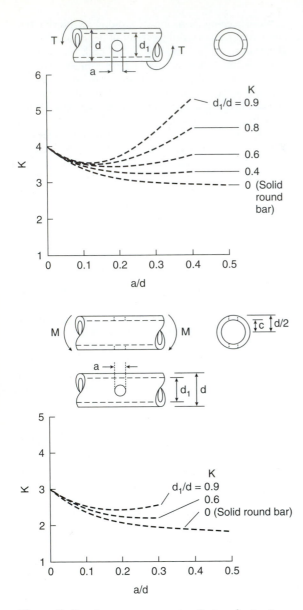

Figure 2–2. Stress concentration factors for torsion (**top**) or bending (**bottom**) of a round bar or tube with a transverse hole, where a = the size of the hole; d = the outside diameter of the tube; d_1 = the inside diameter of the tube; K = the stress concentration factor, defined as the factor by which stress is increased by the hole; M = the bending moment; and T = the torsional load. (Modified and reproduced, with permission, from Peterson RE: Stress Concentration Factors: Charts and Relations Useful in Making Strength Calculations for Machine Parts and Structural Elements. New York: Wiley, 1974.)

C. CLOSURE AND DRESSING

Wound closure should be done quickly and efficiently to minimize total operative and anesthesia time. It should also be accomplished carefully to avoid damage to the skin. When a previous scar has been entered, it is sometimes worthwhile to remove scar tissue from the edge of the skin, as well as from the subcutaneous tissue, to provide a more vascular area for healing. Meticulous subcutaneous wound closure is necessary to avoid tension on the skin in many areas on the extremities. At least four-throw square knots are important for knot security, especially when plans call for use of continuous passive motion machines or early motion, which may apply repetitive stress to the wound before it heals.

Dressings should be padded with cotton or gauze to discourage the formation of hematomas. Tape should be avoided when possible, because it sometimes causes allergic reactions and because the combination of wound swelling and pressure from the tape can lead to blistering and other problems.

Acus RW et al: The use of postoperative suction drainage in total hip arthroplasty. Orthopedics 1992;15:1325.

Batra EK et al: Influence of surgeon's tying technique on knot security. J Appl Biomat 1993;4:241.

POSTOPERATIVE CARE

Inpatient Care

Postoperative care begins in the postanesthesia room and is the same for both inpatients and outpatients. It is imperative that the orthopedic surgeon takes an active and early role in the treatment of the postoperative patient, including pain management, blood management, and DVT prophylaxis. As soon as practicable, neurologic and vascular evaluation of the operated area should be made. Sensory and motor exam of the pertinent upper or lower extremity nerves should be documented as soon as practical. Early vascular surgery consultation is indicated if pulses are absent or diminished. The wound site should be checked for excessive drainage, and, when appropriate, compartment syndrome should be considered. The general medical condition of the patient, although primarily the concern of the anesthesiologist, should be evaluated to be sure that the anesthesiologist is aware of special concerns regarding the individual patient.

During the subsequent postoperative period, orthopedic aspects of care are relatively routine for most procedures. The main responsibility of the orthopedic surgeon is the evaluation of the vascular and neural status of the extremities affected by the surgery, as well as pain control, and vigilance for disorders such as DVT or PE.

The frequency of postsurgical examinations depends on the clinical setting. Hourly examinations may be necessary in the face of a potential compartment syndrome, although daily examinations are usually adequate. Epidural morphine analgesia may significantly mute or alter the pain picture in a compartment syndrome, making clinical evaluation difficult if not impossible in the immediate postoperative period.

A. PAIN MANAGEMENT

Pain management has become a major issue in the United States in recent years. There is a growing concern that patients are undermedicated for pain control and are suffering unnecessarily. The public has embraced this concept, resulting in litigation and disciplinary action by state medical boards for undermedication. Physicians have traditionally been seen as being reluctant to prescribe narcotic medication as a result of concerns that they would be disciplined by state medical boards. This concept has lead to a major initiative by the JCAHO to address pain control as a patient right. JCAHO has mandated that pain control be a factor in the total evaluation of the patient and pain evaluation be performed as the fifth vital sign. The scale that is used is the numeric scale from 0 to 10, similar to the visual analog scale, with 0 being no pain and 10 being unbearable pain. Acceptable pain levels are defined as 4 and below.

Pain is a very subjective sensation that is an emotional response to the process of nociception. Nociception is the sum of four separate components beginning with tissue damage, which results in the first component, transduction to a nerve impulse. The next component is transmission to the spinal cord, where the third component occurs: modulation. This modulated signal is then perceived in the cerebral cortex (perception). Pain perception depends on culture, ethnicity, and gender. It is nonlinear, in that a stimulus two times higher doesn't necessarily result in twice the pain.

Traditional postoperative pain management has included the administration of intravenous (IV) or intramuscular narcotic analgesics, until oral narcotics are able to control the pain. The patient-controlled analgesia (PCA) has been a mainstay. In this system, morphine is used as the analgesic and is typically administered IV at a rate of 1 mg/h with a patient-controlled dose of 1 mg, which can be administered as often as every 10 min. Doses can be increased or decreased to tailor the dose to the patient. Dosing at this level can result in depressed respiration in some patients. On the other hand, more cautious dosing can result in insufficient pain relief that can stress the heart, leading to myocardial ischemia in some patients. Other problems can result from traditional pain management with nar-

cotics. Patient rehabilitation can be delayed; nausea, vomiting, constipation, hallucinations, and disorientation can result in lengthened hospital stay and patient dissatisfaction.

Alternative postoperative analgesic methods have been proposed. These include epidural and intrathecal administration of local anesthetics and analgesics on a continuous and "one-shot" basis. These methods have the potential of providing significant pain relief but must be balanced against the alternatives available and the drawbacks that each presents. The one-shot method of adding morphine to the spinal or epidural anesthetic provides pain relief for a limited time, usually on the order of 12 h. It has the additional problem of limiting additional analgesia by other routes because overdosing may be possible. Long-term use of continuous epidural or intrathecal analgesia has the problem of inhibiting rehabilitation. Nurses and physical therapists tend to not mobilize patients with catheters into the spinal canal, and in some hospitals these patients are mandated to go to the intensive care unit. Nerve blocks and injections into joint cavities are limited by the length of action of the local anesthetic agent. Longer term effect can be achieved by the use of pumps that provide a continuous rate of anesthetic flow into the joint or body cavity. These pumps typically use a long-acting agent such as bupivacaine (0.25% or 0.5%) and infuse at the rate of 2–4 mL/h.

In the past, nonnarcotic pharmacologic treatment of acute postoperative pain has been largely restricted to ketorolac, which can be administered by the IV or IM route in the patient who is restricted in oral intake. Although ketorolac has been shown to be an effective analgesic through the reduction in the need for morphine, it has also been shown to increase the perioperative blood loss. After oral intake is permitted, other NSAIDs can be used for analgesics. Neither ketorolac nor other NSAIDs have played a routine role in the acute pain management for most orthopedic surgical patients because of the effect these drugs have on the platelets and subsequent blood loss. The availability of COX-2 selective NSAIDs has opened up the possibility of using these drugs as major analgesics for postoperative pain control, without fear of bleeding problems. These drugs will act to reduce the need for narcotics with improved pain relief and decreased narcotic side effects. On the horizon are new COX-2 drugs that can be administered parenterally, and these drugs will be of major assistance in the management of early postoperative pain. Such a drug is parecoxib, which is undergoing trials for FDA approval.

Other analgesics and techniques do not get sufficient recognition for their role in pain control. Acetaminophen is thought to be a central prostaglandin synthase inhibitor and thereby achieves significant relief of pain. It can be tolerated in doses up to 4 g/d, and because it does not act in the same pathway as narcotics, its effect is additive to that of morphine or other narcotics and can reduce the requirement for narcotics. Another analgesic that should be used more often for analgesia is tramadol. This analgesic has very low abuse potential but provides significant analgesia, acting through inhibition of norepinephrine reuptake as well as a weak μ-agonist (similar to morphine) action. Again this mechanism of action is additive to that of traditional opioids and acetaminophen in its analgesic effect. Glucocorticoids are naturally increased in periods of stress such as surgery and are provided exogenously for those patients with suppressed adrenal function. Divided doses of about 200 mg of hydrocortisone (8 days normal production) are typically prescribed for such patients. High doses (20 mg) of dexamethasone (equivalent to ~400 mg of hydrocortisone) have been shown to reduce the early postoperative pain in tonsillectomy patients. Although such doses may reduce postoperative nausea, swelling, and pain, as well as create a feeling of well-being, an increased susceptibility to infection may result from longer term dosing. Short courses of relatively high doses of glucocorticoids may be beneficial in reducing postoperative pain. Other methods of pain control may be indirect, such as controlling swelling and pain through hemostasis and cold therapy. Hemostasis may be achieved through the use of bone wax on cancellous bone, or through the use of fibrin glue. Vasoconstriction from cold therapy can reduce swelling and also have a direct effect on nociceptive transduction.

A comprehensive approach to pain management can lead to beneficial effects. Multimodal analgesic regimens have been suggested using several analgesics that address different points in the nociception process. Combinations of medications can include narcotics, acetaminophen, tramadol, COX-2 inhibitors, and local anesthetics administered through the use of pain pumps. Consideration should be given to administering these medications in the preanesthesia room to preempt the pain of surgery. This Can also assist in diminishing peripheral sensitization that occurs with tissue damage.

Mallory TH et al: Pain management for joint arthroplasty: Preemptive analgesia. J Arthoplasty 2002;17:129.

Reuben SS et al: Evaluation of the safety and efficacy of the perioperative administration of rofecoxib for total knee arthroplasty. J Arthoplasty 2001;16:1.

Reuben SS, Sklar J: Pain management in patients who undergo outpatient arthroscopic surgery of the knee. J Bone Joint Surg, Am 2000;82:1754.

Sinatra RS et al: Pain management after major orthopedic surgery: Current strategies and new concepts. J Am Acad Ortho Surg 2002;10:117.

B. Deep Venous Thrombosis/Pulmonary Embolus

Deep venous thrombosis, a potentially life-threatening disorder, frequently accompanies orthopedic surgery. It is much more of a problem for total joint replacements, the spine surgery, and lower extremities immobilized after surgery. This is one of the expected risks after surgery. Venous thromboembolic phenomenon can result in three problems: postphlebitic syndrome, nonfatal PE, and fatal PE. It is necessary to put the risks of PE into appropriate perspective because, contrary to prevailing assumptions in the public and among orthopedic surgeons, PE can occur without surgery (Table 2–2). The risk of having a PE depends on a number of risk factors, including age, weight, the presence of varicose veins, immobility, smoking, previous DVT joint replacement, the season of the year, estrogen therapy, and the location. There is an uncertain relationship between DVT and the probability of having a PE. Obviously one cannot have a PE without having a clot, but which clots are likely to break off and become emboli, and which ones will cause problems are still unresolved issues. It is thought that thigh clots are more important than calf clots because of their size and the potential damage they can do. It is generally conceded, however, that DVT is a marker for PE, and that is the surrogate variable that is used to determine the effectiveness of treatment of PE. A nonfatal PE can cause cor pulmonale, but this is thought to be an unlikely circumstance, and it is speculated that nonfatal PE would result in a residual effect in the range of 0.1 to 0.01% of cases. Deep venous thrombosis itself is thought to be a significant problem, which results in incompetence of the valves in the deep veins of the calf and thigh. This results in persistent edema, which can progress to brawny edema and ulceration over time. However, many things are thought to cause these changes in addition to DVT. There is a uneven geographic distribution of fatal PE without surgery in the United States, with the West Coast census region having the lowest fatal PE rate. The rate of fatal PE increases with age, although age may simply be a marker for health and activity

Table 2–2. Rates of complications associated with total hip replacement at the Mayo Clinic.

Complication	Percentage
Death (overall)	0.5
Myocardial infarction	0.5
Pulmonary embolism	0.4
Deep venous thrombosis	1.1

Reproduced, with permission, from Mantilla et al: Poster presented at the Am Acad of Orthopedic Surgeons Annual Mtg; 2001.

level. The rate of fatal PE in the general population older than 65 is in the range of 0.03%, whereas approximate total joint PE rates are typically about 0.3%, thus there is a 10-fold increase in risk of having a fatal PE with a total hip or knee replacement.

Three classes of drugs can be used for chemoprophylaxis of DVT: warfarin (the vitamin K inhibitor), the low-molecular-weight heparins (dalteparin, enoxaparin, and similar drug fondaparinux), and the platelet aggregation inhibitors (aspirin, naproxen, other NSAIDs). Each approach has its advantages and disadvantages. Sodium warfarin has a slow onset of action, sometimes taking several days to reach therapeutic levels, but its oral route of administration is convenient. However, monitoring of the prothrombin time is necessary to ensure appropriate therapeutic levels. The low-molecular-weight heparins do not affect the prothrombin time or the partial thromboplastin time but do affect factor IIa and Xa levels. These do not have to be monitored because the medications are given in standard doses. These medications are provided parenterally. Both warfarin and the low-molecular-weight heparins have been associated with bleeding problems. Aspirin, naproxen and other NSAIDs, although causing problems with bleeding at the time of surgery, have really not been effective in prevention of DVT. Mechanical means of preventing DVT include compression hose and intermittent pneumatic compression. These have been found to be efficacious as adjunctive therapies.

The American College of Chest Physicians regularly performs and publishes meta-analyses of the data available on DVT with updated recommendations. Generally for orthopedic indications after high-risk surgery, either warfarin with an INR of 2–3, a low-molecular-weight heparin starting 12–24 h after surgery, and elastic stockings and intermittent pneumatic compression are useful as supplemental protection against DVT. The recommended period is a minimum of 7 days. Occasional use of heparin or vena cava filters are recommended in high-risk situations. A listing of current recommendations is given in Table 2–3.

The community standard in orthopedic surgery probably differs somewhat from that recommended by the American College of Chest Physicians. Recent orthopedic literature would seem to suggest that warfarin is the drug of choice but with lower INR values. However, the choice of prophylactic agent is made by the doctor and the patient and is influenced by their interpretation of the risk of thromboembolism and bleeding problems.

Both warfarin and heparin, either low-molecular-weight or regular, have problems that can cause catastrophic side effects in rare cases. Warfarin can cause skin necrosis and venous limb gangrene syndromes un-

Table 2–3. Recommendations for management of DVT prophylaxis for high-risk orthopedic patients.

Procedure	Grade	Recommendation
THA/TKA	1A	LMWH started 12–24 h after surgery Or
	1A	Warfarin started immediately after surgery (Target INR 2.5, range 2.0–3.0)
Hip fractures	1B	LMWH or warfarin As above
Trauma	1A	LMWH when safe to use
	1C	Elastic stockings and intermittent pneumatic compression until LMWH is safe
Acute SCI	1B	LMWH

THA = total hip arthroplasty; TKA = total knee arthroplasty; LMWH = low-molecular-weight heparin; SCI = spinal cord injury; 1A grade = Clear risk benefit ratio based on randomized trials without important limitations; 1B Grade = Same as 1A but with inconsistent results or methodologic flaws; 1C Grade = Clear risk/benefit ratio based on observation studies.

Reproduced, with permission, from Sixth ACCP Consensus Conference.

related to the operative site. Heparin can induce thrombocytopenia. This is apparently an IgG antibody formation that occurs 5–10 days after starting the drug and can result in a hypercoagulable state that can result in serious problems of coagulation in unintended areas. Some new agents are becoming available, some of which are on the market at the present time but are not indicated for DVT prophylaxis. These drugs are related to the antithrombin drug produced by leeches. Two of these are desirudin and bivalirudin and are indicated for anticoagulation in the presence of heparin-induced thrombocytopenia.

In addition, ximelagatran is an antithrombin drug that may soon be available for DVT prophylaxis as an oral prescription. A pentasaccharide (fondaparinux) is approved for DVT prophylaxis and will act in a manner similar to heparin.

1. Diagnosis—DVT is diagnosed with ultrasound in the postsurgical patient with calf swelling, or Homan's sign in the appropriate clinical setting. Several risk factors can be elicited from the history to increase the suspicion of DVT. These include immobilization, lower extremity or pelvic surgery (previous 4 weeks), previous history of DVT, and history of cancer. Ultrasound is a reliable screen for DVT of the thigh veins but is less reliable for calf veins. The gold standard for DVT is the venogram, but this method should be used sparingly because it can be quite uncomfortable for patients.

Testing for PE has evolved. In nonsurgical patients, *d*-dimer can be helpful in the diagnosis of PE, but the risk of PE continues for weeks after surgery so there may be a role for it in the late postoperative period. Previously, ventilation/perfusion scans were the standard method, followed by pulmonary angiography, if the probability was intermediate. Now spiral CT is quite reliable but is still only reported to be 70% sensitive and 91% specific. In outpatients with a normal ultrasound and a normal lung scan, spiral CT has only a 7% false-positive rate and 5% false-negative rate. Furthermore there is evidence from a preliminary study to suggest that fibrin monomer discriminates between total hip arthroplasty patients with PE and those without PE. The *d*-dimer was also higher in PE patients but not significantly until 7 days postoperatively.

Ballard JO: Anticoagulant-induced thrombosis JAMA, 1999;282: 310.

Freedman KB et al: A Meta-analysis of thromboembolic prophylaxis following elective total hip arthroplasty. J Bone Joint Surg Am 2000;82:929.

Geerts WH et al: Prevention of venous thromboembolism. Chest 2001;119(1);132S.

Johnson BF et al: Relationship between changes in the deep venous system and the development of post thrombotic syndrome after an acute episode of lower limb deep vein thrombosis: A one to six-year follow-up. J Vasc Surg 1995;21:307.

Kane RE: Neurodeficits following epidural or spinal anesthesia. Anesth Analg 1981;60:150.

Kubo T et al: Fibrin monomer could be a useful predictor of pulmonary embolism after total hip arthroplasty: Preliminary report. J Orthop Sci 2001;6:119.

Lillienfeld DE, Godbold JH: Geographic distribution of pulmonary embolism with mortality rates in the United States 1980–1984. Am Heart J 1992;124:1068.

Perrier A et al: Performance of helical computed tomography in unselected outpatients with suspected pulmonary embolism. Ann Intern Med 2001;135:88.

Salvati E et al: Recent advances in venous thromboembolic prophylaxis during and after total hip replacement. J Bone Joint Surg Am 2000;82:252.

Turpie AGG et al: A synthetic pentasaccharide for the prevention of deep-vein thrombosis after total hip replacement. N Engl J Med 2001;344:(9)619.

Weitz JI: New anticoagulant drugs. Chest 2001;119(1);955.

Wells PS et al: Excluding pulmonary embolism at the bedside without diagnostic imaging: Management of patients with suspected pulmonary embolism presenting to the emergency department by using a simple clinical model and D-dimer. Ann Intern Med 2001;135:98.

Outpatient Care

Economic realities have mandated earlier discharge from the hospital after some procedures and after outpatient surgery in procedures previously done on an inpatient basis. This trend suggests that patients must take more responsibility for their care, and surgeons must provide outpatient access for patients previously treated as inpatients. The indications for discharge have broadened just as the reasons for admission have narrowed. The reasons for keeping a postoperative patient in the acute-care setting are few. The main indications for hospitalization are pain control requiring parenteral narcotics, presence of hemodynamic instability, a need for traction, or a need for frequent physician observation (drains, infection, etc). Even extended administration of IV antibiotic therapy is not an adequate reason for an acute-care stay. Thus timing of follow-up visits is important, to ensure that the patient is not only unnecessarily inconvenienced but also does not suffer delayed recognition of a complication. In most cases, the first visit should be for suture removal (10–14 days). Again, economic realities mandate a 90-day follow-up as part of the global surgical fee. Follow-up for a total hip replacement patient might be at 2 weeks, 6 weeks, and 12 weeks after surgery. Longer or shorter intervals may be necessary, depending on how the patient is progressing and how much external support the patient is receiving (physical therapy, home nurse visits, home caregivers, and home environment). Joint-replacement patients should be followed up at least yearly on a permanent basis. The American Academy of Orthopedic Surgeons has recommended prophylactic antibiotics for joint-replacement patients for procedures, such as dental cleaning, in which bacteremia may occur, for 2 years after joint replacement, although some surgeons recommend prophylaxis for life, especially when immune compromise is likely, eg, diabetes or renal transplant.

Long-term follow-up for patients with plates, screws, pins, rods, or other fracture devices is not typically necessary after healing of the fracture and rehabilitation of the affected muscles and joints. Antibiotic prophylaxis is not necessary for these patients. In cases of painful hardware, removal may be indicated after healing. Removal of hardware in older patients is generally not indicated. In younger, active patients, hardware removal may be justified to reduce the stress concentration or stress shielding effects of the metal devices to prophylactically prevent fracture. An adequate period (12 weeks or more, depending on activity) of stress protection, especially in torsion, is indicated to reduce the risk of fracture through defects induced in the bone during removal of hardware.

For a detailed discussion of rehabilitation, see Chapter 13.

Montgomery CJ, Ready LB: Epidural opioid analgesia does not obscure diagnosis of compartment syndrome resulting from prolonged lithotomy position. Anesthesiology 1991;75:541.

Strecker WB et al: Compartment syndrome masked by epidural anesthesia for postoperative pain. J Bone Joint Surg Am 1986;68:1447.

Westrich GH et al: Venous haemodynamics after total knee arthroplasty. Evaluation of active dorsal to plantar flexion and several mechanical compression devices. J Bone Joint Surg Br 1998;80:1057.

Blood Loss & Replacement

Because blood replacement has become a complicated issue, it is fortunate that not all orthopedic procedures require blood replacement. In California, the surgeon is obligated to give the patient a brochure from the state that describes the blood management options available to the surgeon and the patient when blood transfusion is likely after surgery. Many California hospitals have now instituted a form for the patient to sign, verifying receipt of this information. Patient involvement in the decision on how to manage blood loss is certainly a good idea. The data on when to transfuse are conflicting, however, and generally the decision is based on the physician's clinical assessment to determine the need for transfusion. Blood volume is approximately 7–8% of body weight, or about 5 L in a 70-kg individual. Normal individuals can be resuscitated from acute blood losses of up to 25% with crystalloid/colloid. Greater blood losses can be tolerated if the euvolemic state is maintained, but transfusion should be considered. The status of the clotting system must be monitored in the acute blood loss phase, to prevent accelerated blood loss. Blood loss in the postoperative subacute phase can be managed with volume replacement and evaluation of symptomatology to determine the need for transfusion of red cell mass. Patients at risk of stroke, myocardial infarction, or those with decreased cardiac output may need transfusion at higher hemoglobin levels. Younger, healthier patients may tolerate lower hemoglobin levels unless they have postural hypotension, tachycardia, dizziness, or fainting.

A. CRITERIA FOR BLOOD TRANSFUSION

The decision to transfuse in the immediate postoperative period is predicated on numerous factors, including age, medical condition and cardiac status, estimated blood loss, projected blood loss, availability of blood (autologous, designated donor, or bank), and the patient's perception of risk. Consideration of all factors argues against transfusion in the younger or healthier patient until the patient has a hematocrit level of 20–22% or has symptoms that include tachycardia, early and postural hypotension, and dizziness or fainting. Older patients at risk of stroke or myocardial infarction would be candidates for transfusion at higher hematocrit levels or with a lower threshold of symptoms.

B. STRATEGIES FOR MINIMIZING THE RISKS ASSOCIATED WITH BLOOD TRANSFUSION

Blood loss is an inevitable part of surgery. With the realization that the banked blood supply is at low risk, but still at risk, of containing infectious agents, strategies to minimize the risk of transmission have been developed.

An obvious method of accomplishing this goal is to reduce blood loss. Anesthetic techniques to reduce mean arterial blood pressure can reduce blood loss by reducing the time of surgery as well as the actual blood loss. The patient has to be counseled to avoid antiplatelet drugs in the period prior to surgery. These medications include baby aspirin but also all of the ubiquitous NSAIDs that are in over-the-counter analgesics, cough and cold remedies, and arthritis medications. In the operative period, topical agents such as bone wax, Gelfoam and similar collagen products, thrombin, tranexamic acid and aminocaproic acid (antifibrinolytic), and fibrin glue should be considered. Surgical technique should be efficient and meticulous to reduce time and therefore blood loss. The patient should be positioned to minimize venous pressure and blood loss such as positioning a postoperative total knee in flexion to reduce blood loss.

Presurgical banking of autologous blood by the patient (with or without hematopoietic growth factors), immediate preoperative autodonation by hemodilution, and salvage of the patient's intraoperative and postoperatively lost blood with infusion of either washed or unwashed red cells can reduce the patient's exposure to the risks of designated donor blood or homologous banked blood. The problems with autologous blood begin with the cost, but there are other issues. Older patients sometimes do not tolerate the anemia from donation. Perhaps the greatest risks are bacterial contamination and clerical error, in which someone gets a potentially fatal ABO-incompatible unit instead of their own. Autologous blood that is not used is discarded and is not put into the general blood bank pool.

Preoperative hemodilution has the cost associated with the operating room time to draw off the blood and that of the anesthesiologist in supervising the process. Preoperative hematocrit can be boosted through parenteral erythropoietin, which can minimize the effect of surgical blood loss. Erythropoietin is estimated to cost $900 per unit of blood saved, which is more than the cost of autologous blood at $300–400/unit. Furthermore there may be risks with abnormally high hematocrits. Thus it is only considered when there is little other choice, such as for surgery on Jehovah's Witnesses who refuse transfusions.

Despite initial resistance and continued questions about cost-effectiveness by blood bank officials, autologous blood donation has achieved considerable acceptability from patients, physicians, and blood bank administrators. Blood can be stored for 35 days or can be frozen as a red cell mass for up to 1 year, but loss in viability of the red cells occurs with both storage methods. Use of autologous blood can eliminate the need for banked blood for many but not all orthopedic patients. Some patients, for example, have marginal laboratory test results (eg, hemoglobin level of 10 g/dL and hematocrit level of 30%) that preclude their predonation of blood. The ability of patients to predonate blood and the amount of blood donated can sometimes be increased through the use of recombinant human erythropoietin therapy. Injections can be given twice weekly and may result in a higher red cell mass collected and a higher hematocrit level at the time of hospital admission. Although expensive, this therapy can be of benefit to patients, especially those who have blood types that are difficult to match or have religious beliefs that conflict with the practice of receiving blood from others.

Red blood cells can be salvaged by suction in the operating room or collected via surgical drains in the recovery room. Adequate loss of blood must be present to make these procedures cost-effective. The salvaged blood is generally washed to remove cell debris, fat, and bone fragments. Newer filtration techniques have permitted the transfusion of blood collected from drains without the washing process.

Birkmeyer JD et al: The cost-effectiveness of preoperative autologous blood donation for total hip and knee replacement. Transfusion 1993;33:544.

Goodnough LT et al: Increased preoperative collection of autologous blood with recombinant human erythropoietin therapy. N Engl J Med 1989;321:1163.

Hirsch J, Levine MN: Low molecular weight heparin. Blood 1992;79:1.

Keating EM: Current options and approaches for blood management in orthopedic surgery. J Bone Joint Surg Am 1998;80:750.

Levine EA et al: Perioperative recombinant human erythropoietin. Surgery 1989;106:432.

Martin JW et al: Postoperative blood retrieval and transfusion in cementless total knee arthroplasty. J Arthroplasty 1992;7:205.

Newman JH et al: The clinical advantages of autologous transfusion. A randomized controlled study after knee replacement. J Bone Joint Surg Br 1997;79:630.

Sparling EA et al: The use of erythropoietin in the management of Jehovah's witnesses who have revision total hip arthroplasty. J Bone Joint Surg Am 1996;78:1548.

Ethics in Orthopedic Surgery

Ethics in medicine started with Hippocrates and was codified by Thomas Percival in 1803, with the publication of his Code of Medical Ethics. This was extended by the American Medical Association in 1847 and has undergone several revisions over time. Ethics basically define the standards of conduct of honorable or moral behavior by the physician. Many areas of medical ethics, such as abortion, or artificial insemination, have little to do with orthopedics. Although many areas of ethics are more restrictive than the law, litigation and legislation have in some cases become the standard by which orthopedists have to abide, with tighter constraints than ethics alone would place. Although ethics as a field is too broad a subject for a text such as this, certain areas that impinge on orthopedics will be addressed.

Clinical Trials

A particularly difficult ethical area is the clinical research study. Although many of these are now more than adequately controlled by institutional review boards (IRB), the federal government's Office for Human Research Protections, and sponsors of research, the single practitioner in a small orthopedic group is still at risk of performing human, or even animal, research without appropriate ethical controls. The three main areas for concern are the use of ionizing radiation for exams that are not clinically indicated, the use of patient or third-party-payer funds for exams that are not clinically indicated, and the use of patient data in a manner that does not maintain confidentiality. Certainly, ionizing radiation can be used, even for control subjects, if adequate IRB review and patient/subject consent is obtained. This must be done in a formal manner. However, the use of third-party-payer funds for research or revealing patient confidentiality is never ethical. Performing unindicated studies (lab, radiographs) at patient expense is certainly unethical. Also, patient confidentiality is fundamental to the doctor-patient relationship. Photos or slides of football injuries in the public domain may be acceptable for presentation, although in some situations this may not be true. Certainly, photos or slides of radiographs with patient identifiers for professional presentations or publications cannot be used without written patient permission.

The typical orthopedic clinical research study is a retrospective review of a surgeon's cases. This model of research is considered to be of modest value by researchers doing multicenter, randomized, controlled, double-blind studies, but until the funding is found to do this type of study on something as common as knee replacement, retrospective reviews will have to serve as the database for decision making. This will especially be true for low-volume procedures. These types of studies raise several issues. The main issues are paying for the study (not through patient or third-party funds), maintaining patient confidentiality, and conflict of interest. The first two issues can be resolved by IRB oversight, and the private practitioner is advised to obtain that help from his hospital. Conflict of interest has at least two aspects. The physician may be a consultant or designer of the prosthesis or drug and have a financial interest in the success of the product, and the physician has ego invested in his surgery, ie, he or she doesn't want to look like a "bad" surgeon and hence may be hesitant to report bad results. Furthermore, he or she may be a professor and need to demonstrate clinical research publications as part of promotion requirements or simply want to "advertise" his or her abilities through publication. The latter aspects are implied conflicts of interest but are probably as important as a financial conflict. The potential financial conflict should be disclosed to the patient and to other parties such as the hospital and to the journal of publication. The surgeon has an ethical obligation to share medical advances and presenting a surgeon's results with a procedure certainly meets that standard.

Gifts from Industry

The concept that gifts from industry may affect the choice of medication, prosthesis, and so on is the concern in this issue. Generally, the guidelines recommended by the American Medical Association allow gifts, other remuneration, subsidies for meetings, etc. if the primary purpose is education or will benefit the patient. Gifts should be of minimal value and related to the physician's work. The pharmaceutical companies have recently been regulated in regard to the type of meetings that they can sponsor. Meetings directly sponsored by the company are only allowed to discuss "label" applications of the drug or device, whereas continuing medical education credit courses, which can only be done through an educational institution, can discuss "off-label" uses of products. Payment for travel costs, lodging, and honoraria to attend such meetings is considered inappropriate unless the physician is performing a service, such as faculty duties, or consulting. Although it seems unlikely that a physician would change his or her prescribing practice based on a free meal, the appearance of impropriety is important and should be kept in mind.

Council on Ethical and Judicial Affairs. Code of Medical Ethics: Current Opinions with Annotations. Chicago: American Medical Association, 2000–2001 edition, 2000.

Musculoskeletal Trauma Surgery ▌3

*Wade R. Smith, MD, John R. Shank, MD, Harry B. Skinner, MD, Edward Diao, MD,
& David W. Lowenberg, MD*

The High Cost of Musculoskeletal Trauma

Trauma is the "neglected disease." It is the leading cause of death for people age 1 to 44 years of all races and socioeconomic levels and the third leading cause of death for all age groups. In 1994, there were 150,956 trauma-related deaths, 61% of which were due to unintentional trauma, half of which were caused by motor vehicle crashes. In 1996, 1 out of 85 people involved in a motor vehicle accident died from injuries sustained in the crash. Overall, there were 3.5 million deaths from motor vehicle trauma. In 1992, approximately 140,000 Americans sustained gunshot injuries. Twenty thousand of these (28%) died as a result. In the pediatric population, 10,000 deaths associated with trauma are recorded annually in the United States. Trauma accounts for 30% of pediatric emergency room visits and is the most common cause of mortality in the noninfant child. This neglected disease costs the nation in excess of $40 billion per year.

Musculoskeletal disorders generated 3.5 million admissions to acute-care hospitals in the United States in 1988, more than 40% of which were trauma-related. Musculoskeletal injuries have a tremendous effect on the patient, the family, and the society in general because of the

(1) physical and psychologic effects of pain, limitation of daily activities, loss of independence, and reduced quality of life;

(2) direct expenditures for diagnosis and treatment; and

(3) indirect economic costs associated with lost labor and diminished productivity.

Musculoskeletal injuries occur frequently, result in significant disability, and consume a major portion of health care resources. An estimated 33 million people in the United States sustained these injuries in 1988, with an incidence of 138 per thousand people. Rates are highest in persons 18–44 years of age, and this has a major socioeconomic effect. Annually, the average number of injuries resulting in restriction of activities is 30.6 million, with 13.4 million of these severe enough to require bed rest. This translates into 1.54 million acute hospitalizations, of an average duration of 7.1 days, and about 45,000 deaths over a 1-year period.

The effect of these injuries on the nation's economy reached $26 billion in 1988, including indirect costs such as lost productivity. For example, the cost of hip fracture is estimated at $8.7 billion, or 43% of the total cost of all fractures. Direct costs are about 80% of the total, of which inpatient hospital care amounts to $3.1 billion and nursing home care $1.6 billion. More recent estimates show an increasing effect on the U.S. economy, including over $150 billion per year in direct and indirect cost from lost labor productivity due to trauma.

Engelhardt S et al: The 15-year evolution of an urban trauma center: What does the future hold for the trauma surgeon? J Trauma 2001;51:633.[PMID: 11586151]

Praemer A, Furner S, Rice DP: Musculoskeletal conditions in the United States. J Am Acad Orthop Surg 1992.

Soderstrom CA, Cole FJ, Porter JM: Injury in America: The role of alcohol and other drugs—an EAST position paper prepared by the injury control and violence prevention committee. J Trauma 2001;50:1.[PMID: 11253757]

Wynn A et al: Accuracy of administrative and trauma registry database. J Trauma 2001;51:464.[PMID: 11535892]

THE HEALING PROCESS

Bone Healing

Bone is a unique tissue because it heals by the formation of normal bone, as opposed to scar tissue. In fact, it is considered a nonunion when a bone heals by a fibroblastic response instead of by bone formation. Whatever part of the skeleton it comes from, bone has a fine fibroid structure. This is true for cortical and cancellous bone from the diaphysis, epiphysis, or metaphysis. Bone will, therefore, heal by the same mechanism wherever it breaks.

Fracture healing can be conveniently divided, based on the biologic events taking place, into the following four phases:

(1) cellular callus,

(2) mineralized callus,

(3) bony callus, and

(4) remodeling

A. Cellular Callus

This is the initial inflammatory phase characterized by an accumulation of mesenchymal cells around the fracture site. The exact origin of these cells remains controversial. In fractures where the periosteum is intact, these cells probably come from the cambium. In higher energy fractures where the periosteum has been compromised, the appearance of spindle-shaped cells that are able to differentiate into osteogenic cells has been found to coincide with the appearance of capillary buds. These cells are possibly derived from the pericytes found around capillaries, arterioles, and venules.

Whatever their origin, these cells ensheathe the fracture and differentiate into chondrocytes or osteoblasts. Low-oxygen tension, low pH, and movement favor the differentiation into chondrocytes; high-oxygen tension, high pH, and stability predispose to osteoblasts. This initial callus acts as an internal splint against bending and rotational deformation and, less effectively, against shearing and axial deformation. Because the stiffness of this callus in bending and torsion varies with the fourth power of the radius, its distribution around the fracture is important; peripheral distribution adds to rigidity. Clinically, the fracture becomes "sticky," and although some motion is detectable, the fracture is stable.

B. Mineralized Callus

Radiologic evidence of mineral formation signals the onset of this phase. Cartilage in callus is replaced by woven bone by a process analogous to the endochondral ossification seen in the fetus. The mechanism of mineralization is poorly understood but is thought to involve active transport of minerals and their precipitation from a supersaturated solution. Mineralization causes the chondrocytes themselves to degenerate and die. Capillary buds then invade the mineralized cartilage, bringing osteoblasts, which resorb part of the calcified cartilage and deposit coarse fibroid bone on its residuum. The proliferating cambium layer of the periosteum also lays down new bone on the exposed surface of the bone, if conditions are favorable.

The phase of mineralized callus leads to a state in which the fracture site is enveloped in a polymorphous mass of mineralized tissues consisting of calcified cartilage, woven bone made from cartilage, and woven bone formed directly.

C. Bony Callus

The woven-bone mineralized callus has to be replaced by lamellar bone arranged in osteonal systems to allow the bone to resume its normal function. Before this stage of remodeling can start, it is necessary to consolidate the fracture site. The concept of consolidation is poorly defined but includes filling the gaps left by the previous phase between the ends of the bone; it is also called **gap-healing bone.** This bone has three major characteristics:

(1) It forms only under conditions of mechanical stability;

(2) It has the ability to replace fibrous or muscle tissue; and

(3) It forms within the confines of the bone defect

Gap-healing bone is essentially coarse fibroid bone and, therefore, is not normal lamellar bone.

D. Remodeling

This final phase, involves the replacement of woven bone by lamellar bone in various shapes and arrangements and is necessary to restore the bone to optimal function. This process involves the simultaneous meticulously coordinated removal of bone from one site and deposition in another.

Two lines of cells, osteoclasts and osteoblasts, are responsible for this process. Osteoclasts are derived from monocytes and are large multinucleated cells that remove bone. They are located on the resorption surfaces of the bone. Osteoblasts are mononuclear and are responsible for the accretion of bone.

Cartilage Healing

Articular cartilage consists of a hydrated glycoprotein gel in which collagen fibrils are interspersed in a unique pattern. This mixture gives the cartilage its unique properties of smoothness, resilience, endurance, and strength.

Chondrocytes are sparse in the adult cartilage, which is not a vascularized tissue. Their nutrition comes from the synovial fluid and depends on the health of the synovial membrane and adequate circulation of the fluid through the spongelike cartilage matrix. Motion of the joint is responsible for most of this circulation. A good part of the rationale behind rigid internal fixation of fractures is to allow early motion of the joints. The same argument can be made for early weight bearing of immobilized joints, which allows cyclical compression of the cartilage and circulation of the synovial fluid.

Articular cartilage has limited reparative capacities because chondrocytes have a low baseline metabolic rate, a small cell-to-matrix ratio, and a restricted mode of nutrition. If the defect in the cartilage does not go through the calcified plate, the body attempts repair with hyaline cartilage. It will be, however, incomplete, except for the smallest defects. If the calcified plate is violated, the subchondral capillaries bring an inflammatory reaction, which fills the defect with granulation tissue and, eventually, fibrocartilage. The quality of this fibrocartilage can be improved by passive or active motion of the joint.

Tendon Healing

Tendons are specialized structures that allow muscles to concentrate or extend their action. The Achilles tendon, for example, concentrates the action of the bulky muscles of the calf over a small area where a large force needs to be applied for pushoff. Tendons consist of long bundles of collagen scattered with relatively inactive fibrocytes. These cells are nourished by the synovial fluid secreted by the one-cell-thick synovial membrane that covers the tendon (endotenon) and the parietal surface of the sheath (epitenon). The flexor tendons are covered by a richly vascularized adventitia (paratenon).

Muscle Healing

Human skeletal muscle is divided into fiber types depending on their metabolic activity and mechanical function. Type 1 fiber, known as **slow twitch, slow oxidative,** or **red,** muscle, has a slow speed of contraction and the greatest strength of contraction. It functions aerobically and, therefore, is fatigue-resistant. Type 2 fiber, known as **fast twitch** or **white** muscle, is subdivided into two types, according to metabolic activity level: fiber that functions by oxidative and glycolytic metabolism (type 2A) and fiber that is largely glycolytic (type 2B). Both subtypes of white fast-twitch muscles are fatigable but have high strength of contraction and high speed of contraction. Fiber type interconversion can occur, but this is generally believed to happen only under extreme conditions. It is generally conceded that the relative proportions of type 1 and type 2 fibers are defined genetically, with little capacity for change. Thus, sprinters are unlikely to become cross-country runners, and vice versa. Interconversion between type 2A and 2B fibers is much more likely, depending on the type of athletic training.

Traumatic injury to muscle can occur from a variety of mechanisms, including blunt trauma, laceration, or ischemia. Recovery occurs through a process of degeneration and regeneration, with new muscle cells arising from undifferentiated cells. Traumatic injuries include muscle laceration, muscle contusion (blunt injury), and strains resulting from excessive stretching. In addition to muscle regeneration, laceration repair requires reinnervation of denervated muscle areas. Muscle contusion frequently results in hematoma. The normal repair process includes an inflammatory reaction, formation of connective tissue, and muscle regeneration. Blunt trauma may result in myositis ossificans and may cause decreased function. Muscle strains go by a variety of names, including **muscle pull** and **muscle tear.** The failure frequently occurs at the myotendinous junction in experimental animals but may also be within the muscle itself rather than at the bone-tendon junction.

Of particular concern to the traumatologist is the effect of immobilization on muscle tissue. As with all tissues, immobilization and lack of activity result in atrophy. Loss of muscle weight initially occurs rapidly and then tends to stabilize, and loss of strength occurs simultaneously. Resistance to fatigue diminishes rapidly. These changes are minimized if immobilization occurs with some stretching of the muscle. Prevention of "fracture disease" after trauma requires an understanding of muscle physiologic principles.

Nerve Healing

Peripheral nerves have a distinct anatomic structure, with multiple nerve fibers combined to form a fascicle surrounded by perineurium. Multiple fascicles are surrounded by epineurium. Nerves fall into patterns of monofascicular, oligofascicular, and polyfascicular structures. The size and distribution of fascicles change as a function of length, reflecting greater or lesser nerve fibers in each fascicle. Around joints, fascicles typically tend to be multiple and small, perhaps to reduce injury from mechanical trauma. In addition, these nerves tend to have thicker epineurium near joints, with many small fascicles, and this may tend to protect the nerve from flexion and extension cycles. Nerve damage may occur through direct compression or stretching injuries. Ischemic damage from stretching may occur at elongation of 15%. Nerve injuries are now rated from 1 to 5 degrees. First-degree injury is the least severe and is equivalent to neurapraxia. The nerve (axon) is in continuity, and loss of function is reversible. Second-degree injury is equivalent to axonotmesis, with degeneration of the axon. The endoneurial sheath remains in continuity, however, and regeneration occurs by growth of the axon down its original endoneurial tube. Third-degree injury is the same as second-degree injury with the addition of loss of continuity of the endoneurial tube. The perineurium is preserved, however. Because of damage to the fascicle, some misdirection of regenerating axons may occur, and the extent of functional return depends on the extent of misdirection. Fourth-degree injuries preserve only the continuity of the nerve trunk but involve much more extensive degeneration of the fascicles. Despite the continuity of the nerve trunk, this injury may require excision of the damaged segment, with reapproximation of the nerve ends to achieve a functional outcome. Fifth-degree injury involves complete loss of continuity of the nerve trunk. Surgical repair, obviously, is required to achieve restoration of function.

Functional recovery after nerve injury depends on a number of variables. The outcome is much more optimistic for children than adults, and the prognosis diminishes with age. Increasing distance from the nerve injury to the distal point of innervation reduces the likelihood of recovery. Other factors include the length of the damage to the nerve, the technical ability of the surgeon, and the length of time prior to repair.

Jackson DW, Scheer MJ, Simon TM: Cartilage substitutes: Overview of basic science and treatment options. J Am Acad Orthop Surg 2001;9:37.[PMID: 11174162]

Browne JE, Branch TP: Surgical alternatives for treatment of articular cartilage lesions. J Am Acad Orthop Surg 2000;8:180. [PMID: 10874225]

Lee SK, Wolfe SW: Peripheral nerve injury and repair. J Am Acad Orthop Surg 2000;8:243.[PMID: 10951113]

Robinson LR: Role of neurophysiologic Evaluation in diagnosis. J Am Acad Orthop Surg 2000;8:190.[PMID: 10874226]

GENERAL CONSIDERATIONS IN DIAGNOSIS & TREATMENT OF MUSCULOSKELETAL TRAUMA

ORTHOPEDIC ASSESSMENT & MANAGEMENT OF POLYTRAUMA PATIENTS

A good understanding of the anatomy, physiology, and physiopathology of the musculoskeletal system is essential for prompt diagnosis and treatment of its injuries. Sound therapeutic principles based on such understanding improve the overall outcome for the patient and optimize the utilization of limited health care resources.

Life-Threatening Conditions: The ABCs of Trauma Care

The patient is assessed and treatment priorities are established according to the type of injury, stability of vital signs, and mechanism of injury. In a severely injured patient, treatment priorities are dictated by the patient's overall condition, with the first goal being to save life and preserve the major functions of the body. Assessment consists of four overlapping phases:

(1) Rapid primary evaluation
(2) Restoration of vital function
(3) Detailed secondary evaluation and
(4) Definitive care

This process, called the **ABCs of trauma care,** identifies and treats life-threatening conditions, and can be remembered as follows:

*A*irway maintenance (with cervical spine control);

*B*reathing and ventilation;

*C*irculation (with hemorrhage control);

*D*isability (neurologic status);

*E*xposure and environmental control (undress the patient but prevent hypothermia).

A brief overview of the treatment of polytrauma patients, with special emphasis on orthopedic aspects, follows:

A. AIRWAY

Great care should be taken while assessing the airway. The cervical spine should be carefully protected at all times and not be hyperextended, hyperflexed, or rotated to obtain a patent airway. A chin lift or jaw thrust maneuver should be used to establish an airway. The history of the trauma incident is essential (ie, anyone with a head bump should be considered at risk). A normal neurologic examination or cross-table lateral radiograph of the cervical spine, including the C7-T1 disk space, does not rule out cervical spine injuries; it only makes them less likely.

B. BREATHING

The trauma surgeon should auscultate and inspect the patient's chest. Remember that the following four conditions, if present, must be addressed:

(1) Tension pneumothorax
(2) Flail chest with pulmonary contusion
(3) Open pneumothorax and
(4) Massive hemothorax

C. CIRCULATION

Level of consciousness and pulses are simple to assess and reliably mirror the hemodynamic status of the patient, especially if recorded serially. Fractures of the femur or the pelvis can cause major blood loss, which can severely compromise the ultimate survival of the patient. (See sections on pelvic and femoral fracture.)

D. DISABILITY (NEUROLOGIC STATUS)

The Glasgow Coma Scale (see Chapter 13) should be used; it is quick, simple, and predictive of patient outcome. An even simpler way to monitor central neurologic status is to check if the patient is

*A*lert and oriented,

or responds to *V*ocal stimuli,

or responds only to *P*ainful stimuli,
or is *U*nresponsive.

E. Exposure and Environmental Control

Recognition of lacerations, contusions, abrasions, swelling, and deformity can only be accomplished in the completely disrobed patient. The safest way to achieve this is to cut off all clothing. This permits complete examination of the patient, prevents further displacement of fractures, and minimizes the risk of overlooking significant problems. Hypothermia must be avoided, as cardiac function may be affected, especially when there is decreased blood volume. Sterile dressings should be applied to any wounds to prevent further contamination.

F. Care of Patient Before Hospitalization

The diagnosis and treatment of musculoskeletal injuries in polytrauma patients should be initiated in the field by the paramedics. Recognition and splinting of major fractures, adequate immobilization of the cervical spine, and proper handling of the injured patient are essential to prevent further damage to the neurovascular elements. In many cases, proper care at this stage will prevent or limit shock as well as avoid catastrophic damage to the spinal cord.

The old saying "splint them where they lie" remains especially true when the exact nature and extent of the fractures remain obscure. As a general rule, the following measures should be taken:

(1) The joints above and below the fracture should be immobilized.

(2) Splints can be improvised with pillows, blankets, or clothing.

(3) Immobilization does not need to be absolutely rigid.

(4) Overt bleeding should be tamponaded with dressing and firm pressure.

(5) Tourniquets should be avoided, unless it is obvious that the patient's life is in danger.

Orthopedic Examination

A. General Examination

The clinical orthopedic examination requires assessment of the axial skeleton, pelvis, and extremities. The extent of this examination depends on the patient's overall central neurologic status. Swelling, hematomas, and open wounds are assessed visually in the undressed patient. It is obligatory to palpate the entire spine, pelvis, and each joint. Examination soon after trauma may precede telltale swelling in joint or long bone injuries. In the unresponsive patient, only crepitation and false motion may be discerned. Patients with a better mental status, however, can provide feedback regarding pain resulting from palpation. The pelvis is examined by compression of the iliac wings in a mediolateral direction and of the pubis.

B. Neurologic Examination

The neurologic examination of the extremities should be documented to the fullest extent possible, in light of the patient's mental status, as it is central to subsequent decision making. This examination includes delineation of sensory function in the major nerves and dermatomes in the upper and lower extremities. Perianal sensation is also important. Thus, in the upper extremity, dermatomes from C5–T1 and radial, ulnar, and median nerve function must be assessed.

C. Muscle Examination

Motor examination can be difficult because of pain or impaired mental status, but even in such cases, useful and relatively complete information can be obtained. In the upper extremity, the function of the deltoid, biceps, brachioradialis, extensor pollicis longus, flexor carpi radialis, and intrinsic muscles (first dorsal interosseus and opponens pollicis muscles) must be examined. A more complete examination is indicated if there is obvious trauma to this area. In the lower extremity, the motor supply to the extensor hallucis longus, tibialis anterior, peroneal muscles, gastrocnemius, and quadriceps muscles must be tested and graded. Muscle strength grading is desirable, but demonstration of a minimum of volitional control (even if withdrawal to painful stimuli) is important in verifying the presence of intact central sensory-motor integration.

Particularly important in the face of spinal cord injury or suspected injury are the reflexes of the anal "wink" and bulbocavernosus muscle. Other spinal reflexes (ie, of the biceps and triceps muscles, of the knee and ankle, and the Babinski reflex) are important in "fine-tuning" the neurologic examination. (These are discussed more fully in Chapter 5, "Disorders, Disease, & Injuries of the Spine.")

Imaging Studies

Radiologic assessment follows the same general hierarchy as the clinical assessment. The severely injured polytrauma patient requires plain films of the chest, abdomen, *and* pelvis to indicate sources of respiratory and circulatory compromise. The second level of examination requires the cervical spine cross-table lateral view. The information obtained from this film dictates treatment and the need for any further evaluation of the cervical spine.

Subsequent evaluation is dependent on clinical findings. Any long bone or joint with a laceration, hematoma, angulation, or swelling must undergo roentgenographic evaluation. Any long bone fracture requires complete evaluation of the joints proximal and distal to the fracture. At the minimum, two views of the extremities are needed, usually the anteroposterior and lateral views. Coordination of more sophisticated studies with other trauma specialties (eg, neurosurgery or urology) is necessary to allow cardiorespiratory monitoring of the patient while efficiently performing these studies. For example, magnetic resonance imaging (MRI) and computed tomographic (CT) scanning should be performed with the fewest changes of position possible that will also provide the necessary information for all surgical subspecialists.

"Clearing" the Cervical Spine

In the evaluation of the trauma patient, an important consideration is the status of the cervical spine. The cervical spine is easily injured because of the large mass of the head relative to the neck, especially in motor vehicle accidents involving rapid acceleration or deceleration. Consequently, the cervical spine can receive significant force and suffer injury. In the conscious and responsive patient, swelling or tenderness on physical examination of the cervical spine is readily apparent. In the unconscious patient, cervical spine injuries can go undetected, and a careful physical examination must be performed with heavy reliance upon radiographic evaluation.

The essential radiographs for evaluation of the cervical spine include anterior-posterior views, lateral views, and an open-mouth odontoid view. It is essential to be able to see to the top of T1. If this level is not visualized through these conventional views, then obtain a swimmer's view, which is a lateral cervical spine radiograph with the arm abducted and elevated.

After the cervical spine x-ray films have been reviewed, the ligamentous stability of the cervical spine can be further evaluated. Lateral cervical spine flexion and extension views can be analyzed to see if the lateral alignment of the anterior cervical spinal segments is correct. If the alert and cooperative trauma patient has any cervical tenderness, these films are often delayed for a several-week period.

On the open-mouth view, the lateral masses of C1 should line up with the body of C2. The amount of total overhang of C1 over C2 should be less than 3 mm. On the lateral view, the anterior border of the bodies of the cervical segments should describe an arc. The posterior border of the anterior arc of C1 should be within 2–3 mm of the anterior border of C2. There should be no diastasis of the spinous processes, and the joints and facet joints should all be visible. If there is a change in orientation from one cervical spine level to another, then cervical fracture, jumped facets, or dislocation should be suspected. Suspected cervical spine fracture should be investigated with appropriate imaging, such as CT scan, to further delineate the injury pattern. Suspected cervical spine injuries should be treated with provisional stabilization using a cervical collar. Rotary subluxation should be managed with evaluation of soft tissues and reduction maneuvers. In the case of neurologic deficit, careful evaluation of the neurologic status is important, and immediate decompression-stabilization must be considered.

Complications

From the orthopedist's viewpoint, the major complications associated with trauma are acute respiratory distress syndrome (fat embolism syndrome), multisystem organ failure, thromboembolic disease, atelectasis, compartment syndrome, sepsis, and ectopic bone formation. The first four disorders involve pulmonary complications and must constantly be kept in mind in managing the polytrauma patient. The institution of early fixation of fractures with concomitant mobilization of the patient has helped to reduce the incidence of these four conditions significantly. They continue to be problems, however, and constant vigilance is necessary to prevent serious consequences.

A. ACUTE RESPIRATORY DISTRESS SYNDROME

Acute respiratory distress syndrome (ARDS) can be a sequela of trauma with subsequent shock. Massive tissue injury releases inflammatory mediators, with subsequent disruption of the microvasculature of the pulmonary system. Pulmonary edema results, with decreased partial pressures of oxygen and arterial oxygen saturation and increased carbon dioxide levels. The onset is frequently within 24 h after trauma and is revealed by hypoxemia, inflammatory reaction, and progressive decrease in arterial oxygen saturation if appropriate treatment is not instituted.

Fat embolism syndrome is a special orthopedic manifestation of ARDS caused by the release of marrow fat into the circulation as may occur following fracture. Pathologic examination of the lungs shows fat droplets, usually diffusely distributed throughout the pulmonary vasculature. This syndrome may also occur in nonfracture situations, as when the medullary canal of a long bone is pressurized during total knee replacement. Fat embolism syndrome occurs frequently as a subclinical occurrence that is insufficient to compromise the patient's pulmonary reserve, but in some cases it can result in severe pulmonary compromise and death.

The clinical diagnosis of ARDS is confirmed by a decrease in arterial P_{O_2}, an increase in systemic P_{CO_2}, infiltrates on chest radiograph, presence of petechiae, and mental confusion in a patient at risk. Relatively minor injuries can result in this syndrome in patients with limited pulmonary reserve. Treatment is directed toward minimizing hypoxemia with ventilatory support as needed. Prevention is enhanced by early mobilization of the patient, which often implies early fracture fixation.

B. ATELECTASIS

Atelectasis, or localized collapse of alveoli, is a frequent postoperative complication in elective patients and can be prominent in trauma patients because of the required immobilization. Significant hypoxemia can result, and the onset may be relatively rapid. This may be the source of postoperative fevers in the early recovery phase. Occasionally, radiograph examination, showing platelike collapse of areas of the lung, will confirm the diagnosis. By encouraging coughing and deep breathing, using incentive spirometry, and, in resistant cases, using respiratory therapy, rapid resolution can be expected.

C. PULMONARY EMBOLISM AND DEEP VENOUS THROMBOSIS

Although ARDS and atelectasis are seen in the early postoperative period, pulmonary embolism (PE) is uncommon sooner than 5 days after the onset of immobilization or bed rest. The trauma patient is at risk for PE, and the patient with spinal cord injury perhaps even more so. Trauma patients without prophylaxis have been shown to have a 1–2% incidence of fatal PA, which appears to decrease with a variety of prophylactic measures. Other groups of patients at risk include the elderly, the obese, and those with malignancy. Although it is uncommon, even a young healthy person can develop deep venous thrombosis (DVT) and be at risk for PE after a long car or airplane trip in which the legs are dependent. Oral contraceptive and smoking use may also increase the risk for a young healthy patient.

Geerts and colleagues examined the incidence of DVT and PE in trauma patients in a prospective series with venography. They found patients to be at significantly increased risk if they had suffered a pelvis or long bone fracture with greater than 5 days immobilization in bed, were obese, had a preexisting coagulopathy or an Injury Severity Score (ISS) greater than 8. The authors noted that fatal PE was the most common yet preventable form of death in the hospitalized trauma patient.

Patients at high risk for PE are those with DVT in the lower extremities. Clinically significant PE usually arise from the large veins proximal to the knee. Prevention of DVT in the venous system in this area reduces the risk of PE. Various strategies used to accomplish this include drug therapy with low-dose heparin, low-molecular-weight heparin, pentasaccharide, or sodium warfarin, and intermittent pneumatic compression.

Clinical diagnosis of DVT is unreliable. Definitive diagnosis is made with venography, duplex ultrasound scanning, impedance plethysmography, or MRI venous scans. Prevention appears to be the best strategy as even routine surveillance screening in a trauma populations is cost-ineffective and does not appear to lower the overall rate of PE.

Pulmonary embolism is suspected in the orthopedic patient suffering an onset of tachypnea and dyspnea usually more than 5 days after an inciting event. The patient frequently reports chest pain and can often point to the painful area. Hemoptysis may also be present. On physical examination, tachycardia, cyanosis, and pleural friction rub can be noted.

Arterial blood gas studies demonstrate hypoxemia, although this is a nonspecific finding. Use of the d-dimer is unreliable in the early trauma patient but may be useful later in the recovery period. Definitive diagnosis is best made with pulmonary angiogram. Perfusion ventilation scanning is less invasive and may help determine whether there is a high or low probability of pulmonary embolus. Spiral CT is becoming useful in diagnosis of PE.

Treatment involves pulmonary support and heparin therapy. The natural history of treated PE is gradual lysis of the emboli, with the return of flow through the pulmonary arterial tree. The natural history of proximal DVT involves recanalization and arborization to bypass the clot. Patients may suffer from postphlebitic syndrome characterized by painful swelling in the extremity.

D. COMPARTMENT SYNDROME

The term **compartment syndrome** refers to pathologic developments in a closed space in the body caused by buildup of pressure. Most commonly, such compartments are circumscribed by fascia and incorporate one or more bones. Pressure rises from edema or bleeding within the compartment, compromising circulation to the contents of the compartment over a period, and can result in necrosis of muscle and damage to nerves.

Compartment syndrome may result from a fracture; a soft-tissue injury; an arterial injury causing ischemia, necrosis, and edema; or from a burn. In an alcohol or drug user, it may be caused by external compression from immobilization that prevents normal postural changes. Failure to redistribute pressure through postural changes results in ischemia of the area under pressure because of collapse of capillaries.

The diagnosis of compartment syndrome must be considered in the postoperative or posttrauma patient who has pain out of proportion to that expected from the inciting injury. As the pain worsens, it can become totally unresponsive to narcotic medication. Epidural narcotics may mask the onset of compartment syndrome in the lower extremity.

The five P's (pulselessness, paresthesia, paresis, pain, and pressure) characteristic of compartment syndrome are helpful, but not diagnostic, for the experienced clinician. Pulses are poor indicators of compartment syndrome as they generally remain intact until late. Paresthesias occur only when the syndrome is significantly advanced. This points to the importance of careful documentation of sensory examination prior to the potential onset of compartment syndrome. Paresis, if present, is an unreliable finding. Subsequent to fracture or injury, pain is likely to induce guarding and thereby is also an unreliable finding. If normal muscle function is present, however, compartment syndrome is unlikely unless it is early. Pain with passive stretching of involved muscles is also a subjective finding and must be differentiated from pain arising from the original injury. To the experienced clinician, pain with passive stretching is a reliable clinical sign. Pressure is a key component of compartment syndrome, but palpitation of a soft compartment does not rule out the diagnosis of compartment syndrome. Patients with equivocal clinical findings or those at high risk but without a reliable clinical examination (eg, those who are comatose, have psychiatric problems, or are under the influence of narcotics) should have compartmental pressure measurements. Intracompartmental pressure readings greater than 30–35 mm Hg or intracompartmental pressures within 30 mm Hg of the diastolic blood pressure are indications for fasciotomy. Prior to fasciotomy, circular dressings including casts should be removed, and the patient should be observed for a short period for signs of improvement. Positive clinical findings may justify fasciotomy even despite normal pressures. Late fasciotomy may result in muscle damage or possible necrosis, with resulting risk of infection.

Although compartment syndrome can occur in almost any portion of the body, the two most common locations are the forearm and calf. In the forearm, an extensile volar incision to permit complete release, including the carpal tunnel distally and the lacertus fibrosis proximally, is necessary. Dorsally, a longitudinal incision is used. In the calf, two incisions are used to release the four compartments of the leg. The anterior and lateral compartments are decompressed using a longitudinal incision approximately over the anterior intermuscular septum. Posteromedially, a second incision is used to approach the superficial and deep posterior compartments.

E. HETEROTOPIC BONE FORMATION

Clinically significant heterotopic ossification occurs as a consequence of trauma in perhaps 10% of cases and may cause pain or joint motion restriction even to the point of ankylosis. Trauma patients without head injuries frequently manifest heterotopic ossification on radiograph 1–2 months following trauma; if the ossification is clinically significant, resection may be indicated when the bone has matured as indicated by radiographs and bone scan. This can take up to 18 months to achieve.

Resection is accomplished by removing the entire piece of heterotopic bone. Selected patients may benefit from low-dose radiation (7 Gy) and oral indomethacin for 3–6 weeks. Further discussion of this topic can be found in Chapter 13, "Rehabilitation." Heterotopic bone is a much more common occurrence in patients with head injuries. This is believed to result from release of humeral modulators that have not yet been characterized.

IMMEDIATE MANAGEMENT OF MUSCULOSKELETAL TRAUMA

The orthopedic injuries in the polytrauma patient are seldom truly emergency situations, except for those involving neural or vascular compromise. For example, fracture-dislocation of the foot or ankle resulting in distal ischemia justifies immediate attempts at reduction to minimize the sequelae of ischemia. Similarly, neural compromise from dislocation of the knee justifies relocation. A more subtle situation requiring emergent treatment would be dislocation of the hip in which vascular compromise of the femoral head may result. Obviously, arterial bleeding from an open fracture should be treated immediately with pressure to minimize blood loss. Other bone and joint injuries, although urgent, may be approached in a more deliberate manner.

Orthopedic management of traumatic injuries requires consideration of the entire individual as well as the entire extremity. It is short-sighted to treat only the area of injury revealed on radiograph, as the soft-tissue envelope around the bone is essential to fracture healing and the ultimate function of the patient. Repair of soft-tissue damage is clearly important in achieving satisfactory function after healing has occurred. A break in the skin is important, but the damage done to the entire extremity is more important than the extent of laceration.

Classification of Open Fractures

A. GUSTILO AND ANDERSON CLASSIFICATION

Gustilo and Anderson made a significant contribution to trauma care of long bones by introducing their classification of open fractures, which includes the degree of open or closed soft-tissue injury. Their system was initially designed for open tibial fractures; however, it has gone on to include all types of long bone fractures. This system uses three grades and divides the third most severe grade into three subtypes.

Grade I fracture is a low-energy injury with a wound less than 1 cm in length, often from an inside-out injury rather than an outside-in injury. These are generally simple transverse or short oblique fractures.

Grade II fracture involves a wound more than 1 cm long and significantly more injury, caused by more energy absorption during the production of the fracture. Grade II fractures usually display some comminution and have a minimal to moderate crushing component.

Grade III open fracture has extensive wounds more than 10 cm in length, significant fracture fragment comminution, and a great deal of soft-tissue damage. It is usually a high-energy injury. This type of injury results typically from high-velocity gunshots, motorcycle accidents, or injuries with contamination from outdoor sites such as with tornado disasters or farming accidents.

Grade III injuries are divided into subtypes A, B, and C. Grade IIIA fractures have extensive soft-tissue laceration with minimal periosteal stripping and have adequate bone coverage. These injuries include some gunshot injuries and segmental fractures and do not require major reconstructive surgery to provide skin coverage. Grade IIIB fractures, in contrast, have extensive soft-tissue injury with periosteal stripping and require a flap for coverage. Grade IIIC injuries involve vascular compromise requiring surgical repair or reconstruction to allow for reperfusion of the limb. The presence of an intact skin envelope may imply somewhat reduced severity of trauma. The soft-tissue and bony damage may be as severe for closed fractures, however, except for the lower risk of infection.

Severe soft-tissue and bony injuries, especially when open, raise the question of immediate amputation. This problem most frequently arises in the lower extremity between the knee and the ankle. The advent of microvascular surgery has reduced the absolute indication for amputation resulting from ischemia. Two years of reconstruction may be necessary to achieve a united tibia fracture without infection, and even then, function may be compromised by muscle or nerve damage. The patient may have also endured multiple operations, loss of work time, and the emotional trauma accompanying an injury of this magnitude. Prosthetic replace-

ments, particularly in the trauma patient at the below-knee level, may well be a viable alternative to a poorly functioning, insensate lower extremity.

It is generally conceded that loss of the posterior tibial nerve, which is responsible for sensation on the plantar aspect of the foot, will likely result in pressure sores and other problems after reconstruction.

B. MULTIPLE TRAUMA TREATMENTS—STRATEGIES AND TRAUMATIC SCORING SYSTEMS

Other factors at the time of injury have a bearing on the decision to amputate, including status of the opposite leg, the time of limb ischemia, and the age of the patient. Many of these factors have been taken into account by Johansen and associates, who have defined a Mangled Extremity Severity Score (MESS). The MESS was previously used as a predictor of eventual amputation; however, recent studies have shown the MESS and other scoring systems to be inaccurate in predicting the functional outcome for mangled limb patients (Table 3–1).

Table 3–1. Factors in evaluation of the mangled extremity severity score (MESS) variables.

	Points
A. Skeletal and soft-tissue injury	
Low energy (stab; simple fracture; "civilian" gunshot wound	1
Medium energy (open or multiple fractures, dislocation)	2
High energy (close-range shotgun or "military" gunshot wound, crush injury)	3
Very high energy (above plus gross contamination, soft-tissue avulsion)	4
B. Limb ischemia[a]	
Pulse reduced or absent but perfusion normal	1
Pulseless; paresthesia, diminished capillary refilling	2
Cool, paralyzed, insensate, numb	3
C. Shock	
Systolic blood pressure almost more than 90 mm Hg	0
Hypotensive transiently	1
Persistent hypotension	2
D. Age	
< 30 years	0
30–50 years	1
> 50 years	2

[a]Score doubled for ischemia more than 6 h.

Adapted and reproduced, with permission, from Johansen K et al: Objective criteria accurately predict amputation following lower extremity trauma. J Trauma 1990;30:369.

Musculoskeletal trauma management, particularly, in polytrauma patients, involves complex interdisciplinary decisions that must account for the needs of the whole patient. Decisions regarding the timing and type of orthopedic surgery must be made in consultation with the trauma and neurosurgery teams to afford the highest chance for survival and preservation of function. The surgeon who has to provide fracture care to patients who have multiple injuries will find that they fall into several categories. In the first are patients with multiple, isolated extremity injuries. In the second are patients with multiple orthopedic injuries who are otherwise medically stable. In a third category are patients with multiple orthopedic injuries and multisystem organ injuries.

Within these categories, orthopedic injuries are either life- or limb-threatening, emergent, urgent, or elective injuries in the timing of treatment. Timing of treatment is also related to the presence and severity of other injuries.

Several classification systems have been used to try to stratify these injuries and to determine severity. The classification systems serve as a guide for both patient treatment and eventual outcomes. The most frequently used include the Glasgow Coma Score (GCS), which is the sum of three related responses: eye opening, verbal response, and best motor response. Patients with a GCS less than 8 are in coma and are considered to have severe head injuries. Patients with a GCS of 9 to 11 are considered to have moderate head injuries, and those with scores of 13 to 15 have only mild injuries.

The Revised Trauma Score (RTS) was developed to help with patient triage. The scores for systolic blood pressure and respiratory rate are separated into five domains with each assigned a point value from 0 to 4. These scores are added to the Glasgow Coma Score to yield a Revised Trauma Score. In the United States, the American College of Surgeons' guidelines directs patients with an RTS of 11 or less to a designated trauma center.

The Abbreviated Injury Scale (AIS) divides injuries into nine body regions and stratifies the injuries from minor to fatal on a 6-point scale. These scores take into account life-threatening aspects of injuries, anticipated permanent impairment, treatment, and injury pattern.

The Injury Severity Score (ISS) is the sum of the squares of the highest AIS scores in the three most severely injured body regions, which are chosen from head and neck, face, chest, abdomen and pelvis, extremities and pelvic girdle, and external. Multiple-trauma patients are defined as patients with ISS greater than or equal to 14. A good prognosis is associated with an ISS of less than 30, whereas an ISS greater than 60 is usually fatal.

The desirability of early and appropriate orthopedic management in multiply injured patients has become well established. Benefits of timely and aggressive treatment include decreased rates of mortality, primarily due to reductions in ARDS and multisystem organ failure (MOF). In one study, 178 patients with femoral fractures were entered into an early fixation group (treatment within 24 h) or a delayed fixation group (treatment after 48 h). The incidence of pulmonary complications, such as ARDS, fat embolism, or pneumonia, was higher, the hospital stay was longer, and the intensive care unit requirements increased when the femoral fixation was delayed. Bone and collaborators did a follow-up retrospective, multicenter study of 676 patients who had an ISS greater than 18 and who had major pelvic or long-bone injuries treated under an early fixation protocol within 48 h at one of six major US trauma centers. These results were compared with historical records of 906 patients from the American College of Surgeons Multiple Trauma Outcomes Study Database. The study, despite shortcomings in methodology, revealed a lower mortality rate for patients whose fractures were stabilized early.

Controversy exists, however, regarding the appropriate timing of orthopedic intervention for specific subsets of injured patients, particularly those with head injury or systemic hypotension. Long bone fracture fixation with reamed intramedullary rods, in particular, may cause intraoperative hypotension or an increased release of inflammatory mediators with deleterious results in specific patients.

In a study by Reynolds, Richards, and Spain, records of 424 consecutive trauma patients were reviewed. Of these, 105 had an ISS of 18 or greater. These patients did not receive definitive early long bone fixation. In general, femur fractures were stabilized on the day of admission if the patients were systemically hemodynamically stable. These authors noticed that progressive surgical delays caused by decline in the patient's condition resulted in a significant increase in pulmonary complications for patients having an ISS less than 18. However, there was no relation between pulmonary complications and timing of femoral fixation when patients had an ISS of 18 or more. The authors concluded that the severity of injuries, not the timing of fracture fixation, tended to determine patient pulmonary outcome.

Soft-Tissue Injuries & Traumatic Arthrotomies

Lacerations of the extremities can result in neural or vascular compromise to an extremity and may also cause traumatic arthrotomies. Compromise of the sterility of any joint requires surgical debridement of that joint. For many joints, arthroscopic irrigation and debridement will minimize trauma and improve the return to function. Other soft-tissue lacerations may require neural or vascular repair. Laceration of a tendon or muscle belly is often involved. Tendon repairs are frequently performed in the foot and the hand. All tendon lacerations of the hand, except for those of the palmaris longus, should be repaired. In the foot, extrinsic tendons are repaired to prevent late imbalance or loss of function. Muscle belly injuries generally require surgical debridement because their subfascial location makes simple irrigation difficult. Laceration involving only the muscle belly requires no surgical repair. Frequently, however, muscle belly laceration involves the continuation of the origin or the insertion tendon of the muscle. In this case, optimal function is obtained by reattaching the lacerated ends. Generally, they can be located by poking into the muscle with a forceps at the site of the blood clot on the surface of the cut end. The tendon portion has retracted and the muscle has expanded because of swelling, leaving a track with a blood clot inside.

In most cases, immediate treatment of open fractures and lacerations consists of surgical debridement. Prior to formal debridement, it is appropriate to splint fractures and cover open wounds with sterile dressings soaked in povidone-iodine. Antibiotic therapy is begun immediately, usually with a cephalosporin bactericidal antibiotic. Tetanus prophylaxis is administered if needed. Antibiotic therapy is continued based on the clinical course.

Irrigation and debridement are intended to convert a clean contaminated wound into a sterile wound. Copious irrigation, using an irrigating solution containing antibiotics, is effective in cleaning the wound. Debridement removes nonviable tissue. Generally, care should be taken to remove only tissue that is necrotic. Skin edges should be debrided, as should muscle that does not respond to a nerve stimulator, and the surface of any contaminated fat or fascia.

After debridement, bone surfaces and exposed tendons should be covered as well as possible with tissue to maintain moistness. Maintain soft tissue attachments to bone whenever possible. Fragments of bone, particularly cortical bone, without attachments, should be removed from the wound. Although the axiom "open fractures should be left open, closed fractures should be left closed" was suitable many years ago, experience has demonstrated that in certain cases minimal risk is assumed in closing the wound. It is acceptable practice, however, to leave any wound open. Grade I wounds may in some cases be closed completely, or the part that was opened to permit debridement may be closed, leaving the original debrided laceration open. This may

close spontaneously. Grade II wounds may be treated in a similar fashion, with somewhat more risk. The possibility of gas gangrene must be entertained whenever such a wound is closed. Primary closure of Grade III wounds is rarely if ever done. Adequate closure to cover bone and other structures that may be damaged by desiccation, without completely closing the wound, may be attempted. Patients with massive wounds should be returned to the operating room in approximately 48 h and then every 48 h until the wound is completely clean and granulating. Smaller wounds that are left open may be closed safely at 3–5 days.

Flaps and Soft-Tissue Coverage for Open Trauma

Soft-tissue wounds in association with skeletal trauma (Gustilo grades I, II, and some IIIA wounds) can be treated by appropriate skeletal fixation, wound debridement, and limited skin grafts or rotation flaps to close the skin successfully. Larger wounds, however, require more aggressive surgical management. These wounds may be treated best by large regional soft-tissue flap reconstruction. Before the advent of microsurgery, the standard of care was pedicle flaps, such as chest wall flaps, applied to the arm for burn contractures around the elbow, cross-leg grafts for lower-extremity trauma, or groin flaps for soft-tissue trauma of the hand. With the advent of microsurgical techniques for skin, muscle, and fascia transplantation, the treatment of large soft-tissue trauma has changed. The classic study by Godina in *Plastic and Reconstructive Surgery* describes the results of immediate free flap reconstruction. Immediate free flap reconstruction is done within the first 48 h after trauma. The requirement for this procedure is radical debridement of the zone of injury, similar to the way one would resect a tumor. Using these techniques, there is little fibrosis of the bed and a fairly large soft-tissue defect for the viability of tissues with which to work and with which to place a free flap.

If radical debridement is not performed, then flap reconstruction should be delayed until soft tissues have healed at the margins, and there is no sign of infection. However, with large wounds, this often becomes a dilemma. Therefore, the use of free flaps gives an overall improved outcome by bringing a new source of vascularity to a compromised extremity, preventing infection and simultaneously providing soft-tissue coverage.

There are many sites that can be harvested for flaps. The most common and the hardiest flaps to use on a large scale include fasciocutaneous flaps from the latissimus dorsi, gracilis, serratus anterior, and rectus abdominis muscles. These are suitable for medium- to large-size wounds in a variety of locations. Additionally, there are a host of smaller tissue transfers designed for more specific uses that have some advantages in the matching of defect to donor and minimizing problems at the donor site. However, the flaps that have been listed are the mainstays of the reconstructive microsurgeon for the extremities.

Gun-Shot Wounds

Optimum treatment of fractures caused by gun-shots relies upon an appreciation of the mechanism of injury, the force, direction, and so on. This is particularly true with regard to soft-tissue injuries. One of the dangers of treating extremity injuries is underestimating the extent of trauma. Visual inspection alone at the time of initial evaluation is not always sufficient because it can cause an underestimation of the extent of damage. This may be true with contusion injuries to the lower extremity, such as a bumper injury to the tibia, in which the soft-tissue envelope is much more injured than is initially appreciated, and later soft-tissue compromise and loss greatly affect the overall outcome. This is particularly true with gun-shot wounds to the musculoskeletal system. These types of injuries result in complex soft-tissue lesions, fractures that are often comminuted, and related nerve, artery, and tendon involvement. Differences between high-velocity and low-velocity weapons and civilian and military settings for these wounds are also important. In general, kinetic energy (KE) associated with an injury is calculated by the formula

$$KE = \frac{M}{2} \times V^2$$

where *M* equals mass and *V* equals velocity. Thus velocity and missile mass are the most significant determinants of resultant tissue damage. Shotgun injuries are different from single gun-shot wounds, because the weight of the shot causes an increase in the kinetic energy, resulting in a more severe injury. Additionally, shotgun shells have wadding that is made of plastic, felt, paper, or cord, between the powder and the shot charge, and this wadding can become embedded in the wound and be another important factor in wound management.

In gun-shot wounds and high-velocity missiles, shock waves occur and can produce injury in areas that are relatively distant from the direct path of the missile.

Low-velocity civilian gun-shot wounds and fractures are relatively simple to treat, because tissue damage is confined to the missile path, and local wound care, with or without antibiotic therapy, can effectively treat the injuries and decrease the incidence of wound sepsis and osteomyelitis. The use of immediate fixation by either internal or external fixator means is somewhat con-troversial. On the one hand, the danger of treatment of these open fractures with foreign material is a deterrent for immediate stabilization. However, in grossly unstable injuries, treatment that would be used for other open fractures appears to be reasonable in selected cases. The impact of gun-shot wounds in ballistic injuries can be significant. In a study by Brown in the *Journal of Orthopaedic Trauma,* a university-affiliated level-1 trauma center conducted a retrospective study through calendar year 1994 in which all patients admitted through the emergency department with a gun-shot wound for which the orthopedic surgery service was consulted were evaluated. These 284 patients were responsible for 24% of all orthopedic admissions, 33% of the average daily orthopedic census, and 14% of all the orthopedic surgery cases. Forty-five percent tested positive for alcohol and 65% for drugs. Eight-seven percent of patients were male; only 4% of patients were privately insured. The authors concluded that during this 1-year study, gun-shot wound injuries required more orthopedic trauma resources than any other surgical areas.

Anglen JO: Wound irrigation in musculoskeletal injury. J Am Acad Orthop Surg 2001;9:219.[PMID: 11476531]

Bae DS, Kadiyala RK, Waters PM: Acute compartment syndrome in children: Contemporary diagnosis, treatment and outcome. J Pediatr Orthop 2001;21:680.[PMID: 11521042]

Bartlett CS: Ballistic and gunshot wounds: Effects on musculoskeletal tissues. J Am Acad Orthop Surg 2000;8:21.[PMID: 10666650]

Biffl WL, Smith WR, Moore EE, et al: Evolution of a multidisciplinary clinical pathway for the management of unstable patients with pelvic fractures. Ann Surg 2001;233(6):843–50.

Bone LB et al: Early vs delayed stabilization of femoral fracture. J Bone Joint Surg Am 1989;71A:336.[PMID: 2925704] Bone LB et al: Mortality in multiple trauma patients with fractures. J Trauma 1994;37:262.[PMID: 8064927]

Bosse MJ et al: Adult respiratory distress syndrome, pneumonia, and mortality following thoracic injury and a femoral fracture treated either with intramedullary nailing with reaming or with a plate. A comparative study. J Bone Joint Surg Am 1997;79:799.

Bosse MJ, Mackenzie EJ, Kellam JF, et al: A prospective evaluation of the clinical utility of the lower-extremity injury-severity scores. J Bone Joint Surg AM. 2001;83-A(1):3–14.

Brown TD et al: The impact of gunshot wounds on an orthopedic surgical service in an urban trauma center. J Orthop Trauma 1997;11:149.

Covey DC, Lurate RB, Hatton CT: Field hospital treatment of blast wounds of the musculoskeletal system during the Yugoslav civil war. J Orthop Trauma 2000;14: 278.[PMID: 10898201]

Dickson K et al: Outpatient management of low-velocity gunshot-induced fractures. Orthopedics 2001;24:951.[PMID: 11688773]

Dunham CM, Bosse MJ, Clancy TV et al: Practice management guidelines for the optimal timing of long-bone fracture stabilization in polytrauma patients: The EAST Practice Management Guidelines Work Group. J Trauma 2001;50(5):958.

Geerts W, Heit JA, Clagett GP et al. Prevention of venous thromboembolism. Chest 2001;119:132S.

Godina M: The tailored latissimus dorsi free flap. Plast Reconstr Surg 1987;80:304.[PMID: 3602183]

Gustilo RB, Anderson JT: Prevention of infection in the treatment of 1025 open fractures of long bones. J Bone Joint Surg Am 1976;58:453.[PMID: 773941]

Gustilo RB, Merkow RL, Templeman D: The management of open fractures. J Bone Joint Surg Am 1990;72:299.[PMID: 2406275]

Hammert WC, Minarchek J, Trzeciak MA: Free-flap reconstruction of traumatic lower extremity wounds. Am J Orthop 2000;29:22.[PMID: 11011776]

Johansen K et al: Objective criteria accurately predict amputation following lower extremity trauma. J Trauma 1990;30:568. [PMID: 2342140]

Koch A et al: Low molecular weight heparin and unfractionated heparin in thrombosis prophylaxis: Meta-analysis based on original patient data. Thromb Res 2001;102:295.[PMID: 11369423]

MacKenzie EJ et al: Characterization of patients with high-energy lower extremity trauma. J Orthop Trauma 2000;14:455. [PMID: 11083607]

Mendelson SA et al: Early versus late femoral fracture stabilization in multiply injured pediatric patients with closed head injury. J Ped Orthop 2001;21:594.[PMID: 11521025]

Mullett H et al: Outcome of compartment syndrome following intramedullary nailing of tibial diaphyseal fractures. Injury 2001;32:411.[PMID: 11382428]

Paiment GD, Mendelsohn C: The risk of venous thromboembolism in the orthopedic patient: Epidemiological and physiological data. Orthopedics. 1997;20:7.

Perrier A et al: Performance of helical computed tomography in unselected outpatients with suspected pulmonary embolism. Ann Int Med 2001;135:88.

Pierce TD, Tomaino MM: Use of the pedicled latissimus muscle flap for upper-extremity reconstruction. J Am Acad Orthop Surg 2000;8:324.[PMID: 11029560]

Reynolds MA et al: Is the timing of fracture fixation important for the patient with multiple trauma? Ann Surg 1995;222:470. [PMID: 7574927]

Scalea TM, Scott JD, Brumback RJ, et al: Early fracture fixation may be "just fine" after head injury: No difference in central nervous system outcomes. J Trauma 1999;46(5):839.

Shorr AF, Ramage AS: Enoxaparin for thromboprophylaxis after major trauma: Potential cost implications. Crit Care Med 2001;29:1659.[PMID: 11546959]

Slutsky AS: The acute respiratory distress syndrome, mechanical ventilation and the prone position. N Engl J Med 2001; 345:610.[PMID: 11529218]

Spain DA et al: Comparison of sequential compression devices and foot pumps for prophylaxis of deep venous thrombosis in high-risk trauma patients. Am Surg 1998;64:522. Discussion:525.[PMID: 9619172]

Stannard JP et al: Mechanical prophylaxis against deep-vein thrombosis after pelvic and acetabular fractures. J Bone Joint Surg Am 2001;83-A:1047.[PMID: 11451974]

Wells PS et al: Excluding pulmonary embolism at the bedside without diagnostic imaging: management of patients with suspected pulmonary embolism presenting to the emergency department by using a simple clinical model and D-dimer. Ann of Int Med 2001;135:98.

FAILURE OF FRACTURE HEALING

Union of a long bone has occurred when the fracture site is not painful or tender, loading produces no pain, there is no motion, radiographs show union, and there has been adequate time for healing. Many variables have an effect on the fracture healing process, including the site of the fracture, the blood supply to the site, whether the fracture is open or closed, the patient's age and nutritional status, and, possibly, medication use (eg, steroids, anticoagulants). In general, fractures will heal when the bone ends are in close apposition and the affected area has been adequately immobilized, has a good blood supply, is surrounded by a muscle envelope, and is not infected.

Nonunion of Fracture

Despite the best efforts and treatment, a certain percentage of fractures will fail to unite. The treatment of nonunited fractures has developed into a subspecialty area of orthopedic surgery. According to the Food and Drug Administration, **delayed union** of a long bone is defined as a fracture that has not gone on to full bony union after 6 months. **Nonunion** is less well defined. Clearly, a fracture that fails to show progressive evidence of healing over a 4- to 6-month period can be considered a nonunion. One can immediately declare a fracture with a 2-in. bony defect, for example, a nonunion, as one knows that bony reconstitution will not occur spontaneously if this fracture is simply left immobilized.

Generally, a fracture has united when there is radiographic evidence of bony bridging of the fracture on multiple projections. For a long bone this is the case if union can be confirmed on at least four projections. Clinical criteria, such as absence of motion and resolution of pain at the fracture site, while helpful, are much less sensitive in confirming that a fracture is healed.

A. REASONS FOR NONUNION

There are many reasons why a fracture might not heal. The two most common reasons are lack of adequate blood supply at the fracture site and inadequate stabilization of the fracture. Other less common reasons include soft-tissue interposition at the fracture site, fractures stabilized in an unacceptable amount of distraction, metabolic abnormalities, and infection. Infection at the fracture site does not in and of itself preclude a fracture from healing, but it can be a contributing cause to the development of nonunion. Rosen has outlined the known causes of nonunion (Table 3–2).

Table 3–2. Causes of nonunion.

1. Excessive motion: inadequate immobilization
2. Diastasis of fracture fragments
   a. Soft-tissue interposition
   b. Distraction from traction or internal fixation
   c. Malposition
   d. Loss of bone
3. Compromised blood supply
   a. Damage to nutrient vessels
   b. Stripping or injury to periosteum and muscle
   c. Free fragments; severe comminution
   d. Avascularity due to internal fixation devices
4. Infection
   a. Bone death (sequestrum)
   b. Osteolysis (GAP)
   c. loosening of implants (motion)
5. General: age, nutrition, steroids, anticoagulants, radiation, burns, predisposure to nonunion
6. Distraction from traction or internal fixation

Adapted and reproduced, with permission, from Rosen H: Treatment of nonunions: General principles. In: Chapman MW (editor): Operative Orthopedics, 2nd ed. Lippincott, 1988.

The location of the fracture is also an important factor in healing. Certain areas of the skeleton are more prone to developing nonunion, even when appropriate treatment is rendered. The distal tibial diaphysis, carpal navicular, and proximal diaphysis of the fifth metatarsal classically have a higher incidence of nonunion than other locations in the body. Fracture pattern also plays a role in the development of nonunion. Segmental fractures of long bones are much more prone to nonunion, as are fractures with large "butterfly" fragments, because of devascularization of the intermediary segment.

B. Classification of Nonunions

Nonunions have been classified according to their radiologic characteristics. The most widely used classification is that developed by Weber and Cech, who classified nonunion of long bones as being either hypertrophic or atrophic. They utilized standard radiographs and strontium isotope studies to differentiate these two categories. **Hypertrophic nonunions** have viable bone ends, whereas **atrophic nonunions** have nonviable bone ends. This differentiation has importance both in prognosis and in determining appropriate treatment. They further subdivided hypertrophic nonunions into "elephant's foot type," "horse's foot type," and oligotrophic nonunions (Figure 3–1). It is somewhat confusing as to what actually causes a viable hypertrophic nonunion to behave by laying down exuberant callus (elephant's foot type) versus no callus (oligotrophic type.) As a generalization, those nonunions with better blood supply and some degree of

micromotion at the fracture site develop more callus, while those with either no motion, excess motion, or distraction and a less rich blood supply produce less callus.

C. Complications of Nonunion

Grossly mobile hypertrophic or atrophic nonunions that are left untreated for an extended period often develop into a pseudarthrosis (false joint) (Figure 3–2). There is an actual synovial-lined capsule enveloping the bone ends. Synovial fluid is present in the cleft. As a joint now exists between the ununited bone ends, surgical intervention is the only treatment option available.

D. Treatment

Once nonunion has been established, the physician must establish treatment goals. The joints above and below the nonunion must be evaluated to determine their function and motion. The degree of shortening or deformity of the affected limb must also be determined. One must also determine the general health of the patient as well as the degree of functional impairment the patient is actually experiencing. This is especially important as some patients are actually asymptomatic and therefore do not warrant treatment. In the sick or elderly, treatment must also be tailored, as these patients may not be able to safely tolerate surgical intervention.

1. Stimulation of osteogenesis by external forces— It is now known that several pathways exist to stimulate healing of nonunion. The pathways can be divided into the type of force required to stimulate osteogenesis. These inductive forces can be categorized as mechanical, electrical, and chemical and can be applied with varying success both operatively and nonoperatively.

   a. Mechanical forces—Application of mechanical forces to achieve bony union has remained the most time-honored, well-tested method to date. Sarmiento has shown that the use of functional bracing incorporated with weight bearing can lead to union of documented tibial nonunions. His results for treating femoral nonunions were less successful using this method. Cyclic mechanical force of ambulation while the fracture reduction is maintained with an external support is the presumed mechanism with which fracture healing is achieved without surgical intervention.

   Mechanical forces can also be generated by surgical means. Mechanical stabilization of a long bone nonunion can be achieved either by placement of an intramedullary rod or compression plating. The rod works by providing mechanical stabilization of the fracture, hence allowing for cyclic axial loading of the limb without shearing forces caused by weight bearing. The compression plate provides stability as well as immediate rigid compression across the fracture fragments.

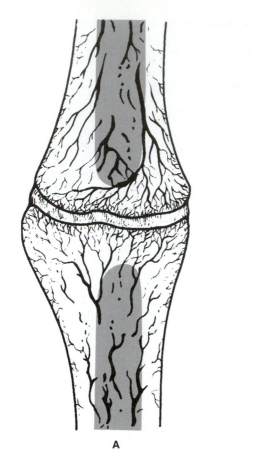 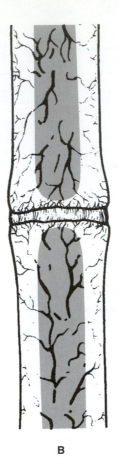 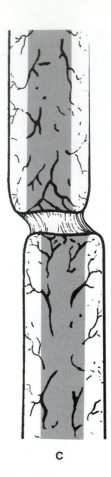

A   B   C

Figure 3–1. Weber and Cech's subclassification of hypertrophic nonunions: elephant's foot (**A**); horse's foot (**B**); oligotrophic (**C**) (This can often resemble atrophic nonunion and is hard to distinguish.) (Reprinted, with permission, from Browner BD et al (editors): Skeletal Trauma, 2nd ed. Philadelphia: WB Saunders, 1998.)

These forms of treatment are often all that is necessary in elephant's foot type nonunions.

b. Electrical forces—Electrical fields have also been shown to stimulate the dormant chondrocytes and mesenchymal cells in the nonunion cleft to "turn on" and produce bone that results in healing. The mechanism of why this occurs has been postulated but to date is not well understood. Currently, most electrical bone growth stimulators used are external devices that are incorporated in a cast or functional brace around the site of nonunion. Surgically implanted devices with internal coils wrapped into the nonunion site have also been used with somewhat equivocal success. Sharrard showed in a controlled double-blind study that application of an external pulsed electromagnetic field led to a statistically significant increase in healing of documented delayed tibial unions as compared with a control group. New

interest in this field is now focusing on the use of nonpulsed electromagnetic fields and ultrasound. Nonunions being treated with adjuvant electrical fields are in fact being treated with mechanical forces as well, as these fractures are usually immobilized and weight bearing is often allowed on the affected limb.

c. Chemical forces—Chemical modulators also play an important role in promoting nonunion healing. Application of autogenous cancellous bone graft (most frequently obtained from the iliac crest) is a potent stimulator of fracture healing. As a rigid nonunion will heal with autogenous bone grafting alone and no internal fixation, it is apparent that chemical modulators from the grafted cancellous bone are responsible for stimulating the healing response. There has been recent intense interest in determining the growth factors present in this cancellous bone responsible for "turning on" the healing process. Some surgeons have even reported success by

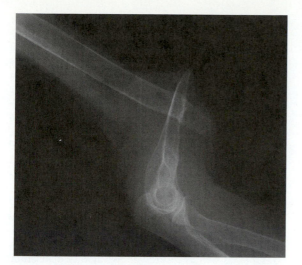

Figure 3–2. Fourteen-year-old distal humeral pseudarthrosis left untreated in an 89-year-old female. All motion about the elbow is occurring through the pseudarthrosis, as the elbow ankylosed.

obtaining bone marrow via a large-bore needle from the iliac crest and injecting this into the nonunion site. In the future, it is likely that the humoral modulator responsible will be isolated, synthesized in sufficient quantities by genetic engineering techniques, and simply injected into nonunion clefts to attain union.

d. Pathways of simulation—It is interesting to note that although three separate forces exist that can stimulate healing, it is unknown whether they act via a common pathway. As often happens in the body, these forces could actually work by different pathways so as to allow for some duplicity to help ensure that most fractures will heal.

2. Atrophic nonunions—Atrophic nonunions are not as easily treated as hypertrophic nonunions, and fewer treatment options are available. Electrical stimulation and nonoperative treatment methods have not been effective. The treatment most commonly utilized, and most successful, is "freshening up" of the avascular bone ends, combined with rigid internal fixation and autogenous bone grafting. This same procedure is used in treating pseudarthroses.

The Ilizarov method has also shown great success in the treatment of complex hypertrophic and atrophic nonunions, sometimes in combination with autogenous bone grafting. This method allows not only for achievement of bony union but also for treatment of any accompanying deformity, segmental bone loss, or shortening that may be present.

Malunion of Fracture

A fracture that has healed with an unacceptable amount of angulation, rotation, or overriding that has resulted in shortening of the limb is defined as malunion. Shortening is better tolerated in the upper than the lower extremity, and angulatory deformities are better tolerated in bones such as the humerus than in the femur or tibia. Hence, no absolute guidelines can be given as to an acceptable versus an unacceptable malunion. Generally, shortening greater than 1 in. is poorly tolerated in the lower extremity. Smaller discrepancies, however, are well treated with just a shoe lift in most situations. When the degree of deformity is sufficient to cause pain (eg, caused by walking on the side of the foot secondary to varus malunion of the distal tibia) or impair normal function, then surgical correction of the malunion is indicated.

When correction of malunion is undertaken, proper preoperative planning is imperative. One must determine the true mechanical axis of the limb to determine the actual site of deformity. If an osteotomy is performed, the surgeon must decide whether to use a closing wedge (where a wedge of bone is removed) or an opening wedge (where a wedge of autogenous or allograft bone is added). This is important, as it will alter the limb length. If the limb is already short, the surgery should also include a limb-lengthening procedure. Proper fixation and often autogenous cancellous bone grafting should be incorporated to ensure that the osteotomy heals, for converting a malunion to a nonunion is only worsening an already bad situation. Special care must be paid to treatment of the soft tissues to prevent wound breakdown and infection.

Determination of the true plane of deformity is essential in planning for the surgical correction. Green and associates have shown in tibial malunions and nonunions that it is rare for the plane of deformity to be in the true sagittal or coronal plane. The true degree of deformity is therefore not fully appreciated on anterior to posterior and lateral radiographs, as the axis is usually in a plane somewhere between these. Thus, treatment of malunions can be appreciated as a difficult task that requires careful planning and execution to achieve anatomic results.

Ilizarov Method

The Ilizarov apparatus and the concepts of distraction osteogenesis have dramatically revolutionized the application of the principles of external fixation in the management of bony defects, nonunions, malunions, pseudarthroses, and osteomyelitis. Since its introduction in Kurgan, Siberia, in 1951 by Gavril A. Ilizarov, surgeons throughout the world have employed this method to pioneer modern limb salvaging and lengthening procedures. This method has numerous advantages, including immediate loading of the limb postoperatively and the use of healthy viable bone to replace devascularized bone in situ by corticotomy, localized transport, and osteogenesis. Accordingly, leg length discrepancy, deformity, nonunions, and infections may all be treated effectively.

The basic premise of the Ilizarov technique is that osteogenesis can occur at a specially controlled osteotomy site (referred to as a **corticotomy**), given the appropriate degree of retained vascularity, fixation, and quantified distraction. Ilizarov realized that healing and neogenesis both required a dynamic state, which could occur in either controlled distraction or compression. This dogma is a function of many principles that Ilizarov classified into three categories: biologic, clinical, and technical. Important biologic concepts include preservation of endosteal and periosteal blood supply via corticotomy and stable fixation. Ilizarov fixation prevents shearing forces but permits axial micromotion with postoperative weight bearing, which enhances bone formation. Distraction osteogenesis occurs at a rate of approximately 1 mm/day. Division of distraction into four equal increments appears to be more physiologically sound than one distraction per day, as used previously in lengthening procedures. At the termination of distraction, neutral fixation is required to allow maturation, calcification, and strengthening of the new bone. In essence, the technique fools the body into believing it is a child again, with the corticotomy site acting as a physis.

Clinical principles such as the geometry of the apparatus once it is constructed, adjustment of the rate of transport, and wound care directly affect the outcome of the procedure. The initial operation for the application of the apparatus is only one small part in the whole treatment scheme. The construct should be as safe and comfortable as possible because it will be worn by the patient for an extended period of time. Pin tract infections are common and must be addressed aggressively with oral antibiotics and local pin care.

From a technical viewpoint, Ilizarov methodology relies on the use of an extremely rigid (in all planes except the axial loading plane), extremely versatile external fixator, employing K-wire fixation under tension. It is this "tension stress" phenomenon of gradually controlled distraction of bone ends at the corticotomy site that makes possible the limb lengthening or osteogenesis required in bone transport. Neogenesis of the accompanying soft tissues, including vessels, nerves, muscle, and skin, also occurs. Likewise, because of the dynamic nature of the apparatus, constant high loads of compression can be maintained across fracture sites to help stimulate fracture healing.

During distraction osteogenesis, the new tissues are aligned parallel to the distraction force vector. Accordingly, the surgeon has fine control over the direction of the regenerating bone. Ilizarov noted that tension stress neogenesis was similar to the natural conditions present in musculoskeletal growth. Mesenchymal cells fill the early distraction gap and soon differentiate into osteoblasts. A hyperemic state exists during distraction osteogenesis, with abundant neovascularization in the distraction gap. The overall blood flow to the affected limb is also increased up to 40%.

As noted earlier, the circular external fixator is attached to the limb using wires under tension. Two diameters of wires are used: 1.5 mm in small children and in upper extremities in adults, and 1.8 mm (twice as stiff in bending) in lower extremities in adults and adolescents. Beaded wires (olive wires) are utilized for bony transport, as well as to provide for rigidity of fixation, to prevent unwanted translation of the bone on the frame. An appropriately applied frame on the lower extremity should allow full weight bearing on the limb, irrespective of the extent of the bony defect present. In fact, Ilizarov felt that ambulation and the restoration of function to the limb were essential to achieve good bone regeneration and union. This cyclic axial loading of the affected limb is a crucial element of the Ilizarov method.

With the incorporation of hinges, plates, rods, and other elements, correction of a deformity can be accomplished in any plane. Hence, the apparatus has become an increasingly useful tool in the treatment of congenital, acquired, and posttraumatic limb deformities, as well as nonunion and malunion. What makes this treatment method unique is that all problems affecting a limb can be managed with the application of one apparatus. For instance, nonunion of the tibia with angulatory deformity and 5 cm of shortening can often be successfully treated with one operation. The surgery would entail application of the Ilizarov apparatus with either acute correction of the angulatory deformity or gradual correction via application of hinges. A corticotomy of the tibia is also performed at the time of surgery to proceed with distraction osteogenesis to restore the 5 cm of limb length. The nonunion is then compressed (once properly aligned) to achieve bony union. The lengthening of the limb is occurring at the same time that the nonunion is being compressed. Ilizarov also found that certain more rigid nonunions could actually heal in distraction. Therefore another treatment approach in the previous example would be primary gradual controlled distraction across the nonunion site for the purpose both of achieving bony union and restoring some of the limb length at the nonunion site. In essence, Ilizarov found that with few exceptions, healing could occur as long as a dynamic force, be it compression or distraction, was properly applied across a nonunion site. This dynamic force, when properly applied, causes the dormant mesenchymal cells in the nonunion gap to differentiate into functioning osteoblasts and allow for bone synthesis and resultant healing.

The Ilizarov method has revolutionized thinking about fracture healing and osteogenesis. It has greatly broadened the scope and indications for limb lengthening and has incorporated limb lengthening as a tool in both fracture and nonunion management. Ilizarov's introduction of the concept of distraction osteogenesis and the tension stress effect have changed Western thinking regarding limb lengthening and fracture healing. Close adherence to Ilizarov's principles makes it now possible to successfully treat a host of orthopedic conditions that previously were fraught with high morbidity rates and poor results. As experience broadens, application of the Ilizarov method will continue to grow.

Bhandari M et al: Reamed versus nonreamed intramedullary nailing of lower extremity long bone fractures: A systematic overview and meta-analysis. J Orthop Trauma 2000;14:2. [PMID: 10630795]

Einhorn TA, Lee CA: Bone regeneration: new findings and potential clinical applications. J Am Acad Orthop Surg 2001; 9:157.[PMID: 11421573]

Hak DJ, Lee SS, Goulet JA: Success of exchange reamed intramedullary nailing for femoral shaft nonunion or delayed union. J Orthop Trauma 2000;14:178.[PMID: 10791668]

Hupel TM et al: Effect of unreamed, limited reamed, and standard reamed intramedullary nailing on cortical bone porosity and new bone formation. J Orthop Trauma 2001;15:18. [PMID:11147683]

Ilizarov GA: The significance of the combination of optimal mechanical and biological factors in the regenerate process of transosseous synthesis. In: Abstracts of First International Symposium on Experimental, Theoretical, and Clinical Aspects of Transosseous Osteosynthesis Method Developed in Kniekot, Kurgan, USSR, September 20–23, 1983.

Ilizarov GA: Transosseous Osteosynthesis. Springer-Verlag, 1992.

Lowenberg DW, Randall RL: The Ilizarov method. In: Braverman MH, Tawes RL (eds): Surgical Technology International II, 1993.

Paley D, Maar DC: Ilizarov bone transport treatment for tibial defects. J Orthop Trauma 2000;14:76.[PMID: 10716377]

Weresh MJ et al: Failure of exchange reamed intramedullary nails for ununited femoral shaft fractures. J Orthop Trauma 2000; 14:335.[PMID: 11029556]

PRINCIPLES OF OPERATIVE FRACTURE FIXATION

Fractures occur when one or more types of stress, in excess of failure strength, are applied to bones. Fractures may occur from axial loading (tension, compression), bending, torsion (a means of applying shearing stress),

or shearing. All of these are observed at one time or another. It is frequently (but not always) helpful to recognize the type of failure in order to treat the fracture. Examples of these mechanisms are shown in Figure 3–3.

Biomaterials Used in Fracture Fixation

Operative fracture fixation requires strength and flexibility of the fixation materials. Two materials found to be useful in these regards are titanium alloy and stainless steel, both of which may be contoured to fit irregularities in bone surfaces at the time of surgery. They provide adequate strength and fatigue resistance to allow fracture healing to occur. The elastic modulus of titanium is half that of stainless steel, resulting in half the flexural rigidity in plates of equal size. Although it is recognized that more flexible devices decrease the disuse osteopenia underneath the plates, a clinical advantage of this difference has not been demonstrated. Other potential materials, including composites, cannot be contoured in the operative suite for particular applications.

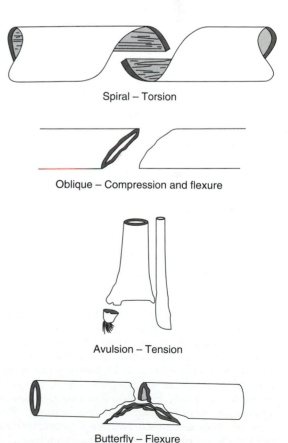

Spiral – Torsion

Oblique – Compression and flexure

Avulsion – Tension

Butterfly – Flexure

Figure 3–3. Mechanisms of failure of bones.

Biomechanical Principles of Fracture Fixation

The principles of operative fracture fixation are demonstrated by several examples described here. These examples illustrate the importance of the location of a bone plate on a bone in relation to the loading applied to the bone and plate composite. They will demonstrate the bending stiffness of bone plates as a function of thickness and the load sharing that goes on between bone plates in bone. In addition, the effect of bending on the composite of an intramedullary rod and bone will be examined.

A. BONE PLATE THICKNESS

One approach to solving the problem of bone plate fractures is to increase the thickness of the plate. If a bone plate is subjected to bending stress, the stress in the plate, assuming no loading is carried by the bone, can be calculated from the flexure formula: $s_{max} = Mc/I$, where M is the bending moment applied to the plate, c is one-half the thickness of the plate, and the area moment of inertia, I, is expressed by

$$\frac{bh^3}{12}$$

where h is the thickness of plate and b is the width of the plate. The maximum stress would then be equal to

$$s_{max} = \frac{6M}{bh^2}$$

because c is equal to one-half of h. Doubling the thickness decreases the stress to

$$\frac{6M}{4bh^2}$$

Thus, increasing the thickness of the plate by a factor of 2 reduces the stress by a factor of 4, meaning that the load would have to be four times higher before the failure stress would be reached. If one considers the area moment of inertia, I, to be proportional to the bending stiffness, then doubling the size of the plate would double h, which would mean that the plate is eight times stiffer (but only four times stronger). Because the endurance limit of steel is approximately one-half the ultimate strength, four times higher cyclic loads can be tolerated without fear of failure caused by fatigue.

B. TITANIUM AND STAINLESS STEEL RODS

The second consideration is the difference in the stress carried by an intramedullary rod made of titanium alloy as compared with one constructed of stainless steel. Assume a tibia is a round bone with a hollow, round intramedullary canal 10 mm in diameter. The flexural rigidity is defined as the area moment of inertia times the elastic modulus. A higher flexural rigidity indicates a greater resistance to bending. The area moment of inertia of a thin tube is

$$p^3 \, r^3_{ave} t$$

where r is the average radius and t is thickness. Assuming this equation holds for bone also, the ratio of the flexural rigidity of the intramedullary rod to the bone is expressed by the equation

$$\frac{E_m I_m}{E_b I_b} = \frac{r^3_m t_m E_m}{r^3_b t_b E_b}$$

The r_{ave} for the metal is 5 mm and for the bone 7.5 mm; t_m is 1 mm and t_b is 5 mm. The ratio E_m/E_b is approximately 10 for stainless steel and 5 for titanium alloy. Thus, the flexural rigidity ratio is

$$\frac{E_m I_m}{E_b I_b} = 0.60 \text{ for stainless steel}$$

$$= 0.30 \text{ for titanium alloy}$$

This indicates that the geometric contribution to stiffness of the construct is greater for bone than for metal. Thus, for a stainless steel rod, the bone and metal rod share the bending stress after healing in a 60:40 ratio, respectively, (75:25 for titanium alloy). It can be seen that the bone is much stiffer than titanium alloy or stainless steel alloy rods. The difference between the two metals is probably not significant for bone remodeling, but maximum strength of the bone would be attained by removal in either case.

C. BONE PLATE

The placement of a plate on a bone has a significant bearing on its function. For example, on a curved bone such as the femur, which bows anteriorly, placement of the plate anteriorly tends to place the plate in tension and the posterior cortex of the femur in compression, owing to muscle action of the hamstrings and quadriceps. Conversely, placement of a plate posteriorly tends to cause the fracture to gap open anteriorly because of muscle action. This means that the bone in posterior placement is bearing none of the bending stress resulting from muscle forces and the bone plate has to resist all of this loading. When the bone plate is placed laterally, the axis of bending bisects the broad aspect of the plate, and thus the bone plate is much more able to tolerate the stress caused by muscle load. The plate, however, is susceptible to high stresses if abduction forces are applied to the femur or lower extremity. Thus, optimal placement of a bone plate is on the tension side of the bone, so that the bone will be placed in compressive loading as a result of muscle action. This stimulates healing and minimizes the stresses on the bone plate.

D. External Fixation

External fixation is an important treatment modality for musculoskeletal injuries. The basic principles are that pins are placed within the musculoskeletal system proximal and distal to the zone of injury. These pins are then placed on an external frame, a frame outside the confines of the bone and soft-tissue envelope to stabilize fractures. These devices can be useful as temporary treatment for musculoskeletal injuries, or as definitive treatment, depending on their location and the type of bone and soft-tissue trauma. In the upper extremity, they play a significant role in treating comminuted distal radius fractures by providing both provisional and definitive stabilization for healing as well as provisional treatment for grade III open fractures with segmental bone loss and large soft-tissue injuries in the forearm, elbow, and humerus.

For the pelvis, rapidly applied external fixation with compression for pelvic injuries can stabilize the pelvis, reduce blood loss, be of assistance in initial resuscitation, and provide definitive treatment of such injuries. In the lower extremity, external fixators are important in the treatment of tibia fractures, particularly open or comminuted fractures, and in the treatment of open forefoot injuries and femur injuries with segmental defects. For femur and tibia fractures, external fixation may provide excellent initial or provisional stabilization, which can then be followed by intramedullary fixation for definitive care.

These specific uses of external fixation will be discussed in the individual sections on specific fractures.

Bone Substitutes Used in Fracture Fixation

A. Autogenous Bone Grafting

The gold standard for bone grafting material to stimulate bone growth is cancellous bone from the iliac crest. Obtaining bone graft is a process with significant morbidity rates, frequently resulting in several hundred milliliters of blood loss, the possibility of infection, hernia, and, of course, discomfort. An alternative to autogenous bone grafting would obviate these problems.

B. Hydroxyapatite and Other Materials

Hydroxyapatite and tricalcium phosphate have been suggested for this process, but they have been found to be only osteoconductive and, by themselves, do not stimulate bone formation. The Food and Drug Administration has recently approved a material that forms hydroxyapatite 15 min after two precursor materials are mixed together. This material can be injected into fracture sites to stabilize them from compressive loads. Another hydroxyapatite material is derived from coral, and has a porous structure that is conducive to osteoconduction. This material may be used to fill gaps, but additional material is necessary to stimulate bone growth. Another material composed of collagen and hydroxyapatite has been made available (Collagraft) for clinical use, but this material also requires autogenous bone marrow to stimulate bone grafting. It also has minimal structural properties.

C. Donor Bone Allografting

The third alternative bone substitute is allograft derived from living or cadaveric donors. Femoral heads obtained at the time of hip replacement provide a source of living donor bone. Bone collected in the same fashion as transplant organs can also be made available for transplantation. It should be noted that all allograft bone is not the same. Immunogenicity, sterility, mechanical properties, and bone stimulation potential are all dependent on the treatment the bone receives from the time of collection until the time of implantation. The highest risk bone, because of occult viral and bacterial contamination, is that collected in a sterile manner from cadaveric donors and delivered in a sterile manner without further sterilization or processing. This bone also has the highest potential for containing bone growth factors and, therefore, the ability to stimulate new bone formation. Sterilization treatments, such as irradiation and ethylene oxide, are known to compromise these qualities to some extent, with ethylene oxide perhaps being worse than irradiation. Freeze-dried bone is convenient for storage at room temperature but must be sterilized secondarily with ethylene oxide. Because ethylene oxide is unable to penetrate to the depths of large pieces, secondary sterilization of large structural allografts is safer with radiation. The accepted dosage of gamma radiation is 2.5 mrad, but even this dose may not be sufficient to eradicate the human immunodeficiency virus.

D. Bone Morphogenetic Proteins

Initially, bone substitutes consisted either of autogenous bone grafts, bone allografts, or material substitutes for bone growth such as hydroxyapatite. However, bone-derived protein extracts or bone morphogenic proteins (BMPs) have been identified as other important components of musculoskeletal repair for bone and cartilage growth. The identification of such specially purified BMPs, which had been shown to induce bone formation in a variety of ectopic and endogenous locations, has been coupled with recent advances in molecular biology and recombinant DNA techniques. Recombinant human bone morphogenic protein has been developed and has been undergoing human trials. These proteins can potentially be coupled with a collagen matrix and the addition of blood products from the patient to stimulate bone healing.

Cobos JA, Lindsey RW, Gugala Z: The cylindrical titanium mesh cage for treatment of a long bone segmental defect: description of a new technique and report of two cases. J Orthop Trauma 2000;14:54.[PMID: 10630804]

El Maraghy AW et al: Influence of the number of cortices on the stiffness of plate fixation of diaphyseal fractures. J Orthop Trauma 2001;15:186.[PMID: 11265009]

Kurdy NG: Serology of abnormal fracture healing: The role of PII-INP, PICP, and BsALP. J Orthop Trauma 2000;14:48. [PMID: 10630803]

MMWR 2002;51:207–210: Update: Allograft-associated bacterial infections—United States,2002. J Am Med Assoc 2002;287 (13):1642.

Radomisli TE et al: Weight-bearing alters the expression of collagen types I and II, BMP 2/4 and osteocalcin in the early stages of distraction osteogenesis. J Orthop Res 2001;19: 1049.[PMID: 11781004]

Spinella-Jaegle S et al: Opposite effects of bone morphogenetic protein-2 and transforming growth factor-beta I on osteoblast differentiation. Bone 2001;29:323.[PMID: 11595614]

Zlotolow DA et al: The role of human bone morphogenetic proteins in spinal fusion. J Am Acad Orthop Surg 2000;8:3. [PMID: 10666648]

I. TRAUMA TO THE UPPER EXTREMITY

FRACTURES & DISLOCATIONS OF THE FOREARM

Anatomy & Biomechanical Principles

The distal radius is shaped to articulate with the proximal carpal bones distally, and along its medial or ulnar border it articulates with the distal ulna. The distal radius therefore has three articular components (Figure 3–4): the scaphoid fossa, which allows articulation with the scaphoid; the lunate fossa, which allows articulation with the lunate; and the sigmoid notch, which allows articulation with the ulna. Between the scaphoid and the lunate fossa is a ridge that corresponds with the scapholunate interval. This entire surface is covered

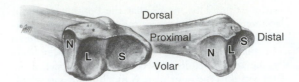

Figure 3–4. Articular components of the distal radius. L = lunate articular surface; N = sigmoid notch; S = scaphoid articular surface. (Reproduced, with permission, from Green DP, Hotchkiss RN, Pederson WC (editors): Operative Hand Surgery, 4th ed. Philadelphia: WB Saunders, 1999.)

with articular cartilage. The radial styloid allows attachment of the brachioradialis tendon. Also, it is the origin of several important wrist ligaments, including the radial scapholunate and radial lunocapitate ligaments.

The third articular component of the distal radius is the sigmoid notch. This convex structure allows the radius to rotate around the distal ulna. The distal ulna itself has an ulnar styloid, which contains attachments to the triangular fibrocartilage complex, including the meniscus homolog, the volar and dorsal ulnar carpal ligaments, and the ulnar collateral ligament at the wrist. The concave elliptical distal radius is oriented in the sagittal plane with an average of 11 degrees of volar tilt. In the frontal plane, the average radial inclination is 23 degrees. Radial length is measured from the tip of the radial styloid to the ulnar articular surface and averages 13 mm.

In addition to the bony surfaces, the articular cartilage, joint capsule, and wrist ligaments, there are other soft tissues within the distal forearm and wrist. On the dorsal surface, six dorsal compartments contain wrist and digital extensor tendons (Figure 3–5). On the volar surface reside the contents of the carpal canal, with nine flexor tendons and the median nerve. On the ulnar surface, the flexor carpi ulnaris tendon can be palpated near its insertion on the pisiform. The boundaries of the ulnar tunnel, or Guyon's canal, are the volar carpal ligament and transverse carpal ligament, the hook of the hamate radially and the pisiform ulnarly. Guyon's canal contains the ulnar artery and nerve. In the most superficial soft tissue layer of the wrist reside the flexor carpi radialis layers, flexor carpi ulnaris, and palmaris longus.

The radius and the ulna structurally support the forearm. The distal radius and ulna have specialized articulations with the carpus and with each other. The shafts of the radius and ulna are approximately parallel. The ulnar shaft, however, remains fixed in its rotation at the ulnohumeral joint, and the radius rotates around the ulna in pronation and supination. The radius has a lateral bow that is crucial to the maintenance of full pronation and supination.

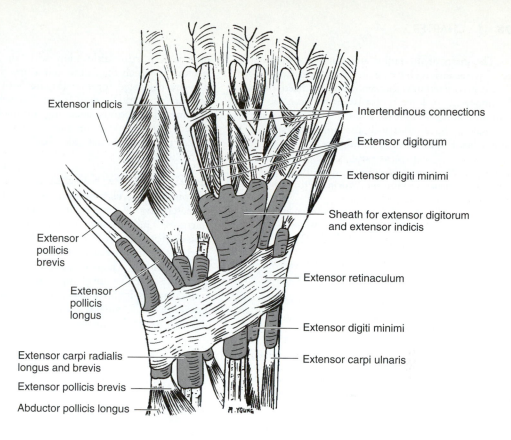

A

- Extensor indicis
- Intertendinous connections
- Extensor digitorum
- Extensor digiti minimi
- Sheath for extensor digitorum and extensor indicis
- Extensor pollicis brevis
- Extensor pollicis longus
- Extensor retinaculum
- Extensor digiti minimi
- Extensor carpi radialis longus and brevis
- Extensor carpi ulnaris
- Extensor pollicis brevis
- Abductor pollicis longus

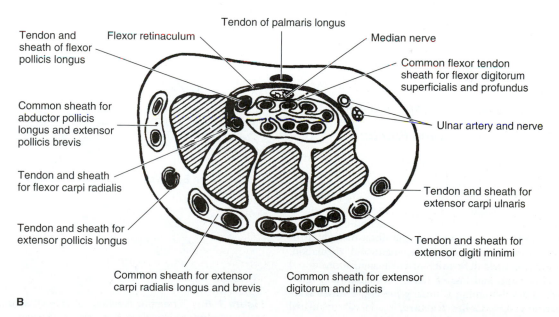

B

- Tendon and sheath of flexor pollicis longus
- Flexor retinaculum
- Tendon of palmaris longus
- Median nerve
- Common flexor tendon sheath for flexor digitorum superficialis and profundus
- Common sheath for abductor pollicis longus and extensor pollicis brevis
- Ulnar artery and nerve
- Tendon and sheath for flexor carpi radialis
- Tendon and sheath for extensor carpi ulnaris
- Tendon and sheath for extensor pollicis longus
- Tendon and sheath for extensor digiti minimi
- Common sheath for extensor carpi radialis longus and brevis
- Common sheath for extensor digitorum and indicis

Figure 3–5. **A:** Dorsal section of the wrist, showing the six dorsal compartments of the extensor tendons. **B:** Cross section of the wrist, showing the tendons, arteries, and nerves. (Reproduced, with permission, from Jenkins DB: Hollinshead's Functional Anatomy of the Limbs and Back, 6th ed. Philadelphia: WB Saunders, 1991.)

The shafts of the radius and ulna are connected by the interosseus membrane in the interosseous space. The central portion is thickened and has been shown to be important in force transmission between the radius and ulna. Origins of flexor and extensor muscles are located along the anterior and posterior surfaces of the radius, ulna, and interosseus membrane.

Berger RA: The anatomy of the ligaments of the wrist and distal radioulnar joints. Clin Orthop 2001;383:32.[PMID: 11210966]

Blazar PE et al: The effect of observer experience on magnetic resonance imaging interpretation and localization of triangular fibrocartilage complex lesions. J Hand Surg Am 2001;26: 742.[PMID: 11466652]

Cober SR, Trumble TE: Arthroscopic repair of triangular fibrocartilage complex injuries. Orthop Clin North Am 2001;32: 279.[PMID: 11331541]

Freeland AE, Geissler WB: The arthroscopic management of intra-articular distal radius fractures. Hand Surg 2000;5:93. [PMID:11301502]

Gupta R, Bozenthka DJ, Osterman AL: Wrist arthroscopy: Principles and clinical applications. J Am Acad Orthop Surg 2001; 9:200.[PMID: 11421577]

Lindau T, Adlercreutz C, Aspenberg P: Peripheral tears of the triangular fibrocartilage complex cause distal radioulnar joint instability after distal radial fractures. J Hand Surg Am 2000; 25:464.[PMID: 10811750]

McGinley JC et al: Mechanics of the antebrachial interosseous membrane: Response to shearing forces. J Hand Surg Am 2001;26:733.(PMID: 11466651)

Nakamura T et al: Origins and insertions of the triangular fibrocartilage complex: A histological study. J Hand Surg Br 2001; 26:446.(PMID: 11560427)

Poitevin LA: Anatomy and biomechanics of the interosseous membrane: Its importance in the longitudinal stability of the forearm. Hand Clin 2001;17:97.(PMID: 11280163)

DISTAL RADIUS & ULNA INJURIES

1. Distal Radius & Ulna Fracture

Classification of Fractures

Fractures of the distal radius account for approximately 14% of all fractures. In 1814, Abraham Colles described distal radius fracture prior to the advent of radiographs. In his purely descriptive definition, the fracture most commonly involves the distal metaphysis of the radius, with dorsal displacement and angulation. The **silver fork deformity** of volar angulation, dorsal displacement, and loss of radial inclination and resultant radial shortening is usually present. **Smith's fracture,** or **reverse Colles' fracture,** is a dorsally angulated fracture of the distal radius, with the hand and wrist displaced volarly with respect to the forearm. The fracture may be extra-articular, intra-articular, or a part of a fracture-dislocation involving the wrist. **Barton's fracture** is a fracture-dislocation with an intra-articular fracture in which the carpus and a rim of the distal radius are displaced together (Figure 3–6). **Chauffeur's fracture** is a radial styloid fracture, which initially was sustained by persons operating automobiles that required hand cranking to start. When the engine engaged, the crank would "kick back," and this fracture would result.

A. FRYKMAN CLASSIFICATION

No one fracture classification system is comprehensive in describing all important variables of distal radius fractures. The Frykman classification has been used to classify distal radius fractures. This system categorizes fractures by the presence or absence of an ulnar styloid fracture and by whether fracture lines are extra-articular, intra-articular involving the radial carpal joint, intra-articular involving the distal radioulnar joint, or intra-articular involving both radiocarpal and distal radioulnar joints (Figure 3–7).

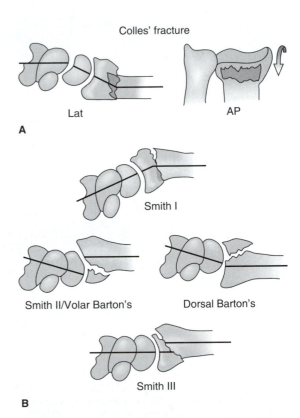

Figure 3–6. Schematic drawings of Colles' fracture (**A**) and Smith's and Barton's fractures (**B**). (Reproduced, with permission, from Green DP, Hotchkiss RN, Pederson WC (editors): Operative Hand Surgery, 4th ed. Philadelphia: WB Saunders, 1999.)

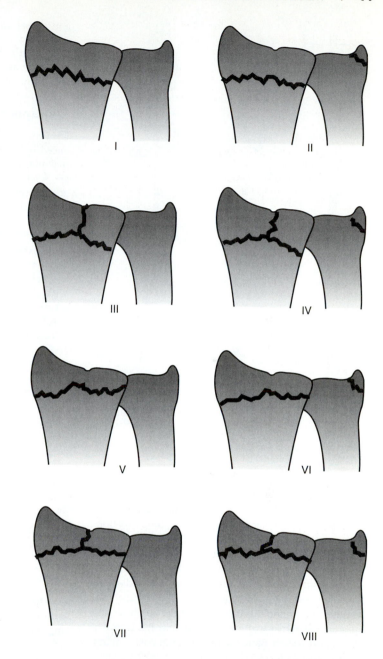

Figure 3–7. Classification of distal radius fractures according to Frykman. (Reproduced, with permission, from Green DP, Hotchkiss RN, Pederson WC, eds: Operative Hand Surgery, 4th ed. Philadelphia: WB Saunders, 1999.)

B. Arbeitsgemeinschaft für Osteosynthesefragen (AO) Association for the Study of Internal Fixation (ASIF) Classification

The AO classification is the most comprehensive system currently used to classify distal radius fractures. Broadly, distal radius fractures are separated into three groups: extra-articular (type A), partial articular (type B), and complete articular (type C). Within these are

subclassifications that relate to the particular amount of displacement and comminution (Figure 3–8).

C. Melone Classification

Another useful classification that addresses intra-articular fractures is that popularized by Melone (Figure 3–9). The Melone classification describes four major fracture components including the shaft, radial styloid,

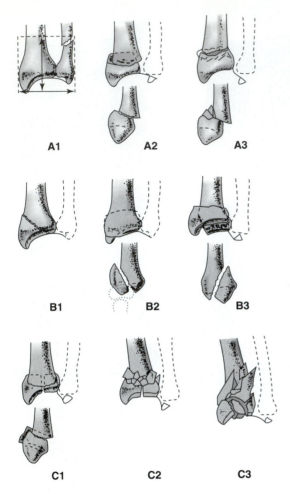

Figure 3–8. AO classification of distal radius fractures. **A:** Extra-articular metaphyseal fracture. Junction of the metaphysis and diaphysis is identified by the "square" or T method (greatest width on frontal plane of distal forearm; illustrated in A1). **A1:** Isolated fracture of distal ulna. **A2:** Simple radial fracture. **A3:** Radial fracture with metaphyseal impaction. **B:** Intra-articular rim fracture (preserving the continuity of the epiphysis and metaphysis). **B1:** Fracture of radial styloid. **B2:** Dorsal rim fracture (dorsal Barton's fracture). **B3:** Volar rim fracture (reverse Barton's 5 Goyrand-Smith type 2, Letenneur). **C:** Complex intra-articular fracture (disrupting the continuity of the epiphysis and metaphysis). **C1:** Radiocarpal joint congruity preserved, metaphysis fractured. **C2:** Articular displacement. **C3:** Diaphyseal-metaphyseal involvement. It should be considered that injury of the distal radioulnar joint is possible in any of these fractures. (Reproduced, with permission, from Green DP, Hotchkiss RN, Pederson WC, eds: Operative Hand Surgery, 4th ed. Philadelphia: WB Saunders, 1999.)

and dorsal and volar medial fragments. Often, the lunate fossa is fractured into dorsal and volar components, with the scaphoid fossa a separate component. Four-part articular fractures can have varying degrees of displacement and comminution.

Treatment

Treatment of distal radius fractures should be influenced by fracture pattern with a goal of restoring normal anatomy and articular surfaces. Factors to consider are fracture displacement, intra-articular components, angulation, and degree of comminution; age of the patient; and functional level.

A. Closed and Open Procedures

1. Closed reduction with splinting and casting—Extra-articular distal radius fractures in certain individuals (classic Colles' fracture) can be treated successfully with closed reduction and splinting with conversion to a cast once swelling subsides. Radial length is generally not fully restored, nor is radial angulation with closed reduction techniques. Small amounts of radial shortening can lead to increased load in the lunate fossa, distal ulna, and triangular fibrocartilage. In most low-demand patients, however, this treatment can be successful, and functional wrist motion can be obtained. If shortening is significant, midcarpal instability may occur. Another potential problem is distal radioulnar joint arthrosis and ulnar carpal abutment, which may necessitate later reconstruction.

2. Percutaneous pin fixation—Percutaneous pins can be an effective adjunct to cast treatment or external fixation. The pins can hold large metaphyseal fragments in good position and prevent collapse or malalignment. Another technique using percutaneous pins is the so-called **intrafocal pin technique,** in which the pin is placed in the fracture site itself. This can be an effective means of achieving anatomic alignment and preventing loss of reduction.

3. Open reduction and internal fixation with plate and screws—This can be extremely effective in achieving reduction. If bone fragments are large, it is also an effective way to maintain reduction. This technique has a tendency to fail, however, if there are multiple fragments and if there is sufficient comminution so that rigid internal fixation is difficult, or impossible, to achieve. Other drawbacks to this technique include creation of an incision, with potential subsequent scarring, and also the possibility of future hardware removal. Additionally, the operative technique involves soft-tissue stripping and potential devascularization of small fragments during the process of open reduction and internal fixation.

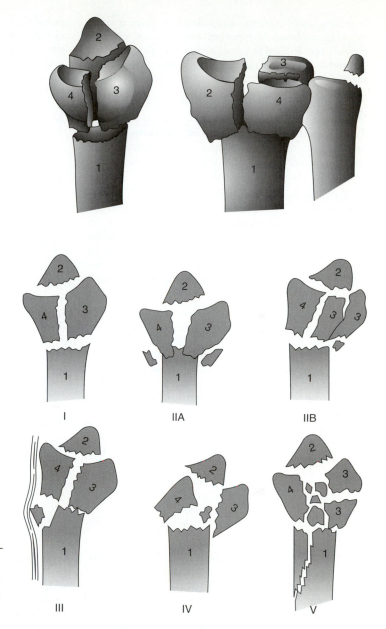

Figure 3–9. Intra-articular fracture classification of Melone. (Reproduced, with permission, from Green DP, Hotchkiss RN, Pederson WC, eds: Operative Hand Surgery, 4th ed. Philadelphia: WB Saunders, 1999.)

Recently, distal radius reconstruction plates have been devised with significant advances for distal radius osteosynthesis. These feature multiple small holes in a T configuration, allowing multiple screws for small fragment fixation. Many recent studies indicate that internal fixation with early postoperative range of motion leads to improved long-term results.

4. External fixation—External fixation is an extremely effective way to handle distal radius fractures.

In particular, it is a much more direct way of controlling the overall length of the distal radius, and to some extent the inclination, compared with cast treatment. Use of indirect traction on fracture fragments, taking advantage of "ligamentotaxis" via the fixator pins, can be effective. There is the additional advantage of not devascularizing the bony fragments and not creating a surgical wound. If there is an open wound that requires care, it can be handled with the external fixator in place. External fixation is effective in preventing loss of reduction and length in situations where there is comminution of bone. In intra-articular fractures, external fixation can be used in combination with percutaneous pin techniques or, if necessary, open reduction and internal fixation.

B. TREATMENT BASED ON CLASSIFICATION OF FRACTURES

1. Extra-articular nondisplaced fractures—Extra-articular nondisplaced fractures can be treated with simple cast immobilization for 6–8 weeks, until fracture healing occurs.

2. Extra-articular displaced fractures—Closed reduction should be attempted on extra-articular displaced fractures. If radial length and volar tilt are restored, then a splint or cast can be effective in holding the reduction. If the reduction is not adequate by closed means then an external fixator (for ligamentotaxis) or percutaneous pins (to manipulate the fracture) may be necessary.

3. Intra-articular rim fractures—Intra-articular rim fractures such as volar Barton's fracture or chauffeur's fracture are ideally treated by open reduction and internal fixation because there is an intact portion of metaphyseal and articular distal radius from which an intra-articular component has been fractured or displaced. If the fracture fragment can be reduced and aligned to the intact portion of distal radius, then articular congruity, length, and bony stability can all be achieved with open reduction and internal fixation. For volar Barton's fractures, the treatment of choice is the volar buttress plate. The only contraindications to this treatment are cases with excessive comminution such that open reduction and internal fixation will fail to achieve a stable bony construct. In these situations, use of an external fixator as a distractor and neutralization device is generally indicated.

4. Intra-articular comminuted fractures—Intra-articular comminuted fractures generally require surgical treatment to prevent shortening and restore the articular surface. The primary modality in most cases would be the external fixator to restore length. Using a fluoroscopy unit to visualize the fracture will help ascertain that both articular alignment and overall radial length have been adequately restored with external fixation alone. If minor adjustments are necessary, percutaneous pins can be an effective adjunct. These maneuvers may fail to achieve the appropriate articular alignment, particularly if some healing has already occurred or if the displacement is severe. In this case, open reduction and internal fixation should be performed. Justification for aggressive treatment of distal radius fractures in young patients comes from several studies. The goal should be articular step-off < 2 mm, radial shortening < 4 mm,

dorsal tilt < 15 degrees, volar tilt < 20 degrees and loss of radial inclination < 10 degrees. Arthroscopically assisted repair of distal radius fractures has been advocated by some as intra-articular step-off and associated injuries such as triangular fibrocartilage, scapholunate, and lunotriquetral tears as well as osteochondral lesions tears can be accurately assessed. Some authors advocate bone grafting in the acute treatment of comminuted fractures.

2. Distal Radioulnar Joint Dislocation

The distal radioulnar joint can be dislocated by a variety of mechanisms, including low- and high-energy trauma. These are associated with disruption of the ulnar soft-tissue triangular fibrocartilage complex, including the articular disk and associated ligaments. There should be a high index of suspicion in order to diagnose this lesion because radiographs that are not taken in the perfect lateral orientation will tend to look relatively normal.

Clinical Findings

The clinical examination is key, with identification of the distal radioulnar joint surface anatomy and clinical evaluation of the joint. The amount of stability should be carefully assessed and compared with that of the opposite wrist. This will help to diagnose subluxation, which is much more common than anterior or posterior dislocation. Limitation of pronation and supination, or pain associated with such motion, would be expected in such a situation. The other common cause of distal radioulnar joint problems is rheumatoid arthritis.

Treatment

Dorsal dislocation, or subluxation, should be treated by reduction of the ulnar head into the sigmoid fossa and placement of the forearm in full supination. The arm should be immobilized in supination, which requires a long-arm cast or splint. Volar dislocation is relatively rare and is usually stable after reduction. If dorsal or volar dislocation or subluxation of the distal ulna cannot be reduced with manipulation in the outpatient setting, closed treatment can be attempted under anesthesia. If this fails, open reduction and soft-tissue reconstruction may be necessary. If this is performed, a retinacular flap may be used to transpose the extensor carpi ulnaris to a more dorsal position to stabilize the distal ulna, as has been described for Darrach reconstruction of the joint.

3. Malunion of Distal Radius

Malunion of the distal radius can have a variety of negative consequences. Alteration of the biomechanical function of the wrist may lead to weakness, limitation of motion, and midcarpal instability. Associated distal radioulnar joint arthrosis may be present, as well as ulnocarpal abutment.

Treatment

The treatment of choice in such a situation, if conservative treatment such as steroid injections and splinting, hand therapy, and nonsteroidal anti-inflammatory agents fails, is reconstructive surgery. The strategy has been elegantly described by Fernandez. An osteotomy of the radius with iliac crest bone grafting and plate fixation is performed (Figure 3–10). The distal radioulnar joint must be addressed and, depending upon the degree of subluxation or arthrosis, may require closed reduction, open reduction, or reconstruction using the Darrach or Sauve-Kapandji procedures (Figure 3–11). In this procedure, instead of distal ulnar resection as in the Darrach procedure, transverse segmental resection of the ulnar metaphysis is followed by creation of an arthrodesis of the distal ulna to the radius, using the resected bone as grafting material. Forearm rotation occurs through the ulnar metaphyseal pseudoarthrosis. Additionally, restoration of the radial length may be difficult with manipulation alone. Useful adjuncts to achieve restoration of appropriate length and orientation in severe malunion include use of laminar spreaders to distract the proximal and distal fragments of the radius after osteotomy. Alternatively, an external fixator may prove useful in helping to achieve appropriate length after osteotomy.

If the distal radius has settled into a position of shortening and significant angulatory deformity but the fracture is not yet fully healed, osteotomy for early or "nascent" malunion is justified. The advantage of taking down a nascent malunion is that the operation is technically simpler to perform, shortens the time of disability, and leads to better long-term results. Additionally, the distal radioulnar joint can be restored more reliably in these early reconstructions than when osteotomy is required for established malunion. The latter often requires adjunctive distal radioulnar joint reconstruction with Darrach resection, Sauve-Kapanji, hemiresection, or matched resection arthroplasty.

Abboudi J, Culp RW: Treating fractures of the distal radius with arthroscopic assistance. Orthop Clin North Am 2001;32: 307.[PMID: 11331543]

Carter PB, Stuart PR: The Sauve-Kapandji procedure for post-traumatic disorders of the distal radio-ulnar joint. J Bone Joint Surg Br 2000;82:1013.[PMID: 11041592]

Chhabra A et al: Biomechanical efficacy of an internal fixator for treatment of distal radius fractures. Clin Orthop 2001;393: 318.[PMID: 11764365]

Goslings JC et al: Kinematics of the wrist with a new dynamic external fixation device. Clin Orthop 2001;386:226.[PMID: 11347841]

Jakob M, Rikli A, Regazzoni P: Fractures of the distal radius treated by internal fixation and early function. J Bone Joint Surg Br 2000;82-B:341.[PMID: 10813166]

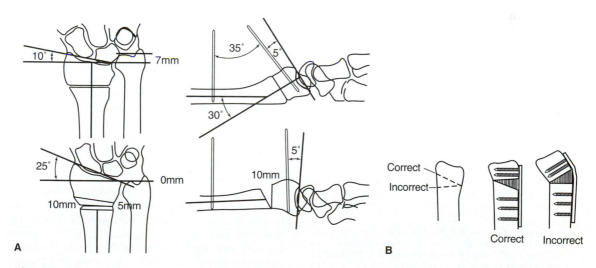

Figure 3–10. Wedge osteotomy of the distal radius with iliac crest bone graft and plate fixation. (Reproduced, with permission, from Green DP, Hotchkiss RN, Pederson WC, eds: Operative Hand Surgery, 4th ed. Philadelphia: WB Saunders, 1999.)

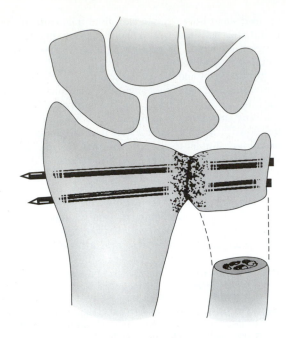

Figure 3–11. Suave-Kapandji reconstruction of the distal radioulnar joint. (Reproduced, with permission, from Green DP, Hotchkiss RN, Pederson WC, eds: Operative Hand Surgery, 4th ed. Philadelphia: WB Saunders, 1999.)

Katz MA et al: Computed tomography scanning of intra-articular distal radius fractures: Does it influence treatment. J Hand Surg Am 2001;26:415.[PMID: 11418901]

Ladd AL, Pliam NB: The role of bone graft and alternatives in unstable distal radius fracture treatment. Orthop Clin North Am 2001;32:337.[PMID: 11331546]

McKay SD et al: Assessment of complications of distal radius fractures and development of a complication checklist. J Hand Surg Am 2001;26:916.[PMID: 11561246]

Mehta JA, Bain GI, Heptinstall RJ: Anatomical reduction of intra-articular fractures of the distal radius. J Bone Joint Surg Br 2000;82-B:79.[PMID: 10697319]

Rogachefsky RA et al: Treatment of severely comminuted intra-articular fractures of the distal end of the radius by open reduction and combined internal and external fixation. J Bone Joint Surg Am 2001;83-A:509.[PMID: 11315779]

Schneeberger AG et al: Open reduction and plate fixation of displaced AO type C3 fractures of the distal radius: Restoration of articular congruity in eighteen cases. J Orthop Trauma 2001;15:350.[PMID: 11436021]

Viso R, Wegener EE, Freeland AE: Use of a closing wedge osteotomy to correct malunion of dorsally displaced extra-articular distal radius fractures. Orthopedics 2000;23:721. [PMID: 10917249]

Wakefield AE, McQueen MM: The role of physiotherapy and clinical predictors of outcome after fracture of the distal radius. J Bone Joint Surg Br 2000;82-B:972.[PMID: 11041584]

DISLOCATION OF THE RADIOCARPAL JOINT

Dislocation of the radiocarpal joint is usually accompanied by significant carpal-ligamentous injury or fracture. Treatment of these injuries involves restoration of the bony architecture through immediate closed reduction, if possible, elective closed reduction, open reduction and internal fixation, or a combination of these procedures. Associated fractures, such as transscaphoid-perilunate or distal radius fracture associated with carpal dislocation, should be treated with open reduction and internal fixation. Ligamentous repair should be performed at this time (see Chapter 10, Hand Surgery). Median nerve evaluation is mandatory, and surgical exploration indicated, if a dense neuropathy is present.

FOREARM SHAFT FRACTURES

In general, any fracture requires evaluation both clinically and radiographically of a joint above and joint below the fracture. It is not uncommon for fractures of the midshaft of the forearm to have significant consequences to either the wrist or elbow

1. Isolated Fracture of the Ulna (Nightstick Fracture)

Nondisplaced or minimally displaced fractures of the ulnar shaft are fairly common and usually result from a direct blow.

Treatment

A variety of treatment options are possible for managing minimally displaced ulnar diaphyseal injuries. The time to union is about 3 months, with union achieved with cast immobilization and early mobilization of the wrist and elbow. Less stringent immobilization protocols have also resulted in satisfactory results. Sarmiento and Lotto achieved excellent results using a functional sleeve for isolated ulnar fractures. After initial long arm cast fixation for immobilization until acute symptoms and swelling have subsided, cast removal is followed by Orthoplast sleeve or cast bracing with Velcro straps, with no limitation of pronation and supination. Some investigators report excellent results with minimal or no immobilization. In general, some sort of immobilization until pain subsides is preferable. With displaced fractures with angulation greater than 10 degrees or displacement greater than 50%, one must be extremely suspicious of an associated injury at the elbow or wrist. In isolated fractures of the ulna in the adult with displacement > 50% or angulation > 10 degrees (or both), open reduction and internal fixation is the treatment of choice. Current recommendations include fixation with a dynamic or limited contact compression plate with six to eight cortices of fixation proximal and distal to the fracture.

2. Isolated Radial Shaft Fractures

A fracture anywhere along the length of the radius with or without associated ulnar fracture with injury to the distal radioulnar joint(DRUJ) is defined as a Galeazzi fracture. Injuries associated with the DRUJ include ulnar styloid fractures, radial shortening > 5 mm, and DRUJ dislocation.

Treatment

Open reduction and internal fixation with plate fixation is recommended in adult patients to ensure a reasonable chance of restoration of the distal radioulnar joint. Hughston's series in 1957 had a 92% incidence of poor results with closed treatment. After open reduction and internal fixation of the radial shaft through a volar Henry approach using compression plating, the distal radioulnar joint should be carefully inspected. If it is unstable, pinning in a position of stability (usually full supination) is required. If it is frankly dislocated and cannot be reduced, closed, and maintained by closed or percutaneous means, then open stabilization with repair of associated ligaments or removal of interposed soft tissue is mandatory.

3. Monteggia Fracture

Classification of Fractures

In 1814, Monteggia of Milan described an injury involving fracture of the proximal third of the ulna, with anterior dislocation of the radial head. This definition was extended by Bado to include the entire spectrum of these fractures with associated radial head dislocations, regardless of the direction of dislocation. They are classified in the following ways:

Type 1: Fracture of the ulnar diaphysis with anterior angulation and anterior dislocation of the radial head (60% of cases)

Type 2: Fracture of the ulnar diaphysis with posterior angulation or posterior or posterolateral dislocation of the radial head (15% of cases)

Type 3: Fracture of the ulnar metaphysis, with lateral or anterolateral dislocation of the radial head (20% of cases)

Type 4: Fracture of the ulna and radius at the proximal third, with anterior dislocation of the radial head (5% of cases)

Other authors have noted that type 3 fractures may be more common than type 2 fractures, but all agree that type 1 lesions are the most common.

Associated lesions include injury to the radial nerve; palsies of both the deep branch of the radial nerve and the posterior interosseous nerve have been described with Monteggia fractures. It is important to perform an adequate neurovascular examination at the time of evaluation. The index of suspicion must be high because radial head dislocation may be missed if appropriate radiographs are not obtained and scrutinized.

Treatment

Closed treatment is usually satisfactory for children, but open reduction and internal fixation is the treatment of choice for Monteggia lesions in an adult. Optimal results require early diagnosis, rigid internal fixation of the fractured ulna, complete reduction of the dislocated radial head, and immobilization for approximately 6 weeks to allow healing with sufficient stability. Internal fixation is best performed with a compression plate technique. The radial head can often be completely reduced by closed means once the ulnar fracture is reduced and rigidly fixed. If this is not possible, open reduction is required; attention should be paid to the relationship between the annular ligament, the lateral epicondyle, and the radial head. Entrapment of the soft tissues is the most common reason for inability to obtain concomitant closed radial head reduction at the time of open reduction and internal fixation of the ulna.

4. Fractures of Both the Radius & Ulna

Fractures of both the radius and ulna (both-bones fractures) usually result from high-energy injuries. These fractures are usually displaced because of the force required to produce such an injury. Careful neurovascular examination and adequate radiographs to show both the wrist and the elbow are mandatory.

Treatment

Treatment of choice for both-bones fractures is open reduction and internal fixation. The volar Henry approach should be used, between the flexor carpi radialis and brachioradialis, with the ulna approached subcutaneously. Open reduction and internal fixation offers the best chance of restoring the normal positions of the radius and ulna, which is critical to forearm function and in particular pronation and supination. For fractures of the proximal half of the radius, the dorsal Thompson approach can be used; however, the risk of iatrogenic injury to the posterior interosseous nerve is increased Technical points to be considered include subperiosteal stripping only of the fracture site. The plates can be placed on top of the periosteum to preserve the blood supply as much as possible. A 3.5-mm dynamic compression plate or limited contact compression plate can be used for AO/ASIF compression plating. Bone grafting can be used for severely comminuted fractures with significant bone loss. Only the skin is closed so as not to cause compartment syndrome or Volkmann's contracture. Splinting of the affected extremity, as in all upper extremity surgery, is recommended, with early digital active and passive motion exercises.

Many authors recommend plate fixation for Gustilo type I, II, and IIIA open both-bones fractures. Use of an external fixator is a viable alternative, however, particularly if severe open wounds are present with skin and soft-tissue loss as in Gustilo type IIIB and IIIC injuries. Criteria for bone grafting include comminution involving more than one third the cortical circumference and comminution that compromises interfragmentary compression; however, the success of acute bone grafting has not been proved in long-term studies.

Chung KC, Spilson SV: The frequency and epidemiology of hand and forearm fractures in the United States. J Hand Surg Am 2001;26:908.[PMID: 11561245]

Dell'Oca AA et al: Treating forearm fractures using an internal fixator. Clin Orthop 2001;389:196.[PMID: 11501811]

Iqbal MJ, Abbas: Distal radioulnar synostosis following K-wire fixation. Orthopedics 2001;24:61.[PMID: 11199355]

Qidwai SA: Treatment of diaphyseal forearm fractures in children by intramedullary Kirschner wires. J Trauma 2001;50:303. [PMID: 11242296]

INJURIES AROUND THE ELBOW

Anatomy & Biomechanical Principles

Accessible surface structures at the elbow that can be inspected and palpated include the medial and lateral condyles and the olecranon. With the elbow in 90 degrees of flexion, these three palpable points form a triangle. Distally, the radial head can be palpated at the lateral aspect of the elbow joint, and the contour can be appreciated with pronation and supination. These bony landmarks are important when clinically assessing the elbow for fractures, dislocations, or effusions. Effusions can be discerned by swelling between the lateral epicondyle and the olecranon. On cross-section, the humerus is circular at the midshaft but flared and flattened at the distal end. Medial and lateral supracondylar columns diverge to increase the diameter of the distal humerus in the mediolateral plane, and each condyle

contains an articulating portion for the radial head, or ulna, and nonarticulating epicondyles, which are terminal portions of the supracondylar ridges on which pronator-flexor muscles and supinator-extensor muscles originate. The three articulations at the elbow are the ulnotrochlear joint, the radiocapitellar joint, and the proximal radioulnar joint. The radial head articulates with the capitellar portion of the lateral condyle. The articular surface of the medial condyle has prominent medial and lateral ridges that aid in stabilizing the articulation with the ulna. Anterior to these two condyles are the coronoid and radial fossa, which receive the coronoid process of the ulna and the radial head when the elbow goes into full flexion. The proximal ulna contains the olecranon process posteriorly, the coronoid process anteriorly, and the sigmoid, or semilunar notch, which articulates with the trochlea. The triceps has a broad tendinous insertion into the olecranon posteriorly; anteriorly, the brachialis inserts on the coronoid process and the tuberosity of the ulna. The radial head lines up in its lesser sigmoid, or radial notch, with the annular ligament surrounding it. Collateral ligaments make up the remainder of the soft-tissue structures of the elbow, with the most important portion being the anterior band of the medial or ulnar collateral ligament arising from the medial epicondyle and attaching to a small process on the medial surface of the coronoid. The lesser posterior portion of the medial collateral ligament attaches to the medial surface of the olecranon process. There is a similarly triangular fan-shaped lateral collateral ligament, whose origin is the lateral epicondyle inserting on the annular ligament of the radius. The ulnar nerve passes through the cubital tunnel at the medial column of the elbow and must be appropriately assessed following injury.

DISTAL HUMERUS FRACTURES

1. Intercondylar-T or -Y Fractures

Intercondylar humerus fractures are among the most challenging fractures treated by the orthopedic surgeon. The usual mechanism of injury is axial loading of the ulna in the trochlear groove. Studies have demonstrated increasing numbers of these injuries in the older population. It is critical to assess the integrity of the medial and lateral column for reconstructible bone fragments and the degree of comminution.

Classification

Jupiter and Mehne classified distal humerus fractures into intra-articular and extra-articular patterns. Intra-articular fractures are divided into the following types:

(1) Single column: Divided into medial or lateral
(2) Bicolumn: Divided into TT, TY, TH, lambda, or multiplane pattern
(3) Capitellum fractures
(4) Trochlea fractures

Extra-articular fractures are classified into intracapsular and extracapsular (Table 3–3).

Treatment

Traditional treatment favored closed techniques because of the difficulty of fracture fixation for intercondylar fractures. Cast immobilization probably represents the worst of all possible worlds: inadequate

Table 3–3. The Jupiter and Mehne classification of distal humerus fractures.

I. Intra-articular fractures
  A. Single-column fractures
    1. Medial
      a. High
      b. Low
    2. Lateral
      a. High
      b. Low
    3. Divergent
  B. Bicolumn fractures
    1. T pattern
      a. High
      b. Low
    2. Y pattern
    3. H pattern
    4. Lambda pattern
      a. Medial
      b. Lateral
    5. Multiplane pattern
  C. Capitellum fractures
  D. Trochlear fractures
II. Extra-articular intracapsular fractures
  A. Transcolumn fractures
    1. High
      a. Extension
      b. Flexion
      c. Abduction
      d. Adduction
    2. Low
      a. Extension
      b. Flexion
III. Extracapsular fractures
  A. Medial epicondyle
  B. Lateral Epicondyle

Reproduced, with permission, from Browner BD et al, eds: Skeletal Trauma, 2nd ed. Philadelphia: WB Saunders, 1998.

reduction plus prolonged immobilization, leading to stiffness and ankylosis. Recent studies recommend open reduction, internal fixation (ORIF) in even the elderly population. Total elbow arthroplasty has similarly given good results in elderly patients with severely comminuted fractures involving osteoporotic bone. The goals of treating intra-articular distal humerus fractures include stable fixation with early motion.

Early operative methods consisted of pins and plaster or limited open reduction and internal fixation. With modern techniques, full ORIF is preferred for most fractures. Surgical exposure is through a transolecranon approach (ie, either transverse osteotomy or chevron osteotomy). A triceps-sparing posterior approach initially used for total elbow replacement but also applicable to fracture fixation has also been described.

Intercondylar T fractures have two distinct components: the intra-articular intercondylar component and the supracondylar one. The intracondylar portion of the fracture can usually be secured surgically with provisional K-wire fixation, followed by definitive screw fixation. After intercondylar fracture, stabilization with restoration of either the medial or lateral column is required to complete the operative fixation. When possible, dual plate fixation can be used. The AO group recommends a posterolateral and a medially applied dynamic compression plate.

In summary, intra-articular distal humerus fractures should in general be treated with (1) anatomic restoration of the articular surface with lag screw fixation of periarticular fragments (2) stable attachment of the metaphysis to the diaphysis with reconstruction plates and (3) early range of motion.

2. Fracture of the Humeral Condyles

Both medial and lateral condyles can be disrupted. These fractures can correspond with the ossification centers of the distal humerus.

Lateral Condylar Fracture

Lateral column fractures are single-column injuries and are divided into "low" and "high." Low fractures have the lateral wall of the trochlea attached to the main mass of the humerus and are generally stable, whereas high fractures involve a majority of the trochlea and are unstable. "Low" and "high" correspond to Milch type I and II injuries, respectively. Stable internal fixation with early range of motion is generally recommended for displaced fractures.

Medial Condylar Fracture

Medial condyle fractures are similarly single-column injuries with low fractures (Milch type I) involving a portion of the trochlea, with preservation of the trochlear ridge and are generally stable. In high medial condyle fractures (Milch type II), the lateral trochlear ridge is included with the fracture portion.

Both fractures, if displaced, should be treated with ORIF and early range of motion.

3. Fracture of the Epicondyles

Although lateral epicondylar fractures are rare, medial epicondylar fractures are fairly common, especially among children or adolescents. They commonly present as avulsion fractures. Treatment depends on the amount of displacement. If displacement is minimal, then closed reduction is appropriate. A displaced fracture may require percutaneous pinning or open reduction. Elbow instability is not generally a problem; however, irritation of the ulnar nerve can result. Early motion seems to be important for restoration and ultimate function. If a displaced fracture results in ulnar symptoms or is itself symptomatic, the fragment can be excised at a later date.

OLECRANON FRACTURES

The olecranon is the most proximal posterior eminence of the ulna. It is on the dorsal subcutaneous border and contains broad attachments for the triceps posteriorly. Anteriorly, the olecranon forms the greater sigmoid (semilunar) notch of the ulna, which articulates with the trochlea. The ulnar nerve passes behind the medial epicondyle at the posterior medial aspect of the elbow and then pierces the volar forearm between the two flexor carpi ulnaris muscle heads.

Fracture of the olecranon commonly occur with a direct blow or as an avulsion injury with triceps contracture. The fractures generally are transverse or oblique in orientation and enter the semilunar notch.

Clinical Findings

Radiographic evaluation consists of a true lateral radiograph of the elbow, and classifications or descriptions generally analyze the fracture based on the percentage of articular surface involved in the fractured proximal fragment. This factor, the amount of comminution, the fracture angle, intra-articular step-off, and the degree of displacement, are all critical in evaluating the injury and selecting the appropriate treatment.

Treatment

Methods of treatment vary from closed treatment to ORIF. Nondisplaced fractures, or fractures with < 2 mm displacement and an intact extensor mechanism, should be immobilized in a long arm cast with the elbow in 90 degrees of flexion.

Displaced transverse or short oblique fractures generally are best treated with ORIF. The optimal method for treating this fracture is tension banding with two longitudinal K-wires placed across the fracture site and stabilized with a figure-of-8 wire loop (Figure 3–12). More oblique fractures can be treated with interfragmentary screws with a neutralization plate. Wire protrusion and pain may sometimes result and may necessitate removal of the hardware.

If the articular surface is significantly comminuted, a low-profile, limited contact compression plate can be applied to the dorsal surface of the ulna. Selected comminuted fractures may be treated by selective bony excision or complete excision of the fragment followed by reattachment of the triceps. All these treatments generally can be accompanied with early protected range-of-motion exercises.

FRACTURE OF THE RADIAL HEAD

The radial head is seated in the lesser sigmoid notch and has contact axially with the capitellum of the distal humerus. The lateral portion contacts the ulna throughout forearm pronation and supination. Gripping or loading forces are transmitted through the interosseous membrane from the radius proximally to the ulnar distally. Load bearing occurs through the radial head.

Radial head fractures are generally caused by longitudinal loading from a fall on an outstretched hand; dislocation of the elbow is another cause.

Clinical Findings

One generally describes these fractures based on their location, percentage of articular involvement, and amount of displacement. Radiographs in the anteroposterior and lateral projections show the injury. The fat pad sign is usually present on the lateral projection (Figure 3–13).

Classification

Mason proposed a classification scheme for radial head fractures: Type I is a nondisplaced fracture; type II is a fracture that is displaced usually involving a single large fragment; type III is a comminuted fracture and type IV is a fracture associated with an elbow dislocation (Figure 3–14).

Treatment

For type I fractures, nonoperative treatment with early motion can generally produce a good outcome.

The treatment of type II fractures is controversial. For fractures with near normal motion, < 2 mm step-

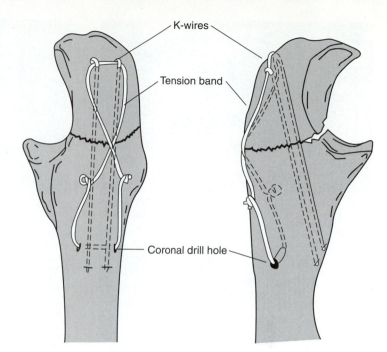

K-wires

Tension band

Coronal drill hole

Figure 3–12. Tension band technique for fixation of olecranon fractures. (Reproduced, with permission, from Browner BD et al, eds: Skeletal Trauma, 2nd ed. Philadelphia: WB Saunders, 1998.)

off and without associated injury, nonsurgical treatment is indicated.

Type II fractures with associated injuries that may compromise elbow stability of fractures with a mechanical block to full motion after injection of anesthetic into the elbow joint are indications for ORIF. Open reduction and internal fixation can be performed with pins, articular screws, or Herbert screws.

Early excision with immediate motion is recommended for type III fractures with no associated elbow instability, coronoid fracture, wrist pain, or injury. If any of these conditions exist, then current literature recommends placement of a metallic radial head prosthesis. The silastic implant has been associated with material failure and particulate synovitis that preclude permanent use of the implant.

Replacement of the radial head becomes most important when there is evidence of soft-tissue disruption involving the interosseous membrane and the distal radioulnar ligaments. This can be determined through the clinical examination. Sometimes radiographic evidence will show proximal migration of the radius and carpus relative to the ulna if the radial head has not been replaced; this is called the Essex-Lopresti injury.

1. Capitellar Fractures

Capitellar fractures frequently accompany and result from the same mechanism that causes radial head fractures. Various levels of injury, from cartilage damage to large os-

teochondral portions of the capitellum, can occur from impaction of the radius against the capitellum. Shearing forces can result in two different, more significant injuries: an osteochondral injury or complete fracture (type 1 or Hahn-Steinthal), an articular-cartilage-only injury (type 2 or Kocher-Lorenz) or a comminuted fracture (type 3). Osteochondral pieces can be overlooked or confused with bone chips from radial head fractures.

Treatment

Today, anatomic reduction and early motion is the standard treatment for these injuries, whether obtained by open or closed means. Open reduction is performed through a lateral approach between the anconeus and extensor carpi ulnaris.

ELBOW DISLOCATION

Dislocations of the elbow occur when loads are placed on the structures about the elbow that exceed the intrinsic stability provided by the anatomic shape of the joint surfaces and soft-tissue constraints. These are potentially limb-threatening, as vascular compromise is a possible sequela. Expeditious reduction of the elbow joint is the goal of treatment.

Although diagnosis of elbow dislocation can be made easily prior to the onset of swelling, the type of dislocation may not be obvious. Elbow dislocations are characterized, like all dislocations, according to direc-

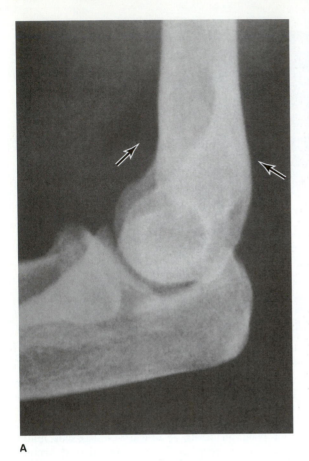
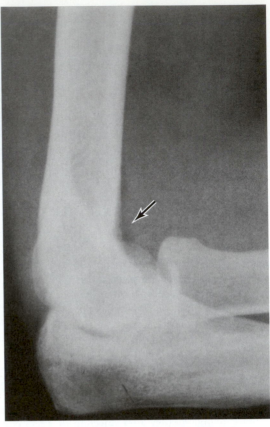

A

B

Figure 3–13. Positive fat pad sign on lateral radiograph of elbow. This finding indicates that fluid is in the elbow joint. In the acute setting, the fluid is blood, most commonly from a fracture.

tion of the distal bone. Thus, pure elbow dislocations are categorized as anterior, posterior, medial, or lateral, depending on the direction of displacement of the radius and ulna. Because two bones are present in the forearm, one more dislocation is possible, the divergent dislocation, but this is rare. This occurs when the radius and ulna are forced apart by the distal humerus. "Partial dislocations" also occur, in which the radial head or the ulna alone dislocate. The ulna has been observed to dislocate anteriorly or posteriorly. The radial head has more latitude and can dislocate laterally as well as in the anterior or posterior direction. Isolated radial head dislocation is rare; it is usually accompanied by an ulnar fracture (Monteggia fracture). When combinations of dislocations with concomitant fractures occur, treatment of the combined injury is usually dictated by the treated fracture. Adequate fracture care will usually cause secondary reduction of the dislocation.

Posterior Elbow Dislocations

Posterior dislocations are the most common type (80%) of elbow dislocations, resulting from an axial force applied to the extended elbow. Both collateral ligaments are disrupted, whether the dislocation is posteromedial or posterolateral.

Diagnosis is made by clinical examination and verified by radiograph to rule out associated fractures. The extremity is typically shortened and the elbow held slightly flexed.

Treatment is initiated after documenting the neurovascular examination. Anesthesia, either injected locally into the joint or administered intravenously is necessary. Traction on the extremity with correction of the medial or lateral displacement usually produces reduction with a "clunk." The elbow is put through a range of motion to ensure that reduction has been obtained and

Type I

Type II

Type III

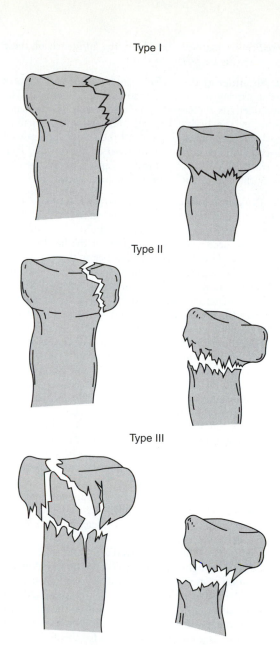

Figure 3–14. Mason classification of radial head fractures. (Reproduced, with permission, from Browner BD et al, eds: Skeletal Trauma, 2nd ed. Philadelphia: WB Saunders, 1998.)

that there is no soft-tissue or bony mechanical blockage to motion. The elbow is generally splinted in flexion and pronation to maintain stability. Postreduction radiographs are necessary to rule out occult fracture.

Anterior Elbow Dislocations

Anterior dislocations are relatively rare. Soft-tissue damage is typically severe. Treatment is similar to that for posterior dislocations, except that the method of reduction is reversed.

Medial & Lateral Elbow Dislocations

The radius and ulna may be displaced medially or laterally. Some semblance of joint motion may be present with lateral dislocations, as the ulna may be displaced into the groove between the trochlea and the capitellum. The anteroposterior radiograph is diagnostic. Medial or lateral force is used, after attempting to distract the joint surfaces, to reduce these dislocations.

Isolated Ulnar Dislocations

Isolated ulnar dislocations occur when the humerus pivots around the radial head, causing the coronoid process to be displaced posterior to the humerus or the olecranon anterior to the humerus. The more common injury is posterior dislocation, which causes cubitus varus deformity of the forearm. Traction in extension and supination reduces the ulna.

General Treatment Procedures

A. EARLY TREATMENT

The elbow is tested for stability to varus and valgus stress and to pronation and supination. Stable dislocations are splinted for comfort at 90 degrees of flexion, and motion is instituted as soon as possible, generally within a few days. Maintenance of reduction is necessary, and radiographs should be taken periodically if any doubt exists. Immobilization does not guarantee maintenance of reduction. Unstable reductions are rare. Immobilization for longer periods may be necessary in these cases, as a stiff but stable elbow is preferable to an unstable elbow.

Uncomplicated elbow dislocations have a favorable long-term prognosis. A loss of extension of 5–10 degrees compared with the contralateral elbow can be expected following this injury. Posterolateral dislocation has been associated with persistent valgus instability in some patients, which is associated with a worse overall clinical result.

B. DELAYED TREATMENT

It would seem impossible for a patient not to seek immediate care for elbow dislocation. Treatment may be delayed, however, because of failure to seek medical attention, altered mental status, or missed diagnosis by the initial physician. Late reduction of elbow dislocations can be accomplished with closed techniques for up to several weeks from the time of injury. Dislocations left untreated for longer periods generally require open reduction techniques. Better function with less flexion contracture after open reduction of posterior dislocations is obtained by lengthening the triceps tendon.

Bailey CS et al: Outcome of plate fixation of olecranon fractures. J Orthop Trauma 2001;15:542.[PMID: 11733669]

Eygendaal D et al: Posterolateral dislocation of the elbow joint. J Bone Joint Surg Am 2000;82-A:555.[PMID: 10761945]

Hak DJ, Golladay GJ: Olecranon fractures: Treatment options. J Am Acad Orthop Surg 2000;8:266.[PMID: 10951115]

Mckee MD et al: Functional outcome following surgical treatment of intra-articular distal humeral fractures through a posterior approach. J Bone Joint Surg Am 2000;82-A:1701.[PMID: 11130643]

Paramasivan ON, Younge DA, Pant R: Treatment of nonunion around the olecranon fossa of the humerus by intramedullary locked nailing. J Bone Joint Surg Br 2000;82-B:332.[PMID: 10813164]

Popovic N, Rodriguez A, Lemaire R: Fracture of the radial head with associated elbow dislocation: Results of treatment using a floating radial head prosthesis. J Orthop Trauma 2000;14: 171.[PMID: 10791667]

Sanchez-Sotelo J, Romanillos O, Garay EG: Results of acute excision of the radial head in elbow radial head fracture-dislocations. J Orthop Trauma 2000;14:354.[PMID: 10926244]

Wainwright AM, Williams JR, Carr AJ: Interobserver and intraobserver variation in classification systems for fractures of the distal humerus. J Bone Joint Surg Br 2000;82-B:636.[PMID: 10963156])

SHOULDER & ARM INJURIES

Anatomy & Biomechanical Principles

A. BONY ANATOMY

1. Humeral shaft—The humeral shaft extends from the level of the insertion of the pectoralis major muscle proximally to the supracondylar ridge distally. The upper portion of the shaft is cylindric and then becomes more flattened in an anteroposterior direction as it proceeds distally. Medial and lateral intermuscular septae divide the arm into anterior and posterior compartments. In the anterior compartment reside the biceps brachii, coracobrachialis, and brachialis muscles, along with the neurovascular bundle coursing along the medial border of the biceps with the brachial artery and vein and the median, musculocutaneous, and ulnar nerves. In the posterior compartment reside the triceps brachii muscle and the radial nerve. Understanding the insertions of the muscle forces around the humerus helps explain the tendency for fractures to displace in predictable patterns, based on the influence of these muscles (Figure 3–15).

2. Shoulder girdle—The shoulder girdle is a complex arrangement of bony and soft-tissue structures. The shoulder has the largest range of motion of any major joint in the body. The glenoid cavity is a shallow socket, approximately one third the size of the humeral head. Stability of the joint depends on capsule, ligament, and muscle. A redundant capsule allows for motion; the rotator cuff controls the joint itself.

3. Proximal humerus—The proximal humerus contains the humeral head, lesser and greater tuberosities, bicipital groove, and proximal humeral shaft. The anatomic neck lies at the junction of the head and the tuberosity. The surgical neck lies below the greater and lesser tuberosities. The major blood supply to the humeral head is through the ascending branch of the anterior humeral circumflex artery, which penetrates the head at the bicipital groove and becomes the arcuate artery. Important structures that lie in the vicinity of the shoulder joint include the brachial plexus and axillary artery, which are anterior to the coracoid process of the scapula and humeral head. Three nerves innervate muscles around the shoulder: the axillary, suprascapular, and musculocutaneous nerves. Fractures of the anatomic neck have a poor prognosis because of complete disruption of the blood supply to the head. Surgical neck fractures are common, and with these the blood supply to the head remains preserved. Within the bicipital groove lies the biceps tendon, which is covered by the transverse humeral ligament. The greater tuberosity provides attachment for the supraspinatus, infraspinatus, and teres minor muscles. The lesser tuberosity contains the attachment of the subscapularis muscle. The neck-shaft inclination angle measures an average of 145 degrees, and the humeral head is retroverted an average of 30 degrees. It is thought that the fusion of the three distinct ossification centers for the humeral head, greater and lesser tuberosities remains an area of weakness, and fractures occur in the areas corresponding to the epiphyseal scars. The acromion protects the superior aspect of the glenohumeral joint, provides origin for the deltoid muscles, and forms the lateral aspect of the acromioclavicular joint. The rotator cuff consists of four muscles: the subscapularis, supraspinatus, infraspinatus, and teres minor muscles. The teres major is not a rotator cuff muscle. The cuff muscles serve as depressors of the humeral head to allow the deltoid to efficiently abduct the humerus. The infraspinatus and teres minor are external rotators, while the subscapularis is an internal rotator of the humerus. Two other important muscles in this region are the deltoid and the pectoralis major muscles. These muscles, along with the rotator cuff, cause predictable displacement of fractures around the proxi-

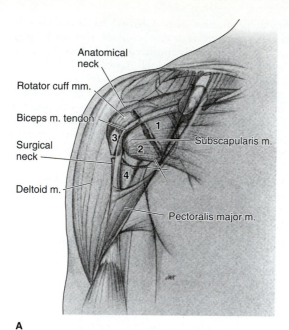

Anatomical neck
Rotator cuff mm.
Biceps m. tendon
Surgical neck
Deltoid m.
Subscapularis m.
Pectoralis major m.

1
2
3
4

A

	2-part	3-part	4-part	Articular surface
Anatomical neck				
Surgical neck	a c b			
Greater tuberosity				
Lesser tuberosity				
Fracture-dislocation	Anterior			
	Posterior			
Head-splitting				

B

Figure 3–15. **A:** Muscle insertions on humerus and fracture displacement. **B:** Neer four-part classification of displaced fractures. (Reproduced, with permission, from Rockwood CA et al, eds: Fractures in Adults, 4th ed. Philadelphia: Lippincott, 1996.)

mal humerus. Additionally, injury to the rotator cuff, independent of injuries to the insertion of the tuberosities, may be encountered and need to be considered when evaluating the shoulder.

B. NERVE SUPPLY

Injuries to the nerves around the shoulders occur with fractures and dislocations. The brachial plexus and axillary artery can also be injured with anterior shoulder dislocations.

The most important evaluation consists of a neurovascular examination after injury around the arm and shoulder girdle. The radial nerve is commonly injured in humeral shaft fractures, particularly at the junction of the middle and distal third (Holstein-Lewis fracture). Careful evaluation of radial nerve sensory and motor function is critical. Evaluation should include sensation of the dorsal web space between the thumb and index finger, independent digital extension, and wrist extension.

Around the shoulder girdle, fractures of the proximal humerus and fracture-dislocations can on occasion result in axillary nerve and artery injuries. An axillary nerve injury from proximal humeral fracture or fracture-dislocation would result in paralysis of the deltoid muscle and anesthesia over the skin patch at the lateral proximal arm. Axillary artery injuries generally result from fractures or fracture-dislocations in which a medial bone spike injures or penetrates the axillary artery. The index of suspicion is high if the arm, upon evaluation, shows significant color differences compared with the uninjured arm or has a bluish or cadaveric appearance. Pulses should be palpated and evaluated by Doppler studies; even if the pulse is present, if it is significantly different from the uninjured side, arterial injury should be suspected. Appropriate arterial studies should be obtained on an emergent basis, or in the operating room, and vascular exploration and repair planned.

More subtle associated injuries involve the rotator cuff. This can generally be expected with fractures of the tuberosities, but it can also result from strictly soft-tissue injuries such as shoulder dislocations. Generally, rotator cuff avulsion is suspected when radiographs reveal no evidence of fracture but the patient is unable to actively externally rotate the shoulder against resistance. Evaluation of the integrity of the rotator cuff may be difficult in the acute setting, and special studies such as MRI or arthrogram may be valuable in making this diagnosis.

HUMERAL SHAFT FRACTURE

Fractures of the shaft of the humerus usually result from a direct blow, a fall, an automobile injury, or a crushing injury. Missiles from firearms or shell fragments may pierce the arm and cause an open fracture.

Other indirect means of injury, such as a fall on an outstretched upper extremity or violent muscle contracture, can cause midshaft fractures.

Classification

Fractures are classified according to whether they are open or closed and according to the level of the fracture in relation to the insertions of the pectoralis major and deltoid muscles. Characteristics of fracture and associated injury are also factors.

Clinical Findings

Clinical signs and symptoms, include a shortened extremity with crepitus and pain at the diaphysis of the humerus. Confirmation should be obtained by radiographs in two planes. Both the shoulder and elbow joints should be thoroughly evaluated, clinically and radiographically, as should the neurovascular status.

Treatment

A. CLOSED TREATMENT

The recommended treatment in isolated diaphyseal humeral fractures involves closed methods. Nonoperative methods lead to good results with very high union rates. Nonoperative methods include traction by hanging casts, coaptation splints, shoulder spica casts, Velcro bracing, abduction humeral bracing, and skeletal traction.

1. Hanging cast—Treatment with a hanging cast involves placement of the arm in a Velcro cast with the elbow flexed to 90 degrees, with a sling fashioned over a loop placed on the radial aspect of the wrist. To correct angulation, loops may be placed on the dorsum or volar aspect of the wrist, and angulation anteriorly and posteriorly can be adjusted by the length of the sling or suspension apparatus. This treatment requires weekly radiographic evaluations; exercises both for shoulder and digital motion are helpful.

Patients with a large body habitus may develop more significant angulation at the time of healing with this technique, compared with slimmer patients. The vertical position must be maintained even at night. Spiral, comminuted, and oblique fractures have additional advantages of large fracture surfaces for ready healing. Transverse fractures may have more difficulty in healing. The musculature of the upper arm will accommodate 20 degrees of anterior angulation, 30 degrees of varus angulation and 3 cm of shortening without apparent deformity.

2. Coaptation splint—A TU-shaped coaptation splint with cuff and collar is another method for treating humerus fractures. The more modern version of this is

functional bracing, as popularized by Sarmiento. The sleeve is ready-made or custom-made from thermoplastic splinting materials and fixed with Velcro straps that can be adjusted to achieve the appropriate level of compression. Stand-alone slings or cuffs are used. Alternatively, a cast brace may be used with a hinge brace at the elbow with upper arm and forearm components. This can control flexion and protect against varus and valgus stresses as well as translational forces; it may be most useful for healing the more distal diaphyseal fractures.

3. Abduction humeral splinting and shoulder casting—Spica casting may be useful in certain unstable fractures, though it is a complex method of immobilization and requires close follow-up.

4. Skeletal traction—In special circumstances, skeletal traction has been used for humeral fractures. When recumbent treatment for other injuries, massive swelling, or open fractures are present, this type of treatment may be indicated. Increasingly, however, multiple trauma patients are treated with aggressive internal fixation to allow early mobilization. The traction pin is inserted through the olecranon, going from a medial to lateral directions to avoid injury to the ulnar nerve. Differential traction on one side of a Steinmann pin bow or Kirschner wire bow can be used to achieve varus and valgus alignment; traction of the humerus longitudinally and flexion of the forearm and hand suspended overhead help to correct angulation. Positioning is checked with portable radiographs.

5. Sling and swathe—Elderly patients may best be treated by reducing fracture motion in a sling and stockinette body swathe for comfort. Aggressive maintenance of anatomic reduction is not a critical goal in this patient population; shoulder exercises should be initiated as early as possible to avoid shoulder contractures.

6. External fixation—External fixation is applicable to the humerus in the case of burns or severe comminuted open injuries with defects of skin, bone, or soft tissue. Because of the soft-tissue envelope around the humerus, one uses external fixation only when other means of management are not applicable or appropriate. Half pins are generally inserted above and below the fracture with access to the soft-tissue defect between the pins.

B. OPEN TREATMENT

Special circumstances may merit ORIF. Selected segmental fractures, inadequate closed reduction, "floating" elbow, bilateral humeral fractures, open fractures, multiple trauma, pathologic fractures, and trauma with associated vascular injuries requiring exploration may benefit from internal fixation. There are two general forms of internal fixation: (1) Compression plate and screw fixation of the AO type may be used, with posterior, modified lateral and anterolateral approaches being used. (2) Recent reports indicate intramedullary nailing to be as successful as other methods of fixation. In multiply injured patients, however, humeral stabilization, permitting mobilization, pulmonary toilet, and pain control, may be beneficial. The incidence of radial nerve palsy with acute fracture is about 16%; however, current literature does not recommend operative fixation and nerve exploration in these injuries.

FRACTURES & DISLOCATIONS AROUND THE SHOULDER

Classification

The classification of shoulder fractures and dislocations developed by Neer in 1970 is based on the work of Codman in 1934 and before that of Kocher in 1896. This comprehensive system considers the anatomy and biomechanical forces resulting in displacement of fracture fragments as they relate to diagnosis and treatment. Although useful, this system has been demonstrated to have significant interobserver variability. Fractures are classified by the number of parts that are displaced more than 1 cm or angulated more than 45 degrees. Displaced parts can include the anatomic neck, surgical neck, or tuberosities; other categories include fracture-dislocations and head-splitting injuries. The relationship of the humeral head to the displaced parts in the glenoid, as well as the blood supply, is also taken into consideration. The incidence of proximal humerus fractures has been estimated at 4–5% of all fractures. The likelihood of proximal humerus fractures increases in the older age groups, especially with concomitant osteoporosis.

Clinical Findings

Clinical presentation is usually with pain, swelling, and ecchymosis.

Radiographic evaluation is a cornerstone for diagnosis and planning of treatment. The recommended series of radiographs is the so-called Neer trauma series, which consists of an (1) anterior-posterior view, (2) lateral view in the scapular plane, and (3) axillary view. The lateral radiograph in the scapular plane is the tangential Y-view of the scapula. The combination of three of these views allows evaluation of the shoulder joint in three separate perpendicular planes. The axillary view is important for evaluating the glenoid articular surface and the relationship of the humeral head anteriorly and posteriorly. It can be obtained even in the traumatized patient, with gentle abduction of the arm, with the

x-ray beam aimed toward the axilla and the plate placed above the patient's shoulder. On occasion, other studies, including CT scanning for detailing bony anatomy and MRI for detailing soft tissues such as the rotator cuff, may prove helpful.

Treatment

A. CLOSED TREATMENT

Approximately 85% of proximal humerus fractures are minimally displaced or nondisplaced and can be treated nonoperatively with a sling for comfort and early motion exercises. The remaining 15% require supplemental techniques. The mainstay of closed treatment is initial immobilization and then early motion. Physical therapy or physician-directed exercises are essential and should be started at 7–10 days if possible. Monitoring of the exercises is important to prevent a program that is either too conservative (thus causing unnecessary contractures) or too aggressive (leading to displacement, with excessive pain and swelling).

B. SURGICAL TREATMENT

Techniques useful for the smaller percentage of fractures include closed reduction, percutaneous pinning, skeletal traction, and ORIF using a variety of techniques and implants. For severe fractures, especially four-part fractures or fracture-dislocations, primary replacement of the injured humeral head by a prosthesis may be the treatment of choice.

C. TWO-PART ANATOMIC NECK FRACTURES

Two-part anatomic neck fractures are rare. No single optimal method of management has been established. Closed reduction is difficult because controlling the articular fragment, which is usually rotated and angulated within the joint capsule, is difficult. The fragment can be preserved in a young patient with ORIF with pins or interfragmentary screws. It may be difficult to obtain adequate screw purchase without violating the articular surface. Additionally, the prognosis for head survival is poor because the blood supply is usually completely disrupted. In general, prosthetic hemiarthroplasty provides the most predictable result in the elderly.

D. TWO-PART GREATER TUBEROSITY FRACTURES

Greater tuberosity fractures generally displace posteriorly and superiorly because of traction by the supraspinatus muscle. This is often associated with anterior glenohumeral dislocation. It is appropriate to attempt closed reduction, which may result in an acceptable position for the greater tuberosity. Neer has reported that displacement of the fragment by more than 1 cm is pathognomonic of a rotator cuff defect. The result of fracture healing in this position is subacromial impingement, with limitation of forward elevation and external rotation. In one series, patients with fractures that healed with more than 1 cm of displacement suffered permanent disability, whereas those with less than 0.5 cm of displacement did well. The group of patients in the midrange, 0.5–1 cm of displacement, had a 20% incidence of revision surgery for persistent pain. Open reduction and internal fixation is recommended if displacement is > 5 mm with some references recommending ORIF with > 3 mm displacement in the high-performance athlete as impingement symptoms may develop in these individuals. A variety of methods, including screws, pins, wires, and suture, can be used to repair the greater tuberosity. Nonabsorbable sutures can be used successfully; the rotator cuff defect can be repaired in a similar fashion. Treatment of this condition should be directed at rotator cuff repair as well as bony reconstruction. Percutaneous pinning tends to be inadequate for preventing redisplacement of greater tuberosity fractures.

E. Two-Part Lesser Tuberosity Fractures

If the displaced fragment is small, closed reduction of this rare injury is satisfactory. This fracture may be associated with posterior dislocation and may be treated by closed reduction in the acute setting. The position of immobilization in this case would be either neutral or slight external rotation. Larger fragments may require internal fixation.

F. Two-Part Surgical Neck Fractures

In these conditions, both tuberosities remain attached to the head, and the rotator cuff in general remains intact. The diaphysis is often displaced anteromedially by the pull of the pectoralis major muscle. Reduction may be blocked by interposition of the periosteum, biceps tendon, or deltoid muscle, or by buttonholing of the shaft in the deltoid, pectoralis major, or fascial elements. One attempt at closed reduction is advisable; if this fails, operative intervention is recommended. If, on the other hand, the reduction is successful, percutaneous pinning under fluoroscopic control may be an excellent choice for the reducible but unstable fracture (Figure 3–16). If open reduction is required to remove displaced soft tissues, internal fixation can be accomplished by means of percutaneous pinning or intramedullary fixation in conjunction with a tension band wiring technique. In the past, an AO buttress plate has been used; however, complications including screw loosening (particularly in osteoporotic patients), retention of the plate, persistent varus, and interference with the blood supply have been reported. In the osteoporotic patient, wire or suture material for tension banding can be passed through the soft tissues and the rotator cuff, which may be superior to bone for fixation.

Another technique for internal fixation utilizes intramedullary devices such as Enders nails or Rush rods, which can be inserted through a limited deltoid-splitting incision. This may serve well to prevent displacement of the head in relation to the shaft; however, the control of rotational alignment is poor. For elderly or debilitated patients, this may be the best solution to achieve overall alignment with minimal surgical morbidity. Hardware removal is often necessary to treat resultant subacromial impingement. For complicated fractures, patients with osteoporotic bone, or other special circumstances, olecranon traction may be incorporated.

G. Three-Part Fractures

Avascular necrosis in three-part fractures has been reported to be as high as 27%. Open reduction and internal fixation is the treatment of choice for displaced

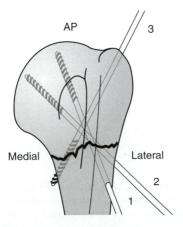
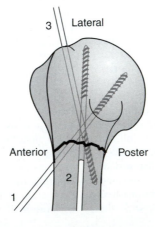

Figure 3–16. Pinning of the unstable surgical neck fracture. (Reproduced, with permission, from Fu FH, Smith WR, eds: Percutaneous pinning of proximal humerus fractures. Oper Tech Orthop 2001;11:235.)

three-part fractures of the proximal humerus. The AO buttress plate has had significant complications, including a high rate of avascular necrosis related in part to extension of soft-tissue displacement and dissection, superior placement of the plate with secondary impingement, loss of plate and screw fixation, malunion, and infections. Recent studies indicate that blade-plate devices tend to have stronger fixation than standard buttress plates. Other studies indicate that Ender nails combined with tension banding are good alternatives in osteoporotic bone.

H. Four-Part Fractures

Open reduction and internal fixation of four-part fractures (as with three-part fractures) has generally produced unsatisfactorily high rates of complications such as avascular necrosis and malunion. Some authors recommend gentle open reduction and limited internal fixation in the active patient. In the less active or elderly patient, the accepted method of treatment is hemiarthroplasty, particularly because the avascular necrosis rate may be as high as 90% and the bone is usually osteoporotic. Appropriate prosthesis level and humeral retroversion, as well as the attachment of greater and lesser tuberosities, are critical in achieving a good result. Repair of any rotator cuff defects is necessary to prevent proximal migration of the humeral component as well as loss of rotator cuff power.

I. Fracture-Dislocations

Fracture-dislocations require reduction of the humeral head, and their management is generally based on the fracture pattern. These injuries usually produce impression defects or head-splitting fractures, with concomitant posterior dislocation. Management is determined by the size of the impression defect and the time of persistent locked dislocation. Fractures of less than 20% will generally be stable with closed reduction and can be treated with immobilization in external rotation for 6 weeks to restore long-term stability. If the defect is 20–50%, however, transfer of the lesser tuberosity with the subscapularis tendon into the defect by open means is indicated. With impression fractures of greater than 50% or chronic dislocations, hemiarthroplasty may be the best treatment. If concomitant glenoid destruction is present, total shoulder arthroplasty may be required.

Reflex Sympathetic Dystrophy

For many years, a constellation of vague painful conditions had been observed as sequelae of infection or trauma that was sometimes relatively minor. These conditions have been described by a variety of terms such as minor causalgia, major causalgia, Sudeck's atrophy, reflex dystrophy, posttraumatic dystrophy, and shoulder-hand syndrome. Attempts have been made to explain all these conditions by a unified theory.

In general, posttraumatic reflex sympathetic dystrophy is produced by an exaggerated response to posttraumatic conditions. Pain, hyperesthesia, and tenderness out of proportion to the physical findings are the predominant features. Skin color, texture, and temperature may vary depending upon the stage of disease, with redness and warmth being common early; pallor, dry shiny skin, and coolness of the involved part are more prevalent later.

Clinically, reflex sympathetic dystrophy has three stages, which are not completely distinct from one another. During the first, or early, stage, a burning or aching pain may be present and may be increased by external stimuli; the pain is out of proportion to the severity of the injury and physical findings. The second stage generally develops at approximately 3 months and is characterized by significant edema, cold glossy skin, and joint limitations. Radiographs may reveal diffuse osteopenia. The third, or atrophic, stage is marked by progressive atrophy of skin and muscle and significant joint contractures.

Sudeck's atrophy is a radiographic term that is extended to a clinical condition. Spotty rarefaction is distinguished from generalized diffuse atrophy of bone and may occur 6–8 weeks after the onset of symptoms. **Shoulder-hand syndrome** is a variation of this phenomenon that often occurs with upper extremity disorders. Stiffness is characteristic, both at the shoulder and at the wrist and hand level.

Because the cause is unclear, the recommended treatment is an aggressive program of physical therapy modalities to help with soft-tissue sensitivity as well as prevention or treatment of joint contractures. Sympathetic blocks may be important. More recently, multidisciplinary pain management services that incorporate counseling, evaluation of orthopedic musculoskeletal neurologic problems, and sympathetic blocks administered typically by anesthesiologists, have proved successful in helping to limit the time and extent of disability associated with these conditions. Progressive loading of the extremity and progressive resistance-type exercises can also be of benefit in the appropriate setting.

Blum J et al: Clinical performance of a new medullary humeral nail: Antegrade versus retrograde insertion. J Orthop Trauma 2001;15:342.[PMID: 11433139]

Chapman JR et al: Randomized prospective study of humeral shaft fracture fixation: Intramedullary nails versus plates. J Orthop Trauma 2000;14: 162.[PMID: 10791665]

Cox MA et al: Closed interlocking nailing of humeral shaft fractures with the Russell-Taylor nail. J Orthop Trauma 2000; 14:349.[PMID: 10926243]

Eberson CP et al: Contralateral intrathoracic displacement of the humeral head. J Bone Joint Surg Am 2000;82-A:105.[PMID: 10653090]

Hintermann B, Trouillier HH, Schafer D: Rigid internal fixation of fractures of the proximal humerus in older patients. J Bone Joint Surg Br 2000;82-B:1107.[PMID: 11132267]

McCormack RG et al: Fixation of fractures of the shaft of the humerus by dynamic compression plate or intramedullary nail. J Bone Joint Surg Br 2000;82-B:336.[PMID: 10813165]

Naranja RJ, Iannotti JP: Displaced three- and four-part proximal humerus fractures: Evaluation and management 2000;8:373. [PMID: 11104401]

Ruch DS et al: Fixation of three-part proximal humeral fractures: A biomechanical evaluation. J Orthop Trauma 2000;14:36. [PMID: 10630801]

Sarmiento A et al: Functional bracing for the treatment of fractures of the humeral diaphysis. J Bone Joint Surg Am 2000;82:478.[PMID: 10761938]

Steinmann SP, Moran EA: Axillary nerve injury: Diagnosis and treatment. J Am Acad Orthop Surg 2001;9:328.[PMID: 11575912]

Strothman D et al: Retrograde nailing of humeral shaft fractures: A biomechanical study of its effects on the strength of the distal humerus. J Orthop Trauma 2000;14:101.[PMID: 10716380]

■ II. TRAUMA TO THE LOWER EXTREMITY

FOOT & ANKLE INJURIES

The appropriate investigation of any foot injury requires obtaining initially a precise history of the mechanism of injury. A thorough physical examination will compare the injured extremity to the uninjured contralateral side (looking for ecchymosis, swelling, or deformity), palpating carefully all points of tenderness, stressing the different joints when indicated, and assessing the neurovascular status. Associated injuries and certain systemic disorders (particularly diabetes and peripheral vascular disease) should be identified. An appropriate radiographic evaluation is mandatory. Anteroposterior and lateral views are standard. Oblique and special views are requested according to clinical suspicion. Although some fracture patterns are still best delineated by conventional tomography, CT scanning has recently proved to be valuable, especially for calcaneus fractures. Radionuclide imaging is helpful to identify occult injuries. MRI is gaining popularity and is particularly helpful in diagnosing soft-tissue damage to the tibialis posterior tendon or gastrocnemius muscle, osteochondral fractures, and avascular necrosis.

Anatomy & Biomechanical Principles

The foot is a complex, highly specialized structure that permits weight bearing in a smooth, energy-conserving pattern. The delicate balance between bones and soft tissues is necessary for optimal function. When planning treatment of an injured foot, both need to be addressed with equal rigor. High-energy injuries, such as crush injuries, generally have a poorer prognosis, even if the bones are anatomically reduced. Scarring of soft tissues, particularly specialized tissues like the heel fat pad or the plantar fascia, prevents normal function and is often painful.

Embryogenetically, the foot develops from proximal to distal into three functional segments: the tarsus, metatarsus, and phalanges. Anatomically, it is divided into the hindfoot (talus and calcaneus), the midfoot (navicular, cuboid, and three cuneiforms), and the forefoot (five metatarsals and 14 phalanges). Besides skin, vessels, and nerves, the soft tissues include extrinsic tendons, intrinsic musculotendinous units, a complex network of capsuloligamentous structures, and some uniquely specialized tissues such as fat pads.

Classically, the plantar aspect of the foot is divided into four layers, from superficial to deep. The first layer consists of the abductor hallucis, flexor digitorum brevis, and abductor digiti minimi. The second layer is made up of the tendons of the flexor hallucis longus and flexor digitorum longus, the quadratus plantae and lumbricales muscles. In the third layer are the flexor hallucis brevis, adductor hallucis, and flexor digiti minimi muscles. The peroneus longus and tibialis posterior tendons, as well as the unipennate plantar and bipennate dorsal interossei muscles, comprise the fourth and deepest layer.

These 28 bones, 57 articulations, and extrinsic and intrinsic soft tissues work harmoniously as a unit resembling functionally a ball and socket to allow walking, running, jumping, and accommodation of irregular surfaces with a minimal expense of energy.

Obviously, the foot is only the distal segment of the lower extremity. Energy-effective gait requires optimal integration of all segments involved in locomotion, and proper coordination involves extremely complex pathways. Fluid motion minimizes energy expenditure, and a lot of the fine-tuning to attain this goal occurs in the foot. For example, the subtalar joint everts at heel strike, unlocking the midtarsal joint. Increasing the flexibility of the foot allows for better energy absorption and foot-to-ground accommodation. Conversely, the subtalar joint inverts at push-off, locking the midtarsal joint. This creates a rigid lever more mechanically advantageous for forward propulsion.

This extremely superficial overview of the anatomy and biomechanical principles of the foot serves only to stress the complex relationship between bone and soft-tissue structures. Restoration of this relationship is the goal of treatment of foot injuries.

FRACTURES COMMON TO ALL PARTS OF THE FOOT

1. Fatigue Fractures

Also known as **stress, march,** or **insufficiency** fractures, fatigue fractures occur when damage from cyclical loading of a bone overwhelms its physiologic repair capacity. Specifically, repetitive stress stimulates an attempt to strengthen areas of bone that are experiencing excessive stress. This process begins with resorption of bone to make room for the deposition of new stronger bone. Continued loading can lead to gross failure of the bone weakened by resorption.

This disorder is commonly seen in young active adults involved in vigorous and excessive exercise. A history of a single significant injury is usually lacking. Sites of fracture are most frequently the metatarsals and the calcaneus, but fatigue fractures can be found anywhere.

Clinical Findings

Incipient pain of varying intensity at rest is then accentuated by walking. Swelling and point tenderness are likely to be present. Depending on the stage of progress, radiographs may be normal or may show an incomplete or complete fracture line or only extracortical callus formation that can be mistaken for osteogenic sarcoma. Radionuclide imaging, CT and MRI can be helpful for occult fractures. Persistent unprotected weight bearing may cause arrest of bone healing and even displacement of the fracture fragment.

Treatment

Treatment is by protection in either a short leg cast, walking boot or a heavy stiff-soled shoe. Weight bearing is restricted until pain has subsided and restoration of bone continuity is confirmed radiographically, usually within 3–4 weeks.

2. Multiple High-Energy Injuries

Violent forces applied to the foot may cause more extensive damage than initially appreciated. Certain mechanisms of injury tend to produce specific patterns of lesions, and a high index of suspicion is necessary so as not to overlook some of the associated bony or ligamentous injuries.

Treatment

High-energy fractures are often open, and the basic principles of open fracture management should be applied. The objectives are to preserve circulation and sensation (particularly of the plantar region), maintain a plantigrade position of the foot, prevent or control infection, preserve plantar skin and fat pads, preserve gross motion of the different joints (both actively and passively), achieve bone union, and, ultimately, preserve fine motion. Fasciotomies of the severely injured foot may be necessary to avoid compartment syndromes and their serious sequelae.

Early stabilization of multiple fractures and dislocations will simplify wound management. This can be accomplished through external fixation or internal fixation with K-wires, plates, or screws. Early soft tissue coverage with local or free flaps is also beneficial.

3. Neuropathic Joint Injuries & Fractures

Fractures and other foot disorders often present in the patient with Charcot arthropathy. Neuropathic fractures are frequently seen with diabetes, tabes dorsalis, syringomyelia, peripheral nerve injury or degeneration, leprosy, and other rare neurologic syndromes.

The potential for bone healing is normal; however, healing of fracture is often delayed in this patient group. Protection, rest, and elevation can result in union without deformity. Open reduction and internal fixation is sometimes necessary. Rarely, arthrodesis is indicated; however, the rate of nonunion is higher than for normal joints.

FOREFOOT FRACTURES & DISLOCATIONS

1. Metatarsal Fractures & Dislocations

Fracture of the metatarsals and dislocation of the tarsometatarsals are frequently caused by a direct crushing or indirect twisting injury to the forefoot. Besides osseous and articular injury, complicating soft tissue lesions are often present. With severe trauma, circulation may be compromised from injury to the dorsalis pedis artery, which passes between the first and second metatarsals.

Metatarsal Shaft Fractures

Nondisplaced fractures of the metatarsal shafts cause only temporary disability, unless failure of bone healing occurs. Displacement is rarely significant when the first and fifth metatarsals are uninvolved because they act as internal splints.

These fractures can be treated with a hard-soled shoe with partial weight bearing, or, if pain is marked, a short leg walking cast.

For displaced fractures of the shaft, it is of paramount importance to correct angulation in the longitudinal axis of the shaft. Residual dorsal angulation causes prominence of the metatarsal head on the plantar surface. The concentrated local pressure may produce a painful skin callus. Residual plantar angulation of the first metatarsal will transfer weight to the heads of the second and third metatarsals. After reduction of angular deformity, a cast should be well molded to the plantar surface to minimize recurrence of deformity and support the transverse and longitudinal arches. If significant angulation or intra-articular displacement persists, open or closed reduction and internal fixation should be considered.

Metatarsal Neck & Head Fractures

Fractures of the metatarsal "neck" are close to the head but remain extra-articular. Dorsal angulation is common and should be reduced to avoid reactive skin callus formation from pressure on the plantar skin. Intra-articular fractures of the metatarsal heads are rare. Even when they heal in a displaced position, some remodeling occurs and the functional outcome is surprisingly good. The indications for open reduction with or without internal fixation remain controversial.

Closed reduction of metatarsal fractures is best achieved by applying traction (Chinese finger traps) to the involved toes. Reduction is evaluated with intraoperative radiographs, and if judged unacceptable, ORIF with K-wires or plates and screws is indicated. Unstable reductions should also undergo percutaneous pinning under fluoroscopic imaging.

Tarsometatarsal (Lisfranc) Dislocations

The stability of the tarsometatarsal joint complex relies in part on strong ligamentous structures and in part on the bony architecture itself. The base of the second metatarsal is recessed proximally to the base of the other metatarsals in a cleft between the first and third cuneiforms, thus "locking" the joint. Injuries to this structure should alert the clinician to the possibility of other injuries along the entire tarsometatarsal complex.

The mechanism of injury is usually and axial load on a hyperplantarflexed foot. Three commonly occurring patterns are identified: total incongruity, partial incongruity, and divergent(Figure 3–17). The medial border of the second and fourth metatarsals should align with the medial borders of the middle cuneiform and the cuboid, respectively. Associated soft-tissue damage is almost always significant, with open wounds, vascular impairment, swelling, and blistering.

An attempt at closed reduction should be made as soon as possible; however, open reduction is often re-

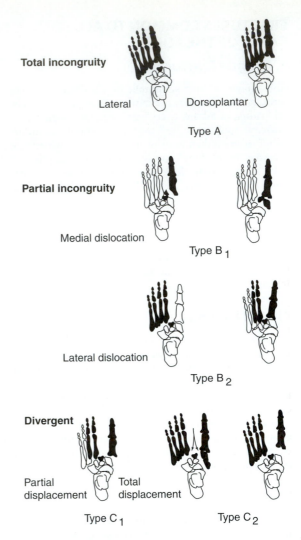

Figure 3–17. Classification of Lisfranc injuries. (Reproduced, with permission, from Coughlin MJ, Mann RA, eds: Surgery of the Foot and Ankle, 7th ed. Philadelphia: WB Saunders, 1999.)

quired. Gentle manipulation can be successful; however, residual instability is common. Postreduction radiographs are obtained, and if anatomic reduction is not obtained, then ORIF with K-wires on the lateral side of the foot to preserve mobility and screws on the medial side of the foot is indicated. The foot is then immobilized and elevated. Timing of hardware removal is controversial with some authors recommending 3 months, with others recommend 6 months.

Some tarsometatarsal injuries present late (> 3–4 weeks), when the healing process will prevent successful closed treatment. If displacement and deformity are significant, open reduction is indicated, but the patient should be advised to expect some residual joint stiffness. If displacement is minimal, it is probably better to defer surgery and direct treatment toward functional recovery. Reconstructive operations can be planned more suitably once residual disability is established.

Complications of this injury include chronic foot swelling, residual deformity making shoe fitting difficult, painful degenerative joint disease, and reflex sympathetic dystrophy.

Fracture of the Base of the Fifth Metatarsal

Two distinct patterns occur: (1) avulsion fracture of a variably sized portion of the tuberosity (styloid process) that may, on rare occasions, involve the joint between the cuboid and the fifth metatarsal and (2) transverse fracture of the proximal metatarsal diaphysis.

Avulsion fractures usually occur after adduction injury to the forefoot. The peroneus brevis muscle may pull and displace the fractured fragment proximally.

Symptomatic treatment is most often successful, and bony healing rarely fails to occur. Nonunions are rarely symptomatic but can be treated by internal fixation or fragment excision. In the rare event of a significant displaced intra-articular component, ORIF may be indicated.

Proximal diaphyseal fractures or "Jones fractures" are most probably secondary to fatigue failure. Again, conservative treatment in a non-weight–bearing short leg cast for 6 weeks will usually bring healing of the fracture. Nonunions do occur and are often symptomatic. If there is no evidence of bone healing at 12 weeks, internal fixation and bone grafting are recommended. Some authors recommend acute ORIF of Jones fractures in the high-performance athlete.

2. Fractures & Dislocations of the Phalanges of the Toes

Fractures of the phalanges of the toes are caused most commonly by a direct force such as a crush injury. Spiral or oblique fractures of the shaft of the proximal phalanges of the lesser toes may occur as a result of an indirect twisting injury.

Treatment

Comminuted fracture of the proximal phalanx of the great toe, alone or in combination with fracture of the distal phalanx, is a disabling injury. Because wide displacement of fragments is not likely, correction of angulation and support by a splint usually suffices. A

weight-bearing removable cast boot may be useful for relief of symptoms arising from associated soft-tissue injury. Spiral or oblique fracture of the proximal or middle phalanges of the lesser toes can be treated adequately by binding the involved toe to the adjacent uninjured toe (buddy taping). Comminuted fractures of the distal phalanx are treated as soft-tissue injuries.

Dislocation of the metatarsophalangeal joints and dislocation of the proximal interphalangeal joints usually can be reduced by closed manipulation. These dislocations are rarely isolated and usually occur in combination with other injuries to the forefoot.

3. Fracture of the Sesamoids of the Great Toe

Fractures of the sesamoid bones of the great toe are rare but may occur as a result of a crushing injury. These injuries must be differentiated from a bipartite sesamoid by comparing radiographs of the contralateral uninvolved foot.

Treatment

Undisplaced fractures require no treatment other than a hard-soled shoe or metatarsal bar. Displaced fractures may require immobilization in a walking boot or cast, with the toe strapped in flexion. Persistent delay of bone healing may cause disabling pain arising from arthritis of the articulation between the sesamoid and the head of the first metatarsal. If conservative modalities have been exhausted excision of the sesamoid may be necessary; however, this should be a last resort treatment.

Kelly IP et al: Intramedullary screw fixation of Jones fractures. Foot Ankle Int 2001;22:585.[PMID: 11503985]

Kuo RS et al: Outcome after open reduction and internal fixation of Lisfranc joint injuries. J Bone Joint Surg Am 2000;82-A:1609.[PMID: 11097452]

Kura H et al: Mechanical behavior of the Lisfranc and dorsal cuneometatarsal ligaments: In vitro biomechanical study. J Orthop Trauma 2001;15:107.[PMID: 11232648]

Larson CM et al: Intramedullary screw fixation of Jones fractures: Analysis of failure. Am J Sports Med 2002;30:55.[PMID: 11798997]

Nunley JA: Fractures of the base of the fifth metatarsal: The Jones fracture. Orthop Clin North Am 2001;32:171.[PMID: 11465126]

Richter M et al: Fractures and fracture dislocations of the midfoot: Occurrence, causes and long-term results. Foot Ankle Int 2001;22:392.[PMID: 11428757]

Rosenberg GA, Sferra JJ: Treatment strategies for acute fractures and nonunions of the proximal fifth metatarsal. J Am Acad Orthop Surg 2000;8:332.[PMID: 11029561]

MIDFOOT FRACTURES & DISLOCATIONS

1. Navicular Fractures

Avulsion Fractures

Avulsion fractures of the tarsal navicular may occur as a result of severe midtarsal sprain and require neither reduction nor elaborate treatment. Avulsion fracture of the tuberosity near the insertion of the posterior tibialis tendon is uncommon and must be differentiated from a persistent ununited apophysis (accessory navicular) from the supernumerary sesamoid bone, or os tibiale externum. Dorsal lip avulsions also occur.

Body Fractures

Body fractures occur either centrally in a horizontal plane or, more rarely, in a vertical plane. They are occasionally characterized by impaction. Noncomminuted fractures with displacement of the dorsal fragment can be reduced. Closed manipulation by strong traction on the forefoot and simultaneous digital pressure over the displaced fragment can restore normal position. If a tendency to redisplace is apparent, this can be counteracted by temporary fixation with a percutaneously inserted Kirschner wire. Non-weight–bearing immobilization in a cast or splint is required for a minimum of 6 weeks. Comminuted and impacted fractures cannot be anatomically reduced. Some authorities offer a pessimistic prognosis for comminuted or impacted fractures. It is their contention that even though partial reduction has been achieved, posttraumatic arthritis supervenes, and that arthrodesis of the talonavicular and naviculocuneiform joints will be ultimately necessary to relieve painful symptoms.

Stress Fractures

The navicular is also a frequent site of fatigue fracture. CT or radionuclide imaging is often necessary to make the diagnosis. Six weeks in a non-weight–bearing short leg cast is usually required for fracture healing.

2. Cuneiform & Cuboid Bone Fractures

Because of their relatively protected position in the midtarsus, isolated fractures of the cuboid and cuneiform bones are rarely encountered. Avulsion fractures occur as a component of severe midtarsal sprains. Extensive fractures usually occur in association with other injuries of the foot and often are caused by severe crushing. A "nutcracker" fracture is a compression fracture of the cuboid and, when associated with lateral column shortening, can be treated by lateral column lengthening, ORIF, and bone grafting.

1. Midtarsal Dislocations

Midtarsal dislocation through the naviculocuneiform and calcaneocuboid joints, or more proximally through the talonavicular and calcaneocuboid joints, may occur as a result of a twisting injury to the forefoot. Fractures of varying extent of adjacent bones are frequently associated.

When acute treatment is administered, closed reduction by traction on the forefoot and manipulation is generally effective. If reduction is unstable and displacement tends to recur upon release of traction, stabilization for 4 weeks by percutaneously inserted Kirschner wires is recommended.

HINDFOOT FRACTURES & DISLOCATIONS

1. Talus Fractures

Three fifths of the talus is covered with articular cartilage. The blood supply enters the neck area and is tenuous. Fractures and dislocations may disrupt this vascularization, causing delayed healing or avascular necrosis.

Major fractures of the talus commonly occur either through the body or the neck. Head fractures involve essentially a portion of the neck with extension into the head. Indirect injury is usually the cause of most fractures of the talus. Compression fracture or impaction of the tibial articular surface may be caused by the initial injury or may occur later in association with complicating avascular necrosis.

Fractures of the Neck of the Talus

The most common mechanism of talar neck fracture is hyperdorsiflexion with an axial load causing impingement between the talar neck and tibia. The most widely used classification is that of Hawkins:

Type 1: Nondisplaced vertical fracture

Type 2: Displaced fracture of the talar neck with subluxation or dislocation of the subtalar joint

Type 3: Displaced fracture of the talar neck with dislocation of the body of the talus from both the tibiotalar and subtalar joints

Type 4: Later, a type 4 fracture was described by Canale and Kelly to include rare variants which are essentially type 3 injuries with talonavicular subluxation or dislocation (Figure 3–18).

This classification is of prognostic value for avascular necrosis of the body: 0–13% for type 1 fractures,

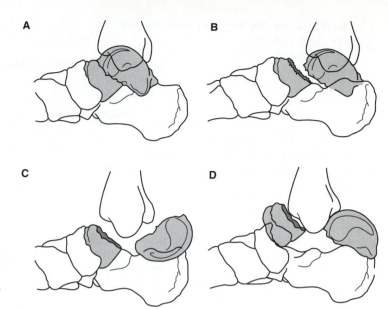

Figure 3–18. Hawkins classification of talar neck fractures. (Reproduced, with permission, from Coughlin MJ, Mann RA, eds: Surgery of the Foot and Ankle, 7th ed. Philadelphia: WB Saunders, 1999.)

25–50% for type 2 fractures, 20–100% for type 3 fractures, and 100% for type 4.

Less frequent complications of talar neck fractures include infection, delayed union or nonunion, malunion, and osteoarthritis of the tibiotalar and subtalar joints.

Treatment is aimed at minimizing the occurrence of these complications. Type 1 fractures are best treated with a non-weight–bearing below-knee cast for 2–3 months until clinical and radiologic signs of healing are present. Closed reduction is first attempted for type 2 fractures and, if this is successful in attaining anatomic alignment, treatment is as for a type 1 fracture. In about 50% of cases, closed reduction is unsuccessful and open reduction and internal fixation with K-wires, pins, or screws is indicated. Closed reduction of types 3 and 4 fractures is almost never successful; ORIF is the rule. The postoperative regimen is the same as above. Progressive weight bearing will be allowed after fracture union if there is no avascular necrosis of the body. This can be determined on the anteroposterior radiograph of the ankle taken out of the cast by the eighth week if there is a subchondral lucency in the dome of the talus. This "Hawkins' sign" is possible only if the talar body is vascularized. The most sensitive method, however, appears to be MRI, which can, as early as 3 weeks, clearly define the extent of osteonecrosis in the body of the talus. When avascular necrosis is evident, revascularization can take up to 3 years. To avoid collapse of the talar dome during this process, partial weight bearing is recommended. One should also remember that there is not a direct correlation between avascular necrosis and permanently disabling symptoms.

Fractures of the Body of the Talus

Minimally displaced fractures of the talar body are not likely to cause disability if immobilization is continued until union is restored. If significant displacement occurs, the proximal fragment is apt to be dislocated from the subtalar and ankle joints. Associated fractures (particularly of the malleoli) occur frequently.

Reduction by closed manipulation is often difficult but is best achieved by traction and forced plantar flexion of the foot. Immobilization in a short leg cast, with the foot in plantar flexion for about 8 weeks, should be followed by further casting with the foot out of equinus until the fracture line has been obliterated and new bone is present on serial radiographs. Even though prompt adequate reduction is obtained by either closed manipulation or open reduction, extensive displacement of the proximal body fragments may be followed by avascular necrosis. If reduction is not anatomic, delayed healing of the fracture may follow, and posttraumatic arthritis is a likely sequela. If this occurs, arthrodesis of the ankle or subtalar joints may be necessary to relieve painful symptoms.

Osteochondral Fractures of the Talar Dome

These can occur with any type of injury to the ankle area, including sprains. A history of trauma is usual, but not always, present. Classically, lesions of the medial aspect of the talar dome are thicker, more extensive, and less likely to displace, whereas the lateral lesions are more shallow, more waferlike, and more prone to be displaced and symptomatic.

Initial radiograph evaluation often does not demonstrate these lesions. Presently, MRI is the best imaging modality for osteochondral talar lesions.

The Berndt and Harty classification is generally used:

Stage 1: Localized compression
Stage 2: Incomplete separation of the fragment
Stage 3: Completely detached but nondisplaced fragment
Stage 4: Completely detached, displaced fracture

Symptomatic stage 1, 2, and 3 lesions are usually initially treated conservatively with immobilization and restricted weight bearing. Healing is monitored radiographically. Lesions that fail conservative treatment and all stage 4 lesions require surgical treatment. Reduction and pinning or fixation with screws and excision with or without drilling have been recommended. Arthroscopic management seems to give as good a result as arthrotomy, with fewer complications. Degenerative disease of the tibiotalar joint is a frequent long-term complication.

Other Talar Fractures

Compression fractures of the talar dome are rare injuries. They cannot be reduced by closed methods. If open reduction, with or without bone grafting, is elected, prolonged protection from weight bearing is the best means of preventing collapse of the healing area.

Other rare fractures include those of the lateral (snowboarders' fracture) or posterior process or its lateral or medial tubercles. These fractures may be difficult to demonstrate. Special radiographs and radionuclide imaging can be very helpful.

Conservative treatment usually gives excellent results; however, consideration should be given to open reduction and fixation of displaced fractures.

Subtalar Dislocation

Subtalar dislocation, also called **peritalar** dislocation, is the simultaneous dislocation of the talocalcaneal and talonavicular joints. Inversion injuries result in medial dislocations (85%), whereas eversion injuries result in lateral dislocations (15%).

Prompt gentle closed reduction is usually successful. Immobilization in a non-weight–bearing short leg cast is usually satisfactory. Soft-tissue interposition, particularly of the posterior tibial tendon, may prevent closed reduction. Open reduction, with or without internal fixation, is then indicated.

Total Dislocation of the Talus

This injury usually results from high-energy trauma, and most are open dislocations. Despite adequate prompt reduction and thorough wound debridement, the complication rate is extremely high, including persistent infection and avascular necrosis. Talectomy and tibiocalcaneal fusion is a frequent final outcome.

2. Calcaneus Fractures

The calcaneus (os calcis) is the tarsal bone most often fractured. The most common mechanism is a fall from a height. Ten percent of calcaneal fractures are associated with compression fractures of the thoracic or lumbar spine, and 5% are bilateral. Comminution and impaction are common features.

Clinical Findings

A. SYMPTOMS AND SIGNS

Pain is usually significant but may be masked by associated injuries. Swelling, deformity, and blistering of the skin occur frequently during the first 36 h as a result of the severe damage to surrounding soft tissues. The heel pad in particular is a highly specialized fatty structure that acts as a hydraulic cushion. Major disruptions of the heel pad lead to persistent pain and deformity and can produce poor functional results in spite of adequate bony healing.

B. IMAGING STUDIES

Initial radiographs include three views: anteroposterior, lateral, and axial projection (Harris view). Disruption of Böhlers angle and the angle of Gissane can be determined from initial radiographs (Figure 3–19). Oblique views, and CT scanning will further delineate fracture

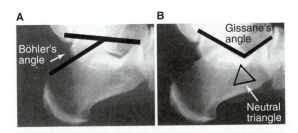

Figure 3–19. Böhler's angle (**A**) and Gissane's angle (**B**), indicating normal anatomical landmarks. (Reproduced, with permission, from Coughlin MJ, Mann RA, eds: Surgery of the Foot and Ankle, 7th ed. Philadelphia: WB Saunders, 1999.)

patterns and occult injuries. Bone scanning may be useful to diagnose a stress fracture.

C. CLASSIFICATION

Various classifications have been advocated. Sanders has developed a classification system based upon coronal CT images (Figure 3–20). This classification has been found to be useful in both treatment and prognosis. Type I fractures are nondisplaced articular fractures. Type II fractures are two-part fractures of the posterior facet and are divided into A, B, and C based upon the location of the fracture line. Type III fractures are three-part fractures with a centrally depressed fragment, also divided into A, B, and C. Type IV fractures are four-part articular fractures with extensive comminution. To simplify classification, calcaneus fractures can be divided into intra-articular and extra-articular fractures. Intra-articular fractures occur frequently (75%), have a poorer prognosis, and are further subdivided into nondisplaced, tongue-type, joint depression and comminuted. Extra-articular fractures are rare (25%) and generally have a better prognosis.

Intra-Articular Fractures

The subtalar joint is almost always involved, and occasionally the fracture line extends into the calcaneocuboid joint. Isolated fractures of the calcaneocuboid joint are rare.

A. TYPES OF FRACTURES

1. Nondisplaced fractures—These fractures are successfully treated by protection from weight bearing, for 4–8 weeks, until clinical and radiographic signs of healing are present.

2. Tongue-type fractures—This fracture pattern (Figure 3–21) involves the subtalar joint with a posterior extension in the transverse plane, creating a dorsal fragment.

3. Joint depression—This fracture pattern (Figure 3–22) creates a separate fragment of the posterior facet with joint incongruity.

4. Comminuted fractures—Some fracture patterns create such comminution and impaction that they defy

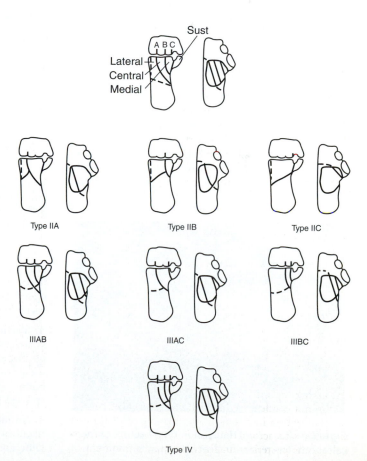

Figure 3–20. Sanders CT classification of calcaneus fractures. (Reproduced, with permission, from Coughlin MJ, Mann RA, eds: Surgery of the Foot and Ankle, 7th ed. Philadelphia: WB Saunders, 1999.)

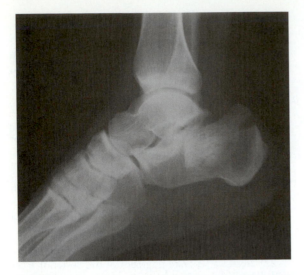

Figure 3–21. Tongue-type fracture of the calcaneus, showing involvement of the subtalar joint.

classification. They all have in common significant soft tissue injury and subtalar joint incongruity.

B. Treatment

Treatment of displaced intra-articular fractures remains controversial. As already stated, the final outcome is much dependent on soft-tissue as well as bony healing. For the severely displaced fracture, the bursting nature of the injury may defy anatomic restoration.

Some surgeons still advise conservative treatment.

Other surgeons advocate early closed manipulation of displaced intra-articular fractures, to at least partially restore the external anatomic configuration of the heel

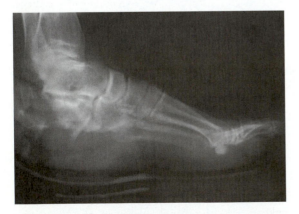

Figure 3–22. Joint depression-type fracture of the calcaneus. The posterior facet is a separate fragment.

region. Internal fixation with percutaneous pins may be performed. This is particularly successful for noncomminuted tongue-type fracture patterns. An axial pin is inserted in the tongue fragment, which is then disimpacted and reduced. The pin is then pushed further to stabilize the fracture (Essex-Lopresti technique). Open reduction and internal fixation with pins, screws, or plates, with or without bone grafting, has gained acceptance. The aim of ORIF is to restore Böhlers angle and improve heel alignment through stable fixation. A recent study has demonstrated a correlation between restoration of Böhlers angle and clinical outcome. Some authors advocate primary subtalar arthrodesis for severely comminuted fractures.

C. Complications

The most significant complication is posttraumatic degenerative arthritis. When only the subtalar joint is involved, talocalcaneal fusion is recommended. When the calcaneocuboid joint is also involved, triple arthrodesis should be performed. The rate of wound complications after ORIF has been reported to range from 0 to 12%.

Extra-Articular Fractures

Because posttraumatic joint disease is usually not a complication of these fractures, the final outcome is usually much better than that for intra-articular fractures. Fractures can affect any part of the bone.

A. Types of Fractures

1. Fracture of the tuberosity—Isolated fractures of the calcaneal tuberosity are rare.

2. Horizontal fracture—These fractures may be limited to the superior portion of the region of the former apophysis (avulsion type) or extend toward the subtalar joint in the substance of the tuberosity (beak type). A pull from the Achilles tendon may displace the fragment proximally, and reduction may be indicated. If the fragment is big enough, the application of skeletal traction can reduce it to the plantar flexed foot, and the pin is incorporated in a long leg cast with the knee flexed at 30 degrees. For smaller fragments or when closed reduction is unsuccessful, ORIF with screws, wires, or pullout sutures is indicated.

3. Vertical fracture—Vertical fracture occurs in the sagittal plane somewhat medially through the tuberosity. Because the minor medial fragment normally is not widely displaced, plaster immobilization is not required but may reduce pain. Limitation of weight bearing with crutches will also be helpful.

4. Nonarticular fracture of the body—Comminuted fractures of the entire tuberosity, sparing the subtalar joint, are rare. Proximal displacement of the fragments may decrease the subtalar joint angle, but symptomatic degenerative arthritis is not an important sequela, even though some joint stiffness may persist permanently. Marked displacement may benefit from closed reduction to improve heel contour.

5. Fracture of the sustentaculum—A rare injury, fracture of the sustentaculum tali should be suspected in the patient with a history of eversion injury and pain below the medial malleolus, which is often accentuated by passive hyperextension of the great toe. Interposition of the flexor hallucis longus tendon may even prevent reduction. Conservative treatment is usually successful. In the rare instance of symptomatic nonunion, careful excision is indicated.

6. Fracture of the anterior process—Usually caused by forced inversion of the foot, it must be differentiated from midtarsal and ankle sprains. The firmly attached bifurcate ligament avulses a bony flake from the anterior process. Maximal tenderness and swelling occurs midway between the tip of the lateral malleolus and the base of the fifth metatarsal. A lateral oblique radiograph will demonstrate the fracture line.

Treatment is by a non-weight–bearing short leg cast in neutral position for 4 weeks.

7. Fracture of the medial process—This process gives origin to the abductor hallucis and part of the flexor digitorum brevis muscle and can be avulsed in eversion-abduction injuries. Conservative treatment with a well-molded short leg walking cast is usually successful.

B. COMPLICATIONS

Posttraumatic arthritis of the subtalar joint has already been mentioned as the most frequent complication of calcaneal fractures. Other complications include peroneal tendinitis, bone spurs, calcaneocuboid arthritis, and nerve entrapment syndromes (medial or lateral plantar branches and sural nerve, either from posttraumatic or postsurgical scarring).

Beals TC: Applications of ring fixators to complex foot and ankle trauma. Orthop Clin North Am 2001;32:205.[PMID: 11465130]

Berlet GC, Lee TH, Massa EG: Talar neck fractures. Orthop Clin North Am 2001;32:53.[PMID: 11465133]

Boon AJ et al: Snowboarder's talus fracture. Mechanism of injury. Am J Sports Med 2001;29:333.[PMID: 11394605]

Brunet JA: Calcaneal fractures in children. J Bone Joint Surgery Br 2000;82-B:211.[PMID: 10755428]

Fortin PT, Balazsy JE: Talus fractures: Evaluation and treatment. J Am Acad Orthop Surg 2001;9:114.[PMID: 11281635]

Harvey EJ et al: Morbidity associated with ORIF of intra-articular calcaneus fractures using a lateral approach. Foot Ankle Int 2001;22:868.[PMID: 11722137]

Juliano P, Nguyen HV: Fractures of the calcaneus. Orthop Clin North Am 2001;32:35.[PMID: 11465132]

Lim EV, Leung JP: Complications of intraarticular calcaneal fractures. Clin Orthop 2001;391:7.[PMID: 11603691]

Longino D, Buckley RE: Bone graft in the operative treatment of displaced intraarticular calcaneal fractures: Is it helpful? J Orthop Trauma 2001;15:280.[PMID: 11371794]

ANKLE FRACTURES & DISLOCATIONS

Fractures and dislocations of the ankle are among the most common injuries treated by orthopedic surgeons. This injury is seen in all age groups, with a slightly different fracture pattern in children and adolescents than with adults. The ankle joint itself is limited to one plane of motion: plantarflexion and dorsiflexion in the sagittal plane. With incorporation of the motion of the subtalar joint (which allows for inversion and eversion in the coronal plane), the foot is able to move in a complex and varied arc in relationship to the leg.

Anatomy & Biomechanical Principles

The distal tibia and fibula are structures easily palpable because of their minimal soft-tissue coverage. The muscles, tendons, and neurovascular structures in the leg are generally grouped into anterior, lateral, and posterior compartments. In the distal leg, the compartments are predominantly tendinous, with little muscle being present. The tibia has a tubular diaphysis with wide flaring metaphyses both proximally and distally. The shape and size of the bone are markedly different in the proximal versus distal metaphysis. A cross-section of the midshaft tibia is approximately triangular, whereas a cross-section of the distal metaphysis is rounder and smaller in diameter. The articular surfaces of the distal tibia and fibula form the ankle mortise, which is the relatively horizontal surface of the distal tibia, including the medial malleolar extension and lateral malleolus of the fibula. The ankle mortise serves as the "roof" over the talus. The articular portions of the lateral and medial malleoli serve as constraining buttresses to allow for controlled plantarflexion and dorsiflexion in the ankle mortise. This geometric configuration resists rotation of the talus in the ankle mortise. Further constraint and stability are provided by the deltoid ligament medially and the lateral ligamentous complex (composed of the anterior talofibular, calcaneofibular, and posterior talofibular ligaments). The syndesmotic ligament connects the tibia to the fibula at the level of the tibial plafond. It allows for 1–2 mm of mortise widening, with ankle plantarflexion and dorsiflexion, to accommodate the geometry of the talar dome. The bony architecture of the mortise also provides some constraint to posterior subluxation of the talus. This is provided by the cup-shaped tibial plafond and the slightly increased width of the talar dome anteriorly as compared with posteriorly.

The distal tibia also serves to absorb the compressive loads and stress placed on the ankle. The internal trabecular pattern of the bone helps transmit, diffuse, and resorb the compressive forces. Cross-sectional studies have shown that reduced activity and old age lead to resorption of cancellous bone, thereby decreasing the compressive resistance of the distal tibia.

Fracture-dislocations of the ankle are frequently referred to as **bimalleolar** (fractures of the medial and lateral malleoli) or **trimalleolar** (fractures of the medial, lateral, and posterior malleoli). Fracture of the lateral malleolus with complete rupture of the deltoid ligament (Dupuytren's fracture) or fracture of the medial malleolus with complete disruption of the syndesmosis and a proximal fibular shaft fracture (Maisonneuve's fracture) are also considered bimalleolar fractures on a functional basis.

Classification

The purpose of any classification scheme is to provide a means to better understand the extent of injury, describe an injury, and determine a treatment plan. Presently, the two most widely used classification schemes for describing ankle fractures are the Lauge-Hansen and Weber classifications.

In 1950, Lauge-Hansen described a classification system based on mechanism of injury that described over 95% of all ankle fractures (Figure 3–23). By stressing freshly amputated limbs in combinations of supination, pronation, adduction, abduction, and external rotation, he was able to describe nearly all fracture patterns. Pronation and supination refer to the position of the patient's foot at the instance of injury, while adduction, abduction, and external rotation refer to the vector of the force that is applied. Thus, four mechanisms of injury were described for ankle fractures: (1) supination adduction, (2) supination-external rotation, (3) pronation abduction, and (4) pronation-exter-

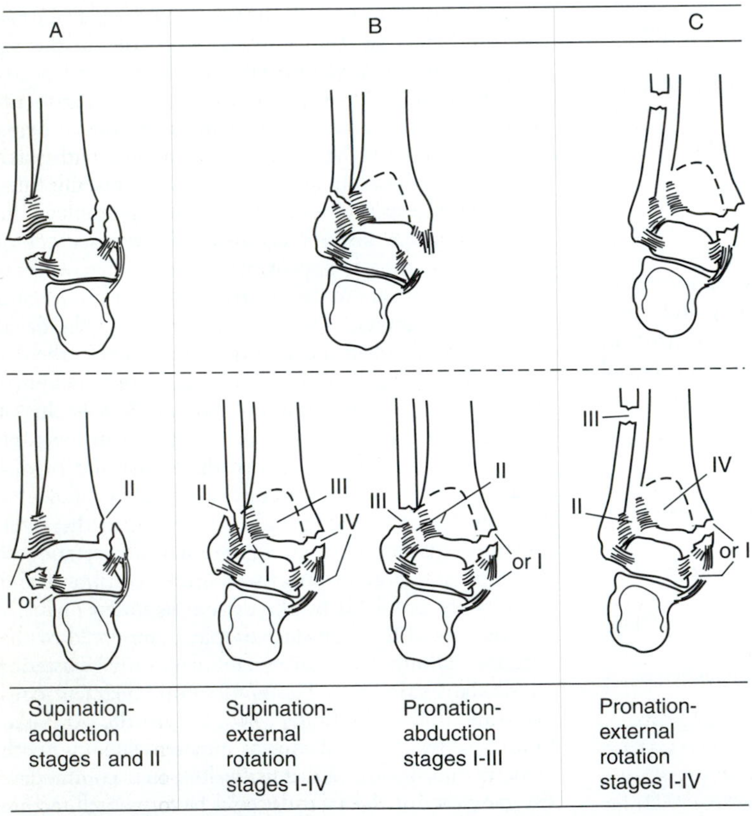

Figure 3–23. Comparison of Lauge-Hansen and Danis-Weber ankle classifications. (Reproduced, with permission, from Browner BD et al, eds: Skeletal Trauma, 2nd ed. Philadelphia: WB Saunders, 1998.)

nal rotation. Lauge-Hansen later added a fifth type of injury, the pronation dorsiflexion injury, in order to include a mechanism for tibial plafond fractures. This fifth type is caused by a compression-type injury.

The Weber classification is much simpler, and is based on the level at which the fibular fracture occurs.

Type A: Fracture in which the fibula is avulsed distal to the joint line. The syndesmotic ligament is left intact, and the medial malleolus is either undamaged or is fractured in a shear-type pattern, with the fracture line angulating in a proximal-medial direction from the corner of the mortise.

Type B: Spiral fracture of the fibula beginning at the level of the joint line and extending in a proximal-posterior direction up the shaft of the fibula. Parts of the syndesmotic ligament complex can be torn, but the large interosseous ligament is usually left intact so that no widening of the distal tibiofibular articulation occurs. Complete syndesmotic disruptions, however can result from this fracture pattern.

The medial malleolus can either be left intact or sustain a transverse avulsion fracture. If the medial malleolus is left intact there can be a tear of the deltoid ligament. Avulsion fracture of the posterior lip of the tibia (posterior malleolus) can also occur.

Type C: Fracture of the fibula proximal to the syndesmotic ligament complex, with consequent disruption of the syndesmosis. Medial malleolar avulsion fracture or deltoid ligament rupture is also present. Posterior malleolar avulsion fracture can also occur. Figure 3–23 shows a comparison of the Weber and Lauge-Hansen schemes.

Treatment

Four criteria should be met for the optimal treatment of ankle fractures: (1) dislocations and fractures should be reduced as soon as possible; (2) all joint surfaces must be precisely restored; (3) the fracture must be held in a reduced position during the period of bony healing, and (4) joint motion should be initiated as early as possible. If these treatment goals are met, a good outcome can be expected, keeping in mind that disruption of the articular cartilage results in permanent damage.

Previous studies have demonstrated that the ankle has the thinnest articular cartilage but the highest ratio of joint congruence to articular cartilage thickness of any of the large joints. This suggests that loss in congruity of the ankle joint following fracture will be poorly tolerated and lead to posttraumatic arthritic changes. Thus, it is important to obtain anatomic reduction of the articular surfaces of the ankle after a fracture. A lateral talar shift of as little as 1 mm will decrease surface contact at the tibiotalar joint by 40%.

Initial treatment of ankle fractures should include immediate closed reduction and splinting, with the joint held in the most normal position possible to prevent neurovascular compromise of the foot. An ankle joint should never be left in a dislocated position. If the fracture is open, the patient should be given appropriate intravenous antibiotics and taken to the operating room on an emergent basis for irrigation and debridement of the wound, fracture site, and ankle joint. The fracture should also be appropriately stabilized at this time.

With the advent of excellent results obtained from the techniques of open reduction and rigid internal fixation as developed by the AO group, the standard of care for displaced ankle fractures has become operative intervention. Exceptions to this rule are nondisplaced, isolated Weber type B lateral malleolar fractures (supination eversion stage 2), nondisplaced medial malleolar fractures, distal fibular avulsion fractures, fractures in nonambulatory (ie, paraplegic) patients, and fractures in patients for whom the surgical risks are greater than the consequences of nonanatomic reduction of the fracture. The isolated previously described lateral or medial malleolar fractures may be treated in a well-molded short leg walking cast for 6 weeks. Unstable ankle fractures treated by immobilization should be placed in a long leg cast with the knee flexed to prevent weight bearing on the involved limb. Most nondisplaced medial malleolar fractures should be treated with internal fixation because of the risk of nonunion, when these fractures are treated nonoperatively.

When performing ORIF of ankle fractures, several principles must be followed. It is important to gently handle the soft tissues about the ankle so as to minimize the risks of infection and wound-healing problems. In the treatment of bimalleolar and trimalleolar fractures, the lateral malleolus should usually be reduced and internally fixed first. This has two benefits: (1) it helps to correctly restore the original limb length, and (2) because of the strong ligamentous connections between the lateral malleolus and talus (anterior and posterior talofibular ligaments), initial fixation of the lateral malleolus will correctly position the talus in the mortise. If a long oblique fracture of the lateral malleolus is present, fixation can sometimes be adequately obtained with two interfragmentary screws. More commonly, however, further fixation, in the form of a neutralization plate and screws, is required.

When performing ORIF of the medial malleolus, it is important to remove any soft tissue or periosteum interposed in the fracture site. It is also preferable to fix the medial malleolus with either two cancellous-type screws or a screw and a K-wire to provide rotational control of the medial malleolar fragment.

The necessity for fixation of the posterior malleolar fragment is dependent on several factors. After the lateral and medial malleolar fractures have been internally fixed, ligamentotaxis often will anatomically reduce the posterior malleolar fragment. If this fragment represents less than 25% of the articular surface of the tibial plafond and there is less than 2 mm of displacement, internal fixation is not always required. If the fragment does not reduce on the intraoperative radiograph with ligamentotaxis, or if the fragment represents more than 25% of the articular surface, most authors agree that it should be internally fixed. Several methods have been described for this, utilizing either direct fixation posteriorly via the lateral or medial incisions, or a lag screw from anterior to posterior.

Following surgery, the limb is placed in a bulky sterile dressing with plaster splints from the ball of the foot to the proximal calf to allow for wound healing. The ankle is kept in neutral position to prevent equinus deformity. After the sutures are removed at 1–2 weeks, the surgeon must decide whether to begin early mobilization of the ankle joint. If the patient is reliable and stable fixation was achieved at the time of surgery, then early range of motion may be initiated, keeping the patient on crutches and not allowing weight bearing. If there is a question about patient reliability or stability of fixation, the limb can be placed in a short leg cast for added protection. Usually at 6 weeks all immobilization is discontinued and weight bearing is slowly advanced. Physical therapy often helps promote ankle motion, strengthening, and regained ankle proprioception.

Egol KA, Dolan R, Koval KJ: Functional outcome of surgery for fractures of the ankle. J Bone Joint Surg Br 2000;82-B:246. [PMID: 10755435]

Hintermann B et al: Arthroscopic findings in acute fractures of the ankle. J Bone Joint Surg Br 2000;82-B:345.[PMID: 10813167]

Kay RM, Matthys GA: Pediatric ankle fractures: Evaluation and treatment. J Am Acad Orthop Surg 2001;9:268.[PMID: 11476537]

Obremskey WT et al: Change over time of SF-36 functional outcomes for operatively treated unstable ankle fractures. J Orthop Trauma 2002;15:30.[PMID: 11782630]

Pankovich AM: Acute indirect ankle injuries in the adult. J Orthop Trauma 2002;15:58.[PMID: 11782638]

Saltzman R, French BG, Mizel MS: Ankle fracture with syndesmotic injury: case controversies. J Orthop Trauma 2000; 14:113.[PMID: 10716383]

Tabrizi P et al: Limited dorsiflexion predisposes to injuries of the ankle in children. J Bone Joint Surg Br 2000;82-B:1103. [PMID: 11132266]

Tornetta P: Competence of the deltoid ligament in bimalleolar ankle fractures after medial malleolar fixation. J Bone Joint Surg;82-A:843.[PMID: 10859104]

Tornetta P, Creevy W: Lag screw only fixation of the lateral malleolus. J Orthop Trauma 2001;15:119.[PMID: 11232650]

TIBIA & FIBULA INJURIES

Anatomy & Biomechanical Principles

The tibial diaphysis is straight and triangular in cross-section. Its anteromedial border and anterior crest are palpable throughout the entire length of the bone, and are useful landmarks for closed reduction techniques and cast molding with pressure relief, as are the palpable fibular head, distal third of the fibula, and patellar tendon. The distal half of the leg has more tendons and less muscle than the proximal half, and thus soft tissue coverage and blood supply of the distal tibia is more precarious than its proximal portion. The fibula transmits approximately one sixth of the axial load from the knee to the foot and the tibia five sixths.

From a surgical standpoint, the leg has been divided into four compartments. A compartment is defined by the unyielding boundaries, such as bone and fascia, enclosing a given content. The anterior compartment is limited medially by the tibia, posteriorly by the interosseous membrane, laterally by the fibula, and anteriorly by the crural fascia. It contains the tibialis anterior, extensor hallucis longus, extensor digitorum longus, and peroneus tertius muscles, as well as the anterior tibial artery and the deep branch of the peroneal nerve. It is responsible for ankle and toe extension. The lateral compartment contains the peroneus brevis and longus muscles responsible for ankle flexion and foot eversion and the superficial branch of the peroneal nerve. The superficial posterior compartment contains the gastrocnemius, soleus, plantaris, and popliteus muscles and the sural nerve. It is responsible for plantar flexion of the foot and ankle. The deep posterior compartment is enclosed by the tibia, the interosseous membrane, and the deep transverse fascia. It contains the tibialis posterior, flexor hallucis longus, and flexor digitorum longus muscles, and also the posterior tibial and peroneal arteries and the tibial nerve.

1. Tib-Fib Fractures

Fractures of the tibial or fibular diaphysis are the result of direct or indirect trauma, with some of these injuries being open fractures. A thorough assessment of the surrounding soft tissues is mandatory. One must remember that the size of the skin wound does not necessarily correlate with the amount of underlying soft tissue damage. A Gustilo grade 1 skin laceration can be associated with a grade 3 muscle and periosteal injury and have a much poorer prognosis.

When the fracture is displaced, the clinical diagnosis is usually evident. All compartments should be palpated, and a thorough distal neurovascular examination should be recorded.

Radiographs in the anteroposterior and lateral projections are taken of the entire leg, including the knee and ankle joints. Oblique views are sometimes necessary. Fractures of the distal end of the tibia (pilon or plafond fractures) can be better visualized with CT scanning.

Fibula Diaphysis Fractures

Isolated fibula fractures can be associated with other injuries of the leg, such as fracture of the tibia or fracture-dislocation of the ankle joint. One should pay particular attention to the medial malleolus to rule out deltoid ligament rupture or medial malleolus fracture. Isolated fibula fracture can be the result of a direct or "tapping" mechanism; however, it can also coincide with syndesmosis disruption. If reduction of the mortise is congruent, radiographic follow-up needs to be careful to ensure maintenance of reduction.

Tibia Diaphyseal Fractures

Isolated fractures of the tibial diaphysis are usually the result of torsional stress. There is a tendency for the tibia to displace into varus angulation because of an intact fibula.

Fractures of both the tibia and fibula are more unstable, and displacement can recur after reduction. The fibular fracture usually heals independently of the reduction achieved. The same does not apply to the tibia. There is some controversy as to what is an acceptable reduction of a tibial shaft fracture in the adult. The following criteria are generally accepted: apposition of 50% or more of the diameter of the bone in both anteroposterior and lateral projections, no more than 5 degrees of varus or valgus angulation, 5 degrees of angulation in the anteroposterior plane, 10 degrees of rotation, and 1 cm of shortening. It is assumed that fracture healing in an unacceptable position (ie, malunion) will affect the mechanics of the knee or ankle joint and possibly lead to premature degenerative joint disease.

Acceptable reduction can be obtained in one of many ways, and this is another area of ongoing controversy: closed versus open treatment. The goal of any treatment is to allow the fracture to heal in an acceptable position with minimal negative effect on the surrounding tissues or joints. Closed reduction is obtained under general anesthesia if necessary, and the patient is immobilized in a long leg non-weight–bearing cast. Weekly radiographs for the first 4 weeks will help ensure that displacement does not occur. If it does, angulation can be corrected by "wedging" the cast. This involves dividing the plaster circumferentially and inserting wedges in the appropriate direction after corrective manipulation. At 6 weeks, some shaft fractures are stable enough to be put in a short leg weight-bearing cast, usually a patellar tendon-bearing cast or brace as recommended by Sarmiento. Protected weight bearing should be continued until clinical and radiologic healing is evident.

If acceptable and stable reduction cannot be obtained by closed means, other methods are required. Skeletal traction via a calcaneal transfixing pin is rarely used, although it is an acceptable short-term option in the polytraumatized patient. An external fixator with an outer frame is extremely useful for open fractures, as it provides rigid fixation and still allows access for wound care. This is still the initial treatment for some Gustilo type 3 injuries and in the unstable patient. A reamed intramedullary nail is the recommended treatment for most displaced closed fractures. There are proponents of reamed and unreamed nails in the treatment of open injuries. Intramedullary nails are introduced from a proximal starting point anterior to the tibial tubercle and across the fracture site under fluoroscopic control without opening the fracture site. Dynamic or static interlocking can be achieved with transfixing screws in one or both ends of the nail, and this maintains length and provides rotational control.

Open reduction and internal fixation with plates and screws requires opening of the fracture site and results in extensive soft-tissue dissection, devascularization of the bone with increased risk of infection, and delayed union. Such treatment should be reserved for the multiply injured child and is rarely indicated in adults.

Recent studies comparing tibia fractures treated with cast immobilization with those treated with intramedullary nailing indicate that the intramedullary nail group has a shorter time to healing, a better rate of healing, and an improved functional score. Disadvantages of operative treatment include infection, wound problems, and possible contractures. The advantages of closed treatment are early mobilization with or without weight bearing and a short hospital stay, with less risk of infection from the operative approach. Closed treatment does not preclude further surgical treatment. Disadvantages include residual deformity, knee or ankle joint stiffness, and more difficult wound care. Sound clinical judgment is needed in the decision-making process. An isolated closed tibial fracture in a compliant patient is a much different problem than the same tibial injury in a polytraumatized comatose patient.

Fracture of the Distal End of the Tibia

Also referred to as **pilon** or **plafond** fractures, these fractures involve the distal articular surface of the tibia at the tibiotalar joint. Ruedi and Allgower classified these injuries into I, II, and III based upon the amount of articular displacement and comminution, which represents a wide spectrum of injury (Figure 3–24).

As for any intra-articular fracture, the goal of treatment is to restore an anatomic articular surface. This can be difficult and sometimes impossible. Closed reduction of displaced fractures is almost never successful and external fixation spanning the injury, with or without ORIF of the fibula can be initially performed. Once soft-tissue swelling subsides, minimally invasive open reduction and percutaneous techniques should be attempted. Bone graft can be added to metaphyseal defects to support the articular surface. When the fracture is so comminuted that internal fix-

ation is impossible, an attempt at indirect reduction by ligamentotaxis should be done: ORIF of the fibular fracture to restore length, and closed reduction and external fixation of the tibia with a external fixator. This can usually restore normal contours and alignment of the distal leg and make an eventual tibiotalar fusion easier should disabling posttraumatic arthritis occur.

These fractures are notorious for associated soft-tissue damage. Swelling can be impressive, and prolonged leg elevation is often necessary, especially to prevent surgical wound problems after open reduction. Healing is likely to be slow, and weight bearing should be carefully started only when radiologic evidence of bone healing is present.

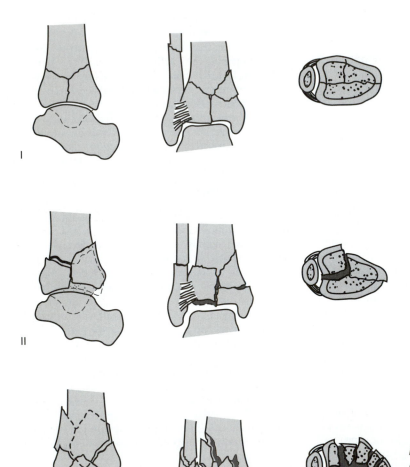

Figure 3–24. Ruedi and Allgower classification of Pilon fractures. (Reproduced, with permission, from Browner BD et al, eds: Skeletal Trauma, 2nd ed. Philadelphia: WB Saunders, 1998.)

Compartment Syndrome

Compartment syndrome is a frequent concern in tibia fractures and is caused by increased pressure in any of the four closed osteofascial spaces, compromising circulation and perfusion of the tissues within the involved compartment. Nerves and muscle tissue are particularly susceptible.

Fasciotomies are performed through a lateral and a medial incision in the skin and fascia of all four compartments. Compartment pressure measurements are taken after decompression to ensure adequate pressure reduction. Tissue debridement is kept to a minimum. The wounds are left open, sterilely dressed, and then treated by delayed primary closure or split-thickness skin grafting 5 days later. Delaying treatment of any compartment syndrome by more than 6–8 h can lead to irreversible nerve and muscle damage.

Complications

Complications are common after tibia and fibula fractures and may be related to the nature of the injury itself or to its management.

A. Delayed Union or Nonunion

Because of its relatively poor soft-tissue coverage, the tibia, particularly its distal third, is prone to delayed union or nonunion. This occurs more frequently in high-energy, open, and segmental fractures. Pain and motion at the fracture are noted to be present more than 6 months after the injury. Radiographs show the persistence of the fracture line without bridging callus. Sclerosis and flaring of the bone ends characterize the hypertrophic nonunion, whereas osteopenia and thinning of the fragments are seen in atrophic nonunions. Early weight bearing is thought to stimulate bone healing. If nonunion develops in spite of this, rigid fixation or bone grafting may be required in order for the nonunion to heal. Electrical stimulation has limited efficacy but may achieve union in selected cases.

B. Malunion

Malunion may lead to premature degenerative joint disease. Corrective osteotomies may be required. When associated with shortening, multiple-plane correction and lengthening can be obtained after corticotomy and external fixation with Ilizarov-type devices, which allow progressive correction of the deformity.

C. Infection

Infection of the tibia following open fracture or surgical treatment remains the most severe complication, especially when associated with nonunion. Perioperative prophylactic antibiotic therapy and adequate debridement and irrigation of open fractures are not always successful in preventing this dreaded complication. Recently, the generous utilization of free muscle flaps to increase the local blood supply has significantly improved the overall results of treatment, although amputation is still occasionally required.

D. Reflex Sympathetic Dystrophy

Reflex sympathetic dystrophy is a fortunately rare complication of unknown cause. It is seen most often in those comminuted fractures associated with significant soft-tissue damage treated with prolonged cast immobilization without weight bearing. Swelling, pain, and vasomotor disturbances are the hallmarks of this syndrome. Gradual increase in weight bearing and early joint mobilization will minimize the occurrence of this complication. Chemical or surgical sympathetic blockade may be helpful for the more severe forms of this disease.

E. Other Complications

Posttraumatic arthritis is a frequent occurrence after pilon fractures or as a complication of tibial shaft malunion. Joint stiffness and ankylosis may occur after prolonged immobilization. Soft-tissue injuries, including those of nerve, vessels, or muscles, have been discussed in the compartment syndrome section. Sequelae may include dropfoot and clawtoe deformities and may require further soft-tissue or bone procedures.

Blauth M et al: Surgical options for the treatment of severe tibial pilon fractures: A study of three techniques. J Orthop Trauma 2001;15:153.[PMID: 11265004]

Brinker MR et al: Tibial shaft fractures with an associated infrapopliteal arterial injury: A survey of vascular surgeons' opinions on the need for vascular repair. J Orthop Trauma 2000;14:194.[PMID: 10791671]

Finkemeier CG et al: A prospective, randomized study of intramedullary nails inserted with and without reaming for the treatment of open and closed fractures of the tibial shaft. J Orthop Trauma 2000;14:187.[PMID: 10791670]

Gaston P et al: Analysis of muscle function in the lower limb after fracture of the diaphysis of the tibia in adults. J Bone Joint Surg Br 2000;82-B:326.[PMID: 10813163]

Gopal S et al: Fix and flap: The radical orthopaedic and plastic treatment of severe open fractures of the tibia. J Bone Joint Surg Br 2000;82-B:959.[PMID: 11041582]

Hernigou P, Cohen D: Proximal entry for intramedullary nailing of the tibia. J Bone Joint Surg Br 2000;82-B:33.[PMID: 10697311]

Keating JF et al: Reamed nailing of Gustilo grade-IIIB tibial fractures. J Bone Joint Surg Br 2000;82-B:1113.[PMID: 11132268]

Lin J, Hou SM: Unreamed locked tight-fitting nailing for acute tibial fractures. J Orthop Trauma 2001;15:40.[PMID: 11132268]

McQueen MM, Gaston P, Court-Brown CM: Acute compartment syndrome. J Bone Joint Surg Br 2000;82-B:200.[PMID: 10755426]

Meffert RH et al: Distraction osteogenesis after acute limb-shortening for segmental tibial defects. J Bone Joint Surg Am 2000;82-A:799.[PMID: 10859099]

Nassif JM et al: Effect of acute reamed versus undreamed intramedullary nailing on compartment pressure when treating closed tibial shaft fractures: A randomized prospective study. J Orthop Trauma 2000;14:554.[PMID: 11149501]

Samuelson MA, McPherson EJ, Norris L: Anatomic assessment of the proper insertion site for a tibial intramedullary nail. J Orthop Trauma 2002;16:23.[PMID: 11782628]

Sarmiento A: On the behavior of closed tibial fractures: Clinical/radiological correlations. J Orthop Trauma 2000;14:199.

Skoog A et al: One-year outcome after tibial shaft fractures: Results of a prospective fracture registry. J Orthop Trauma 2001;15:210.[PMID: 10791672]

Thordarson DB: Complications after treatment of tibial pilon fractures: Prevention and management strategies. J Am Acad Orthop Surg 2000;8:253.[PMID: 10951114]

Vives MJ et al: Soft tissue injuries with the use of safe corridors for transfixion wire placement during external fixation of distal tibia fractures: An anatomic study. J Orthop Trauma 2001; 15:555.[PMID: 11733671]

INJURIES AROUND THE KNEE

Anatomy & Biomechanical Principles

The knee is a synovial joint formed by three bones: the distal femur, the proximal tibia, and the patella. It is often divided into three compartments: medial, lateral, and patellofemoral.

The distal femoral diaphysis broadens into two curved condyles at the metaphyseal junction. Each condyle is convex and articulates distally with its corresponding tibial plateau. Their articular surfaces join anteriorly to articulate with the patella. Posteriorly, they remain separate to form the intercondylar notch. The lateral condyle is wider in the anteroposterior plane and extends further proximally. The medial condyle is narrower but extends further distally. This difference in length of both condyles allows for the distance between both knees, when weight bearing, to be smaller than the distance between both hips. Both condylar surfaces form a horizontal plane parallel to the ground and create an anatomic angle (physiologic valgus position) of 5–7 degrees with the femoral shaft. Normally, the centers of the hip, knee, and ankle joints are all aligned to form a mechanical angle of 0 degrees. The supracondylar area of the femur is defined as the distal 9 cm. Fractures proximal to this are considered femoral shaft fractures and carry a different prognosis.

As for the distal femur, the proximal tibia widens proximally at the diaphyseal-metaphyseal junction to form the medial and lateral tibial plateaus (condyles). There is a 7–10 degrees slope from anterior to posterior of the tibial plateaus. The tibial eminence, with its me-dial and lateral spines, separates both compartments and is the attachment for the cruciate ligaments and the menisci. Distal to the joint itself, the tibia has two prominences: the tibial tubercle anteriorly, where the patellar tendon attaches, and Gerdy's tubercle anterolaterally, where the iliotibial band inserts. Posterolaterally, the undersurface of the tibial plateau articulates with the fibular head to form the proximal tibiofibular joint.

The patella is the biggest sesamoid bone in the body. It lies within the substance of the quadriceps tendon. The distal third of the undersurface is nonarticular and provides attachment for the patellar tendon. The proximal two thirds articulates with the anterior surface of the femoral condyles and is divided into medial and lateral facets by a longitudinal ridge. The area of contact at the patellofemoral joint varies according to the degree of knee flexion. On each side of the patella are the medial and lateral retinacular expansions formed by fibers of the vastus medialis and vastus lateralis muscles. These expansions bypass the patella to insert directly on the tibia. When intact, they can allow active knee extension even in the presence of a fractured patella. The blood supply to the patella generally goes from the distal pole proximally. Avascular necrosis of a proximal fracture fragment is not uncommon.

The main plane of motion of the knee is flexion and extension, but internal and external rotation, abduction and adduction (varus and valgus), and anterior and posterior translation also all occur physiologically as well. The intrinsic bony configuration of the joint affords little stability. A complex soft-tissue network provides joint stability under physiologic loading. It includes passive stabilizers such as medial and lateral collateral ligaments, medial and lateral menisci, anterior and posterior cruciate ligaments, joint capsule, and active stabilizers such as the extensor mechanism, the popliteus muscle, and the hamstrings with their capsular expansions. All these soft tissue components work together in an extremely complex and finely tuned way to prevent excessive displacement of the joint surfaces throughout the full arc of motion under physiologic loading. When abnormal stresses that exceed the soft tissues' ability to resist them are transmitted across the joint, an infinite range of injuries can occur. These may be isolated or combined, partial or complete, or associated or unassociated with bony injuries. An accurate diagnosis, although sometimes difficult, is essential before the appropriate treatment can be decided upon.

LIGAMENTOUS INJURIES

As already stated, a wide spectrum of ligamentous injuries, from partial sprain of an isolated ligament to major soft-tissue disruption are seen in knee dislocations. Associated injuries to bone, cartilage, and menisci are common.

Knowledge of the mechanism of injury is of paramount importance, as certain injury patterns may be anticipated. Dashboard injuries may cause posterior translation of the tibia under the femur with posterior cruciate ligament damage. Hyperextension injuries, as seen in skiers, volleyball players, or basketball players, often involve the anterior cruciate ligament. Tackles at knee level in football often create a valgus flexion external rotation injury with damage to the medial collateral ligament, medial meniscus, and anterior cruciate ligament (The Terrible Triad). A good clinical examination is sometimes difficult, particularly in a young muscular athlete with a large lower extremity, but it is essential and will usually provide key diagnostic information.

Plain radiograms are of limited benefit. They will show fractures, bony avulsions at ligament attachment sites, or capsular avulsion signs such as the lateral capsular sign (Segund fracture), which is diagnostic of anterior cruciate ligament disruption (Figure 3–25).

Tomograms and contrast arthrograms have only limited indications because MRI has become so widely accepted. MRI is now by far the imaging tool of choice for ligamentous injuries of the knee, with an accuracy rate above 95%. Diagnostic arthroscopy is now reserved for cases when MRI is inconclusive or the surgeon is fairly sure that surgical treatment of a lesion will be necessary.

1. Medial (Tibial) Collateral Ligament Injury

This ligament normally resists valgus angulation at the knee joint. A history of abduction injury, often with a torsional component, is usually obtained. Examination reveals tenderness over the site of the lesion and often some knee effusion. When compared with the contralateral knee, valgus stressing with the knee flexed at 20–30 degrees will show exaggerated laxity at the joint line, signaling a complete tear. Stress radiographs can, on rare occasions, be useful in confirming the diagnosis.

Grade 1 and 2 sprains (incomplete) are treated with protective weight bearing in a hinged brace or cast to prevent further injury while healing progresses. Grade 3 sprains (complete) are rarely isolated. Known associated injuries, such as medial meniscus damage, anterior cruciate ligament tear, or lateral tibial plateau fractures, should be systematically ruled out. Most surgeons now favor conservative treatment of isolated grade 3 medial collateral ligament tears in a long leg hinged-knee brace for 4–6 weeks because surgical repair has not proved to provide any long-term benefit.

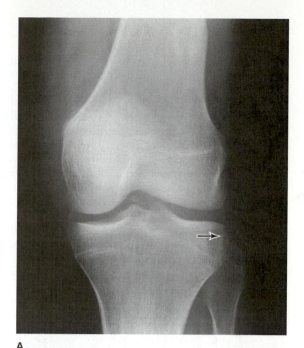

A

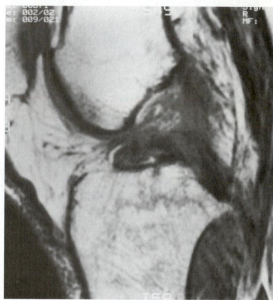

B

Figure 3–25. Lateral capsular sign, diagnostic of anterior cruciate ligament injury, as demonstrated by radiograph (**A**) and MRI studies (**B**).

2. Lateral (Fibular) Collateral Ligament Injury

This ligament originates from the lateral femoral condyle and inserts on the fibular head. It resists varus angulation at the knee joint. Isolated injuries are extremely rare. Most often, there is a combination of varying degrees of injury to the posterolateral corner, which includes the biceps tendon, posterolateral capsule, popliteus tendon, and iliotibial band. Injury to the peroneal nerve is not uncommon. Pain and tenderness are present over the lateral aspect of the knee, usually with some intra-articular effusion. In severe injuries, there is abnormal laxity on varus stressing compared with the other knee.

Radiographs often show avulsion of the fibular head. When this fragment is of sufficient size, internal fixation with a screw gives excellent results. Conservative management involves protected weight bearing in a long leg hinged-knee brace for 4–6 weeks. Most injuries require operative treatment, although conservative treatment may be indicated for the low-demand patient with mild laxity.

3. Anterior Cruciate Ligament Injury

This ligament originates at the posteromedial aspect of the lateral femoral condyle and inserts near the medial tibial spine. Because it is composed of at least two distinct fiber bundles, part of it remains taut throughout the normal flexion-extension arc of motion. It prevents anterior translation (gliding) of the tibia under the femoral condyles. Isolated injuries are frequent, especially with hyperextension mechanism, but associated medial collateral ligament, medial meniscus, posteromedial capsule, and even posterior cruciate ligament injuries are more common. When the tear is complete, it most often occurs within the substance of its fibers. Rarely, bony avulsion at the femoral or tibial attachment will be seen on plain radiograms.

Clinical Findings

The patient usually recalls the mechanism of injury, and classically feels a popping or snapping sensation in the knee. Moderate effusion over the next few hours is usually the rule. The only clinical finding in acute anterior cruciate ligament deficiency may be a positive Lachman's test, which is the anterior drawer test performed with 20–30 degrees of knee flexion. The classic drawer test, done with the knee flexed at 90 degrees and the foot resting on the table, is not as reliable. The injured knee should always be compared with the uninjured contralateral knee. In chronic anterior cruciate ligament deficiency, secondary restraints have stretched out and other clinical signs, such as the pivot shift and the active drawer sign, become more apparent.

Treatment

Treatment remains controversial despite the abundance of literature on this topic over the last 20 years. Most surgeons feel that surgical reconstruction affords the best long-term results. When bony avulsions from the femur or tibia are present, surgical repair is indicated as bone-to-bone healing and good long-term results have been demonstrated.

Primary repair of the ligament stumps without reconstruction is likely to fail. The trend presently seems to reserve surgical reconstruction for young high-demand athletes. For others, conservative management with rehabilitation therapy and bracing can give satisfactory results. Those patients who remain unacceptably unstable after conservative treatment can still benefit from delayed reconstructive surgery. Favored techniques at the present include the arthroscopically assisted use of the middle third of the patellar tendon or harvest of a autogenous hamstrings graft.

4. Posterior Cruciate Ligament Injury

The posterior cruciate ligament is a broad thick ligament that extends from the lateral aspect of the medial femoral condyle posteriorly and inserts extra-articularly over the back of the tibial plateau approximately 1 cm below the joint line. It resists posterior translation (gliding) of the tibia under the femoral condyle. It usually ruptures after a posteriorly directed force on the proximal tibia as is sometimes seen in dashboard injuries. Posterior cruciate ligament ruptures can also occur as the end stage of severe hyperextension injuries.

Clinical Findings

The posterior drawer test will be positive, as will the sag test, showing posterior sagging of the tibia with the knee flexed to 90 degrees compared with the opposite side. As for the anterior cruciate ligament, the rupture may be at the bone-ligament junction or more often in the middle substance of the ligament.

Treatment

Reattachment of bony avulsions should restore functional competency of the ligament. Repair of the middle substance tear alone is of no value. Complex reconstructions have been described but remain of unproved value for nonathletic patients. Conservative treatment with rehabilitation (particularly of the extensor mechanism), and even bracing, of isolated posterior cruciate ligament injuries is currently recommended.

5. Meniscal Injury

The meniscus is a fibrocartilage that allows a more congruous fit between the convex femoral condyle and the flat tibial plateau. Both medial and lateral menisci are attached peripherally and have a central free border. They are wedge-shaped and thicker at the periphery. The medial meniscus is C-shaped and the lateral meniscus is O-shaped, with both anterior and posterior horns almost touching medially. They are vascularized only at their peripheral third. Tears involving that vascularized portion have a better repair potential. The menisci spread the load more uniformly on the underlying cartilage, thus minimizing point contact and wear. They are secondary knee stabilizers but are more important in the ligament-deficient knee.

Clinical Findings

Tears can be secondary to trauma or attrition. The medial meniscus is more often involved. Symptoms include pain, swelling, a popping sensation, and occasionally locking. Examination usually reveals nonspecific medial or lateral joint-line pain, and occasionally grinding or snapping can be felt with tibial torsion and the knee flexed to 90 degrees (McMurray's sign). Radiographs are of minimal value but may rule out other disorders; contrast arthrography has been replaced by MRI.

Treatment

Initial conservative management with immobilization, bracing, protective weight bearing, and exercises can give good results. Arthroscopic evaluation and treatment is recommended for recurrent or persistent locking, recurrent effusion, or disabling pain. If the tear is large enough and in the vascularized portion, repair should be attempted. For other tears, the affected area should be removed, leaving as much as possible of the healthy meniscus. Routine total meniscectomy has been abandoned.

6. Chondral & Osteochondral Injuries

The hyaline articular cartilage is avascular and has no intrinsic capability to repair superficial lacerations. Deep injuries involve the bone in the subchondral plate, and extrinsic repair occurs first with a fibrin clot replaced by granulation tissue, which is then transformed to fibrocartilage. Repetitive injury, can cause abnormal motion with shearing stresses that can loosen chondral or osteochondral fragments. Compression injuries to the cartilage can lead to posttraumatic chondromalacia.

Clinical Findings

Chondral injuries usually give nonspecific symptoms that mimic meniscal injury. Plain radiographs will often reveal a loose body if the osteochondral fragment is big enough. Tunnel views and patellar tangential views can be helpful. Pure chondral fragments will only be seen with contrast arthrograms or MRI, both of which can easily miss the smaller fragments. Arthroscopy remains the most accurate diagnostic procedure.

Treatment

Removal of the free fragment, debridement of the donor site, and drilling of the underlying subchondral bone to promote fibrin clot formation is the most accepted treatment. Rarely, an osteochondral fragment involving weight-bearing cartilage is large enough to warrant reduction and internal fixation.

7. Knee Dislocation

Traumatic dislocation of the knee is a rare injury that almost always results from high-energy trauma. It is classified according to the direction of displacement of the tibia: anterior, posterior, lateral, medial, or rotatory. Complete dislocation can occur only after extensive tearing of the supporting ligaments and soft tissues. Injury to the neighboring neurovascular bundle is common and should be looked for systematically.

Treatment

Knee dislocations require prompt reduction. This is most easily accomplished in the emergency room by applying axial traction on the leg. Rarely, reduction can only be obtained under general anesthesia. Even if the pedal pulses return after reduction, angiography is still indicated to rule out an intimal tear of the popliteal artery. Any vascular injury should be repaired as soon as possible. Ischemia of more than 4 h implies a poor prognosis for salvage of a functional limb. Prophylactic fasciotomies should be performed at the time of vascular repair to prevent compartment syndrome caused by postrevascularization edema.

Once vascular patency has been restored, treatment of the ligamentous damage can be addressed. Most authors now agree that surgical repair of all ligaments is indicated in relatively young active patients. Others still prefer closed management in a cast or braces. Whatever method is used, close follow-up is essential, especially at the beginning, to prevent subluxation, usually posteriorly. If subluxation occurs, the knee should be maintained in a reduced position using a femorotibial external fixator. After 6–8 weeks of immobilization, the knee is protected in a long leg brace and motion is started. Intensive quadriceps and hamstring rehabilitation is necessary to minimize functional loss. The need for a brace for strenuous activities may be permanent.

Severity of limb injury, as measured by the MESS, is predictive of amputation. In a study conducted to evaluate factors associated with popliteal artery injuries, which influence the decision to amputate, with emphasis on factors a surgeon can control, the authors concluded that minimizing ischemia is the most important factor in maximizing limb salvage. To minimize ischemia, they recommend intraoperative use of systemic heparin or local urokinase, or both, during repair of popliteal artery injuries.

PROXIMAL TIBIA FRACTURES

1. Tibial Plateau Fractures

Proximal tibia fractures account for 1% of all fractures. There is a wide spectrum of fracture patterns that involve either the medial tibial plateau (10–23%), the lateral tibial plateau (55–70%), or both (11–31%). These fractures occur through metaphyseal bone. Like all metaphyseal fractures, the spongiosa is impacted and once reduced, there can be a void with functional bone loss. These fractures usually result from axial loading, as seen in falls from a high place, combined most often with some varus and valgus forces. It is reported that at

least 20% of unilateral tibial plateau fractures are associated with ligament rupture of the opposite compartment. The bone fails in compression and shear, with the ligament in tension. This is not easy to determine clinically, because of pain and motion at the fracture site. A thorough neurovascular evaluation should be recorded.

Classification

Many different classification systems have been proposed, none with universal acceptance. The system most widely used today is the Schatzker classification; type I: split fracture of the lateral plateau, type II: split-depression of the lateral plateau, type III: depression of the lateral plateau, type IV: medial plateau fracture, type V: bicondylar fracture, and type VI: a fracture with metaphyseal-diaphyseal dissociation (Figure 3–26). Proper classification is based on quality radiographs, including oblique views if necessary. If fat is present in the knee aspirate and plain films fail to show any obvious fractures, occult injury needs to be ruled out. CT and more recently, MRI have all been used successfully for this purpose.

Treatment

The goal of treatment is to restore anatomic contours to the articular surface, to prevent posttraumatic degenerative joint disease, allow soft-tissue healing in optimal position, and prevent knee stiffness. Both closed and open treatment can achieve these goals. The choice will depend on multiple factors, including the patient's age and general medical condition, the degree of displace-

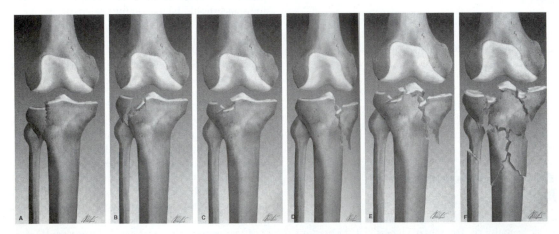

Figure 3–26. Schatzker classification of tibial plateau fractures: **A** (type I-lateral split), **B** (type II-lateral split depression), **C** (type III-lateral depression), **D** (type IV-medial plateau), **E** (type V-bicondylar), **F** (type VI-bicondylar with separation of metaphysis from diaphysis). (Reproduced, with permission, from Rockwood CA et al, eds: Fractures in Adults, 4th ed. Philadelphia: Lippincott, 1996.)

ment and comminution of the fracture, associated local soft-tissue and bony injuries, local skin condition, residual knee stability, and fracture configuration.

Closed treatment with a cast or fracture brace is appropriate for minimally displaced fractures with no ligament instability. Definite varus and valgus laxity at full extension is a poor prognostic sign for closed treatment. Articular step-off of 3 mm or less and condylar widening of 5 mm or less can be treated conservatively. Lateral or valgus tilt up to 5 degrees is well tolerated. Medial plateau fractures with any significant displacement should be surgically stabilized. Articular step-off > 3 mm should be anatomically fixed. Bicondylar fractures with any medial displacement, valgus tilt > 5 degrees or with significant articular step-off should be surgically stabilized. Range of motion is usually allowed after 6 weeks and weight bearing after 3 months. Noncomminuted fractures can undergo closed reduction with fluoroscopic imaging and percutaneous pinning with cannulated screws.

Recently, reduction of the articular fragment under arthroscopic visualization has become more popular, particularly for Schatzker type I, II, III, and IV injuries. The depressed fragment is elevated and bone graft packed underneath to prevent loss of reduction.

Open reduction and internal fixation with plates and screws remains the traditional approach of operative treatment. Reduction should be as anatomically precise as possible, and fixation should be solid enough to allow early mobilization. More recently, minimally invasive plate osteosynthesis (MIPO) and less invasive stabilization systems (LISS) are being used in the treatment of these injuries. Bone defects should be grafted with either autograft or allograft. Early range of motion is allowed according to the stability of the construct. Weight bearing is occasionally allowed at 6–8 weeks and more frequently after 12 weeks.

The external fixator can be used for definitive treatment of fractures and provisional fixation in a variety of settings.

Recently, the advent of hybrid ring external fixators has improved treatment of tibial plateau fractures, particularly Schatzker V and VI patterns.

Bai B et al: Effect of articular step-off and meniscectomy on joint alignment and contact pressures for fractures of the lateral tibial plateau. J Orthop Trauma 2001;15:101.[PMID: 11232647]

Ballmer FT, Hertel R, Notzli HP: Treatment of tibial plateau fractures with small fragment internal fixation: A preliminary report. J Orthop Trauma 2000;14:467.[PMID: 11083608]

Bono CM et al: Nonarticular proximal tibia fractures: Treatment options and decision making. J Am Acad Orthop Surg. 2001;9:176.[PMID: 11421575]

Chen FS, Rokito AS, Pitman MI: Acute and chronic posterolateral rotatory instability of the knee. J Am Acad Orthop Surg 2000;8:97.[PMID: 1075373]

Collinge CA, Sanders RW: Percutaneous plating in the lower extremity. J Am Acad Orthop Surg 2000;8:211.[PMID: 10951109]

Geller J et al: Tension wire position for hybrid external fixation of the proximal tibia. J Orthop Trauma 2000;14:502.[PMID: 11083613]

Griffin LY et al: Noncontact anterior cruciate ligament injuries: Risk factors and prevention strategies. J Am Acad Orthop Surg 2000;8:141.[PMID: 10874221]

Kumar A, Whittle AP: Treatment of complex (Schatzker type VI) fractures of the tibial plateau with circular wire external fixation: A retrospective case review. J Orthop Trauma 2000;14:339.[PMID: 10926241]

Lonner JH, Dupuy DE, Siliski JM: Comparison of magnetic resonance imaging with operative findings in acute traumatic dislocations of the adult knee. J Orthop Trauma 2000;14:183.[PMID: 10791669]

Lundy DW, Johnson KD: "Floating knee" injuries: Ipsilateral fractures of the femur and tibia. J Am Acad Orthop Surg 2001;9:238.{PMID: 11476533]

Stevens DG et al: The long-term functional outcome of operatively treated tibial plateau fractures. J Orthop Trauma 2001;15:312.[PMID: 11433134]

Complications

Early complications include infection, deep vein thrombosis, compartment syndrome, loss of reduction, and hardware failure. Late complications include residual instability and posttraumatic degenerative joint disease that may require total knee replacement arthroplasty or arthrodesis.

2. Tibial Tuberosity Fracture

Tibial tuberosity fractures can occur with a violent quadriceps muscle contraction causing avulsion of the tibial tuberosity. When the fracture is complete, the extensor mechanism is disrupted and active knee extension is impossible.

Although conservative treatment of a nondisplaced avulsion fracture with a cylinder cast in extension for 6–8 weeks will allow it to heal, rigid fixation with percutaneous screws allows much earlier knee mobilization. Closed or open reduction and solid internal fixation is recommended for all fractures displaced by 5 mm or more.

3. Tibial Eminence (Spine) Fracture

A tibial eminence fracture occurs as an isolated injury or as part of the comminution of tibial plateau fractures. The isolated type of injury occurs mostly in the pediatric age group before physeal closure and is believed to be an avulsion fracture at the tibial attachment of the anterior cruciate ligament.

Myers has classified this lesion into three stages and has recommended open reduction for the displaced type 3 fractures. Type 1 and 2 fractures should be treated with a cylinder cast with the knee in extension for 4–6 weeks. When associated with other fractures of the tibial plateau, the tibial eminence fragment usually keeps its attachment to the anterior cruciate ligament, and anatomic reduction with rigid fixation should be obtained.

DISTAL FEMUR FRACTURES

These fractures involve the distal metaphysis and epiphysis of the femur. It is important to distinguish between extra-articular (supracondylar) and intra-articular (condylar or intercondylar) fractures. The distal fragment is usually rotated into extension from traction by the gastrocnemius muscle. The distal end of the proximal fragment is apt to perforate the overlying quadriceps and may penetrate the suprapatellar pouch, causing hemarthrosis.

The distal fragment may impinge on the popliteal neurovascular bundle, and an immediate thorough neurovascular examination is mandatory. Absence or marked decrease of pedal pulsations is an indication for immediate reduction. If this fails to restore adequate circulation, an arteriogram should be obtained immediately and the vascular lesion repaired as indicated. Injuries to the tibial or peroneal nerves are less frequent.

1. Extra-Articular Fractures

For simple fracture patterns, closed reduction under general anesthesia is occasionally successful. Most of these fractures, however, are best treated with internal fixation, which allows early mobilization of the patient and of the neighboring joints. Most fractures are best treated with fixed-angle plates, MIPO, or retrograde intramedullary nailing. Skeletal traction treatment is reserved for patients for whom surgery is contraindicated and is fraught with all the previously mentioned complications that can accompany prolonged recumbency.

2. Intra-Articular Fractures

As for any intra-articular fracture, maximal functional recovery of the knee joint requires anatomic reduction of the articular components. Closed reduction of displaced fragments is almost never successful. Displaced intra-articular fractures can be treated with a variety of methods including AO buttress plating, LISS, and percutaneous or minimally invasive plate osteosynthesis.

3. Intercondylar Fracture

A comminuted fracture of the distal femoral epiphysis is classically described as a T or Y fracture, according to the configuration of the articular fragments. Displaced fractures are best treated by open reduction, to restore anatomic alignment of the articular surface, and by internal fixation using screws and condylar plates or screws. Even if the fracture heals in anatomic position, joint stiffness, pain, and posttraumatic arthritis are not uncommon outcomes.

4. Condylar Fracture

Isolated fractures of the lateral or medial femoral condyles are rare. They usually result from varus or valgus stress to the knee joint, and associated ligament injuries should be looked for systematically. Fractures of the posterior portion of one or the other condyle in the frontal plane can also be seen.

Closed reduction of displaced fragments is rarely successful. Open reduction and internal fixation is usually indicated. Associated ligamentous ruptures are repaired as needed. If fixation is solid, postoperative immobilization is kept at a minimum, and the patient can start moving the knee joint early. Weight bearing is usually allowed at 3 months when clinical and radiologic evidence of bone healing is present.

PATELLAR INJURIES

1. Transverse Patellar Fracture

Transverse fractures of the patella (Figure 3–27) are the result of an indirect force, usually with the knee in flexion. Fracture may be caused by sudden voluntary contraction of the quadriceps muscle or sudden forced flexion of the leg with the quadriceps contracted. The level of fracture is commonly in the middle. Associated tearing of the patellar retinacula depends upon the force of the initiating injury. The activity of the quadriceps muscle causes upward displacement of the proximal fragment, the magnitude of which depends on the extent of the retinacular tear.

Clinical Findings

Swelling of the anterior knee region is caused by hemarthrosis and hemorrhage into the soft tissues overlying the joint. If displacement is present, the defect in the patella can be palpated, and active extension of the knee is lost. A straight leg raise may be preserved if the retinacula is intact.

Treatment

Nondisplaced fractures can be treated with a walking cylinder cast or brace for 6–8 weeks followed by knee rehabilitation. Open reduction is indicated if the fragments are displaced > 3 mm or if articular step-off is > 2 mm. The fragments must be accurately repositioned

If comminution is not severe and displacement is insignificant, immobilization for 8 weeks in a cylinder extending from the groin to the supramalleolar region is sufficient.

Severe comminution can often be treated with ORIF with addition of a cerclage wire, but on rare occasions excision of the patella and repair of the defect by imbrication of the quadriceps expansion is the only viable alternative. Excision of the patella can result in decreased strength, pain in the knee, and general restriction of activity. No matter what the treatment, high-energy injuries are frequently complicated by chondromalacia patella and patellofemoral arthritis.

3. Patellar Dislocation

Acute traumatic dislocation of the patella should be differentiated from episodic recurrent dislocation, as the latter condition is likely to be associated with occult organic lesions. When dislocation of the patella occurs alone, it may be caused by a direct force or activity of the quadriceps, and the direction of dislocation of the patella is almost always lateral. Spontaneous reduction is apt to occur if the knee joint is extended. If so, the clinical findings may consist merely of hemarthrosis and localized tenderness over the medial patellar retinaculum. Gross instability of the patella, which can be demonstrated by physical examination, indicates that injury to the soft tissues of the medial aspect of the knee has been extensive.

Reduction is maintained in a brace or cylinder cast with the knee in extension for 2–3 weeks. Isometric quadriceps exercises are encouraged. Physical therapy should be initiated to maximize the strength of the vastus medialis. Dynamic bracing may be helpful. Recurrent episodes require operative repair for effective treatment.

4. Tear of the Quadriceps Tendon

Tear of the quadriceps tendon occurs most often in patients over the age of 40. Apparent tears that represent avulsions from the patella occur in patients with renal osteodystrophy or hyperparathyroidism. Preexisting attritional disease of the tendon is apt to be present, and the causative injury may be minor. The tear commonly results from sudden deceleration, such as stumbling or slipping on a wet surface. A small flake of bone may be avulsed from the superior pole of the patella, or the tear may occur entirely through tendinous and muscular tissue.

Pain may be noted in the anterior knee region. Swelling is caused by hemarthrosis and extravasation of blood into the soft tissues. The patient is unable to extend the knee completely. Radiographs may show a bony avulsion from the superior pole of the patella.

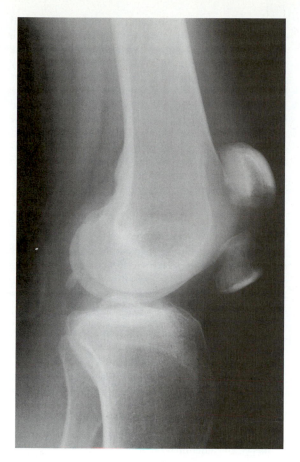

Figure 3–27. Transverse fracture of the patella.

to prevent early posttraumatic arthritis of the patellofemoral joint. If the minor fragment is small (no more than 1 cm in length) or severely comminuted, it may be excised and the quadriceps or patellar tendon (depending upon which pole of the patella is involved) sutured directly to the major fragment. Whenever possible, internal fixation of anatomically reduced fragments should be done, allowing early motion of the knee joint. This is best achieved by figure-of-eight tension banding over two longitudinal parallel K-wires.

Accurate reduction of the articular surface must be confirmed by lateral radiographs taken intraoperatively.

2. Comminuted Patellar Fracture

Comminuted fractures of the patella are usually caused by a direct force. Most often, little or no separation of the fragments occurs because the quadriceps retinaculum is not extensively torn. Severe injury may cause extensive destruction of the articular surface of both the patella and the opposing femur.

Operative repair is recommended for complete tear. Postoperative immobilization should be encouraged in a walking cylinder cast or brace for 6 weeks, at which time knee mobilization is started.

5. Tear of the Patellar Tendon

The same mechanism that causes tears of the quadriceps tendon, transverse fracture of the patella, or avulsion of the tibial tuberosity may also cause the patellar ligament to tear. The characteristic finding is proximal displacement of the patella. A bony avulsion may be present adjacent to the lower pole of the patella if the tear takes place in the proximal patellar tendon.

Operative treatment is necessary for a complete tear. The ligament is resutured to the patella, and any tear in the quadriceps mechanism is repaired. The extremity should be immobilized for 6–8 weeks in a cylinder cast extending from the groin to the supramalleolar region. Guarded exercises may then be started.

Jutson JJ, Zych GA: Treatment of comminuted intraarticular distal femur fractures with limited internal and external tensioned wire fixation. J Orthop Trauma 2000;14:405.[PMID: 1100141])

Meyer RW et al: Mechanical comparison of a distal femoral side plate and a retrograde intramedullary nail. J Orthop Trauma 2000 14;398.[PMID: 11001413]

Stahelin T, Hardegger F, Ward JC: Supracondylar osteotomy of the femur with use of compression. J Bone Joint Surg 2000;82-A;712.[PMID: 10819282]

Woo SL et al: Healing and repair of ligament injuries in the knee. J Am Acad Orthop Surg 2000;8:364.[PMID: 11104400]

FEMORAL SHAFT FRACTURES

DIAPHYSEAL FRACTURES

Fracture of the shaft of the femur usually occurs as a result of severe trauma. Indirect force, especially torsional stress, is likely to cause spiral fractures that extend proximally or, more commonly, distally into the metaphyseal regions. Most are closed fractures; open fracture is often the result of compounding from within.

Clinical Findings

Extensive soft-tissue injury, bleeding, and shock are commonly present with diaphyseal fractures. The most significant features are severe pain in the thigh and deformity of the lower extremity. Hemorrhagic shock may be present, as multiple units of blood may be lost into the thigh, though only moderate swelling may be apparent. Careful radiographic examination in at least two planes is necessary to determine the exact site and configuration of the fracture pattern. The hip and knee should be examined and radiographs obtained to rule out associated injury. A femoral neck fracture may occur in association with a femur fracture and if overlooked can increase patient morbidity.

Injuries to the sciatic nerve and the superficial femoral artery and vein are uncommon but must be recognized promptly. Hemorrhagic shock and secondary anemia are the most important early complications. Later complications include those of prolonged recumbency, joint stiffness, malunion, nonunion, leg-length discrepancy, and infection.

Classification

No classification is universally accepted for fractures of the femoral diaphysis. Classically, the fracture is described according to its location, pattern, and comminution. Winquist has proposed a comminution classification that is now widely used.

Type 1: Fracture that involves no, or minimal, comminution at the fracture site, and does not affect stability after intramedullary nailing

Type 2: Fracture with comminution leaving at least 50% of the circumference of the two major fragments intact

Type 3: Fracture with comminution of 50–100% of the circumference of the major fragments. Non-locked intramedullary nails do not afford stable fixation.

Type 4: Fracture with completely comminuted segmental pattern with no intrinsic stability

Treatment

Treatment depends upon the age and medical status of the patient as well as the site and configuration of the fracture.

A. CLOSED TREATMENT

This remains a treatment option for some skeletally immature patients. Depending on the age of the pediatric patient and the amount of initial displacement at the fracture site, treatment may consist of immediate immobilization in a hip spica cast, or skin or skeletal traction for 3–6 weeks, until the fracture is "sticky," and then spica casting.

Closed treatment of femoral shaft fractures in the adult is rarely indicated. Acceptable alignment may be difficult to maintain, and joint stiffness is frequent. Other rarer complications of prolonged recumbency, like pressure sores and deep vein thrombosis, can have disastrous consequences.

B. OPERATIVE TREATMENT

Most fractures in the middle third of the femur can be internally fixed by an intramedullary rod. Intramedullary fixation of femoral shaft fractures allows early mobilization of the patient (within 24–48 h if the fracture fixation is stable), which is of particular benefit to the polytraumatized patient; more anatomic alignment; improved knee and hip function by decreasing the time spent in traction; and a marked decrease in the cost of hospitalization.

Although open nailing procedures have been described, intramedullary fixation is routinely performed closed.

In closed nailing, the fracture is reduced by closed manipulation on a fracture table under fluoroscopic control. An small incision is made proximal to the greater trochanter, and the nail is inserted through the piriformis fossa down into the intramedullary canal, after reaming to the appropriate size. The fracture site is not opened. Closed nailing decreases the chance of infection by decreasing the amount of soft-tissue dissection necessary and by limiting access to the fracture site to the medullary canal. It also does not disturb the periosteal circulation. Some authors feel that bone reamings at the fracture site further promote bone healing.

More recently, interlocking nails have gained popularity. Screws are inserted percutaneously through holes in one or the other end of the nail (or both ends) in the frontal plane. Dynamic interlocking (screws at only one end of the nail) relies on interference friction of fracture fragments and muscle action to prevent rotation of the unlocked fragment. It allows axial compression at the fracture site. Static interlocking (screws at both ends of the nail) provides rotational control and prevents shortening of the bone at the fracture site; this is the preferred technique. It is recommended to routinely use static interlocking, unless the fracture line does not involve the isthmus of the shaft and the fracture pattern is intrinsically stable (uncomminuted transverse or short oblique fracture). Reamed interlocked nailing is recommended for most grade 1, 2, and 3a open fractures. When associated with extensive soft-tissue loss, as in grade 3b and 3c open fractures, temporary bony stability may be achieved with external fixation devices.

Complications of this procedure can arise from technical problems at the time of surgery (eg, choice of a rod that is too short or too narrow) and result in malalignment or shortening. Comminution of the fracture can occur during placement of the rod. Late bone fracture (weeks or months) can occur through interlocking screws, and severely comminuted fractures with weight bearing can suffer rod or screw breakage. Infection can occur after any open procedure but is uncommon with closed nailing. Occasionally, a painful bursa or heterotopic calcification may develop over the proximal end of the nail, causing discomfort when the patient sits or walks. The rod may be removed after healing is complete, usually at 12–16 months. The healing rate of femoral shaft fractures in general is high and approaches 100% after closed nailing techniques.

Other fixation devices are seldom used. Flexible intramedullary rods of the Ender type do not provide sufficient stability in the adult; however, they are routinely used in the pediatric population. Plates and screws require significant soft-tissue dissection and opening of the fracture hematoma and are usually reserved for special cases such as ipsilateral femoral neck and diaphyseal fractures. External fixation remains indicated in some open fractures. It has also recently gained acceptance as treatment for closed femoral shaft fractures in children to allow earlier mobilization and decreased hospital stays. The distal fragment pins should always be inserted with the knee in flexion to avoid quadriceps tenodesis that will prevent knee flexion. Superficial pin tract infection is common but rarely involves the bone. A course of oral antibiotics, proper pin care, and eventual pin removal, when the fracture is sufficiently healed, are usually all that are needed to control this problem.

SUBTROCHANTERIC FRACTURES

Subtrochanteric fractures occur below the level of the lesser trochanter and are usually the result of high-energy trauma in young to middle-aged adults. They are often comminuted, with distal or proximal extension toward the greater trochanter. Associated soft-tissue damage can be extensive.

The Russell and Taylor classification (Figure 3–28) is a treatment based classification system that incorporates involvement of the piriformis fossa. Type Ia Russell-Taylor fractures do not involve the piriformis fossa, with the lesser trochanter attached to the proximal fragment. These fractures may be treated with a first-generation intramedullary nail. Type Ib fractures do not involve the piriformis fossa; however, the lesser trochanter is detached from the proximal fragment. These fractures require a second-generation nail, with screw fixation into the head and neck. Type II fractures have fracture extension into the piriformis fossa and are best treated with a sliding hip screw or fixed angle plate. The patient usually presents with a swollen painful proximal thigh with or without shortening or malrotation. If the lesser trochanter is intact, the proximal fragment will tend to displace in flexion, external rotation,

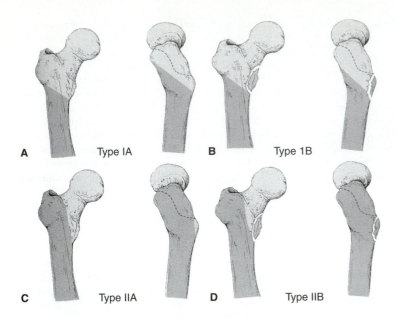

A   Type IA   **B**   Type 1B

C   Type IIA   **D**   Type IIB

Figure 3–28. Russell and Taylor classification of subtrochanteric femur fractures. (Reproduced, with permission, from Browner BD et al, eds: Skeletal Trauma, 2nd ed. Philadelphia: WB Saunders, 1998.)

and abduction because of the unopposed pull of the iliopsoas and abductor muscles.

In the vast majority of cases, internal fixation (by closed or open methods) is now widely favored. Temporary skeletal traction will maintain femoral length until the definitive surgical procedure can be performed. A variety of devices are available.

Closed intramedullary interlocking nails have gained more popularity recently. Devices with intracephalic proximal interlocking are now available for those cases where conventional intertrochanteric proximal interlocking is contraindicated. Fixation can be obtained with first-generation intramedullary nails, "gamma nails," intramedullary hip screws, or with a variety of intracephalic nails or blades and long sideplates based upon the fracture pattern.

Postoperative activity depends on the adequacy of internal fixation. If fixation is solid, an agile cooperative patient can be out of bed within a few days after surgery and ambulating on crutches with toe-touch weight bearing on the affected side. The fracture is usually healed at 3–4 months, but delayed union and nonunion are not uncommon. Hardware failure in these cases are frequent. Repeat internal fixation with autogenous bone grafting is then the treatment of choice.

Brumback RJ, Virkus WW: Intramedullary nailing of the femur: Reamed versus nonreamed. J Am Acad Orthop Surg 2000; 8:83.[PMID: 10799093]

Dora C et al: Entry point soft tissue damage in antegrade femoral nailing: A cadaver study. J Orthop Trauma 2001;15:488. [PMID: 11602831]

Giannoudis PV et al: Nonunion of the femoral diaphysis. J Bone Joint Surg Br 2000;82-B:655.[PMID: 10963160]

Herscovici D et al: Treatment of femoral shaft fracture using unreamed interlocked nails. J Orthop Trauma 2000;14:10. [PMID: 10630796]

Nowotarski PJ et al: Conversion of external fixation to intramedullary nailing for fractures of the shaft of the femur in multiply injured patients. J Bone Joint Surg Am 2000;82-A:2000.]PMID: 1085909]

Ostrum RF et al: Prospective comparison of retrograde and antegrade femoral intramedullary nailing. J Orthop Trauma 2000;14:496.[PMID: 11083612]

Patton JT et al: Late fracture of the hip after reamed intramedullary nailing of the femur. J Bone Joint Surg Br 2000;82-B:967. [PMID: 11041583]

Ricci WM et al: Angular malalignment after intramedullary nailing of femoral shaft fractures. J Orthop Trauma 2001;15:90. [PMID: 11232660]

Ricci WM et al: Retrograde versus antegrade nailing of femoral shaft fractures. J Orthop Trauma 2001;15:161.[PMID: 11265005]

Shepherd LE et al: Prospective randomized study of reamed versus undreamed femoral intramedullary nailing: An assessment of procedures. J Orthop Trauma 2001;15:28.[PMID: 11147684]

Tornetta P, Tiburzi D: Antegrade or retrograde reamed femoral nailing. J Bone Joint Surg Br 2000;82-B:652.[PMID: 10963159]

Tornetta P, Tiburzi D: Reamed versus nonreamed anterograde femoral nailing. J Orthop Trauma 2000;14:15.[PMID: 10630797]

HIP FRACTURES & DISLOCATIONS

Epidemiology & Social Costs

Hip fractures include intertrochanteric fractures and femoral neck fractures and constitute a major problem in the United States because of the disabling nature of these injuries. Ambulation is almost impossible in all fractures except femoral neck fractures until they have been treated surgically. These fractures primarily occur in older patients, unable in many cases to care for themselves. Although relatively few in number, hip fractures accounted for 3.5 million hospital days, more than the total for tibial fractures, vertebral column fractures, and pelvic fractures combined. These hip fractures account for nearly half of the total hospital costs of all fractures and more than half of the nursing home care costs. Further, prompt and effective care is necessary to avoid the all too frequent occurrence of death in the elderly patient with a hip fracture (20–30% of patients in the first year after fracture). Thus, this injury justifies state-of-the-art care to minimize not only the cost but the human suffering.

Anatomy & Biomechanical Principles

The hip joint is the articulation between the acetabulum and the femoral head. The trabecular pattern of the femoral head and neck, and that of the acetabulum, is oriented to optimally accept the forces crossing the joint. The total force across the joint is the vector sum of body weight and active muscle force. When the concept of lever arm is factored in, surprising forces across the hip joint are attained: 2.5 times body weight when standing on one leg, five times body weight when running, and 1.5 times body weight when lifting the leg from the supine position with the knee in extension. Using a cane in the opposite hand reduces the force to body weight when standing on that leg. For the same reasons, forces across the joint when the ipsilateral leg is kept in the air are significantly greater than when toe-touch weight bearing is allowed.

The hip capsule is a strong thick fibrous structure that attaches on the intertrochanteric line anteriorly and somewhat more proximally posteriorly. The intracapsular portion of the neck is not covered with periosteum, and fractures of the intracapsular part of the neck cannot heal with periosteal callus formation, only with endosteal union. Interposition of synovial fluid between fracture fragments, as in any joint, can delay or altogether prevent bony union.

The vascular supply of the femoral head is also of paramount importance. There are three main sources of vascular supply: (1) the retinacular vessels arising from the lateral femoral circumflex artery and the inferior metaphyseal artery and then running beneath the synovium along the neck, which they penetrate proximally both anteriorly and posteriorly; (2) the interosseous circulation crossing the marrow spaces from distal to proximal; and (3) unreliably, the ligamentum teres artery. Fractures of the femoral neck always disrupt the interosseous circulation; the femoral head then relies only on the retinacular arteries, which may also be disrupted or thrombosed. Secondary avascular necrosis of part or all of the femoral head can result. Union of a fracture can occur in the presence of an avascular fragment, but the incidence of nonunion is higher. Revascularization of the necrotic fragment occurs through the process of creeping substitution. Part of this process involves replacement of necrotic bony substrate with a "softer" granulation tissue and sets the stage for delayed segmental collapse.

Intertrochanteric fractures usually do not suffer this same fate. The capsule (and vessels) are still attached to the proximal fragment after fracture, and thus the blood supply remains patent.

1. Femoral Neck Fractures

Femoral neck fractures are intracapsular fractures. Because of the already mentioned unusual vascularization of the femoral head and neck, these fractures are at high risk of nonunion or avascular necrosis of the femoral head. The incidence of avascular necrosis increases with the amount of fracture displacement and the amount of time before the fracture is reduced.

Fractures of the femoral neck occur most commonly in patients over age 50. The involved extremity may be slightly shortened and externally rotated. Hip motion is painful, except in the rare cases of nondisplaced or impacted fractures, where pain may be evident only at the extremes of motion. Good quality anteroposterior and lateral radiographs are mandatory.

Classification

The Garden classification for acute fractures is the most widely used system:

Type 1: Valgus impaction of the femoral head

Type 2: Complete but nondisplaced

Type 3: Complete fracture, displaced less than 50%

Type 4: Complete fracture displaced greater than 50%

This classification is of prognostic value for the incidence of avascular necrosis: The higher the Garden number, the higher the incidence. Once the diagnosis is confirmed, the patient should be placed in gentle skin traction while awaiting definitive treatment.

Stable Femoral Neck Fractures

These include stress fractures and Garden type 1 fractures. Stress fractures may be difficult to diagnose. Physical examination, as well as the initial radiographs, may be normal. Repeat radiographs, radionuclide imaging, and MRI may be necessary to confirm the diagnosis.

Toe-touch weight bearing (with crutches) until radiologic evidence of healing is usually successful for the compliant patient. Healing is usually complete in 3–6 months. Rarely, prophylactic internal fixation is necessary and is indicated by failure of pain resolution with toe-touch weight bearing or by displacement.

The Garden type 1 fracture is impacted in valgus position and is usually stable. Impaction must be demonstrated on both anteroposterior and lateral views. The risk of displacement is nevertheless significant; most surgeons recommend internal fixation to maintain reduction and allow earlier ambulation and weight bearing. If surgery is contraindicated, closed treatment with toe-touch crutch ambulation and frequent radiographic follow-up until healing can be successful.

Unstable Femoral Neck Fractures

Although nondisplaced, a Garden type 2 femoral neck fracture is unstable because displacement is probable under physiologic loading. Garden type 3 and 4 fractures are displaced and often comminuted. They can be life-threatening injuries, especially in elderly patients.

Treatment is directed toward preservation of life and restoration of hip function, with early mobilization. This is best attained by rigid internal fixation or primary arthroplasty as soon as the patient is medically prepared for surgery. Closed treatment in a spica cast is almost always bound to fail. Definitive treatment by skeletal traction requires prolonged recumbency with constant nursing care and is associated with numerous complications, including malunion, nonunion, pressure sores, deep vein thrombosis and pulmonary embolus, osteoporosis, and hypercalcemia, to name a few. If for some reason surgery is not possible, it is probably better to mobilize the patient just as soon as pain permits, and accept a nonunion that can be treated at a later stage if symptoms justify it. Surgical options are internal fixation or primary arthroplasty. In general, the younger the patient, the greater the effort is justified to save the femoral head.

Treatment

A. INTERNAL FIXATION

The goal of internal fixation is to preserve a viable femoral head fragment and provide the optimal setting for bony healing of the fracture while allowing the patient to be as mobile as possible. Because persistent displacement and motion at the fracture site may further jeopardize the femoral head blood supply, surgery should be performed as soon as possible. General or spinal anesthesia is used. The fracture is reduced under fluoroscopic imaging as anatomically accurately as possible. Gentle manipulation is usually sufficient. Rarely, open reduction may be necessary before fixation. Open reduction, if performed, should be approached anteriorly as this results in less disruption of blood supply than a posterior approach. Rigid internal fixation is obtained using multiple parallel partially threaded screws, a sliding hip screw and plate, or a combination of both. The patient can usually be mobilized the following day, and weight bearing is allowed according to the stability of the construct.

B. PRIMARY ARTHROPLASTY

This procedure is indicated in the elderly patient for Garden type 4 fractures, in which avascular necrosis is highly probable, and for Garden type 3 fractures that cannot be satisfactorily reduced or for femoral heads with preexisting disease. The femoral head is sacrificed, but a definitive procedure is performed, whereas internal fixation of Garden type 4 fractures frequently fails and repeat surgery is required. When the acetabulum is undamaged, the most commonly accepted technique is hemiarthroplasty, using a femoral stem stabilized with methyl methacrylate or a surface that allows biologic fixation with bony ingrowth. If the hip joint itself is already damaged by preexisting disease, total hip replacement may be indicated. Primary head and neck resection (Girdlestone arthroplasty) may be rarely indicated in the presence of infection or local malignant growth.

Complications

The most common sequelae of femoral neck fractures are loss of reduction and hardware failure, nonunions or malunions, and avascular necrosis of the femoral head. This latter complication can appear as late as 2 years after injury. According to different series, the incidence of avascular necrosis for Garden type 1 fractures varies from 0 to 15%, for type 2 fractures 10–25%, for type 3 fractures 25–50%, and for type 4 fractures 50–100%. Secondary degenerative joint disease appears somewhat later. The most disabling complication, infection, is fortunately rare.

2. Trochanteric Fractures

Lesser Trochanter Fracture

Isolated fracture of the lesser trochanter is rare. When it occurs, it is the result of the avulsion force of the iliopsoas muscle. Rarely, a symptomatic nonunion may require fragment fixation or excision.

Greater Trochanter Fracture

Isolated fracture of the greater trochanter may be caused by direct injury or may occur indirectly as a result of the activity of the gluteus medius and gluteus minimus muscles. It occurs most commonly as a component of intertrochanteric fracture.

If displacement of the isolated fracture fragment is less than 1 cm and there is no tendency to further displacement (as determined by repeated radiographic examinations), treatment may be bed rest until acute pain subsides. As rapidly as symptoms permit, activity can increase gradually to protected weight bearing with crutches. Full weight bearing is permitted as soon as healing is apparent, usually in 6–8 weeks. If displacement is greater than 1 cm and increases on adduction of the thigh, extensive tearing of surrounding soft tissues may be assumed, and ORIF is indicated.

Intertrochanteric Fractures

By definition, these fractures usually occur along a line between the greater and the lesser trochanter. They typically occur at a later age than do femoral neck fractures. They are most often extracapsular and occur through cancellous bone. Bone healing within 8–12 weeks is the usual outcome, regardless of the treatment. Nonunion and avascular necrosis of the femoral head are not significant problems.

Clinically, the involved extremity is usually shortened and can be internally or externally rotated. The degree of displacement and comminution will determine the instability of the fracture. A wide spectrum of fracture patterns is possible, from the nondisplaced fissure fracture to the highly comminuted fracture with four major fragments (head and neck, greater trochanter, lesser trochanter, and femoral shaft). The Muller/ AO system is useful in classifying intertrochanteric femur fractures and has gained more popularity in recent years (Figure 3–29).

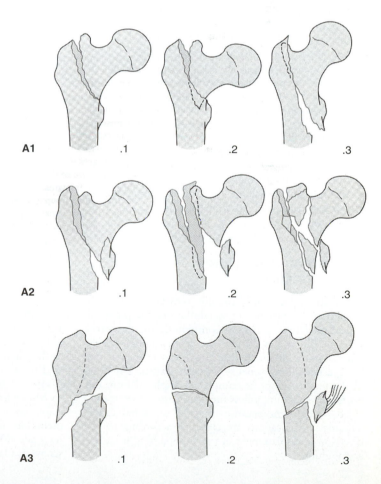

Figure 3–29. Muller/AO system for intertrochanteric femur fracture classification. (Reproduced, with permission, from Browner BD et al, eds: Skeletal Trauma, 2nd ed. Philadelphia: WB Saunders, 1998.)

The selection of definitive treatment depends upon the general condition of the patient and the fracture pattern. Rates of illness and death are lower when the fracture is internally fixed, allowing early mobilization. Operative treatment is indicated as soon as the patient is medically able to tolerate surgery. Initial treatment in the hospital should be by gentle skin traction to minimize pain and further displacement. Skeletal traction as the definitive treatment is rarely indicated and is fraught with complications such as pressure sores, deep vein thrombosis and pulmonary embolus, deterioration of mental status, and varus malunion. When surgery is contraindicated, it may be preferable to mobilize the patient as soon as pain permits and accept the eventual malunion or nonunion.

The great majority of these fractures are amenable to surgery. The goal is to obtain a fixation secure enough to allow early mobilization and provide an environment for sound fracture healing in a good position. Reduction of the fracture is usually accomplished by closed methods, using traction on the fracture table, and monitored using fluoroscopic imaging. Some surgeons do not attempt to anatomically reduce comminuted fractures but instead prefer to keep the distal fragment medially displaced, to enhance mechanical stability. Internal fixation is most widely obtained with a sliding screw and sideplate. The screw can slide in the barrel of the sideplate, allowing the fracture to impact in a stable position. The patient can be taken out of bed the next day, and weight bearing with crutches or a walker is begun as soon as pain allows. The fracture usually heals in 6–12 weeks. Other devices used to treat intertrochanteric fractures include second-generation interlocked nails and prosthetic replacement.

Complications include infection, hardware failure, loss of reduction, and irritation bursitis over the tip of the sliding screw.

3. Traumatic Dislocation of the Hip Joint

Traumatic dislocation of the hip joint may occur with or without fracture of the acetabulum or the proximal end of the femur. It is most common during the active years of life and is usually the result of high-energy trauma, unless there is preexisting disease of the femoral head, acetabulum, or neuromuscular system. The head of the femur cannot be completely displaced from the normal acetabulum, unless the ligamentum teres is ruptured or deficient because of some unrelated cause. Traumatic dislocations are classified according to the direction of displacement of the femoral head from the acetabulum.

Posterior Hip Dislocation

Usually, the head of the femur is dislocated posterior to the acetabulum when the thigh is flexed, for example, as may occur in a head-on automobile collision when the knee is driven violently against the dashboard.

The significant clinical findings are shortening, adduction, and internal rotation of the extremity. Anteroposterior, lateral and, if fracture of the acetabulum is demonstrated, oblique radiographic projections (Judet views) are required. Common associated injuries include fractures of the acetabulum or the femoral head or shaft and sciatic nerve injury. The head of the femur may be displaced through a rent in the posterior hip joint capsule. The short external rotator muscles of the femur are commonly lacerated. Fracture of the posterior margin of the acetabulum can create instability.

If the acetabulum is not fractured or if the fragment is small, reduction by closed manipulation is indicated. General anesthesia provides maximum muscle relaxation and allows gentle reduction. Reduction should be achieved as soon as possible, preferably within the first few hours after injury, as the incidence of avascular necrosis of the femoral head increases with time until reduction. The main feature of reduction is traction in the line of deformity followed by gentle flexion of the hip to 90 degrees with stabilization of the pelvis by an assistant. While manual traction is continued, the hip is gently rotated into internal and then external rotation to obtain reduction.

The stability of the reduction is evaluated clinically by ranging the extended hip in abduction and adduction and internal and external rotation. If stable, the same movements are repeated in 90 degrees of hip flexion. The point of redislocation is noted, the hip is reduced, and an anteroposterior radiograph of the pelvis is obtained. Soft tissue or bone fragment interposition will be manifested by widening of the joint space as compared to the contralateral side. Irreducible dislocations, open dislocations, and those that redislocate after reduction despite hip extension and external rotation (usually because of associated posterior wall fracture of the acetabulum) are indications for immediate open reduction and internal fixation if necessary. Most authors agree that a widened joint space on radiograph, despite a stable reduction, is also an indication for immediate arthrotomy. Others prefer obtaining a CT scan first, to further delineate the incarcerated fragments and associated injuries before surgery. Recently, hip arthroscopy has gained popularity, but it remains controversial.

Minor fragments of the posterior margin of the acetabulum may be disregarded, but larger displaced fragments are not usually successfully reduced by closed methods. Open reduction and internal fixation with screws or plates is indicated.

Postreduction treatment will vary according to the type of initial surgery. A strictly soft-tissue injury with a stable concentric reduction may be treated with light skin or skeletal traction for a few days to a week before exercises are begun. A motivated patient can then start crutch ambulation, progressing to full weight bearing at 6 weeks. An unstable reduction can be immobilized in a spica cast for 4–6 weeks. Securely fixed fractures are treated as soft-tissue injuries, but weight bearing is allowed when radiologic signs of bone healing are present. When fixation is tenuous, skeletal traction for 4–6 weeks or hip spica immobilization is recommended.

Complications include infection, avascular necrosis of the femoral head, malunion, posttraumatic degenerative joint disease, recurrent dislocation, and sciatic nerve injury. Avascular necrosis occurs because of the disruption of the retinacular arteries providing blood to the femoral head. Its incidence increases with the duration of the dislocation. It can occur as late as 2 years after the injury. MRI studies enabling early diagnosis and protected weight bearing until revascularization has occurred are recommended. Sciatic nerve injury is present in 10–20% of patients with posterior hip dislocation. Although usually of the neurapraxia type, these lesions leave permanent sequelae in about 20% of cases. The rare patient who is neurologically intact before reduction but has a deficit after reduction should be explored surgically to see if the nerve has been entrapped in the joint. Associated injuries also, on rare occasions, include fracture of the femoral head. Small fragments or those involving the non-weight–bearing surface should be ignored if they do not disturb hip mechanics; otherwise they should be excised. Large fragments of the weight-bearing portion of the femoral head should be reduced and fixed if at all possible.

Anterior Hip Dislocation

Anterior dislocation of the hip is much rarer than its posterior counterpart. It usually occurs when the hip is extended and externally rotated at the time of impact. Associated fractures of the acetabulum and the femoral head or neck occur rarely. Usually, the femoral head remains lateral to the obturator externus muscle but can be found rarely beneath it (obturator dislocation) or under the iliopsoas muscle in contact with the superior pubic ramus (pubic dislocation).

The hip is classically flexed, abducted, and externally rotated. The femoral head is palpable anteriorly below the inguinal flexion crease. Anteroposterior and transpelvic lateral radiographic projections are usually diagnostic.

Closed reduction under general anesthesia is generally successful. Here also the surgeon must make sure of a concentric reduction comparing both hip joints on the postreduction anteroposterior radiograph. The patient starts mobilization within a few days when pain is tolerable. Active and passive hip motion, excluding external rotation, is encouraged, and the patient is usually fully weight bearing by 4–6 weeks. Skeletal traction or spica casting may rarely be useful for uncooperative patients.

4. Rehabilitation of Hip Fracture Patients

The goal of rehabilitation after hip injuries is to return the patient as rapidly as possible to the preinjury functional level. Factors influencing rehabilitation potential include age, mental status, associated injuries, previous medical status, myocardial function, upper extremity strength, balance, and motivation.

For the rare patient treated conservatively, rehabilitation focuses early at preventing stiffness and weakness of the other extremities, and at eventually mobilizing the patient out of bed when pain is tolerable. Because the great majority of these injuries are now treated with internal fixation or prosthetic replacement, rehabilitation efforts are focused toward early range of motion, muscle strengthening, and weight bearing. Early full weight bearing as tolerated is encouraged for patients with prosthetic replacements, cemented or not, and for patients with stable fixation of an intertrochanteric fracture to allow compression of the fracture fragments. Most authors now agree that the same applies for femoral neck fractures with stable internal fixation, although some still prefer partial weight bearing until radiologic evidence of bone healing is present to prevent hardware failure. When internal fixation does not provide stable fixation of the fracture fragments, supplemental protection may be added with a spica cast or brace. If not, restricted range of motion or weight bearing may be allowed according to the surgeon's specifications.

Barquet A et al: Intertrochanteric-subtrochanteric fractures: treatment with the long gamma nail. J Orthop Trauma 2000; 14:324.[PMID: 10926238]

Gotfried Y: Percutaneous compression plating of intertrochanteric hip fractures. J Orthop Trauma 2000;14:490.[PMID: 11083611]

Gruson et al: The relationship between admission hemoglobin level and outcome after hip fracture. J Orthop Trauma 2002; 15:39.[PMID: 11782632]

Hernigou P, Charpentier P: Routine use of adjusted low-dose oral anticoagulants during the first three postoperative months after hip fracture in patients without comorbidity factors. J Orthop Trauma 2001;15:535.[PMID: 11733668]

Jaglal S, Lakhani Z, Schatzker J: Reliability, validity and responsiveness of the lower extremity measure for patients with a hip fracture 2000; J Bone Joint Surg Am;82-A:955.[PMID: 10901310]

McLoughlin SW et al: Biomechanical evaluation of the dynamic hip screw with two-and four-hole side plates. J Orthop Trauma 2000;14:318.[PMID: 10926237]

Palmer SJ, Parker MJ, Hollingworth W: The cost and implications of reoperation after surgery for fracture of the hip. J Bone Joint Surg Br 2000;82-B:864.[PMID: 10990312]

Rosen JE et al: Efficacy of preoperative skin traction in hip fracture patients: a prospective randomized study. J Orthop Trauma 2001;15:81.[PMID: 11232658]

Shah MR et al: Outcome after hip fracture in individuals ninety years of age and older. J Orthop Trauma 2001;15:34.[PMID: 11147685]

Tidermark J et al: Quality of life related to fracture displacement among elderly patients with femoral neck fractures treated with internal fixation. J Orthop Trauma 2002;15:34.[PMID: 11782631]

Zuckerman JD et al: A functional recovery score for elderly hip fracture patients I. Development. J Orthop Trauma 2000; 14:20.[PMID: 10630798]

Zuckerman JD et al: A functional recovery score for elderly hip fracture patients II. Validity and reliability. J Orthop Trauma 2000;14:26.[PMID: 10630799]

PELVIC FRACTURES & DISLOCATIONS

Both pelvic bones articulate with the sacrum through the sacroiliac joints and between themselves through the symphysis pubis. Upper body weight is transmitted across the hip joint to the lower limbs via the sciatic buttress and the acetabulum. The mechanism and severity of trauma will determine the pattern of injury. Osteoarticular structures and adjacent soft tissues will be involved in varying degrees and combinations. Treatment may require a multidisciplinary approach.

Clinical Findings

Knowledge of the injury mechanism is of prime importance and should be assessed in the cooperative patient. The physical examination includes palpation of the pelvic bony landmarks, compression maneuvers to assess stability, and rectovaginal examination looking for bony spikes protruding through the mucosa and contaminating the fracture hematoma. The mortality rate of open pelvic fractures is as high as 30–50%, compared with 8–15% for closed fractures. Associated injuries should also be systematically sought: lower urinary tract injuries, distal vascular status, and a thorough recorded neurologic examination.

An anteroposterior pelvic radiograph will be complemented as needed by inlet and outlet views and Judet's oblique views for the acetabulum. Eventually, CT scanning will further delineate the lesions. Vascular and urologic imaging may also be required.

Treatment

Significant forces, either directly or indirectly through the lower extremities, are required to destabilize the pelvic ring. A systematic search of associated injuries is mandatory. Hemorrhage may be important. Treatment of associated abdominal, thoracic, vascular, or urinary tract injuries should take precedence over treatment of the pelvic fracture.

General resuscitation principles are applied to provide adequate tissue perfusion. Hypovolemia may not be corrected by fluid and blood replacement alone. Once the patient is admitted and other sites of hemorrhage have been ruled out, active bleeding from a pelvic fracture may be controlled by the use of an external fixator device, pelvic C-clamp or pelvic stabilizer. Major fracture fragments are stabilized, and the pelvic and retroperitoneal space available for fluids is decreased or at least prevented from increasing. If this fails to control the hemorrhage and stabilize the patient, arterial embolization under fluoroscopic imaging is then indicated. Surgical exploration for bleeding control is indicated only on extremely rare occasions, if ever.

When used in this fashion to control pelvic fracture motion, the pelvic external fixator is a useful tool to manage volume depletion. It does not provide stable enough fixation to treat complex fractures or most unstable pelvic fractures. It usually resists stresses imposed by sitting but not those from weight bearing, and further internal fixation is often required at a later stage.

A. ASSOCIATED INJURIES

1. Hemorrhage—The bleeding associated with pelvic ring fractures usually comes from the small to medium-sized arteries and veins in the surrounding soft tissues and from the bone itself. Occasionally, large vessels such as the femoral artery or the common iliac artery or vein are lacerated or torn. An arteriogram is diagnostic, and surgery for repair or bypass is urgently required if there is distal ischemia.

2. Thrombosis—It is now well recognized that patients with pelvic fractures have a high incidence of thrombosis of the pelvic veins and, less frequently, of the femoral vein. Those treated with bed rest compound the risk of deep vein thrombosis and secondary pulmonary embolus. More trauma centers now use prophylactic anticoagulation once the acute hemorrhagic phase has passed (24–48 h).

3. Neurologic injury—Neurologic injuries are common. They involve either the roots as they travel in or around the sacral foramen, or the peripheral nerve itself (sciatic, femoral, obturator, pudendal, or superior gluteal). Neurologic injury following closed or open reduction is not uncommon. It is thus of paramount importance that a thorough neurologic examination be performed and recorded as soon as possible, searching for sensory or motor deficits in the distribution of all previously mentioned nerves. Peripheral nerve injuries have, overall, a better prognosis than root injuries. Partial nerve injuries also have a better outcome than complete ones. Most of the lesions are of the neurapraxia type, with favorable outcome. It is still accepted that nearly 10% have clinically significant permanent neurologic sequelae.

4. Urogenital injuries—Urogenital injuries are also common, especially in men. The incidence of bladder rupture and urethral disruption is estimated at 5–10% for each. These injuries should be suspected in the conscious patient who is unable to void or who has gross hematuria. Other signs include bloody urethral discharge, swelling or ecchymosis of the penis or perineum, or a high-riding or "floating" prostate on rectal examination. A retrograde urethrogram should be obtained before attempting to introduce a Foley catheter. If negative, catheterization can be safely undertaken and a cystogram obtained later. When a partial or complete urethral disruption is diagnosed, a suprapubic cystostomy should be performed. Late sequelae are common and include urethral strictures, sexual dysfunction, and impotence.

1. Injuries to the Pelvic Ring

Pelvic ring fractures account for 3% of all fractures. There is an extremely wide spectrum between the innocuous avulsion fracture and the life-threatening severely unstable pelvic ring disruption. The choice between different treatment modalities revolves around one key issue: Is the fracture pattern stable or unstable?

From the anatomic standpoint, the posterior sacroiliac ligamentous complex is the single most important structure for pelvic stability. Injuries involving the pelvic ring in two or more sites create an unstable segment. The integrity of the posterior sacroiliac ligamentous complex will determine the degree of instability. Inlet and outlet views and CT scanning are necessary imaging techniques to make this determination. When intact, the hemipelvis will be rotationally unstable but vertically stable. When disrupted, the hemipelvis will be both rotationally and vertically unstable.

Classification & Treatment

Tile devised a dynamic classification system based on the mechanism of injury and residual instability (Table 3–4).

Type A: Fractures that involve the pelvic ring in only one place and are stable.

Type A1: Avulsion fractures of the pelvis, which usually occur at muscle origins such as the anterosuperior iliac spine for the sartorius, anteroinferior iliac spine for the direct head of the rectus femoris, and ischial apophysis for the hamstring muscles. These fractures occur most often in the adolescent, and conserva-

Table 3–4. The Tile classification of pelvic ring disruptions.

Type A: Stable, posterior arch intact
A1: Posterior arch intact, fracture of innominate bone (avulsion)
   A1.1 Iliac spine
   A1.2 Iliac crest
   A1.3 Ischial tuberosity
A2: Posterior arch intact, fracture of innominate bone (direct blow)
   A2.1 Iliac wing fractures
   A2.2 Unilateral fracture of anterior arch
   A2.3 Bifocal fracture of anterior arch
A3: Posterior arch intact, transverse fracture of sacrum caudal to S2
   A3.1 Sacrococcygeal dislocation
   A3.2 Sacrum undisplaced
   A3.3 Sacrum displaced
Type B: Incomplete disruption of posterior arch, partially stable, rotation
B1: External rotation instability, open-book injury, unilateral
   B1.1 Sacroiliac joint, anterior disruption
   B1.2 Sacral fracture
B2: Incomplete disruption of posterior arch, unilateral, internal rotation (lateral compression)
   B2.1 Anterior compression fracture, sacrum
   B2.2 Partial sacroiliac joint fracture, subluxation
   B2.3 Incomplete posterior iliac fracture
B3: Incomplete disruption of posterior arch, bilateral
   B3.1 Bilateral open-book
   B3.2 Open-book, lateral compression
   B3.3 Bilateral lateral compression
Type C: Complete disruption of posterior arch, unstable
C1: Complete disruption of posterior arch, unilateral
   C1.1 Fracture through ilium
   C1.2 Sacroiliac dislocation and/or fracture dislocation
   C1.3 Sacral fracture
C2: Bilateral injury, one side rotationally unstable, one side vertically unstable
C3: Bilateral injury, both sides completely unstable

Reproduced, with permission, from Browner BD et al, eds: Skeletal Trauma, 2nd ed. Philadelphia: WB Saunders, 1998.

tive treatment is usually sufficient. On rare occasions, symptomatic nonunion occurs, and this is best dealt with surgically.

Type A2: Stable fractures with minimal displacement. Isolated fractures of the iliac wing without intraarticular extension usually result from direct trauma. Even with significant displacement, bony healing is to be expected, and treatment is, therefore, symptomatic. On rare occasions, the soft tissue injury and accompanying hematoma may heal with significant heterotopic ossification.

Type A3: Obturator fractures. Isolated fractures of the pubic or ischial rami are usually minimally displaced. The posterior sacroiliac complex is intact, and the pelvis is stable. Treatment is symptomatic, with bed rest and analgesia, early ambulation, and weight bearing as tolerated.

Type B: Fractures that involve the pelvic ring in two or more sites. They create a segment that is rotationally unstable but vertically stable.

Type B1: Open-book fractures occur from antero-posterior compression. Unless the anterior separation of the pubic symphysis is severe (> 6 cm), the posterior sacroiliac complex is usually intact and the pelvis relatively stable. Significant injury to perineal and urogenital structures is often present and should always be looked for. One should remember that fragment displacement at the time of injury might have been significantly more than what is apparent on radiograph. For minimally displaced symphysis injuries, only symptomatic treatment is needed. The same applies for the so-called straddle (four rami) fracture. For more displaced fracture-dislocations, reduction is done by lateral compression using the intact posterior sacroiliac complex as the hinge on which "the book is closed." Reduction can be maintained by external or internal fixation. "Closing the book" decreases the space available for hemorrhage. It also increases patient comfort, facilitates nursing care, and allows earlier mobilization, which is beneficial to the polytrauma patient.

Type B2 and B3: Lateral compression fractures. A lateral force applied to the pelvis causes inward displacement of the hemipelvis through the sacroiliac complex and the ipsilateral (B2) or, more often, contralateral pubic rami (B3, bucket-handle type). The degree of involvement of the posterior sacroiliac ligaments will determine the degree of instability. The posterior lesion may be impacted in its displaced portion, affording some relative stability. The hemipelvis is infolded, with overlapping of the symphysis. Major displacement requires manipulation under general anesthesia. This should be done soon after injury because disimpaction becomes difficult and hazardous after the first few days. Reduction can be maintained with external or internal fixation, or both. External fixation alone decreases pain and makes nursing care easier but is not strong enough for ambulation if the fracture is unstable posteriorly.

Type C: Fractures that are both rotationally and vertically unstable. They often result from a vertical shear mechanism, like a fall from a height. Anteriorly, the injury may fracture the pubic rami or disrupt the symphysis pubis. Posteriorly, the sacroiliac joint may be dislocated or there may be a fracture in the sacrum or in the ilium immediately adjacent to the sacroiliac joint, but there is always loss of the functional integrity of the posterior sacroiliac ligamentous complex. The hemipelvis is completely unstable. Three-dimensional displacement is possible, particularly proximal migration. Massive hemorrhage and injury to the lumbosacral nerve plexus are common. Indirect radiologic clues of pelvic instability should be looked for such as avulsion of the sciatic spine or fracture of the ipsilateral L5 transverse process. Reduction is relatively easy, with longitudinal skeletal traction through the distal femur or the proximal tibia. If chosen as definitive treatment, traction should be maintained for 8–12 weeks. Bony injuries heal quicker than ligamentous injuries. External fixation alone is insufficient to maintain reduction in highly unstable fractures, but it may help control bleeding and eases nursing care. Open reduction and internal fixation is often required. The surgical technique is demanding, and there is a significant risk of complications. It is best left to experienced pelvic surgeons.

Complications

Long-term complications of unstable pelvic ring disruptions are more frequent and disabling than once thought. Of those patients with residual displacement of more than 1 cm, fewer than 30% are pain free at 5 years. Chronic low back pain and posterior sacroiliac pain is the most frequent long-term complaint, approaching 50% in some series. Nearly 5% of type C injuries are left with a leg length discrepancy of more than 2–5 cm. Residual gait abnormalities are present in 12–32% of cases. The overall nonunion rate is around 3%.

Clinically significant neurologic deficit is present in 6–10% of patients, but abnormal electromyographic findings are present in up to 46%. Long-term urologic complications include urethral strictures in 5–20% of cases and impotence in 5–30% of cases.

2. Fractures of the Acetabulum

The acetabulum is the portion of the pelvic bone that articulates with the femoral head to form the hip joint. It results from the closure of the Y or triradiate cartilage and is covered with hyaline cartilage.

Fractures of the acetabulum occur through direct trauma on the trochanteric region or indirect axial loading through the lower limb. The position of the limb at the time of impact (rotation, flexion, abduction, or adduction) will determine the pattern of injury. Comminution is common.

Classification

Letournel has classified acetabular fractures based on which column is involved. The anterior column comprises the anterior iliac crest, the anterior half of the acetabulum, and the pubic ramus. The posterior column includes the sciatic buttress and the sciatic notch, the posterior half of the acetabulum, and the ischial tuberosity. These two columns unite in an inverted Y pattern, the center of which articulates with the femoral head. Fractures may involve one or both columns in a simple or complex pattern.

Proper fracture classification requires good-quality radiographs. Two oblique views (Judet views) taken 45 degrees toward and away from the involved side complement the standard anteroposterior view of the pelvis. CT scanning gives further information on the fracture pattern, the presence of free intra-articular fragments, and the status of the femoral head and the rest of the pelvic ring.

Letournel has classified acetabular fractures into 10 different types: 5 simple patterns (one fracture line) and 5 complex patterns (the association of two or more simple patterns) (Figure 3–30). This is the most widely used classification system, as it allows the surgeon to choose the appropriate surgical approach.

Treatment

The goal of treatment is to attain a spherical congruency between the femoral head and the weight-bearing acetabular dome, and to maintain it until bones are healed. As with other pelvic fractures, acetabular fractures are frequently associated with abdominal, urogenital, and neurologic injuries, which should be systematically sought and treated. Significant bleeding is often present and should be addressed as soon as possible.

The stabilized patient should be put in longitudinal skeletal traction through a distal femoral or proximal tibial pin pulling axially in neutral position. A trochanteric screw for lateral traction is contraindicated, as it will create a contaminated pin tract and thus preclude possible further surgical treatment. Postreduction radiographs are obtained. In general, a displaced

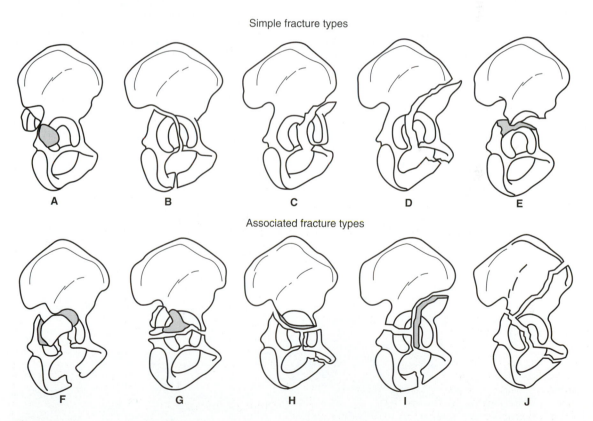

Figure 3–30. Letournel classification of acetabular fractures. (Reproduced, with permission, from Canale ST, ed. Campbells operative orthopaedics, 9th ed. Philadelphia: Lippincott, 1998.)

acetabular fracture is rarely reduced adequately by closed methods. If the reduction is judged acceptable, traction is maintained for 6–8 weeks until bone healing is evident. Another 6–8 weeks is necessary before full weight bearing can be attempted. Surgical indications include intra-articular displacement of 2 mm or more, an incongruous hip reduction, marginal impaction > 2 mm, or intra-articular debris. The choice of approach is of primary importance, and sometimes more than one approach will prove necessary. Acetabular surgery uses extensile approaches and sophisticated reduction and fixation techniques and is best performed by trained pelvic surgeons. Other surgical indications include free osteochondral fragments, femoral head fractures, irreducible dislocations, or unstable reductions.

Complications

Complications inherent to the injury include posttraumatic degenerative joint disease, heterotopic ossification, femoral head osteonecrosis, deep vein thrombosis, and other complications related to conservative treatment. Surgery is performed to prevent or delay osteoarthritis, but increases the possibility of complications such as infection, iatrogenic neurovascular injury, and increased heterotopic ossification. When the reduction is stable and fixation is solid, the patient can be mobilized after a few days with non-weight–bearing ambulation, and weight bearing may begin as early as 6 weeks. Most pelvic surgeons now routinely use postoperative prophylactic anticoagulation and heterotopic bone formation prophylaxis with irradiation or indomethacin, or both.

Bellabarba C, Ricci WM, Bolhofner BR: Distraction external fixation in lateral compression pelvic fractures. J Orthop Trauma 2000;14:475.[PMID: 11083609]

Carlson DA et al: Safe placement of S1 and S2 iliosacral screws: the vestibule concept. J Orthop Trauma 2000;14:264.[PMID: 10898199]

Ertel W et al: Control of Severe hemorrhage using C-clamp and pelvic packing in multiply injured patients with pelvic ring disruption. J Orthop Trauma 2001;15:468.[PMID: 11602828]

Routt ML, et al. Circumferential pelvic antishock sheeting: A temporary resuscitation aid. J Orthop Trauma 2002;15:45.[PMID: 11782633]

Saterbak AM et al: Clinical failure after posterior wall acetabular fractures: The influence of initial fracture patterns. J Orthop Trauma 2000;14:230.[PMID: 10898194]

Switzer JA, Nork SE, Routt ML: Comminuted fractures of the iliac wing. J Orthop Trauma 2000;14:270.[PMID: 10898200]

Tornetta P: Displaced acetabular fractures: Indications for operative and nonoperative management. J Am Acad Orthop Surg 2001;9:18.[PMID: 11174160]

Sports Medicine

4

Patrick J. McMahon, MD, & Harry B. Skinner, MD

Introduction

Sports medicine developed in the 1970s as an orthopedic specialty focusing on competitive athletes. Today, sports medicine includes the overall care of athletes from many skill levels. Increasingly, care of recreational athletes has risen to that common for professional athletes. Initial sports medicine focused on knee injuries; now its purview also includes other musculoskeletal injuries including the shoulder, elbow, and ankle. In addition to the musculoskeletal system, emphasis is placed on the cardiovascular and pulmonary systems, and on training techniques, nutrition, and women's athletics. This wide range of care requires a multidisciplinary team of medical personnel, including athletic trainers, physical therapists, cardiologists, pulmonologists, orthopedic surgeons, and general practitioners.

■ KNEE INJURIES

Anatomy

The bones of the knee are the distal femur, the proximal tibia, and the patella. These bones depend upon supporting ligaments, the joint capsule, and the menisci to provide stability for the joint.

A. MENISCI AND JOINT CAPSULE

The menisci, or semilunar cartilage, are C-shaped fibrocartilaginous disks in the knee that provide shock absorption, allow for increased congruency between joint surfaces, enhance joint stability, and aid in distribution of synovial fluid.

The medial and lateral menisci provide a concave surface with which the convex femoral condyles can articulate. If the menisci are not present, the convex femoral condyles articulate with the relatively flat tibial plateaus, and the joint surfaces are not congruent. This decreases the surface area of contact and increases the pressure on the articular cartilage of the tibia and femur, which may lead to rapid deterioration of the joint surface. The medial meniscus is firmly attached to the joint capsule along its entire peripheral edge. The lateral meniscus is attached to the anterior and posterior capsule, but there is a region posterolaterally where it is not firmly attached (Figure 4–1). Therefore, the medial meniscus has less mobility than the lateral meniscus and is more susceptible to tearing when trapped between the femoral condyle and tibial plateau. The lateral meniscus is larger than the medial meniscus and carries a greater share of the lateral compartment pressure than the medial meniscus carries for the medial compartment.

B. LIGAMENTS

Within the knee, the anterior cruciate ligament travels from the medial border of the lateral femoral condyle to its insertion site anterolateral to the medial tibial spine. This ligament prevents anterior translation and rotation of the tibia on the femur (Figure 4–2). The posterior cruciate ligament prevents posterior subluxation of the tibia on the femur. It runs from the lateral aspect of the medial femoral condyle to the posterior aspect of the tibia, just below the joint line (Figure 4–3). On the medial side, the medial collateral ligament has superficial and deep portions (Figure 4–4), which stabilize the knee to valgus stresses. The lateral collateral or fibular collateral ligament runs from the lateral femoral condyle to the head of the fibula. It is the main stabilizer against varus stress (Figure 4–5). The lateral collateral ligament is part of the posterolateral "complex" or "corner" of the knee that also resists external rotation. An important component is the poplitofibular ligament, present in 90% of knees that runs from the tendon of the popliteus muscle to the styloid on the posterior fibular head.

History and Physical Examination

A. GENERAL APPROACH

The history of the knee injury may be obtained by asking the patient the questions listed in Table 4–1. The physical examination begins with observation of the patient's gait. The uninjured knee is then examined as a basis of comparison with the injured knee. Any swelling or effusion should be noted. A small effusion will cause obliteration of the recesses on the medial and lateral aspects of the patellar tendon; with a larger effusion, diffuse swelling is present in the region of the suprapatellar pouch. Then, a fluid wave can be palpated on the sides of the patella. Active and then passive range of motion is tested carefully. The knee is palpated to define areas

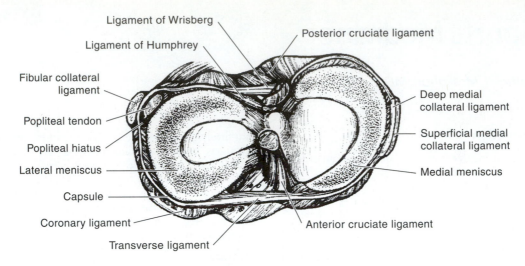

Figure 4–1. The medial and lateral menisci with their associated intermeniscal ligaments. *Note*: The lateral meniscus is not attached in the region of the popliteus tendon. (Reproduced, with permission, from Scott WN: Ligament and Extensor Mechanism Injuries of the Knee: Diagnosis and Treatment. St. Louis: Mosby-Year Book, 1991.)

of localized tenderness. The joint lines are located at the level of the inferior pole of the patella when the knee is flexed to 90 degrees.

B. LIGAMENT LAXITY EVALUATION

To determine varus and valgus stability (Table 4–2), the patient's foot is held between the examiner's elbow and hip, with both hands free to palpate the joint (Figure 4–6). Stability should be determined at both full extension and 30 degrees of knee flexion. Grading of laxity is based on the amount of opening of the joint (grade 1, 0–5 mm; grade 2, 5–10 mm; and grade 3, 10–15 mm). Laxity in full extension to varus or valgus angulation is an ominous sign of disruption of key ligamentous structures. If significant valgus laxity is present in full extension, the posteromedial capsule and medial collateral ligament are torn. With varus laxity in full extension, the posterolateral capsular complex is torn, in addition to the lateral collateral ligament. With either varus or valgus laxity at full extension, anterior and posterior cruciate ligament tears are likely. At 30 degrees of flexion, the posterior capsule and cruciate ligaments are relaxed and the medial and lateral collateral ligaments can best be isolated. Pain with varus or valgus stress is more suggestive of ligament damage than a meniscal tear.

C. LACHMAN'S TEST

Lachman's test is the most sensitive test for anterior cruciate ligament tears. It is done with the knee flexed

at 20 degrees, stabilizing the distal femur with one hand and pulling forward on the proximal tibia with the other hand (Figure 4–7). With an intact ligament, minimal translation of the tibia occurs and a firm end point is felt. With a torn anterior cruciate ligament, more translation is noted, and the end point is soft or mushy. The hamstring muscles must be relaxed during this maneuver to prevent false-negative findings. Comparison of the injured and uninjured knees is essential.

D. ANTERIOR DRAWER TEST

The anterior drawer test is done with the knee at 90 degrees of flexion and is not as sensitive as Lachman's test but serves as an adjunct in the evaluation of anterior cruciate ligament instability (Figure 4–8). With the patient supine and the knee flexed to 90 degrees (hip flexed to about 45 degrees), the foot is restrained by sitting on it and the examiner's hands are placed around the proximal tibia. Then while the hamstrings are felt to relax and the tibia is pulled forward, the displacement and the end point are evaluated.

E. LOSEE'S TEST

The pivot shift phenomenon demonstrates the instability associated with an anterior cruciate ligament tear. Once demonstrated, it is often difficult to repeat because the patient may find this maneuver uncomfortable and will guard against having it done again. As described by Losee, a valgus and internal rotation force is applied to the tibia (Figure 4–9). Starting at 45 degrees

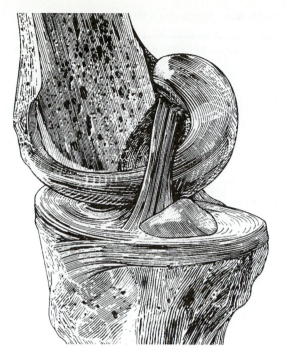

Figure 4–2. Drawing of the anterior cruciate ligament with the knee in extension, showing the course of the ligament as it passes from the medial aspect of the lateral femoral condyle to the lateral portion of the medial tibial spine. (Reproduced, with permission, from Girgis FG et al: The cruciate ligaments of the knee joint: Anatomical, functional, and experimental analysis. Clin Orthop 1975;106:216.)

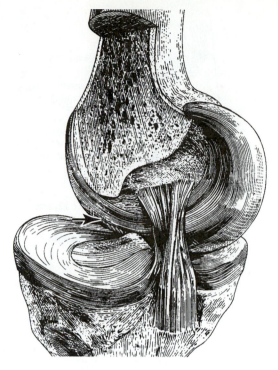

Figure 4–3. Drawing of the posterior cruciate ligament, showing the course of the ligament as it passes from the lateral aspect of the medial femoral condyle to the posterior surface of the tibia. (Reproduced, with permission, from Girgis FG et al: The cruciate ligaments of the knee joint: Anatomical, functional, and experimental analysis. Clin Orthop 1975;106:216.)

of flexion, the lateral tibial plateau is reduced. Extending the knee causes the lateral plateau to subluxate anteriorly with a thud at about 20 degrees of flexion. It reduces quietly at full extension. Many other ways of doing this test have been described, but the phenomenon and significance of the different tests are similar.

F. POSTERIOR DRAWER TEST

The posterior drawer test evaluates the integrity of the posterior cruciate ligament. It is performed with posterior pressure on the proximal tibia with the knee flexed at 90 degrees (Figure 4–10). Normally, the tibial plateau is anterior to the femoral condyles, and a step-off to the tibia is palpated when the thumb is slid down the femoral condyles. With a posterior cruciate ligament injury, sagging of the tibial plateau may be appreciated and no step-off is palpated (Figure 4–11). An associated contusion on the anterior tibia suggests a posterior cruciate ligament injury.

G. MCMURRAY'S TEST

With McMurray's test, forced flexion and rotation of the knee may elicit a click or clunk along the joint line when a meniscal injury is present (Figure 4–12). Found in less than 10% of patients with a meniscus injury, joint line pain with the McMurray's test is much more common.

Arthroscopic Examination

A. INDICATIONS FOR KNEE INJURIES

Indications for arthroscopic examination in the knee include the following:

(1) acute hemarthrosis
(2) meniscus injuries
(3) bodies
(4) selected tibial plateau fractures

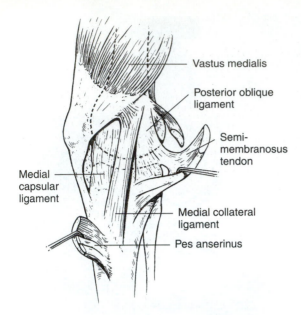

Figure 4–4. Medial capsuloligamentous complex. (Reproduced, with permission, from Feagin JA Jr: The Crucial Ligaments. New York: Churchill Livingstone, 1988.)

(5) patellar chondromalacia or malalignment (or both)
(6) chronic synovitis
(7) knee instability
(8) recurrent effusions
(9) chondral and osteochondral fractures

Partly because of experience with arthroscopy, a specific diagnosis of the type of knee injury can now usually be made preoperatively. A specific diagnosis can then be confirmed, expanded, or revised, and treatment can be rendered as needed.

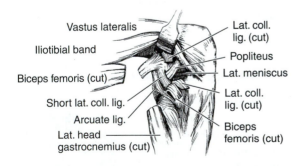

Figure 4–5. The lateral supporting structures of the knee. (Reproduced, with permission, from Rockwood CA Jr et al: Fractures in Adults. New York: Churchill Livingstone, 1988.)

Table 4–1. History of a knee injury.

Did an injury occur?	Yes: possible ligament tear or meniscus tear. No: overuse problem or degenerative condition.
Was it a noncontact injury?	Yes: often the ACL is the only ligament torn.
Was it a contact injury?	Yes: possible multiple ligament injuries, including ACL and MCL, ACL and LCL, ACL, PCL, and a collateral ligament.
Did the patient hear or feel a pop?	Yes: a pop often occurs with ACL tears.
How long did it take to swell up?	Within hours: often an ACL tear. Overnight: often a meniscus tear.
Does the knee lock?	Yes: often a meniscus tear flipping into and out of the joint.
Does it buckle (trick knee)?	Yes: not specific; may arise from quadriceps weakness, trapped meniscus, ligament instability, or patella dislocating.
Is climbing or descending stairs difficult?	Often patellofemoral problems.
Are cutting maneuvers difficult?	ACL tear.
Is squatting (deep knee bends) difficult?	Meniscus tear.
Is jumping difficult?	Patellar tendinitis.
Where does it hurt?	Medial joint line: medial meniscus tear or medial compartment arthritis. MCL: MCL sprain. Lateral joint line: lateral meniscus tear, injury, iliotibial band tendinitis, popliteus tendinitis.

ACL = anterior cruciate ligament; MCL = medial collateral ligament; LCL = lateral collateral ligament; PCL = posterior cruciate ligament.

B. TECHNIQUE

Examination under anesthesia is very helpful in diagnosing ligament injuries and instability, so it should be performed before the beginning of the procedure, before preparing and draping the extremity. For diagnostic arthroscopy, the knee joint is distended with irrigating fluid (usually saline or lactated Ringer's solution), which washes away blood and debris from the joint. A lateral

Table 4–2. Anatomic correlation of clinical ligament instability examination of the knee.

Direction of Force	Position	Ligament Instability
Varus or valgus	Full extension	Posterior cruciate, posterior capsule
Varus	Flexion at 30 degrees	Lateral collateral ligament/complex
Valgus	Flexion at 30 degrees	Medial collateral ligament
Anterior	Flexion at 30 degrees neutral position (AP)	Anterior cruciate ligament
Anterior	Flexion at 90 degrees neutral internal or external rotation	Anterior cruciate ligament
Posterior	90 degrees (sag test)	Posterior cruciate ligament

AP = anteroposterior.

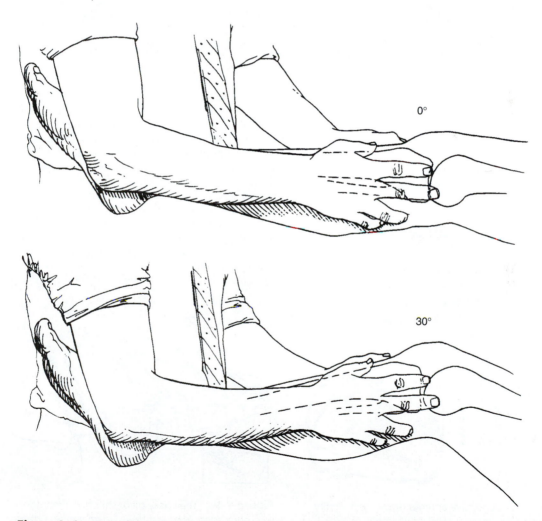

Figure 4–6. The collateral ligaments being tested in extension and 30 degrees of flexion with the foot held between the examiner's elbow and hip. (Reproduced, with permission, from Feagin JA Jr: The Crucial Ligaments. New York: Churchill Livingstone, 1988.)

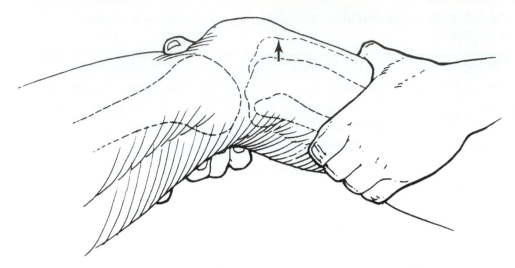

Figure 4–7. Lachman's test. (Reproduced, with permission, from Feagin JA Jr: The Crucial Ligaments. New York: Churchill Livingstone, 1988.)

portal, for the arthroscope, is placed about a thumb's breadth above the joint line and just lateral to the patellar tendon. The medial portal is placed at about the same level but just medial to the patellar tendon for introducing arthroscopic tools such as a probe. One approach to the general inspection of the joint is to start in the suprapatellar pouch. Loose bodies and plicas are sought. The patellofemoral joint is then inspected and observed for tracking problems and cartilage damage. The lateral gutter, the popliteus tendon, and the medial gutter are examined. Then with flexion and valgus stress to the leg, the medial compartment is entered. The medial meniscus is probed using a nerve hook through the medial por-

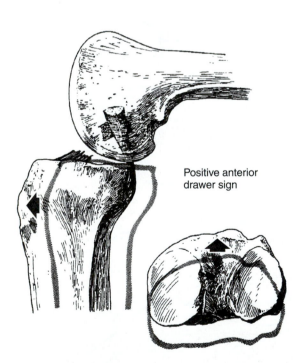

Positive anterior drawer sign

Figure 4–8. A positive anterior drawer test signifying a tear of the anterior cruciate ligament. (Reproduced, with permission, from Insall JN: Surgery of the Knee. New York: Churchill Livingstone, 1984.)

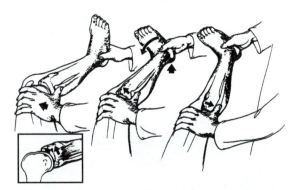

Figure 4–9. The Losee pivot shift test. (Reproduced, with permission, from Scott WN: Ligament and Extensor Mechanism Injuries of the Knee: Diagnosis and Treatment. St. Louis: Mosby-Year Book, 1991.)

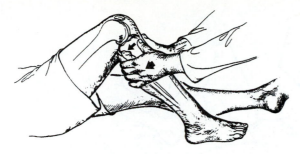

Figure 4–10. The posterior drawer test is done in the same fashion as the anterior drawer test, except that the examiner exerts a posterior force. (Reproduced, with permission, from Scott WN: Ligament and Extensor Mechanism Injuries of the Knee: Diagnosis and Treatment. St. Louis: Mosby-Year Book, 1991.)

tal. The intercondylar notch, including the anterior cruciate ligament, is inspected. The lateral compartment is then examined in a similar manner. Documentation of findings and procedures performed is important and may be done by videotape, photographs, and diagrammatic sketches. With assessment of the pathologic changes treatment can be initiated, such as debridement and repair of meniscal tears, removal of loose bodies, or anterior cruciate ligament reconstruction.

Imaging & Other Studies

A. MAGNETIC RESONANCE IMAGING

Magnetic resonance imaging (MRI) is a powerful technique for evaluation of the knee joint. Although the di-

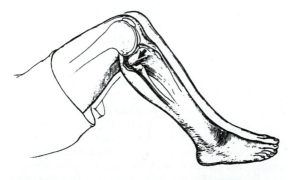

Figure 4–11. The posterior sag seen in posterior cruciate disruption. (Reproduced, with permission, from Scott WN: Ligament and Extensor Mechanism Injuries of the Knee: Diagnosis and Treatment. St. Louis: Mosby-Year Book, 1991.)

agnosis is usually evident from the history and physical examination, MRI can confirm the suspected injury. Other times, when a physical examination is impossible because of pain, or the diagnosis remains elusive, MRI can aid in proper diagnosis. In one study, the specificity, sensitivity, and accuracy of MRI were compared with the same factors in arthroscopic examination and were found to vary depending on the structure under consideration. It was found to be greater than 90% for the medial and lateral menisci and the anterior and posterior cruciate ligaments. Therefore, MRI is appropriate for ruling out the need for diagnostic arthroscopic examination. It is less helpful for the diagnosis of problems in knees with previous arthroscopy.

B. IMAGING STUDIES

Roentgenographic examination of the knee is indicated in the evaluation of traumatic injury. In cases of minimal trauma, radiographs may not be needed if the injury proves to be self-limited. MRI is very helpful in diagnosis of the injured knee, especially when pain makes physical examination difficult. Arthrographic examination can be helpful in patients who are unable to undergo MRI because of claustrophobia, metal in the body that may be dislodged, or other contraindications.

C. LABORATORY TESTS

Laboratory tests may be helpful in ruling out nonmechanical disorders such as inflammatory arthritis as described in Chapter 7.

Kocher MS et al: Diagnostic performance of clinical examination and magnetic resonance imaging in the evaluation of intraarticular knee disorders in children and adolescents. Am J Sports Med 2001;29(3):292.

Lonner JH et al: Comparison of magnetic resonance imaging with operative findings in acute traumatic dislocations of the adult knee. J Trauma 2000;14(3):183.

Scholten RJ et al: The accuracy of physical examination diagnostic tests for assessing meniscal lesions of the knee: A meta-analysis. J Fam Pract 2001;50(11):938.

Solomon DH et al: Does the patient have a torn meniscus of ligament of the knee?: Value of the physical examination. JAMA 2001;286(13):1610.

MENISCUS INJURY

Meniscal injuries are the most common reason for arthroscopy of the knee. The medial meniscus is more frequently torn than the lateral because the medial meniscus is securely attached around the entire periphery of the joint capsule, whereas the lateral has a mobile area where it is not attached. Meniscus injury is rare in childhood, occurs in the late teens, and peaks in the third and fourth decades. After the age of 50, meniscus tears are more often the result of arthritis than trauma.

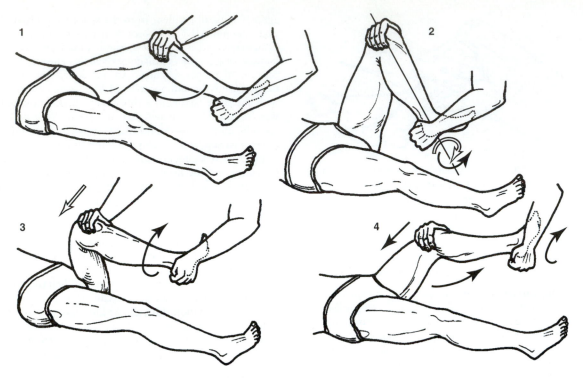

Figure 4–12. The McMurray test to produce click. (Reproduced, with permission, from American Academy of Orthopaedic Surgeons: Athletic Training and Sports Medicine, 2nd ed, 1991.)

Clinical Findings

Symptoms of meniscal injury include joint line pain, catching, popping and locking. Examination elicits tenderness along the joint line, and an effusion is present. There is pain and occasionally clicking along the joint line with forced flexion and rotation of the knee (McMurray's test) (see Figure 4–12). A deep squat and duck-walking are usually painful.

The anatomy of meniscus tears varies widely (Figure 4–13) and includes incomplete tears, bucket-handle tears, flap tears, radial tears, and complex tears. The tears may be isolated or associated with other injuries to the knee (eg, anterior cruciate ligament tears). If the meniscus tear is in the avascular portion of the meniscus and acute hemarthrosis does not develop, a synovial fluid effusion may slowly develop.

The meniscus may become completely displaced and locked between the femur and tibia, preventing full extension of the knee (Figure 4–14). More frequently, the torn meniscus will cause pain, intermittent catching and occasionally locking as it flips into and out of the region of contact between the femur and the tibia.

Treatment and Prognosis

Small stable asymptomatic meniscus tears do not need to be treated surgically. Those causing persistent symptoms should be addressed arthroscopically. Before the importance of the meniscus was understood and arthroscopy became available, the meniscus was often removed, even when normal, when the preoperative diagnosis was "internal derangement of the knee." Attempts are now made to remove only the torn portion of the meniscus or repair the meniscus, if possible.

During arthroscopy, the meniscus should be visualized and palpated with a hooked probe. The inner two thirds of the meniscus is avascular and usually requires resection. A punch-basket forceps is often used to complete the resection of the torn portion of the meniscus, and the meniscal fragment is removed with a grasping instrument. Power shavers are used to smoothly contour the remaining meniscus to prevent further tearing from a jagged edge. Return to full function may be expected in 4–6 weeks.

Tears in the peripheral third of the meniscus, if small (less than 15 mm), may heal spontaneously because this portion of the adult meniscus has a blood supply. Larger

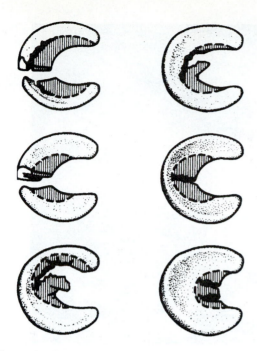

Figure 4–13. Patterns of meniscal tears: bucket-handle, flap, horizontal cleavage, radial, degenerative, and double radial tear of a discoid meniscus. (Reproduced, with permission, from Scott WN: Arthroscopy of the Knee. Philadelphia: WB Saunders, 1990.)

tears require repair. Patients who undergo meniscectomy at a young age are at risk of early osteoarthritis. These changes were first described by Fairbanks and include flattening of the femoral condyle, joint space narrowing, and osteophyte formation. Therefore, if a meniscus can be saved, it should be.

Suturing of the tears may be done by four different techniques: inside-out, outside-in, all-inside, or open. In the inside-out technique, the needles are passed through special cannulas under arthroscopic guidance. An incision is made where the needles will exit the skin, the subcutaneous tissue is undermined, and an instrument (spoon, disassembled vaginal speculum, or special meniscus repair retractor) is inserted to catch the needle, protecting the neurovascular structures. The outside-in technique involves placing long needles through the skin and into the torn meniscus within the knee joint. Sutures are placed through the needles from outside, then grasped within the knee and tied. The sutures are then also tied outside the knee. With both of these techniques, neurovascular damage is possible. On the medial side, the structure most often damaged is the saphenous nerve. Laterally, the peroneal nerve is at risk. Posteriorly, the popliteal vessels and the tibial and per-

oneal nerves are all at risk. In the all-inside technique, sutures are passed through the torn meniscus, and special instruments are used to tie the sutures within the knee. This technique has recently become more popular as bioabsorbable devices have become available for meniscus repair. Unfortunately, loosening of the devices has been reported, and the biomechanical properties of the repaired meniscus are less than that after suture repair. Open repair is also possible for tears of the peripheral portion of the meniscus.

Repairable meniscus tears often occur with an anterior cruciate ligament tear. Stabilizing the knee with anterior cruciate ligament reconstruction protects the repaired meniscus from abnormal knee motion; this method has a higher rate of success than if the knee is left unstable.

An alternative to leaving the patient with a meniscus-deficient knee, and almost certain early osteoarthrosis, is meniscal transplantation. This technique yields satisfactory results in about two thirds of patients after a short-term follow-up. In the future, biologic scaffolds may enable menisci to be regenerated after meniscectomy.

Englund M et al: Patient-relevant outcomes fourteen years after meniscectomy: Influence of the type of meniscal tear and size of resection. Rheumatology (Oxford) 2001;40(6):631.

Hulet CH et al: Arthroscopic medial meniscectomy on stable knees. J Bone Joint Surg 2001;83B(1):29.

McNicholas MJ et al: Total meniscectomy in adolescence A thirty-year follow-up. J Bone Joint Surg 2000;82B(2):217.

Noyes FR, Barber-Westin SD: Arthroscopic repair of meniscus tear extending into the avascular zone with or without anterior cruciate ligament reconstruction in patients 40 years of age and younger. Arthroscopy 2000;16(8):822.

Rodeo SA: Meniscal allografts—Where do we stand? Am J Sports Med 2001;29(2):246.

KNEE FRACTURE

Articular cartilage injuries of the knee are infrequent, and the examiner must have a high index of suspicion to detect them. Arthroscopy is very helpful with these injuries, especially pure chondral injuries, where radiographs will be normal.

1. Osteochondral Lesions

Osteochondral Fracture

Chondral and osteochondral fractures have been thought to arise from shear stress, with lower speed and applied energy causing the deeper osteochondral fractures. Osteochondral fractures usually occur in adolescents and young adults, before the tidemark layer appears in the articular cartilage. The most common sites

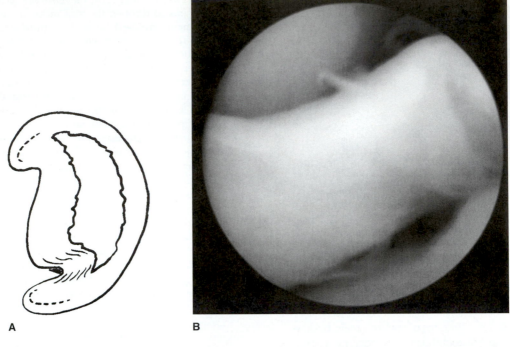

A   **B**

Figure 4–14. **A:** Diagram of a typical bucket-handle tear of the medial meniscus. **B:** Arthroscopic view of a bucket-handle fragment displaced into the intercondylar notch. (Reproduced, with permission, from McGinty JB: Operative Arthroscopy. New York: Raven Press, 1991.)

of osteochondral fracture are the patella and the femoral condyles, and infrequently, the tibial surface. Osteochondral fractures occur with patellar dislocations, direct blows to the knee, and twisting and shearing forces on the extended knee. The symptoms are very similar to those of meniscus tears, with pain, swelling, and locking. Careful examination of radiographs and use of MRI are helpful, yet the diagnosis may still be missed. Arthroscopy is the best procedure for establishing the diagnosis and treating the lesion. If one or two large fragments are present, they may be replaced and secured with pins or screws. If multiple small pieces are found, they should be removed. Transplantation of articular cartilage from one region of the knee to the injured area is now possible. In the short term, this procedure has promising results; however, long-term results are not yet available.

Peterson L et al: Two- to 9-year outcome after autologous chondrocyte transplantation of the knee. Clin Orthop 2000;374:212.

Osteochondritis Desiccans

Osteochondritis desiccans is a focal osteochondral separation on the weight-bearing portion of the femoral condyles. The cause is unknown, but it may be caused by repetitive trauma or localized avascular necrosis, among other possibilities. It most often occurs in boys between the ages of 10 and 20 years. Before physeal closure, the prognosis for spontaneous healing is good; after physeal closure, surgical intervention is more often needed for pinning, bone grafting, removing the fragments, or osteochondral autograft transplantation.

Bertlet GC et al: Treatment of unstable osteochondritis desiccans lesions of the knee using autologous osteochondral grafts (mosaicplasty). Arthroscopy 1999;15(3):312.

Cain EJ, Clancy WG: Treatment algorithm for osteochondral injuries of the knee. Clin Sports Med 2001;20(2):321.

2. Chondral Fracture

Chondral fractures are very difficult to diagnose even with the use of MRI. They occur in skeletally mature people, with the fracture line at the tidemark, the weak zone occurring between the calcified and uncalcified cartilage. Patients appear with meniscal symptoms of locking, catching, and "giving way" of the knee. An effusion may be present, but hemarthroses are not common, unless the subchondral bone is violated. Arthroscopic diagnosis and treatment are recommended for patients with persistent symptoms.

All loose and overhanging pieces of cartilage must be removed back to a stable base. The base may be either drilled or abraded to bleeding bone that will allow healing with fibrocartilage. This fibrocartilage does not have the biomechanical properties of the original hyaline cartilage and will not last as long, but hyaline cartilage has minimal, if any, repair capabilities. Osteochondral autograft transplantation should be considered.

Restoration of the joint surface after acute or chronic chondral fractures or damage can be attempted through several modalities. These include subchondral drilling, abrasion, or microfractures, which presumably recruit pluripotential stem cells to regenerate cartilage. The early results of these techniques are sufficient to generate some enthusiasm for continuing to use them, but are generally controversial. These methods are unlikely to harm the patient and offer some chance for improvement. Regeneration of new cartilage with isolated cells or tissue with the potential to generate cartilage is an attractive option for treating cartilage defects. Periosteum and perichondrium have been used in animals and in limited studies in humans. Some studies have yielded largely unpredictable but promising results, with technical problems. Isolated, autogenous cartilage cell transplants were recently touted as giving a high percentage of healed medial femoral cartilage defects. All of these techniques should probably be considered investigational and evaluated by controlled studies before entering routine clinical application.

Bobic V, Noble J: Annotation: Articular cartilage—To repair or not to repair. J Bone Joint Surg 2000;82B(2):165.

Farmer JM et al: Chondral and osteochondral injuries: Diagnosis and management. Clin Sports Med 2001;20(2):299.

KNEE LIGAMENT INJURY

Knee injuries occur during both contact and noncontact athletic activities. Advances in the diagnosis and treatment of ligament injuries have allowed athletes at all levels of ability to return to sports at their preinjury level of activity. The ligaments and menisci of the knee work in concert with one another, and frequently more than one structure is damaged when an acute injury occurs.

Ligament injuries are graded as follows: grade 1, stretching of the ligament with no detectable instability; grade 2, further stretching of the ligament with detectable instability, but with the fibers in continuity; and grade 3, complete disruption of the ligament.

1. Medial Collateral Ligament Injury

The medial collateral ligament has a superficial and a deep (capsular) layer. The superficial layer provides the main restraint to valgus stress. The deep layer is attached to the medial meniscus and adds stability to valgus stress. Injury to the medial collateral ligament is the most common knee ligament injury.

With isolated medial collateral ligament injuries, there will be tenderness along the ligament, localized swelling, pain with valgus stress of the knee, and absence of hemarthrosis. When testing the medial collateral ligament, valgus stress should first be applied with the knee flexed at 30 degrees. When the knee is examined in full extension, an intact posterior capsule will prevent valgus instability. It is important to evaluate the rest of the knee, especially the cruciate ligaments and the medial meniscus, when a medial collateral ligament injury is suspected.

If indeed the injury is an isolated one, treatment with early functional motion, strengthening, and a valgus stabilizing brace is usually successful and may return an athlete to sports rapidly. Surgical treatment of these injuries is rarely necessary.

Woo SL et al: Healing and repair of ligament injuries of the knee. J Am Acad Orthop Surg 2000;8(6):364.

2. Lateral Collateral Ligament Injury

Injuries to the lateral collateral ligament are less common than those to the medial ligaments. They are usually more severe and are seldom isolated injuries because the cruciate ligaments and the posterolateral complex are often also damaged. Valgus stress should first be applied with the knee flexed at 30 degrees and then with the knee in full extension. External rotation of the knee should be assessed and compared with the contralateral knee at both 30 and 90 degrees of knee flexion. The peroneal nerve may sustain a stretch injury in severe varus injuries of the knee; the examiner should always perform a neurologic examination of the lower extremity.

Treatment of these injuries is often difficult. In combined injuries, the posterolateral complex including the lateral collateral ligament should be repaired and the cruciate ligaments reconstructed. Significant stiffness or residual instability are often disabling sequelae of such an injury.

Covey DC: Injuries of the posterolateral corner of the knee. J Bone Joint Surg. 2001;83A(1):106.

Latimer HA et al: Reconstruction of the lateral collateral ligament of the knee with patellar tendon allograft. Report of a new technique in combined ligament injuries. Am J Sports Med 1998;26(5):656.

3. Anterior Cruciate Ligament Injury

Injuries to the anterior cruciate ligament are most common in sports in which the foot is planted solidly on the ground and the leg is twisted by the rotating body (ie, football, soccer, basketball, skiing). With twisting of the knee, the patient may hear a pop when the injury occurs and is unable to continue the activity. The incidence of anterior cruciate ligament injury peaks during the third decade of life.

Acute hemarthrosis, the extravasation of blood into the knee, commonly occurs within a few hours of an anterior cruciate ligament tear. As with any acute hemarthrosis, other injuries, such as a peripheral meniscal tears, patella dislocation, osteochondral fracture, and posterior cruciate ligament tear, must be looked for. Repeat examination of the knee within the ensuing few weeks, after the hemarthrosis and stiffness have resolved, may be beneficial. If a diagnosis is needed immediately, aspiration of the acute hemarthrosis and injection of lidocaine into the joint may increase comfort, making the examination more reliable.

In childhood, anterior cruciate ligament injury is usually associated with an avulsion of bone from the tibial insertion site.

Clinical Findings

A. Acute Injury

In acute injuries, examination is often hindered by pain and muscle spasm. The presence of a hemarthrosis should make the examiner very suspicious of an anterior cruciate ligament injury. The finding of a positive Lachman's test with either increased anterior translation or a soft end point confirms suspicion of this injury. The pivot shift phenomenon may not be apparent with the patient awake but becomes apparent when the knee is examined under anesthesia.

The knee should be evaluated for meniscal injuries, which are common with anterior cruciate ligament injury. The other knee ligaments should also be carefully evaluated for injury. Comparison of the injured and uninjured knees is crucial to ensuring that subtle instability is not overlooked. Examination under anesthesia and arthroscopy of the knee with an acute hemarthrosis has aided in detection of these injuries.

B. Chronic Injury

Not uncommonly, patients will present with chronic anterior cruciate ligament deficiency, complaining that the knee "gives way." These patients either did not consult a physician after the initial injury, the diagnosis was missed, or nonoperative care of a recognized anterior cruciate ligament tear was unsuccessful. Increasing instability, a meniscus tear, or muscle weakness might contribute to their decision to seek care. Laxity is often obvious on examination, and pivot shift phenomenon is positive. The longer the deficiency has been present the more likely it is to have an abnormal appearance on

radiograph examination. This is also true when an associated meniscus tear is present. A radiograph may reveal peaking of the tibial spines, spurs in the intercondylar notch, and medial tibial osteophyte formation.

With chronic anterior cruciate ligament instability, the examiner must ascertain whether there is associated injury to the posterolateral complex; symptomatic meniscus tears must also be ruled out.

Treatment

A. Criteria for Treatment

1. Acute injury—The treatment of anterior cruciate ligament tears needs to be individualized for each patient. The outcome from nonoperative treatment depends on the degree of knee instability, associated knee injuries, the patient's activity level, age, job demands, and general medical condition (Figure 4–15). The most common associated knee injuries are meniscus tears and MRI-detected bone bruises. As reconstruction techniques for this injury improve and complications decrease, the trend is toward surgical repair of the knee.

Early reconstruction is indicated for high-performance athletes. A knee that "gives way" during daily activities is also a strong indication for surgery. The presence of a meniscus tear that can be repaired is a relative indication for surgery.

Young, active individuals in whom the knee gives way may also benefit from reconstruction to minimize the chance of future meniscus tears and osteoarthritis. Surgery may also allow return to a preinjury activity level, impossible in the knee with an anterior cruciate ligament rupture.

The skeletally immature patient with an anterior cruciate ligament injury presents special problems for the orthopedic surgeon. The long-term adverse effects on knee function of immediately returning to athletic activities should be explained to the patient. Anterior cruciate ligament injuries in skeletally immature patients are as disabling as they are in adults. Thus, anterior cruciate ligament reconstruction should be considered when instability is not controlled with activity modification and bracing, using similar criteria as in adults. A reconstruction that does not violate the physis should be considered. Recent studies have indicated that transphyseal tunnels may be used, but a graft composed entirely of collagen, such as hamstring tendons, should be used.

2. Chronic injury—With chronic injury, the physician must determine if the patient's biggest problem is pain or the knee giving way. If giving way is more of a problem and there is good strength in the quadriceps and hamstring muscles, reconstruction of the torn anterior cruciate ligament may be considered. Even in a patient with mild osteoarthritis, significant improvement may

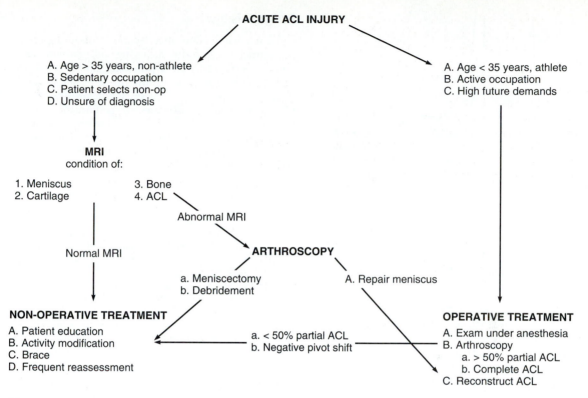

Figure 4–15. Flow chart that summarizes the current management of acute anterior cruciate ligament injuries. (Reproduced, with permission, from Marzo JM, Warren RF: Results of nonoperative treatment of anterior cruciate ligament injury: Changing perspectives. Adv Orthop Surg 1991;15:59.)

be expected. If the knee is painful, the examiner must determine whether the cause is a meniscus tear or osteoarthritis. If giving way is not a significant component of the patient's complaint, then ligament reconstruction would not be expected to relieve the symptoms.

B. Methods of Treatment

1. Acute injury—Primary repair of the torn anterior cruciate ligament has not been successful. Numerous operations have been described for reconstruction of, or substitution for, the anterior cruciate ligament. The middle third of the patellar tendon with a block of bone on each end may be used as a graft. This is passed through tunnels to the original origin and insertion sites of the anterior cruciate ligament (Figures 4–16 and 4–17), simulating as closely as possible the proper anatomic position of the ligament. Interference-fit fixation of the bone plugs in the tunnels yields the highest ultimate tensile loads. Adequate reconstruction allows for immediate postoperative rehabilitation of the knee. New surgical equipment has made this operation easier to perform and more precise, so that more surgeons are

able to perform it. Most postoperative problems are related to harvesting of the patellar tendon graft. Anterior knee pain and patellofemoral dysfunction are the most common complications; patellar tendon rupture and patellar fracture may also occur, but are infrequent. The gracilis and semitendinosus hamstring tendons may be harvested with fewer complications and used as an anterior cruciate ligament graft. Long-term follow-up, as that with the patellar tendon grafts, will soon be available. Allografts of patellar tendon may be used, but their unknown longevity, and a small concomitant risk of disease transmission make them less desirable. So far, synthetic substitutes for the anterior cruciate ligament have been unsuccessful.

2. Chronic instability—Patients with chronic anterior ligament instability and recurrent giving way are best treated initially with quadriceps and hamstring strengthening rehabilitation; a derotational brace and activity modification is probably the best treatment. If this treatment fails, then ligament reconstruction is indicated.

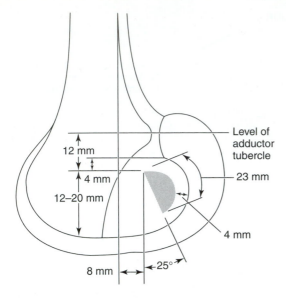

Figure 4–16. Drawing of the medial surface of the right lateral femoral condyle showing the average measurements and body relations of the femoral attachment of the anterior cruciate ligament. (Reproduced, with permission, from Arnoczky SP: Anatomy of the anterior cruciate ligament. Clin Orthop 1983;172:19.)

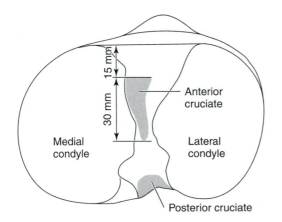

Figure 4–17. The upper surface of the tibial plateau to show average measurements and relations of the tibial attachments of the anterior cruciate ligament. (Reproduced, with permission, from Girgis FC et al: The cruciate ligaments of the knee joint: Anatomical, functional, and experimental analysis. Clin Orthop 1975;106:216.)

Prognosis

Current rehabilitation after anterior cruciate ligament reconstruction includes achieving full motion very quickly postoperatively. Open-chain kinetic exercises such as knee extension against resistance are avoided initially, to prevent excessive strain on the graft. Closed-chain kinetic exercises are performed, such as the leg press, bicycling, and stair-climbing machines. About 90% of all patients can be expected to have a normal or nearly normal knee after anterior cruciate ligament reconstruction.

Anderson AF et al: Anterior cruciate ligament reconstruction: A prospective randomized study of three surgical methods. An J Sports Med 2001;29(3):272.

Deehan DJ et al: Endoscopic reconstruction of the anteriocruciate ligament with an ipsilateral patella tendon autograft: A prospective longitudinal five-year study. J Bone Joint Surg 2000;82B(7):984.

Harner CD et al: Evaluation and treatment of recurrent instability after anterior cruciate ligament reconstruction. J Bone Joint Surg 2000;82A(11):1652.

Johnson DL et al: Articular cartilage changes seen with magnetic resonance imaging-detected bone bruises associated with anterior cruciate ligament rupture. Am J Sports Med 1998;26 (3):409.

Kouyoumjian A, Barber FA: Management of anterior cruciate ligament injuries in skeletally immature patients. Am J Orthop 2001;30(10):771.

Natsu-ume T et al: Endoscopic reconstruction of the anterior cruciate ligament with quadrupled tendons. A correlation between MRI changes and restored stability of the knee. 2001;83B (6):834.

4. Posterior Cruciate Ligament Injury

The posterior cruciate ligament is the primary restraint to posterior translation of the tibia on the femur. It is about twice as strong as the anterior cruciate ligament and runs from the lateral portion of the medial femoral condyle to the posterior aspect of the tibia below the joint line (see Figure 4–3). Injury to the posterior cruciate ligament is much less common than to the anterior cruciate ligament. Isolated injury usually results from a fall on the tibial tubercle, or from hitting the tibial tubercle on the dashboard in a motor vehicle accident.

Clinical Findings

Often, clinical findings are minimal and the injury is misdiagnosed. Careful examination of the posterior drawer, making sure that the tibia is not situated in a posteriorly subluxed starting position, is essential in making the diagnosis. Posterior laxity is maximal at 90 degrees of flexion. Lateral radiographs of the knees with posterior stress on the tibia may be helpful. MRI is a good way of confirming the diagnosis. Unlike with anterior cruciate ligament injuries, the menisci are rarely damaged. Combined injuries of the posterior cruciate ligament, collateral ligaments, and anterior cruciate ligament may occur and are essentially variants of knee dislocation.

Treatment

A. CRITERIA FOR TREATMENT

Nonoperative treatment of isolated posterior cruciate ligament injuries is recommended for the majority of posterior cruciate ligament injuries. Some authors recommend reconstruction for acute isolated posterior cruciate ligament injuries that demonstrate more than 15 mm of posterior instability. Vigorous quadriceps strengthening may often compensate for loss of the posterior cruciate ligament, so that athletes can continue their activities.

Patients with symptomatic posterior cruciate ligament instability after rehabilitation are candidates for surgical reconstruction. This is more difficult and less predictable than anterior cruciate ligament reconstruction. If the posterior cruciate ligament is avulsed from the tibia with a piece of bone and significant posterior instability exists, these defects should be repaired primarily. Good stability and function may be expected. Patients with chronic symptomatic posterior cruciate ligament instability have a higher than normal incidence of degeneration of the medial compartment of the knee and should undergo reconstruction of the posterior cruciate ligament.

B. METHODS OF TREATMENT

In posterior cruciate ligament reconstruction, the graft should be about twice as large as the graft most often used for anterior cruciate ligament reconstruction. The necessary size and strength of the graft may cause some difficulty. Two thirds of a patellar tendon allograft, or an Achilles tendon allograft, may be used.

Prognosis

The results of surgical reconstruction of the posterior cruciate ligament have not been as reproducible as the results for reconstruction of the anterior cruciate ligament.

Cosgarea AJ, Jay PR: Posterior cruciate ligament injuries: Evaluation and management. J Am Acad Orthop Surg 2001;9(5): 297.

5. Patella Dislocation

Dislocation of the patella is a potential cause of acute hemarthrosis and must be considered when evaluating a patient with an acute knee injury. The injury occurs when the knee is bent and encounters valgus force and external rotation of the tibia. It is most common in females in the second decade of life.

Clinical Findings

The patella almost always dislocates laterally. The patient may notice the patella sitting laterally or might say that the rest of the knee has shifted medially. It is unusual to see actual dislocation of the patella except at the time of injury. Reduction occurs when the knee is extended.

Examination will demonstrate tenderness over the medial retinaculum and adductor tubercle, which is the origin of the medial patellofemoral ligament. The patient will also have pain and apprehension when the patella is pushed laterally with the knee slightly bent. Radiographs, including an axial patellar view, should be obtained to determine whether osteochondral fractures are present. Often, a small fleck of bone is avulsed by the capsule on the medial aspect of the patella. This is not intraarticular and does not require removal. A displaced osteochondral fracture will require excision or internal fixation. Examination of the uninjured knee is recommended to determine whether any factors, such as patella alta, genu recurvatum, increased Q angle, and patellar hypermobility, predispose for dislocation. Patella alta, or high-riding patella, is identified by measuring the length of the patellar tendon and dividing by the length of the patella. The upper limit of normal is 1.2. The Q angle is formed by a line through the patellar tendon intersecting a line from the anterior superior iliac spine in the center of the patella. A normal Q angle is about 10 degrees, with a range of about plus or minus 5 degrees. Patients with generalized hypermobility have increased extension of the knee, or genu recurvatum, which in effect gives them patella alta. They also often have hypermobility of all the capsular ligamentous structures, including the static stabilizers of the kneecap, giving them significant patellar hypermobility.

Treatment & Prognosis

A wide variety of treatment options have been recommended for patellar dislocations, including immediate mobilization and strengthening exercises, immobilization in a cylinder cast for 6 weeks followed by rehabilitation, arthroscopy with or without retinacular repair, surgical repair of the torn retinaculum, or immediate patellar realignment.

Treatment is based on which predisposing factors are present. Little is lost by functional treatment, similar to the treatment of isolated medial collateral ligament sprains, which is often successful. If dislocation recurs, realignment may be performed. A long-term study showed that patients treated surgically for patellar malalignment problems had a higher incidence of osteoarthritis than those treated nonoperatively.

Atkin DM et al: Characteristics of patients with primary acute lateral patella dislocation and their recovery within the first 6 months of injury. Am J Sports Med 2000;28(4):472.

Bensahal H et al: The unstable patella in children. J Pediatr Orthop 2000;9(4):265.

KNEE TENDON INJURY

Ruptures of the quadriceps and patellar tendons usually result from a tremendous eccentric contraction of the quadriceps muscle, as may occur when an athlete stumbles and tries not to fall.

1. Rupture of the Quadriceps Tendon

Quadriceps tendon ruptures occur most frequently in patients over 40 years old. Biopsies of fresh rupture sites showed local degenerative changes already present, consistent with the theory that normal tendons do not rupture. Rarely the injury occurs bilaterally, showing the degree of pre-existing disease process. When it does occur bilaterally with only a small amount of trauma, the diagnosis may be difficult to make because of the small amount of swelling or symptoms of injury.

The cardinal symptom is inability to extend the knee. When extension is attempted, a gap develops in the suprapatellar region. The patella rides at a slightly lower level, and the anterior margin of the femoral condyles may be palpated.

Acute complete quadriceps tendon ruptures should be repaired surgically. If left untreated, proximal migration and scarring of the quadriceps muscle will occur. Direct-end repair produces excellent results. Neutralizing the forces across the repair is difficult, and immobilization in extension is recommended. Repair of ruptures more than 2 months old may be difficult and may require quadriceps lengthening, muscle or tendon transfers, or a combination of these procedures.

Konrath GA et al: Outcomes following repair of quadriceps tendon ruptures. J Orthop Trauma 1998;12(4):273.

2. Rupture of the Patellar Tendon

Rupture of the patella tendon occurs more frequently in patients younger than 40. The patient cannot actively extend the knee, the patella is high-riding, and a defect is palpable beneath the patella. Surgical repair is the treatment of choice. The tendon, along with the medial and lateral retinaculum, should be sewn end to end. A stress-relieving wire or suture may be placed around the patella and through the tibial tubercle. The wire should be removed in 6–8 weeks. Chronic patellar tendon ruptures are very hard to treat. The quadriceps must be freed up from the femur and the patella pulled down to the proper location. The gracilis and semitendinosus tendons can be used to substitute for the patellar tendon.

The extensor mechanism may also be disrupted at the inferior pole of the patella where the patellar tendon originates. This usually occurs in a child between the ages of 8 and 12 years. The distal pole of the patella plus a large sleeve of articular cartilage is pulled off (Figure 4–18). This may be easily misdiagnosed if the fragment of bone is small. Reestablishment of an intact extensor mechanism is necessary. With displaced fractures, open reduction and internal fixation with tension band wiring are recommended.

KNEE PAIN

Pain in the knee region is a very common complaint of athletes. If there is no history of an acute injury, then overuse is commonly the cause. The patient is often able to point to the area of pain. The history of activity must be obtained as well as overall evaluation of the extremities.

1. Anterior Knee Pain

Clinical Findings

A. SYMPTOMS AND SIGNS

This is a common complaint and is frequently bilateral. It is most common in females during the second decade of life. The patellofemoral joint is often the source of pain. Entities such as chondromalacia patella, patellofemoral arthralgia, and lateral patellofemoral compression syndrome are diagnostic considerations.

Patellar pain is often felt when going up or down hills or stairs, and there may be complaints of instability during walking, running, or other sports activities. These activities may create a joint reaction force of several times the body weight on the patella with each step. Swelling is seldom a complaint. If the pain is in one knee only, the patient may alter the way of climbing and descending stairs so that the affected leg is kept straight and each step leads with the same foot. This strategy significantly decreases the joint reaction force on the patellofemoral joint.

Many of these problems arise because the patellofemoral joint is semiconstrained, in the range of 0–20 degrees of flexion, and the constraint increases as flexion increases. The degree of constraint is also dependent on a number of other factors, including the angle

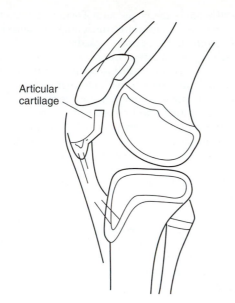

of the sulcus of the femur, the presence or absence of patella alta, and the generalized ligamentous laxity of the patient. In addition, femoral anteversion and increased Q angle (Figure 4–19) may lead to increased instability of the patellofemoral joint. This lack of constraint may predispose the patella to dislocation, although subluxation is a much more common finding. The degree of congruity is anatomically variable and may lead to high-contact stresses caused by anatomic configuration and static and dynamic constraints on the patella. Increased pressure may cause pain and patellofemoral osteoarthritis.

On physical examination of the patient with patellofemoral subluxation, minimal findings in relation to complaints may be present. Occasionally, crepitance, a crackling or clicking sound or feeling, is found with flexion and extension. Quadriceps strength, tone, and bulk are usually reduced. Pain may be elicited at a particular angle of flexion by putting the knee through its range of motion with resistance. Subluxation may

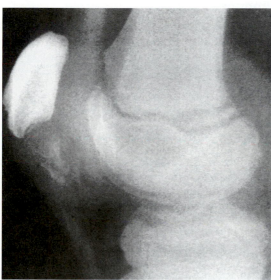

Figure 4–18. Sleeve fracture of the patella. **A:** A small segment of the distal pole of the patella is avulsed with a relatively large portion of the articular surface. **B:** Lateral radiograph of the knee with a displaced sleeve fracture of the patella. Note that the small osseous portion of the displaced fragment is visible, but the cartilaginous portion is not seen. (Reproduced, with permission, from Rockwood CA Jr (editor): Fractures in Children, 3rd ed. Baltimore: Lippincott, 1991.)

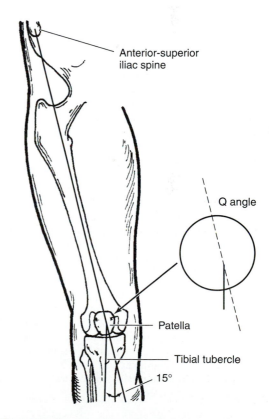

Figure 4–19. Q angle and valgus angulation. (Reproduced, with permission, from American Academy of Orthopaedic Surgeons: Athletic Training and Sports Medicine, 2nd ed., 1991.)

often be diagnosed with the apprehension sign, a rapid contraction of the quadriceps when the patella is passively moved laterally by the examiner.

B. IMAGING STUDIES

Roentgenographic examination will frequently show a valgus angulation of the knee on anteroposterior views. Occasionally, patella alta may be identified on the lateral view, and tangential views of the patella at various knee flexion angles will reveal a lack of contact of the medial facet of the patella with the medial facet of the trochlear groove of the femur. Lateral subluxation of the patellofemoral joint may also be observed.

This syndrome with a normal roentgenographic examination is frequently called chondromalacia patellae, or with subluxation identified on radiograph is referred to as patellofemoral subluxation. A more accurate term would be patellofemoral arthralgia because patellofemoral subluxation was probably present prior to the onset of pain and because chondromalacia patellae (softening of the patellar cartilage) is an arthroscopic or pathologic diagnosis.

Treatment

A. CHONDROMALACIA PATELLAE

Initially, treatment is conservative, with the intent of improving quadriceps strength and stamina to stabilize the patellofemoral joint. Weight loss is prescribed to decrease the stress on the patellofemoral joint; reduction in loading the knee in the flexed position also accomplishes pressure reduction. Knee orthotics may be beneficial. When subluxation and fear of dislocation are major concerns, an orthotic that limits extension of the knee may be beneficial because the patella becomes inherently more stable with knee flexion. Nonsteroidal anti-inflammatory drugs (NSAIDs) may be beneficial.

B. PATELLOFEMORAL ARTHRALGIA

Only when conservative treatment has been exhausted is surgical treatment considered. Alteration in the alignment of the patellofemoral joint may be beneficial in patellofemoral arthralgia. Lateral retinacular release followed by a period of rehabilitation be beneficial in some cases. Distal realignment may be necessary to achieve appropriate alignment and reduction in pain in those cases with an abnormality such as valgus knee or increased femoral anteversion.

C. PATELLOFEMORAL COMPRESSION SYNDROME

With lateral patellofemoral compression syndrome, tenderness occurs along the lateral facet of the patella or along the femoral condyle. Without cartilage damage,

an effusion is rarely present. Treatment includes decreasing the activity level, including avoiding hills or step aerobics. Ice-massage, quadriceps and hamstring stretching, and short-arc quadriceps exercises against resistance are recommended to strengthen the vastus medialis obliquus muscle without aggravating the pain. Patellar supports or neoprene sleeves may also be helpful. Most patients will respond to this regimen and be able to gradually resume their activities. If nonoperative treatment is unsuccessful, a lateral retinacular release may be helpful to minimize symptoms.

D. PATELLAR TENDINITIS

Patellar tendinitis, or jumper's knee, is seen in basketball and volleyball players. Tenderness along the tendon, usually at the inferior pole of the patella, is noted. Treatment with ice and avoiding jumping usually suffices. In refractory cases, debridement of mucinous degenerative material from the tendon may be successful.

Prognosis

The prognosis for jumper's knee is quite good. The condition is often persistent but self-limiting. The patient can always avoid the symptoms by avoiding the situation that causes the problem.

Csintalan R et al: Gender effects on the biomechanical properties of the peripatellar retinaculum. Clin Orthop Rel Res 2001:accepted.

Grelsamer RP: Current concepts review: Patellar malalignment. J Bone Joint Surg 2000;82A(11):1639.

Holmes SW Jr, Clancy WG Jr: Clinical classification of patellofemoral pain and dysfunction. J Orthop Sports Phys Ther 1998;28(5):299.

Thomee R et al: Patellofemoral pain syndrome: A review of current issues. Sports Med 1999;28(4):245.

2. Lateral Knee Pain

Lateral knee pain that is not located on the joint line may result from iliotibial band friction syndrome. This is a form of bursitis caused by rubbing of the iliotibial band against the lateral epicondyle. Tenderness over the lateral epicondyle at about 30 degrees of flexion when the knee is being extended is indicative of this diagnosis. Runners and cyclists are commonly afflicted. Crossover gait or running on banked terrain is thought to be a causative factor.

Treatment involves decreasing the athlete's activities, ice-massage, stretching of the iliotibial tract, and use of a lateral wedge orthotic in those patients with heel varus. Running on flat terrain and changing the gait pattern may be helpful. In cyclists, lowering the seat height so the full extension of the knee is not reached and adjusting the pedals so that the toes are not internally rotated should help. Steroid injections are infrequently needed, and release of the inflamed portion of the iliotibial band is seldom necessary. As for other overuse syndromes of the knee, the prognosis is good.

Kirk KL et al: Iliotibial band friction syndrome. Orthopaedics 2000;23(11):1209.

■ ANKLE OR FOOT PAIN

Evaluation of foot and ankle injuries is described in Chapter 9. Injury specific to athletics includes chronic Achilles tendonitis, heel pain, plantar fascitis, and posterior tibial syndrome.

Clinical Findings

Achilles tendonitis is a frequent complaint in runners. This may result from a contracted gastrocsoleus, or hyperpronation may cause overpulling of the medial insertion. Additionally, a bony prominence may be evident on the superior-posterior aspect of the calcaneus, causing retrocalcaneal bursitis.

Heel pain is a common problem in runners and is difficult to treat because of the uncertainty as to cause. Theories include painful heel spurs, bursitis, fat-pad atrophy, stress fracture, plantar fasciitis, or entrapment of the terminal branches of the posterior tibial nerve.

Many patients have pain localized in the posteromedial surface of the foot just distal to the attachment of the plantar fascia to the calcaneus (plantar fasciitis). This pain is often most severe on initially getting up in the morning and decreases as the day goes on.

Posterior tibial syndrome occurs in runners with hyperpronation. As the longitudinal arch flattens out, the posterior tibial musculotendinous unit that normally elevates the flattened arch has abnormal strain placed upon it.

Treatment

Treatment depends on the cause of the injury but includes decreasing running activities, using a heel lift, and performing stretching exercises. If hyperpronation is thought to be the cause, an orthotic may be used. Steroid injections are not recommended as they could lead to weakening and subsequent rupture of the tendon.

Surgical intervention for chronic Achilles tendinitis or retrocalcaneal bursitis is seldom needed. This would be done to remove areas of fibrosis or calcium within the tendon and possibly some bone from the posterior process of the calcaneus. The treatment for plantar fasciitis includes rest, ice-massage, and possibly NSAIDs. A small shock-absorbing type of heel cup often is helpful, and a steroid injection may be given in recalcitrant cases. Acute rupture of the plantar fascia may occur. The pain is usually quite sharp and may cause significant disability for 6–12 weeks.

Hyperpronation may also cause fibular stress fractures. A semirigid orthosis may be recommended for this to decrease the amount and angular velocity of pronation. Using an orthosis while running actually increases the work of running, but if it decreases abnormal stresses in those whom hyperpronate, it may be quite helpful.

Myerson MS, McGarvey W: Instructional Course Lecture. Disorders of the insertion of the Achilles tendon and Achilles tendonitis. J Bone Joint Surg Am 1998;80:1814.

■ OTHER INJURIES OF THE LOWER BODY

Many disorders seen while caring for athletes may be difficult to diagnose with certainty. The differential diagnosis must be carefully made to rule out more severe injuries. Often, a period of rest followed by gradual return to activities is the best treatment. During convalescence, application of ice packs, stretching exercises, and gradual strengthening of the injured limb will facilitate return to sports activities.

OVERUSE SYNDROMES OF THE LOWER EXTREMITIES

Many athletes such as runners, cyclists, aerobics enthusiasts, volleyball players, and basketball players have developed painful disorders of the lower extremities without an acute injury. History taking is very important, and the examiner should ask specific questions about the circumstances in which the discomfort occurs. In a runner, for example, the examiner should ask whether there was an increase in the distance run or a change in the running surface, at what point the pain was felt, and what home remedies have been tried before the runner sought advice from a physician.

The physical examination should include not only the affected area, but also evaluation of the back, pelvis, leg lengths, genu varum or valgum, femoral and tibial torsion, and cavus or flatfoot deformities. The presence of hamstring and heel cord contracture should be determined, and the gait pattern should be observed. Running shoes should be inspected for wear patterns, which may be quite helpful.

1. Muscle Strains

Muscle strains of the lower extremity are one of the most frequent and disabling muscle injuries, with strain of the distal muscle tendon junction being most common. Muscles may stretch to about 125% of their resting length before tearing. Strains are graded as mild, moderate, or severe, based upon the degree of pain, spasm, and disability the strain causes. A severe strain would be complete disruption of the muscle, with a palpable defect and balling up of the muscle proximally.

In spite of the frequency of muscle strains and the disability they produce, little scientific information is available on their pathologic basis. Muscles susceptible to more stretching are more susceptible to strains. In the lower extremity, the muscles most frequently injured are the hamstring, quadriceps, and gastrocnemius muscles. These muscles all cross two joints, and they may be unable to resist full stretching across both of them. The most powerful muscles are more likely to be strained, and strains are more common in "explosive" type athletics. Eccentric contraction, (muscle contraction while the muscle is lengthening) is often thought to be causative in muscle strains.

Clinical Findings

The diagnosis is relatively easy. Often the athlete will feel the muscle "grab" while he or she is accelerating. There is localized tenderness over the muscle and pain on stretching of the muscle. Because the two joint muscles are most frequently involved, the muscles should be stretched over both of the joints during examination.

Treatment & Prognosis

Muscle strains should be treated with ice in the immediate postinjury period. Flexibility and strength should be regained prior to return to activity. This may take many months, and patients who return to activity too early may experience a setback to the level of the original injury.

Strengthening of the muscles might make them less susceptible to being torn. It is commonly believed that flexibility will help prevent muscle strains, but reports regarding this are conflicting , and it is still unproved.

Funk D et al: Efficacy of moist heat pack application over static stretching on hamstring flexibility. J Strength Cond Res 2001;15(1):123.

Levine WN et al: Intramuscular corticosteroid injection for hamstring injuries. A 13-year experience in the National Football League. Am J Sports Med 2000;28(3):297.

2. Shin Pain

Clinical Findings

A. Shin Splints

The term *shin splints* is widely used for shin pain, but it is not a diagnostic term. A more specific diagnosis should be made if possible. Shin splints are usually defined as pain associated with activity in the beginning of training after a relatively inactive period. The pain and tenderness are usually located over the anterior compartment and disappear in 1–2 weeks as the athlete becomes conditioned to the exercise. Care must be taken to differentiate shin splints from stress fractures of the tibia, which cause more localized pain and have many more potential complications if not cared for properly.

B. Medial Tibial Syndrome

Medial tibial syndrome is also seen in runners, occurring along the medial border of the distal tibia. After 3–4 weeks, some hypertrophy of the cortical bone and periosteal new bone formation may be seen on radiograph. It is thought to be either a periostitis or possibly an incomplete stress fracture. The pull of the tibialis posterior muscle from its origin on the tibia and posterior tibial tendinitis are also thought to be possible causes.

Treatment

Treatment for shin splints and medial tibial syndrome is rest and resumption of athletic activities in a graduated fashion.

3. Stress Fractures

Stress fractures may occur in the pelvis, femoral neck, tibia, navicular, and metatarsals. They are usually the result of a significant increase in training and activity. In the female athlete, poor nutrition, low bone density, and a history of menstrual disturbance are associated with a higher prevalence of stress fractures. The history is important in differentiating these injuries from infection or neoplasm. Plain radiographs are often normal at first. MRI or technetium bone scans are then the best diagnostic tests. If symptoms persist for over a month, radiographs may become positive.

Treatment of stress fractures involves rest and avoidance of high-impact activities until healing has occurred. This includes resolution of the tenderness and signs of fracture healing on plain radiographs. Continuous activity with stress fractures may lead to complete fractures.

Patients must be made aware of this and all the complications that may develop with a complete fracture.

Korpelainen R et al: Risk factors for recurrent stress fractures in athletes. Am J Sports Med 2001;29(3):304.

Perron AD et al: Principles of stress fracture management. The whys and hows of an increasingly common injury. Postgrad Med 2001;110(3):115.

4. Exertional Compartment Syndromes

Exertional compartment syndromes may result from muscle hypertrophy within the confining osseofascial compartment. As the muscles hypertrophy and the amount of edema within the compartment increases, the blood supply to the nerves and muscles within the involved compartment is diminished, and the pressure continues to increase.

The syndrome presents as recurrent claudication during exertional activity and is relieved by rest. After exercise, the findings of localized pain, pain on passive motion, and hypesthesia are indicative.

Treatment consists of activity modification, including gradual onset of training. If unsuccessful, compartment pressures may be measured while the patient is exercising on a treadmill, and if the pressures are elevated, surgical fasciotomy is usually effective.

Blackman PG: A review of chronic exertional compartment syndrome in the lower leg. Med Sci Sports Exerc 2000;32(3 Suppl):S4.

CONTUSIONS & AVULSIONS OF THE LOWER BODY

1. Contusion to the Quadriceps Muscle

Clinical Findings

A severe contusion to the quadriceps muscle (charley horse), is a disabling condition that results in prolonged inactivity. These injuries frequently occur in football players. The resultant significant bleeding into the muscle inhibits movement. Rarely, a compartment syndrome will occur.

Myositis ossificans may occur after these injuries. It may be apparent 2–4 weeks after the injury. Radiographically and histologically, myositis ossificans may be similar to osteogenic sarcoma; therefore, the history of contusion is very important. Radiographs should be obtained after such a contusion to minimize the myositis ossificans being confused with cancer.

Treatment & Prognosis

Quadriceps contusions should be treated with elevation of the leg and the hip and knee flexed to tolerance to minimize bleeding. After a few days the knee can be moved with continuous passive motion or "drop-and-dangle," gravity-assisted exercises. For the latter, the patient is seated on a table high enough to keep the feet off the floor. The patient then hooks the uninjured foot behind the ankle of the injured leg. The uninjured leg extends the knee of the injured leg, and gravity flexes the injured knee. The average length of disability is a few weeks.

If heterotopic ossification is present, no specific treatment is recommended other than treatment for the contusion. Normal function may be obtained, but the recovery period is longer. Because early surgery may exacerbate the heterotopic ossification, it should be avoided.

Alonso A et al: Predicting a recovery time from the initial assessment of a quadriceps contusion injury. Aust J Physiother 2000;46(3):167.

2. Contusion about the Hip and Pelvis

Clinical Findings

Contusions about the pelvis and hip region may be very painful and disabling. Because of the subcutaneous location of the iliac crests and the greater trochanters, these regions are at risk in contact sports.

A contusion over the greater trochanter may cause persistent bursitis, tenderness directly over the greater trochanter, and increased pain with adduction of the leg. Females are more prone to trochanteric bursitis because of their broader pelvis.

A hip pointer is a very painful contusion over the iliac crest that occurs from many contact sports. It must be differentiated from an avulsion fracture in the skeletally immature athlete and from a tear of the muscle aponeurosis in an adult. Profuse bleeding may occur and be very painful.

Treatment & Prognosis

For a contusion over the greater trochanter, treatment consists of ice applications and decreased activities. Padding may be helpful to prevent recurrent injuries. The prognosis is good. For hip pointer injuries, initial treatment with ice is helpful. Protective pads are useful in returning the athlete to activities sooner.

Busconi B, McCarthy J: Hip and pelvic injuries in the skeletally immature athlete. Sports Med Arthroscopy Rev 1996;4;132.

3. Avulsion of the Tibial Tubercle

Clinical Findings

Tibial tubercle avulsions occur in adolescent athletes, most often in males between the ages of 14 and 16 years. They result from a powerful contraction of the quadriceps muscle against a fixed tibia, as in jumping, or with forced passive flexion of the knee against a powerful quadriceps contraction, as in an awkward landing at the end of a jump or fall. Avulsion of the tubercle may occur with either a sudden acceleration or deceleration of the knee extensor mechanism. The patellar tendon must pull hard enough to overcome the strength of the growth plate, the surrounding perichondrium, and the adjacent periosteum.

Swelling and tenderness are located over the proximal anterior tibia. A tense hemarthrosis may be present. A palpable defect in the anterior tibia is associated with a severely displaced avulsion. Proximal migration of the patella occurs, and the patella may seem to float off the anterior aspect of the femur. The knee is held flexed; with displaced fractures, the patient is unable actively to extend the knee.

Watson-Jones defined three types of avulsion fractures, which were subsequently refined as the following three types (Figure 4–20): Type 1 fracture, in which the fracture line lies across the secondary center of ossification at the level of the posterior border of the patellar ligament; type 2 fracture, in which a separation breaks out at the primary and secondary ossification centers of epiphysis; and type 3 fracture, in which the separation propagates upward through the main portion of the proximal tibial epiphysis. The degree of displacement depends upon the severity of injury to the surrounding soft-tissue moorings. A lateral radiograph with the tibia slightly internally rotated is the best view to see the fracture and the degree of displacement.

Differential Diagnosis

Osgood-Schlatter disease, or osteochondrosis of the tuberosity of the tibia, should not be confused with acute avulsion of the tibial tubercle. In the former, the patient is usually between the ages of 11 and 15 years and is involved in athletics. Pain is located at the tibial tubercle, and it has usually been present intermittently over a period of several months. Walking on a flat surface is not difficult, but ascending or descending stairs causes difficulty. Radiograph examination may show slight separation of the tibial tubercle with new bone formation beneath it (Figure 4–21).

Treatment recommendations vary from decreasing the amount of running and jumping but continuing participation in athletics, to cylinder cast immobilization for a short time. The long-term prognosis is excellent. Although symptoms are often present for 2 years, early short-term cast immobilization may shorten this period of discomfort to 9 months. In most children, casting is not necessary. Explaining the benign nature of the problem to both the patient and the parents, reassuring them that the long-term prognosis is good, and modifying activities usually allows continued participation in athletics. Hamstring stretching and ice-

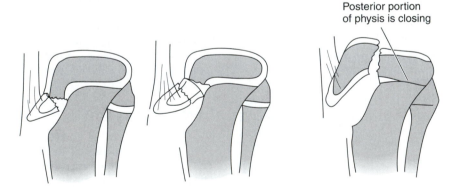

Figure 4–20. Classification of avulsion fractures of the tibial tubercle. Type 1 fracture (**left**) across the secondary ossification center at level with the posterior border of the inserting patellar ligament. Type 2 fracture (**center**) at the junction of the primary and secondary ossification centers of the proximal tibial epiphysis. Type 3 fracture (**right**) propagates upward across the primary ossification center of the proximal tibial epiphysis into the knee joint. This fracture is a variant of the Salter-Harris III separation and is analogous to the fracture of Tillaux at the ankle, because the posterior portion of the physis of the proximal tibia is closing. (Reproduced, with permission, from Odgen JA et al: Fractures of the tibial tuberosity in adolescents. J Bone Joint Surg Am 1980;62:205.)

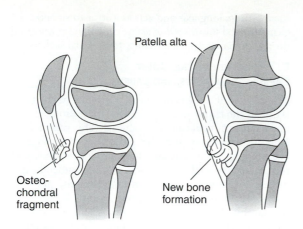

Patella alta

Osteo-
chondral
fragment

New bone
formation

Figure 4–21. Development of Osgood-Schlatter lesion. (**Left**) Avulsion of osteochondral fragment that includes surface cartilage and a portion of the secondary ossification center of the tibial tubercle. (**Right**) New bone fills in the gap between the avulsed osteochondral fragment and the tibial tubercle. (Reproduced, with permission, from Rockwood CA Jr (editor): Fractures in Children, 3rd ed. Baltimore: Lippincott, 1991.)

massage may decrease symptoms during the time needed for maturation of the tibial tubercle. The pain will go away when the tubercle unites with the tibia. In a very small number of cases, chronic pain will be present if the ossicle fails to unite. Painful ossicles in the adult are successfully treated with simple excision.

Treatment

Tibial tubercle avulsion fractures must be treated to maintain full functioning of the extensor mechanism. If the fracture is minimally displaced, and the patient is able to fully extend the knee against gravity, nonoperative treatment is acceptable. A cylinder cast should be applied with the knee extended and worn for 4 weeks. Active range-of-motion and strengthening exercises should then commence. At 6 weeks, quadriceps exercises against resistance are initiated. For displaced fractures, open reduction and internal fixation are recommended, with screws if the piece or pieces are large enough. If rigid fixation of large fragments is obtained, early active flexion and passive extension may be initiated. If a tenuous repair is obtained, protection in a cast is advisable.

Prognosis

Because the injury occurs in children who are close to skeletal maturity, meaningful growth abnormalities at the proximal tibial physis do not occur. Return to activities is allowed after the athlete develops quadriceps mass and strength equal to the contralateral side.

4. Avulsions about the Pelvis

Clinical Findings

In the skeletally immature athlete, the apophysis, or growth plate where the muscle attaches to bone, is the weak link in the bone-muscle-tendon unit. Therefore, just as the growth plate is prone to breaking in children's fractures, the bony origin of muscles may be pulled off. This most commonly occurs in athletes between the ages of 14 and 25 years. Comparison radiographs may be helpful to make sure the avulsion fracture is not just a normal anatomic variant. In the pelvis, this may occur at the iliac crest (abdominal muscles), anterior superior iliac spine (sartorius origin), anterior inferior iliac spine (rectus femoris origin), ischial tuberosity (hamstring origin), and lesser trochanter of the femur (iliopsoas insertion).

Treatment & Prognosis

Symptomatic care with a few days of rest followed by ambulation with crutches for about a month is recommended. It is usually 6–10 weeks before athletic activities may be resumed. Long-term athletic activity will probably not be affected. Open reduction and internal fixation have not shown superior results and therefore are usually not warranted. Abundant calcification may occur in the ischial tuberosity region and may be the cause of chronic bursitis and pain. Excision of the exuberant callous should cure this problem. Another indication for surgery is a painful fibrous nonunion, which also may be cured with excision of the fragment.

Rossi F, Dragoni S: Acute avulsion fractures of the pelvis in adolescent competitive athletes: Prevalence, location and sports distribution of 203 cases collected. Skeletal Radiol 2001;30 (3):127.

■ SHOULDER INJURIES

The shoulder is the third most commonly injured joint during athletic activities, after the knee and the ankle. Sports-related injury of the shoulder may result from a direct traumatic event or repetitive overuse. Any activity that requires arm motion, particularly overhead arm motion such as throwing, may stress the soft tissues surrounding the glenohumeral joint to the point of injury. The shoulder is the most mobile joint in the body partly as a result of minimal containment of the large humeral head by the smaller glenoid fossa. The trade-off for this mobility is less structural restraint to undesirable and potentially damaging movements. Thus, a fine balance must be struck to maintain full range of shoulder motion and normal glenohumeral joint stability.

Dawson J et al: The benefits of using patient-based methods of assessment. Medium-term results of an observational study of shoulder surgery. J Bone Joint Surg 2001;83B(6):877.

Anatomy

A. The Bony Articulation of the Glenohumeral Joint

The glenohumeral joint is a modified ball-and-socket joint. The glenoid fossa is an inverted, comma-shaped, articular surface one fourth the size of the humeral head. The articular surface of the humeral head is retroverted approximately 30 degrees relative to the transverse axis of the elbow. Because the scapula is oriented anterolaterally about 30 degrees on the thorax, relative to the coronal plane of the body, the face of the glenoid fossa matches the humeral head retroversion. The scapula rotates to direct the glenoid superiorly, inferiorly, medially, or laterally to accommodate changing humeral head positions. As a result, the humeral head is centered in the glenoid throughout most shoulder motions. When this centered position is disturbed, instability may result.

B. The Clavicle and Its Articulations

The clavicle articulates medially with the sternum at the sternoclavicular joint and laterally with the acromion of the scapula at the acromioclavicular joint. The clavicle rotates on its long axis and acts as a strut to stabilize the glenohumeral joint, serving as the only bone connecting the appendicular upper extremity to the axial skeleton.

C. The Glenohumeral Joint Capsule, Ligaments, and Labrum

The capsule of the glenohumeral joint may be the most lax of all the major joints, yet in certain positions it has important contribution to stability. The capsuloligamentous structures and the glenoid labrum share a common insertion. The anterior capsule is composed of the coracohumeral and superior glenohumeral ligaments, the middle glenohumeral ligament, and the inferior glenohumeral ligament (Figure 4–22). The relationship between the anterior capsuloligamentous structures and the labrum, making certain anatomic variations to be associated with joint instability more often than others may. For example, an anterosuperior sublabral hole is variably present within the glenohumeral joint, connecting with the subscapularis bursa between the subscapularis tendon and the capsule.

The glenoid labrum not only acts as an attachment site for the capsuloligamentous structures but also as an extension of the articular cavity. Its presence deepens the glenoid socket by nearly 50%, and removal of the labrum decreases joint stability to shear stress. In this way, the triangular cross-section of the labrum acts as a chock-block to help prevent subluxation.

D. The Shoulder Musculature

The muscles around the shoulder may be divided into three functional groups: glenohumeral, thoracohumeral, and those that cross both the shoulder and elbow.

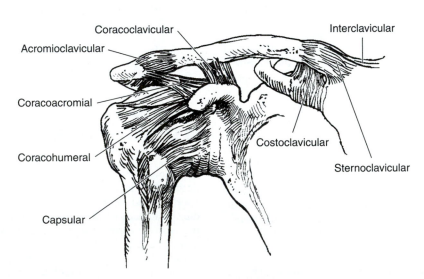

Figure 4–22. Ligaments about the shoulder girdle.

1. Glenohumeral muscles—Four muscles compose the rotator cuff: the supraspinatus, subscapularis, infraspinatus, and teres minor. The supraspinatus has its origin on the posterosuperior scapula, superior to the scapular spine. It passes under the acromion, through the supraspinatus fossa, and inserts on the greater tuberosity with an extended attachment of fibrocartilage. The supraspinatus is active during the entire arc of scapular plane abduction; paralysis of the suprascapular nerve results in an approximately 50% loss of abduction torque. The infraspinatus and the teres minor muscles originate on the posterior scapula, inferior to the scapular spine, and insert on the posterior aspect of the greater tuberosity. Despite their origin below the scapular spine, their tendinous insertions are not separate from the supraspinatus tendon. These muscles function together to externally rotate and extend the humerus. Both account for approximately 80% of external rotation strength in the adducted position. The infraspinatus is more active with the arm at the side, and the teres minor activates mainly with the shoulder in 90 degrees of elevation. The subscapularis muscle arises from the anterior scapula and is the only muscle to insert on the lesser tuberosity. The subscapularis is the sole anterior component of the rotator cuff and functions to internally rotate and flex the humerus. The tendinous insertion of the subscapularis is continuous with the anterior capsule so that both provide anterior glenohumeral stability.

The deltoid is the largest of the glenohumeral muscles. It covers the proximal humerus on a path from its tripennate origin at the clavicle, acromion, and scapular spine to its insertion midway on the humerus at the deltoid tubercle. Abduction of the joint results from activity of the anterior and middle portions. The anterior portion is also a forward flexor. The posterior portion does not abduct the joint, but instead adducts and extends the humerus. The deltoid is active throughout the entire arc of glenohumeral abduction; paralysis of the axillary nerve results in a 50% loss of abduction torque. The deltoid muscle can fully abduct the glenohumeral joint with the supraspinatus muscle inactive.

The teres major muscle originates from the inferior angle of the scapula and inserts on the medial lip of the bicipital groove of the humerus, posterior to the insertion of the latissimus dorsi. The axillary nerve and the posterior humeral circumflex artery pass superior to it through the quadrilateral space also bordered by the teres minor, the triceps, and the humerus. It contracts with the latissimus dorsi muscle and the two muscles function as a unit in humeral extension, internal rotation, and adduction.

2. Thoracohumeral muscles—The pectoralis major and the latissimus dorsi muscles are powerful movers of the shoulder and, hence, contribute to the joint force that in turn usually stabilizes the glenohumeral joint. The pectoralis major muscle arises as a broad sheet of two distinct heads with the lowermost fibers of the sternal head inserting most proximally on the humerus.

Muscles that originate on the thorax contribute to glenohumeral stability and may have roles in instability as well. When the shoulder is placed in horizontal abduction, similar to the apprehension position, the lowermost fibers of the sternal head of the pectoralis major muscle are stretched to an extreme. Because anterior instability also occurs from forcible horizontal abduction of the shoulder, the humeral head can be pulled out of the glenoid by passive tension in the pectoralis major and latissimus dorsi muscles.

3. Biceps brachii muscle—Both heads of the biceps brachii muscle have their origin on the scapula. The short head originates from the coracoid and with the coracobrachialis muscle forms the conjoined tendon. The long head of the biceps has its origin just superior to the articular margin of the glenoid from the posterosuperior labrum and the supraglenoid tubercle and is inside the synovial sheath of the glenohumeral joint. It traverses the glenohumeral joint, passing over the anterior aspect of the humeral head to the bicipital groove where it exits the joint under the transverse humeral ligament.

Its origin on the scapula and insertion of the radius leaves the long head of the biceps brachii muscle with potential for function at both the shoulder and the elbow. Its function at the elbow has been well established to include both flexion and supination. Long considered a depressor of the humeral head, the role of the active biceps has been recently questioned because electromyographic studies have shown little or no activity of the biceps when elbow motion was controlled. This does not preclude a passive role or an active role associated with elbow motion because tension in the tendon may then contribute to glenohumeral joint stability.

E. The Neurovascular Supply

The axillary artery traverses the axilla, extending from the outer border of the first rib to the lower border of the teres minor muscle, forming the brachial artery. The axillary artery lies deep to the pectoralis muscle but is crossed in its midregion by the pectoralis minor tendon, just before the tendon inserts on the coracoid process. The axillary vein travels with the axillary artery, and branches of the axillary artery supply most of the shoulder girdle. The brachial plexus consists of the ventral rami of the fifth through eighth cervical nerves and the first thoracic nerve. This network of nerve fibers begins with the joining of the ventral rami proximally in the neck and continues anteriorly and distally, crossing into the axillary region obliquely underneath the clavicle at about the junction area of the distal one third and proximal two thirds. Clavicular fractures in this area have the potential of injuring the brachial plexus. The plexus then lies inferior to the coracoid process, where its cords form the peripheral nerves that continue down the arm. Muscles of the shoulder girdle are supplied by the nerves arising at all levels of the brachial plexus.

Eberly VC et al: Variation in the glenoid origin of the anteroinferior capsulolabrum. Clin Orthop 2002;400,58.

History & Physical Examination

A. General Approach

The history of shoulder complaints must include age, arm dominance, location, intensity, duration, temporal occurrence, aggravating and alleviating factors, radiation of discomfort, physical activity level, occupation, and the mechanism of injury. Previous responses to treatment will help to characterize their efficacy and establish a pattern of disease or injury progression. The physical examination begins with the patient undress-

ing so that both shoulders are fully exposed. Patients should be examined first in the standing position. The surface anatomy should be checked for asymmetry, atrophy, or external lesions. It is especially important to examine the supraspinatus and infraspinatus fossae for any signs of atrophy. The area of pain should be pointed out by the patient prior to the physician manipulating the shoulder to avoid causing the patient any unnecessary pain. A thorough neurovascular examination of the upper extremity should be performed.

B. Shoulder Range of Motion

1. Types of movement—Many terms may be used to describe movements of the shoulder joint (Figure 4–23, Table 4–3). Flexion occurs when the arm begins at the side and elevates in the sagittal plane of the body anteriorly. Extension occurs when the arm starts at the side and elevates in the sagittal plane of the body posteriorly. Adduction occurs when the arm moves toward the midline of the body, with abduction occurring as the arm moves away from the midline of the body. Internal rotation occurs when the arm rotates medially, inward toward the body, and external rotation occurs as the arm rotates laterally or outward from the body. Horizontal adduction occurs as the arm

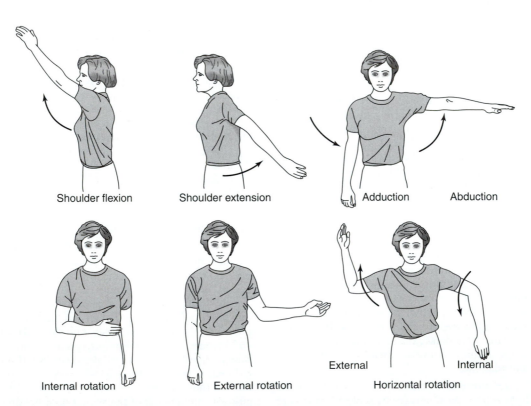

Shoulder flexion Shoulder extension Adduction Abduction

Internal rotation External rotation External Internal Horizontal rotation

Figure 4–23. Description of shoulder motion.

Table 4–3. Movements at the shoulder joint.

Movement	Muscles[b]	Nerve Supply[c]
Flexion	Pectoralis major, clavicular part	Pectoral nerves
	Deltoid, clavicular part	Axillary
	Biceps, short head	Musculocutaneous
	Coracobrachialis	Musculocutaneous
Extension	Deltoid, posterior part	Axillary
	Latissimus dorsi (if shoulder flexed)	Thoracodorsal
	Teres major (if shoulder flexed)	Subscapular
Abduction	Deltoid, acromial part	Axillary
	Supraspinatus	Suprascapular
Adduction	Pectoralis major, sternocostal part	Pectoral
	Latissimus dorsi	Thoracodorsal
	Teres major	Subscapular
Lateral rotation of humerus	Deltoid, posterior part	Axillary
	Infraspinatus	Suprascapular
	Teres minor	Axillary
Medial rotation of humerus	Pectoralis major	Pectoral
	Latissimus dorsi	Thoracodorsal
	Deltoid, clavicular part	Axillary
	Teres major	Subscapular
	Subscapularis	Subscapular
Stabilization[a]	Subscapularis	Subscapular
	Supraspinatus	Suprascapular
	Infraspinatus	Suprascapular
	Teres minor	Axillary
	Triceps, long head	Radial
	Biceps, long head	Musculocutaneous

[a]All the muscles of stabilization are attached close to the shoulder joint, have a poor mechanical advantage over it, and are more effective in holding the joint than in moving it.
[b]The actions of muscles shown in this table presuppose a fixed scapula. If the arm is fixed, muscles passing from the shoulder girdle to the arm will move the girdle on the trunk. If the shoulder joint is fixed, muscles passing from the trunk to the humerus will move the girdle on the trunk at the sternoclavicular joint.
[c]At the shoulder joint no movement is controlled by one never alone. However, some movements have their major muscle (or muscles) innervated by a single nerve and so are severely affected by damage to that nerve, eg, the axillary nerve in abduction, extension, and lateral rotation. Thus, destruction of the axillary nerve leads to the shoulder being held in a position of adduction, medial rotation, and flexion.

starts at 90 degrees of abduction and adducts forward and medially toward the center of the body, and horizontal abduction happens as the arm starts at 90 degrees of abduction and moves outward, away from the body. Elevation is the angle made between the thorax and arm, regardless if it is in the abduction plane, flexion plane, or in between.

2. Evaluation of movement—Range of motion of the injured shoulder should be compared with that in the opposite shoulder, along with the strength during abduction and rotation. This should be done both passively and actively. The shoulder should be inspected for any changes in synchrony, such as scapular winging, elevation of the scapula, and any other irregular or asymmetric movements of the scapula. Information may be gained on loss of flexibility and instability resulting from contractures of muscle, tendon, capsule, or ligament. Loss of flexibility most commonly occurs in the capsular tissues of the glenohumeral joint. Sudden pain or clicking may indicate an intra-articular problem.

3. Provocative tests—Specific tests are then performed that aid in making the correct diagnosis. The specific tests for instability, impingement syndrome, bicipital tendonitis, and superior capsulolabral/biceps anchor lesions are discussed in a later section.

Arthroscopic Evaluation

A. INDICATIONS FOR SHOULDER INJURIES

Indications for arthroscopic examination of the shoulder include the following:

(1) impingement syndrome, including subacromial bursitis, rotator cuff tendonitis, and rotator cuff tears

(2) acromioclavicular joint osteoarthritis

(3) loose bodies

(4) chronic synovitis

(5) glenohumeral instability

(6) superior capsulolabral/biceps anchor lesions

(7) adhesive capsulitis (frozen shoulder)

B. TECHNIQUE

With the patient either in the lateral decubitus or the beach chair position, the arthroscope is inserted into a posterior portal, medial and inferior to the posterolateral corner of the acromion. With visualization of the glenohumeral joint, an anterior portal immediately lateral to the coracoid allows additional inflow and entrance of additional instruments. Distal clavicle excision, removal of loose bodies, and capsular release of adhesive capsulitis can be performed. An additional anterior portal inferior to the first is required for instability repair with an arthroscopic technique. The arthroscope is then removed from the joint and placed into the subacromial bursa. Portals lateral to the acromion allow subacromial decompression and rotator cuff repair to be carried out with arthroscopic techniques.

C. STEPS IN EVALUATION

Examination of shoulder range of motion and stability is helpful in treatment of shoulder injuries. The steps in arthroscopic examination should include the following:

(1) glenohumeral articular surfaces

(2) rotator cuff from inside the joint

(3) labrum including the biceps anchor

(4) anterior capsuloligamentous structures

(5) rotator cuff from the subacromial bursa

(6) coracoacromial ligament

(7) acromion

(8) acromioclavicular joint

Imaging & Other Studies

Many varieties of radiologic views and projections are available for examining shoulder injuries. An initial radiographic evaluation of the shoulder should consist of an anteroposterior view of the glenohumeral joint in both internal and external rotation, and an axillary lateral. Additional plain radiographic views depend on the underlying pathologic factors. MRI may be indicated in evaluation of rotator cuff disorders recalcitrant to conservative treatment. For instance, a rotator cuff tear that has retracted to the level of the glenoid is usually irreparable. Arthrography is rarely indicated because it is invasive and has little or no advantage over MRI. Ultrasonography is also useful in diagnosis of rotator cuff injury, but its effectiveness is operator-dependent. Electromyographic examination can be useful in identifying shoulder pain of cervical origin.

Lintner SA, Speer KP: Traumatic anterior glenohumeral instability: The role of arthroscopy. J Am Acad Orthop Surg 1997;5 (5):233.

GLENOHUMERAL JOINT INSTABILITY

To make the correct diagnosis the glenohumeral joint must be tested for anterior, posterior, and inferior instability. Different classifications of glenohumeral joint instability have been proposed, based on etiology, the direction of the instability, or on various combinations. TUBS is an acronym describing instability caused by a *t*raumatic event, which is *u*nidirectional, associated with a *B*ankart lesion, and often requires *s*urgical treatment. AMBRI is *a*traumatic, *m*ultidirectional instability that may be *b*ilateral and is best treated by *r*ehabilitation. In this classification, the cause of multidirectional instability is thought to be enlargement of the capsule from genetic or microtraumatic origin.

The positive sulcus sign has been used as the diagnostic hallmark for multidirectional instability, but we now know that the sulcus sign is sometimes found in asymptomatic shoulders of individuals with increased laxity. Laxity or joint play is a trait of body constitution that differs from one individual to another. Individuals may be loose- or tight-jointed. A shoulder is hyperlax if the examiner can easily subluxate the humeral head out of the glenoid in the anterior, posterior, and inferior directions without eliciting symptoms. Unfortunately, this makes classification of instability based on cause, or on direction alone, extremely difficult. Instead, classification is best based on the direction of instability that elicits symptoms and the presence or absence of hyperlaxity (Table 4–4).

Gerber C, Nyffeler RW: Classification of glenohumeral instability. Clin Orthop Rel Res 2002;400:65.

A. GLENOHUMERAL JOINT INSTABILITY EVALUATION

1. Anterior instability—The apprehension test is performed to assess anterior instability. The test applies an anterior directed force to the humeral head from the back with the arm in abduction and external rotation (Figure 4–24). A positive test results from the patient's

Table 4-4. Classification of glenohumeral instability based on the direction of instability and the presence or absence of hyperlaxity.

Direction / Laxity	UDI (Unidirectional Instability)	MDI (Multidirectional Instability)
Normal laxity	Very common 60%	Very rare 3%
Increased laxity	Common 30%	Rare 7%

Adapted, with permission, from Gerber C. Observations of the classification of instability. In Warner JJP et al (eds). Complex and Revision Problems in Shoulder Surgery. Philadelphia: Lippincott-Raven, 1997:9–18.

apprehension that the joint will dislocate. This maneuver mimics the position of subluxation, or dislocation, and causes reflex guarding. Conversely, the relocation test is positive if relief is obtained by applying a posterior directed force to the humeral head (Figure 4–25).

2. Posterior instability—No single test has high sensitivity and specificity for posterior instability. The posterior apprehension test is performed by applying a posterior directed force to the forward flexed and internally rotated shoulder. To perform the circumduction test the patient is instructed to actively move the shoulder in a large circle starting from a flexed, internally rotated and cross-body position, then to forward flexion, then to an abducted and externally rotated position and lastly to the arm at the side. The examiner stands behind the patient and palpates the posterior shoulder. If

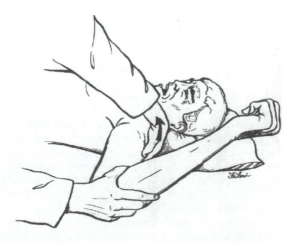

Figure 4-24. The apprehension test for anterior instability.

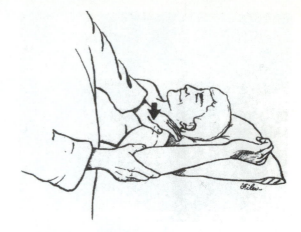

Figure 4-25. The relocation test is positive if relief is obtained by applying a posterior directed force to the humeral head.

positive, the joint subluxes in the flexed, internally rotated and cross-body position and reduces as the shoulder is moved. For the Jahnke test, a posterior directed force is applied to the forward flexed shoulder. The shoulder is then moved into the coronal plane as an anterior directed force is applied to the humeral head. A clunk occurs as the humeral head reduces from the subluxed position (Figure 4–26).

3. Inferior instability—The sulcus sign is used to evaluate laxity and inferior instability. The test is performed with the athlete in a sitting position with the arm at the side or abducted 30 degrees. A distraction force is applied longitudinally along the humerus. If positive, discomfort or apprehension of instability are experienced as the skin just distal to the lateral acromion hollows out (Figure 4–27).

1. Glenohumeral Dislocation

When the shoulder is forced beyond the limit of its normal range of motion, the articular surface of the humeral head may displace from the glenoid to varying degrees. The majority of glenohumeral dislocations, or subluxations, are in the anteroinferior direction (Figure 4–28).

Anterior Dislocation

Anterior glenohumeral dislocation occurs from either an external rotation, or horizontal abduction force on the humerus, a direct posterior blow to the proximal humerus, or a posterolateral blow on the shoulder large

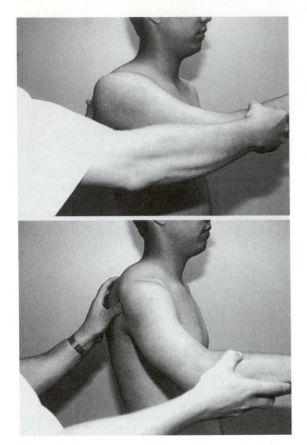

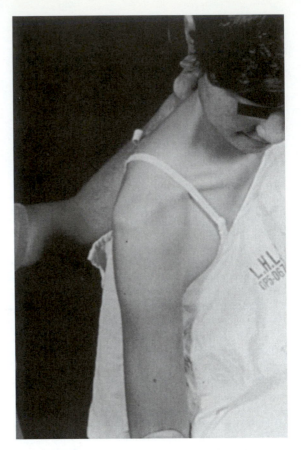

Figure 4–26. The Jahnke test for posterior instability. (**A**) A posterior directed force applied to the forward flexed shoulder. (**B**) The shoulder is then moved into the coronal plane as an anterior directed force is applied to the humeral head. A clunk occurs as the humeral head reduces from the subluxed position. (Reprinted, with permission, from Hawkins RJ, Bokor DJ: Clinical evaluation of shoulder problems. In Rockwood CA et al (editors): The Shoulder. Philadelphia: WB Saunders, 1998, p. 186.)

Figure 4–27. The sulcus test for inferior instability (Reprinted, with permission, from Hawkins RJ, Bokor DJ: Clinical evaluation of shoulder problems. In :Rockwood CA et al (editors): The Shoulder. Philadelphia: WB Saunders, 1998, p. 189.)

enough to displace the humeral head. The anterior capsule is either stretched or torn within its attachment to the anterior glenoid. The head may be displaced into a subcoracoid, subglenoid, subclavicular, or intrathoracic position. Two major lesions are typically seen in patients with recurrent anterior dislocations. First is the Bankart lesion, an anterior capsular injury associated with a tear of the glenoid labrum off the anterior glenoid rim. The Bankart lesion may occur with fractures of the glenoid rim. Such fractures are often minimally displaced, and treatment is usually dictated by the joint instability. The second major lesions associated with recurrent anterior dislocations is the Hill-Sachs lesion, a compression fracture of the posterolateral articular surface of the humeral head. It is created by the sharp edge of the anterior glenoid as the humeral head dislocates over it. When large, both the Bankart and the Hill-Sachs lesions predispose to recurrent dislocations when the arm is placed in abduction and external rotation. If the glenoid rim fracture involves greater than 20% of the glenoid diameter, then the joint becomes prone to instability and treatment with open reduction and internal fixation is best. If the fracture is old, or the glenoid rim is worn to a similar level, then corticocancellous bone grafting of the glenoid rim is indicated.

ANATOMICAL LESIONS

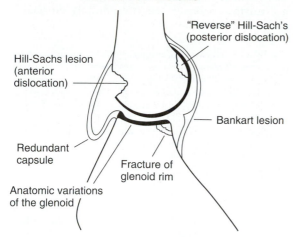

Figure 4–28. Anatomic lesions producing shoulder instability.

Other injuries associated with anterior dislocation may occur. These include avulsion of the greater tuberosity from the humerus, caused by traction from the rotator cuff, and injury to the axillary nerve, which may be stretched, or torn. Permanent loss of axillary nerve function results in denervation of the deltoid muscle and loss of sensation over the proximal lateral aspect of the arm. Axillary nerve palsy may also occur during reduction of the dislocation and therefore should be tested both before and after reduction. The deltoid extension lag sign, described later in the section on Axillary Nerve Injury may be the best way to assess function of this nerve. Lastly, the "dead arm" syndrome may occur after anterior joint instability. For example, a pitcher may report sudden inability to throw, with the arm going numb and becoming extremely weak after the ball release. The symptoms are transient, resolving within a few seconds to minutes.

Athletes who sustain a shoulder dislocation will try to hold the injured extremity at the side, gripping the forearm with the opposite hand. Most athletes know their shoulder is dislocated and will immediately seek help. On physical examination of an anterior dislocation, the examiner will note a space underneath the acromion where the humeral head should lie and a palpable anterior mass representing the humeral head in the anterior axilla.

One must distinguish between acute and recurrent anterior glenohumeral dislocations because an acute dislocation sustains severe trauma with the increased probability of associated injuries. The recurrent dislocation may occur with minimal trauma, and reduction

may be accomplished with much less effort. Anterior dislocations may be reduced by one of several techniques. Longitudinal traction may be exerted on the affected arm with external rotation, followed by internal rotation of the arm. Care must be taken to avoid direct pressure on the neurovascular structures. Another method is to have the patient lie face down on the table and tie or tape a bucket to the injured arm and slowly fill it with water. This allows the musculature around the shoulder to relax from the force of the weight and effect a spontaneous reduction.

Following reduction of an initial dislocation, the shoulder should be immobilized in internal rotation for 2–6 weeks. Healing will generally take at least 6 weeks. Before returning to athletics, the patient should have normal range of motion without pain and normal strength in the shoulder. Emphasis must be placed on strengthening the rotator cuff muscles to compensate for the laxity of the ligamentous support. When weight training is begun, military press, fly exercises, a narrow grip while bench pressing, and deep shoulder dips must be excluded until considerable time has elapsed and complete healing is realized.

Recurrent dislocations should be treated with minimal immobilization until the pain subsides, followed by range-of-motion and muscle-strengthening exercises. Many restraining devices are available to help prevent recurrent dislocations during sporting activities, focusing on keeping the arm from going into abduction and external rotation. These orthotics may be effective, but because they limit the athlete's range of shoulder motion, their use is limited for certain competitive activities.

If an athlete has sustained multiple dislocations that are unresponsive to conservative treatment, surgical reconstruction of the shoulder joint may be indicated. There are a wide variety of procedures to correct the instability, with most involving repair of the labral defect and tightening of the anterior capsule and ligamentous structures through an anterior incision (Table 4–5).

For most surgical procedures, aggressive range-of-motion exercises do not start until at least 3 weeks postoperatively. The goal is to have full abduction and 90 degrees of external rotation. By 12 weeks, patients have often progressed well into their initial programs and may begin a variety of weight-training exercises. Return to sports activities takes a minimum of 6 months.

Posterior Dislocation

Posterior glenohumeral dislocations result from the posterior capsule being torn, stretched, or disrupted from the posterior glenoid. A reverse Hill-Sachs lesion may appear on the anterior articular surface of the

Table 4–5. Repair of capsule and labrum back to the glenoid rim.

Bankart procedure
duToit procedure
Viek procedure
Eyre-Brook procedure
Moseley procedure
Muscle and capsule plication
Putti-Platt procedure
Symeonides procedure
Muscle and tendon sling procedures
Magnuson-Stack procedure
Bristow-Helfet-Latarjet procedure modifications
Boytchev procedure
Nicola procedure
Gallie-LeMesurier procedure
Boyd transfer of long head of biceps (for posterior
    dislocation)
Bone block
Eden-Hybbinette procedure
DeAnquin procedure (through a superior approach to the
    shoulder)
Osteotomies
Weber (humeral neck)
Saha (humeral shaft)

---

humerus. With a posterior dislocation, the subscapularis, or its insertion on the lesser tuberosity, may be injured. Posterior dislocations are often difficult to diagnose because the patient may have a normal contour to the shoulder or the deltoid of a well-developed athlete may mask signs of a displaced humeral head. The patient holds the injured shoulder in internal rotation and the examiner cannot externally rotate it. Anteroposterior and axillary radiographs must be obtained to diagnose a posterior dislocation.

Applying traction in the line of the adducted humerus, with an anteriorly directed force to the humeral head, reduces a posterior dislocation. Anesthesia often helps decrease the trauma of reduction. Following reduction, the shoulder is immobilized for 2–6 weeks in external rotation and a small amount of abduction. Surgical treatment should be considered if these measures fail to provide the desired results.

Multidirectional Instability

Some patients will have instability in both the anterior and posterior directions, most often subluxation and not dislocation. This may result in a painful shoulder, especially if rotator cuff strength decreases. The pain is often primarily a result of rotator cuff inflammation,

likely from attempts to stabilize the humeral head during activity. A rotator cuff strengthening program is often successful treatment.

Cole BJ et al: Comparison of arthroscopic and open anterior shoulder stabilization: A two to six-year follow-up study. J Bone Joint Surg 2000;82A(8):1108.

Fuchs B et al: Posterior-inferior capsular shift for treatment of recurrent, voluntary posterior subluxation of the shoulder. J Bone Joint Surg 2000;82A(1):16.

Hovelius LK et al: Long-term results with the Bankart and the Bristow-Latarjet procedures: Recurrent shoulder instability and arthroplasty. J Shoulder Elbow Surg 2001;10(5):445.

Itoi E et al: The effect of a glenoid defect on anteroinferior stability of the shoulder after Bankart repair: A cadaveric study. J Bone Joint Surg 2000;82A:35.

Pollock RG et al: Operative results of the inferior capsular procedure for multidirectional instability of the shoulder. J Bone Joint Surg 2000;82A(7):919.

Sperber A et al: Comparison of an arthroscopic and an open procedure for posttraumatic instability of the shoulder: A prospective, randomized multicenter study. J Shoulder Elbow Surg 2001;10(2):105.

2. Glenoid Labrum Injury

The glenoid labrum is a fibrocartilaginous rim around the glenoid fossa that deepens the socket and provides stability for the humeral head. It also is a connection for the surrounding capsuloligamentous structures. Glenoid labrum tears may occur from repetitive shoulder motion or acute trauma. In the athlete with repeated anterior subluxation of the shoulder, tears of the anteroinferior labrum may occur, leading to progressive instability.

Weight lifters may also develop glenoid labrum tears from repetitive bench pressing and overhead pressing. Weakness in the posterior rotator cuff may aggravate this condition. Tears of the glenoid labrum may also occur from acute trauma such as falling on an outstretched arm but is also seen in the leading shoulders of golfers and batters when they ground their clubs or bats.

Patients with glenoid labrum injuries may describe their pain as interrupting smooth functioning of the shoulder during their specific activity. On examination, they may have discomfort on forced external rotation at 90 degrees of abduction, with the pain typically not increasing as the arm goes into further abduction. Frequently, a labrum disruption may be felt as a "pop" or "click" on forced external rotation. The patient may also experience discomfort on forced horizontal adduction of the shoulder. Manual muscle testing may show associated weakness in the rotator cuff muscles. Diagnostic tests such as a computed tomographic scan and

MRI following injection of contrast dye into the shoulder joint may allow early detection of glenoid labrum lesions. If range-of-motion exercises and gradual return to activity are not successful in relieving symptoms, arthroscopic intervention may be indicated to debride a torn, symptomatic labrum. During arthroscopy, care must be taken not to debride the inferior labrum because this may result in increased anterior shoulder instability, thus escalating the probability of anterior shoulder dislocation. Immediately following surgery, range-of-motion exercises and strengthening training begin. Usually within 2–3 weeks following surgery, the athlete may begin a throwing program. Baseball pitchers may be ready to throw 3 months postoperatively.

SLAP LESIONS

The use of shoulder arthroscopy in the diagnosis and treatment of shoulder disorders has led to increased awareness of superior labrum anterior posterior (SLAP) lesions. Their potential role in shoulder pain and pathology has also recently increased. SLAP lesions involve the origin of the long head of the biceps brachii, (biceps anchor) and the superior capsulolabral structures. A type I lesion exhibits degeneration or fraying of the labrum without instability. Type II lesions are most common, accounting for over 50% of patients with a SLAP lesion, and involve detachment of the superior labrum from the glenoid. A type III lesion has a bucket-handle tear of the superior labrum with firm attachment of the remainder of the labrum. Type IV lesions also remain attached to the labrum but have an associated bucket-handle tear of the labrum that extends into the biceps tendon (Figure 4–29).

Types V–VII SLAP lesions were later added to this initial four-part classification. A type V lesion is an anterior-inferior Bankart lesion that continues superiorly to include separation of the biceps tendon. A type VI lesion included a biceps separation with an unstable flap tear of the labrum. Finally, a type VII is a superior labrum-biceps tendon separation that extended anteriorly beneath the middle glenohumeral ligament.

Clinical Findings

Patients present with nonspecific shoulder pain associated with activity. A complicating factor in making the diagnosis is that the majority of SLAP lesions are associated with other shoulder pathology, such as rotator cuff tears, acromioclavicular joint pathology, and instability. Less than 28% of SLAP lesions are isolated.

No single test is both sensitive and specific for diagnosis of SLAP lesions. Diagnostic arthroscopy remains the best means to definitively diagnose SLAP lesions.

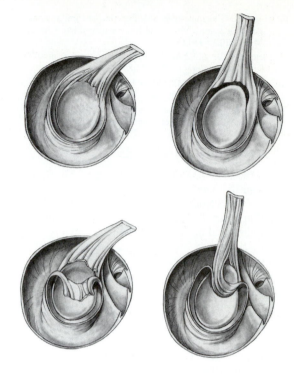

Figure 4–29. The five types of the SLAP lesion include fraying of the superior capsulolabrum (type 1), detachment of the superior capsulolabrum and the biceps anchor (type 2), bucket-handle tearing of the superior capsulolabrum (type 3), detachment of the superior capsulolabrum and tearing into the biceps anchor (type 4), and combinations of these (type 5).

Yet, the active compression test may prove to be the most useful single test. The internally rotated shoulder is forward flexed to 90 degrees and then brought across the body in horizontal abduction about 10 degrees. The test is positive if the patient has pain with resisted forward flexion that is relieved by external rotation of the shoulder.

Treatment

Treatment of SLAP lesions can be simplified by noting whether or not the lesion would contribute to detachment of either the biceps anchor or the anterosuperior capsulolabrum. Lesions producing meaningful detachment of the anterior capsuloligamentous structures generally require repair of these structures back to the bony glenoid rim. Lesions producing significant defects extending into the biceps tendon may require biceps tenotomy, with or without tenodesis.

Gartzman GM, Hammerman SM: Superior labrum, anterior and posterior lesions: When and how to treat them. Clin Sports Med 2000;19(1):115.

Handelberg F et al: SLAP lesions: A retrospective multicenter study. Arthroscopy 1998;14(8):856.

Musgrave DS, Rodosky MW: SLAP lesions: Current concepts. Am J Sports Med 2001;30(1):29.

Parentis MA et al: SLAP Lesions in the New Millennium: Review and treatment guidelines. Clin Orthop Rel Res 2002;400:77.

CLAVICULAR FRACTURE

The clavicle is one of the most commonly fractured bones in the body, with direct trauma being the usual cause in athletic events (Figure 4–30). Football, wrestling, and ice hockey are the sports most commonly involved in clavicular fractures, which is not surprising as all three are associated with high-speed contact between players.

Clinical Findings

Despite the proximity of vital structures, clavicular fractures that occur during athletic activities are rarely associated with neurovascular damage, and accompanying soft-tissue disorders are uncommon. The patient will usually give a history of falling in the area of the shoulder or receiving a blow to the clavicle, experiencing immediate pain and inability to raise the arm. Radiography will usually confirm the clinical impression and must show the entire clavicle, including the shoulder girdle, upper third of the humerus, and sternal end of the clavicle. Midclavicular fractures account for 80% of clavicular fractures, with distal fractures at 15% and proximal fractures at 5%. Most fractures of the shaft of the clavicle heal well. The potential for a rare but serious neurovascular complication, such as a tear of the subclavian artery or brachii plexus injury, must be kept in mind when evaluating and treating clavicular fractures, and a neurovascular examination on initial evaluation is very important. Pulses in the distal part of the upper extremity, strength, and sensation must be carefully evaluated.

Because the clavicle is the single bony structure that fixes the shoulder girdle to the thorax, a fracture through the clavicle causes the shoulder to sag forward and downward. The pull of the sternocleidomastoid muscle may displace the proximal fragment superiorly. These forces tend to hinder the initial reduction and maintenance of that reduction. In addition, distal fractures, which are more common in older age groups, may involve tears in the coracoclavicular ligament, which allows the proximal clavicle to ride up superiorly, mimicking an acromioclavicular dislocation. Delayed union in this type of fracture is a much greater possibility than with other clavicular fractures.

Treatment & Prognosis

Mid and proximal clavicular fractures are usually treated using figure-of-eight strapping, with tightening periodically to maintain good shoulder position. Even with the strap, athletes must be instructed to keep the shoulder from sagging forward. The strap should not be applied so tightly that it puts pressure on the axilla. In the first few days after injury, a sling may also be used on the affected side to support the extremity.

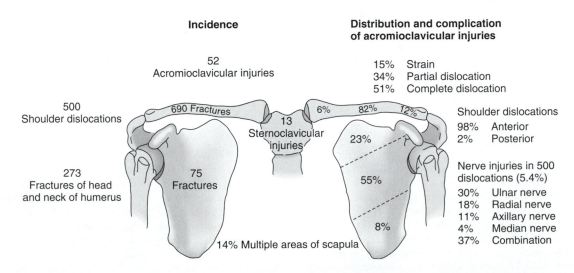

Figure 4–30. Analysis of 1603 shoulder girdle injuries, showing the frequency and location of fractures and dislocations.

Immobilization is usually discontinued at 3–4 weeks, and once the clavicular fracture has healed, range-of-motion and strengthening exercises should begin. Onset of exercises prior to healing may result in nonunion. Athletes should not be allowed to return to play until achieving their preinjury shoulder strength and range of motion. Generally, no special braces or pads are required when the athlete returns to play.

Grassi FS et al: Management of midclavicular fractures: Comparison between nonoperative treatment and open intramedullary fixation in 80 patients. J Trauma 2001;50(6):1096.

Robinson CM: Fractures of the clavicle in the adult. Epidemiology and classification. J Bone Joint Surg Br 1998;80:476.

PROXIMAL HUMERUS EPIPHYSEAL INJURY

Proximal Humerus Epiphyseal Fracture

In young athletes, epiphyseal fractures of the proximal humerus may occur. The separate growth centers of the articular surface, greater tuberosity, and lesser tuberosity coalesce at approximately age 7 years, with the remaining growth plates closing as late as 20–22 years of age. Therefore, fracture separations may occur at any age until the growth plates have closed, though fractures in this area usually do not arrest growth.

Injury can occur to the shoulder of the growing musculoskeletal system from overhead throwing sports. Proximal humerus pain, especially while throwing and associated with widening of the proximal humerus epiphysis has been termed "little league shoulder." Although widening of the proximal humerus epiphysis can be an adaptive change to throwing, when painful it may represent an overuse fracture.

Kocher MS et al: Upper extremity injuries in the paediatric athlete. Sports Med 2000;30(2):117.

ACROMIOCLAVICULAR JOINT INJURY

Clinical Findings

Acromioclavicular dislocations or subluxations, commonly referred to as separations, vary in severity depending on the extent of injury to the stabilizing ligaments and capsule. The typical mechanism of injury is a direct downward blow to the tip of the shoulder. Clinically, pain at the top of the shoulder over the acromioclavicular joint is the predominant symptom, with varying decreases in motion depending on the severity of the injury. The athlete who has sustained this type of injury will typically leave the field holding the arm close to the side.

When checking for instability of the acromioclavicular joint, the examiner should manipulate the midshaft of the clavicle, rather than the acromioclavicular joint to rule out pain from contusion to the acromioclavicular area. For milder acromioclavicular injuries, the patient should put the hand of the affected arm on the opposite shoulder, and the examiner may then gently apply downward pressure at the patient's affected elbow, noting if this maneuver causes pain at the acromioclavicular joint.

Acromioclavicular joint injuries were initially divided into grades I–III (Figure 4–31). Grade I injuries are typically produced by a mild blow causing a partial tear of the acromioclavicular ligament. When the acromioclavicular ligament is completely torn but the coracoclavicular ligament remains intact, a grade II injury that involves subluxation or partial displacement results. When the force of injury is severe enough to tear the coracoclavicular and acromioclavicular ligaments in addition to the capsule, a grade III injury occurs.

Three additional injuries were later added to the classification. In grade IV injuries, the clavicle is displaced posteriorly and buttonholed through the fascia of the trapezius muscle. Grade V injuries demonstrate severe inferior displacement of the glenohumeral joint, with the clavicle often 300% superior to the acromion.

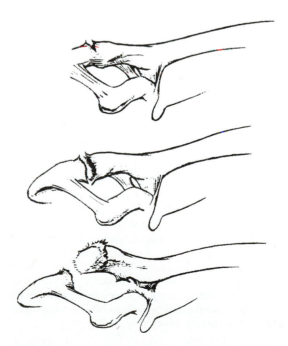

Figure 4–31. Grades of acromioclavicular joint separations.

Lastly, in grade VI injuries the distal end of the clavicle is locked inferior to the coracoid.

Acromioclavicular joint displacement is often obvious on physical examination, but it is best classified by radiography. An anteroposterior radiograph that is aimed 10 degrees cephalad allows visualization of the acromioclavicular joint. A radiograph of the entire upper thorax allows the vertical distance between the coracoid and the clavicle on both the involved and uninvolved sides to be compared. Anteroposterior radiographs with weights applied to the upper extremities are usually unnecessary. An axillary lateral radiograph is also essential for proper classification.

Monig SP et al: Treatment of complete acromioclavicular dislocation: Present indications and surgical technique with biodegradable cords. In J Sports Med 1999;20(8):560.

Treatment & Prognosis

Management of acromioclavicular joint injuries depends on their severity. Grade I and grade II injuries may be treated with a sling until discomfort dissipates, usually within 2–4 weeks. Next a rehabilitation program starts and normal range of motion and strength to the upper extremity begins to be restored. The treatment of grade III injuries or complete dislocations in athletes is controversial. Although most clinicians feel that grade III injuries are best managed nonoperatively, others advocate operative treatment. Grade IV–VI injuries are best treated with open reduction and internal fixation along with reconstruction of the coracoclavicular ligaments.

Nonsurgical treatment is a sling for comfort. Ice and other support modalities are used for the acute acromioclavicular injury to reduce soreness and swelling. Pain is the limiting factor in beginning range-of-motion and isometric muscle-strengthening exercises. It should be used as a guide for gradual initiation and escalation of these physical therapy regimes. Isotonic exercises may then follow because isometric exercises are more effective earlier when range of motion is limited.

Before resuming athletic activities, the patient must have full range of pain-free motion and no tenderness upon direct palpation of the acromioclavicular joint or pain when manual traction is applied. Athletes who do not require elevation of the arm, such as soccer or football players, tend to return to sports earlier than players who require overhead arm activity, such as tennis, baseball, and swimming athletes.

Eskola A et al: The results of operative resection of the lateral end of the clavicle. J Bone Joint Surg Am 1996;78:584

Rawes ML, Dias JJ: Long-term results of conservative treatment for acromioclavicular dislocation. J Bone Joint Surg Br 1996; 78:410.

Fractures of the coracoid process are rare, usually seen in professional riflemen and skeet shooters, though they have also been reported in baseball and tennis players. They are identified radiographically, and conservative treatment, including cessation of activity, usually results in uncomplicated healing after 6–8 weeks.

STERNOCLAVICULAR JOINT INJURY

In the skeletally mature adult athlete, injury to the sternoclavicular joint usually consists of the surrounding soft tissue and capsule tearing, leading to subluxation or dislocation. The mechanism of injury is either a blow to the point of the shoulder, which predisposes to anterior dislocation, or a direct blow to the clavicle or chest with the shoulder in extension, which predisposes to posterior dislocation. The injury may range from a symptomatic sprain to a complete sternoclavicular dislocation with disruption of the capsule and its restraining ligaments.

Anterior Dislocation

The most common type of sternoclavicular dislocation is anterior dislocation. This is recognized clinically by an anterior prominence of the proximal clavicle on the involved side. Radiographic documentation of an anterior sternoclavicular dislocation is difficult because of overlapping of the rib, sternum, and clavicle at the joint but may be confirmed by oblique views. A computed tomographic scan is usually very sensitive and should be done if radiographic appear normal but the diagnosis is suspected.

Although dislocation of the anterior sternoclavicular joint may cause considerable distress initially, the symptoms usually subside rapidly, with no loss of shoulder function. A variety of surgical and nonsurgical approaches have been advocated, but most feel that surgery for anterior dislocations results in significant complications. Closed treatment modalities vary from a sling alone to attempted closed reduction, which may be successful initially but is difficult to maintain.

Posterior Dislocation

Posterior sternoclavicular dislocation is much less common, but has more complications because of the potential for injury to the esophagus, great vessels, and trachea. Presenting symptoms range from mild to moderate pain in the sternoclavicular region to hoarseness, dysphagia, severe respiratory distress, and subcutaneous emphysema from tracheal injury.

In most instances, closed reduction of posterior dislocations, if performed early, are successful and stable. To effect reduction, a pillow is placed under the upper back of the supine patient and gentle traction is applied with the shoulder held in 90 degrees of abduction and at maximum extension (Figure 4–32). Rarely, closed reduction under general anesthesia or open reduction is required.

After reduction, the patient is put in an immobilization splint, instructed to use ice and NSAIDs. Once the joint has healed sufficiently, usually within 2–3 weeks, range-of-motion exercises may begin. Elevation of the arm should not be attempted until 3 weeks after injury.

Clavicular Epiphyseal Fracture

In athletes younger than 25 years, sternoclavicular injuries may not result in true dislocations but rather in fractures through the growth plate of the proximal clavicle. These clavicular epiphyseal fractures may appear clinically as dislocations, especially if some displacement is present, and may be treated conservatively. Typically, these are not associated with growth deformities, and reduction of the fracture is not needed unless severe displacement occurs. Symptomatic treatment for pain will usually suffice. Sometimes an adolescent

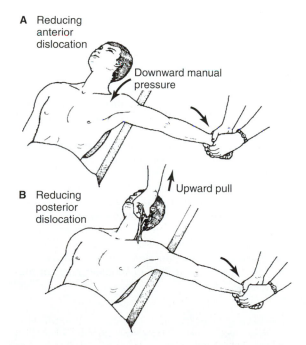

A Reducing anterior dislocation

Downward manual pressure

B Reducing posterior dislocation

Upward pull

Figure 4–32. Method for reducing (**A**): anterior sternoclavicular dislocation and (**B**): posterior sternoclavicular dislocation.

presents with an enlarging mass at the sternoclavicular joint, and parents become concerned about the possibility of cancer. A careful history reveals trauma several weeks earlier and the mass represents the callus of a healing clavicular epiphyseal fracture that can be demonstrated radiographically.

3. Shoulder Stiffness (Adhesive Capsulitis, Frozen Shoulder)

Often called adhesive capsulitis or frozen shoulder, shoulder stiffness is a painful condition characterized by significant restriction in both active and passive range-of-motion. The shoulder is characterized as being stiff when the articular surfaces are normal and the joint is stable, yet range of motion is restricted. Stiffness may also result from pathologic connections between the articular surfaces, soft-tissue contracture, bursal adhesions, or a shortened muscle-tendon unit. Often of uncertain cause, the restrictions of shoulder motion are global. That is, none of the shoulder planes of motion is spared.

Shoulder stiffness may be separated into idiopathic and post-traumatic causes. Idiopathic shoulder stiffness is most common in older individuals, especially women between 40 and 60 years of age. Other factors that predispose to idiopathic shoulder stiffness include cervical, cardiac, pulmonary, neoplastic, neurologic, and personality disorders. Patients with diabetes mellitus are also at a high risk of developing shoulder stiffness, with 10–35% of diabetics having restriction of shoulder motion. Diabetics who have been insulin-dependent for many years have the greatest incidence and bilateral involvement. The pathophysiology of idiopathic shoulder stiffness remains uncertain, but the pathoanatomy is commonly limited to contracture of the glenohumeral capsule (Figure 4–33). Most prominently involved is the rotator interval that includes the coracohumeral ligament.

Although all patients can recall some traumatic event that preceded their shoulder stiffness, those with distinct trauma such as a prior fracture, rotator cuff tear, or surgical procedure have a post-traumatic cause. Stiffness after shoulder surgery is typical and typically resolves with time and appropriate rehabilitation. But the shoulder should not be neglected after any surgery about the shoulder girdle. This includes axillary or cervical lymph node dissections especially when combined with radiation therapy, cardiac catheterization in the axilla, coronary artery bypass grafting with sternotomy and thoracotomy. All surgeons should be aware that these procedures may result in restricted shoulder motion.

The clinical presentation of idiopathic shoulder stiffness is classically described as having three phases.

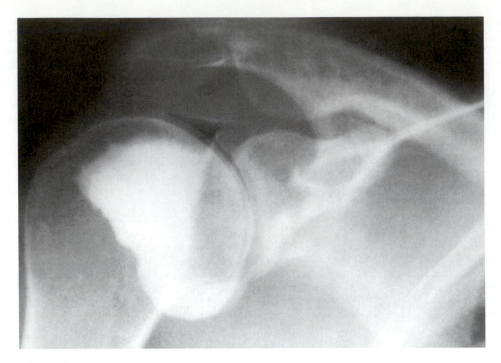

Figure 4–33. Adhesive capsulitis of the shoulder. Note the small irregular joint capsule with addition of contrast material.

The first phase is the painful, freezing phase. The pain is typically achy in nature and sudden jolts or attempts at rapid motion exacerbate the chronic discomfort. The pain may begin at night and shoulder motion becomes progressively limited. Patients often hold their arm at their side and in internal rotation with the forearm across the belly. They may also be treated for nonspecific shoulder pain with a sling in this position. This inflammatory phase often lasts between 2 and 9 months.

The second phase of progressive stiffness lasts between 3 and 12 months. Stiffness progresses to the point where shoulder motion is restricted in all planes. Essentially, the shoulder has undergone fibrous arthrodesis. Fortunately, pain progressively decreases from the initial, inflammatory phase. With time, patients are able to use the shoulder with little or no pain, within the restricted range of motion, but attempts to exceed this range are accompanied by pain. The patient's symptoms then plateau. Unfortunately, this phase may be persistent with symptoms lasting for extended periods. In the resolution, or thawing phase, the shoulder slowly and progressively becomes more supple. This phase can be as short as a month, but typically lasts 1–3 years.

On clinical examination, loss of both active and passive range of shoulder motion is evident. Often the first motion to be affected is internal rotation demonstrated by an inability to bring the arm up the back to the same level as the normal shoulder. Radiographic confirmation of adhesive capsulitis may be done by arthrography, which will demonstrate marked reduction in the capacity of the joint. Often the affected shoulder will not take more than 2–3 mL of dye, although normal capacity is 12 mL.

Treatment varies, but conservative modalities and progressive range-of-motion exercises seem effective. Range-of-motion exercises for external rotation and abduction will help minimize the length of restriction in motion and dysfunction. Manipulation under anesthesia, long the mainstay of intervention, is being replaced by selective arthroscopic capsular release. Short-term results indicate a quicker return of motion. Whether treated with rehabilitation alone, or with capsular release, a return of about 80% of shoulder range of motion is usual.

Griggs SM et al: Idiopathic adhesive capsulitis: A prospective functional outcome study of nonoperative treatment. J Bone Joint Surg 2000;82A(10):1398.

Harryman DT et al: The stiff shoulder. In Rockwood CA, Matsen FA, editors: The Shoulder. Philadelphia: WB Saunders, 1998, pp. 1064–1112.

Omari A, Bunker TD: Open surgical release for frozen shoulder: Surgical findings and results of the release. J Shoulder Elbow Surg 2001;10(4):353.

Warner JJP: Frozen shoulder: Diagnosis and management. J Am Acad Orthop Surg 1997;5:130.

SHOULDER TENDON & MUSCLE INJURY

1. Rotator Cuff Tendon Injuries

Injury to the rotator cuff, a common cause of shoulder pain and disability, has a high prevalence during athletic activities. Injury of the rotator cuff may result in pain, weakness, and decreased range of motion. Symptoms are often worsened by activity, especially when the hand is positioned overhead. Night pain is also common, and many complain of awakening after rolling onto the affected shoulder. Although shoulder weakness and decreased range of motion usually result from a rotator cuff tendon tear, pain alone from subacromial bursitis or rotator cuff tendonitis may also be the cause. Each of these entities most often results from impingement syndrome.

A. IMPINGEMENT SYNDROME

Any prolonged repetitive overhead activity such as tennis, pitching, golf, or swimming may compromise the space between the humeral head and the coracoacromial arch that includes the acromion, coracoacromial ligament, and the coracoid process. Impingement causes microtrauma to the rotator cuff, resulting in local inflammation, edema, cuff softening, pain, and poor function. These problems may even cause greater impingement, producing a continuous vicious cycle (Figure 4–34). This cycle may be precipitated by acute injury to the rotator cuff tendon itself. Blood supply to this tendon is precarious, thus decreasing its capacity for healing.

1. Subacromial bursitis—Bursitis of the shoulder refers to the inflammation of the subacromial bursa. It has the mildest signs and symptoms of shoulder impingement. Pain is present with overhead activity, and when the arm is at the side pain is usually absent or mild.

Active range of shoulder motion is limited by pain. No atrophy of the shoulder muscles is present, and manual muscle testing demonstrates mild weakness (Figure 4–35). Passively, when the internally rotated shoulder is moved into forward flexion, the patient will experience discomfort (Neer impingement sign). This pain then resolves, and with the Neer impingement test (10 mL of lidocaine injected into the subacromial space) strength and range of motion dramatically increase.

Radiographs of the subacromial space, such as the supraspinatus outlet view, may show a spur on the undersurface of the acromion, causing narrowing of the subacromial space. In recent years, advances in imaging methods such as ultrasonography and MRI have aided in diagnosis of subacromial bursitis, rotator cuff tendonitis, and rotator cuff tendon tear (Figure 4–36).

Treatment for impingement syndrome starts with conservative measures such as activity modification, physical therapy, and administration of oral NSAIDs. Activity modification is necessary to minimize overhead arm motion and effect a return to normal overhead throwing biomechanics. Therapeutic modalities such as use of heat and cold, iontophoresis or phonophoresis, and microelectric nerve stimulation may also be helpful. Only with normal function of the rotator cuff tendons will glenohumeral mechanics be improved and the impingement syndrome cease. If this treatment fails, a subacromial injection of corticosteroids may be helpful. Nevertheless, few injections should be given, as multiple injections may cause weakening of the cuff tissue itself and predispose it to tearing.

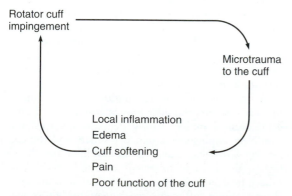

Figure 4–34. The cycle of injury and reinjury resulting from rotator cuff impingement.

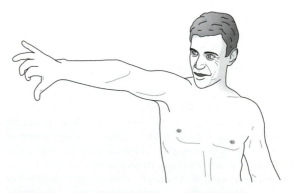

Figure 4–35. Evaluating for impingement of the supraspinatus tendon with the "empty can" test.

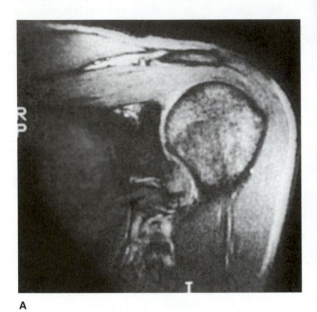

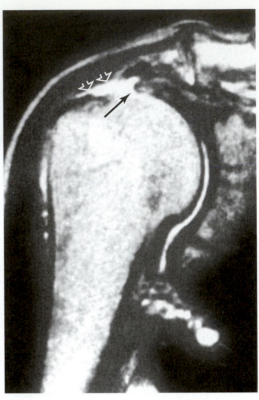

A   **B**

Figure 4–36. MRI demonstrating (**A**) normal shoulder anatomy and (**B**) cystic changes at the greater tuberosity with rotator cuff tear (*arrow*).

Surgical intervention is indicated only after failure of a prolonged conservative treatment program (a minimum of 3 months). If the subacromial space is narrow, release of the coracoacromial ligament combined with shaving the undersurface of the acromion may result in relief of symptoms. This procedure can be done arthroscopically to decrease postoperative discomfort and minimize the complication of deltoid muscle rupture from the acromion.

2. Rotator cuff tendonitis—Of the four rotator cuff muscles, the supraspinatus tendon is most often initially involved. Rotator cuff tendonitis also results from impingement syndrome and is characterized by pain with overhead activity. The patient may be occasionally awakened by pain at night. Active shoulder range of motion is limited by pain. Typically, no atrophy of the shoulder muscles is present, and manual muscle testing demonstrates mild weakness. The Neer impingement sign is positive, and the pain resolves with subacromial injection of lidocaine. Radiologic evaluation and treatment are similar to that for subacromial bursitis man-

agement. An exception is the young athlete with glenohumeral instability and secondary tendonitis. In this case, the instability should be treated first and the rotator cuff tendonitis will then resolve.

3. Rotator cuff tendon tear—A rotator cuff tendon tear most often results from impingement syndrome. Characterized by pain with overhead activity, the patient is often awakened at night with pain. The athlete with a chronic rotator cuff tear may describe a gradual loss of strength. Pain may be persistent, occurring even with the arm at the side.

Active range of shoulder motion is limited, and if the tear is severe, shoulder muscle atrophy will be evident. Manual muscle testing demonstrates weakness. The Neer impingement sign is positive, and the pain resolves with subacromial injection of lidocaine. Radiologic evaluation and treatment are similar to that for subacromial bursitis management. Unlike acute tears, chronic rotator cuff tears often present insidiously, with slow progression from subacromial bursitis to rotator cuff tendonitis and eventual tendon tear. Differentiating severe rotator cuff tendonitis from partial or small full-thickness chronic rotator cuff tears may be difficult.

Tears are most common at the humeral insertion site of the supraspinatus tendon, where stress is greatest with the joint in abduction. Tears may involve either the partial or full thickness of the tendon. The size may be small (< 1 cm), medium (1–3 cm), large (3–5 cm), or massive (> 5 cm). Chronic rotator cuff tears may result partly from degeneration within the rotator cuff tendon (Figure 4–37). Poor vascularity and repetitive activity, especially in the athlete with a restricted subacromial space, may be contributing factors. A minor traumatic event may also cause a full-thickness tear in an athlete with mild or moderate tendon degeneration.

If the tear is small, a prolonged period of rest, lasting 4–9 months, may relieve symptoms. Range-of-motion exercises are also recommended, unless they cause significant discomfort. If this fails to control the symptoms, surgical repair of the tear is recommended. The thin degenerated tissue of a chronic rotator cuff tear makes surgical repair more difficult than repair of an acute tear. Surgical decompression of the subacromial space to remove spurs should also be performed.

Rehabilitation lasts from 6 months to a year, with gradual exercise progression needed to restore normal, or near normal, function and strength. This varies with the tear size repaired and type of surgery performed. Typically, immediately after the procedure, passive motion and isometric strengthening exercises start, along with elbow, hand, and grip-strengthening exercises. At 6 weeks, the athlete may be able to begin low-intensity active strengthening exercises against gravity. The goals are to bring the athlete to normal strength with a functional, pain-free range of motion.

Although the lesion location and size is helpful in describing the rotator cuff tear, symptoms do not correlate with these factors alone. Both epidemiologic and imaging studies indicate a high incidence of partial-thickness rotator cuff tears at younger ages and a high incidence of full-thickness rotator cuff tears at older ages. Small full-thickness rotator cuff tears may be asymptomatic as long as the force couple of the anterior and posterior rotator cuff is preserved. Instead, a number of other factors influence the severity of symptoms, including: acute/chronic nature of injury; patient age; activity level; humeral head superior migration; shoulder muscle strength; arthritis; pain tolerance, and a claim for workman's compensation.

A partial articular-sided tendon avulsion is much more common than a bursal-sided tear of the rotator

ROTATOR CUFF TEARS

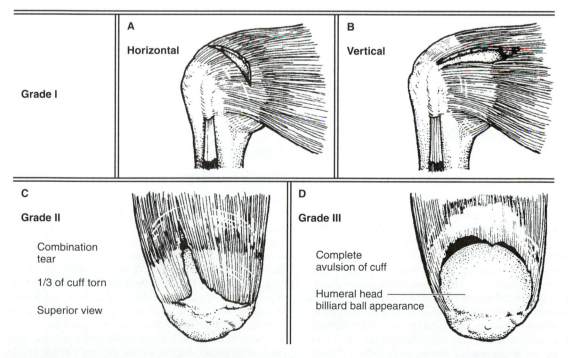

Figure 4–37. Classification of rotator cuff tears.

cuff. As with other rotator cuff injuries, symptoms may resolve with appropriate physical therapy and analgesics. Yet, some individuals with a partial-thickness tear have persistent or recurrent symptoms. If a conservative program of exercise and gradual return to activity does not lead to steady improvement, then further diagnostic evaluation with an ultrasonography, MRI, or arthroscopy may be helpful. Arthroscopic debridement of the abnormal cuff may promote healing in athletes with partial-thickness post-traumatic tears. Following debridement, immediate resumption of range-of-motion and muscle-strengthening exercises begins. Typically, it requires 6–12 months for a throwing athlete to return to athletics following arthroscopic debridement of a partial-thickness rotator cuff tear.

Budoff JE et al: Current concepts review. Debridement of partial thickness tears of the rotator cuff without acromioplasty. Long-term follow-up and review of the literature. J Bone Joint Surg Am 1998;80:733.

Gartsman GM et al: Arthroscopic repair of full-thickness tears of the rotator cuff. J Bone Joint Surg Am 1998;80:832.

Gartsman GM: Instructional course lecture. Combined arthroscopic and open treatment of tears of the rotator cuff. An outcome analysis. J Bone Joint Surg Am 1998;80:33.

Gerber C et al: The results of repair of massive tears of the rotator cuff. J Bone Joint Surg 2000;82A(4):505.

Jost B et al: Clinical outcome after structural failure of rotator cuff repairs. J Bone Joint Surg 2000;82A(3):304.

McKee MD, Yoo DJ: The effect of surgery for rotator cuff disease on general health status: Results of a prospective trial. J Bone Joint Surg 2000;82A(7):970.

Soslowsky LJ et al: Neer Award 1999: Overuse activity injures the supraspinatus tendon in an animal model: A histological and biomechanical study. J Shoulder Elbow Surg 2000;9(2):79.

Tifford C, Plancher K: Nonsurgical treatment of rotator cuff tears. In: Orthopaedic Knowledge Update, Shoulder and Elbow. Park Ridge, IL: AAOS; 1999; pp. 135–150.

2. Bicipital Tendinitis

The long head of the biceps muscle is an intra-articular structure deep in the rotator cuff tendon as it passes under the acromion to its insertion at the top of the glenoid. The same mechanism that initiates impingement syndrome symptoms in rotator cuff injuries may inflame the tendon of the biceps in its subacromial position, causing bicipital tendinitis. Tendinitis may also result from subluxation of the tendon out of its groove in the proximal humerus, which occurs with rupture of the transverse ligament. The symptoms of bicipital tendinitis, whether the result of impingement or tendon subluxation, are essentially the same. Pain is localized to the proximal humerus and shoulder joint, with resisted supination of the forearm aggravating the pain. Pain may also occur on manual testing of the elbow flexors and on palpation of the tendon itself. The Yergason test

is used to test for instability of the long head of the biceps in its groove.

If the tendinitis is associated with shoulder impingement, then therapy aimed at treating the impingement syndrome will relieve the bicipital tendinitis. If subluxation of the tendon within its groove is the cause of the irritation, conservative therapy includes administration of NSAIDs and restriction of activities, followed by a slow resumption of activities after a period of rest. Strengthening of the muscles that assist the biceps in elbow flexion and forearm supination is also beneficial. Steroid injections into the sheath of the biceps tendon are helpful, but they may be hazardous if placed into the substance of the tendon because they will promote tendon degeneration. Persistent symptoms may warrant tenodesis of the biceps tendon directly into the humerus. Recovery from this procedure is difficult, and it is doubtful if a competitive athlete could return to peak performance after such a procedure.

3. Pectoralis Major Rupture

Rupture of the pectoralis major tendon is an uncommon injury, usually occurring during bench press exercises in weight lifting caused by sudden unexpected muscle contraction during pulling or lifting. The athlete usually experiences sudden pain and develops local ecchymosis and swelling. As the swelling subsides, a sulcus and deformity may be visible, and the patient notices weakness of the arm in adduction and internal rotation. The rupture may be partial or complete, and nonoperative treatment usually results in satisfactory function for the activities of daily life. Surgery may be considered if the athlete wishes to return to heavy weight lifting.

Arciero RA, Cruser DL: Pectoralis major rupture with simultaneous anterior dislocation of the shoulder. J Shoulder Elbow Surg 1997;6:318.

4. Biceps Tendon Rupture

Clinical Findings

The long head of the biceps tendon may rupture proximally, either from the supraglenoid tubercle of the scapula at the entrance of the bicipital groove proximally or at the exit of the tunnel at the musculotendinous junction. The muscle mass moves distally, producing a bulging appearance to the arm. Rupture of the long head of the biceps is predictive of a rotator cuff tear. Rupture of the biceps distally involves both heads, and the muscle mass moves proximally. The mechanism is usually a forceful flexion of the arm and is more common in older athletes, or with direct trauma. Microtears probably serve to render the tendon vulnerable to an acute tearing event. The degree of ecchymosis is dependent on the location of the tear, with avascular areas having less and the musculotendinous junction producing quite a noticeable amount of ecchymosis. Diagnosis is usually easily accomplished because the deformity is obvious.

Treatment & Prognosis

Surgical treatment of proximal ruptures, if indicated, is usually reserved for younger patients. Open surgical repair leaves a long scar and usually does not completely restore the underlying anatomy. The coiled-up distal end of the tendon is usually found beneath the attachment of the pectoralis major. A correlation exists between proximal biceps tendon rupture and rotator cuff tears in middle-aged and older athletes. Rupture of the distal biceps tendon warrants surgical repair, regardless of age, due to loss of forearm flexion and supination strength. In this case, the tendon is usually found about 5–6 cm above the elbow joint, and care must be taken to avoid damage to the lateral antebrachial cutaneous nerve.

Berstein AD et al: Distal biceps tendon ruptures: A historical perspective and current concepts. Am J Sports Med 2001;30 (3):193.

Vardakas DG et al: Partial rupture of the distal biceps tendon. J Shoulder Elbow Surg 2001;10(4):377.

SHOULDER NEUROVASCULAR INJURY

1. Brachial Plexus Injury

Brachial plexus injuries are typically caused by a fall on the shoulder as seen in acromioclavicular joint injuries. Most brachial plexus injuries do not involve motor loss and exhibit paresthesias, which resolve in a period of minutes to weeks, although some cases may persist for months or years. Early in the course of the injury, a transient slowing of conduction across the plexus or a mild prolongation of nerve latency may be seen. The "burner" or "stinger" is one of the most common brachial plexus injuries encountered in athletes. The key to diagnosis is short duration of upper extremity paresthesias and shoulder weakness, with pain-free range of motion of the cervical spine. Players may return to competition after shoulder strength and full, pain-free range of motion has returned.

Rarely, a severe injury will occur (eg, from motorcycle racing). Chronic injuries result in instability of the shoulder that may be treated with trapezius transfer. Arthrodesis is an alternative, initially or after failed muscle transfer.

Alpar EK, Killampalli VV: Symptoms and signs of irritation of the brachial plexus in whiplash injuries. J Bone Joint Surg (Br) 2001;83B(6):931.

Feinberg JH: Burners and stingers. Phys Med Rehabil Clin North Am 2000;11(4):771.

2. Peripheral Nerve Injury

Long Thoracic Nerve Injury

Traction incidents may cause a long thoracic nerve palsy, with subsequent serratus anterior paralysis and winging of the scapula. Traction and blunt trauma may also cause injury to the spinal accessory nerve, another cause of winging of the scapula. These can be differentiated on physical examination by the position of the scapula. With serratus anterior palsy, the inferior portion of the scapula tends to go medially, whereas the opposite occurs with spinal accessory nerve palsy. Treatment is usually conservative, with return of function in weeks if the nerve has not been divided.

Aquino SL et al: Nerves of the thorax: Atlas of normal and pathologic findings. Radiographics 2001;21(5):1275.

Atasoy E, Majd M: Scapulothoracic stabilization for winging of the scapula using strips of autogenous fascia lata. J Bone Joint Surg (Br) 2000;82B(6):813.

Suprascapular Nerve Injury

Entrapment of the suprascapular nerve is often associated with activities such as weight lifting, baseball pitching, volleyball, and backpacking. Traction and repetitive shoulder use are the mechanisms of injury. Compression of the nerve may occur from entrapment at the anterior suprascapular notch of the scapula or at the level of the spinoglenoid notch. The latter occurs in volleyball players and baseball players and is likely caused by rapid overhead acceleration of the arm. Compression is associated with poorly localized pain and weakness in the posterolateral aspect of the shoulder girdle. This may be followed by atrophy of the supraspinatus or infraspinatus muscles. Eventually, forward flexion and external rotation of the shoulder is weakened. The diagnosis is confirmed by electromyography and nerve conduction studies.

Conservative therapy consists of rest, NSAIDs, and physical therapy designed to increase muscular tone and strength. If this is unsuccessful, then surgical exploration is indicated, which may reveal hypertrophy of the transverse scapular ligament, anomalies of the suprascapular notch, and ganglion cysts. Results of surgery vary with the lesion discovered, but many patients return to full function postoperatively.

Romeo AA et al: Suprascapular neuropathy. J Am Acad Orthop Surg 2001;7(6):372.

Shishido H, Kikuchi S: Injury to the suprascapular nerve in shoulder surgery: An anatomic study. J Shoulder Elbow Surg 2001;10(4):372.

Musculocutaneous Nerve Injury

This nerve is susceptible to direct frontal blows or surgical procedures. Injury is associated with numbness in the lateral forearm to the base of the thumb and weak to absent biceps muscle function. Most injuries seen in sports are transient and respond to conservative treatment in a matter of days to weeks.

Klepps SJ et al: Anatomic evaluation of the subcoracoid pectoralis muscle transfer in human cadavers. J Shoulder Elbow Surg 2001;10(5):453.

Axillary Nerve Injury

The usual mechanism of injury is trauma either by direct blow to the posterior aspect of the shoulder or following dislocation of the shoulder or fracture of the proximal humerus. Axillary nerve injury occurs in many sports such as football, wrestling, gymnastics, mountain climbing, rugby, and baseball. The degree of injury to the nerve varies because the initial presentation may be mild weakness during elevation and abduction of the arm with or without numbness of the lateral arm. The deltoid extension lag sign is indicative of axillary nerve injury. To perform this test the examiner elevates the arm into a position of near full extension and then releases the arm while asking the patient to hold the arm in this position. If the deltoids are completely paralyzed, the arm will drop. For partial nerve injuries, the magnitude of the angular drop, or lag, is an indicator of deltoid strength. Approximately 25% of all dislocated shoulder injuries are associated with axillary nerve traction injuries, which respond well to rest, physical therapy, and time. If recovery is not complete within 3–6 months, surgical intervention is recommended with exploration, utilizing neurolysis or grafting, or both, as necessary. Results of surgery are usually favorable, with sensory recovery occurring before motor recovery.

Hertel R et al: The deltoid extension lag sign for diagnosis and grading of axillary nerve palsy. J Shoulder Elbow Surg 1998;7 (2):97.

Steinmann SP, Moran EA: Axillary nerve injury: Diagnosis and treatment. J Am Acad Orthop Surg 2001;9(5):328.

3. Thoracic Outlet Syndrome

The symptoms resulting from thoracic outlet compression may be neurologic, venous, or arterial in nature. Obstruction of the subclavian vein may lead to stiffness, edema, and even thrombosis of the limb. Arterial obstruction may be the result of direct compression and manifests with pallor, coolness, and forearm claudication. Doppler ultrasound examination reveals changes in arterial and venous flow. Electromyography and nerve conduction studies are also helpful in diagnosis.

Nonoperative treatment is recommended for less severe forms of this syndrome and, once the pain subsides, an exercise program to strengthen the pectoral girdle muscles is beneficial. Special exercises to strengthen the upper and lower trapezius, along with the erector spinae and serratus anterior muscles, yield good results. Correcting poor posture and an ongoing maintenance program are mandatory once improvement is reached. Progression of symptoms or failure of nonoperative treatment are indications for surgical exploration and correction of the pathologic factors encountered.

Leffert RD: Thoracic outlet syndrome. J Am Acad Orthop Surg 1994;2:317.

■ ELBOW INJURIES

EPICONDYLITIS (TENNIS ELBOW)

Tennis elbow is an eponym given to many painful conditions about the elbow. An anatomic location may usually be found and specific diagnosis made.

Lateral Epicondylitis

Lateral tennis elbow involves the common tendon to the extensor muscles of the wrist and hand. Patients who perform repetitive wrist extension against resistance (such as the backhand stroke in tennis) are at risk. The pain they have is usually chronic in nature and more bothersome than disabling. Tenderness is located over the lateral humeral epicondyle, and pain is produced by extending the wrist against resistance. The tendon of the extensor carpi radialis brevis has been identified as the most common site of the lesion. Other causes for lateral elbow pain should be considered, including radiocapitellar arthritis and posterior interosseous nerve compression. Radiographs only rarely reveal soft-tissue calcification near the lateral humeral epicondyle, and MRI is of questionable aid in making the diagnosis.

Treatment includes decreasing specific activities and using a tennis elbow band to distribute the tension of the muscular pull over a larger area, thereby decreasing the force per unit area. A lighter racquet, smaller grip on the racquet, and correcting poor backhand technique are also helpful. Exercises to strengthen the wrist extensor muscles should be included in the treatment plan. If this approach fails, an injection of local anesthetic and cortisone into the most tender region is often curative. Surgical treatment is needed in recalcitrant cases. Multiple procedures have been described to take care of this malady. Commonplace in all procedures is release of the common extensor origin. Histologic studies of the afflicted tendon show degenerative changes with angiofibroblastic proliferation. These are thought to be similar to the pathologic changes of the torn rotator cuff, with diminished vascularity, an altered nutritional state, and tearing of the susceptible tendon.

Medial Epicondylitis

Medial epicondylitis involves the common flexor pronator origin. Treatment is similar to that for management of lateral tennis elbow. Ulnar nerve compression at the elbow may occur in conjunction with medial tennis elbow. In about 60% of the cases treated surgically, ulnar nerve compression was present. The common flexor origin is an important medial stabilizer of the elbow, so if surgical treatment is indicated, the debrided tendon should be reattached rather than released from the medial epicondyle.

Jobe FW, Ciccotti MG: Lateral and medial epicondylitis of the elbow. J Am Acad Orthop Surg 1994;2:1.

Kurvers H, Verhaar J: The results of operative treatment of medial epicondylitis. J Bone Joint Surg Am 1995;77:134.

Pasternack I et al: MR findings in humeral epicondylitis: A systematic review. Acta Radiol 2001;42:5434.

Stahl S, Kaufman T: The efficacy of an injection of steroids for medial epicondylitis: A prospective study of sixty elbows. J Bone Joint Surg (Am) 1997;79:1648.

ELBOW INSTABILITY

Rupture of the collateral ligaments of the elbow occurs most commonly from elbow dislocation. This can result from excessive valgus force, and initially the ulnar collateral ligament ruptures. Excessive posterolateral rotatory force may also result in rupture of the lateral ulnar collateral ligament. In either case, the elbow may dislocate, and typically the direction is posterior. Treatment after relocation and brief immobilization consists of active range-of-motion exercises. Recurrent instability is rare, and instead a small loss of elbow extension, usually less than 10 degrees, commonly results.

Valgus Instability

Valgus instability may result from overuse in overhead throwing sports such as baseball, football, and javelin throwing. With acute medial collateral ligament rupture, a pop may be felt during a throw. Tenderness is present on the medial side of the elbow, usually just distal to the medial epicondyle. Instability can then be appreciated when a valgus force is applied to the elbow. This must be done with the elbow flexed 20 degrees because failure to unlock the olecranon from within the olecranon fossa in full extension creates a false sense of stability. Comparison to the contralateral side aids in making the correct diagnosis. If the ulnar collateral ligament has been injured but remains intact, then the valgus stress test may elicit pain but no instability. Then the "milking maneuver" (Figure 4–38) will also elicit pain along the medial side of the elbow.

A stress radiograph may aid in making the diagnosis. An anteroposterior radiograph can be taken while the examiner performs the valgus stress test. Alternatively,

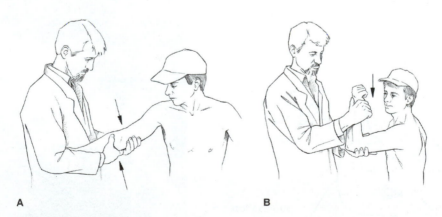

A　　　　　　　　　　　　　　　　　**B**

Figure 4–38. The valgus stress and milking maneuver tests for medial ulnar collateral ligament injury. (Reprinted, with permission, from Chen FS et al: Medial elbow problems in the overhead-throwing athlete. J Am Acad Orthop Surg 2001;9(2):102.)

gravity can be used to apply the valgus stress. For this, an anteroposterior radiograph of the elbow is taken with the shoulder externally rotated at 90 degrees with the elbow flexed at approximately 20 degrees. When instability is present, there will be a wider medial opening than on the contralateral normal side. MRI may also be useful, especially if an arthrogram is performed concurrently, as dye leaking through the ulnar collateral ligament is diagnostic of a rupture.

Surgical repair may be indicated in athletes engaged in sports requiring overhead throwing who suffer an acute rupture of their ulnar collateral ligament and still want to continue to participate in their sport. Soccer and basketball players and other athletes participating in sports that do not require overhead throwing may be treated with a program of early active range-of-motion exercises with the expectation of full return to their sport. Chronic ulnar collateral ligament injuries resulting from overuse are best treated with rehabilitation, NSAIDs, and avoidance of throwing for as long as 3 months. Only those with residual pain and instability after participation in such a program should undergo reconstruction of the anterior band of the ulnar collateral ligament. In this surgery, pioneered by Dr. Frank Jobe, the palmaris longus tendon is woven through drill holes in the medial humeral epicondyle and olecranon. Nearly 70 of athletes are able to return to highly competitive throwing after such surgery.

Chen FS et al: Medial elbow problems in the overhead-throwing athlete. J Am Acad Orthop Surg 2001;9(2):99.

Singh H et al: Valgus laxity of the ulnar collateral ligament of the elbow in collegiate athletes. Am J Sport Med 2001;29(5):558.

Thompson WH et al: Ulnar collateral ligament reconstruction in athletes: Muscle-splitting approach without transposition of the ulnar nerve. J Shoulder Elbow Surg 2001;10(2):152.

Posterolateral Rotatory Instability

Posterolateral rotatory instability of the elbow may result from a fall on the outstretched upper extremity, surgery of the lateral side of the elbow, or chronic varus stress as may occur in long-term crutch walkers. The instability covers a spectrum of severity from mild subluxation to recurrent dislocation. Those with mild forms complain of intermittent symptoms on the lateral side of the elbow associated with supination of the forearm, such as pain, snapping, or catching. More severe symptoms include locking or sensations of elbow instability. To perform the posterolateral rotatory instability test, a valgus stress is applied to the supinated elbow with the patient supine and the upper extremity over the head. Subluxation of the radial head occurs with the elbow in extension and resolves when the elbow is flexed. This maneuver also reproduces the patient's symptoms. A lateral stress radiograph, done with the elbow in extension as described for the posterolateral rotatory instability test, may also demonstrate the instability (Figure 4–39). Treatment for acute cases consists of an elbow brace to hold the forearm in pronation and restrict terminal elbow extension for 6 weeks. Chronic cases are best treated with reconstruction of the lateral ulnar collateral ligament. Postoperatively the patient is put in

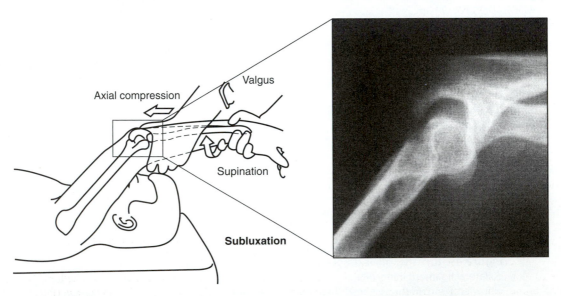

Figure 4–39. The posterolateral rotatory instability test reproduces the patient's symptoms

the same brace as used for acute posterolateral rotatory instability for 6–12 weeks.

O'Driscoll SW et al: Tardy posterolateral rotatory instability of the elbow due to cubitus varus. J Bone Joint Surg (Am) 2001; 83A(9):1358.

Smith JP et al: Posterolateral instability of the elbow. Clin Sports Med 2001;20(1):47.

OTHER ELBOW OVERUSE INJURIES

Posterior Elbow Impingement

Impingement may result from mechanical abutment of bone and soft tissues in the posterior elbow. This may or may not be associated with injury of the ulnar collateral ligament. Hyperextension injuries with an intact ulnar collateral ligament occur in gymnasts, football lineman, and weight lifters among others. The lesion is usually located in the center of the posterior elbow, and the pain is reproduced by forcible extension of the elbow. If the ulnar collateral ligament is insufficient, as is often the case when posterior elbow impingement occurs in athletes performing overhead-throwing maneuvers, the lesion is posteromedial. In this case, the impingement is between the medial aspect of the olecranon and the lateral side of the medial wall of the olecranon fossa (Figure 4–40). Pain may be reproduced with the valgus stress test as described in Figure 4–38 for valgus instability, but the pain is posteromedial and medial. Radiographs may demonstrate osteophytes of the olecranon of the olecranon fossa.

As with most injuries caused by repetitive trauma, treatment begins with prevention. The number of innings pitched is probably the most important factor relating to injury in baseball players. If symptoms persist, removal of osteophytes is successful, providing no ulnar collateral ligament injury is present. Treatment of the valgus instability is also required for successful outcome.

Moskal MJ et al: Arthroscopic treatment of posterior elbow impingement. Instr Course Lect 1999;48:399.

Fatigue Fracture of the Medial Epicondyle

In children, fatigue fractures of the medial epicondyle cause pain and swelling. This has been blamed on throwing curve balls, but some studies have shown that a properly thrown curve ball causes no more injuries than the traditional fast ball. Prevention or minimization of damage involves several steps. First, it is important to maintain proper conditioning by continuing pitching practice in the off-season or beginning the

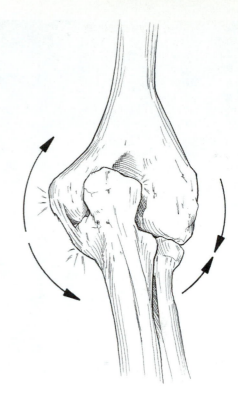

Figure 4–40. Mechanism of posteromedial impingement between the medial aspect of the olecranon and the lateral side of the medial wall of the olecranon fossa. (Reprinted, with permission, from Chen FS et al: Medial elbow problems in the overhead-throwing athlete. J Am Acad Orthop Surg 2001;9(2):105.)

baseball season slowly and progressively fashion. Second, pain and inflammation should be avoided, and if the elbow becomes painful, the athlete should stop throwing immediately. An accurate pitching count should be kept during a game, and a stopping point should be planned in advance. If the pitcher begins having pain or shows loss of control, pitching should be temporarily terminated and treatment to decrease the swelling and inflammation should begin. No competitive throwing is allowed until full range-of-motion returns and no pain or tenderness is associated with throwing.

Osteochondritis Dissecans of the Capitellum

Osteochondritis dissecans of the capitellum usually affects pitchers older than 10 years of age (Figure 4–41). Changes in the radiocapitellar joint are very worrisome

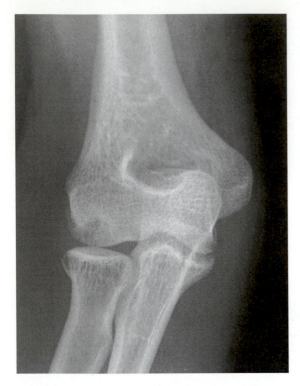

Figure 4–41. AP view of an elbow with osteochondritis dissecans of the capitellum.

because of possible permanent loss of function. If fragmentation occurs, loose bodies may require excision.

Stubbs MJ et al: Osteochondritis desiccans of the elbow. Clin Sports Med 2001;20(1):1.

■ SPINE INJURIES

CERVICAL SPINE INJURY

Cervical spine injuries in athletes are relatively infrequent, but the potential for serious injury to the nervous system exists. If spine injury is suspected, it is wise to be extremely cautious until a proper diagnosis can be made. This is the best way to prevent conversion of a repairable injury to a catastrophic outcome. Most often, a spine injury results from a collision and sometimes includes associated head injuries. The head and neck must be immobilized, the patency of the airway established, and level of consciousness ascertained immediately.

1. Brachial Plexus Neuropraxia

The most common cervical injury is pinching or stretching neuropraxia of the nerve root and brachial plexus. The injury is of short duration, and the patient has a full pain-free range of motion of the neck. These injuries are commonly called "stinger" or "burner" injuries. They result from lateral impact of the head and neck with simultaneous depression of the shoulder. This may cause stretching and pinching of the nerves of the brachial plexus, with burning pain, numbness, and tingling extending from the shoulder down into the hand and arms. Symptoms frequently involve the C5 and C6 root levels. Usually, recovery is spontaneous within a few minutes after the acute episode.

Patients who demonstrate full muscle strength of the intrinsic muscles of the shoulder and upper extremity and have full pain-free range of motion of the cervical spine may return to their activities. If they have residual weakness or numbness, they should not be allowed to re-enter the game. Absence of neck pain should alert one to the possibility of a cervical spine injury because neck pain is not part of the syndrome.

Persistence of paresthesia or weakness requires further evaluation, including neurologic, electromyographic, and radiographic methods, before allowing the athlete to return to play. The athlete should not participate in contact sports until full muscle strength has been achieved and a repeat electromyogram shows evidence of axonal regeneration, usually at least 4–6 weeks.

Stinger injuries are prevented chiefly through correct head and neck techniques and strengthening of the neck musculature. Additionally, the use of cervical rolls may eliminate extremes of motion during impact.

2. Cervical Strain

Acute strains of the muscles of the neck are probably the most frequent cervical injuries in athletes. The word *strain* implies injury to a muscle, whereas a sprain is a ligamentous injury. A strain happens when a muscletendon unit is overloaded or stretched. The clinical picture is common to all musculotendinous injuries. Motion of the neck becomes painful, reaching a peak after several hours or the next day. NSAIDs, heat, massage, and other therapeutic modalities are beneficial.

3. Cervical Sprain

In a cervical sprain, the ligamentous and capsular structure connecting the facet joints and vertebra have been damaged. This condition is often difficult to differentiate from a strain. Movement is limited, and the area of the injury and along the muscle groups overlying the area of the injury are painful. Ligamentous disruption may be extensive enough to result in instability with associated neurologic involvement. Routine cervical spine radiographs are indicated. In those athletes with diminished motion as well as pain, stability of the cervical spine should be documented. This may be done with flexion and extension radiographs.

Treatment of a cervical sprain consists of immobilization, rest, support, and NSAIDs. Return to participation is permitted when motion and muscle strength normalize.

4. Cervical Spinal Cord Neuropraxia with Transient Tetraplegia

The phenomenon of cervical spinal cord neuropraxia with transient tetraplegia is a distinct clinical entity. Sensory changes include a burning pain, numbness, tingling, or loss of sensation. Motor changes include weakness or complete paralysis, which is usually transient, with complete recovery occurring in 10–15 min, although in some cases gradual resolution occurs over 36–48 h. Complete motor function and full pain-free cervical motion returns. Routine radiographs of the cervical spine are negative for fractures or dislocations. Some radiographic findings include spinal stenosis, congenital fusions, cervical instability, and intervertebral disk disease. To determine whether cervical spinal stenosis is present, the anteroposterior diameter of the spinal canal is measured, and this figure is divided by the anteroposterior diameter of the vertebral body (Figure 4–42). If the ratio is less than 0.80, stenosis is present.

Athletes who have suffered transient tetraplegia are not known to be at any greater risk for permanent tetraplegia. Patients who have this syndrome and associated instability of the cervical spine or cervical disk disease should be precluded from further participation in contact sports. Those who have spinal stenosis alone should be treated on an individual basis.

More severe injuries, including fractures and dislocation of the cervical spine, may occur. Treatment of these begins on the playing field, with immobilization of the spine. A face mask, if worn, may be cut off with bolt cutters. After thoroughly stabilizing the spine, the patient is moved to a spine board. Sandbags are used to immobilize the head and neck. The patient may then be transported to a local emergency room for further evaluation and treatment. Fractures and dislocations with or without permanent neurologic injury are treated like other spine injuries.

Torg JS et al: The relationship of developmental narrowing of the cervical spinal canal to reversible and irreversible injury of the cervical spinal cord in football players. An epidemiological study. J Bone Joint Surg Am 1996;78:1308.

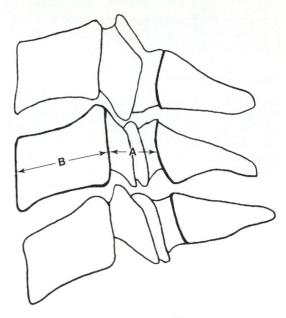

Figure 4–42. The ratio of the spinal canal to the vertebral body is the distance from the midpoint of the posterior aspect of the vertebral body to the nearest point on the corresponding spinolaminar line (**A**) divided by the anteroposterior width of the vertebral body (**B**). (Reproduced, with permission, from Torg JS et al: Neuropraxia of the cervical spinal cord with transient quadriplegia. J Bone Joint Surg (Am) 1986;68:1354.)

Torg JS et al: Neuropraxia of the cervical spinal cord with transient quadriplegia. J Bone Joint Surg Am 1986;68:1354.

LUMBAR SPINE INJURY

Clinical Findings

Spondylolysis is a disruption of the pars interarticularis, whereas spondylolisthesis involves anterior slippage of one vertebral body over the next. Spondylolysis is most often found at L5 and L4 but may occasionally be seen at L3 and L2. It is believed to result from repeated stress around the pars interarticularis during hyperextension of the lumbar spine. If continued hyperextension activity occurs, spondylolysis may become spondylolisthesis. Sports in which spondylolisthesis is commonly found include gymnastics, football, and weight lifting. Teenage female gymnasts, for example, often have back pain but normal radiographs. Approximately 3–6 weeks later, a stress response may be seen around the pars interarticularis, with increased density developing. At this time, the bone scan will be positive, indicating an impending stress fracture that will show up on plain radiographs in 2–4 weeks. A physician who is aware of which sports put stress on the pars inter-articularis should consider a bone scan to rule out spondylolisthesis.

Treatment & Prognosis

The treatment of spondylolisthesis involves cessation of all aggravating sports and other actions producing spinal hyperextension. A certain percentage of these fractures will heal spontaneously. Healing time for spondylolysis of the lumbar spine is usually about 6 months. If after that period of time no significant signs of healing are apparent, it is unlikely that sponta-neous healing will take place. At this point, spinal fusion should be considered, or the patient should be willing to confine his or her activities to less stressful, pain-free sports.

Many patients with spondylolisthesis engage in high-level sporting activities without significant pain or neurologic deficit. Only a small percentage actually present for evaluation and care. Complete evaluation and treatment recommendations for spondylolisthesis and spondylolysis are found in the section on the spine.

Muschik M et al: Competitive sports and the progression of spon-dylolisthesis. J Pediatr Orthop 1996;16:364.

Disorders, Diseases, & Injuries of the Spine

5

Serena S. Hu, MD, Clifford B. Tribus, MD, Bobby K-B Tay, MD, & Gregory D. Carlson, MD

■ OSTEOMYELITIS OF THE SPINE

Osteomyelitis of the spine constitutes approximately 1% of all cases of pyogenic skeletal infections. Pathogenic organisms can infect the vertebra, the intervertebral disc, or the spinal canal from multiple mechanisms including local spread from an adjacent infection or as a result of seeding from a noncontiguous source of infection either hematogenously or through the lymphatics. Bacteria can also be introduced directly to compromised tissues as a result of trauma, surgery, discography, or intravenous or intradural catheterization. Although many organisms have been implicated, the most frequently cultured organisms are *Staphylococcus aureus* and *Pseudomonas aeruginosa*. *Salmonella* should be strongly considered as a potential pathogen in patients with sickle cell disease, and infection with *Mycobacterium tuberculosis* is often seen in less developed countries and in prison populations. Spinal sepsis is most common in adolescents, the elderly, intravenous drug abusers, patients with diabetes or renal failure, and patients who have undergone spinal surgery. Osteoporosis has also been implicated as a predisposing factor secondary to increased blood flow. Eismont and Bohlman reported several risk factors for neurologic deterioration, including patients with diabetes, rheumatoid arthritis, steroid use, age older than 50 years, a cephalad level of infection, and infection with *Staphylococcus aureus*.

Clinical Findings

A. SYMPTOMS AND SIGNS

Patients with osteomyelitis of the spine may or may not present with symptoms relating to their spine. Pyogenic osteomyelitis is fundamentally different from tubercular osteomyelitis. In the latter, patients generally complain of indolent, chronic back pain. In pyogenic osteomyelitis, the symptoms of acute spontaneous back pain, fever, and weight loss are common but are not always present. On physical examination, patients with discitis or pyogenic osteomyelitis of the spine often ex-

hibit significant percussion tenderness posteriorly over the affected vertebral segments. Paraspinal muscle spasm may be seen is over 90% of patients. A history of fevers is found in less than 50% of affected patients. Neurologic involvement, fortunately, affects less than 10% of all patients with spinal infections. When the infection involves the cervical spine, patients may develop a Horner's syndrome, or dysphagia. Pyogenic osteomyelitis should be suspected in any patient that presents with back pain and a recent history of an acute systemic infection (eg, appendicitis, perinephritic abscess, pneumonia, genitourinary tract infection, or meningitis).

B. LABORATORY STUDIES

The results of laboratory tests can be equivocal. The white cell count will be elevated in only 42% of patients and often will be normal. Both blood and spinal cultures may also be negative. Blood cultures are accurate in only 25% of cases and closed biopsy techniques are diagnostic in only 70% of cases. The sedimentation rate is usually elevated in over 90% of patients, and the C-reactive protein level will also be elevated at an earlier timepoint in the infectious process. However, both of these tests are systemic indicators of inflammation and are relatively nonspecific. Thus, there is often a significant delay in diagnosis because many of the signs and symptoms of pyogenic vertebral osteomyelitis are subtle. Clearly, the diagnosis relies on having a high index of suspicion in at-risk patients as well as initiating the appropriate evaluation that will identify the organism and determine the extent of infection.

C. IMAGING STUDIES

Radiographic signs of osteomyelitis typically lag behind symptomatic progression of the disease. Magnetic resonance imaging (MRI) with vascular-based contrast enhancement (gadolinium) has become the gold standard for early neurodiagnostic imaging. Radiographic findings may appear normal.

In pyogenic osteomyelitis, early radiographic changes may include loss of disc space height, erosion of the vertebral end plates, and vertebral destruction and collapse (Figure 5–1). In advanced cases, the vertebral bodies

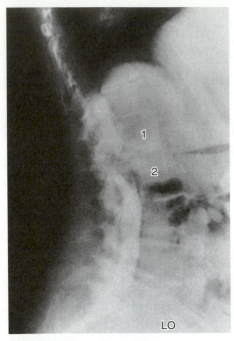

A

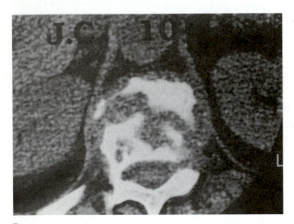

B

Figure 5–1. Imaging studies in patients with osteomyelitis of the spine. **A:** Radiograph showing an epidural abscess and advanced collapse between L1 and L2. **B:** CT scan showing destruction of the vertebral body.

may become fused due to the inflammation and destruction of the intervertebral disc.

In tubercular osteomyelitis, radiographic studies typically demonstrate anterior vertebral body destruction with sparing of the intervertebral disc. Loss of bone stability in the cervical or thoracic spine may lead to kyphotic deformity and paralysis. Progression to solid fusion may occur but usually later than that seen in pyogenic osteomyelitis.

Treatment

Early diagnosis and identification of the responsible organism is the cornerstone of treatment. Once the organism has been confirmed by biopsy or blood culture, appropriate intravenous antibiotics should be initiated and continued for at least 6 weeks. Short-term bed rest for pain management is appropriate. Spinal column bracing is often necessary for pain relief, immobilization of the affected segments, and to minimize the progression of spinal deformity. Success of nonoperative treatment has been linked to patient age less than 60 years, immunocompetency, infection with *Staphylococcus aureus,* and a decreasing erythrocyte sedimentation rate with appropriate medical treatment. Indications for surgery other than tissue diagnosis include moderate to advanced destruction of the spine with instability, neurologic compromise, sequestrum formation, and failure to respond to intravenous antibiotics. Paraspinal abscesses may be managed conservatively with intravenous antibiotics unless the patient meets one of the above-mentioned surgical criteria.

Pediatric discitis often responds to spinal column bracing, immobilization, and rest. Although controversial, antibiotic therapy in the pediatric discitis patient appears to improve nonoperative resolutions of symptoms.

The incidence of epidural abscesses may be on the rise, associated with older patients and chronic illness. Epidural abscesses are best treated with early recognition, antibiotic therapy, and immediate surgical decompression. Preoperative paralysis and neurologic deterioration are poor prognostic factors of the disease. MRI is as sensitive as myelography with computed tomography. For diagnostic purposes, MRI offers the advantage of being noninvasive and being able to delineate other disease entities, making it the imaging modality of choice.

For surgical candidates with osteomyelitis or discitis, the treatment of choice consists of anterior surgical debridement and stabilization with an autogenous structural bone graft. Often posterior instrumentation and spinal fusion over the affected segments is necessary to prevent collapse of the anterior graft and to prevent late deformity. Foreign bodies, such as methylmethacrylate, are relatively contraindicated in spinal stabilization. However, antibiotic impregnated polymethylmethacrylate cement used as a temporary spacer may be useful in grossly contaminated sites. New minimally invasive surgical techniques that use laparoscopy and thoracoscopy appear to be an excellent alternative for operative management of spinal infections. These techniques employ similar surgical principles with expanding surgeon experience, and a thorough decompression of the spinal canal is not currently possible with the minimally invasive technique.

Carragee EJ: Pyogenic vertebral osteomyelitis. J Bone Joint Surg Am 1997;79:874.

Emery SE et al: Treatment of hematogenous pyogenic vertebral osteomyelitis with anterior debridement and primary bone grafting. Spine 1989;14:284.

Eismont FJ et al: Pyogenic and fungal vertebral osteomyelitis with paralysis. J Bone Joint Surg Am, 1983;65(1):19.

Glazer PA, Hu SS: Pediatric spinal infections. Orthop Clin North Am 1996;27:111.

Graziano GP, Sidhu KS: Salvage reconstruction in acute and late sequelae from pyogenic thoracolumbar infection. J Spinal Disord 1993;6:199.

Hlavin ML et al: Spinal epidural abscess: A 10-year perspective. Neurosurgery 1990;27:177.

Kornblum MB et al: Computed tomography-guided biopsy of the spine. A review of 103 patients. Spine 1998;23(1):81.

Parker LM et al: Minimally invasive surgical techniques to treat spine infections. Orthop Clin North Am 1996;27:183.

Ring D et al: Pyogenic infectious spondylitis in children: The convergence of discitis and vertebral osteomyelitis. J Pediatr Orthop 1995;15:652.

Sampath P, Rigamonti D: Spinal epidural abscess: A review of epidemiology, diagnosis, and treatment. J Spinal Disord 1999; 12(2):89.

■ TUMORS OF THE SPINE

PRIMARY TUMORS OF THE SPINE

Primary tumors of the spine account for 0.04% of all tumors and 10% of all primary tumors of bone. The overwhelming majority of spinal tumors are metastatic. As with tumors elsewhere in the musculoskeletal system, primary lesions in the spine may be osteogenic, chondrogenic, fibrogenic, hematopoietic, neurogenic, or vascular. Generally, benign tumors typically occur in the younger age group (< 21 y), whereas up to 70% of malignant tumors are found in patients older than 21 years of age.

Principles of Diagnosis

A. History and Physical Examination

If the presence of a spinal tumor is suspected, a thorough history and physical examination must be performed. Pain is the common presenting symptom. Persistent pain, especially at night, is the chief complaint in more than 80% of cases. The average time from onset of symptoms until diagnosis in patients with benign lesions is 19 months, whereas that in patients with metastatic disease is 4 months. The age of the patient is important in establishing the differential diagnosis. In adults, malignant lesions of bone occur twice as frequently as benign lesions. In children younger than 10 years, however, only 15–20% of tumors are malignant. Location within the spinal column also aids in establishing the diagnosis. Although 75% of tumors located in the vertebral bodies or pedicles are malignant, only 35% of those in the posterior elements are malignant.

On examination, the patient may complain of tenderness over the involved region of the spine. Although rare initially, radiculopathy secondary to nerve root compression may be the only finding. Signs and symptoms may mimic a herniated nucleus pulposus and may progress to localized weakness, sensory loss, and bowel or bladder dysfunction. Up to 70% of patients may develop motor weakness by the time the diagnosis is made. Pathologic fractures may present with acute onset of pain and paraparesis. Examination of the spine may reveal scoliosis, as occurs with osteomas or osteoblastomas, or may reveal a painful kyphosis.

B. Imaging Studies

The workup begins with high-quality plain radiographs, followed by computed tomographic (CT) scanning, radioisotope bone scanning, and MRI as necessary. The routine anteroposterior (AP) view may reveal the presence of the so-called winking owl sign, which is indicative of early pedicle destruction. As with other bony tumors, the more slowly expanding bony tumors of the spine are well circumscribed with reactive ossification. More aggressive lesions have a "moth-eaten" or erosive appearance. It is important to realize that radiographic evidence of bony destruction is not apparent until 30–50% of the trabecular bone has been lost. Vertebral collapse with preservation of the disc space is a common finding.

Early on it is often difficult on plain radiographs to distinguish a neoplastic process from an infectious one. Technetium bone scans are an accurate and sensitive modality for detecting metastatic disease. False-positive results are acceptably low and are usually a result of osteoarthritis. If the osteoblastic response is impaired, as in multiple myeloma or in highly lytic lesions, false-negative results may occur. However, with the advent of MRI, bone scanning has been largely limited in its usefulness to staging of the tumor.

CT scanning with or without myelography is of great benefit in detecting and evaluating osseous lesions and dural impingement. CT scanning also allows an accurate assessment of the extent of bony destruction to help in preoperative planning. Evaluation of soft tissue and marrow has improved immensely with the advent of MRI. Tumor resolution is outstanding (Figure 5–2), and preoperative planning is greatly enhanced.

Arteriography enables the surgeon to evaluate the vascular supply to the tumor and the extent of vascular neogenesis. Highly vascular tumors such as metastatic renal cell tumors, thyroid carcinoma, hemangiosarcoma, and aneurysmal bone cysts are well visualized. Partial or complete embolization of highly vascular tumors may make operative resection significantly easier and safer. In addition, identification of feeder vessels in tumors in the lower thoracic spine may help to identify possible vascular supply to the tumor from the artery of Adamkiewicz. Inappropriate ligation of this major vessel may result in spinal cord ischemia and paralysis.

MRI is the method of choice for diagnosing and evaluating primary neoplasms of the spine. Its advantages include superior soft-tissue visualization, the availability of multiplanar images, and its ability to evaluate the extent of neural compression or infiltration.

C. BIOPSY

An open or closed percutaneous biopsy may be necessary for establishing the diagnosis. If the workup is consistent with a benign symptomatic tumor such as an osteoid osteoma, an excisional biopsy may be appropriate. When malignancy is suspected, needle biopsy should be performed prior to resection. Because the accuracy rate for needle biopsy is 75% or less, several specimens should be obtained. Open biopsy is necessary if aspiration is nondiagnostic.

D. SURGICAL TREATMENT

The surgical treatment of spinal tumors depends on (1) biologic tumor type, (2) location within the spine, (3) percentage of vertebral involvement, (4) neurologic involvement, (5) potential for spine failure and instability, and (6) anticipated life expectancy of the patient.

If removal of the tumor is necessary, the surgeon must determine the best approach for excision. Tumoral excision can be broadly categorized into intralesional and en-bloc excision. Curettage describes the piecemeal removal of the tumor and is always considered to be intralesional. En-bloc excision is an attempt to remove the entire tumor, which on pathologic examination can be intralesional, marginal, or wide, in one piece. If the surgeon has cut into the tumor mass, the excision is intralesional. Marginal excision occurs when the tumor has been removed by dissection along its pseudocapsule. Wide excision is accomplished if the tumor is removed along with a continuous shell of normal tissue.

Barbieri E et al: Radiotherapy in vertebral tumors. Indications and limits: A report on 28 cases of Ewing's sarcoma of the spine. Chir Organi Mov 1998;83:105.

Boriani S et al: Primary bone tumors of the spine—Terminology and surgical staging. Spine 1997;22(9):1036.

Perrin RG, McBroom RJ: Thoracic spine tumors. Clin Neurosurg 1992;38:353.

Shi HB et al: Preoperative transarterial embolization of spinal tumor: embolization techniques and results. AJNR 1999;20 (10):2009.

Weinstein JN, McLain RF: Primary tumors of the spine. Spine 1987;12:843.

Weinstein JN, McLain RF: Tumors of the spine. In Rothman RH, Simeone FA (editors): The Spine, 4th ed. Philadelphia: WB Saunders, 1998.

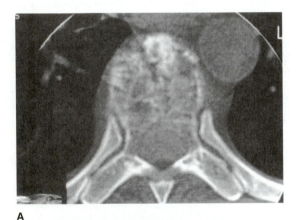

A

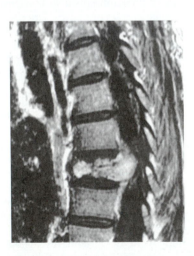

B

Figure 5–2. Imaging studies in a patient with a hemangioendothelioma. **A:** CT scan showing the tumor invading the spinal canal. **B:** MRI of the thoracic spine, demonstrating tumor extension.

1. Benign Tumors

Benign primary tumors of the spine include osteoid osteoma, osteoblastoma, osteochondroma, aneurysmal bone cyst, hemangioma, eosinophilic granuloma, and giant cell tumor.

Osteoid Osteoma

Osteoid osteoma and osteoblastoma are osteoblastic lesions that are differentiated from each other by size. Lesions that are smaller than 2 cm are arbitrarily named osteoid osteomas, and those larger than 2 cm are called osteoblastomas. Osteoid osteoma affects males more frequently than females and is generally seen in patients between the ages of 10 and 20 years. This benign tumor is usually located in the posterior elements and most frequently involves the lumbar spine, followed by the cervical and then the thoracic spine.

The patient presents with a complaint of a progressive localized ache that may or may not have a radicular component but is usually relieved by the use of salicylates. Tenderness, muscle spasm, neurologic abnormalities, and even scoliosis may be present on examination. Torticollis may be associated with scoliosis of the cervical spine. Pelvic tilt may be seen in conjunction with lumbar spine scoliosis. Minimal correctability is seen with side bending. In the majority of cases, the tumor is located on the concave side of the curve.

Osteoid osteomas appear radiographically as a nidus surrounded by densely sclerotic bone. Tumors that grow close to the periosteum may cause a fusiform thickening of the overlying cortex secondary to hyperemia. Both the nidus and periosteal reaction can sometimes be seen on plain radiographs but is most easily delineated on the axial cuts of a CT scan.

Although spontaneous resolution has been reported in some cases, treatment of osteoid osteoma generally requires thorough local excision of the lesion because recurrence is likely. Indications for surgical excision include pain that is unresponsive to medical treatment, neurologic compromise, and progressive enlargement of the tumor mass. Spinal fusion is usually not indicated at the time of excision. In most cases, any scoliosis present preoperatively will improve over the next 6–12 months. If the scoliosis is severe (> 40 degrees) or the spine has been rendered unstable by resection of the articular facets and pedicle, fusion should be considered.

Osteoblastoma

Osteoid osteomas that have grown larger than 2 cm are called osteoblastomas. Benign osteoblastomas account for fewer than 1% of all bone tumors. Although cases are rare, more than 40% of them involve the spine, and half of these spinal cases are associated with scoliosis. Osteoblastomas are more common in males than females and are seen most frequently in patients younger than 30 years.

Patients generally complain of localized pain or scoliosis. Fifty-three percent of spinal osteoblastomas are found in the lumbar spine and the rest were equally distributed in the thoracic and cervical spine.

Radiographic examination may reveal an expanded, sclerotic cortex, although there are no classic characteristics. Rarely is the lesion lobulated. The posterior elements and pedicles are more frequently involved than the vertebral body. Vertebral involvement almost always occurs due to secondary expansion from the pedicle and an associated soft-tissue mass may be present.

Curettage can offer a high rate of disease remission when the lesions are well contained within the vertebral bone. Wide excision of the lesion is always curative and may also provide reliable pain relief and resolution of the spinal deformity. However, marginal excision is safer and also provides an excellent cure rate. Thus marginal excision is the treatment of choice for these tumors. Even partial excision may offer symptom resolution if the nidus is removed. This can be aided by the use of adjuvant radiotherapy. The local recurrence rate can be up to 10% for some osteoblastomas, but malignant degeneration is a rare occurrence.

Osteochondroma

Osteochondromas result when metaplastic cartilage cells in the periosteum undergo progressive endochondral ossification. Multiple osteochondromatosis is the most common of all skeletal dysplasias, and about 7% of these patients have vertebral involvement. Spinal cord compression may occur and is the main indication for excision, which is almost always curative

Aneurysmal Bone Cyst

Aneurysmal bone cysts result from an expansile hyperemic osteolytic process that erodes through bone. Approximately 80% of patients are under the age of 20. Twelve to thirty percent of these neoplasms occur in the spine, especially the lumbar areas. The tumor involves the posterior elements 60% of the time. Symptoms and signs include a rapid evolution of pain in the spine and radiculopathy. Radiographs reveal the presence of an osteolytic tumor with poor demarcation, peripheral ballooning, and cortical erosion with osseous septa within its substance. Like the chordoma but unlike most other tumors, the aneurysmal bone cyst may cross the intervertebral space. Scoliosis or kyphosis may be present.

The differential diagnosis includes giant cell tumors and cavernous hemangiomas. Giant cell tumors usually occur in an older patient population and tend to involve the sacrum. Cavernous hemangiomas are usually located in the vertebral body.

Appropriate treatment of aneurysmal bone cysts requires an understanding that it may arise from or coexist with a pre-existing neoplasm. For the isolated lesion the treatment of choice for aneurysmal bone cyst is aggressive debulking. If the size and location of the tumor preclude complete surgical removal, incomplete curettage can be undertaken and usually eradicates the lesion. Bone grafting is often necessary. Spinal instrumentation, fusion, or both may be necessary, depending on the extent of the lesion.

Profound hemorrhage is a risk with primary surgical resection and may be controlled with preoperative embolization. Although aneurysmal bone cysts are sensitive to radiation, complications of irradiation-induced myelopathy and sarcoma have been noted.

Hemangioma

Hemangioma, a common tumor of the vertebral column, arises from embryonic angioblastic tissue. They comprise about 7% of all benign tumors. It is much more common in females than in males and has a predilection for the lower thoracic and upper lumbar spine.

Hemangiomas are frequently asymptomatic. In some cases, they are found serendipitously on screening radiographs. In other cases, they are associated with a compression fracture, with the patient presenting with pain and neurologic symptoms. Radiographically, they present with classic vertebral striations resulting from the abnormally thickened bony trabeculae. CT scans easily delineate the lesion, and MRI shows high signal intensity on T_2-weighted images and low signal intensity on T_1-weighted images.

If the patient presents with pain without neurologic deficit, low-dose irradiation is extremely effective in ameliorating the symptoms. If the patient shows signs of neurologic dysfunction, treatment should consist of anterior decompression, mass excision, and anterior fusion. Preoperative embolization of the feeding artery may facilitate surgical management.

Eosinophilic Granuloma (Langerhans' Cell Histiocytosis)

Eosinophilic granuloma is a proliferative disorder of the Langerhans' cells that is commonly seen in young children younger than age 10 years and rarely in adults. The disease has a male preponderance. Vertebral involvement is seen in 7–15% of cases and typically presents with the sudden onset of neck pain and torticollis.

Patients frequently present with localized pain. Spinal cord compression is a rare but reported event.

Eosinophilic granuloma can present with a spectrum of radiographic manifestations depending on the stage of the tumor. Early on, the tumor presents as a central, lytic lesion with poorly defined margins. On plain radiographs, permeative bony destruction is evident, with a marked periosteal reaction. At this stage, the tumor is difficult to distinguish from a high-grade sarcoma such as Ewing's sarcoma. Later in the evolution of the tumor, vertebral body collapse occurs, leading to a flattening the vertebral bone between the adjacent intact discs. This phenomenon results in the classic "coin on end" appearance and "vertebra plana."

The differential diagnosis includes Ewing's sarcoma and infection, and biopsy may be necessary to confirm the diagnosis.

Eosinophilic granuloma usually resolves spontaneously. If the patient suffers from disseminated Langerhans' cell histiocytosis, chemotherapy may be appropriate. Local infiltration with corticosteroids has been of some benefit. Low-dose irradiation (500–1000 rads) is used in cases associated with neurologic compromise. The use of anterior decompression and anterior fusion is the treatment of choice in patients with neurologic symptoms.

Giant Cell Tumor

Giant cell tumors constitute about 10% of all primary bone tumors. These tumors occur in people between the ages of 20 and 40, with a slight female predominance (70.8%). Spinal involvement is seen in patients in the third and fourth decades of life. This tumor is locally aggressive and presents most commonly in the anterior vertebral structures. The presenting complaint is typically pain; however, as many as 50% of patients may present with neurologic deficits. Plain radiographs will show a lytic lesion with matrix calcification and sclerosis. Aggressive surgical curettage or en-bloc excision depending on the location and extent of tumor yield the best results. Because of the risk of sarcomatous transformation, radiation therapy should be reserved for patients with incomplete excision or local recurrence. The recurrence rate is higher in those patients with soft-tissue extension, anterior and posterior tumor, and spinal canal involvement.

Beer SJ: Primary tumors of the spine in children. Natural history, management and long-term follow-up. Spine 1997;22(6): 649.

Biorani S et al: Osteoblastoma of the spine. Clin Orthop 1992; 278:37.

Hart RA et al: A system for surgical staging and management of spine tumors. A clinical outcome study of giant cell tumors of the spine. Spine 1997;22(15):1773.

Kak VJ et al: Solitary osteochondroma of the spine causing spinal cord compression. Clin Neurol Neurosurg 1985;87:135.

Mammano S et al: Cast and brace treatment of eosinophilic granuloma of the spine: Long-term follow-up. J Pediatr Orthop 1997;17:821.

Papagelopoulos PJ et al. Aneurysmal bone cyst of the spine. Management and outcome. Spine. 1998;23:621.

Sanjay BK et al: Giant-cell tumors of the spine. J Bone Joint Surg Br 1993;75 (1):148.

Shikata J et al: Surgical treatment of giant cell tumors of the spine. Clin Orthop 1992;278:29.

Weinstein JN, McLain RF: Primary tumors of the spine. Spine 1987;12:843.

Weinstein JN, McLain RF: Tumors of the spine. In Rothman RH, Simeone FA (editors): The Spine, 4th ed. Philadelphia: WB Saunders, 1992.

2. Malignant Tumors

Primary malignant tumors of the spine are rare and carry a poor prognosis. Multiple myeloma is the most common. Osteosarcoma, Ewing's sarcoma, chondrosarcoma, and chordoma occur much less frequently.

Solitary Plasmacytoma & Multiple Myeloma

Multiple myeloma and solitary plasmacytoma are B-cell lymphoproliferative diseases composed of abnormal aggregates of plasma cells. The neoplasm has a peak occurrence between the ages of 50 and 60, with an equal sex distribution. Multiple myeloma is a multifocal plasma cell cancer of the osseous system whose neoplastic cells produce complete or incomplete immunoglobulins. The annual incidence of myeloma is about 2–3 per 100,000 among the general population. Genetic analysis of the tumor cells have demonstrated abnormalities in band q32 of chromosome 14. The diagnosis is made on serum and urine evaluation for abnormal immunoglobulin levels. Serum protein electrophoresis will show increases in the levels of one of the immunoglobulin classes. The M-component is IgG in 55% of cases, IgA in 25% of cases, and rarely IgE, IgD, or IgM. Urine protein electrophoresis may detect the presence of immunoglobulin light chains called Bence-Jones proteins in up to 99% of patients. In 60% of patients afflicted with multiple myeloma, both Bence-Jones proteins and abnormal serum immunoglobulin levels will be detected.

The initial treatment of myeloma consists of chemotherapy and irradiation. Chemotherapy is an effective means of controlling the advancement of the disease process but may increase the risk of secondary leukemia. The commonly employed agents include melphalan and prednisone. Newer agents such as gallium nitrate may attenuate the rate of skeletal bone loss from the disease and from steroid treatment. Radiation to affected osseous sites may reduce pain and prevent vertebral collapse, deformity, and neural compression. Patients with solitary plasmacytoma have a 5-year survival rate of 60%. In contrast, patients with multiple myeloma have only an 18% 5-year survival rate and a median survival of 24 months.

Osteosarcoma

Primary osteosarcoma is a malignant tumor of mesenchymal cells characterized by the direct formation of osteoid or bone by the tumor cells. After myeloma, it is the second most common primary neoplasm of bone. Most appear in persons younger than 20 years before epiphyseal closure. There is a slight male preponderance. In a series of osteosarcoma cases, Barwick noted that 1–2% arose initially in the spine.

Patients with retinoblastoma (caused by a hereditary mutation in the q14 band of chromosome 13, which codes for a tumor suppressor gene) have a 500-fold greater risk of developing osteosarcoma. The overall consensus is that these tumors have a multifactorial origin involving genetic, constitutional, and environmental influences.

Radiographically, osteosarcomas present as mixed lytic and sclerotic lesions that cause cortical destruction and soft-tissue calcification. In advanced stages, vertebral collapse occurs from replacement of the structural elements of the spine with tumor.

Traditional therapy has involved limited tumor resection and radiotherapy. A more aggressive approach as described by both Sundaresan and Weinstein with wide resection, combination chemotherapy, and local radiotherapy demonstrated promising early results.

Secondary spinal osteosarcoma caused by malignant transformation of pagetoid or previously irradiated bone is extremely aggressive and is associated with early metastasis. A 5-year survival rate of 17% is reported in cases involving pagetoid bone, and the prognosis is even poorer in cases involving irradiated bone.

Ewing's Sarcoma

Ewing's sarcoma is a malignant round cell tumor with a peak incidence in the second decade of life. The sarcoma was first described in 1921 by James Ewing who called it an "endothelial myeloma." The neoplasm occurs twice as often in men than in women. Spinal involvement is seen in 3.5% of all Ewing's sarcomas and a large proportion of these arise in the sacrum.

Metastatic involvement of the spine is more common in the late stage of the disease. The vertebral body involvement seen on radiographs in patients with Ewing's sarcoma can mimic the vertebra plana seen in patients with eosinophilic granuloma.

When the lesion is localized to the sacrum, the prognosis is worse because these particular lesions tend to be more aggressive and less responsive to chemotherapy and irradiation.

Chondrosarcoma

Chondrosarcoma is the third most common primary bone tumor behind myeloma and osteosarcoma. Although chondrosarcoma rarely affects the spine, it does so more often than osteosarcoma or Ewing's sarcoma. The peak incidence of chondrosarcoma is in the fourth to sixth decade, with males affected four times more often than females. Six to ten percent of all chondrosarcomas arise in the spine.

Pain in the area of involvement is the first symptom. Fifty percent of patients will have a palpable mass before being diagnosed. About 4.5% will have some form of neurologic deficit varying from sensory deficits to frank paraplegia.

Radiographs show typical cortical destruction and paraspinal soft-tissue calcification. MRI will help to delineate the extent of soft-tissue and bony involvement.

Chondrosarcomas are radioresistant. Thus, the mainstay of treatment is wide excision. Survival is closely related to obtaining a clear surgical margin at the time of surgical excision. In the Mayo clinic series, 15/20 (75%) of the patients with chondrosarcoma died of local progression. Their 5-year survival rate was 21–55%, with a median survival of 6 years. High-dose irradiation therapy may have limited benefit for inoperable lesions.

Chordoma

A chordoma is a slow-growing tumor that arises from notochordal cells in the vertebral body. Physaliferous cells, containing abundant vacuoles filled with glycogen and oxidative enzymes, are the distinctive cells of this neoplasm. Molecular analysis has shown that chordoma cells express galectin-3, a carbohydrate-binding protein that plays a role in cell differentiation, morphogenesis, and cancer biology. The neoplasm usually occurs in the fifth and sixth decades of life and afflicts men twice as often as women. Chordomas are found in the sacrum and coccyx in 55% of cases, in the basilar skull in 30%, and in the lumbar and cervical spine in 15%. The clinical course is indolent, and detection is often delayed until after metastasis has occurred. Symptoms and signs include local pain, radiculopathy, and bowel or bladder dysfunction. Patients with cervicothoracic tumors can present with progressive dyspnea. Rectal examination can reveal a presacral mass.

After wide surgical resection, the local recurrence rate varies from 28 to 64%. Great care must be taken to prevent tumor spillage during resection since this can increase the local recurrence rate from 28 to 64%. Adjuvant radiation therapy is indicated when complete resection is impossible or when tumor spillage occurs at the time of resection. Radiation therapy may allow an increased continuous disease-free survival. The 5-year survival rate in patients treated with irradiation alone is about 50%, whereas that in patients treated with irradiation plus surgical resection is 71%. Virtually all patients eventually die from tumor recurrence.

Barwick KW et al: Primary osteogenic sarcoma of the vertebral column: A clinicopathologic correlation of ten patients. Cancer 1980;46:595.

Biorani S et al: Chondroma of the spine above the sacrum. Treatment and outcome in 21 cases. Spine 1996;21:1569.

Cheng EY et al: Lumbosacral chordoma. Prognostic factors and treatment. Spine 1999;24:1639.

Fujita T et al: Chordoma in the cervical spine managed with en bloc excision. Spine 1999;24:1848.

Gotz W et al: Detection and distribution of the carbohydrate binding protein galectin-3 in human notochord, intervertebral disc and chordoma. Differentiation 1997;62:149.

Hester TO et al: Cervicothoracic chordoma presenting as progressive dyspnea and dysphagia. Otolaryngol Head Neck Surg 1999;120:97.

Lecouvet F et al. Long-term effects of localized spinal radiation therapy on vertebral fractures and focal lesions appearance in patients with multiple myeloma. Br J Haematol 1997;96:743.

McLain RF, Weinstein JN: Solitary plasmacytomas of the spine: A review of 84 cases. J Spinal Dis 1989;2:69.

Munzenrider JE, Liebsch NJ: Proton therapy for tumors of the skull base. Strahlenther Onkol 1999;175 Suppl 2:57.

Perrin RG, McBroom RJ: Thoracic spine tumors. Clin Neurosurg 1992;38:353.

Rich TA et al: Clinical and pathological review of 48 cases of chordoma. Cancer 1985;56:182.

Samson IR et al: Operative treatment of sacrococcygeal chondroma. A review of twenty-one cases. J Bone Joint Surg Am 1997;75:1476.

Shives TC et al: Chondrosarcoma of the spine. J Bone Joint Surg Am 1989;71:1158.

Shives TC et al: Osteosarcoma of the spine. J Bone Joint Surg Am 1986;68:660.

Sundaresan N et al: Combined treatment of osteosarcoma of the spine. Neurosurgery 1988;23:714.

Valderrama JA, Bullough PG: Solitary myeloma of the spine. J Bone Joint Surg Br 1988;50:82.

Weinstein JN, McLain RF: Primary tumors of the spine. Spine 1987;12:843.

METASTATIC DISEASE OF THE SPINE

Although the skeleton is the third most common site for metastatic disease, the spine, especially the thoracic spine, is the most frequently involved region of the skeleton. Approximately 70% of patients who die of cancer have evidence of vertebral metastasis on postmortem examination.

Lung, breast, prostate, renal, thyroid, and gastrointestinal carcinomas have all been reported to metastasize to the spine, where lesions can lead to multilevel spinal instability and cord compression. Unfortunately, 30–50% of the bone must be destroyed before the metastatic involvement becomes evident on radiographs.

Many patients with spinal metastasis are asymptomatic. Symptoms, when they do occur, are typically a result of invasion of the tumor into the paravertebral soft tissues, compression of the spinal cord or nerve roots, or pathologic fracture and spinal instability. In these cases, patients will frequently complain of severe, unrelenting back pain with or without neurologic sequelae. The pain will typically wake the patient up at night. The course may be rapid, leading to paraplegia or quadriplegia.

Technetium bone scanning will reveal multiple sites of radioisotope uptake. MRI is the imaging study of choice to assess the extent of the tumor. Biopsy is necessary when the primary tumor is unknown and typically can be performed under CT guidance.

Most patients who do not develop progressive instability or neurologic compromise can be managed nonoperatively with systemic chemotherapy, local irradiation, and bracing.

Radiation therapy and chemotherapy protocols will depend on the primary source of carcinoma. From 80 to 90% of patients suffering from spinal metastatic disease are reported to gain significant relief with radiation therapy. Irradiation can be started as early as 2 weeks after surgical decompression and fusion. Surgical intervention is warranted in patients who have severe pain and have failed to respond to conservative treatment. It is also indicated in patients who have significant neurologic dysfunction or spinal instability. Factors found to affect survival include preoperative neurologic status, anatomic site of primary carcinoma, and number of vertebral bodies involved. Patients with a slower onset of neurologic compromise have a better prognosis for recovery of neurologic function than patients with acute onset of neurologic compromise. Stabilizing constructs can consist of bone, metal, or methylmethacrylate (Figure 5–3).

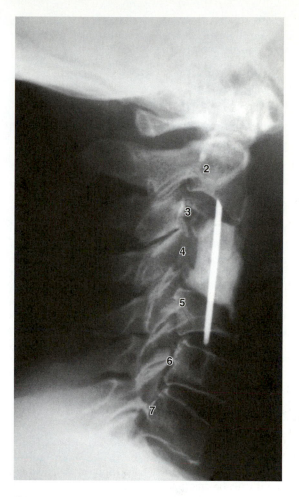

Figure 5–3. Radiograph showing metastasizing adenocarcinoma of C4 and C5, treated with excision, methylmethacrylate, and Kirschner wire.

Abe E et al: Total spondylectomy for solitary spinal metastasis of the thoracolumbar spine: A preliminary report. Tohoku J Exp Med, 2000;190(1):33.

Barr JD et al: Percutaneous vertebroplasty for pain relief and spinal stabilization. Spine 2000;25(8):923.

Bauer HC: Posterior decompression and stabilization for spinal metastases. Analysis of 67 consecutive patients. J Bone Joint Surg Am 1997;79:514.

Chataigner H, M Onimus: Surgery in spinal metastasis without spinal cord compression: Indications and strategy related to the risk of recurrence. Eur Spine J 2000;9(6):523.

Chong CC et al: Managing malignant spinal cord compression. Aust Fam Physician 2001;30(9):859.

Jeremic B: Single fraction external beam radiation therapy in the treatment of localized metastatic bone pain. A review. J Pain Symptom Manage 2001;22(6):1048.

Mink J: Percutaneous bone biopsy in the patient with known or suspected osseous metastases. Radiology 1986;161:191.

Perrin RG, McBroom RJ: Thoracic spine tumors. Clin Neurosurg 1992;38:353.

Sioutos PJ et al: Spinal metastases from solid tumors. Analysis of factors affecting survival. Cancer 1995;76:1453.

Sundaresan N et al: Indications and results of combined anterior-posterior approaches for spine tumor surgery. J Neurosurg 1996;85:438.

Weinstein JN, McLain RF: Tumors of the spine. In Rothman RH, Simeone FA (editors): The Spine, 4th ed. Philadelphia: WB Saunders, 1992.

EXTRADURAL TUMORS

Extradural tumors include hemangiomas, lipomas, meningiomas, and lymphomas. Surgical management usually involves laminectomy and tumor excision. This is often all that is needed for symptomatic relief in these slow-growing tumors.

Cappellani G et al: Primary spinal epidural lymphoma. J Neurosurg Sci 1986;30:147.

■ INFLAMMATORY DISEASES OF THE SPINE

RHEUMATOID ARTHRITIS

Rheumatoid arthritis is the most common form of inflammatory arthritis. It affects 3% of women and 1% of men. The disease frequently affects the spine. The same inflammatory cells that destroy peripheral joints affect the synovium of apophyseal and uncovertebral joints, causing painful instability and neurologic compromise. Up to 71% of patients with rheumatoid arthritis show involvement of the cervical spine. The most common patterns of involvement are C1-2 instability, basilar invagination, and subaxial subluxation. Sudden death associated with rheumatoid arthritis, most probably secondary to brain stem compression, has been reported.

Clinical Findings

A. SYMPTOMS AND SIGNS

From 7 to 34% of patients present with neurologic problems. Documentation of neurologic function can be difficult because loss of joint mobility leads to general muscle weakness. Although many patients complain of nonspecific neck pain, atlantoaxial subluxation is the most common cause for pain in the upper neck, occiput, and forehead in patients with rheumatoid arthritis. Symptoms are aggravated by motion. Increasing compression of the spinal cord will result in severe myelopathy with gait abnormalities, weakness, paresthesias, and loss of dexterity. Findings may also include Lhermitte's sign (a tingling or electrical feeling that occurs in the arms, legs, or trunk when the neck is flexed), increased muscle tone of the upper and lower extremities, and pathologic reflexes.

B. IMAGING STUDIES

Instability of the upper cervical spine is determined on lateral flexion-extension radiographs. An atlanto-dens interval (ADI) that exceeds 3.5 mm is abnormal. Subluxation with an ADI of 10–12 mm indicates disruption of all supporting ligaments of the atlantoaxial complex (transverse and alar ligaments). The spinal cord in this position is compressed between the dens and the posterior arch of C1. Although the ADI is an important measurement for traumatic instability of the C1-2 complex, the posterior atlanto-dens interval (PADI) is more prognostic for assessing neurologic compromise. The PADI is a direct measure of the space available for the spinal cord at the C1-2 level. The PADI is measured from the posterior aspect of the odontoid process to the nearest posterior structure (the foramen magnum or the posterior ring of the atlas). If the space available for the spinal cord is less than 13 mm, the likelihood that the patient will develop myelopathy is extremely high.

Cranial settling is present in from 5 to 32% of patients. The odontoid process should not project more than 3 mm above Chamberlain's line, which is a line between the hard palate and the posterior rim of the foramen magnum. The tip of the dens should not project more than 4.5 mm above McGregor's line, which is a line connecting the posterior margin of the hard palate to the occiput. The Clark classification divides the axis into thirds in the sagittal plane. In severe cases of cranial settling, the anterior arch of C1 moves from station 1 (the upper third of C2) to station 3 (the lower third of C2). Neurologic compromise occurs as a result of impingement of the dens into the brain stem and the upper cervical spinal cord. The vertebral arteries can also become occluded as they course between the dens and the foramen magnum to enter the skull.

Lateral subluxation and posterior atlantoaxial instability are less frequent. From 10 to 20% of patients with rheumatoid arthritis present with subaxial subluxation. Erosion of the facet joints and narrowing of the discs leads to subtle anterior subluxations often found on several levels. This results in a characteristic "stepladder" deformity that occurs most commonly at the C2-3 and C3-4 levels.

C. LABORATORY STUDIES

Rheumatoid factor is positive in up to 80% of patients. The erythrocyte sedimentation rate is elevated and the hemoglobin is decreased in the active phase of the disease.

After plain radiographs which should include lateral flexion-extension views, MRI is the study of choice to evaluate the degree of neural compression and deformity.

Treatment

Indications for surgery are severe neck pain and increasing loss of neurologic function. Most commonly, a posterior arthrodesis between C1 and C2 is performed. A Gallie type or Brooks type of fusion can be done, or posterior transarticular screw fixation can be used. The latter obviates the need for postoperative halo immobilization. In cases of basilar invagination (cranial settling), extension of the fusion to the occiput is necessary. Preoperative halo traction is often required to reduce the subluxation or pull the odontoid process out of the foramen magnum. Often a suboccipital craniectomy is necessary to adequately decompress the brainstem. Good fixation can be obtained through the use of plate-screw and rod-screw constructs.

Alberstone CD, Benzel EC: Cervical spine complications in rheumatoid arthritis patients. Awareness is the key to averting serious consequences. Postgrad Med, 2000;107(1):199, 205.

Boden SD et al: Rheumatoid arthritis of the cervical spine. A long-term analysis with predictors of paralysis and recovery. J Bone Joint Surg Am 1993;75A:1282.

Christensson D et al: Cervical spine surgery in rheumatoid arthritis. A Swedish nation-wide registration of 83 patients. Scand J Rheumatol 2000;29(5):314.

Clark CR et al: Arthrodesis of the cervical spine in rheumatoid arthritis. J Bone Joint Surg Am 1989;71:381.

Dvorak J et al: Functional evaluation of the spinal cord by magnetic resonance imaging in patients with rheumatoid arthritis and instability of the upper cervical spine. Spine 1989; 14:1057.

Faraj AA et al: Surgical treatment for rheumatoid neck arthritis bilateral occipitospinal fusion with plate fixation. Acta Orthop Belg 2001;67(2):164.

Graziano GP et al: The use of traction methods to correct severe cervical deformity in rheumatoid arthritis patients: A report of five cases. Spine 2001;26(9):1076.

Grob D: Posterior occipitocervical fusion in rheumatoid arthritis and other instabilities. J Orthop Sci 2000;5(1):82.

Haid RW, Jr et al: C1-C2 transarticular screw fixation for atlantoaxial instability: A 6-year experience. Neurosurgery 2001;49(1):65, discussion 69.

Matsunaga S et al: Results of a longer than 10-year follow-up of patients with rheumatoid arthritis treated by occipitocervical fusion. Spine 2000;25(14):1749.

Santavinta S et al: Ten-year results of operations for rheumatoid cervical spine disorders. J Bone Joint Surg Am 1991;73B:116.

van Asselt KM et al: Outcome of cervical spine surgery in patients with rheumatoid arthritis. Ann Rheum Dis 2001;60(5):448.

Yaszemski MJ, Shepler TR: Sudden death from cord compression associated with atlantoaxial instability in rheumatoid arthritis: A case report. Spine 1990;15:338.

Zygmut S et al: Reduction of rheumatoid periodontoid pannus following posterior occipitocervical fusion visualized by magnetic resonance imaging. Br J Neurosurg 1988;2:315.

ANKYLOSING SPONDYLITIS

Ankylosing spondylitis is a chronic seronegative inflammatory disease that affects the axial skeleton, especially the sacroiliac joints, hip joints, and spine. Extraskeletal involvement is found in the aorta, lung, and uvea. The incidence of ankylosing spondylitis is 0.5–1 per 1000 people. Although males are affected more frequently than females, mild courses of ankylosing spondylitis are more common in the latter. The disease usually has its onset during early adulthood. However, juvenile ankylosing spondylitis affects adolescents (those younger than 16 years of age) and has a predisposition toward hip involvement. The HLA-B27 surface antigen is found in 88 to 96%% of patients, and investigators have postulated that an endogenic component (ie, HLA-B27) and an exogenic component (eg, *Klebsiella* or *Chlamydia*) are responsible for triggering of the disease process. The erythrocyte sedimentation rate is elevated in up to 80% of the cases but does not accurately reflect disease activity. The serum creatine phosphokinase level, however, is a good indicator of the severity of the disease process.

Clinical Findings

A. SYMPTOMS AND SIGNS

The onset is insidious, with early symptoms including pain in the buttocks, heels, and lower back. Patients complain typically of morning stiffness, the improvement of symptoms with activity during the day, and the return of symptoms in the evening. The earliest changes involve the sacroiliac joints and then extends upward into the spine. Spinal disease results in loss of motion and subsequent loss of lordosis in the cervical and lumbar spine. Synovitis in the early stages leads to progressive fibrosis and ankylosis of the joints during the reparative phase. Enthesitis occurs at the insertion of the annulus fibrosus on the vertebral body with eventual calcification that results in the characteristic "bamboo spine." The pain from the inflammatory process subsides after full ankylosis of the affected joints occur. About 30% of patients develop uveitis, and 30% have chest tightness. Limited chest expansion indicates thoracic involvement. Fewer than 5% of patients have involvement of the aorta, characterized by dilation and possible conduction defects. In addition, patients may suffer from renal amyloidosis and pulmonary fibrosis.

B. IMAGING STUDIES

The earliest radiographic changes are visible in the sacroiliac joints. Symmetric bilateral widening of the joint space is followed by subchondral erosions and ankylosis. Bony changes in the spine affect the vertebral body. Changes include loss of the anterior concavity of the vertebral body, squaring of the vertebra, and marginal syndesmophyte formation, which give the spine the appearance of a bamboo spine. Ankylosis of the apophyseal joints also develops. The disease generally starts in the lumbar spine and migrates cephalad to the cervical spine. Atlantoaxial instability is seen occasionally.

Treatment

The natural history of ankylosing spondylitis, with its slow progression over several decades, has to be considered in planning treatment. Initially, treatment consists of exercises and indomethacin and phenylbutazone. About 10% of patients develop severe bony changes that eventually require surgical intervention. These changes characteristically include a fixed bony flexion deformity that limits their ambulatory potential. Hip disease should be addressed before correction of spinal deformities because correction of hip flexion deformities may allow significant compensation of the spinal kyphosis to allow adequate horizontal gaze.

Loss of lumbar lordosis can be treated by multilevel posterior closing wedge osteotomies (the Smith-Peterson procedure), by a decancellation procedure (the Heinig procedure) of L3 or L4, or by pedicle subtraction osteotomy based at L3 or L4 (Figure 5–4). The spine is then fused in the corrected position. Utilization of modern fixation systems such as a pedicle screw system allows for early mobilization of the patient. Thorough preoperative assessment of the deformity and measuring of the chin-eyebrow-to floor angle are helpful for the exact planning of the corrective osteotomy. Relative contraindications to surgery are poor general health and significant scarring of the major vessels that may be injured when the spine is extended.

The cervical osteotomy is performed between C7 and T1. This approach avoids injury to the vertebral artery that usually enters the transverse foramen of C6. The procedure is usually performed with the patient under local anesthesia. However with the evolution of somatosensory and motor-evoked potential monitoring of the spinal cord, the procedure can be safely performed under general anesthesia. After removal of the posterior elements and neural decompression, the kyphotic deformity is corrected with gentle extension of the head. The head is held in the corrected position using internal fixation with plate-screw constructs or plate-rod constructs with adjunctive halo-vest immobilization.

Berven SH et al: Management of fixed sagittal plane deformity: Results of the transpedicular wedge resection osteotomy. Spine 2001;26(18):2036.

Chen IH et al: Transpedicular wedge osteotomy for correction of thoracolumbar kyphosis in ankylosing spondylitis: Experience with 78 patients. Spine 2001;26(16):E354.

Danisa OA et al: Surgical correction of lumbar kyphotic deformity: Posterior reduction "eggshell" osteotomy. J Neurosurg 2000; 92(1 Suppl):50.

Fox MW et al: Neurological complications of ankylosing spondylitis. J Neurosurg 1993;78:871.

Haslock I: Ankylosing spondylitis. Baillieres Clin Rheumatol 1993; 7:99.

Kumar A et al: Long-term outcome of undifferentiated spondyloarthropathy. Rheumatol Int 2001:20(6):221.

Lehtinen K: Mortality and causes of death in 398 patients admitted to hospital with ankylosing spondylitis. Ann Rheum Dis 1993;52:174.

Savolaine ER et al: Aortic rupture complicating a fracture of an ankylosed thoracic spine: A case report. Clin Orthop 1991; 272:136.

Simmons EH: Kyphotic deformity of the spine in ankylosing spondylitis. Clin Orthop 1977;128:65.

Taggard DA, Traynelis VC: Management of cervical spinal fractures in ankylosing spondylitis with posterior fixation. Spine 2000;25(16):2035.

van der Linden S, van der Heijde D: Clinical aspects, outcome assessment, and management of ankylosing spondylitis and postenteric reactive arthritis. Curr Opin Rheumatol 2000;12 (4):263.

DISEASES & DISORDERS OF THE CERVICAL SPINE

Principles of Diagnosis

In evaluating the cervical spine, the use of appropriate imaging studies is critical to a timely and precise diagnosis. Available imaging techniques include plain radiography, tomography, myelography, CT, CT with myelography, three-dimensional reconstruction CT, MRI, and scintigraphy. An understanding of the advantages and disadvantages of each technique is necessary for the proper selection of imaging studies and interpretation of results.

A. Plain Radiography

In evaluating the patient with neck pain, cervical spine radiographs are important in the initial search for a possible lesion. In the trauma setting, when a head or neck injury is suspected, radiographic studies must be carried out appropriately or a life-threatening lesion may be overlooked. The trauma series includes AP, right oblique, left oblique, and open-mouth (odontoid) views in addition to an initial cross-table lateral view. When all five views are taken, sensitivity is 92%. It is extremely important that cervical spine precautions be implemented throughout the radiographic evaluation (see General Principles of Managing Acute Injuries of the Cervical Spine). In the absence of a history of trauma, the oblique and odontoid views are not always required.

If performed correctly, the lateral view will reveal the majority of traumatic lesions. Inadequate views can miss more than 20% of cervical spine injuries, however.

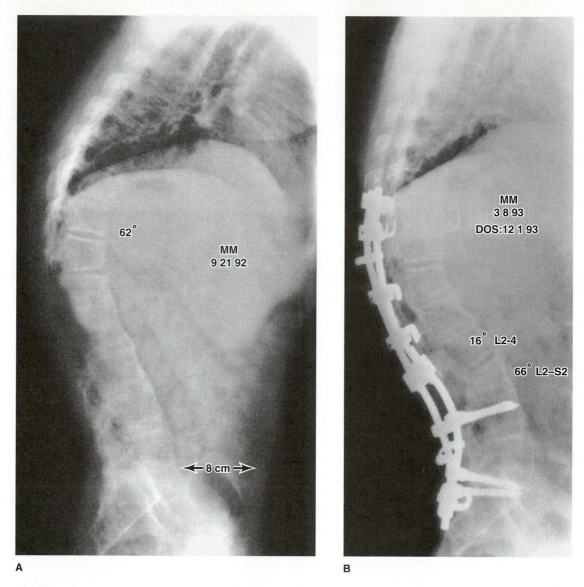

Figure 5–4. Imaging studies in a patient with ankylosing spondylitis. **A:** Radiograph demonstrating flat back deformity, junctional kyphosis, and sagittal decompensation. **B:** Radiograph taken after a decancellation procedure of L3 and posterior fusion were performed to correct the alignment.

All seven vertebrae should be clearly visible. Gentle traction on the upper extremities may be necessary to view C7. If this is unsuccessful, a swimmer's view may be necessary. The prevertebral soft tissue, the anterior border of the vertebral bodies, the vertebral bodies themselves, the posterior border of the bodies, the spinal canal proper, and the posterior elements must all be carefully scrutinized.

The prevertebral region may reveal swelling consistent with a hematoma, and this may serve as the only clue to a traumatic lesion. The upper limits for the prevertebral space are 10 mm at C1; 5 mm at C2; 7 mm at C3 and C4; and 20 mm at C5, C6, and C7. The contours of the cervical bony structures are regular, and subtle incongruities may indicate significant instability. Variations in normal cervical anatomy do exist, however, and a familiarity with them may prevent an overzealous workup. The atlanto-dens interval normally measures less than 3 mm in adults and less than 4 mm in children.

In reviewing the AP radiograph, the interspinous distance must be carefully assessed. Vertical widening at a given level greater than 1.5 times the level above and below indicates a hyperflexion injury with posterior instability or interlocking of the posterior facets. Traumatic tilting may also be noted in the AP plane but not be appreciated on the lateral view.

Oblique views taken at 45 degrees allow visualization of the articulations of the facet joints. The open-mouth view permits evaluation of the odontoid process, the lateral masses, and the articulations of the lateral masses, and it also permits assessment of the distance between each lateral mass and the odontoid process. In atlantoaxial rotatory subluxation, the lateral mass of the atlas that is rotated forward is closer to the midline (medial offset), whereas the opposite mass is farther away from the midline (lateral offset). Burst fractures of the C1 ring will cause overhang of the C1 lateral masses on C2. A combined overhang exceeding 6.9 mm is highly correlated with insufficiency of the transverse ligament and C1-2 sagittal instability.

This radiographic series is equally important in evaluating infants and children with suspected congenital or developmental defects and adults with insidious neck pain. Arthritic changes may be subtle or readily apparent with osteophytes, disc space narrowing, and facet sclerosis. Bone quality can also be assessed on plain radiographs.

B. COMPUTED TOMOGRAPHY

CT scans allow excellent visualization of the bony architecture and the paravertebral soft tissues of the cervical spine. The pedicles, laminae, spinous processes, and bony spinal canal can be examined with significantly better resolution when CT is used than when conventional radiographs are taken. CT with myelography or intrathecal contrast enhancement permits a visualization of the spinal canal contents that otherwise could not be appreciated.

CT is an appropriate modality for evaluating congenital variations and malformations, including spinal canal stenosis and spina bifida. Pars defects, atlantoaxial joint diseases, primary tumors, and metastatic carcinoma are well appreciated with CT. Subtle inflammatory changes, such as those seen in early rheumatoid arthritis or degenerative osteoarthritis, and their potential neurologic sequelae can be evaluated with CT. Although cervical disc disease is detectable when thin cuts and contrast enhancement are used with CT, it is better visualized with MRI.

In the trauma patient with questionable findings on plain radiographs, CT has proved integral in evaluating possible fractures or instability. Intrathecal contrast may be necessary to detect spinal cord impingement caused by disc or cartilage material. Atrophy, deformity, and displacement of the spinal cord from acute or chronic injury are all appreciable with the use of intrathecal contrast. With the advent of MRI, however, CT has been reserved for the assessment of the bony architecture, which it does better than MRI.

Three-dimensional reconstruction of CT images has gained wide clinical acceptance with the advancement of computer graphics. The reconstructions can be rotated in space to evaluate the anatomy from almost any perspective. This technique is valuable in the understanding of atlantoaxial rotatory subluxations or complex fractures of the spinal column.

C. MAGNETIC RESONANCE IMAGING

MRI permits axial, sagittal, coronal, or oblique plane analysis of the anatomy. It is routinely noninvasive, requiring contrast material in only selected cases.

MRI is the standard for assessing cervical spinal cord damage. Spinal cord tumors and trauma as well as central disc herniation can be easily visualized. In the preoperative evaluation of patients with spondylosis or disc herniation, MRI has replaced CT and CT myelography as the neuroimaging test of choice.

Intravenous paramagnetic agent gadolinium is commonly used to differentiate tissues receiving higher blood flow. This is helpful in the diagnosis of infection, tumor, and postsurgical scar.

D. SCINTIGRAPHY

Bone scans that employ technetium-99m phosphate permit assessment of physiologic processes within the musculoskeletal system. Metabolic, metastatic, and inflammatory abnormalities can be detected. Technetium-99m phosphate is incorporated into the hydroxyapatite crystals in bone and reflects increased bone osteogenesis in a given region of bone. Early phase imaging with technetium-99m gives blood flow information. Accordingly, subtle fractures, avascular necrosis, and osteomyelitis can be detected. Other radioisotopes used in scintigraphy include gallium-67 citrate, which labels serum proteins, and indium-111, which labels white blood cells. These labeling techniques are helpful in discerning areas of neoplasia or acute infection.

Bachulis BL et al: Clinical indications for cervical spine radiographs in the traumatized patient. Am J Surg 1987;153:473.

Blahd WH Jr et al: Efficacy of the posttraumatic cross-table lateral view of the cervical spine. J Emerg Med 1985;2:243.

Doris PE, Wilson RA: The next logical step in the emergency radiographic evaluation of cervical spine trauma: The five-view trauma series. J Emerg Med 1985;3:371.

Larsson EM et al: Comparison of myelography, CT with myelography, and magnetic resonance imaging in cervical spondylosis and disk herniation. Acta Radiol 1989;30:233.

Mace SE: Emergency evaluation of cervical spine injuries: CT versus plain radiographs. Ann Emerg Med 1985;14:973.

O'Malley KF, Ross SE: The incidence of injury to the cervical spine in patients with craniocerebral injury. J Trauma 1988;28:1476.

Reid DC et al: Etiology and clinical course of missed spine fractures. J Trauma 1987;27:980.

Ross SE et al: Clearing the cervical spine: Initial radiologic evaluation. J Trauma 1987;27:1055.

CONGENITAL MALFORMATIONS

The atlanto-occipital region is a frequent location for abnormalities. Various combinations involving bone and nerve structures are possible. During embryologic development, 42 somites are formed from the paraxial mesoderm. The somites divide into sclerotomes, which form the vertebral bodies after separation into a caudal and cephalad portion. The middle portion builds the intervertebral disc. The second, third, and fourth somites fuse and become the occiput and posterior part of the foramen magnum. The fate of the first somite is unclear. The development of the neural tube progresses simultaneously with that of the cartilaginous skeleton.

Disturbances of embryologic development can result in incomplete development or absence of a tissue or part, as found in dysraphism, aplasia of the odontoid process, incomplete closure of the atlas, or absence of the atlas facet. Lack of segmentation results in atlanto-occipital fusion, block vertebrae, and possible instability at adjacent cervical levels. A disturbance of neurologic development, alone or in combination with bony defects, can lead to basilar impression, Arnold-Chiari malformation, and syringomyelia, all of which manifest in myelopathy.

1. OS Odontoideum

Os odontoideum is an uncommon type of pseudarthrosis between the odontoid process and the body of the axis. It can cause significant atlantoaxial instability and myelopathy and can result in sudden death. The development of cervical myelopathy is thought to be a function of the amount of space available for the spinal cord. Because of the instability between C1 and C2, the spinal cord can become compressed against the anterior portion of the axis or the posterior ring of the atlas. In some cases, extrinsic compression of the vertebral arteries results in ischemic insult to the brain.

Clinical Findings

A. SYMPTOMS AND SIGNS

Patients with os odontoideum may be asymptomatic or may present with symptoms and signs that relate to atlantoaxial instability, such as ill-defined neck complaints or focal or diffuse neurologic deficits. A careful history may be needed to rule out trauma, although congenital os odontoideum may come to the attention of the surgeon secondary to a reported but inconsequential neck injury.

B. IMAGING STUDIES

The radiographic findings may be extremely subtle and difficult to distinguish. In the mature skeleton, os odontoideum appears as a radiographic lucency. In children younger than 5 years, however, an anomalous gap may be confused with a normal neural synchondrosis. Flexion-extension views must therefore be obtained to demonstrate motion between the odontoid process and the body of the axis. The ossicle in os odontoideum is either round or ovoid, with a smooth surface and uniform cortical thickness. It is usually about half the size of the normal odontoid process. In traumatic nonunion, the edge is irregular with a narrow gap. The fracture line may involve the body of C2 as well. An additional radiologic finding in os odontoideum is hypertrophy of the anterior ring of the atlas with a corresponding hypoplastic posterior ring. In flexion-extension views, the ossicle travels with the anterior ring of the atlas (Figure 5–5). In cases that are difficult to diagnose, further studies include open-mouth views, tomograms, and CT reconstructions.

Treatment

Patients diagnosed with os odontoideum must be warned of the gravity of the situation because minimal trauma can be fatal. Patients with cervical myelopathy can be treated with traction, immobilization, or both, but they often require subsequent posterior fusion. Sometimes symptoms are reversible with or without intervention. Treatment of asymptomatic patients with instability is controversial. The benefits of surgical stabilization in an attempt to avoid potentially lethal injury from relatively minor trauma are counterbalanced by the possible complications of surgery.

If fusion is indicated, usually a posterior fusion of C1-2 is adequate. Different fusion techniques are available. Most surgeons use the Gallie technique or the Brooks technique. The Gallie technique involves the use of a single block-shaped bone graft between the posterior ring of C1 and the spinous process of C2. A single sublaminar wire holds the graft in place. The Brooks technique uses from two to four sublaminar wires, and

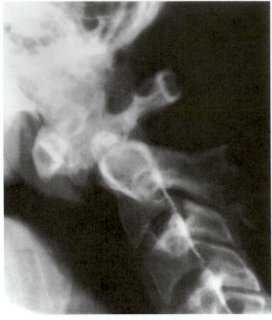
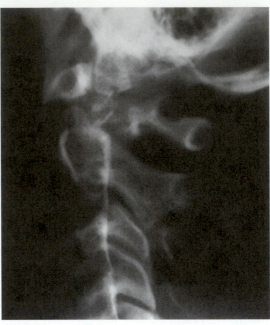

A   B

Figure 5–5. Imaging studies in a patient with os odontoideum. **A:** Radiograph in flexion. The ossicle moves with the anterior ring of the atlas. **B:** Radiograph in extension.

two bone grafts are wedged between the laminae of C1 and C2. More recent screw fixation techniques, such as the one proposed by Magerl for facet screw fixation between C1 and C2, are more stable in rotation and show an increased fusion rate. The loss of motion between atlas and axis results in an overall decrease of 50% of cervical rotation. Use of transarticular screws or screw-rod constructs that purchase into the lateral masses of C1 and the pedicle of C2 are rigid enough to allow the patient to mobilize without a halo-vest.

Grob D et al: Atlantoaxial fusion with transarticular screw fixation. J Bone Joint Surg Br 1991;73:972.

Hensinger RN: Congenital anomalies of the atlantoaxial joint. In Cervical Spine Research Society (editor): The Cervical Spine, 3rd ed. Baltimore: Lippincott, 1989.

2. Klippel-Feil Syndrome

Klippel-Feil syndrome refers to an array of clinical disorders associated with congenital fusion of one or more cervical vertebrae. The fusion, which may be multilevel, results from a failure of the normal division of the cervical somites during the third through eighth weeks of embryogenesis. The cause of this failure is unknown. The syndrome was first described in 1912 by M. Klippel and A. Feil as a triad of clinical features: a short "web" neck, a low posterior hair line, and limited cervical neck motion. Interestingly, only 50% of patients with the syndrome that now bears the names of Klippel and Feil present with this classic triad.

Various conditions have subsequently been seen in association with congenitally fused cervical vertebrae. These include scoliosis (seen in about 60% of cases), renal abnormalities (in 35%), deafness (in 30%), Sprengel's deformity (in 30%), synkinesis or mirror movement (in 20%), congenital heart defects (in 14%), brain stem anomalies, congenital cervical stenosis, adrenal aplasia, ptosis, Duane's contracture, lateral rectus palsy, facial nerve palsy, syndactyly, and upper extremity diffuse or focal hypoplasia.

Clinical Findings

A. SYMPTOMS AND SIGNS

Decreased range of motion is the most frequent finding in patients with cervical spine involvement. Involvement of only the lower cervical spine or fusion of fewer than three vertebrae will result in minimal loss of motion, however. Patients may also be able to compensate at other cervical interspaces, masking any loss of motion.

Neck shortening is difficult to detect unless extreme. Webbing of the neck (pterygium colli), facial asymmetry, or torticollis is seen in fewer than 20% of patients. Webbing of the neck can nevertheless be dramatic, with underlying muscle involvement extending from the mastoid to the acromion. Sprengel's deformity, which results from a failure of either or both scapulae to descend from their embryologic origin at C4, is seen in about 30% of patients. Sometimes an omovertebral bone bridges the cervical spine to the scapulae and limits the neck and shoulder motion.

Cervical spine symptoms in Klippel-Feil syndrome are related to the secondary hypermobility of the unfused vertebrae. Except for atlantoaxial joint involvement, resulting in a significant decrease in occipital rotation, the fused joints at a given level are asymptomatic. Because of the increased mechanical demands placed upon the uninvolved joints, secondary osteoarthritis, disc degeneration, spinal stenosis, and instability may result at these levels. Neurologic sequelae, usually confined to the head, neck, and upper extremities, result from impingement of the cervical nerve roots. With progressive cervical instability, the spinal cord may become involved, leading to spasticity, weakness, hyperreflexia, and even quadriplegia or sudden death from minor trauma.

B. Imaging Studies

Radiographic findings (Figure 5–6) of congenital cervical vertebral fusion are diagnostic of Klippel-Feil syndrome. This may present as synostosis of two vertebral bodies or as a multilevel fusion, as originally described in 1912. Other noteworthy findings are flattening of the involved vertebral bodies and the absence of disc spaces. Hypoplastic cervical discs in a child are often hard to appreciate radiographically. If suspected, flexion-extension views can be taken. CT scanning and MRI have improved the assessment of bony and nerve root involvement.

Spinal canal stenosis is not usually seen until adulthood. Although anterior spina bifida is infrequent, the posterior form is not. Enlargement of the foramen magnum with fixed hyperextension often accompanies the cervical spina bifida. Hemivertebrae have also been noted.

Involvement of the upper thoracic spine can occur and may be the first sign of an undiagnosed cervical synostosis.

Because of the potential for multiorgan involvement in patients with Klippel-Feil syndrome, an electrocardiogram and renal ultrasound are also recommended.

Treatment

Treatment of the cervical spine abnormalities is limited. Multilevel involvement leads to hypermobility at uninvolved joints, so affected patients should be cautious in their activities. Prophylactic surgical stabilization is not routinely performed in asymptomatic patients, because the risk-benefit ratio has not been well defined. In some cases, however, surgical fusion is performed.

Secondary osteoarthritis may be treated in the usual manner, including use of a cervical collar, traction, and anti-inflammatory agents. Nerve root impingement requires careful evaluation before surgical decompression, because more than one level may be involved and central abnormalities may also occur.

Surgical correction of the aesthetic deformities has been only moderately successful. Carefully selected candidates may benefit from soft-tissue Z-plasty or tenotomies. This may improve the patient's appearance but will not affect cervical motion.

Prognosis

Children with mild involvement can be expected to grow up to lead healthy, normal lives. Patients with more severe involvement can do comparably well if the associated conditions are successfully treated at an early age.

Ducker TB: Cervical myeloradiculopathy: Klippel-Feil deformity. J Spinal Dis 1990;3:439.

Elster AD: Quadriplegia after minor trauma in the Klippel-Feil syndrome. J Bone Joint Surg Am 1984;66:1473.

Hall JE et al: Instability of the cervical spine and neurological involvement in the Klippel-Feil syndrome. J Bone Joint Surg Am 1990;72:460.

Herring JA, Bunnell WP: Klippel-Feil syndrome with neck pain. J Pediatr Orthop 1989;9:343.

Prusick VR et al: Klippel-Feil syndrome associated with spinal stenosis: A case report. J Bone Joint Surg Am 1985;67:161.

CERVICAL SPONDYLOSIS

Cervical spondylosis is defined as a generalized disease process affecting the entire cervical spine and related to chronic disc degeneration. In about 90% of men older than 50 years and 90% of women older than 60 years, degeneration of the cervical spine can be demonstrated by radiographs. Initial disc changes are followed by facet arthropathy, osteophyte formation, and ligamentous instability. Myelopathy, radiculopathy, or both may be seen secondarily. Cervical myelopathy is the most common form of spinal cord dysfunction in people older than 55 years of age. People over the age of 60 are more likely to have multisegmental disease. The incidence of cervical myelopathy is twice as great in men as in women.

Pathophysiology

The relationship between the spinal cord and its bony arcade has been studied extensively. The first publica-

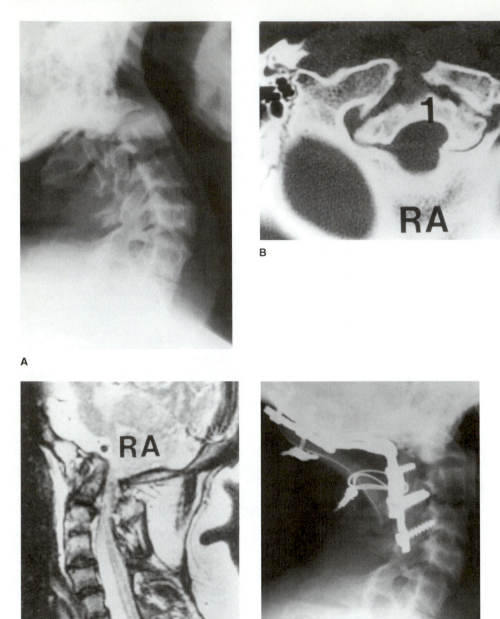

A

B

C

D

Figure 5–6. Imaging studies in a patient with Klippel-Feil syndrome and cervical myelopathy. **A:** Radiograph showing fusion of the atlas and the occiput and autofusion of the posterior elements of C3 and C4. **B:** CT scan demonstrates this as well. **C:** MRI demonstrating severe stenosis of the spinal canal. The odontoid process is above the level of the foramen magnum. **D:** Radiograph following posterior decompression and fusion between the occiput and C4.

tion on the subject was written in the early 1800s and gave the first account of a "spondylotic bar," which was actually a thickened posterior longitudinal ligament protruding into the canal secondary to disc degeneration. Subsequent work revealed that disc degeneration and osteoarthritis could lead to spinal cord and nerve root impingement.

Acute traumatic disc herniation was distinguished from the chronic spondylotic process in the mid 1950s. Concurrently, anterior spinal artery impingement by the disc or osteophyte was proposed as part of the pathogenesis. As indicated in these studies, disc degeneration starts with tears in the posterolateral region of the annulus. The subsequent loss of water content and proteoglycans in the nucleus then leads to a decrease of disc height. The longitudinal ligaments degenerate and form bony spurs at their insertion into the vertebral body. These so-called hard discs have to be distinguished from soft discs, which represent acute herniation of disc material into the spinal canal or into the neural foramen. The most frequently involved levels are the more mobile segments C5-6, C6-7, and C4-5. The converging of the cervical disc space may result in buckling of the ligamentum flavum, with further narrowing of the spinal canal. Segmental instability will result in hypertrophic formation of osteophytes by the uncovertebral joint of Luschka and by the facet joints. These prominent spurs result in compression of both the exiting nerve roots and the spinal cord.

Further work revealed that the sagittal cervical canal diameter was appreciably smaller (3 mm on average) in the myelopathic spondylotic spine than in the normal spine. The AP dimensions of the cervical spinal canal measure between 17–18 mm in normal individuals. Spinal canal stenosis is present when the canal diameter becomes less than 13 mm. With extension of the neck, both the spinal canal diameter and the neuroforaminal diameter decrease.

Clinical Findings

A. SYMPTOMS AND SIGNS

Headache may be the presenting symptom of cervical spondylosis. Usually, the headache is worse in the morning and improves throughout the day. It is commonly located in the occipital region and radiates toward the frontal area. Infrequently, patients complain of a painful, stiff neck. Signs include decreased range of motion, crepitus, or both. With more advanced cases, radicular or myelopathic symptoms may be present.

1. Cervical spondylotic radiculopathy—Cervical radiculopathy in spondylosis can be quite complex, with nerve root involvement seen at one or more levels and occurring either unilaterally or bilaterally. The onset may be acute, subacute, or chronic, and impingement on the nerve roots may be from either osteophytes or disc herniation. With radiculopathy, sensory involvement in the form of paresthesias or hyperesthesia is more common than motor or reflex changes. Several dermatomal levels may be involved, with radiation of pain into the anterior chest and back. The chief complaint is radiation of pain into the interscapular area and into the arm. Typically, patients have proximal arm pain and distal paresthesias.

2. Cervical spondylotic myelopathy—Cervical myelopathy has a variable clinical presentation, given the complex pathogenic mechanisms involved. These include static or dynamic canal impingement, facet arthropathy, vascular ischemia, and the presence of spondylotic transverse bars. In addition, given its neuronal topography, the cord may be affected in dramatically different ways by relatively minor differences in anatomic regions of compression. The clinical course of myelopathy is usually progressive, leading to complete disability over a period of months to years with stepwise deteriorations in function.

Patients often present with paresthesias, dyskinesias, or weakness of the hand, the entire upper extremity, or the lower extremity. Deep aching pain of the extremity, broad-based gait, loss of balance, loss of hand dexterity, and general muscle wasting are found in patients with advanced myelopathy. Impotence is not uncommon in male patents.

Hyperextension injuries of the spondylotic cervical spine can precipitate a central cord syndrome in which motor and sensory involvement is typically greater in the upper extremities than the lower extremities. Recovery from this injury is usually incomplete. Complete quadriplegia can also occur if the preexisting stenosis is severe. In this setting, the 1-year mortality rate approaches 80%.

Deep tendon reflexes can be either hyporeflexic or hyperreflexic, with the former seen in anterior horn cell (upper extremity) involvement and the latter seen in corticospinal tract (lower extremity) involvement. Hyporeflexia is found at the level of compression, and hyperreflexia occurs on the level below. Long-tract signs, such as the presence of Hoffmann's reflex or Babinski's reflex, indicate an upper motor neuron lesion. Clonus is often present though asymmetric. Upper extremity involvement is often unilateral, whereas lower extremities are affected bilaterally. High cervical spondylosis (C3-5) leads to complaints of numb and clumsy hands, whereas myelopathy of the lower cervical spine (C5-8) presents with spasticity and loss of proprioception in the legs.

Abdominal reflexes are usually intact, enabling the clinician to differentiate spondylosis from amyotrophic lateral sclerosis, in which reflexes are often absent. Multiple compressions of the spinal cord cause more severe deterioration functionally and electrophysiologically than a single level compression does.

B. IMAGING STUDIES

Although spondylosis results from cervical spine degeneration, not every patient with radiographic evidence of cervical disc degeneration will have symptoms. Furthermore, patients with all the radiographic stigmas of cervical spondylosis may be asymptomatic, whereas others with clinical evidence of myelopathy may show only modest radiographic changes. This paradox is explainable by canal size differences, with the smaller diameter canal having less space to buffer the degenerative lesion.

The average AP diameter of the spinal canal measures 17 mm from C3 to C7. The space required by the spinal cord averages 10 mm. The dural diameter increases by 2–3 mm in extension. The smallest sagittal AP diameter is measured between an osteophyte on the inferior aspect of the vertebral body to the base of the spinous process of the next vertebra below. An absolute spinal canal stenosis exists with a sagittal diameter of less than 10 mm. The stenosis is relative if the diameter measures 10–13 mm.

Plain film findings will also vary according to the stage of spondylosis at which they were taken. X-ray films may appear normal in early disc disease. Alternatively, they may show single or multilevel disc space narrowing with or without osteophytes. C5-6 and C6-7 are the two most commonly involved segments (Figure 5–7). Vertebral body sclerosis at the adjacent base plates may also be seen. Cortical erosion is uncommon and indicates an inflammatory process such as rheumatoid arthritis.

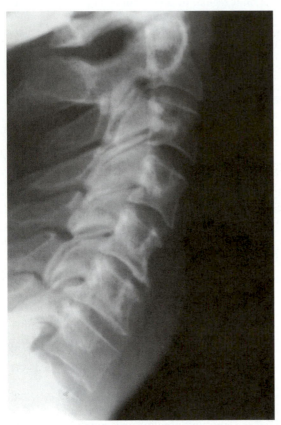

A

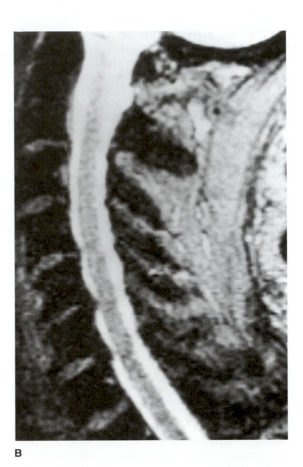

B

Figure 5–7. Imaging studies in a patient with cervical spondylosis and chronic neck pain. **A:** Radiograph showing collapsed disc space between C5 and C6 and a large posterior osteophyte at the inferior end plate of C6. **B:** MRI showing collapsed disc spaces, a mild stenosis of the spinal canal, and effacement of the spinal cord by an osteophyte at C6.

Oblique views permit evaluation of the facet joints and detection of osteophytosis and sclerosis. The superior facets undergo degeneration more frequently than their inferior counterparts. The superior joints may then subluxate posteriorly and erode into the lamina below. Inferior osteophytes, however, may prevent significant slippage. If instability seen on flexion-extension views is significant (greater than 3.5 mm when measured at the posteroinferior corner of the vertebral body), foraminal stenosis as well as vertebral artery impingement may result.

MRI permits visualization of the entire cervical canal and spinal cord by showing the spinal cord and nerve roots in two planes. The use of a contrast-enhanced CT scan is occasionally required in elderly patients with advanced degenerative bony changes of the cervical spine. Accurate identification of the location and extent of pathologic changes is necessary to determine the optimal approach for decompression. Selective nerve root blocks and electromyography may be useful in identifying the level of involvement.

Differential Diagnosis

Inflammatory, neoplastic, and infectious conditions can mimic cervical spondylotic radiculopathy and myelopathy.

Rheumatoid arthritis affects the cervical spine in most patients. Atlantoaxial subluxation or subaxial instability can cause symptoms similar to those seen in degenerative cervical myelopathy. A primary tumor or metastatic disease can present with unremitting neck pain, which is often more intense at night. MRI should easily distinguish the neoplastic condition from a pure degenerative disorder. Infections of the cervical spine occur in children and in elderly or immunocompromised individuals. Neurologic deficits vary depending on spinal canal involvement. Multiple sclerosis should be considered in the differential diagnosis. It occurs in younger patients but can present with similar motor signs. Pancoast tumors may invade the brachial plexus, resulting in upper extremity symptoms. Syringomyelia presents with tingling sensations plus motor weakness. A low protein concentration in the cerebrospinal fluid and characteristic changes on MRI are found. Disorders of the shoulder, especially rotator cuff tendinitis, can imitate cervical radiculopathy. Compressive peripheral neuropathies such as thoracic outlet syndrome also have to be ruled out.

Treatment

Patients should be divided into three groups, according to the predominance of their symptoms: neck pain alone, radiculopathy, and myelopathy. The duration and progression of symptoms need to be considered in the planning of treatment. Several studies suggest that patients with cervical radiculopathy or myelopathy have better long-term results from surgery if symptoms are of short duration.

A. CONSERVATIVE TREATMENT

Initial management of cervical spondylosis may involve a soft collar, anti-inflammatory agents, and physical therapy consisting of mild traction and the use of isometric strengthening and range-of-motion exercises. The soft cervical collar should be worn only briefly, until the acute symptoms subside. Analgesics are important in the acute phase, and muscle relaxants are helpful in breaking the cycle of muscle spasm and pain. Diazepam should be avoided because of its side effects as a clinical depressant. Epidural corticosteroid injections may be efficacious in patients with radicular pain. Trigger point injections are an empirical form of therapy that seems to work well in patients with chronic neck pain.

The value of cervical traction remains unclear. It is contraindicated in patients with cord compression, rheumatoid arthritis, infection, or osteoporosis. A careful screening of roentgenograms before treatment is mandatory. There is no evidence that home traction is more effective than manual traction. Isometric strengthening exercises of the paravertebral musculature should be started after the acute symptoms have resolved. The patient should be instructed to start a home exercise program early, to avoid long-term dependency on passive therapy modalities. Although ice, moist heat, ultrasound, and transcutaneous electrical nerve stimulation are safe to use, there is no scientific proof of their efficacy.

B. SURGICAL TREATMENT

Surgical intervention should be considered if the patient does not respond to a conservative treatment protocol or shows evidence of deteriorating myelopathy or radiculopathy. The spinal cord can be effectively decompressed by anterior, posterior, or combined approaches.

The anterior approach allows multilevel discectomy, vertebrectomy, foraminotomy, and fusion with tricortical iliac crest bone grafts or strut grafts. Newer instrumentation techniques, such as cervical plates (Figure 5–8), alleviate the need for halo immobilization. Supplemental posterior fixation and fusion should be added, however, if more than three vertebral levels are decompressed anteriorly. The posterior fixation minimizes the risk of anterior dislodgement of the graft even in the presence of solid anterior fixation. Anterior interbody fusion after decompression for a herniated cervical disc (Figure 5–9) has a high success rate.

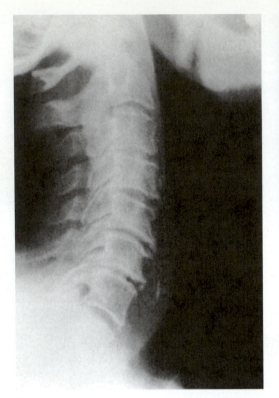

A

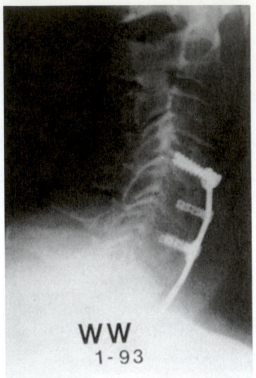

B

C

Figure 5–8. Imaging studies in a patient with cervical spondylotic myelopathy. **A:** Radiograph showing degenerative changes between C4 and C7. **B** and **C:** Radiographs taken after anterior vertebrectomy of C5 and C6, iliac crest strut graft, and anterior plate fixation.

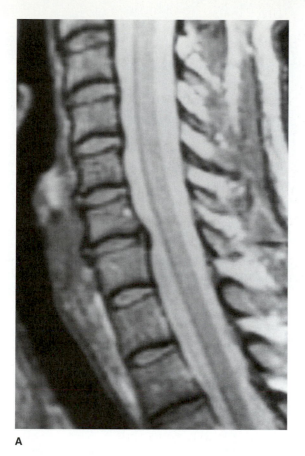

A

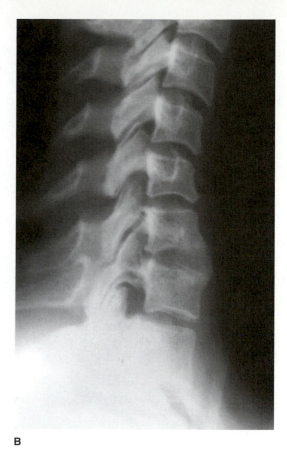

B

Figure 5–9. Imaging studies in a patient with cervical disc herniation. **A:** MRI showing herniation at C6-7. **B:** Radiograph taken after anterior cervical fusion with a tricortical graft from the pelvis.

The number of involved levels may be important in deciding which of the surgical approaches to use. Patients with cervical myelopathy and involvement of more than three levels may be best treated using a posterior approach. Multilevel laminectomy or laminaplasty has shown excellent results. If laminectomies are performed, the facet joints and capsules should be preserved to minimize the chance of postlaminectomy deformity. Late swan-neck deformities after laminectomy can be avoided with simultaneous posterior fusion utilizing lateral mass plates. Laminaplasty has the advantage over in that the cervical spinal cord can be decompressed without the high risk of developing late deformity. In addition, the morbidity associated with instrumentation and fusion can be avoided.

Operative treatment in cases of cervical spondylotic radiculopathy and myelopathy must be individualized for every patient.

Prognosis

Cervical spondylosis is generally a progressive, chronic disease process. In a study of 205 patients with neck pain, Gore and coworkers found that many patients had decreased pain at the 10-year follow-up, but those with the most severe involvement did not improve. Conservative measures may retard the disease process in its early stages. If myelopathy or radiculopathy becomes clinically evident, surgical intervention is often necessary. For disease involving less than three vertebral levels, early anterior decompression and fusion has improved the clinical outcome, particularly in the elderly individual who suffers from cervical myelopathy.

Bell GR, Ross JS: Diagnosis of nerve root compression. Myelography, computed tomography, and MRI. Orthop Clin North Am 1992;23:405.

Emery SE: Cervical spondylotic myelopathy: diagnosis and treatment. J Am Acad Orthop Surg 2001;9(6):376.

Epstein N: Anterior approaches to cervical spondylosis and ossification of the posterior longitudinal ligament: Review of operative technique and assessment of 65 multilevel circumferential procedures. Surg Neurol 2001;55(6):313.

Gore D et al: Neck pain: A long-term follow-up of 205 patients. Spine 1987;12:1.

Heller JG et al: Laminaplasty versus laminectomy and fusion for multilevel cervical myelopathy: An independent matched cohort analysis. Spine 2001;26(12):1330.

Herkowitz HN: The surgical management of cervical spondylotic radiculopathy and myelopathy. Clin Orthop 1989;239:94.

Lestini WF, Wiesel SW: The pathogenesis of cervical spondylosis. Clin Orthop 1989;239:69.

Onari K et al: Long-term follow-up results of anterior interbody fusion applied for cervical myelopathy due to ossification of the posterior longitudinal ligament. Spine 200126(5):488.

Wada E et al: Subtotal corpectomy versus laminaplasty for multilevel cervical spondylotic myelopathy: A long-term follow-up study over 10 years. Spine 2001;26(13):1443; discussion 1448.

Yoo JU et al: Effect of cervical spine motion on the neuroforaminal dimensions of human cervical spine. Spine 1992;17:1131.

OSSIFICATION OF THE POSTERIOR LONGITUDINAL LIGAMENT

Ossification of the posterior longitudinal ligament is a relatively common cause of spinal canal stenosis and myelopathy in the Asian population. Its overall incidence is 2–3% in Japan, compared with 0.6% in Hawaii and 1.7% in Italy. Males are affected more often than females, and the peak age at onset of symptoms is the sixth decade. Although the cause of the disorder is unknown, it may be controlled by autosomal-dominant inheritance because it is found in 26% of the parents and 29% of the siblings of affected patients. The disorder has been associated with several rheumatic conditions, including diffuse idiopathic skeletal hyperostosis, spondylosis, and ankylosing spondylitis.

Clinical Findings

Almost all patients have only mild subjective complaints at the onset, although 10–15% of them complain of clumsiness and spastic gait. Nevertheless, minor trauma can lead to acute deterioration of symptoms and can result in quadriplegia. Spastic quadriparesis is the most common neurologic presentation.

Ossification of the posterior longitudinal ligament can easily be diagnosed on plain lateral radiographs. The levels most frequently involved are C4, C5, and C6. A segmental type of disorder is distinguished from the continuous, local, and mixed type on the basis of the distribution of lesions behind the vertebral bodies. CT scanning is helpful in assessing the thickness, lateral extension, and AP diameter of the ossified ligament.

More than 95% of the ossification is localized in the cervical spine although extension into the thoracic spine has been reported to be a cause of persistent myelopathy following cervical decompression.

Enchondral ossification is mainly responsible for the formation of the ossified mass, which connects to the upper and lower margins of the vertebral bodies. In many cases, the ossified material adheres closely to the underlying dura and makes excision quite hazardous. Compression of the spinal cord results in atrophy and necrosis in the gray matter and demyelinization of the white substance.

Treatment

Neurologic improvement with either conservative or surgical treatment is achieved in a significant proportion of patients. The patients with severe myelopathy require neural decompression by an anterior, posterior, or combined approach. Sophisticated posterior decompression techniques, such as the open-door laminaplasty, have yielded excellent long-term results.

Hirabayashi K, Satomi K: Operative procedure and results of expansive open-door laminaplasty. Spine 1988;13:870.

Kawaguchi Y et al: Progression of ossification of the posterior longitudinal ligament following en bloc cervical laminaplasty. J Bone Joint Surg Am 200183-A(12):1798.

Koyanagi I et al: Magnetic resonance imaging findings in ossification of the posterior longitudinal ligament of the cervical spine. J Neurosurg 1998;88:247.

Macdonald RL et al: Multilevel anterior cervical corpectomy and fibular allograft fusion for cervical myelopathy. J Neurosurg 1997;86:990.

Matsuoka T et al: Long-term results of the anterior floating method for cervical myelopathy caused by ossification of the posterior longitudinal ligament. Spine 2001;26(3):241.

Smith MD et al: Postoperative cerebrospinal-fluid fistula associated with erosion of the dura. Findings after anterior resection of ossification of the posterior longitudinal ligament in the cervical spine. J Bone Joint Surg Am 1992;74:270.

■ DISEASES & DISORDERS OF THE LUMBAR SPINE

LOW BACK PAIN

Low back pain is a very common symptom in the general population. According to the Quebec Task Force on Spinal Disorders, over 80% of the population experiences some low back pain at some time. The overall prevalence of low back pain the United States is estimated to be around 18%. The annual incidence of low back pain is 15–20%. Males are affected as often as females, and the pain is usually self-limiting, with 50% of affected patients recovering by 2 weeks and 90% recovering by 6 weeks. Only 1% of the population in the United States is chronically disabled by back symptoms. If a patient stays off work for more than 2 years because of problems of the lower back, he or she is unlikely to return to work at all.

The socioeconomic impact of back problems is enormous. Over 14% of all new patient visits to physicians are for complaints of low back pain. Low back pain is the most common reason for visits to the orthopedic surgeon. Costs are estimated to range from $20 billion to $50 billion annually, with 10% of the patients accounting for 85–90% of the costs. Investigators have shown that patients with chronic low back pain tend to be dissatisfied with their vocation, viewing it as boring and repetitive. They also have an increased divorce rate, more problems with headaches and gastrointestinal ulcers, and a higher rate of alcoholism than the average population. The extensive use of the Minnesota Multiphasic Personality Inventory (MMPI) in the assessment of patients with chronic low back pain has demonstrated an association between chronic pain, somatization, and hypochondriasis.

Etiology & Pathophysiology

The exact cause of symptoms is found in only 12–15% of patients. A thorough understanding of the lumbar anatomy and its function is important because lower back pain might originate from the disc, vertebral body, or posterior elements or might be unrelated to the spine. The earlier concept of a motor segment has been superseded by the concept of a functional spinal unit or motion segment. This unit consists of two adjacent vertebrae and the intervertebral disc, which together form a three-joint complex with the disc in front and two facet joints posteriorly. The motion segment involves joint capsules, ligaments, muscles, nerves, and vessels as well. Changes in one joint affect the other two. Disc degeneration leads to disc space narrowing, end-plate sclerosis, abnormal stress on facet joints, and, ultimately, facet degeneration.

Significant emphasis has been placed recently on the idea of the intervertebral disc as a pain generator. These axial pain syndromes of discogenic origin have been roughly categorized as internal disc disruption, degenerative disc disease, and disc degeneration as a sequela of segmental instability. The overriding principle is that the posterior portion of the annulus fibrosus is innervated by fibers of the sinuvertebral nerve, which is a branch of the dorsal root ganglion. Irritation of the sinuvertebral nerve is thought to be responsible for axial back pain. In the rat, Suseki has shown that these pain fibers are not innervated segmentally. Sensory information from the lumbar intervertebral discs are conducted to other spinal levels via the paravertebral sympathetic trunks. These data suggest that decompression of the nerve root at one level is unlikely to help with low back pain symptoms.

Principles of Diagnosis

A. HISTORY AND PHYSICAL EXAMINATION

A focused history and physical examination of the patient are crucial for the appropriate diagnosis and treatment. Typical initial questions include the following: What is the problem? Which areas are affected? How much does the pain interfere with sitting, standing, and walking? Were there previous episodes? If so, how long did they last? Are there bowel or bladder symptoms? The presence of bowel or bladder symptoms may indicate a cauda equina syndrome. Leg and buttock pain are usually indicative of nerve root irritation from a herniated disc or neuroforamenal stenosis, whereas axial low back pain is often mechanical. Drawing a diagram of the areas affected by pain may be of help, and a history of other medical problems may provide additional clues.

The physical examination is subjective and requires the patient's interpretation and cooperation. The diagnostic significance of range-of-motion measurements of the spine is questionable. Although a positive result in the straight leg-raising test is highly suggestive of nerve root irritation in a young patient, use of this test is less reliable in an older patient. In addition to noting a general impression of the patient and testing for sensory and motor deficits, the clinician should check the patient's response to local touch, axial loading, and simulated rotation and should record the presence of other nonorganic signs (Waddell's signs). Patients with chronic low back pain demonstrate illness behavior and score high in nonorganic signs.

The pain is considered acute if it lasts less than 6 weeks and chronic if it lasts longer than 12 weeks. The most common cause is a lumbar strain after a lifting or twisting event or without known trauma. Patients usually present with localized pain in the lumbosacral area, in some cases with pain radiating into the buttocks. Palpation of the paraspinal muscles reveals spasms, and motion is limited. Results of the neurologic examination are normal, and the straight leg-raising test is negative. Sensation and reflexes are symmetric.

B. IMAGING STUDIES

1. Radiography—Radiographs are not necessary during the initial evaluation. If a patient's symptoms do not resolve, x-ray films may be obtained. They are indicated in patients who are older than 50 years and have a history of trauma, cancer, weight loss, pain at rest, drug abuse, neurologic deficit, or fever. Radiographs may appear normal or demonstrate disc space narrowing, osteophyte formation, or localized instability on lateral flexion-extension views. No association has been established between low back pain and the presence of disc space narrowing, transitional vertebrae, Schmorl's nodes, the disc vacuum sign, claw spurs, lumbar lordosis, or spina bifida occulta. Routine flexion-extension views of the lumbar spine are not indicated and rarely demonstrate obvious segmental instability.

2. Other studies—If plain radiographs are unsuccessful in establishing the cause of the patient's problem and the patient has not responded to conservative therapy, additional imaging studies may be helpful.

MRI of the lumbar spine is noninvasive and excellent in assessing compromise of neural structures. For example, MRI with gadolinium enhances the imaging of intraspinal tissue and can help distinguish scar formation after previous surgery from new encroachment on neural structures by disc material. CT scanning, with and without enhancement by myelography, can be helpful if MRI studies are not possible or do not yield positive results. CT myelography is especially useful in assessing patients who have had spinal instrumentation. If an infection of the spine is suspected, a gadolinium-enhanced MRI is an extremely sensitive and specific test for discitis, spinal osteomyelitis, and epidural abscess.

Disc degeneration is common in adults with low back pain. Caution in interpreting the results of MRI and CT is necessary, however, because studies have shown that positive findings are seen in asymptomatic patients who undergo MRI or CT evaluation of the lumbar spine. When MRI was used to examine the lumbar spines of asymptomatic volunteers, disc herniation was found in 17% of those younger than 40 years, 22% of those between 40 and 59 years, and 36% of those older than 60 years. In the oldest group, 21% showed lumbar stenosis without symptoms. When CT was used to examine the lumbar spines of asymptomatic volunteers, disc herniation was found in 35.4% of the volunteers.

If disc degeneration is suspected to be the cause of lower back pain, a discogram may be indicated. In this provocative test, dye is injected into the nucleus pulposus, and then a CT scan of the injected segment is taken. The pain response of the patient seems to be the most accurate indication that the injected disc might be responsible for the patient's pain. However, the use of provocative discography in the evaluation of axial back pain continues to be controversial. The results are subjective and depends greatly on the patient's psychologic status at the time of the procedure. Discography is more sensitive than MRI in assessing internal disc disruption, although questions about the value of using discography, facet blocks, and other invasive tests remain to be answered.

Principles of Treatment

Management of low back pain has to be tailored to the individual. The goal is early return to work. Most patients can simply modify their activities during the acute phase. If a serious pathologic condition has been ruled out, a more aggressive approach is warranted because bed rest for more than 2 days has serious side effects: the body is in a catabolic state; 3% of muscle bulk is lost daily; 6% of bone is demineralized in 2 weeks; and restriction of social activities leads to illness behavior, depression, and loss of interest and motivation. Iatrogenic disability must be avoided. Patients with acute low back pain should avoid sitting and lifting. Mild analgesics and anti-inflammatory agents are useful in the acute phase of the disease. Educational programs, aerobic endurance exercises, and abdominal conditioning have also proved to be helpful.

There is no evidence that the following treatment modalities are useful in the management of acute low back pain: transcutaneous electrical nerve stimulation, traction, manipulation in the presence of radicular signs, acupuncture, biofeedback, narcotics for longer than 2 weeks, trigger point injections, and muscle relaxants.

Patients who have low back pain that persists for more than 3 months occasionally benefit from antidepressant medication. If narcotic analgesics are not needed and if surgery has been ruled out, they may be candidates for a functional restoration program involving an interdisciplinary approach with physical therapists, occupational therapists, psychologists, and medical professionals. One study showed that 87% of program participants returned to work, whereas only 41% of control subjects did so.

A subgroup of patients who have persistent, disabling axial low back pain of discogenic origin in the absence of other psychologic or organic pathologies may benefit from complete discectomy and interbody fusion. This can be performed through an anterior open or laparoscopic approach or via the posterior approach. Good to excellent outcomes have been reported in up to 70–80% of patients.

Disc replacement surgery was first introduced in the early 1950s with variable results. As spinal fusion demonstrated itself to be a relatively efficacious procedure, surgeons quickly lost their initial enthusiasm for spinal arthroplasty. However, as the limitations of spinal fusion have become evident and as technology has improved to design better bearing surfaces, disc replacement has enjoyed a new resurgence in interest. The theoretical advantages include preserving or restoring motion after removal of the painful disc, preventing late adjacent segment degeneration, and improving function without the need for fusion. Currently FDA-approved clinical trials are under way to examine the efficacy of these devices.

Other less invasive therapies for discogenic axial back pain have also been introduced. One of these, an intradiscal electrothermal therapy, attempts to thermally ablate the painful nerve fibers in the posterior annulus. The reported outcomes on this procedure have varied and it is unclear whether the results are a significant improvement over the natural history of axial low back pain.

Bernard TJ: Lumbar discography followed by computed tomography: Refining the diagnosis of low back pain. Spine 1990;15: 690.

Birney TJ et al: Comparison of MRI and discography in the diagnosis of lumbar degenerative disc disease. J Spinal Dis 1992; 5:417.

Boden SD et al: Abnormal magnetic resonance scans of the lumbar spine in asymptomatic patients: A prospective investigation. J Bone Joint Surg Am 1990;72:403.

Carette S et al: A controlled trial of corticosteroid injections into facet joints for chronic low back pain. N Engl J Med 1991; 325:1002.

Derby R et al: The ability of pressure-controlled discography to predict surgical and nonsurgical outcomes. Spine 1999;24(4): 364; discussion 371.

Faas A et al: A randomized, placebo-controlled trial of exercise therapy in patients with acute lower back pain. Spine 1993;18: 1388.

Humphreys SC et al: Comparison of posterior and transforaminal approaches to lumbar interbody fusion. Spine 2001;26(5): 567.

Saal JS, Saal JA: Management of chronic discogenic low back pain with a thermal intradiscal catheter. A preliminary report. Spine 2000;25(3):382.

Suseki K et al: Sensory nerve fibers from lumbar intervertebral discs pass through rami communicantes. A possible pathway for discogenic low back pain. J Bone Joint Surg Br 1998;80(4): 737.

LUMBAR DISC HERNIATION

Symptomatic disc herniations are seen in all age groups but have their peak in patients between the ages of 35 and 45 years. Although smoking is a general risk factor for disc degeneration and herniation, occupational risk factors include sedentary work and motor vehicle driving. Sciatica, characterized by pain radiating down the leg in a dermatomal distribution, is the most common symptom and is found in 40% of patients with disc herniation. About 50% of patients recover within 1 month, and 96% function normally by 6 months. The rate of surgical treatment in the United States is three times higher than that in Sweden.

Pathophysiology

A disc herniation is usually preceded by degenerative changes inside the disc. Circumferential tears in the an-

nulus progress to radial tears, and these in turn frequently cause internal disruption or frank herniation. Two pathologic patterns can be distinguished. In a contained disc protrusion, the annulus fibers are intact. In a noncontained disc herniation, the annulus is completely disrupted. Disc material can be subligamentous or sequestered as a free fragment. The pain accompanying disc herniation may be caused by direct pressure on the nerve root or may be induced by breakdown products from a degenerated nucleus pulposus or by an autoimmune reaction. Disc material has been shown to be a direct source of chemically irritative substances such as phospholipase A_2, prostaglandin E, substance P, and lactic acid. Biochemical studies in operated disc fragments demonstrate an advanced aging process. The hydration of the disc changes from 90% during childhood to 70% by the sixth decade, and the ability of proteoglycans to aggregate decreases with advancing age.

Clinical Findings

A. SYMPTOMS AND SIGNS

The typical sciatica is commonly preceded by back pain for a period of days or weeks. This suggests that a compression of nerve fibers in the outer layers of the annulus preceded the rupture of the disc material into the spinal canal and the advent of leg pain. A complete physical examination is necessary. Although the dominating symptom is pain, patients often present with scoliosis or a sciatic list. The mobility of the lumbar spine is diminished more in flexion than in extension. Coughing, sneezing, or a voluntary Valsalva's maneuver commonly aggravates the radiating pain. Prolonged sitting also accentuates the pain.

In more than 90% of cases, lumbar disc herniations are localized at L4-5 and L5-S1. Herniations can occur in the central portion of the posterior annulus (central disc herniation), adjacent to the central portion of the posterior annulus (right or left paracentral disc herniation), or within or just lateral to the neural foramen (far lateral disc herniation). Most disc herniations that cause unilateral radicular symptoms are paracentral disc herniations. Paracentral disc herniations typically affect the traversing nerve root at the affected level, whereas lateral and foraminal herniations affect the exiting nerve root at the affected level. This occurs because of the particular path of the nerve roots as they emerge from the dural sleeve and enter the intervertebral foramen. A lumbar nerve root typically exits at its corresponding disc level (ie, the L4 root will exit through the L4-5 intervertebral foramen). This course will allow it to exit the spinal canal just above the L4-5 disc space. However, the traversing nerve root (in this case the L5 root) emerges from the dural sleeve just above the disc space and must cross the posterior portion of the annulus in order to reach and exit at the intervertebral foramen at the next level (in this case the L5-S1 level). Thus a paracentral disc herniation at L4-5 will compress the traversing L5 nerve root instead of the L4 nerve root, which will exit just above the level of the herniation. Compression of the L4 nerve root, which leads to pain and numbness in the L4 dermatome, can occur in a central disc herniation at L3-4 or in a lateral herniation at L4-5. When the L4 nerve root is affected, there may be weakness of the quadriceps muscle, and the patella tendon reflex may be depressed or absent. Central or paracentral disc herniations at L4-5 usually compromise the L5 nerve root, where they may cause numbness in the L5 dermatome and weakness of the foot and toe dorsiflexors. A disc herniation at L5-S1 usually compromises the S1 nerve root, causing numbness or pain in the S1 dermatome, weak plantarflexion of the foot, loss of the Achilles tendon reflex, or tingling in the nerve distribution.

The straight leg-raising test should be performed. The Lasègue sign (pain when the affected leg is elevated) is positive in 98% of patients with lumbar disc herniation, and the cross-Lasègue sign (pain radiating to the affected leg when the contralateral leg is elevated) is positive in 20%. This test is less accurate in older patients and in patients with chronic lumbar disc herniation. For lesions involving the L3 or L4 nerve root, the femoral nerve stretch test should be applied. The radicular pain is reproduced when the knee is flexed while the hip is slightly extended.

B. Imaging Studies

MRI is the study of choice for diagnosis of a herniated disc (Figure 5–10). Because 28% of asymptomatic patients show a disc herniation on MRI, it is important to correlate the level of spinal involvement with the peripheral nerve deficit. CT scanning and myelography are less frequently used to confirm the diagnosis.

Differential Diagnosis

Radicular pain is typical and should be distinguished from referred pain, which commonly radiates from the lower back into the posterior thigh and ends at the knee level. The posterior spinal elements are frequently a source of this pain. Anterior thigh pain may indicate a retroperitoneal process, such as renal disease or a tumor of the uterus or bladder. Hip disorders, including trochanteric bursitis and coxarthrosis, must be ruled out. The presence of incontinence, perianal numbness, and bilateral leg pain associated with numbness suggests a cauda equina syndrome and requires immediate surgical attention. A primary tumor or metastatic disease involving the spine can present with radiculopathy, and

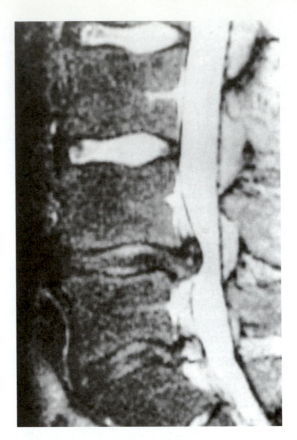

Figure 5–10. MRI in a patient with disc herniation at L4L5 and L5-S1. Both discs are markedly desiccated as compared with discs of the upper lumbar spine.

symptoms and signs such as pain at night, a previous history of cancer, and loss of weight should raise the suspicion of the examiner.

Treatment

In cases of lumbar disc herniation, the goal of treatment is to return the patient to normal activities as quickly as possible. Unnecessary surgery should be avoided. In determining the proper treatment plan, a knowledge of the natural history of lumbar disc herniation is important. In a prospective study of 280 patients with lumbar disc herniations, Weber compared the outcome of a group treated conservatively with the outcome of a group treated with discectomy. Although better results were seen in the surgically treated patients at 1-year follow-up, the groups showed nearly equal results in terms of function 4 and 10 years later. The study demonstrated a slight tendency to a more favorable outcome with surgery.

A. CONSERVATIVE TREATMENT

Two days of bed rest followed by a good physical therapy program will often lead to significant alleviation of symptoms within 2 or 3 weeks. Analgesics and nonsteroidal medication may also be included in the regimen. Chiropractic adjustments should be avoided in patients with documented disc herniation. Although the role of epidural corticosteroids is unclear, they seem to be successful in decreasing the acute sciatic pain.

B. SURGICAL TREATMENT

About 10% of patients with lumbar disc herniation will ultimately require surgery. Surgery is recommended if the sciatica is severe and disabling and tension signs are positive, if symptoms persist without improvement for longer than 1 month, or if findings on clinical examination and in diagnostic tests are consistent with nerve root compromise.

When a standard discectomy is used, the overall success rate is 85%, and 95% of the patients with successful surgery return to work. Microdiscectomy minimizes the dissection and has an equally high success rate. With this technique, only removal of the extruded part of the disc or of the free fragment is necessary. Risks of surgery include dural tear, wrong level exploration, hemorrhage, infection, and nerve deficit.

In cases of contained disc protrusion, percutaneous automated discectomy or chemonucleolysis may be considered. Each of these approaches has a success rate of about 75%. When percutaneous discectomy is used, a cannula is placed into the disc space under fluoroscopic control, a cutting instrument is fitted inside the cannula, and disc material is then cut and suctioned at the same time. Insertion of an optical device through an extra portal has made direct visualization of the disc possible. Although a multicenter analysis of percutaneous discectomy showed that only 55% of patients returned to work following treatment, the success rate appears to be higher in the centers with the greatest experience.

Chemonucleolysis of herniated discs is used extensively in Europe. Chymopapain is injected into the nucleus of the contained herniated disc, and it enzymatically degrades the nucleus pulposus but leaves the annulus intact. This procedure fell into disfavor in the United States after a series of deaths occurred secondary to anaphylaxis. Other complications associated with the procedure include transverse myelitis, discitis, seizures, and subarachnoid hemorrhage. Many of the previous bad results have been linked with poor patient selection or technical error.

Because experience with laser discectomy is limited, this extradural approach must still be viewed as experimental. Thus far, its success rate is slightly lower than that of percutaneous discectomy.

Asch HL et al: Prospective multiple outcomes study of outpatient lumbar microdiscectomy: Should 75 to 80% success rates be the norm? J Neurosurg, 2002;96(1 Suppl):34.

Atlas SJ et al: The Quebec Task Force Classification for Spinal Disorders and the severity, treatment, and outcomes of sciatica and lumbar spinal stenosis. Spine 1996;21:2885.

Atlas SJ et al: Long-term disability and return to work among patients who have a herniated lumbar disc: the effect of disability compensation. J Bone Joint Surg Am 2000;82(1):4.

Burton AK, et al: Single-blind randomised controlled trial of chemonucleolysis and manipulation in the treatment of symptomatic lumbar disc herniation. Eur Spine J 2000;9(3): 202.

Ito T et al: Types of lumbar herniated disc and clinical course. Spine 2001;26(6):648.

Marks RA: Transcutaneous lumbar diskectomy for internal disk derangement: A new indication. South Med J 2000;93(9):885.

Nygaard OP et al: Duration of leg pain as a predictor of outcome after surgery for lumbar disc herniation: A prospective cohort study with 1-year follow up. J Neurosurg 2000;92(2 Suppl): 131.

Weber H: Lumbar disc herniation: A controlled, prospective study with 10 years of observation. Spine 1983;8:131.

Yorimitsu E et al: Long-term outcomes of standard discectomy for lumbar disc herniation: a follow-up study of more than 10 years. Spine 2001;26(6):652.

FACET SYNDROME

The facet joint is probably not a common source of pain. The term *facet syndrome* was introduced in 1933 by Ghormley, who thought that a narrow disc space would lead to increased facet joint degeneration and serve as a potential source for sciatica. In the following decades, a distinction was made between radicular pain, which resulted from direct pressure on exiting nerve roots, and referred pain, which originated from the posterior spinal elements and the facet joints in particular.

Later research showed innervation of the facet joint by the medial branch of the posterior ramus of the spinal nerve. This nerve and its branches will innervate the facet joints of a three-joint complex, making it virtually impossible to denervate a single joint by the injection of an agent at a single level.

The lumbar facet joints are biomechanically important. They absorb significant loads in extension and are a valuable part of the three-joint complex. Their role is to restrain excessive mobility of a spinal segment and to distribute axial loading over a broad area. In patients with symptomatic facet syndrome, biopsies have revealed cartilage changes that are similar to findings in chondromalacia patellae.

Clinical Findings

A. SYMPTOMS AND SIGNS

Although patients with facet syndrome tend to have problems localizing the exact source of their pain, they usually complain of low back pain that often increases on extension. The pain may radiate into the posterior thigh and commonly ends at the knee level. When patients wake up with low back pain, they frequently can alleviate the pain by changing position.

B. IMAGING STUDIES

Plain radiographs will demonstrate a narrowed disc space. Oblique views of the lumbar spine may show osteophyte formation of the superior and inferior facet. A more accurate study is a CT scan, which allows axial cuts and demonstration of arthritic changes involving the facets.

Treatment

Conservative care with anti-inflammatory medication, an external back support, and physical therapy should alleviate symptoms in most cases of facet syndrome. Intra-articular injections might be helpful as a diagnostic tool and buy time in these often difficult cases. The result of facet joint injections has been shown to be unreliable, however. A low back fusion might be successful in extreme degenerative cases that have failed to respond to conservative care, but the selection of fusion levels should not be based on the outcome of previous facet joint injections.

Esses SI, Moro JK: The value of facet joint blocks in patient selection for lumbar fusion. Spine 1993;18:185.

Jackson RP: The facet syndrome: Myth or reality? Clin Orthop 1992;279:110.

Jackson RP et al: Facet joint injection in low back pain: A prospective statistical study. Spine 1988;13:966.

STENOSIS OF THE LUMBAR SPINE

Stenosis of the lumbar spine is a clinical entity that is responsible for a variety of complaints ranging from low back pain to lower extremity dysfunction. The condition has been defined as any developmental or acquired narrowing of the spinal canal, nerve root canals, or intervertebral foramina that results in compression of neural elements.

Pathophysiology

Some physiologic narrowing of the canal occurs with age. There are also normal variations in the cross-sectional areas and shapes of the lumbar spinal canal, with the narrowest area found between L2 and L4. The canal volume increases in flexion and decreases in extension. Narrowing of the spinal canal can further occur by bulging of the disc anteriorly, by buckling of

the ligamentum flavum posteriorly, and by encroachment of the articular facets. Degeneration of the intervertebral disc causes increased stress on the facet joint and can lead to arthrosis and hypertrophy of facets and adjacent structures. This will ultimately compromise the spinal canal. The decrease in canal volume occurs at such a slow and gradual pace that the neurologic structures in most patients accommodate to it, with the result that there may be surprisingly few neurologic symptoms even in patients with advanced degenerative stenosis.

The cause of pain experienced by patients with stenosis is perplexing and has been attributed to mechanical, ischemic, inflammatory, and various other mechanisms. The simplest explanation, of course, is pure mechanical compression of cord and adjacent roots. The "hourglass" configuration and bulging of the dura as it is decompressed attests to the increased pressures within the stenotic canal. According to the neuroischemic explanation, the nerve fibers are nutritionally deprived by compression of the small nutrient vessels. Inflammatory conditions of the dura and exiting nerve roots are equally suspect. Common surgical findings are an adhesive arachnoiditis of the pia and the presence of friction neuritis, and these may constrict or tether the neural elements. The hypertrophic membranes also have reduced permeability and may obstruct the free flow of cerebrospinal fluid (CSF) from perfusing the root tissues. This can compromise the metabolism of nerve fibers because nearly 50% of their nutrients are derived from CSF.

According to a recent vascular and nutritional explanation for the onset of pseudoclaudication, the nerve fibers in the resting state have diminished metabolic requirements that enable them to conduct sufficient impulses for minimal activity of the muscles. With increases in exertion, however, the metabolic requirements of the compromised nerve rise rapidly. The tension of root fixation and the reduced permeability to CSF hamper the delivery of necessary nutrients and the removal of noxious accumulations. The resulting relative neuroischemia renders the nerve more mechanosensitive, causing ectopic impulses to be conducted and to produce pain, paresthesias, and pseudoclaudication.

Gross morphologic changes include a compressed caudal sac, diffuse ligamentous and facet joint hypertrophy, disc space narrowing with or without concomitant protrusion, encroachment of the lamina, and occasional degenerative spondylolisthesis. Microscopic changes include quantitative losses of neurons with numerous empty axons, various degrees of demyelinization, diffuse interstitial fibrosis with venous congestion, and coiled arterial "pigtails" on either side of the compressed lesion.

Classification

Spinal stenosis is classified as congenital or acquired. The congenital type is caused by developmental spinal anomalies that compromise the neural elements. This type is seen, for example, in patients with achondroplasia (Figure 5–11). The acquired type is more common and has been further divided into the degenerative, olisthetic-scoliotic, posttraumatic, and postoperative subtypes. Although the original shape of the spinal canal may be round, oval, or trefoil, the trefoil shape is most commonly associated with stenosis and may be a predisposing factor.

The location of stenosis can be central or lateral. In central stenosis, hypertrophied structures cause circumferential pressure of the spinal cord. Lateral stenosis is associated with narrowing of the foraminal canal, which is divided into three separate zones: the entrance zone, the middle zone, and the exit zone.

Clinical Findings

A. SYMPTOMS AND SIGNS

In degenerative spinal stenosis, which occurs primarily in elderly individuals and is seen more commonly in men than in women, the lower lumbar segments are affected the most severely. The pattern of complaints varies among patients. In many cases, onset is insidious and progression of pain in the lower back, buttock, and thigh is slow. The pain is generally diffuse rather than neurosegmental and is episodic. Nearly all patients report that their lower extremity pain is altered by changes in position. It generally occurs with standing or walking and is relieved by rest, lying, sitting, or adopt-

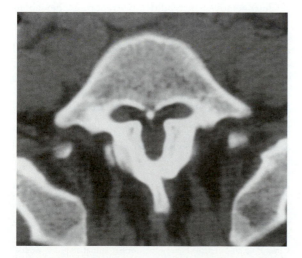

Figure 5–11. CT scan showing severe stenosis and typical trefoil shape of the lumbar spine in a patient with achondroplasia.

ing a position of flexion at the waist. In addition, the patient may find it easier to walk uphill (when their trunk is flexed) than downhill (when their trunk is extended). They may also have greater walking tolerance pushing a shopping cart because they are able to ambulate in a more flexed position. These are the hallmarks of pseudoclaudication. Neurogenic and vascular claudication may be difficult to distinguish from each other. Thus all patients should have their distal pulses examined as a part of the overall neurologic evaluation. Mistaken diagnoses are not uncommon.

In a recent study of 172 patients with symptoms of claudication who were found on myelogram and CT to have lumbar stenosis and were treated operatively, investigators found that 65% of the patients demonstrated objective weakness and 25% exhibited diminished deep tendon reflexes. Only 10% had positive results in the straight leg-raising test, indicating entrapment of a nerve root. Nine patients had peripheral vascular disease identified by ultrasound and arteriography, and six of these nine required additional vascular bypass surgery for persistent symptoms of lower extremity claudication.

B. IMAGING STUDIES

Findings on plain radiographs include degenerative disc disease, osteoarthritis of the facets, spondylolisthesis, and narrowing of the interpedicular distance as seen on the AP view. Although myelography was commonly used in the past to evaluate spinal cord or root compression, it is an invasive procedure with possible side effects and is no longer routinely used. CT scanning is commonly used to evaluate the spinal elements and allows for accurate measurement of the canal dimensions when combined with contrast enhancement. A dural sac with an AP diameter of less than 10 mm correlates with clinical findings of stenosis.

MRI is comparable to contrast-enhanced CT scanning in its ability to demonstrate spinal stenosis and is now the imaging modality of choice for assessing the spinal canal and the neural structures (Figure 5–12).

Differential Diagnosis

A complete physical examination is essential to exclude other causes of referred pain in the low back, such as retroperitoneal tumors, aortic aneurysms, peptic ulcer disease, renal lesions, and pathologic processes of the hips or pelvis.

Psychologic factors of low back pain often give rise to symptoms independent of spinal canal narrowing and can lead to confusing differential diagnoses. Depression is common in the elderly, and prompt recognition and treatment of underlying depression as the cause of somatic complaints may result in marked diminution of symptoms.

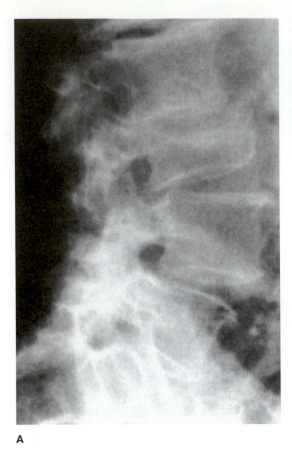

A

B

Figure 5–12. Imaging studies in a patient with degenerative stenosis of the lumbar spine. **A:** Radiograph showing degenerative spondylolisthesis between L4 and L5, as well as an old compression fracture of L3. **B:** MRI showing severe stenosis of the spinal canal at L4L5, marked facet hypertrophy and ligamentous hypertrophy resulting in central canal stenosis, and lateral recess stenosis.

Treatment

A. CONSERVATIVE TREATMENT

Initial treatment of the patient with symptoms suggestive of spinal stenosis should consist of salicylates or nonsteroidal agents and an exercise program tailored to the patient's goals or life-style. Surprisingly, many patients show an appreciable response to this form of treatment. Narcotics may induce dependency and should be avoided. Epidural corticosteroid injections have a short-term success rate of 50% and a long-term success rate of 25%.

B. SURGICAL TREATMENT

If conservative methods fail, the patient's quality-of-life must be a key factor in deciding when to proceed with surgery. Decompressive laminectomy has a short-term success rate between 71% and 85%. About 17% of older patients require reoperation for recurrent stenosis or instability. The disc should be preserved under any circumstances, to avoid postoperative instability. The best surgical results are seen in patients without coexisting morbid conditions (Figure 5–13).

Postoperative instability is reported in about 10–15% of patients treated. Preoperative risk factors for developing instability include disc space narrowing, osteoporosis, preexisting spondylolisthesis, and multilevel decompression. Late instability can occur when 50% of bilateral facets have been resected, when 100% of one facet joint has been resected. In these cases, a prophylactic instrumented lateral fusion should be performed.

Amundsen T et al: Lumbar spinal stenosis: Conservative or surgical management?: A prospective 10-year study. Spine 2000;25 (11):1424; discussion 1435.

Atlas SJ et al: Surgical and nonsurgical management of lumbar spinal stenosis: Four-year outcomes from the Maine lumbar spine study. Spine 2000;25(5):556.

Barrick WT et al: Anterior lumbar fusion improves discogenic pain at levels of prior posterolateral fusion. Spine 2000;25(7):853.

Cirak B et al: Surgical therapy for lumbar spinal stenosis: Evaluation of 300 cases. Neurosurg Rev 2001;24(2-3):80.

Cornefjord M et al: A long-term (4- to 12-year) follow-up study of surgical treatment of lumbar spinal stenosis. Eur Spine J 20009(6):563.

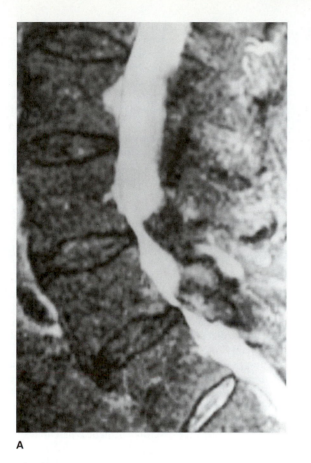

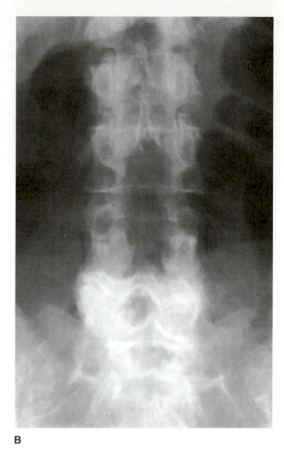

A

B

Figure 5–13. Imaging studies in a patient with stenosis of the lumbar spine and leg pain. **A:** MRI showing stenosis at L3-4. **B:** Radiograph taken after two-level laminectomy, which led to resolution of the preoperative leg pain.

Iguchi T et al: Minimum 10-year outcome of decompressive laminectomy for degenerative lumbar spinal stenosis. Spine 2000;25(14):1754.

Stromqvist B et al: The Swedish National Register for lumbar spine surgery: Swedish Society for Spinal Surgery. Acta Orthop Scand 2001;72(2):99.

Vaccaro AR, Garfin SR: Degenerative lumbar spondylolisthesis with spinal stenosis, a prospective study comparing decompression with decompression and intertransverse process arthrodesis: A critical analysis. Spine 1997;22:368.

Whitehurst M et al: Functional mobility performance in an elderly population with lumbar spinal stenosis. Arch Phys Med Rehabil 2001;82(4):464.

OSTEOPOROSIS AND VERTEBRAL COMPRESSION FRACTURES

Osteoporosis is characterized by a decline in overall bone mass in the axial and appendicular skeleton. The disease affects between 15 and 20 million people in the United States. Peak bone mass, attained between the ages of 16 to 25 years, slowly declines with age as the rate of bone resorption exceeds that of bone formation. This phenomenon occurs in both men and women and is known as senile osteoporosis. Women are also susceptible to postmenopausal osteoporosis that occurs during the 15 to 20 years after the onset of menopause and is directly linked to estrogen deficiency. Environmental factors also play a role in accelerating the rate of skeletal bone loss. These include, chronic calcium deficiency, smoking, excessive alcohol intake, hyperparathyroidism, and inactivity. Genetic influences may also play a role.

Vertebral compression fractures are one of the most frequent manifestations of osteoporosis in the elderly. Over 700,000 vertebral compression fractures occur each year. Fortunately, the overwhelming majority of patients are asymptomatic.

Clinical Findings

Patients with symptomatic vertebral compression fractures typically complain of axial pain localized to the fractured level. Occasionally, the patient's family will notice that the patient's back is becoming increasingly rounded and significant loss of height has occurred. This spinal deformity is known as the "dowager's hump." In general, no neurologic dysfunction and no radiation of the pain in any dermatomal distribution. There is often no history of significant trauma or an inciting event.

Imaging

Plain radiographs and densitometric scans are the major imaging modalities in the assessment of osteoporotic bone and their pathologic counterparts (insufficiency fractures). Dual-energy x-ray absorptiometry has been the most useful of the densitometric imaging techniques because it carries a high degree of precision (0.5–2%) and subjects the patient to minimal amounts of radiation. It is also quite accurate for assessing osteoporosis in both the axial and appendicular skeleton. Other imaging modalities include single-energy x-ray absorptiometry, quantitative computed tomography, and radiographic absorptiometry.

AP and lateral radiographs of the affected area of the spine will likely reveal the location and severity of the osteoporotic fracture(s). In the thoracic spine, wedge compression fractures are most commonly encountered. In the lumbar spine, both compression and burst fractures can occur. Other imaging modalities include technetium bone scans and MRI scans. These studies should be reserved for the evaluation of fractures that remain symptomatic or progress after a course of conservative treatment. MRI is extremely useful in differentiating nonunited fractures from those that have healed and in differentiating osteoporotic fractures from those cause by malignancy.

Bone biopsy is indicated if a metabolic bone disease or a malignancy is suspected as the cause of the osteoporosis. The sample is typically retrieved from the anterior iliac crest and is examined using bone histomorphometry.

Treatment

Prevention still remains the best treatment for osteoporosis. Maximizing bone mineral density prior to the onset of bone loss and minimizing the bone loss that occurs is the optimal regimen for preventing the painful sequelae of the disease. In women, estrogen replacement therapy can be initiated if there is no history of breast cancer, thromboembolic disease, endometrial disease, or heart disease. Routine gynecologic examination is necessary once therapy is initiated. Calcitonin therapy can be used if estrogen therapy is contraindicated. Parathyroid hormone is currently under clinical trials for the treatment of osteoporosis. Early evidence suggests that it may help to significantly increase skeletal bone mass and may be useful as a first-line treatment for severe osteoporosis.

The bisphosphonates, etidronate and alendronate, prevent osteoclastic resorption of bone. They are the only FDA-approved compounds in widespread use that have been shown to increase bone mineral density. However, the increase is relatively small.

The initial treatment of symptomatic vertebral compression fractures involves a trial of analgesic therapy and bracing for comfort. Evaluation and treatment for osteoporosis can be initiated if not done already. Conservative therapy should be attempted for at least 6–12 weeks or longer if the patient is improving.

Surgical Treatment

Patients with fractures that cause neurologic deficit or significant spinal cord compression should be treated with anterior decompression and fusion followed by posterior segmental instrumentation and fusion. The poor bone quality makes correction of deformity and maintenance of posterior constructs a challenging task.

Patients who have recalcitrant back pain from a nonunited vertebral compression fracture who have failed a course of conservative management can obtain excellent symptomatic relief from fracture stabilization through injection of polymethylmethacrylate (PMMA) bone cement into the fracture through a percutaneous technique. The two most popular procedures, vertebroplasty and kyphoplasty, have been shown to be both safe and efficacious. In both techniques, a cannula is inserted transpedicularly or extrapedicularly (lateral to the pedicle) into the anterior portion of the affected vertebral body, and acrylic cement is instilled into the fractured bone under fluoroscopic control. Once the cement has cured, the fracture is immediately stabilized. In the kyphoplasty technique, a balloon is inflated in the vertebral body in an attempt to compress the existing bone, create a void for instillation of more viscous cement under lower pressure, and to correct the wedge deformity. This technique has the theoretical advantage of allowing some deformity correction and preventing high-pressure–related extrusion of PMMA into the spinal canal.

Why vertebroplasty and kyphoplasty relieve the pain is unclear. Multiple mechanisms may play a role, including fracture stabilization, denervation of pain fibers by the heat generated during the cement curing process, and neurotoxicity of the PMMA monomer. In addition, longer follow-up has raised concerns over predisposing the adjacent segment to fracture by over-stiffening the affected level. These concerns are currently under active investigation.

Barr JD et al: Percutaneous vertebroplasty for pain relief and spinal stabilization. Spine 2000;25(8):923.

Dudeney S, Lieberman I: Percutaneous vertebroplasty in the treatment of osteoporotic vertebral compression fractures: An open prospective study. J Rheumatol 2000;27(10):2526.

Garfin SR et al: New technologies in spine: Kyphoplasty and vertebroplasty for the treatment of painful osteoporotic compression fractures. Spine 2001;26(14):1511.

Kaufmann TJ et al: Age of fracture and clinical outcomes of percutaneous vertebroplasty. AJNR Am J Neuroradiol 2001;22 (10):1860.

Lieberman IH et al: Initial outcome and efficacy of "kyphoplasty" in the treatment of painful osteoporotic vertebral compression fractures. Spine 2001;26(14):1631.

Peh WC et al: Percutaneous vertebroplasty: A new technique for treatment of painful compression fractures. Mo Med 2001; 98(3):97.

Ryu KS et al: Dose-dependent epidural leakage of polymethylmethacrylate after percutaneous vertebroplasty in patients with osteoporotic vertebral compression fractures. J Neurosurg 2002;96(1 Suppl):56.

■ DEFORMITIES OF THE SPINE

SCOLIOSIS

Scoliosis is an abnormal curvature of the spine when viewed in the coronal plane. It is also generally associated with a rotational deformity, and it is the rotational component, manifested as a rib hump, prominent scapula, or lumbar fullness, that is most likely to call attention to the spinal curvature.

Etiology, Classification, & Pathophysiology

Scoliosis is classified according to its cause, with the most common causes summarized in Table 5–1. For example, if the curvature is secondary to a structural bony abnormality, it is described as congenital scoliosis. If it is caused by a neurologic disturbance or muscle disease (myopathy), it is described as neuromuscular scoliosis. If no cause can be determined, it is described as idiopathic scoliosis. The idiopathic type is the most common. Although experimental and observational data have suggested that posterior column abnormalities (ie, impaired proprioception and vibratory sensibility) and other abnormalities of the central nervous system are causally related in cases of idiopathic scoliosis, these data are not conclusive.

Particularly in idiopathic cases, scoliosis can also be classified according to the patient's age at onset. The age ranges for infantile, juvenile, adolescent, and adult scoliosis are shown in Table 5–1.

Table 5–1. Classification of scoliosis by cause.

I. Idiopathic scoliosis
  A. Infantile (under 3 years of age)
  B. Juvenile (from 3 to 10 years of age)
  C. Adolescent (from 10 years of age to skeletal maturity)
  D. Adult
II. Neuromuscular scoliosis
  A. Neuropathic
    1. Upper motor neuron
      a. Cerebral palsy
      b. Charcot-Marie-Tooth disease
      c. Syringomyelia
      d. Spinal cord trauma
    2. Lower motor neuron
      a. Poliomyelitis
      b. Spinal muscular atrophy
      c. Myelomeningocele
  B. Myopathic
    1. Arthrogryposis
    2. Muscular dystrophy
III. Congenital scoliosis
  A. Failure of formation
  B. Failure of segmentation
  C. Mixed failure of formation and segmentation
IV. Neurofibromatosis
V. Connective tissue scoliosis
  A. Marfan's syndrome
  B. Ehlers-Danlos syndrome
VI. Osteochondrodystrophy
  A. Diastrophic dwarfism
  B. Mucopolysaccharidosis
  C. Spondyloepiphyseal dysplasia
  D. Multiple epiphyseal dysplasia
  E. Achondrodysplasia
VII. Metabolic scoliosis
VIII. Nonstructural scoliosis
  A. Postural, hysterical
  B. Secondary to nerve root irritation

Modified and reproduced, with permission, from Winter RB: Classification and terminology of scoliosis. In: *Moe's Textbook of Scoliosis and Other Spinal Deformities*, 3rd ed. Lonstein JE et al (editors). WB Saunders, 1994.

The curvature is named according to the side of the convexity, as well as the level of the apex, which is the most rotated vertebral body in the curve. For a cervical curve, the apex is at C1 through C6; for a cervicothoracic curve, C7 through T1; for a thoracic curve, T2 through T11; for a thoracolumbar curve, T12 or L1; for a lumbar curve, L2 through L4; and for a lumbosacral curve, L5 or lower.

The most common types of curves in cases of idiopathic scoliosis are the right thoracic curve, followed by the double curve (right thoracic and left lumbar) and the right thoracolumbar curve. A secondary curve, known as a compensatory curve, may occur that permits the head to be centered over the pelvis. Compensatory curves are of lesser magnitude, more flexible, and less rotated; when they become less flexible and rotation is evident, it may be difficult to determine which curve is the primary one.

The natural history of spinal curvatures is affected by factors such as the magnitude of the curve, the age of the patient, and the underlying cause of the problem. With curve progression, the deformity can become severe, leading in some cases to a "razor-back" deformity secondary to rib rotation. With curves measuring more than 60 degrees, cardiopulmonary function is compromised, and a secondary restrictive lung disease may result from the chest deformity. Curve progression is most common during continued skeletal growth; however, it has become evident that moderate curves of 40–50 degrees should be observed for progression in adulthood. Although the extent of progression in adulthood varies widely among patients, the average amount is 1 degree per year. Taking radiographs every 2–5 years appears to be satisfactory for adults who have idiopathic scoliosis without other clinical signs of progression. The likelihood of progression is greater in patients whose scoliosis is associated with conditions such as neurofibromatosis or connective tissue diseases, including Marfan's syndrome and Ehlers-Danlos syndrome.

Principles of Diagnosis

A. History and Physical Examination

In a patient with a spine deformity, the history should include the age when the deformity was first noted; the manner in which it was noted (by the patient or family member, by the pediatrician or other health professional during examination or school screening, etc); the perinatal history; developmental milestones; other illnesses; and family history of scoliosis or other diseases that may affect the musculoskeletal system. Although the incidence of scoliosis in the general population is about 1%, the incidence is greater in the children of women with scoliosis and particularly in the daughters of these women. For this reason, the children of women with scoliosis should be screened repeatedly throughout their preadolescent and adolescent years. Idiopathic scoliosis of the adolescent type (see Table 5–1) is more common in females, whereas that of the infantile type is more common in males.

In children and adolescents, the curvature is generally not painful. If the patient complains of pain, appropriate diagnostic tests should be performed to determine whether the curvature is secondary to the presence of a bony or spinal tumor, herniated disc, or other abnormality.

The patient's skin, habitus, and back should be carefully inspected. The presence of café au lait spots, skin tags, or axillary freckles is suggestive of neurofibromatosis. The presence of hairy patches or dimples over the spine is suggestive of spinal dysraphism. Numerous clinical syndromes are associated with scoliosis (see Table 5–1), and some of these include unusual facies. Tall, long-limbed patients may have Marfan's syndrome and should be examined for high-arched palate, cardiac murmur, and dislocated lenses. Dwarfs have a high incidence of spinal deformity, both kyphosis (see section on Kyphosis) and scoliosis, as well as spinal instability.

In patients with scoliosis, the shoulders or pelvis may not be level, or waist asymmetry may be noted. Most commonly, these patients have scapular prominence, with rotational deformity and rib prominence. The rib hump, or the lumbar prominence of a lumbar curve, can be accentuated by having the patient lean forward from the waist, permitting the arms to hang down; the examiner then views the spine from above or below (Figure 5–14). The rib hump can be quantified by direct measurement of its height or by using a scoliometer, which permits measurement of angular deformity. Also important in the patient's examination is measurement of decompensation, if present. This can be determined by dropping a plumb bob from the prominence of the C7 spinous process and measuring where it falls with respect to the gluteal line (Figure 5–15).

Flexibility of the curve can be qualitatively assessed by having the patient bend in the direction that effects curve correction. The spinous processes within the curve as well as the rib hump can then be assessed for correctability of the deformity.

B. Neurologic Tests

Patients should demonstrate a normal gait and be able to walk on their toes and heels, unless other concomitant conditions are present. Motor and sensory testing of the lower extremities should be performed, and testing of the upper extremities should also be done if the curve pattern is atypical or if a neuromuscular condition is suspected. Reflexes should be tested, and the presence of asymmetry or a pathologic reflex (eg, clonus, a positive Babinski sign, or a positive Hoffmann sign) should be noted.

An asymmetric abdominal reflex is the most common neurologic abnormality noted with an intracanal lesion, such as a syrinx, diastematomyelia, or spinal cord tumor. The abdominal reflex is assessed by gently scratching each of the four quadrants of the abdomen, just a few centimeters away from the umbilicus. The response is considered normal if the umbilicus moves slightly toward the direction scratched.

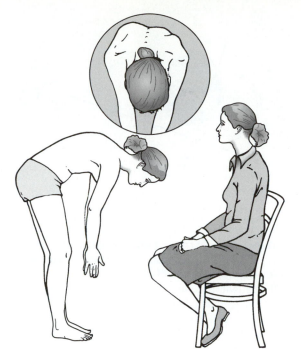

Figure 5–14. The rotational deformity of scoliosis is manifested by a rib hump, which is accentuated by having the patient bend forward. (Reproduced, with permission, from Day LJ et al: Orthopedics. In Way LW [editor]: *Current Surgical Diagnosis & Treatment*, 9th ed. Stamford: Appleton & Lange, 1991.)

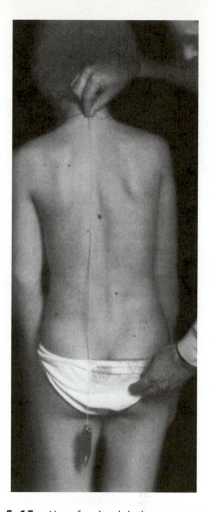

Figure 5–15. Use of a plumb bob to measure coronal decompensation in a patient with scoliosis. (Reproduced, with permission, from McCarthy RE: Evaluation of the patient with deformity. In Weinstein SL [editor]: *The Pediatric Spine*. New York: Raven, 1994.)

Abnormal neurologic test results are an indication for further workup, such as a spine MRI, particularly if the patient has an atypical curve (eg, a left thoracic curve) or a rapidly progressive spinal deformity.

C. Imaging Studies

AP and lateral radiographs of the entire length of the spine should be taken, and this generally requires the use of an extra-long x-ray cassette. When the radiographs are taken, the patient should be in the standing position. If neuromuscular problems make it impossible for the patient to stand, however, radiographs can be taken with the patient sitting.

Curves are measured using the Cobb method, as shown in Figure 5–16.

Views taken with the patient bending away from the concavity may be helpful or necessary, particularly if levels for fusion are being selected. These bend views allow for the assessment of the maximal correction of the curve. If the patient cannot perform the bending movement, traction films can be obtained by having two assistants exert longitudinal traction on the patient, either by grasping the legs and arms or via application of a head halter.

For severe curves (> 90 degrees), the rotational deformity of the spine may distort the detail on an AP view. For this reason, a special Stagnara view should be obtained. The x-ray cassette is positioned parallel to the rib hump, and the x-ray beam is directed perpendicular to this to obtain an AP view of the spine, rather than of the patient (Figure 5–17).

For patients with abnormal results in the neurologic examination, atypical curve patterns, rapidly progressive curvatures, or congenital scoliosis, evaluation of the spinal

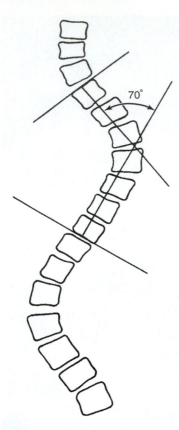

Figure 5–16. Use of the Cobb method to measure the scoliotic curve. First, lines are drawn along the end plates of the upper and lower vertebrae that are maximally tilted into the concavity of the curve. Next, a perpendicular line is drawn to each of the earlier-drawn lines. The angle of intersection is the Cobb angle. (Reproduced, with permission, from Day LJ et al: Orthopedics. In Way LW [editor]: *Current Surgical Diagnosis & Treatment,* 9th ed. Stamford: Appleton & Lange, 1991.)

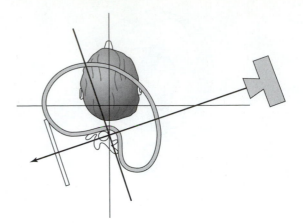

Figure 5–17. In cases of severe curvature, the x-ray beam and cassette are positioned as shown to obtain an anteroposterior view of the curve itself, rather than of the patient. This view is known as the Stagnara view. (Reproduced, with permission, from Lonstein JE: Patient evaluation. In Bradford DS et al [editors]: *Moe's Textbook of Scoliosis and Other Spinal Deformities,* 2nd ed. Philadelphia: WB Saunders, 1987.)

canal is indicated. MRI or myelograms with CT scanning can be used. For young patients, sedation is often required. The radiologist should be advised to look for the following: a syrinx (a fluid-filled cyst within the spinal cord); a tethered cord (a fibrous band that is located distally and can prevent the normal cephalad migration of the cord); a diastematomyelia (a bony or fibrous defect that divides the spinal cord and may cause a tether); or a diplomyelia (a reduplication of the spinal cord).

D. OTHER STUDIES

If the patient has a finding of intracanal abnormalities, particularly if surgical correction of the deformity is contemplated, neurosurgical evaluation may be indi-

cated. In many cases, the release of a tethered cord or decompression of a syrinx can be performed prior to or at the same time as the scoliosis surgery.

Patients with curves greater than 60 degrees, those with respiratory complaints, and those with scoliosis resulting from a neuromuscular cause should undergo pulmonary function testing, particularly if surgery is being considered. In cases in which pulmonary function test values are less than 30% of predicted values based on the age, sex, and size of the patient, some clinicians have recommended an aggressive approach with preoperative tracheostomy placement. We prefer, however, to caution patients about the possibility of tracheostomy placement if postoperative weaning from the respirator is prolonged, and we have rarely found tracheostomy to be necessary.

Principles of Treatment

Although general principles of treatment are discussed here, additional details about treatment of idiopathic scoliosis in adults, neuromuscular scoliosis, neurofibromatosis, and congenital scoliosis are given in subsequent sections of this chapter.

A. CONSERVATIVE TREATMENT

Mild curves (< 20 degrees) can generally be managed conservatively. In most cases, curves less than 10 degrees require observation only, except in very young patients who have neuromuscular scoliosis and a high risk of progression in their collapsing-type curves.

Although some skeletally immature patients with curves greater than 20 degrees require bracing, others do not. If an adolescent has less than 2 years of skeletal growth remaining, has not demonstrated progression, and has a curve that is still less than 30 degrees, the clinician may consider observation even at this point; however, considerations such as rotational deformity or a positive family history may suggest a more aggressive treatment for certain patients in this group. Any skeletally immature patient with a significant curve who shows progression of the curvature should be referred to an orthopedic surgeon with experience in treating scoliosis for possible brace treatment. Because the error of measurement of the Cobb angle is 3–5 degrees, progression of more than 5 degrees is considered significant.

Several types of braces are available for the treatment of scoliosis. The Milwaukee brace, which is also called the **cervical thoracolumbosacral orthosis,** can be used for nearly all curvatures, but its high profile makes it less desirable, particularly for a self-conscious adolescent. This brace (Figure 5–18) has a pelvic mold to which upright metal struts are attached. The struts are then joined to a neck ring. Corrective pads can be fastened to the metal struts, applying pressure to the rib at the apex of the convexity. If shoulder asymmetry is significant, a shoulder ring can be applied.

The thoracolumbosacral orthosis is a more cosmetically acceptable brace, but its use is limited to patients whose curves have an apex at T8 or below. The thoracolumbosacral orthosis is an external shell orthosis that is generally constructed of copolymer (largely polypropylene but with a small portion of polyethylene to prevent cracking). The shell is molded to the patient, and corrective pads are placed. One pad applies pressure at the apical rib, at the most prominent area. A second pad can be applied over the lumbar prominence if a double curve pattern is present. If the patient shows significant decompensation to the left or right, a trochanteric extension can be included on that side to correct this tendency.

Because of the corrective forces being placed posteriorly, bracing may aggravate thoracic lordosis. For this reason, particular care should be made to place pads as laterally as possible. A decrease of normal thoracic kyphosis is common in idiopathic scoliosis and in fact contributes to the cardiovascular problems seen in patients because of the resultant decreased AP diameter of the thoracic cage.

For isolated lumbar curves, a lumbosacral orthosis can be used (Figure 5–19). Although the Boston brace is the most well-known type of lumbosacral orthosis, others are available. The various types of lumbosacral orthosis all use the corrective effect of flattening of lumbar lordosis to facilitate curve correction.

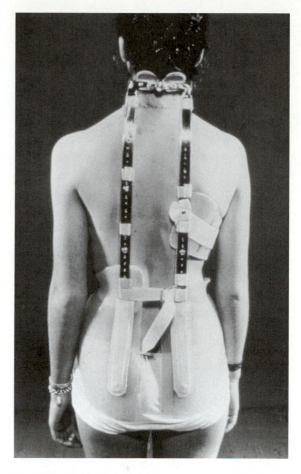

Figure 5–18. The Milwaukee brace, which is also known as the cervical thoracolumbosacral orthosis (CTLSO), can be used to treat scoliosis.

Although braces are designed to apply corrective forces to the spinal curvature and although corrective effects are frequently noted on follow-up radiographs taken with the patient in the brace, it is important to note that braces do not afford long-term correction. Success may be achieved in preventing curve progression during the growth period of the patient and improvement may even be noted, but the curvature generally returns to the preorthotic level of severity.

Unlike most braces, the Charleston night bending brace is worn only during the night. When this brace was used in the treatment of idiopathic scoliosis, with patients braced in maximal correction only at night, early results suggested that it was as effective as full-time brace wear; however, most of the patients had not yet achieved skeletal maturity.

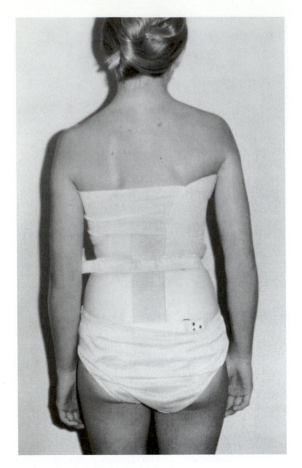

Figure 5–19. The underarm brace, which is also known as the lumbosacral orthosis (LSO), can be used to treat lumbar scoliosis.

Infants may require casting for management of severe curves. When the patients become large enough in size, a Milwaukee brace may be used.

Patients who are wearing braces for the treatment of scoliosis should be reexamined at intervals ranging from 4 to 6 months, depending upon how close they are to their growth spurt. Some clinicians prefer that patients wear their braces during follow-up radiographs, but others prefer that the braces be removed on the day of the office visit and while radiographs are taken. Generally, it is felt that full-time brace wear (23 h a day) is best, and some studies have indicated that compliance with brace wear is correlated with the success of braces. Patients may be permitted to remove the brace during athletic activities. As children grow, corrective pads may not be applying force at the appropriate area, and this should be checked clinically as well as with confirming radiographs where appropriate.

If an idiopathic curvature can be controlled with bracing, bracing should be continued until the end of skeletal growth. This can be assessed clinically by measuring the patient's height during each office visit as well as by following the patient's history (in female patients, for example, growth generally continues for approximately 2 years after menarche). Skeletal growth can be assessed radiographically by evaluating the iliac apophysis (Risser's sign, as shown in Figure 5–20) or by taking radiographs of the various physes in the wrist and comparing them with radiographs published in *Gruelich and Pyle's Radiographic Atlas of Skeletal Development of the Hand and Wrist*. Weaning from the brace can be begun as the patient nears the end of skeletal growth. Depending on the severity of the final curvature, follow-up radiographs may be necessary to assess the loss of correction. Some loss of correction should be expected; again, it is important to remember that permanent curve correction cannot be anticipated.

B. Surgical Treatment

Curves greater than 40 degrees are difficult to control with bracing because of the greater pressures that must be exerted to effect correction. Moreover, such curves are at risk for progression, even in adulthood. When conservative treatment is not possible, several options are available for surgical intervention.

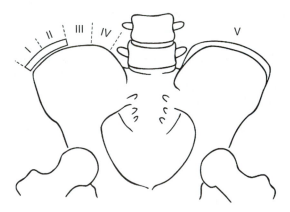

Figure 5–20. The Risser sign for skeletal maturity. The iliac apophysis first appears laterally and grows medially. Risser I is less than 25% ossification; Risser II is 50% ossification; Risser III is 75% ossification; Risser IV is completion of ossification; and Risser V denotes that the apophysis has fused with the iliac crest or complete skeletal maturity has occurred. (Reproduced, with permission, from McCarthy RE: Evaluation of the patient with deformity. In Weinstein SL [editor]: *The Pediatric Spine*. New York: Raven, 1994.)

The standard treatment has historically consisted of posterior fusion and Harrington rod instrumentation. This involves placing hooks on a ratcheted rod in distraction at the ends of the curve to be fused and then performing a fusion and bone grafting. Segmental wire fixation through the spinous processes (also known as the Wisconsin wire technique, devised by Drummond) or sublaminar wiring (also known as Luque wiring) may be added to gain additional correction as well as better fixation and can decrease the need for postoperative bracing or casting. Sublaminar wiring, because of the passage of each wire around the lamina and therefore into the spinal canal, carries an increased risk of neurologic complications. The sublaminar wiring technique is generally reserved for neuromuscular scoliosis patients, because of the need for better fixation in the generally osteoporotic bone, as well as for other patients who may have significant osteoporosis, such as older patients.

Recent years have seen the advent of variable hook-rod constructs, including the Cotrel-Dubousset system, the Texas Scottish Rite Hospital (Danek) system, and the Isola system. These systems permit placement of hooks at multiple selected sites along the deformity and the application of distraction or compression, as appropriate, to correct the curve (Figure 5–21). Detailed descriptions of the various hook patterns are beyond the scope of this chapter, but the basic principle is to distract on the concavity of a curve and compress across the convexity. The patient's sagittal contours can also be corrected, if needed, by applying compression to decrease kyphosis or maintain lordosis and by applying distraction to increase kyphosis. The sagittal contours can also be improved by carefully bending the rod prior to insertion so that rotation of the rod converts the coronal curve to the sagittal kyphosis if desired. Originators of the Cotrel-Dubousset system felt that rod rotation had the effect of untwisting the rotated spine; however, several studies have challenged this claim. The system uses a concave and a convex rod. These two rods are cross-linked, and they provide rigid fixation so that postoperative brace wear is not needed for most young patients.

For more rigid curves, such as may be found in older patients, it may be necessary to perform an anterior release and fusion as well. With an anterior approach, the disc material can be removed completely, gaining additional mobility and correction and, because an anterior fusion is then performed as well, increasing the fusion rate through this region. Additional factors that may suggest the need for anterior release and fusion include rigid kyphosis, prior failed fusion, and the presence of severe spasticity, as would be found in some cases of neuromuscular scoliosis. When possible, the two operations are performed at the same surgical sitting because this appears to decrease the perioperative complications.

Certain thoracolumbar and lumbar curves can be treated with an anterior approach alone (rather than with a combined posterior and anterior approach) if desired by the surgeon. In some cases, this can decrease the number of levels fused, which is particularly desirable in the lumbar spine. Instrumentation may be applied anteriorly in such cases. Screws are placed into the vertebral body on the convex side of the curve, connected to a rod, and compression is applied to gain correction (Figure 5–22). They are generally not used lower than the level of L4 because the common iliac vessels would then lie over them and face potential erosion. The newer systems are more rigid than the traditional Zielke system but are also more difficult to apply to more severe curves. If the surgeon is planning posterior instrumentation, application of anterior instrumentation can limit the correction obtained at the time of the posterior procedure. For this reason, combined instrumentation is generally used only if the patient lacks posterior elements for attachment of posterior instrumentation, such as with myelomeningocele.

Complications & Risks of Surgery

The risk of major complications in adult scoliosis surgery has been reported to be upward of 30%, with increased rates found in association with more complex cases, older patients, and patients with coexisting medical conditions.

A. NEUROLOGIC COMPROMISE

Among the risks faced by patients who undergo major spine fusion are paralysis and death. The incidence of paralysis, however, according to reports of the Scoliosis Research Society, is 0.4%, including both temporary and permanent deficits. Some of the neurologic risk appears to have been greater in the earlier days of using the variable hook-rod systems. These systems are powerful, and overcorrection and overdistraction can result. Because this is better understood today, the risk appears to have decreased.

B. CARDIOPULMONARY PROBLEMS

Cardiopulmonary complications are unusual in adolescents, but the incidence increases in older individuals. In patients with severe pulmonary disease or a history of cigarette smoking, prolonged intubation may be required. In older patients with a preexisting disease, the risk of cardiac ischemia is increased, particularly with long surgeries, significant blood loss, and controlled hypotension as might be induced by the anesthesia team. Controlled hypotension is used to minimize blood loss during many procedures but should be tailored to what can be tolerated by a given patient.

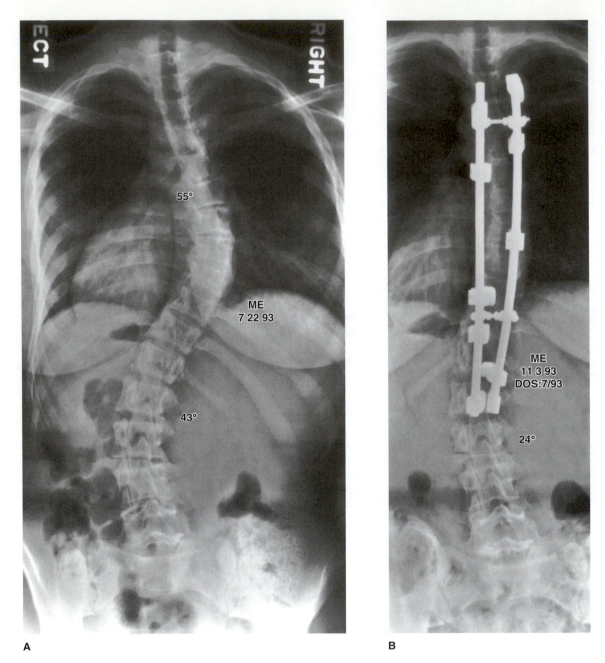

Figure 5–21. Imaging studies in a patient with scoliosis. **A:** Radiograph showing preoperative curvature. **B:** Radiograph taken after treatment using Cotrel-Dubousset instrumentation.

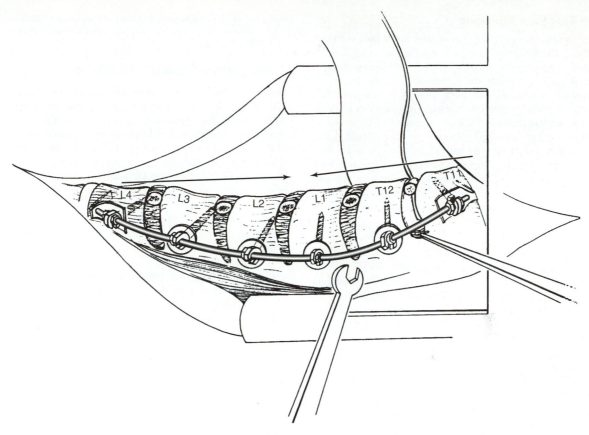

Figure 5–22. **A, B:** Preoperative AP and lateral radiographs demonstrating thoracolumbar curve in healthy 38-year-old female. The patient noted increasing deformity and increasing pain. Note slight lateral slippage of L3 relative to L4 on AP view. **C, D:** Postoperative AP and lateral radiographs demonstrating excellent correction of scoliosis after anterior instrumentation and fusion. The slight coronal lean corrected itself over a few months, and at 3 years postoperatively, she is doing well, with only rare back discomfort and able to do all activities.

The risk of thromboembolic complications after spine surgery has been reported to range from 0.5% to 50%. Many surgeons use antithromboembolic hose, sequential compression boots, or low-molecular-weight heparin during and after surgery. Although their efficacy has been well documented with hip and knee arthroplasty, benefits have not yet been demonstrated for spinal surgery patients.

C. Infection

Although perioperative antibiotics are given, patients undergoing spinal surgery are at risk for infection.

D. Pseudarthrosis

Rarely occurring in the adolescent but seen occasionally in adults is pseudoarthrosis, or the failure of fusion. This can result in persistent pain or loss of curve correction. Although tomograms or bone scans are difficult to interpret because of the presence of metallic artifacts, they may help delineate suspicious areas. High suspicion for pseudarthrosis may necessitate reexploration and refusion, sometimes supplemented by anterior fusion.

E. Decompensation

In cases of decompensation, the patient leans with the trunk shifted to one side more after surgery than before. Decompensation, particularly in the coronal plane, can generally be attributed to overcorrection of the instrumented curves such that the flexibility of the compensatory curves is insufficient to allow righting of the patient. Again, increased familiarity with the currently used instrumentation systems has resulted in fewer cases of decompensation.

F. Flat Back Syndrome

Seen less frequently now that contoured rods are used, flat back syndrome can be a debilitating complication and reinforces the need to restore or maintain the normal sagittal contours of the spine. The distraction required to achieve curve correction by Harrington rods, when applied across the lumbar spine, flattens the normal lumbar lordosis. Patients may need to hyperextend their hips to stand fully upright, or a hip-flexed, knee-flexed gait may be adopted. At an average of 14 years after spine fusion, affected patients note increasing back fatigue or pain and the inability to stand up straight. Surgical correction of flat back syndrome has a high rate of complications, although patient satisfaction is generally high.

G. Low Back Pain

Lower distal levels of fusion appear to correlate with increasing risk of low back pain. This raises the concern of late degeneration below the spine fusion. If the clinician can attribute a patient's symptoms to a specific unfused level, extension of the fusion may be indicated.

Berven SH et al: Management of fixed sagittal plane deformity results of the transpedicular wedge resection osteotomy. Spine 2001;26:2036.

Connolly PG et al: Adolescent idiopathic scoliosis: Long term effect of instrumentation extending into the lumbar spine. J Bone Joint Surg Am 1995;77:1210.

Danielsson AJ, Nachemson AL: Radiologic findings and curve progression 22 years after treatment for adolescent idiopathic scoliosis. Spine 2001;26:516.

Dickson RA, Weinstein SL: Bracing (and screening)—Yes or no? J Bone Joint Surg Br 1999;80:193.

Gruelich W, Pyle S: Radiographic Atlas of Skeletal Development of the Hand and Wrist. Stanford: Stanford University Press, 1959.

Lagrone MO et al: Treatment of symptomatic flat back after spinal fusion. J Bone Joint Surg Am 1988;70:569.

Lenke LG et al: Radiographic results of arthrodesis with Cotrel-Dubousset instrumentation for the treatment of adolescent idiopathic scoliosis: A 5 to 10-year follow-up study. J Bone Joint Surg Am 1998;80:807.

Logue E, Sarwick JF: Idiopathic scoliosis: New instrumentation for surgical management. J Am Acad Orthop Surg 1994;2:67

Luk KD et al: The effect on the lumbosacral spine of long spinal fusion for idiopathic scoliosis. Spine 1987;12:996.

Majd ME et al: Anterior fusion for idiopathic scoliosis. Spine 2000;25:696.

Nachemson AL, Petersen P-E, and members of the Brace study group of the Scoliosis Research Society. Effectiveness of treatment with a brace in girls who have adolescent idiopathic scoliosis. J Bone Joint Surg Am 1995;77:815.

Petersen L-E, Nachemson AL, and members of the Brace Study of the Scoliosis Research Society. Prediction of Progression of the curve in girls who have adolescent idiopathic scoliosis of moderate severity. J Bone Joint Surg Am 1995:77:823.

Rowe DE et al: A meta-analysis of the efficacy of nonoperative treatments for idiopathic scoliosis. J Bone Joint Surg Am 1997;79:664.

1. Idiopathic Scoliosis in Adults

Indications for intervention in adults with scoliosis are pain and progression. Painful scoliosis can be treated with conservative measures, including anti-inflammatory agents and physical therapy, in an approach similar to the treatment of low back pain without a deformity. Bracing of the curvature is rarely indicated because these patients have no skeletal growth remaining; however, a patient who cannot tolerate surgery for medical reasons may be braced as a salvage measure. In an otherwise reasonably healthy patient, if progression greater than 5 degrees can be documented or if symptoms are refractory to conservative measures, surgical correction may be indicated.

The same surgical principles apply to adults as younger patients. Adults are more likely to have rigid curves, which may require a combined anterior and posterior approach. Depending on the deformity and region of pain, fusion to the sacrum may be indicated. Patients with significant leg pain should have preoperative CT scanning or MRI to assess whether spinal stenosis accounts for the symptoms and warrants surgical decompression.

In adulthood, previously compensatory curves are often structural. It is important to consider the flexibility of all curves present in adult patients, including the fractional curve between L4 and the sacrum. (A fractional curve is one that does not cross the midline, such as that measured between a tilted L4 end-plate and the horizontal and midline sacrum.) The preoperative bend films of all curves should be reviewed and the following question addressed: If correction of the major curve or curves is achieved as would be predicted by the curve flexibility, will the patient still be able to stand centered head over pelvis? If not, the clinician may need to consider fusing a lesser curve to balance the spine.

Another concern is the need to correct sagittal plane deformity, particularly kyphosis, or maintain normal sagittal contours.

Anterior release and fusion may be indicated prior to posterior instrumentation in some cases to permit the patient to stand upright with the head over the sacrum and the knees and hips straight.

For older patients, particularly women, osteoporosis may prevent optimal fixation of the instrumentation to the spine. Sublaminar wires, as previously mentioned, can improve the rigidity of the fixation because the multiple sites of attachment spread the load over more bony attachments. There is, however, a theoretical increase in risk of neurologic damage during surgery when this approach is used.

Because of the complexity of spinal reconstructive procedures in adult patients, it may be useful to employ hybrid instrumentation techniques. For example, an older female patient with a significant double major curvature, a stiff fractional curve, leg pain, and evidence of spinal stenosis may require decompression and fusion. An anterior spinal fusion should be considered to improve the curve correction and the likelihood of solid fusion, especially across the lumbosacral junction. Instrumentation may require pedicle screws through the decompressed area because removal of laminae precludes placement of hooks or sublaminar wires there. Nevertheless, sublaminar wires may be preferred through the remaining spine to be fused because of the relative osteoporosis. The Galveston technique or iliac screws placed in the same manner as a Galveston rod segment would be preferred for pelvic fixation (Figure 5–23) because it appears best at resisting flexion moments that are experienced at the lumbosacral junction. The Galveston technique apparently has a lower failure rate in this type of surgery. In complex and difficult cases such as the one discussed here, surgery should only be undertaken for relatively healthy patients who have failed to respond to nonoperative intervention and who have a clear understanding of the goals and the significant perioperative risks of surgery.

Postoperative care in the adult patient undergoing major reconstructive surgery requires detailed attention to the patient's systemic needs, much more so than is generally required by patients undergoing other orthopedic procedures. Those patients who require thoracotomy or thoracoabdominal approaches will have postoperative chest tubes and are at higher risk for pulmonary complications.

Fluid shifts can be significant after lengthy procedures, particularly those with large blood losses. Anterior approaches, although largely retroperitoneal, can lead to prolonged ileus, a problem compounded by the use of postoperative narcotics that all orthopedic patients require.

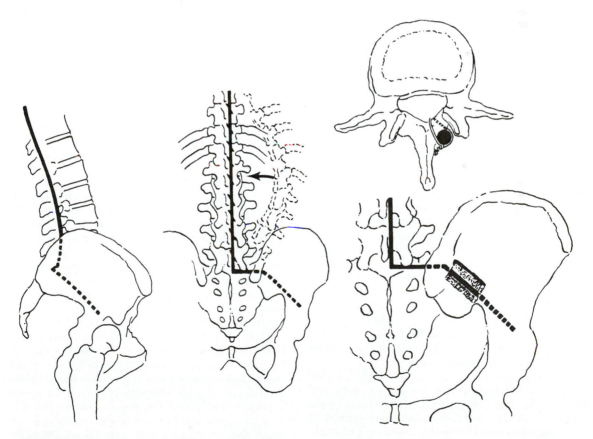

Figure 5–23. Use of the Galveston technique to obtain pelvic fixation. (Reproduced, with permission, from Shook JE, Lubicky JP: Paralytic spinal deformity. In Bridwell KH, DeWald RL [editors]: *The Textbook of Spinal Surgery.* Philadelphia: Lippincott, 1991.)

Bradford DS et al: Adult scoliosis: Surgical indications, operative management, complications, and outcomes. Spine 1999;24 (24):2617.

Connolly PJ et al: Adolescent idiopathic scoliosis. J Bone Joint Surg Am 1995;77A:1209.

Dickson JH et al: Results of operative treatment of idiopathic scoliosis in adults. J Bone Joint Surg Am 1995;77A:513.

Eck KR et al: Complications and results of long adult deformity fusions down to L4, L5 and the sacrum. Spine 2001;26(9): E182.

Grubb SA et al: Results of surgical treatment of painful adult scoliosis. Spine 1994;19(14):1619.

Nachemson AL et al: Effectiveness of treatment with a brace in girls who have adolescent idiopathic scoliosis. J Bone Joint Surg Am 1995;77A:815.

Peterson LE et al: Prediction of progression of the curve in girls who have adolescent idiopathic scoliosis of moderate severity. J Bone Joint Surg Am 1995;77A:823.

Weinstein SL, Ponseti IV: Curve progression in idiopathic scoliosis. J Bone Joint Surg Am 1983;65:447.

2. Neuromuscular Scoliosis

Neuromuscular conditions that are frequently associated with scoliosis include muscular dystrophy, cerebral palsy, poliomyelitis, spinal cord tumor, spinal cord trauma, spinal muscular atrophy, Friedreich's ataxia, syringomyelia, familial dysautonomia, and myelomeningocele (spina bifida). Spinal deformities tend to present early in life in patients with these conditions and often progress to severe deformities because of muscle weakness and the many years of ensuing growth. Although neuromuscular scoliosis can be subdivided into neurogenic and myogenic types (see Table 5–1), the principles of treatment for the two types are the same.

The assessment of patients should be detailed and should include an evaluation of overall function, mental status, motor strength, ambulatory status, and sitting tolerance as well as a search for the presence of problems such as joint contractures, pelvic obliquity, and pressure sores. Joint contractures can lead to pelvic obliquity or can limit the patient's ambulatory or sitting ability. Pelvic obliquity can be primary and lead to scoliosis or can be secondary to the spinal deformity. The primary condition should be determined, and if corrected sufficiently early, this may obviate or delay the need for further corrective surgery.

With neuromuscular scoliosis, as with idiopathic scoliosis, curvatures affecting the thoracic spine and therefore the chest cage can have adverse effects on the pulmonary system, which is already compromised in most neuromuscular scoliosis patients owing to weakness of the respiratory musculature. Truncal imbalance or pelvic obliquity, or both, are often associated with neuromuscular scoliosis and can impair ambulatory ability or sitting balance in affected patients. Before treatment of neuromuscular scoliosis is undertaken, the goals should be understood by the clinician as well as the patient and family. In many cases, the conditions are progressive, and the long-term prognosis for the patient and the patient's curvature should be considered. Stabilization of a curvature clearly does not affect the disease process and therefore does not affect the life expectancy of the patient.

Studies have shown, however, that in patients with Duchenne-type muscular dystrophy, thoracic curvatures contribute in themselves to loss of pulmonary function, beyond that which would be experienced by the generalized loss of pulmonary function associated with the progressive weakness of the respiratory muscles. In patients with Duchenne-type muscular dystrophy, an increase of 10 degrees in thoracic scoliosis will result in a loss of 4% of functional vital capacity.

The neuromuscular condition associated with scoliosis in each case should be well delineated and understood, as the curvatures in neuromuscular scoliosis have a higher likelihood of progression than those in idiopathic scoliosis, given the factors of muscle weakness, muscle imbalance, progression of disease, and the generally younger age at which the curves in patients with neuromuscular conditions are diagnosed. Particularly as pulmonary function is also progressively lost in many neuromuscular conditions, a more aggressive surgical approach is generally recommended, with intervention performed once the probable curve progression is established (by history, diagnosis, or degree of curvature) and preferably while the pulmonary function is still relatively good.

Unlike patients with idiopathic scoliosis, patients with neuromuscular scoliosis do not experience the active corrective effect of a brace. Instead, the brace functions as a shell of support, counteracting the effect of gravity on the collapsing spine. Bracing may adversely affect the breathing of these compromised patients but may slow progression in very young patients or while the course of the disease is being determined.

If surgery is recommended in cases of neuromuscular scoliosis, special concerns include whether the bone is osteoporotic, whether pelvic obliquity is present, and whether the patient has sitting balance. Osteoporotic bone often necessitates the use of sublaminar wiring, despite the theoretically increased neurologic risk associated with the multiple fixation sites when this technique is employed. If pelvic obliquity exists or if the patient has poor sitting balance, fusion to the pelvis is advisable. This is best performed with the Galveston technique, in which the ends of a specially bent rod are placed between the inner and outer tables of the iliac wing. The proximal rod ends are then placed on either side of the spine after being bent to appropriate sagittal contours.

The rods are subsequently attached to the spine with the sublaminar wires. Because of the collapsing nature of the spine in cases such as those described here, it is necessary to extend the fusion proximally to T3 or T4 to prevent kyphosis from developing above the fusion.

The perioperative management of neuromuscular scoliosis can be complex, and these patients often benefit from a multidisciplinary approach involving the orthopedic surgeon, pulmonologist, pediatrician, anesthesiologist, physical and occupational therapists, and additional specialists, depending on other system involvement. Patients with Duchenne-type muscular dystrophy, for example, may also develop cardiomyopathy. Those with Friedreich's ataxia have a high incidence of cardiomyopathy and diabetes mellitus.

With aggressive medical and surgical management and a supportive family, the longevity and quality-of-life for patients with neuromuscular scoliosis can be optimized.

Benson ER et al: Results and morbidity in a consecutive series of patients undergoing spinal fusion for neuromuscular scoliosis. Spine 1998;23:2308.

Boachie-Adjei O et al: Management of neuromuscular spinal deformities with Luque segmental instrumentation. J Bone Joint Surg Am 1989;71:548.

Lee DY et al: Fixed pelvic obliquity after poliomyelitis. Classification and management. J Bone Joint Surg Br 1997;77B:190.

Miller F et al: Pulmonary function and scoliosis in Duchenne dystrophy. J Pediatr Orthop 1988;8:133.

Miller RG et al: The effect of spine fusion on respiratory function in Duchenne muscular dystrophy. Neurology 1991;41:38.

Yazici M et al: The safety and efficacy of Isola-Galveston instrumentation and arthrodesis in the treatment of neuromuscular spinal deformities. J Bone Joint Surg Am 2000;82:524.

3. Neurofibromatosis

Spinal deformity associated with neurofibromatosis poses some special considerations. Curvatures seen in affected patients may be of the idiopathic type or the dysplastic type. Curvatures of the first type exhibit the same curve patterns as seen in patients with idiopathic scoliosis and are most commonly right thoracic curves. Curvatures of the second type can be much more malignant in behavior.

Dysplastic curves can be identified by evidence of dysplastic bone: penciling of the ribs or transverse processes, enlargement of the foramina, erosion of the vertebrae, and evidence of a shorter, more abrupt curve than that seen in idiopathic scoliosis. Usually, dysplastic curves are associated with kyphosis, which also exists through a fairly short sharp segment. They may occur in the thoracic, thoracolumbar, or lumbar spine.

Dysplastic curves in patients with neurofibromatosis can progress rapidly and can lead to severe deformity.

Bony erosion can occur secondary to neurofibromas or to dural ectasia (expansions of the dural sac, which can account for enlargement of the foramina or erosion of the vertebrae). The short, kyphotic curves and erosion of bone can in severe cases result in neurologic impairment, including paraplegia.

Surgery in patients with dysplastic curves is associated with a high incidence of pseudarthrosis. If surgery is indicated, it is often necessary to perform both an anterior and a posterior fusion. This combined approach results in a satisfactory fusion rate of up to 80%. Because of the dysplastic bone stock, it may be necessary to use a hybrid instrumentation system, such as one consisting of sublaminar wire use in association with hook placement. Preoperative MRI may be useful in assessing the extent of dural ectasia. Fusion levels are selected according to the end vertebra of the curvature. The end fusion level must lie centered over the middle of the sacrum, much like the selection for idiopathic scoliosis. Clearly, however, the fusion should not end above or below a dysplastic vertebra, although it would be rare for such a level to not be within the curve.

Akbarnia BA et al: Prevalence of scoliosis in neurofibromatosis. Spine 1992;17:S244.

Funasaki H et al: Pathophysiology of spinal deformities in neurofibromatosis: An analysis of 71 patients who had curves associated with dystrophic changes. J Bone Joint Surg Am 1994;76:692.

Winter RB et al: Spine deformity in neurofibromatosis. A review of one hundred and two patients. J Bone Joint Surg Am 1979;61A:677.

4. Congenital Scoliosis

Congenital scoliosis is caused by one of two types of structural bony abnormality (Figure 5–24). Type I is a failure of formation, such as that seen with hemivertebrae. Type II is a failure of segmentation, such as that seen with block vertebrae and that seen with unsegmented bars, where there is a tether to growth on one side of the spine. Mixed abnormalities are also found in patients with congenital scoliosis. Unilateral unsegmented bars with contralateral hemivertebrae have the greatest tendency for rapid progression and should be surgically fused as soon as the bony abnormality is evident. Unilateral unsegmented bars also tend to progress.

With respect to progression, hemivertebrae have a variable prognosis, depending on whether a contralateral hemivertebra is present that results in overall balance of the spine, whether multiple hemivertebrae are on one side of the spine, and how much growth potential is predicted for each end-plate of the hemivertebra. Hemivertebrae at the cervicothoracic junction and the

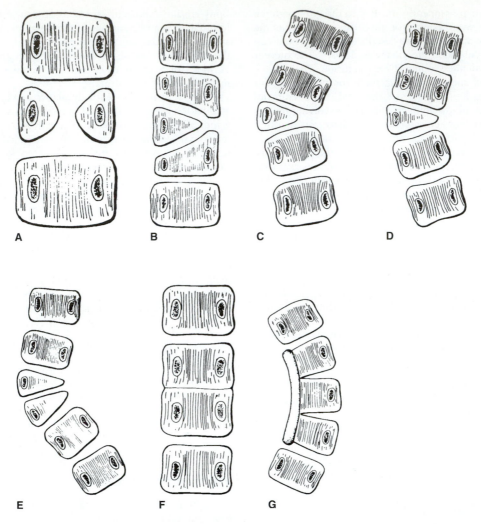

Figure 5–24. The major types of congenital scoliosis are failure of formation, as shown in diagrams A through E, and failure of segmentation, as shown in diagrams F and G. (Reproduced, with permission, from Hall JE: Congenital scoliosis. In Bradford DS, Hensinger RN [editors]: *The Pediatric Spine.* Thieme, 1985.)

lumbosacral junction have a relatively poor prognosis because the spine above or below the abnormality cannot compensate. Hemivertebrae should be observed so as to delineate their growth potential and progression.

Bracing is ineffective in treating congenital scoliosis because the curves are inflexible. Bracing is sometimes used to prevent progression of the compensatory curve, however.

In patients with congenital scoliosis, the incidence of cardiac abnormalities is increased, as is the incidence of renal abnormalities (20–30%) and intracanal abnormalities (10–50%). Abdominal ultrasound or other imaging tests should be used to rule out absent or abnormal kidneys. Intracanal abnormalities may include a syrinx (cyst within the cord), diastematomyelia or diplomyelia (division or reduplication of the cord, respectively), and tethered cord (presence of a tight filum terminale that does not permit the conus medullaris to migrate upward normally with growth).

If surgical intervention in patients with congenital scoliosis is indicated, several options are available. Fusion in situ is the simplest procedure. For very young patients, however, a posterior fusion alone will result in tethering of the posterior elements while the anterior elements continue to grow. This may lead to the crankshaft phenomenon, whereby the anterior growth in the spine results in a twisting deformity around the fused posterior elements. For this reason, combined anterior and posterior fusion is usually recommended for very young patients, halting growth circumferentially about the spine. (The crankshaft phenomenon can also occur in very young patients with noncongenital forms of scoliosis that have been treated by posterior fusion.)

In some cases of hemivertebra, hemiepiphysiodesis may be performed, arresting growth on the curve convexity but permitting continued growth on the curve concavity, with resultant gradual curve correction. This procedure has had good results in selected patients but can be unpredictable with respect to the amount of actual correction that can be achieved.

In cases in which a hemivertebra is accompanied by significant coronal decompensation and compensatory growth would not be adequate to result in spinal balance, consideration can be given to hemivertebra excision via a combined anterior and posterior approach. Although this procedure is technically more demanding and has greater potential risks, it allows for better overall curve correction and improvement of coronal balance. Hemivertebra excision may be the preferred option in the lumbar spine or lumbosacral junction, where the neurologic risk is to the cauda equina rather than the spinal cord and where oblique takeoff of the vertebra above the hemivertebra can result in significant truncal decompensation.

Bradford DS: Partial epiphyseal arrest and supplemental fixation for progressive correction of congenital spinal deformity. J Bone Joint Surg Am 1982;64:610.

Bradford DS, Boachie-Adjei O: One-stage anterior and posterior hemivertebral resection and arthrodesis for congenital scoliosis. J Bone Joint Surg Am 1990;72:536.

Deviren V et al: Excision of hemivertebrae in the management of congenital scoliosis of the thoracic and thoracolumbar spine. J Bone Joint Surg Br 2001;83:496.

Holte DC et al: Excision of hemivertebrae and wedge resection in treatment of congenital scoliosis. J Bone Joint Surg Am 1995;77A:159.

Thompson AG et al: Long term results of combined anterior and posterior convex epiphysiodesis for congenital scoliosis due to hemivertebrae. Spine 1995;20:1380.

KYPHOSIS

The normal sagittal contour of the spine includes cervical lordosis, thoracic kyphosis, and lumbar lordosis (Figure 5–25). Increases or decreases in any of these can be seen. If they are severe enough, they can cause disability, as discussed later in the cases of congenital kyphosis and Scheuermann's kyphosis.

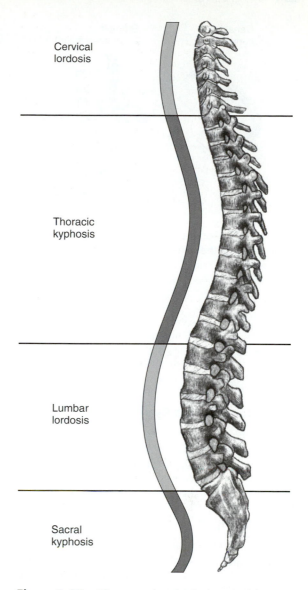

Figure 5–25. The normal sagittal contour of the spine. (Reproduced, with permission, from Bullough PG, Boachie-Adjei O: *Atlas of Spinal Diseases*. Gower, 1988.)

Labels in figure: Cervical lordosis; Thoracic kyphosis; Lumbar lordosis; Sacral kyphosis

1. Congenital Kyphosis

As in congenital scoliosis (see previous discussion), congenital kyphosis can result from a failure of formation or a failure of segmentation. In congenital kyphosis, however, failures of formation have a much more dangerous clinical prognosis. These can lead to congenital or progressive "dislocation" of the spinal column (Figure 5–26) and paralysis if not treated appropriately. If

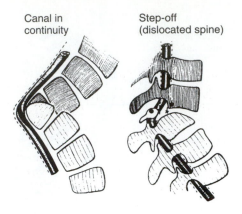

Canal in continuity

Step-off (dislocated spine)

Figure 5–26. Congenital kyphosis and congenital "dislocation" of the spinal column. (Reproduced, with permission, from Dubousset J: Congenital kyphosis. In Bradford DS, Hensinger RN [editors]: *The Pediatric Spine.* Thieme, 1985.)

performed early enough, posterior fusion may be sufficient to prevent neurologic problems. Severe deficiencies, however, may require anterior and posterior fusion to achieve stability.

2. Scheuermann's Kyphosis

Normal thoracic kyphosis ranges from 25 to 45 degrees. Postural kyphosis can increase this curvature, but if no abnormalities are present, the curve is flexible and the posture can be easily corrected by the child. If endplate abnormalities are present and three or more vertebral bodies are wedged as seen on the lateral radiograph, the diagnosis of Scheuermann's kyphosis can be made. Schmorl's nodes, characterized by herniation of the disc material at the vertebral end-plates, and increased thoracic kyphosis are also seen. Clinically, patients with this type of kyphosis have a curvature that is more abrupt than that observed in people with postural roundback, and this type is only partly correctable by forced extension. This can be demonstrated either by having the patient hyperextend or by taking a lateral radiograph with the patient lying over a pad at the apex of the kyphosis so that the Cobb angle can be measured. Thoracic curves may cause pain and discomfort, although some report that pain is more commonly seen in thoracolumbar curves.

Bracing can be instituted if the kyphosis measures more than 45 or 55 degrees in a skeletally immature patient, particularly if the curvature is progressive or accompanied by pain. If lesser degrees of deformity are symptomatic, they can be treated with physical therapy exercises and observed for progression. Brace treatment

requires the use of the Milwaukee brace, with two paraspinal pads placed over the apical ribs posteriorly. Radiographs should be taken with the patient in the brace to confirm that adequate correction is being effected. The brace can be removed for sports and bathing but should otherwise be worn 23 h a day. Repeat lateral radiographs should be taken at intervals of 4–6 months. If bracing is successful at controlling the curve, then it should be continued until the patient nears skeletal maturity. Weaning should be performed slowly, so as to maintain correction. Although some correction may be lost, proper use of the Milwaukee brace can result in long-lasting improvement in many patients with kyphosis (this is not the case with brace treatment of adolescent idiopathic scoliosis).

Surgical treatment of kyphosis may be indicated if the curve magnitude increases despite bracing, if the patient has significant associated symptoms, or if the patient who is nearing skeletal maturity has a severe curvature. Posterior spinal fusion with a variable hook-rod system such as the Cotrel-Dubousset system is the treatment of choice in these cases. If the curve flexibility does not permit adequate correction as demonstrated on a hyperextension lateral radiograph, an anterior release and fusion prior to the posterior spinal fusion is indicated.

Recent reports have described the natural history of Scheuermann's kyphosis, suggesting some functional limitations but little actual interference with life-style. The deformity can worsen over time. It appears clear, however, that many patients have their symptoms of back pain and deformity improved by surgery. Proper patient education and selection are essential for appropriate treatment of these patients.

Lowe TG, Kasten MD: An analysis of sagittal curves and balance after Cotrel-Dubousset instrumentation for kyphosis secondary to Scheuermann's disease. Spine 1994;19:1680.

Murray PM et al: The natural history and long-term follow-up of Scheuermann's kyphosis. J Bone Joint Surg Am 1993;75:236.

MYELODYSPLASIA

Neural tube defects can result in complex spinal deformities secondary both to the neuromuscular collapsing nature of the spine and to the vertebral anomalies that can give rise to congenital kyphosis or congenital scoliosis. Myelomeningocele or meningocele will be present at birth in a patient whose neural tube failed to close in utero. Sac closure is usually performed shortly after birth. In many cases, the affected infant also requires placement of a ventriculoperitoneal shunt because of hydrocephalus. The level of neurologic function usually corresponds to the level of the defect. For example, a low thoracic myelomeningocele patient has no lumbar nerve roots functioning and therefore no lower extremity function. An L4 myelomeningocele patient has a functioning tibialis anterior but no extensor hallucis and no gastrocnemius and usually no voluntary bowel and bladder control.

Neurologic function in patients with myelodysplasia is static and should not deteriorate with growth. Neurologic changes, especially during growth spurts, require evaluation for tethered cord, a common occurrence in affected children.

Orthopedic management includes maximizing the function of patients through the use of braces, ambulatory aids, wheelchairs, or surgery. The degree of spinal deformity is related to the neurologic level, with spinal collapse more likely in those with a higher neurologic level of involvement than in those with a lower level. The presence of bony abnormalities can affect this prognosis, of course.

As with many neuromuscular spinal deformities, curvatures may present early in life. If the clinician elects to treat a patient with bracing, it is important to remember that bracing in the presence of insensate skin can result in pressure sores if the brace is not adequately padded and the parents are not instructed regarding skin care.

In many cases, the curvature eventually requires surgical stabilization. Because of the magnitude and stiffness of the curvature as well as the absence of posterior elements, the preferred treatment is anterior and posterior fusion. Anterior instrumentation may improve rigidity of the surgical construct. In patients with myelodysplasia, fusion to the sacrum is invariably required because of pelvic obliquity or lack of sitting balance. Luque-Galveston instrumentation to the proximal thoracic spine is preferred, as with many neuromuscular deformities.

The lack of posterior elements in the myelodysplastic spine can lead to congenital kyphosis. Although kyphosis in these patients will not compromise neurologic function, it can lead to pressure sores over the prominent area. The treatment of choice for this problem is posterior kyphectomy and fusion.

SPONDYLOLISTHESIS & SPONDYLOLYSIS

Spondylolisthesis is the slipping forward of one vertebra upon another. Spondylolysis is characterized by the presence of a bony defect at the pars interarticularis, which can result in spondylolisthesis.

The classification system most commonly used in spondylolisthesis was originated by Wiltse and coworkers in 1976 and subsequently modified by others. Type I, the dysplastic form of spondylolisthesis, is a congenital deficiency of the superior sacral facet, the inferior fifth lumbar facet, or both. Type II, the isthmic form, is caused by a defect in the pars interarticularis but can

also be seen with an elongated pars. Types I and II are most commonly seen in younger patients and most likely to occur at the L5-S1 level. Type III, the degenerative form of spondylolisthesis, is seen in older patients and most frequently involves the L4-5 level. Type IV, the traumatic form, is located other than at the pars. Type V, the pathologic form, is caused by conditions such as a neoplasm. The Wiltse classification of spondylolisthesis is shown in Figure 5–27.

More recently, Marchetti and Bartolozzi have proposed a classification of spondylolisthesis that separates developmental and acquired types of spondylolisthesis. Developmental spondylolisthesis is divided into high dysplastic and low dysplastic types, with each of these being subdivided into those with lysis of the pars interarticularis or elongation of the pars interarticularis. Acquired types include degenerative, traumatic, postsurgical, and pathologic.

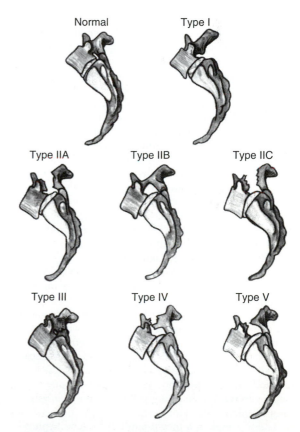

Figure 5–27. Classification of spondylolisthesis. (Reproduced, with permission, from Bradford DS, Hu SS: Spondylolysis and spondylolisthesis. In Weinstein SL [editor]: *The Pediatric Spine*. New York: Raven, 1994.)

Marchetti PG, Bartolozzi P: Classification of spondylolisthesis as a guideline for treatment. In Bridwell KH, DeWal RL (editors): The Textbook of Spinal Surgery, 2nd Edition. Philadelphia: Lippincott-Raven Publishers, 1997, pp. 1211-1254.

Wiltse LL et al: Classification of spondylolisthesis and spondylolysis. Clin Orthop 1976;117:23.

1. Isthmic Spondylolisthesis

The cause of isthmic spondylolisthesis may be developmental, with a congenital defect of dysplasia predisposing some individuals to spondylolysis. The overall incidence of spondylolysis is about 6%. The high incidence of spondylolysis in gymnasts, football players, weight lifters, and other athletes who place their lumbar spines in hyperextension suggests that repetitive injury may be a contributing mechanism. Biomechanical studies have also suggested that the pars interarticularis is under the greatest stress in extension.

Clinical Findings

Spondylolysis and spondylolisthesis may be asymptomatic, or they may present with back pain and leg pain. Rarely, they present with radicular symptoms or bowel and bladder symptoms. Isthmic spondylolisthesis most commonly presents during the preadolescent growth spurt, between the ages of 10 and 15 years. The extent of slippage may not be correlated with the severity of pain. The L5 pars interarticularis defect, with resultant slippage of L5 forward on the sacrum, is most commonly seen.

In young patients, regardless of the extent of slippage, there may be tight hamstrings and a knee-bent, hips-flexed gait, the classic Phalen-Dickson sign. Careful palpation of the spine of the patient with spondylolisthesis may reveal a step-off secondary to the prominent spinous process of L5. With more severe slippage, the lumbosacral junction becomes more kyphotic and the trunk appears shortened, with the rib cage approaching the iliac crests (Figure 5–28).

Radiographic examination will show the defect on the lateral view, with the percentage of slippage measurable from this view. Meyerding's classification is most commonly used (Figure 5–29). Oblique radiographs will demonstrate the "collar" or "broken neck" on the "Scottie dog" (Figure 5–30). If a unilateral defect is present, the contralateral pars or lamina may show sclerosis. If the history is suggestive of an early stress fracture and radiographic findings are negative, bone scans may be useful. CT scanning will show spondylolysis as an incomplete ring.

The slip angle is a measure of lumbosacral kyphosis and has been found to be useful in determining the likelihood of progression to higher grades of slippage in young patients. A line is drawn along the posterior cortex of the sacrum, and the angle between its perpendic-

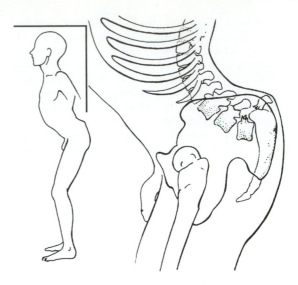

Figure 5–28. Diagram showing how high-grade spondylolisthesis results in a short trunk, with the rib cage approaching the iliac crests. (Reproduced, with permission, from Bradford DS, Hu SS: Spondylolysis and spondylolisthesis. In Weinstein SL [editor]: *The Pediatric Spine*. New York: Raven, 1994.)

ular and a line drawn along the inferior border of L5 is measured (Figure 5–31). If the slip angle is greater than 50 degrees, the likelihood of progression is high.

In patients with radicular symptoms or bowel or bladder impairment, CT scanning or MRI is essential if surgical intervention is considered.

Treatment

A. CONSERVATIVE TREATMENT

Low-grade spondylolisthesis (Meyerding grade I or II) can usually be managed with conservative measures, including restriction of the aggravating activity, bracing to reduce lumbar lordosis, and physical therapy. Patients with grade I slips who respond to conservative therapy may be permitted to resume all activities. For those with grade II slips who are improved with conservative treatment, it is usually recommended that they refrain from activities that hyperextend the spine. Skeletally immature patients with grade III or higher slips are at significant risk for progression and are recommended for fusion.

B. SURGICAL TREATMENT:

1. Fusion and decompression—Fusion is indicated for patients who fail to respond to conservative measures, demonstrate progression, or have greater than 50% slippage and are skeletally immature. For most pa-

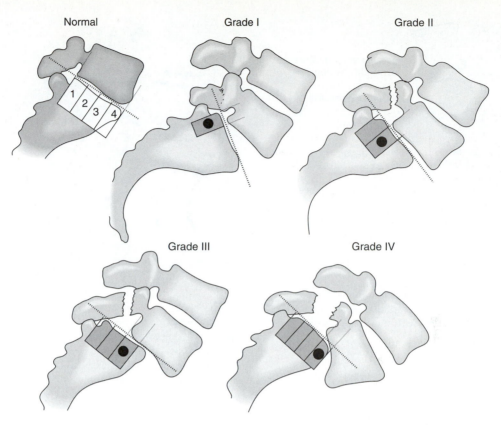

Figure 5–29. Meyerding's classification of degree of slippage in spondylolisthesis. Grade I is 1–25% slippage; grade II is 26–50% slippage; grade III is 51–75% slippage; and grade IV is 76–100% slippage. (Reproduced, with permission, from Bradford DS, Hu SS: Spondylolysis and spondylolisthesis. In Weinstein SL [editor]: *The Pediatric Spine*. New York: Raven, 1994.)

tients, fusion in situ is indicated. If slippage is less than 50%, fusion from L5 to S1 is sufficient. If slippage is greater than 50%, it is necessary to fuse from L4 to S1 to achieve a fusion bed that is under compression. Intertransverse fusion can result in fusion rates of 95% and good to excellent clinical outcomes in 75–100% of patients. This technique can be performed through two parallel paraspinal skin incisions. Alternatively, a midline skin incision with paraspinal fascial incisions, approximately two fingerbreadths off the midline, can be employed. The sacrospinalis fibers can be split, and access to the transverse processes is obtained. The transverse processes, pars interarticularis, facet joint, and adjacent lamina are exposed and decorticated. Iliac crest bone graft is harvested and placed in corticocancellous strips over the fusion bed (Figure 5–32).

If neurologic findings such as numbness, leg pain, leg weakness, or bowel and bladder compromise are present, decompression may be needed. Central and foraminal stenosis can be evaluated with a CT scan or MRI. In many cases, fibrocartilaginous scarring at the site of the pars defect accounts for the compressive symptoms. Particularly for young patients, an isolated decompression without fusion is likely to result in slip progression, so decompression should be combined with fusion. Some reports indicate that signs of nerve root irritation, including hamstring tightness, will resolve when fusion is used without surgical decompression. It may take up to 18 months for these signs to resolve after fusion alone.

Bracing or casting may be indicated after fusion and may consist of the use of a lumbar corset, a thoracolumbar orthosis, or a thoracolumbosacral orthosis with leg extension or pantaloon spica cast, depending on the preference of the surgeon. Once the patient's fusion is solid, full activities are permitted.

2. Pars repair—Pars repair may be indicated for young patients who have single-level or multiple-level

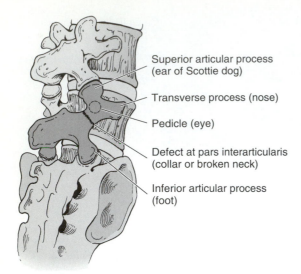

Figure 5–30. Diagram showing the "Scottie dog" (dark shaded area) seen on oblique radiographs of the lumbar spine in patients with spondylolisthesis.

Superior articular process (ear of Scottie dog)

Transverse process (nose)

Pedicle (eye)

Defect at pars interarticularis (collar or broken neck)

Inferior articular process (foot)

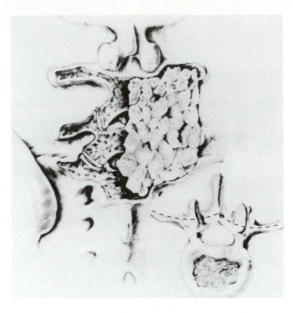

Figure 5–32. Schematic diagram of fusion for spondylolisthesis, as described by Wiltse. (Reproduced, with permission, from Bradford DS, Hu SS: Spondylolysis and spondylolisthesis. In Weinstein SL [editor]: *The Pediatric Spine*. New York: Raven, 1994.)

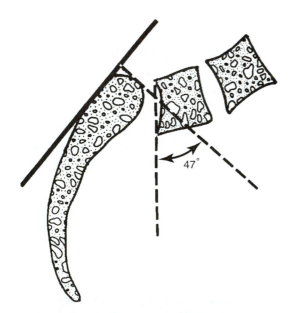

Figure 5–31. Measurement of the slip angle as a predictor of progression in spondylolisthesis. (Reproduced, with permission, from Bradford DS, Hu SS: Spondylolysis and spondylolisthesis. In Weinstein SL [editor]: *The Pediatric Spine*. New York: Raven, 1994.)

L1 to L4 pars defects without evidence of disc damage. Screw fixation or wiring of the transverse process to the spinous process (Figure 5–33) has yielded good results in appropriately selected patients.

3. Fibular strut graft—Bohlman and Cook have described a technique for one-stage posterior decompression and interbody fusion for treatment of grade V spondylolisthesis (spondyloptosis). After wide decompression, a drill hole is prepared between the L5 and S1 nerve roots, passing through the sacrum to the L5 vertebral body that has slipped in front of the sacrum. The configuration is similar to that diagrammed in Figure 5–34 for anterior strut graft fusion. Autograft or allograft fibula is inserted and then countersunk to avoid dural impingement. Posterolateral fusion is also performed at this time.

4. Anterior fusion—Another option for achieving fusion is via an anterior transperitoneal or retroperitoneal approach. The surgeon can either perform disc space grafting with tricortical iliac crest or place a fibular graft through a drill hole from the L5 vertebral body to the sacrum (see Figure 5–34). For high-grade slips, anterior fusion places the graft in compression. Clearly, there are significant risks with the anterior approach, including the risk of vascular damage in male and female pa-

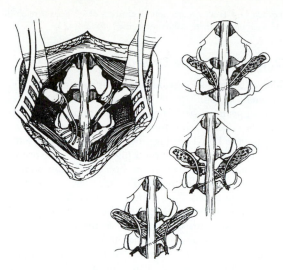

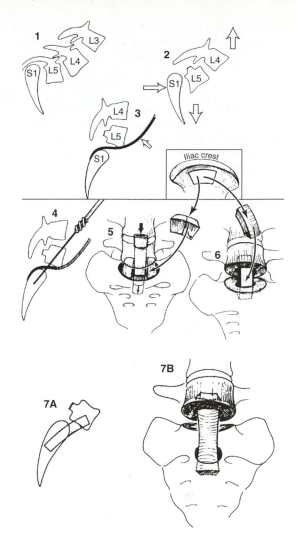

Figure 5–33. Illustration of pars repair, which can be performed in younger patients with minimal slippage, particularly above L5. Wires are placed around the transverse process and wired around the spinous process. The pars defect itself must be cleared of fibrous tissue and then bone grafted. (Reproduced, with permission, from Bradford DS, Hu SS: Spondylolysis and spondylolisthesis. In Weinstein SL [editor]: *The Pediatric Spine.* New York: Raven, 1994.)

tients and the risk of retrograde ejaculation secondary to damage of the sympathetic nervous system in male patients. Because of these risks and because good results can generally be achieved with posterolateral fusion, anterior fusion is best reserved for patients with high-grade slippage or patients who have undergone unsuccessful posterior arthrodesis treatment.

5. Reduction—Reduction of high-grade spondylolisthesis remains controversial but may be considered in patients who have high-grade slippage and are unable to stand balanced with their head over the sacrum while keeping their knees straight. Reduction can improve the patient's overall trunk appearance, which is characterized by a short waist, transverse abdominal skin fold, and heart-shaped pelvis, all of which become more prominent with high-grade spondylolisthesis. Improvement of the slip angle may prevent slip progression.

Although even fusion in situ of high-grade slips can lead to neurologic compromise and cauda equina syndrome, concern is raised over the neurologic risk with reduction techniques. Closed reduction using halo-pelvic or halo-femoral traction allows for gradual reduction while permitting the awake patient to have repeated neurologic assessments. It is less commonly used because

Figure 5–34. Diagram showing the steps involved in an anterior strut grafting procedure for high-grade spondylolisthesis. This approach permits grafting of iliac crest or fibula from the L5 vertebra to the sacrum, with the graft being placed under compression. (Reproduced, with permission, from Bradford DS, Hu SS: Spondylolysis and spondylolisthesis. In Weinstein SL [editor]: *The Pediatric Spine.* New York: Raven, 1994.)

of the availability of smaller pedicle screws. A posterolateral fusion can be performed after traction is completed or initially at the time of decompression. Anterior fusion may or may not be indicated, depending on the particular patient and on the reduction achieved.

Pedicle screw instrumentation can be used by experienced surgeons to distract and then posteriorly translate the slipped vertebra. Neurologic complications have occurred but in most cases are temporary. Supplemental techniques, such as intrasacral rods with iliac buttressing, or iliac screws, appear to improve distal fixation as does performing an interbody fusion.

For severe slips, L5 vertebrectomy with reduction of L4 onto S1 has been successfully performed. The technique shortens the spine and therefore theoretically poses less neurologic risk, but surgical manipulation of the nerve roots and posterior translation of L4 can result in neurologic compromise such as footdrop.

Complications

As noted earlier, neurologic compromise sometimes results even after fusion in situ. Particularly with decompression alone (which is rarely indicated) but also with high-grade slips even after fusion, progression of the slip can occur. This happens if there is pseudarthrosis (failure of fusion), but slippage can also occur postsurgically before the fusion becomes solid, or the fusion mass can bend if the forces across it are sufficiently great.

Incomplete pain relief is rare in adolescents but is sometimes a complaint of adults. The reasons for this are not entirely clear, but it has been noted that secondary degenerative changes can occur either at the level of the spondylolisthesis or at the level above.

Bohlman H, Cook SS: One-stage decompression and posterolateral and interbody fusion for lumbosacral spondyloptosis through a posterior approach. J Bone Joint Surg Am 1990;64:415.

Dubousset J: Treatment of spondylolysis and spondylolisthesis in children and adolescents. Clin Orthop 1997;337:77.

Hu SS et al: Reduction of high-grade spondylolisthesis using Edwards instrumentation. Spine 1996;21:367.

Frederickson BE et al: The natural history of spondylolysis and spondylolisthesis. J Bone Joint Surg Am 1984;66:699.

Frennered AK et al: Natural history of symptomatic isthmic low-grade spondylolisthesis in children and adolescents: A seven-year follow-up study. J Pediatr Orthop 1991;11:209.

Gill GG: Long-term follow-up evaluation of a few patients with spondylolisthesis treated by excision of the loose lamina with decompression of the nerve roots without spinal fusion. Clin Orthop 1984;182:215.

Hu SS et al: Reduction of high-grade spondylolisthesis using Edwards instrumentation. Spine 1996;21:367.

Kakiuchi M: Repair of the defect in spondylolysis. J Bone Joint Surg Am 1997;79:818.

Laursen M et al: Functional outcome after partial reduction and 360° fusion in grade III-V spondylolisthesis in adolescent and adult patients. J Spinal Dis 1999;12:300.

Lehmer SM et al: Treatment of L5-S1 spondyloptosis by staged L5 resection with reduction and fusion of L4 onto S1. Spine 1994;19:1916.

Muschil M et al: Surgical management of severe spondylolisthesis in children and adolescents. Spine 1997;22:2036.

Petraco DM et al: An anatomic evaluation of L5 nerve stretch in spondylolisthesis reduction. Spine 1996;21:1133.

2. Degenerative Spondylolisthesis

Unlike isthmic spondylolisthesis, degenerative spondylolisthesis is found more commonly at the L4-5 level. This appears to be secondary to a number of factors. This level sees more stresses than other lumbar levels because the L5-S1 level is protected by the strong transverse-alar ligaments that run from the transverse process of L5 to the sacral ala and also because the lumbosacral junction usually lies below the iliac crest and is additionally protected from motion. Other lumbar levels have more motion segments above and below to disperse stress. With degeneration at the disc and facet joints occurring at a somewhat greater rate, narrowing of the disc can occur. Because of the configuration of the facet joints and the lumbar lordosis, this results in some slippage forward of the vertebral body upon the one below. Note that without iatrogenic removal of the posterior elements, degenerative spondylolisthesis rarely reaches the severity that can be seen in severe isthmic spondylolisthesis.

The narrowing at the disc level can lead to increased stresses at the facet joints, with resultant degenerative facet disease, including joint narrowing and hypertrophy of the facets. As this cycle continues, the hypertrophied facets and the redundant ligamentum flavum can result in spinal stenosis. The forward displacement of one vertebra upon the other can further narrow the canal.

Most patients with degenerative spondylolisthesis demonstrate an element of spinal stenosis symptomatology with dysesthesias or leg pain. The spinal stenosis pattern of pain when walking beyond a well-defined distance (neurogenic claudication) is often present, relieved only by sitting down or bending over.

If degenerative spondylolisthesis is refractory to conservative measures (described earlier for isthmic spondylolisthesis), surgery may be indicated. Surgical intervention should consist of decompression. Fusion has been shown to enhance surgical results after decompression for degenerative spondylolisthesis. Instrumentation such as pedicle screws may enhance fusion rates and prevent further slippage during the postdecompression period before the fusion has consolidated.

Boden SD et al: Orientation of the lumbar facet joints: Association with degenerative disc disease. J Bone Joint Surg Am 1996; 78:403.

Fischgrund JS et al. Degenerative lumbar spondylolisthesis with spinal stenosis: a prospective randomized study comparing decompressive laminectomy and arthrodesis with and without spinal instrumentation. Spine 1997; 22:2807.

Herkowitz HN: Spine update. Degenerative spondylolisthesis. Spine 1995;20:1084.

Herkowitz HN, Kurz LT: Degenerative lumbar spondylolisthesis with spinal stenosis. A prospective study comparing decompression with decompression and intertransverse process arthrodesis. J Bone Joint Surg Am 1991;73A:802.

Love TW et al: Degenerative spondylolisthesis. J Bone Joint Surg Br 1999;81:670.

Nork SE et al: Patient outcomes after decompression and instrumented posterior spinal fusion for degenerative spondylolisthesis. Spine 1999;24:561.

Zdeblick TA: A prospective randomized study of lumbar fusion. Preliminary results. Spine 1993;18:983.

3. Thoracic Disc Disease

Disc herniation is found much less commonly in the thoracic spine than in the cervical and lumbar spine, presumably because of the decreased mobility seen in this region with the rib cage and sternum. Herniated thoracic discs account for 1–2% of operative discs, although the reported incidence in autopsy series is 7–15%.

Patients with thoracic disc disease may present with radicular symptoms at the level of involvement and complain of back or lower extremity pain, extremity weakness, numbness corresponding to the level of the disc herniation or below, and bowel or bladder dysfunction. They may demonstrate a spastic gait, with long-tract signs, if the disc is more central. Diagnosis is made by myelography, sometimes in conjunction with CT scanning or MRI.

In the absence of long-tract signs and paraparesis, conservative measures may include rest, anti-inflammatory medications, and physical therapy, with a 70–80% success rate.

Surgical treatment is recommended for patients with signs of myelopathy, including paraparesis or hyperreflexia. Decompression is most safely performed via an anterior approach. The anterior extrapleural approach has been advocated and has yielded good results.

When an anterior approach is used, 58–86% of patients show neurologic improvement and 72–87% experience pain relief. Neurologic deterioration has been reported in up to 7% of patients who have undergone surgery via an anterior or anterolateral approach and in 28–100% of patients who have undergone posterior decompression. Posterior laminectomies are associated with a high rate of complications, including worsening neurologic function from manipulation of the cord and incomplete decompression of an inadequately visualized disc.

Bohlman H, Zdeblick T: Anterior excision of herniated thoracic discs. J Bone Joint Surg Am 1988;70:1038.

Brown CW et al: The natural history of thoracic disc herniation. Spine 1992;17:97.

Maiman DJ et al: Lateral extracavitary approach to the spine for thoracic disc herniation: Report of 23 cases. Neurosurgery 1984;14:178.

Otani K et al: Thoracic disc herniation. Spine 1988;13:1262.

Regan JJ et al: A technical report on video-assisted thoracoscopy in thoracic spinal surgery. Spine 1995;20:831.

Rosenbloom SA: Thoracic disc disease and stenosis. Radiol Clin North Am 1991;29:765.

Vanichkachorn JS, Vaccaro AR: Thoracic disk disease: Diagnosis and treatment. J Am Acad Orthop Surg 2000;8:159.

■ INJURIES OF THE CERVICAL SPINE

The cervical spine is the most mobile area of the spine, and as such it is prone to the greatest number of injuries. Injuries to the cervical spine and spinal cord are also potentially the most devastating and life-altering of all injuries compatible with life. In the United States, about 10,000 spinal cord injuries occur each year. Approximately 80% of the victims are younger than 40 years, with the highest proportion of injuries reported in those between the ages of 15 and 35 years. About 80% of all people who suffer from spinal column injuries are male. Falls account for 60% of injuries to the vertebral column in patients older than 75 years. In younger patients, 45% of injuries result from motor vehicle accidents, 20% from falls, 15% from sports injuries, 15% from acts of violence, and the remainder from other causes.

With the use of seat belts and air bags in motor vehicles and the advent of trauma centers and improved emergency service awareness of potential cervical injuries, fewer patients with cervical spine injuries are dying secondary to respiratory complications. The approach in treating these patients is early recognition of cervical spine injuries with rapid immobilization to prevent neurologic deterioration while the evaluation and treatment of associated injuries are carried out. After the patient has been stabilized, the goals are restoration and maintenance of spinal alignment to provide stable weight bearing and facilitate rehabilitation.

Identification & Stabilization of Life-Threatening Injuries

Eighty-five percent of all neck injuries requiring medical evaluation are a result of a motor vehicle accident. Many of the affected patients are multiple-trauma victims and therefore may have more urgent, life-threatening conditions. The ABCs of trauma are followed in order of priority, with airway, ventilation, and circulation being secured before further evaluation proceeds. Throughout the evaluation of other body systems, the cervical spine should be presumed injured and thus immobilized. Approximately 20% of patients with cervical trauma are hypotensive upon presentation. The hypotension is neurogenic in origin in about 70% of cases and is related to hypovolemia in 30%. Concomitant bradycardia is suggestive of a neurogenic component. Another finding suggestive of cervical spine injury is an altered sensorium secondary to head trauma or lacerations and facial fractures. Appropriate diagnosis and fluid management are critical in the early hours of postinjury management. After all life-threatening injuries have been identified and stabilized, the secondary evaluation, including an extremity examination and neurologic examination, can be safely carried out.

History & General Physical Examination

Details of the history of the injury should be obtained. If the patient is conscious, much of the information can be obtained directly from him or her. If not, family members or witnesses of the injury should be questioned. In the case of a motor vehicle accident, for example, pertinent questions would include the following: Which part of the patient's body was the point of impact? Was the patient thrown from the car? Was there head trauma or a loss of consciousness? Were there any transient signs of paresis? Was the patient able to move any of his or her extremities at any time following the accident and before loss of function? What were the speeds of the involved motor vehicles? Was the patient restrained with a seat belt? Did an air bag deploy?

The history taken from the patient or family members should also include information about preexisting conditions such as epilepsy or seizures and about preexisting injuries. If the patient had any previous radiographic examinations, the x-ray films might be useful for comparison.

It is helpful to question patients about what they are experiencing at the time of the examination. Are there areas of numbness, paresthesia, or pain? Can they move their extremities? The examiner should then proceed with the physical evaluation, beginning by observing the face and head of the patient for any areas of potential injury and attempting to determine the potential mechanism of injury. For instance, any lacerations or contusions to the forehead might indicate a hyperextension type injury. Observation should next include watching the extremities for any signs of motion. A genital examination should be performed because a sustained penile erection may be indicative of severe spinal cord injury. Then without moving the patient, palpa-

tion can be performed. Although palpation can be helpful in identifying potential levels of injury of the spine, it should not be used as the sole screening examination, because false-negative results are possible.

Neurologic Evaluation

A meticulous neurologic examination should be performed following the history and general physical examination.

A. NEUROLOGIC TESTS

The neurologic evaluation should start with documentation of the function of the cranial nerves, working proximally to distally. Observation is particularly important in the unconscious patient. Spontaneous motion in an extremity may be a sole source of information regarding spinal cord function. Respiratory efforts made with intrathoracic musculature versus abdominal musculature are also significant. In the conscious patient who is able to follow commands, a motor examination should be fairly straightforward. Rectal and perirectal sensations should be documented because these may be the sole signs for distal spinal cord function.

An extensive sensory examination should also be performed with careful attention to dermatomal innervation. In the acute setting, it is useful to document sharp and dull sensations as well as proprioception. Sharp and dull sensations are carried via the lateral spinothalamic tract, whereas proprioception is carried through the posterior columns. Sharp and dull sensations are effectively tested with the sharp and blunt ends of a pen, and proprioception is tested by having the patient verify the position of the large toe and other joints as the examiner places them in dorsiflexion and plantarflexion. It proves helpful to make ink markings directly on the patient's skin to show the level of the dermatomal deficit, and this decreases the chance for intraobserver or interobserver error over sequential examinations.

Reflexes should be checked bilaterally. In the upper extremity, the biceps reflex at the flexor side of the elbow evaluates the C5 nerve root, and the brachioradialis stretch reflex at the radial aspect of the forearm just proximal to the wrist checks the C6 nerve root. The triceps reflex is innervated by C7. In the lower extremity, the knee jerk reflex is innervated by L4, and the ankle jerk is innervated by S1.

The presence or absence of the four reflexes listed in Table 5–2 should be checked. The Babinski reflex (plantar reflex) is evaluated by firmly stroking the lateral plantar aspect of the foot distally and then medially over the metatarsal heads and then observing the toes. If the toes flex, the response is considered negative (nor-

Table 5–2. Evaluation of reflexes in patients with injuries of the cervical spine.

Reflex	Root	Positive Response	Significance
Babinski	Upper motor neurons	Extension and spread of toes	Upper motor neuron lesion is present
Bulbocavernosus	S3 and S4	Contraction of anal sphincter	Spinal shock is over
Cremasteric	T12 and L1	Retraction of scrotal sac	Spinal shock is over
Anal wink	S2, S3, and S4	Contraction of anal sphincter	Spinal shock is over

mal). If the toes extend and spread, the response is considered positive (abnormal) and is indicative of an upper motor neuron lesion. The bulbocavernosus reflex has its root in the S3 and S4 nerves and is evaluated by squeezing on the glans in a male patient or applying pressure to the clitoris in a female patient. This action should elicit a contraction of the anal sphincter. If a Foley catheter is in place, simply pulling on the Foley catheter can stimulate the anal sphincter contraction. The cremasteric reflex is evaluated by stroking the inner thigh and observing the scrotal sac, which should retract upward secondary to contraction of the cremasteric muscle. This function is innervated by T12 and L1. Finally, the anal wink, innervated by S2, S3, and S4, is elicited by stimulating the skin about the anal sphincter and eliciting a contraction.

The presence of spinal shock causes the absence of all reflexes and typically lasts up to 24 h after the injury. The bulbocavernosus reflex is the reflex that returns first (see Table 5–2), thus marking the end of spinal shock. This point has prognostic importance because recovery from a complete neurologic deficit that is still present at the end of spinal shock is extremely unlikely. A complete neurologic examination should be repeated over time as the patient is manipulated and treated.

B. ANATOMIC CONSIDERATIONS

The ability to appropriately interpret the results of a patient's neurologic examination is contingent upon a thorough knowledge of the anatomy of the spinal cord and peripheral nerves.

Peripheral nerves are a combination of afferent fibers, which carry information from the periphery to the central nervous system, and efferent fibers, which carry information away from the central nervous system. As the peripheral nerve approaches the spinal cord, it becomes known as the spinal nerve. Proximal to the spinal cord, the fiber splits, with the afferent fibers becoming the dorsal root or sensory root and the efferent fibers becoming the ventral root. The afferent fibers are often regrouped in various plexuses that are located between the spinal cord and the periphery. This regrouping takes place before the fibers enter the dorsal root, therefore leading to significant overlap between the dorsal root and the respective dermatomes. The im-

plications of this anatomic fact should be kept in mind by the clinician when performing a sensory examination. For example, a sectioned peripheral nerve is demonstrated by a highly specific sensory loss in that particular dermatome, whereas the clinical findings are more variable for a sectioned dorsal root.

The spinal cord is a caudal continuation of the brain, extending in an organized fashion from the foramen magnum at the base of the skull down to the proximal lumbar spine. The spinal cord has three primary functions: it provides a relay point for sensory information; it serves as a conduit for ascending sensory information and descending motor information; and it mediates body and limb movements because it contains both interneurons and motor neurons. Headed from caudal to rostral, the spinal cord is highly organized with a central butterfly-shaped area of gray matter and surrounding white matter.

The overall diameter of the spinal cord varies as a relative percentage of the spinal canal. The cord fills about 35% of the canal at the level of the atlas but increases to about 50% of the canal in the lower cervical spine. This variation results from the relative increasing and decreasing size of the spinal gray matter and spinal white matter. As the spinal roots become larger, as occurs at the base of the cervical spine, the size of the gray matter increases relative to the white matter, whereas the size of the white matter decreases linearly from cephalad to caudal.

The gray matter, so called because it appears gray on unstained cross sections, is divided into three zones: the dorsal horn, the intermediate zone, and the ventral horn. It is made up predominantly of lower motor neurons and is prominent in the cervical swellings and lumbar swellings, where axons concentrate before exiting to innervate the upper extremities and lower extremities, respectively.

The white matter derives its name from the fact that the axons in this area are myelinated, casting a white hue on unstained sections. White matter is functionally and anatomically divided into three bilaterally paired columns: the ventral columns, the lateral columns, and the dorsal columns.

The two major ascending systems that relay somatic sensory information are the dorsal columns and the anterolateral system. The ascending axon has its cell body located in the dorsal root ganglion before proceeding without synapsing through the dorsal horn at that level and then ascending along the dorsal column before synapsing at the approximate level of the medulla and crossing over to the contralateral side before proceeding to the cerebral cortex. The topography of the dorsal column is such that the sacrum and lower extremities are medial, with the trunk and cervical region being lateral. The anterolateral system carries pain and temperature sensorium. The afferent fibers have a cell body in the dorsal root ganglion and then synapse at that given level in the dorsal horn before crossing directly to the contralateral side and traveling up the spinothalamic tract.

Motor pathways originate in the cerebral cortex and travel distally to the contralateral side approximately at the level of the medulla and travel down the lateral corticospinal tract before synapsing with the lower motor neuron in the ventral horn of the gray matter. The topography of the corticospinal tract is such that the sacrum and legs lie lateral to the trunk and cervical axons. Thus, at the level of the cervical spine, the spinal cord contains both lower motor neurons traversing to the upper extremities and upper motor neurons being transmitted to the lower extremities. Therefore, injury in this area can give both upper and lower motor findings.

The anatomy of the reflex arc and especially its relationship to spinal shock should be kept in mind. The basic reflex circuitry is an afferent nerve coming from a stretch receptor through the dorsal horn of gray matter before synapsing with the lower motor neuron in the ventral horn of the gray matter, which sends a positive signal to the same muscle via an alpha motor neuron. This simple arc, however, is modulated by input from higher centers. If all descending influence is interrupted, such as would occur in a traumatic transection of the spinal cord, all reflexes are lost. This is also seen during spinal shock. If the local circuitry of the reflex arc is not disturbed, reflexes will return at the end of spinal shock. The earliest reflex to return is the bulbocavernosus reflex, which typically returns within 24 h of injury. Peripheral reflexes may take several months before they return.

C. Risk of Neurologic Damage

As mentioned earlier, the spinal cord varies in its diameter from cephalad to caudad. In the upper cervical spine, it occupies about one third of the spinal canal. In the lower cervical spine, it occupies about one half of the canal. As inferred from this anatomy, the risk of neurologic damage from injury is greater in the lower cervical spine.

Cord compromise extends from two causes, the first of which is mechanical destruction resulting directly from the trauma and the second of which is vascular insufficiency. With vascular insufficiency, hypoxia and edema follow and result in further tissue damage. By about 6 h after the trauma, axonal transport has ended, and by 24 h, cord necrosis has begun.

D. Classification of Neurologic Status

1. Intact—Approximately 60% of injuries to the cervical spine result in no neurologic sequelae. In most of these cases, the injuries are in the upper cervical spine, where the ratio of the spinal cord to the spinal canal is smaller. It is obviously critical to identify unstable injuries of the cervical spine in the intact patient because the evolution of neurologic deficits is both potentially catastrophic and preventable.

2. Nerve root injuries—Eight cervical nerve roots correspond to the seven cervical vertebral bodies. Each of the first seven nerve roots exits above its respective body (the C1 nerve exiting above the C1 vertebral body, the C2 nerve exiting above the C2 body, and so forth), whereas the C8 nerve root exits through the foramen between the C7 and T1 vertebral bodies. Nerve root injuries can happen either in isolation or in conjunction with more severe spinal cord injuries. Injury to the nerve root alone may result from a compression or fracture of the lateral bone mass and thus impingement on the neural foramen. The clinical findings of a root injury would be those of a lower motor neuron lesion. If the nerve root is still intact and the ongoing pressure to the root is removed, the prognosis for recovery of nerve root function is good.

3. Incomplete versus complete neurologic injury— In the acute setting, any evidence of neurologic function distal to the level of injury is significant and defines the lesion as being incomplete rather than complete. As Lucas and Ducker reported in a prospective study published in 1979, "The less the injury, the greater the recovery," and "partial lesions partially recover, whereas complete lesions do not."

According to the Frankel system, which is the most widely used system for classifying sensory and motor deficits in patients with spinal cord lesions, there are five categories of injury: (A) sensory function absent, motor function absent (complete injury); (B) sensation present, motor absent; (C) sensation present, motor active but not useful; (D) sensation present, motor active and useful; and (E) normal sensory function, normal motor function.

In the acutely injured spinal cord patient, the documentation of sacral nerve root function by testing perianal sensation, rectal tone, and flexion of the great toe is critically important. Intact sacral function may be the only sign of an at least partially functioning spinal cord. In contrast, the absence of sacral function may be the only finding on physical examination in patients with an injury to the conus medullaris or cauda equina at the distal spinal column. Because these patients can move their lower extremities, a cursory examination might easily miss these significant deficits.

E. CLINICAL FEATURES OF SPINAL CORD SYNDROMES

Combining the findings on examination with knowledge of the cross-sectional anatomy of the spinal cord allows the examiner to identify specific injury patterns (Figure 5–35).

1. Central cord syndrome—The most common of the incomplete cord syndromes is the central cord syndrome, which occurs most frequently in elderly people with underlying degenerative spondylosis but can also be found in younger people who have had a severe hyperextension injury with or without evidence of a fracture. Central cord syndrome is defined by the American Spinal Injury Association (ASIA) as a clinical presentation characterized by "dissociation in degree of motor weakness with lower limbs stronger than upper limbs and sacral sensory sparing." The syndrome typically occurs following a hyperextension injury and is thought to be caused by an expanding hematoma or edema forming in the central aspect of the spinal cord. Central cord syndrome can be quite variable in presentation and in recovery. A mild presentation may consist of a slight burning sensation in the upper extremities, while a severe central cord syndrome would include motor impairment in both the upper and lower extremities, bladder dysfunction, and a variable sensory deficit below the level of injury. The pattern of clinical presentation is directly related to the cross-sectional anatomy of the spinal cord. Because the lower extremity and sacral tracts of the spinothalamic and corticospinal tracts are lateral, these areas are often spared in central cord syndrome. In cases in which they are involved, they are the areas whose function returns first. The upper extremity deficit is caused by a lesion in the gray matter, and the damage here is largely irreversible.

From 50% to 75% of patients with central cord lesions show some neurologic improvement, but the amount of improvement varies considerably among patients. The usual order in which motor function recovery occurs is as follows: return of lower extremity strength, return of bladder function, return of upper extremity strength, and return of intrinsic function of the hand.

2. Anterior cord syndrome—The patient with an anterior cord syndrome typically presents with immediate paralysis and loss of pain and temperature sensation. Both the spinothalamic and corticospinal tracts are located in the anterior aspect of the spinal cord and are therefore involved. With the dorsal columns preserved, the patient still has intact proprioception and vibratory sense as well as intact sensation to deep pressure. This clinical presentation is the most common in the younger trauma victim. The mechanism of injury is typically a flexion injury to the cervical spine. It is usually associated with an identifiable lesion of the cervical spine, most commonly a vertebral body burst fracture or a herniated disc. Return of useful motor function is reported in only 10–16% of patients with anterior cord syndrome. The prognosis is slightly improved, however, if evidence of spinothalamic tract function is present early.

3. Brown-Séquard syndrome—Patients with this syndrome have a motor weakness on the ipsilateral side of the lesion and a sensory deficit on the contralateral side. This is caused by a functional hemisection of the spinal cord. For example, a cervical lesion on the right side of the spinal cord would disrupt the ipsilateral corticospinal tract, which is the tract that would carry motor function to the right side of the body distal to the level of the lesion. The right spinothalamic tract would also be disrupted. This tract carries pain and temperature fibers from the contralateral side of the body distal to the level of injury. Position sense and vibratory sense, which are carried in the posterior column, have not yet crossed the midline; therefore, these sensory functions would be disrupted on the ipsilateral side of the injury.

Brown-Séquard syndrome may result from a closed rotational injury such as a fracture-dislocation or may result from a penetrating trauma such as a stab wound. The prognosis in cases resulting from a closed injury is quite favorable, with 90% of patients regaining function of the bowel and bladder as well as the ability to walk.

4. Posterior cord syndrome—The posterior cord syndrome is the least common of the incomplete syndromes and is typically a result of an extension type injury. Its clinical presentation is one of loss of position and vibratory sense below the level of injury secondary to disruption of the dorsal columns. With these deficits as isolated findings, the prognosis for recovery of ambulation and function of the bowel and bladder is excellent.

5. Complete spinal cord injury—A complete neurologic deficit is characterized by a total absence of sensation and voluntary motor function caudal to the level of spinal cord injury in the absence of spinal shock. Initial evaluation must rule out any evidence of sacral sparing and the presence of a bulbocavernosus reflex. In the absence of sacral sparing and with the return of the bulbocavernosus reflex, which typically occurs within 24 h, the spinal cord injury is termed complete and there is virtually no likelihood of functional spinal cord recovery.

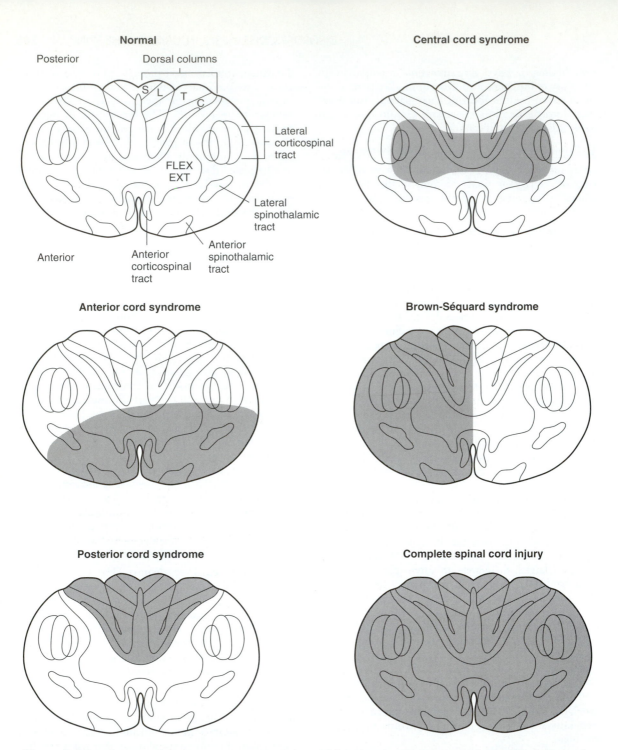

Figure 5–35. Diagrams illustrating cross-sectional views of the normal and injured spinal cord. The diagram of the normal spinal column shows the segmental arrangement (S = sacral, L = lumbar, T = thoracic, and C = cervical) and the area of flexors and extensors (FLEX and EXT). Central cord syndrome, anterior cord syndrome, Brown-Séquard syndrome, and posterior cord syndrome are incomplete injuries, with affected areas shaded. In complete spinal cord injury, all areas are affected.

Affected patients may gain some root function about the level of the injury—a phenomenon called root escape, because this damage to nerve roots is a peripheral nerve injury. Although the presence of root escape should not be taken as a potential return of spinal cord function, it can significantly improve the patient's rehabilitation efforts because vital function of the upper extremities may be regained.

Imaging Studies

A. RADIOGRAPHY

1. Screening radiograph—A lateral radiograph of the cervical spine may be the only screening tool obtained upon initial radiographic evaluation of the multiple-trauma patient. This radiograph must be carefully reviewed. Should a patient present with a complete neurologic injury or a densely affected incomplete neurologic injury indicating a traumatically malaligned cervical spine, closed reduction of the cervical spine should be urgently attempted with axial traction through Gardner Wills tongs. Once the patient has been fully evaluated and life-threatening injuries stabilized, secondary diagnostic studies can then be undertaken.

2. Subsequent plain radiographs—Full radiographic evaluation of the cervical spine with plain x-ray films includes lateral, AP, open-mouth (odontoid), right oblique, and left oblique views. The lateral radiograph, if adequate, will visualize approximately 85% of significant cervical spine injuries. It must display the base of the skull with all seven cervical vertebrae, as well as the proximal half of the T1 vertebral body. If the C7-T1 junction is not visualized, a repeat radiograph should be done with axial traction on the upper extremities caudally to attempt to visualize the C7-T1 junction. If this is unsuccessful, a swimmer's view, which is a transthoracic lateral with the patient's arm fully abducted, should be taken. If this plain radiograph is not satisfactory and if suspicion of injury is still high, a CT scan must be obtained.

When evaluating a lateral cervical spine radiograph, the clinician should first evaluate the bony anatomy. Four lines or curves should be kept in mind (Figure 5–36). The anterior spinal line and the posterior spinal line are imaginary lines drawn from the anterior cortex and posterior cortex, respectively, of the cervical vertebral body from C2 all the way down to T1. The spinal laminar curve is an imaginary line drawn from the posterior aspect of the foramen magnum connecting the anterior cortex of each successive spinous process. These three lines (labeled A, B, and C in Figure 5–36) should have a gentle, continuous lordotic curve with no areas of acute angulation. The fourth line (labeled D in

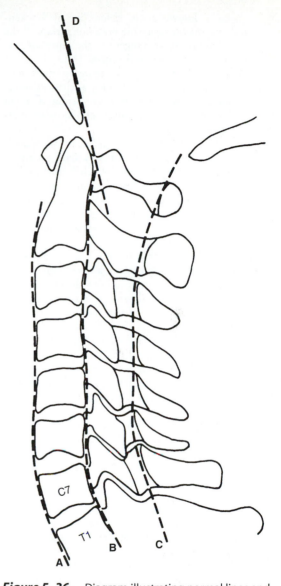

Figure 5–36. Diagram illustrating normal lines and curves in the bony anatomy of the cervical spine. The anterior spinal line (line A), the posterior spinal line (line B), and the spinal laminar curve (line C) should have a gentle, continuous lordotic curve. The basilar line of Wackenheim (line D) is drawn along the posterior surface of the clivus and should thus be tangent to the posterior cortex of the tip of the odontoid process. (Reproduced, with permission, from El-Khoury GY, Kathol MH: Radiographic evaluation of cervical spine trauma. Semin Spine Surg 1991;3:3.)

Figure 5–36) is known as the basilar line of Wackenheim, and it is drawn along the posterior surface of the clivus and should thus be tangent to the posterior cortex of the tip of the odontoid process. After the clinician examines the radiograph in terms of these four lines or curves, he or she should look at the individual vertebral bodies to see if there is loss of height of any of them or if a rotational deformity is present with alterations in the alignment of the facets.

The evaluation of soft tissues can also prove valuable diagnostically. Prevertebral soft tissues have an upper limit of normal width beyond which a prevertebral hematoma indicative of vertebral injury can be suspected. The upper ends of normal are 11 mm at C1, 6 mm at C2, 7 mm at C3, and 8 mm at C4. The measurements below C4 become more variable and therefore less reliable clinically.

The AP view of the cervical spine is at first a confusing projection to those who are unfamiliar with cervical anatomy, yet careful attention to bony detail in the AP view can be of significant diagnostic aid in picking up subtle injuries. The bony and soft-tissue anatomy seen on the AP projection should be symmetric. The spinous processes should be equally spaced because a single level of increased intraspinous process distance suggests posterior instability. Abrupt malalignment of the spinous processes suggests a rotatory injury such as a unilateral facet dislocation. After checking for these problems, the clinician should inspect the lateral masses. The facet joints are typically angled away from the vertical and are therefore not clearly seen on the AP projection. If, however, the facet joint can be seen at a particular level, this is indicative of a fracture through the lateral masses and a rotational malalignment of the facet.

The open-mouth (odontoid) view is the projection most useful for looking at C1-2 anatomy. It permits visualization of both the dens in the AP plane, and the lateral masses of C1 on C2.

The right and left oblique views can be taken of the cervical spine with the patient in the supine position. These views are useful as confirmatory studies in ruling in or out lateral mass injuries.

3. Stress radiographs—Two techniques are used in obtaining cervical stress radiographs. The first is to apply axial distraction to the cervical spine through a halo or traction device and obtain a lateral radiograph. This technique should be carefully performed in the presence of a physician and only after gross instabilities of the cervical spine have been ruled out. Serial lateral radiographs are taken as weight is sequentially added, reaching an amount equivalent to about one third of body weight or 30 kg, depending on the level of suspected injury. Occult instability can be inferred by not-

ing an interspace angulation of at least 11 degrees or an interspace separation of at least 1.7 mm (Figure 5–37).

The second technique, which should only be performed in a fully alert and cooperative patient, is used to obtain flexion-extension lateral radiographs that are helpful in the diagnosis of late instability. The technique is to have the patient flex his or her head forward as far as possible while a lateral radiograph is taken and then to have the patient put his or her head in full extension while another radiograph is taken. Findings presumptive of instability are facet subluxation, forward subluxation of 3.5 cm of one vertebral body on the next, and interbody angulation of greater than 11 degrees.

B. COMPUTED TOMOGRAPHY

CT scanning is the most useful means for definitive delineation of bony fracture anatomy. Its advantages are its ready availability and its ability to be performed with a minimal amount of patient manipulation. CT scans provide excellent axial detail, and if the sections are taken with close enough cuts, the computer can reconstruct images in sagittal, coronal, or oblique planes. CT scans can now even be reformatted into a three-dimensional construct for excellent visualization of the bony anatomy.

C. MAGNETIC RESONANCE IMAGING

MRI is the most effective means by which to evaluate the soft-tissue component of cervical trauma. The major advantage of MRI is that it can visualize occult disc herniation, hematoma, or edema about the spinal cord, as well as ligamentous injury. Current disadvantages are that MRI is disrupted by metallic objects, so these should be removed from the area of examination, and it also requires a prolonged amount of time to perform, therefore making close monitoring of the acutely ill patient difficult.

Diagnostic Checklist of Spinal Instability

The concept of spinal stability is central to the understanding and treatment of cervical spine injuries. In a broad sense, patients with injuries that are deemed unstable require surgical intervention, whereas those deemed to have stable injury patterns can be treated nonoperatively. Spinal injuries, however, are not readily divided into unstable and stable injuries and in actuality fall along a spectrum of spinal instability.

White and Panjabi's diagnostic checklist of spinal instability (Table 5–3) has nine categories, each of which is assigned a point value. If a total of 5 points is present in a given patient, the injury is deemed unstable.

Holdsworth's two-column theory of spine stability as well as Denis's three-column theory, proposed for

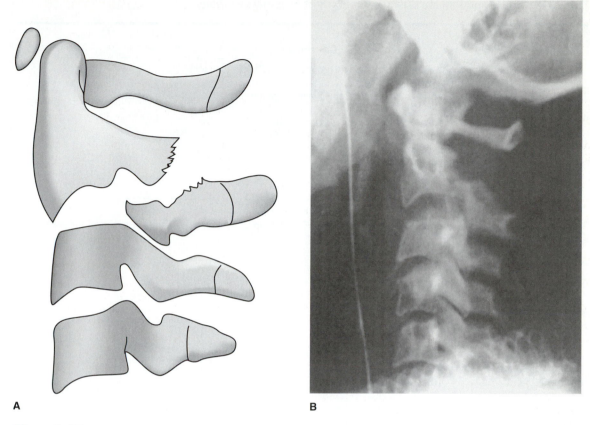

A   **B**

Figure 5–37. **A:** Diagram illustrating an increase of the C2-3 interdisc space in a patient with type IIA traumatic spondylolisthesis. **B:** Radiograph demonstrating an increased space. (Reproduced, with permission, from Levine AM, Rhyne AL: Traumatic spondylolisthesis of the axis. Semin Spine Surg 1991;3:47.)

application to the thoracolumbar spine, have also been applied to the cervical spine in an attempt to better predict stability in the neck.

General Principles of Managing Acute Injuries of the Cervical Spine

Management of acute cervical spine injury is predicated upon two principles: protection of the uninjured spinal cord and prevention of further damage to the injured spinal cord. This is accomplished by following spine precaution principles from the very onset of medical care, starting at the accident scene. The cervical spine should be considered injured until proven otherwise and should be securely immobilized before the patient is transported to a medical center. The equipment for initial immobilization should not be removed until the definitive means of immobilization can be put in place or the cervical spine is cleared of injury. Use of a spinal

board, with the patient's head taped to the board and held between two sandbags, is the most secure form of immobilization that is readily available in the field. This can be supplemented by a Philadelphia collar. When the medical center is reached, if a definitive cervical spine injury is identified and deemed unstable, skeletal traction for immobilization, reduction, or both may be applied. Gardner-Wells traction is easily applied and is adequate for axial traction. Halo traction affords the added advantage of four-point fixation and thus controlled traction in three planes. Halo traction can also be easily converted at a later time to halo-vest immobilization.

Among the various agents that have shown potential benefits in laboratory studies of models of spinal cord injury are corticosteroids, opiate receptor antagonists (such as naloxone or thyrotropin-releasing hormone), and diuretics (such as mannitol). Many trauma centers now routinely give corticosteroids as soon as possible

Table 5–3. White and Panjabi's diagnostic checklist of spinal instability.

Checklist Category	Description	Point Value[a]
1	Disruption of the anterior elements, with greater than 25% loss of height	2
2	Disruption of the posterior elements	2
3	Sagittal plane translation of greater than 3.5 mm or greater than 20% of the anteroposterior diameter of the vertebral body	2
4	Intervertebral sagittal rotation of greater than 11 degrees	2
5	Intervertebral distance of greater than 1.7 mm on a stretch test	2
6	Evidence of cord damage	2
7	Evidence of root damage	1
8	Acute intervertebral disk space narrowing	1
9	Anticipated abnormally large stress	1

[a]If a total of 5 points is present in a given patient, the injury is deemed unstable.

Modified and reproduced, with permission, from White AA III, Panjabi MM: Update on the evaluation of instability of the lower cervical spine. Instr Course Lect 1987;36:513.

because data from the Second National Acute Spinal Cord Injury Study suggest that it may improve neurologic recovery. The recommended dosage of methylprednisolone in an acute setting is 30 mg/kg given as a bolus and followed by 5.4 mg/kg/h for 23 h. The methylprednisolone must be begun within 8 h of the injury to be effective. This protocol is not without complications but is followed widely. The Third National Acute Spinal Cord Injury Study was recently published modifying existing recommendations. If a patient is treated within 3 h of injury, the standard 24-h protocol of methylprednisolone is still recommended. If methylprednisolone is begun within 3–8 h after injury, it should be continued for 48 h.

Bracken MB et al: Administration of methylprednisolone for 24 or 48 hours or tirilazad mesylate for 48 hours in the treatment of acute spinal cord injury; Results of the Third National Acute Spinal Cord Injury Randomized Control Trial. JAMA 1997;277:1597.

Denis F: The three-column spine and its significance in the classification of acute thoracolumbar spinal injuries. Spine 1983; 8:817.

El-Khoury GY, Kathol MH: Radiographic evaluation of cervical spine trauma. Semin Spine Surg 1991;3:3.

Glaser JA et al: Variation in surgical opinion regarding management of selected cervical spine injuries. A preliminary study. Spine 1998;23(9):975. [PMID: 9589534]

Harris J Jr.: The cervicocranium: Its radiographic assessment. Radiology 2001;218(2):337. [PMID: 11161145]

Holdsworth F: Fractures, dislocations, and fracture-dislocations of the spine. J Bone Joint Surg Br 1970;52:1534.

Johnson RM et al: Cervical orthoses: A guide to their selection and use. Clin Orthop 1981;154:34.

Stauffer ES: Spinal cord injury syndromes. Semin Spine Surg 1991;3:87.

Wagner FC, Cheharzi B: Neurologic evaluation of cervical spinal cord injuries. Spine 1984;9:507.

White AA III, Panjabi MM: Update on the evaluation of instability of the lower cervical spine. Instr Course Lect 1987;36:513.

INJURIES OF THE UPPER CERVICAL SPINE

With the exception of occipitoatlantal dissociation, traumatic injuries to the upper cervical spine are less frequently associated with significant neurologic injury than are traumatic injuries to the lower cervical spine. This is secondary to the fact that the spinal cord occupies only one third of the upper spinal canal versus one half of the lower spinal canal.

Occipitoatlantal Dissociation

Occipitoatlantal dissociation is a disruption of the cranial vertebral junction, and it implies a subluxation or complete dislocation of the occipitoatlantal facets. This injury is typically fatal, yet the clinician must be aware of it because unrecognized occipitoatlantal dissociation may have catastrophic results. The mechanism of dissociation is poorly understood, but it most likely results from either a severe flexion or distraction type of injury. Anterior translation of the skull on the vertebral column is a common presentation and is most likely a hyperflexion injury. Bucholz, however, presented the pathologic anatomic findings of fatal occipitoatlantal dissociation and proposed a mechanism of hyperextension with resultant distractive force applied across the craniovertebral junction.

When the dissociation is a frank dislocation, the findings are clear on a lateral radiograph. When the dissociation is a subluxation, however, findings may be more subtle. In normal individuals, the distance between the tip of the dens and the basion (the anterior aspect of the foramen magnum) should be no greater than 1.0 cm, and the previously described Wackenheim line should run from the base of the basion tangentially to the tip of the dens. If the dens penetrates this line, anterior translation of the cranium is implied. Calculation of the Powers ratio can also be helpful in securing the diagnosis. Powers and his colleagues described a ratio of two lines (Figure 5–38), the first of which runs from the tip of the basion to the midpoint of the posterior lamina of the atlas (line BC) and the second of which runs from the anterior arch of C1 to the opisthion (line AO). When the ratio of BC to AO is greater than 1:1, anterior occipitoatlantal dissociation is present. Other radiographic signs include marked soft-tissue swelling and the presence of avulsion fractures at the occipitovertebral junction.

Early recognition and surgical stabilization are the mainstays of treatment in cases of occipitoatlantal dissociation.

Fractures of Vertebra C1 (Atlas Fractures)

The mechanism of injury in the fracture of the atlas is most typically axial compression with or without exten-

sion force, and the anatomic findings of the fracture are indicative of the specifics of the force and the position of the head at the time of impact. In 1920, Jefferson presented his classic description of the four-part fracture of the atlas following an axial injury. This fracture is a burst type that occurs secondary to the occipital condyles being driven into the interior portions of the ring of the atlas and driving the lateral masses outward, resulting in a two-part fracture of the anterior ring of the atlas as well as a two-part fracture of the posterior ring. More common than the classic four-part atlas fracture, however, are the two-part and three-part fractures. Isolated anterior arch fractures are the least common and are typically associated with fractures of the dens, whereas the more common posterior arch fracture is typically the result of a hyperextension injury.

A fracture of the atlas is typically diagnosed on plain radiographs. Findings may be subtle on the lateral cervical spine radiograph. The open-mouth (odontoid) view may show asymmetry of the lateral masses of C1 on C2 with overhang (Figure 5–39). A bilateral overhang totaling more than 6.9 mm is presumptive evidence of a disruption to the transverse ligament and suggests potential late instability. Presumptive evidence for transverse ligament disruption can also be seen on the lateral radiograph if the atlanto-dens interval is greater than 4 mm.

The treatment for fractures of the atlas as isolated injuries is typically nonoperative (Figure 5–40). If there are signs of transverse ligament disruption, halo traction is indicated with later transfer to halo-vest immobilization for a total of 3–4 months. Immediate halo-

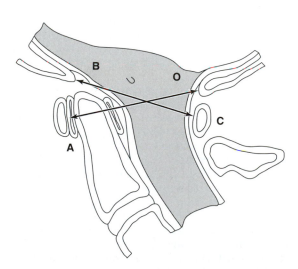

Figure 5–38. Diagram showing lines used in the calculation of the Powers ratio, which is helpful in diagnosing occipitoatlantal dissociation. The distance between the basion (point B) and the posterior arch (point C) is divided by the distance between the anterior arch of C1 (point A) and the opisthion (point O). The normal ratio of BC to AO is 1:1. A ratio of greater than 1 suggests that the head is dislocated anteriorly on the spine.

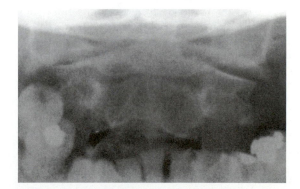

Figure 5–39. Open-mouth (odontoid) radiographic view demonstrating asymmetry of the lateral masses of C1 on C2 with overhang in a patient with a Jefferson fracture. (Reproduced, with permission, from El-Khoury GY, Kathol MH: Radiographic evaluation of cervical spine trauma. Semin Spine Surg 1991:3:3.)

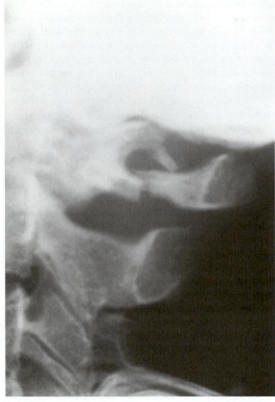

A

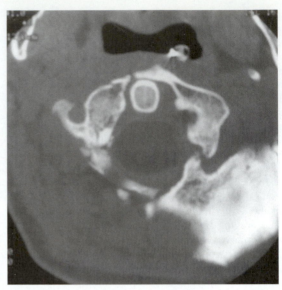

B

Figure 5–40. Imaging studies in a patient who was in a motor vehicle accident and sustained a distractive extension injury to his cervical spine and a three-part fracture of his atlas (a Jefferson fracture). **A:** Lateral radiographic view showing a fracture of the posterior arch. **B:** Axial section of a CT scan further delineating the fracture anatomy. This injury was deemed stable and was treated nonoperatively in a halo-vest.

vest application is indicated in cases involving a moderately displaced fracture with lateral mass overhang up to 5 mm, although collar immobilization is preferred in cases involving a minimally displaced fracture of the atlas. At completion of bony union, flexion-extension views should be obtained to rule out any evidence of late instability. If late instability is present and the bony elements have been allowed to heal, a limited C1-2 fusion can address the instability. If a nonunion is present or if the posterior arch remains disrupted, an occiput to C2 fusion is necessary to control the late instability.

Dislocations & Subluxations of Vertebrae C1 & C2

A. ATLANTOAXIAL ROTATORY SUBLUXATION

Atlantoaxial rotatory subluxation is most common in children and may be associated with minimal trauma or even occur spontaneously. Although some patients are asymptomatic, others present with neck pain or torticollis (a position in which the head is tilted toward one side and rotated toward the other). Inasmuch as the mechanism of injury is often unclear, the propensity for

the C1-2 location is based on anatomic factors. In about 50% of cases, cervical spine rotation occurs at the C1-2 junction, where the facet joints are more horizontal and less inherently stable in rotation.

The diagnosis of atlantoaxial rotatory subluxation is typically suspected on the basis of radiographs taken in several views. The odontoid view may show displacement of the lateral masses with respect to the dens; a lateral view may show an increased atlanto-dens interval; and the AP view may show a lateral shift of the spinous process of C1 on C2. CT scanning can be used to confirm the diagnosis, and a dynamic CT scan with full attempted right and left rotation can demonstrate a fixed deformity.

There are four types of atlantoaxial rotatory subluxations. In type I, the atlanto-dens interval is less than 3 mm, which suggests that the transverse ligament is still intact. In type II, the interval is 3–5 mm, which suggests that the transverse ligament is not structurally intact. In type III, the interval exceeds 5 mm, which is indicative of disruption of the transverse ligament as well as secondary stabilization of the alar ligament. In type IV, there is a complete posterior dislocation of the atlas on the axis, a finding that is typically associated with a hypoplastic odontoid process such as that seen in several forms of mucopolysaccharidosis (eg, Morquio's syndrome).

Treatment of atlantoaxial subluxation is typically conservative, consisting of traction followed by immobilization. About 90% of patients will respond to this treatment regimen. There is a high incidence of recurrence, however. For patients who do not respond to conservative measures and for patients with recurrent problems, C1-2 arthrodesis may be required to control the deformity.

B. Disruption of the Transverse Ligament

The transverse ligament and secondarily the alar ligament are the main constraints to anterior displacement of C1 on C2. It was previously presumed that because anterior subluxation of C1 on C2 typically involved a fracture through the dens, the transverse ligament was in fact stronger than the bony elements of the dens. Fielding and his colleagues, however, showed that experimentally this was not the case, yet clinically the higher association of anterior dislocation of dens fractures still holds true.

The mechanism of disruption is typically a flexion injury, and the diagnosis is made on lateral radiographs. The atlanto-dens interval should not exceed 3 mm in the adult. If the interval is 4 mm or larger and the dens is intact, a rupture of the transverse ligament is presumed.

High-resolution CT scan can be used to categorize this injury into two types. Type 1 is a disruption in the substance of the transverse ligament, whereas type 2 involves an avulsion fracture of the insertion of the transverse ligament on the lateral mass of C1. Type 1 injuries will predictably fail conservative treatment and should be managed with a C1-2 arthrodesis. A trial of nonoperative care in type 2 injuries using a rigid cervical orthosis may be a reasonable alternative. A 74% success rate can be anticipated, with surgery reserved for patients who have failed nonoperative care, showing persistent instability after 12 weeks in mobilization.

C. Fracture of the Odontoid Process

Fracture of the odontoid process is typically associated with high-velocity trauma, and the mechanism of injury is flexion in most cases. Depending on the fracture pattern, extension may be the predominant force in a smaller subset of cases. Associated injuries, particularly fractures of the ring of the atlas, should be ruled out. Neurologic involvement is relatively rare with odontoid fractures. In a study of 60 patients with acute fractures of the odontoid process, Anderson and D'Alonzo reported that 15 had some neurologic deficit on presentation, but only 5 of the 15 had major neurologic involvement and only 2 of this group of 5 remained quadriparetic at follow-up.

Odontoid fractures may be suspected on the basis of clinical presentation and confirmed on plain radiographs, although spasm and overlying shadows can obscure the diagnosis. AP and lateral conventional tomography is the best method by which to confirm the diagnosis. CT scanning is less helpful because the axial sectioning may miss a horizontal fracture line.

Both the risk of nonunion with delayed instability and the method of treating odontoid fracture will depend on the classification of the fracture. Reported rates of nonunion range from 20% to 63%. According to the classification system proposed in 1974 by Anderson and D'Alonzo, there are three types of fracture of the odontoid process (Figure 5–41).

Type I is a fracture through the tip of the odontoid process. In this configuration, the blood supply is maintained through the base of the odontoid process and through the attachment of the alar transverse ligaments. The mechanical stability of this fracture pattern is left intact. Symptomatic care and immobilization are the treatment of choice.

Type II, the most common type, is a fracture through the base of the odontoid process at its junction with the body of the axis. In this configuration, soft-tissue attachments to the fracture fragment cause distrac-

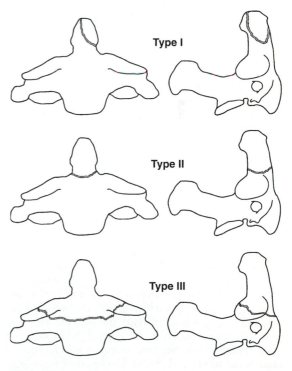

Figure 5–41. Diagram showing the three types of fractures of the odontoid process.

tion at the fracture site. Because the amount of cancellous bone available for opposition is limited, a high nonunion rate is expected, particularly if displacement is significant or the patient is older. In this case, primary surgical treatment may be indicated. Anterior screw fixation of the odontoid process has evolved to become the treatment of choice for most type 2 odontoid fractures. Although it is technically demanding, it does allow for the maintenance of motion at C1-2 (Figure 5–42).

Type III is a fracture through the body of the axis. The blood supply is maintained through soft-tissue attachments, and abundant cancellous bone opposition at the fracture site facilitates a high rate of union. The treatment, therefore, is conservative, consisting of halo traction or halo-vest immobilization until bony union occurs.

D. HANGMAN'S FRACTURE (TRAUMATIC SPONDYLOLISTHESIS OF VERTEBRA C2)

Hangman's fracture occurs when a fracture line passes through the neural arch of the axis. The anatomy of the axis is such that the superior facets are anterior and the inferior facets are posterior, thus concentrating stress through the neural arch. Because of the high ratio of spinal canal size to spinal cord size at this level, neurologic damage associated with hangman's fracture should be unusual. Bucholz reported, however, in his postmortem studies that traumatic spondylolisthesis was second only to occipitoatlantal dislocations in cervical injuries leading to fatalities.

According to the scheme proposed by Levine and Rhyne, hangman's fractures can be classified on the basis of anatomic factors and the presumed mechanism of injury. Treatment depends on the type of fracture. Imaging studies in a patient with Hangman's fracture are shown in Figure 5–43.

Type I is typically caused by hyperextension with or without additional axial load. There is no angulation of the deformity, and the fracture fragments are separated by less than 3 mm. Treatment should consist of immobilization in a cervical collar or halo-vest until union occurs, which is typically 12 weeks.

Type II is thought to be caused by hyperextension and axial load with a secondary flexion component leading to displacement of the fracture. Reduction of the anterior angulation in this type of fracture is necessary and is typically obtained by traction therapy and then followed by placement of a halo-vest until union occurs. An atypical type II hangman's fracture has been described. This fracture occurs through the posterior aspect of the vertebral body, potentially resulting in cord compromise as the anterior aspect of the vertebral body flexes forward. A higher likelihood of neurologic injury with this atypical pattern is seen, and halo-vest immobilization is recommended.

Type IIA has the same fracture pattern as type II but with a component of distraction that also occurred at the time of injury and led to disruption of the C2-3 disc space, rendering this injury inherently unstable. Traction should be avoided in cases of type IIA fracture because it will exacerbate the injury. Treatment should consist of immediate halo-vest application, with the patient's head positioned in slight extension to afford a reduction.

Type III includes a fracture through the neural arch, a facet dislocation, and a disruption of the C2-3 disc space that renders the injury highly unstable. Treatment generally consists of early closed reduction of the facet dislocation and application of a halo-vest to maintain the reduction. If the reduction cannot be obtained in a closed fashion or cannot be maintained conservatively, then treatment with open reduction of the dislocation and anterior or posterior fusion is indicated.

Anderson LD, D'Alonzo RT: Fractures of the odontoid process of the axis. J Bone Joint Surg Am 1974;56:1663.

Chiba K et al: Treatment protocol for fractures of the odontoid process. J Spinal Disord 1996;9:267.

Dickman CA et al: Injuries involving the transverse atlantal ligament: Classification and treatment guidelines based on experience with 30 injuries. Neurosurgery 1996;38:44.

Govender S et al: Fractures of the odontoid process. J Bone Joint Surg Br 2000;82(8):1143. [PMID: 11132275]

Levine AM, Rhyne AL: Traumatic spondylolisthesis of the axis. Semin Spine Surg 1991;3:47.

Powers B et al: Traumatic anterior atlanto-occipital dislocation. Neurosurgery 1979;4:12.

Vieweg U, Schultheiss R: A review of halo vest treatment of upper cervical spine injuries. Archives of Orthopaedic & Trauma Surgery 2001;121(1-2):50. [PMID: 21034862]

Zhu Q et al: Traumatic instabilities of the cervical spine caused by high speed axial compression in a human model. An in vitro biomechanical study. Spine 1999;24(5):440. [PMID: 99183926]

Ziai WC, Hurlbert RJ: A six year review of odontoid fractures: The emerging role of surgical intervention. Can J Neurol Sci 2000;27(4):297.[PMID: 11097519]

INJURIES OF THE LOWER CERVICAL SPINE

As stated earlier, fractures and dislocations of the lower cervical spine have a greater frequency of catastrophic neurologic involvement. This is attributed to the decreased ratio of spinal canal to spinal cord in the lower levels. Treatment of affected patients again relies upon early recognition of the injury, recognition of inherent stability or instability of the injury pattern, and institution of appropriate definitive care.

In 1982, Allen and colleagues developed a classification system for closed indirect fractures and dislocations

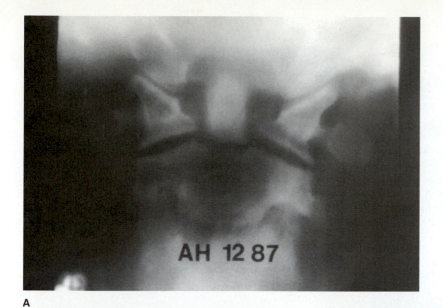

A

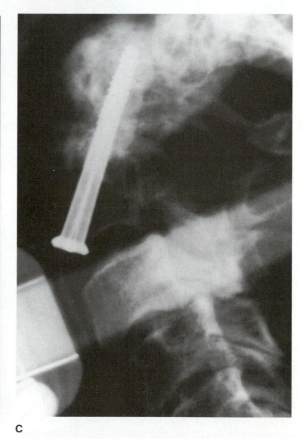

B

C

Figure 5–42. Imaging studies in a patient with a type II odontoid fracture nonunion. **A:** Open-mouth radiographic view showing the fracture line at the base of the odontoid process. **B:** Sagittal reconstruction using CT scanning to better delineate the fracture anatomy. **C:** Radiograph taken after the patient underwent anterior placement of two odontoid screws under fluoroscopic control using a cannulated screw system.

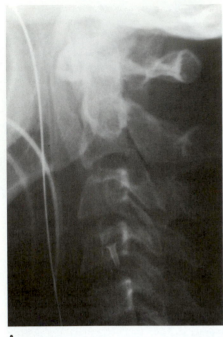

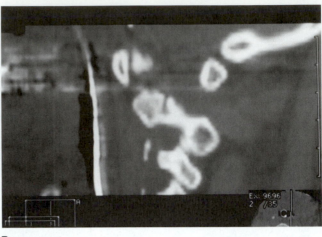

Figure 5–43. Imaging studies in a patient who was in a motor vehicle accident and sustained a hangman's fracture, or traumatic spondylolisthesis of C2. **A:** Lateral radiographic view, which is largely unremarkable. **B:** Sagittal reconstruction using CT scanning to better delineate the fracture site at the base of the posterior elements. The patient was treated nonoperatively.

of the lower cervical spine. After reviewing numerous cases previously described by other authors as well as 165 of their own cases, they grouped the injuries into six categories, based on the position of the cervical spine at the time of impact and on the dominant mode of failure. The six categories were compressive flexion, vertical compression, distractive flexion, compressive extension, distractive extension, and lateral flexion. Of these, the distractive flexion injuries were the most common, followed by the compressive extension injuries and the compressive flexion injuries. Some of the categories were further divided into stages, as described below.

Compressive Flexion Injury

There are five stages of compressive flexion injuries, which are labeled compression flexion stage (CFS) I through V (Figure 5–44). CFS I shows a slight blunting and rounding to the anterior superior vertebral margin, without any evidence of posterior ligamentous damage. CFS II shows some additional loss of height of the anterior vertebral body, again sparing the posterior elements. CFS III has an additional fracture line passing from the anterior surface of the vertebral body through to the infe-

rior subchondral plate, with minimal displacement. CFS IV has less than 3 mm of displacement of the inferior posterior vertebral fragment into the neural canal. CFS V has severe displacement of the inferior posterior fragment into the canal, with widening of the spinous processes posteriorly, indicative of three-column disruption.

Within the compressive flexion category, there are two types of fractures more commonly referred to as the **compression fracture** and the **teardrop fracture.** Most compression fractures without disruption of the posterior elements are thought to be stable, so that no surgical intervention is required. The more severe compression fracture injuries, however, can result in displacement of bone into the spinal canal, and if a neurologic injury is present, these require anterior decompression and stabilization. All patients should be carefully checked with flexion-extension views at the completion of their treatment to rule out any evidence of late instability.

Vertical Compression Injury

Vertical compression (VCS) injuries occur secondary to axial loading and are divided into three stages. VCS I consists of an end-plate central fracture with no

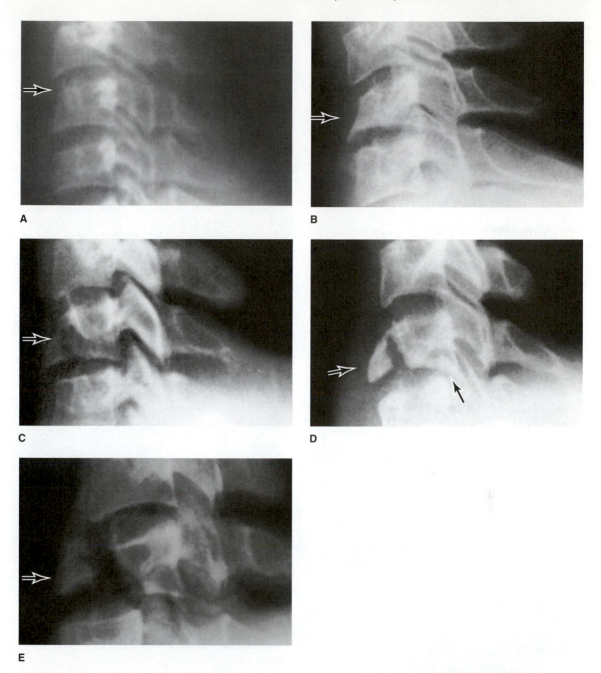

Figure 5–44. Radiographs showing the five stages of compressive flexion injury. **A** shows CFS I. **B** shows CFS II. **C** shows CFS III. **D** shows CFS IV. **E** shows CFS V. (Reproduced, with permission, from Allen BL et al: A mechanistic classification of closed, indirect fractures and dislocations of the lower cervical spine. Spine 1982;7:1.)

evidence of ligamentous failure. VCS II is a fracture of both vertebral end-plates, again with only minimal displacement. VCS III is the more commonly termed **burst fracture** with a spectrum of fragmentation of the vertebral body, with or without posterior element disruption.

The treatment for vertical compression injuries is typically nonoperative. Traction is applied to obtain and maintain alignment, and bony union is generally complete after 3 months of halo-vest immobilization. Flexion-extension views should be obtained at the completion of healing because a posterior ligamentous injury can result in late instability.

Distractive Flexion Injury

The category of distractive flexion injury was the most common injury category reported by Allen and colleagues, and it includes both unilateral and bilateral facet subluxation and dislocation. There are four stages of distractive flexion (DFS) injury. DFS I, which is termed a **flexion sprain,** is characterized by subluxation of the facet joint, with possible interspinous process widening. This injury has subtle radiographic findings and may easily be missed during initial evaluation and therefore result in late symptomatic instability (Figure 5–45). DFS II is a unilateral facet dislocation, the diagnosis of which can be confirmed on plain radiographs. The lateral radiograph would reveal an anterior subluxation of one vertebra of approximately 25% of vertebral body width at the affected level. The facet itself may be perched or fully dislocated. DFS III is a bilateral facet dislocation with approximately 50% anterior dislocation at the affected level. DFS IV, which is also termed a **floating vertebra,** is a bilateral facet dislocation with displacement of a full vertebral width.

Treatment of distractive flexion injuries depends on the severity of the injury. Achievement of anatomic

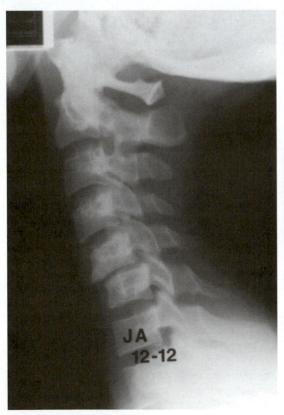
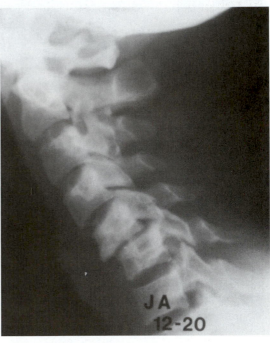

Figure 5–45. Imaging studies in a patient with a distractive flexion injury of the cervical spine. **A:** This lateral radiographic view demonstrates anterior subluxation of C5 on C6. **B:** The follow-up radiograph shows progression of the subluxation. The patient was treated with a posterior spinal fusion of C5-6.

alignment and spinal stability yields the best results. Patients with unilateral facet dislocation should be treated with closed reduction in the acute phase, followed by immobilization. If closed reduction is not possible, open reduction and fusion are indicated (Figure 5–46). Bilateral facet dislocations are associated with a higher incidence of both neurologic injury and instability. Treatment consisting of closed reduction and immobilization is feasible, but because it results in a high percentage of late instability and this eventually requires posterior fusion, the use of early posterior fusion is indicated.

Another fracture pattern that should be included in the discussion on flexion injuries is the clay shoveler's fracture, which is a fracture of the spinous process, typically at level C6, C7, or T1. This is an avulsion injury that generally occurs in flexion by the counteractive forces of the muscular attachments. As an isolated in-

jury, it is considered stable and is usually treated nonoperatively.

Compressive Extension Injury

The category of compressive extension (CES) injury was the second most common injury category reported by Allen and colleagues. It is divided into five stages. CES I is a fracture of the vertebral arch unilaterally, with or without displacement, and CES II is a bilateral fracture. CES III and CES IV were not encountered in the series reported by Allen and colleagues but were theoretic interpolations between CES II and CES V. CES III would be a bilateral fracture of the vertebral arch articular processes, lamina, or pedicle without vertebral displacement, whereas CES IV would be the same fracture pattern but with moderate vertebral body

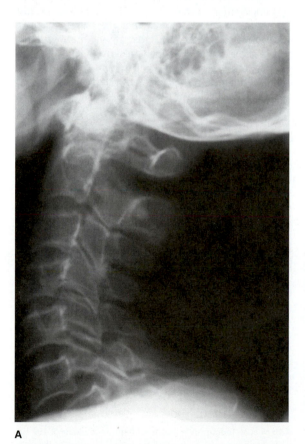

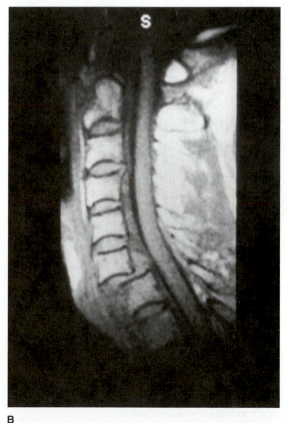

A

B

Figure 5–46.   Imaging studies in a man who fell from a height and suffered a C6-7 fracture-dislocation with a perched facet but remained neurologically intact. **A:** Lateral radiographic view demonstrating the fracture-dislocation at C6-7. **B:** MRI demonstrating the anterior subluxation of C6 on C7, with the intervertebral disc retropulsed behind the C6 vertebral body. The patient was treated with an anterior discectomy, reduction, and fusion.

displacement. Three patients in Allen and colleagues' series had CES V injuries, which were bilateral vertebral arch fractures with 100% anterior displacement.

Treatment of compressive extension injuries is related to the three-column theory. Stabilization with a posterior, anterior, or combined approach is indicated if there is significant disruption of the middle column or of two of the three columns.

Distractive Extension Injury

Distractive extension (DES) injuries are typically soft-tissue lesions and are divided into two stages. DES I is a disruption of the anterior ligamentous complex or, rarely, a nondisplaced fracture of the vertebral body. Radiographs may appear entirely normal. One clue to the diagnosis is widening of the disc space, which is sometimes present. DES II is a disruption of the posterior soft-tissue complex, which can allow posterior displacement of the upper vertebral body into the spinal canal. This lesion is often reduced at the time of lateral radiographs and may show only subtle or no changes on routine radiographs. When neurologic involvement is present, it is most commonly a central cord syndrome, and provided that any no coexisting compression lesions are present, some neurologic recovery is expected.

The distractive extension injury is usually stable and does not require surgical intervention. Late flexion-extension views, however, are indicated to rule out any evidence of late instability.

Lateral Flexion Injury

Allen and colleagues included the injuries of five patients in the category of lateral flexion (LFS) injury. This category is further divided into two stages. LFS I is an asymmetric compression fracture of the vertebral body and ipsilateral posterior arch, with no displacement in the coronal plane. LFS II has a similar fracture pattern but with displacement in the coronal plane, which suggests ligamentous disruption on the tension side of the injury. This mechanism can lead to brachial plexus injuries of varying degrees on the distracted side.

Because of the rarity of LFS injuries, treatment protocols are not well established. Surgical stabilization should be considered if late instability is expected or if there is a neurologic deficit.

Cervical Strains & Sprains (Whiplash Injury)

Cervical strains and sprains, which are commonly referred to as a **whiplash injury** when associated with motor vehicle accidents, can produce a protracted and confusing clinical picture. Pain is typically the one unifying feature, yet there may be numerous other complaints, including local tenderness, decreased range of motion, headaches that are typically occipital, blurred or double vision, dysphagia, hoarseness, jaw pain, difficulty with balance, and even vertigo. It is often difficult for the physician to correlate radiographic findings, diagnostic test results, and other objective findings with the subjective complaints of the patient. The constellation of symptoms is fairly uniform, however, and should certainly not be discounted, and many investigators have proposed an anatomic basis for the clinical complaints. McNabb proposed that paresthesias in the ulnar distribution may be secondary to spasm of the scalenus muscle, and certainly symptoms such as hoarseness and dysphagia can be related to retropharyngeal hematoma. The cervical zygapophysial joint and facet capsule have been implicated as a source for chronic pain after whiplash injury.

Figure 5–47 presents an algorithm for management of cervical strain. Radiographs should be taken because the amount of neck trauma that the patient has sustained may be significant. Radiographic findings, however, may be subtle or entirely negative. Cervical lordosis may be reversed, indicating spasm. Subtle signs of instability may also be present, and these can be further delineated on flexion-extension views if symptoms persist. The prevertebral soft-tissue window should be within normal limits to rule out any prevertebral hematoma.

Once the stability of the spine has been ensured, the care of the cervical sprain or whiplash injury should be symptomatic. Initial rest, bed rest if necessary, and soft collar immobilization are indicated, along with the use of anti-inflammatory medications. Early mobilization with progressive range of motion and weaning from external supports should be encouraged, however. Frequent reassurance is often necessary because the symptoms may be long-lasting.

About 42% of patients have persistent symptoms beyond 1 year, with approximately one third having persistent symptoms beyond 2 years. Most patients who do improve do so within the first 2 months. Factors associated with a poor prognosis include the presence of occipital headaches, interscapular pain, or reversal of cervical lordosis. Women have a worse prognosis than men, and hyperextension injuries are thought to have a worse prognosis than hyperflexion injuries.

Aebi M et al: Indication, surgical technique, and results of 100 surgically treated fractures and fracture-dislocations of the cervical spine. Clin Orthop 1986;203:244.

Allen BL et al: A mechanistic classification of closed, indirect fractures and dislocations of the lower cervical spine. Spine 1982;7:1.

Gertzbein SD: Scoliosis Research Society multicenter spine fracture study. Spine 1992;17:528.

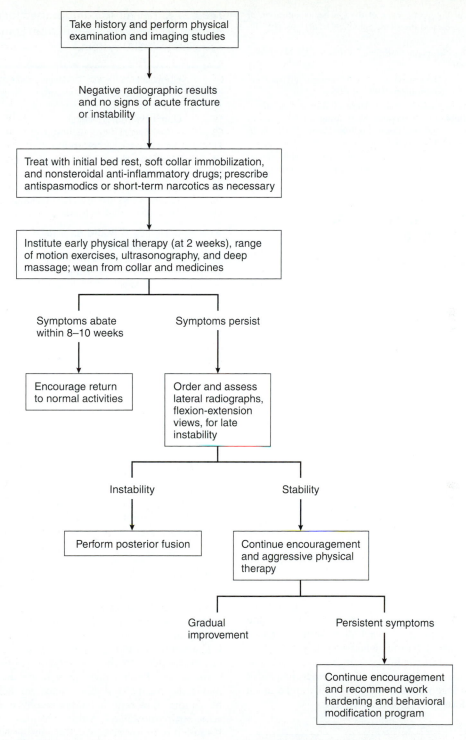

Figure 5–47.   Algorithm for management of patients with cervical strain.

Hartling L et al: Prognostic value of the Quebec classification of whiplash associated disorders. Spine 2001;26(1):36. [PMID: 11148643]

McNabb I: The "whiplash syndrome." Orthop Clin North Am 1971;2:389.

Parent AD et al: Lateral cervical spine dislocation and vertebral artery injury. Neurosurgery 1991;31:501.

Siegmund GP et al: Mechanical evidence of facet capsule injury during whiplash—A cadaveric study using combined shear, compression, and extension loading. Spine 2001;26(19):2095. [PMID: 11698885]

Yoganandan N et al: Whiplash injury determination with conventional spine imaging and cryomicrotomy. Spine 2001;26(22):2443. [PMID: 11707708]

INJURIES OF THE THORACIC & LUMBAR SPINE

Principles of Diagnosis

The management of fractures of the thoracolumbar spine is intended to maximize neurologic recovery, optimize spinal stability, restore the anatomy, maintain motion, and decrease the likelihood of pain.

A. NEUROLOGIC EVALUATION

Although both the Frankel grading system and the ASIA motor scoring system have been used to assess patients from a neurologic and structural standpoint, the ASIA system provides more detail in most cases.

The Frankel grading system classifies injuries as follows: grade A indicates complete paralysis; grade B indicates sensory sparing alone; grade C indicates that motor function is present but is not useful; grade D indicates that motor function is present and useful; and grade E indicates that motor function is present and normal.

The ASIA motor scoring system delineates key muscle groups for root levels. Each muscle group is graded on a standard 5-point scale in which 5 denotes normal function and 3 denotes motion against gravity. The grades are totaled for the right and left sides in each group (Table 5–4).

Results of sensory, reflex, and motor tests should be recorded, and a rectal examination must be performed to assess perirectal sensation, rectal tone, anal wink, and the presence or absence of a bulbocavernosus reflex. The last will help determine whether or not the patient is in spinal shock if the injury is at the cord level. The presence of any sacral sparing will mean that the patient may have an incomplete spinal cord injury and a much better prognosis for neurologic recovery.

B. IMAGING STUDIES

Once the neurologic examination has been carefully reviewed, appropriate radiographs should be obtained. If the patient is unconscious, if back pain or calcaneal

Table 5–4. Key muscle groups used for motor grading according to the American Spinal Injury Association (ASIA) system.[a]

C5	Elbow flexors (biceps, brachialis, and brachioradialis)
C6	Wrist extensors (extensors carpis radialis longus and brevis)
C7	Elbow extensors (triceps)
C8	Finger flexors (flexor digitorum profundus)
T1	Hand intrinsics (interossei)
L2	Hip flexors (iliopsoas)
L3	Knee extensors (quadriceps)
L4	Ankle dorsiflexors (tibialis anterior)
L5	Toe extensors (extensor hallucis longus)
S1	Ankle plantarflexors (gastrocnemius and soleus)

[a]Each muscle group is graded on a standard 5-point scale in which 5 denotes normal function and 3 denotes motion against gravity. The grades are totaled for the right and left sides in each group. While a patient with normal function would score 100 points, a complete paraplegic would score 50 points.

fractures are present, or if the patient has a history of an axial loading injury, the log-rolling technique should be used while the patient is being evaluated and until adequate radiographs have been obtained.

1. Radiography—Plain radiographs in both the posteroanterior and lateral planes should be reviewed. The lateral radiograph should be inspected for fracture lines, alignment, angulation, and translation. The posterior cortex of a vertebral body that is suspected of fracture can be viewed to see if bone is retropulsed into the spinal canal. The posteroanterior view can also show the fracture or abnormalities in alignment, angulation, and translation. The spacing of the pedicles of each vertebral body should be carefully measured. Normally, there is very slight widening as one proceeds more distally along the thoracolumbar spine. If the pedicles of one vertebral body are wider apart than those of the vertebral body below, a burst type of fracture should be suspected (see section on Burst Fracture).

2. Computed tomography and magnetic resonance imaging—If a neurologic deficit is present or a burst fracture is suspected, additional studies such as MRI or CT scanning should be performed. CT scanning can give better detail of the bony anatomy, but MRI gives better detail of soft tissues, particularly the neural elements, ligaments, and discs, and can help detect a hematoma. It is rare that myelography is done in the acute setting nowadays, with or without CT scanning, because it is an invasive procedure and usually does not give any information that cannot be obtained through MRI. It should be noted that CT scanning can miss a shear type of fracture or a distractive flexion injury because the plane of the fracture may be in the plane of the sections. Sagittal reformatting and a high clinical index of suspicion can help avoid this problem.

C. Assessment of Spinal Stability

According to the arguments set forth by Holdsworth in 1970, the two-column spine is the key to stability. The anterior column comprises the vertebral body, disc, and anterior and posterior longitudinal ligaments; the posterior column comprises the posterior bony arch, interspinous and intertransverse ligaments, and facet joints; and the injured spine is not unstable unless both of these columns are disrupted.

In 1983, Denis refined these concepts and described the three-column spine, in which the middle column comprises the posterior half of the vertebral body and disc as well as the posterior longitudinal ligament. According to Denis, a middle column that is not disrupted is the key to stability of the thoracolumbar spine.

Critics of the three-column theory point out that not all fractures with disruption of the middle column are unstable either acutely or chronically. Biomechanical studies suggest that the middle column structures do not significantly affect stability. In some cases, burst fractures progressively become deformed and painful, but the risk that this will occur is difficult to predict. Some investigators have suggested that fractures with greater than 50% canal compromise, greater than 30-degree angulation, or greater than 50% loss of anterior vertebral height are at increased risk for painful post-traumatic deformity. Others have suggested that high degrees of comminution and spreading of the fracture fragments predispose the spine to collapse.

Although evidence of neural compression by the bone or disc in the presence of a neurologically incomplete injury may be an indication for surgical decompression, and the surgeon should in such cases stabilize the patient at the time of decompression, the presence of middle column disruption per se is not an indication for operative intervention.

Principles of Treatment

A. Criteria for Conservative or Surgical Treatment

The type of treatment depends on whether the patient has a neurologic injury, whether the neurologic injury is complete or incomplete, whether the spine is unstable in the acute setting or is expected to be unstable chronically, and whether other injuries are present in the spine or musculoskeletal system or in the chest or abdomen. The medical stability of the patient and rehabilitation considerations also influence the treatment options.

1. Incomplete versus complete neurologic injury— A neurologically complete injury is one in which no motor or sensory function is present below the level of injury once the period of spinal shock is over (ie, once the bulbocavernosus reflex has returned). Note that this delineation only applies for spinal cord injuries; it does not apply for injuries below the end of the cord, which is usually at L1. In contrast to the complete injury, the neurologically incomplete injury is one in which function or sensation is present below the level of injury.

Patients with neurologically complete injuries have virtually no chance of recovering function, although occasionally some recovery occurs at the level of injury, termed **root escape.** Patients with neurologically incomplete injuries may recover some function, sometimes even a great deal, over the months or even up to 2 years after injury.

2. Stable versus unstable spine—Patients who have suffered multiple trauma benefit from early mobilization, which facilitates pulmonary toilet, decreases the incidence of thromboembolic phenomena and pressure sores, and helps prevent other sequelae of prolonged bed rest. If a patient has a spinal injury that is acutely unstable and is at high risk for developing the complications associated with prolonged bed rest, it may be necessary to use protective bracing or casting or to perform spinal fusion. These measures have also been shown to facilitate rehabilitation for patients who have neurologic deficits secondary to their spinal injury and will require weeks to months of rehabilitative services to learn to use ambulatory aids or wheelchairs and to undertake self-care.

Examples of patients who may have neurologically complete injuries but stable spines include those who have suffered from gunshot wounds to the spine. Examples of patients who may have incomplete injuries that are stable and do not usually require decompression are those who have suffered lower energy penetrating injuries to the spine, such as stab wounds.

3. Indications for decompression—If a patient has an incomplete spinal cord injury and evidence of continued neural element compression, decompression may be indicated. At the time of surgery, stabilization in the form of fusion, accompanied by instrumentation, may be performed.

Although emergency decompression is indicated if a patient demonstrates a worsening neurologic deficit in the acute setting, the timing of decompression in most patients with incomplete injuries may not be so crucial. On the one hand, two findings concerning patients with incomplete injuries support this argument: First, these patients often demonstrate significant neurologic recovery if the neural elements are protected from additional damage (by bed rest, bracing, or surgical stabilization). Second, neurologic recovery in these patients can take place even if decompression is performed up to 2 years after the injury. On the other hand, no studies specifically compare the effects that early and late decompression have on neurologic outcome in humans. Studies in animals seem to suggest that earlier decompression is preferable. Several studies have also shown that bony canal encroachment remodels over time. In general, it is agreed that for a patient with a stable neurologic examination who is indicated for surgery, it is appropriate to perform the surgery in a timely fashion when an optimized team is available, including anesthesia and nursing staff.

B. Surgical Procedures

1. Decompression—If decompression is felt to be indicated, the surgical approach used should depend on where the compression lies. Similar neurologic outcomes can be achieved by anterior decompression or posterolateral decompression, if one can achieve adequate decompression. Laminectomy as a definitive procedure alone is absolutely contraindicated for fractures. A posterolateral approach to decompression, in which the retropulsed bone can be removed or pushed back into place, can be performed and permits the application of posterior instrumentation for realignment and stabilization. The posterolateral decompression may require removal of the pedicle to avoid undue manipulation of the spinal cord. Intraoperative ultrasound or postoperative CT scanning should be performed in these cases to assess adequacy of decompression. If a patient has a burst fracture with neurologic deficit and an accompanying laminar fracture, there is a significant probability that that patient may have nerve roots entrapped at the site of the laminar fracture. This can sometimes be seen with the imaging studies of MRI or CT/myelogram. These patients should have a posterior decompression with decompression of the entrapped nerve roots and posterior instrumentation. Follow-up studies to determine the adequacy of decompression and long-term structural integrity of the anterior elements will determine whether the patient needs anterior reconstruction or decompression.

If the majority of the neurologic compression is from the anterior elements, as is the case with most burst fractures, an anterior corpectomy provides the most direct visualization for decompression. The fractured vertebra can be reconstructed with iliac crest structural graft, allograft supplemented by autograft or a mesh cage filled with autograft. The removed vertebra serves as a good source of bone graft, although structural support should be obtained via the other options noted.

2. Instrumentation—If the spine is unstable, either from the injury itself or from decompression, instru-

mentation and fusion should be performed. Currently, most surgeons use variable hook-rod systems including pedicle screw fixation for posterior instrumentation. Harrington rods are the time-tested device, but their reliance on distraction for correction flattens the spine's sagittal curves and can result in secondary changes and flatback syndrome, particularly in the lumbar spine.

In the acute setting, the presence of an intact posterior longitudinal ligament can allow the surgeon to use the distraction of the spine and its realignment to realign the retropulsed bone from the vertebral body. This **ligamentotaxis** can be helpful, but its results vary, depending on how old the fracture is, whether the posterior longitudinal ligament is indeed intact, and how large or small the fracture fragments are.

Initially, when pedicle screw fixation was used in the treatment of spine fractures, fixation of one level above and below the fracture was often performed. There appears, however, to be a significant risk of screw breakage or loss of correction with this technique. With significant loss of anterior column support, posterior instrumentation alone may not be sufficient, and anterior reconstruction may be indicated. Biomechanical studies and clinical experience indicate that placement of a sublaminar hook at the ends of the construct above and below the screws protects the screws and decreases the risk. At the thoracolumbar junction, variable hook-rod systems can be used in combination, with hooks placed in the thoracic spine and pedicle screws and the protective hook or hooks placed within the lumbar spine.

If an anterior decompression is elected, anterior instrumentation may applied. Depending on whether the posterior elements are intact and how good the bone quality is at the screw attachments of this instrumentation, this may be adequate for stabilization, although many surgeons do recommend bracing for a few months until initial healing is complete.

Anterior instrumentation may be placed at the time of anterior decompression if desired for improved stability. Among the available systems are the Kaneda device, Z-plate, Danek instrumentation, and I-plate. This last merely contains the bone graft material and reinforces its strength; it is not rigidly fixed to the vertebral body above and below. The other systems use screws through the vertebral bodies above and below, and these screws are connected to or through a plate or rods to afford stability. These devices are load-sharing devices, and supplementing their use with a brace postoperatively is typically recommended.

Denis F: The three-column spine and its significance in the classification of acute thoracolumbar spine injuries. Spine 1983;8: 817.

Holdsworth F: Fractures, dislocations, and fracture dislocations of the spine. J Bone Joint Surg Am 1970;52:1534.

McCormack T et al: The load-sharing classification of spine fractures. Spine 1994;19:1741.

McLain RF et al: Early failure of short-segment pedicle instrumentation for thoracolumbar fractures. J Bone Joint Surg Am 1993;75A:162.

Panjabi MM et al: Graded thoracolumbar spinal injuries: Development of multidirectional instability. Eur Spine J 1998;7:332.

Panjabi MM et al: Validity of the three-column theory of thoracolumbar fractures. Spine 1995;20:1122.

Parker JW et al: Successful short-segment instrumentation and fusion for thoracolumbar spine fractures. Spine 2000;25:1157.

Stambough JL: Posterior instrumentation for thoracolumbar trauma. Clin Orthop Rel Res 1997;335:73.

COMPRESSION FRACTURE (WEDGE FRACTURE)

Compression fractures, or wedge fractures, involve buckling or fracture of the anterior cortex of the vertebral body. Axial loading with a flexion moment is the mechanism of injury. The degree of angulation may be very slight or severe. Multiple compression fractures may occur with the same trauma, often contiguous. (With all types of spine fractures, other spine fractures can coexist.) Compression fractures can occur in the osteoporotic or elderly patient with minimal trauma. Neurologic deficit does not result.

Treatment is generally symptomatic. Bracing may be used if the deformity is significant or for comfort until the fracture heals and pain diminishes.

BURST FRACTURE

The burst type of fracture has been the subject of much debate concerning the assessment of spinal stability (see previous section on Principles of Diagnosis). A burst fracture occurs when the axial and flexion load has been sufficient to retropulse bone into the neural canal. The fracture may have a lateral bend, flexion, or rotational component as well, and it is sometimes accompanied by a laminar fracture.

On AP radiographs, the fracture will demonstrate interpedicular widening, suggestive of the bursting-type injury that has occurred and spread the pedicles apart. Lateral radiographs will show kyphotic angulation, and careful review may suggest how much bone has been retropulsed.

The quantification of retropulsed bone is important, particularly if the patient shows a neurologic deficit. As discussed earlier, evidence of neural compression in the face of an incomplete neurologic injury may be an indication for surgical decompression. It is unclear how much canal compromise is significant, and this may be related to the level of injury. Narrowing to T12 at the cord level is more crucial than at the conus level (at L1) or at the cauda equina level (below L1) both because the nerve roots can tolerate more compression and because the ratio of canal size to neural element size is greater. Many investigators believe that a canal compromise of 50% is an indication for decompression, but a canal compromise upward of 80% has been shown to be tolerated by occasional patients.

Burst fractures associated with laminar fractures, particularly in cases of neurologic deficit, have a high risk of dural tear with entrapment of the nerve roots. Because this cannot be addressed via an anterior approach and vertebrectomy, a posterior procedure may be selected.

Cammisa FP et al: Dural laceration occurring with burst fractures and associated lamina fractures. J Bone Joint Surg Am 1989; 71A:1044.

Ghanayem AJ, Zdeblick TA: Anterior instrumentation in the management of thoracolumbar burst fractures. Clin Orthop Rel Res 1997;335:89.

Kim N-H et al: Neurologic injury and recovery in patients with burst fracture of the thoracolumbar spine. Spine 1999;24: 290.

DISTRACTIVE FLEXION INJURY (CHANCE FRACTURE)

In a distractive flexion injury, or Chance fracture, the vertebral body fails in flexion and the posterior elements fail in distraction. The injury generally results in acute instability. This type of injury frequently occurs when an automobile passenger wearing a seat belt over the lap is thrown forward, and for this reason it is also known as a seat belt type of injury. In some cases, the fracture occurs entirely through one vertebral body. In other cases, it occurs either through the bone and the adjacent disc or through the posterior elements of one vertebra and the body of another.

Distractive flexion injuries occurring entirely through bone generally heal well with hyperextension casting or bracing. Those occurring entirely through disc and ligament are not likely to heal and therefore are recommended for surgical stabilization, which involves the use of posterior compression, instrumentation, and fusion as described earlier (see previous section on Principles of Treatment).

FRACTURE-DISLOCATION INJURY

Fracture dislocations involve a rotatory or shear component and result in complete disruption of the spinal column structures. They are often associated with complete neurologic injuries and clearly are unstable injuries. In many cases, the fracture will eventually heal adequately, but prolonged bed rest and casting may be required. Surgical stabilization may be indicated to permit early mobilization of the patient and facilitate rehabilitation.

Tumors in Orthopedics

6

R. Lor Randall, MD

Tumors of the musculoskeletal system are an extremely heterogeneous group of neoplasms consisting of well over 200 benign types of neoplasms and approximately 90 malignant conditions. The relative incidence of benign to malignant disease is 200:1. They uniformly arise from embryonic mesoderm and are categorized according to their differentiated or adult histology, with current classification schemes being essentially descriptive. Each histologic type of tumor expresses individual, distinct behaviors with great variation between tumor types. Benign disease, by definition, behaves in a nonaggressive fashion with little tendency to recur locally or to metastasize. Malignant tumors or sarcomas, such as osteosarcoma and synovial cell sarcoma, are capable of invasive, locally destructive growth with a tendency to recur and to metastasize.

Neoplastic processes arise in tissues of mesenchymal origin far less frequently than those of ectodermal and endodermal origin. Soft-tissue and bone sarcomas have an annual incidence in the United States of over 6000 and 3000 new cases, respectively. When compared with the overall average cancer mortality of 550,000 cases per year, sarcomas are a small fraction of the problem. However, although a relatively uncommon form of cancer, these mesenchymal tumors behave in an aggressive fashion with reported current mortality rates in some series greater than 50%. According to the National Cancer Institute's Surveillance, Epidemiology, and End Results (SEER) Program, approximately 5700 new soft-tissue sarcomas developed in the United States in 1990 with 3100 sarcoma-related deaths. More recent epidemiologic studies support this. The associated morbidity is much higher. These tumors inflict a tremendous emotional and financial toll on individuals and society alike. Furthermore, sarcomas are more common in older patients, with 15% percent affecting patients younger than 15 years of age and 40% percent affecting persons older than 55. Accordingly, as the population ages, as it is doing at a rapid rate, the incidence of these tumors will increase.

■ ETIOLOGY OF MUSCULOSKELETAL TUMORS

It is a central theorem in tumor biology that a tumor arises from an initial monoclonal expansion of a single cell whose genetic regulatory machinery has gone awry. This results in unchecked cellular proliferation. This tumorigenesis is a complex, multiple-step pathway by which healthy tissue progressively transforms from a normal phenotype into an abnormal colony of proliferating cells. Such a process may progress beyond the controlled state of benign disease to become a dedifferentiated, aggressive, and immortal phenotype via a pathway of genomic instability. It is this instability that allows the cell to progress to fulminant malignancy. DNA regulation and correspondingly, integrity, is ultimately lost and a cancer is born.

Accordingly, to appreciate the way in which a bone or soft-tissue tumor develops, one must have a basic understanding of the cell cycle. The cell cycle is the process by which a given cell replicates its cellular machinery and divides into two daughter cells. This process is orchestrated by a complex array of cellular proteins and is separated into four distinct phases: G1 (gap 1), S (DNA synthesis), G2 (gap 2), and M (mitosis). DNA synthesis occurs during the S phase, with chromosomal separation and cell division occurring in the M phase. The majority of cell growth takes place during G1. The mature state for mesenchymal tissues is normally in a resting, nonproliferative phase designated G0. It is the factors that affect the exit of the cell from G0, with entrance into G1, that is the hallmark of neoplastic disease.

Control of this process is a function of numerous regulatory proteins and checkpoints, These checkpoints allow for the monitoring and correction in the genetic sequence. These proteins are encoded by two basic gene types: oncogenes and suppressor genes. Oncogenes, encoding a variety of growth factors, promote progression of the cell through G1, effecting a mitogenic signal. Suppressor genes, such as wild-type *TP53,* act to arrest the cell cycle. Specifically, *TP53* acts to stop the cell cycle at the G1/S border as a final attempt to abort proliferation. Other suppressor genes work earlier to keep reproduction at bay. A complex array of molecules can serve as either an induction or suppressor function. Cyclins and cyclin-dependent kinases are being studied actively to elucidate their role in regulation of the cell cycle.

When this pathway is not orchestrated properly, a given cell obtains the potential for limited or even immortal proliferation. A normal cell progresses through a preneoplastic state on its way to becoming neoplastic via the accumulation of mutations. A critical step in this process of mutagenesis is the loss of suppressor gene function. This occurs by a variety of defects, including deletions, translocations, amplifications, loss of heterozygosity, point mutations, microsatellite changes, and telomeric associations. The degree to which the daughter cells dedifferentiate into a malignant phenotype is a function of the amount of genomic instability that arises with each subsequent mitosis. Mutation begets mutation as the checkpoints and regulatory machinery continually fail to repair the genetic code.

Factors that influence these mechanisms include both inheritable genetic conditions (eg, Li-Fraumeni syndrome, retinoblastoma) or environmental factors. It is well established that oncogenic viruses, radiation, and chemical carcinogens can affect these processes, ultimately compromising genomic stability.

The neoplastic process may arrest in the "benign" state, with further genomic instability curtailed, or it can almost progress to a sarcomatous state. For example, if the cell type of origin is a lipocyte then a lipoma or liposarcoma may develop. Furthermore, a liposarcoma can progress in its dedifferentiation such that its phenotype, as a high-grade lesion, minimally reflects its lipocytic origin. It is important to point out that this does not imply that all benign lesions are necessarily at risk for malignant degeneration. It is not a surgical indication to remove a lipoma because of concern over developing a liposarcoma.

Although a plethora of molecular markers are being studied, understanding the details of genomic instability and subsequent tumor formation is lacking. The initiation of the neoplastic process and subsequent disease progression is a complex, multistep process in gene expression and deregulation. There is no single pathway by which all neoplasms arise but instead multiple genetic targets are altered in a variety of sequences with the common result of cellular proliferation that is tumorigenesis.

■ EVALUATION & STAGING OF TUMORS

History & Physical Examination

When evaluating a new patient with a possible tumor, the workup must commence with a careful and thorough history and physical. Prior to ordering any diagnostic studies, particular questions must be answered and the physical characteristics of the mass in question must be assessed. This will prevent the ordering of unnecessary tests and better enable the physician to determine which tests will be most helpful in diagnosing the condition as well as facilitating therapeutic interventions if needed.

The clinical history is of paramount importance (Table 6–1). The age of the patient will permit the gen-

Table 6–1. Questions that must be asked in the workup of a possible tumor.

1. **The patient's age.** Certain tumors are relatively specific to particular age groups.
2. **Duration of complaint.** Benign lesions generally have been present for an extended period (years). Malignant tumors usually have been noticed for only weeks to months.
3. **Rate of growth.** A rapidly growing mass, as in weeks to months is more likely to be malignant. Growth may be difficult to assess by the patient if it is deep-seated, as can be the case with bone. Deep lesions may be much larger than the patient thought ("tip-of-the-iceberg" phenomenon).
4. **Pain associated with the mass.** Benign processes are usually asymptomatic. Osteochondromas (see text) may cause secondary symptoms because of encroachment on surrounding structures. Malignant lesions may cause pain.
5. **History of trauma.** With a history of penetrating trauma, one must rule out osteomyelitis. With a history of blunt trauma, healing fracture must be entertained.
6. **Personal or family history of cancer.** Adults with a history of prostate, renal, lung, breast, or thyroid tumors are at risk for developing metastatic bone disease. Children with neuroblastoma are prone to bony metastases. Patients with retinoblastoma are at an increased risk for osteosarcoma. Secondary osteosarcomas and other malignancies can result from treatment of other childhood cancers. Family history of conditions such as Li-Fraumeni syndrome must raise suspicion of any bone lesion. Furthermore, certain benign bone tumors can run in families (eg, multiple hereditary exostoses; see text).
7. **Systemic signs or symptoms.** Generally there should be no significant findings on the review of systems with benign tumors. Fevers, chills, night sweats, malaise, change in appetite, weight loss, etc should alert the physician that an infectious or neoplastic process may be involved.

eration of a list of potential diagnoses (Table 6–2) that when combined with the history and a few additional studies should permit establishing a diagnosis. The duration of symptoms, rate of growth, the presence of pain, and a history of trauma can help to elucidate the diagnosis. A careful past medical history, family history, and review of systems must not be overlooked either.

A thorough physical exam is also critical (Table 6–3). The clinician must assess the location and size of the mass, the quality of the overlying skin, the presence of warmth, any associated swelling, the presence of tenderness, and the firmness of the lesion. Range of motion of all joints in proximity to the tumor, above and below, must be recorded as well as a complete neurovascular exam. An assessment of the related lymph node chains as well as an examination for an enlarged liver or spleen should be performed.

The clinician must also consider pseudotumors in addition to true neoplastic conditions. A history of trauma suggests a possible stress fracture or myositis ossificans as a diagnosis. The history of stress-related physical activity and the exact timing of symptom presentation and variations of symptoms with the passage of time are important considerations in establishing a differential diagnosis.

Imaging Studies

A. RADIOGRAPHY

Initial evaluation should begin with plain radiography. In every patient with a suspected tumor, orthogonal anteroposterior and lateral views of the affected area should be taken. This includes soft-tissue masses as well. In many cases, radiographic examination will be diagnostic, and no further imaging studies will be indicated. However, in the case of a more aggressive process the diagnosis may be able to be determined on the plain radiographs but further evaluation with advanced studies is usually indicated to determine the extent of local soft-tissue involvement as well as to assess the extent of disseminated disease (staging).

The initial radiographic images must be scrutinized. For bone lesions, the location within the bone (eg, epiphyseal, metaphyseal, or diaphyseal) must be considered and will facilitate the diagnosis. Epiphyseal tumors are usually benign. The more malignant primary sarcomas, such as osteosarcoma, are typically seen in a metaphyseal location; however, round cell tumors, such as Ewing's sarcoma, multiple myeloma, and lymphomas, are usually medullary diaphyseal lesions. A tumor arising from the surface of a long bone may be a benign lesion, such as an osteochondroma, or may be a low-grade sarcoma, such as a parosteal osteosarcoma.

Terms such as "geographic," "well circumscribed," "permeative," and "moth-eaten" are used to describe the appearance of radiographic abnormalities. Geographic or well circumscribed implies that the lesion has a distinct boundary and is sharply marginated, suggesting a benign tumor (Figure 6–1). A poorly defined, infiltrative process is described as permeative or moth-eaten and reflects a more aggressive process such as a malignancy (Figure 6–2) although aggressive but benign processes can have this radiographic quality as well (Figure 6–3). An exception to this rule is multiple myeloma, which frequently demonstrates a punched-out, well demarcated appearance but in multiple locations.

With a careful history, physical, and appropriate radiographs, the physician can reach a working diagnosis of the lesion. Although benign and malignant tumors can mimic each other, some tumors can be ruled out on the basis of the history, the age of the patient, the location of the tumor (in which bone and where in the bone), and the radiographic appearance of the tumor, as shown in Tables 6–1 through 6–6. For example, a 20-year-old man with a 3-month history of pain in the knee is found to have an epiphyseal lesion in the distal femur. The lesion has a benign, geographic appearance. If the tumor is benign, the criteria of the patient's age (see Table 6–2) eliminates only solitary bone cyst and osteofibrous dysplasia, but all other benign tumors remain possibilities. If the tumor is malignant, it is likely to be an osteosarcoma (various types), Ewing's sarcoma, fibrosarcoma, vascular sarcoma, or, possibly, chondrosarcoma, according to the age criterion. The most common site for bone tumors is about the knee, especially the distal femur. The likely benign tumors are giant cell tumor, nonossifying fibroma, chondroma, osteochondroma, and chondroblastoma. The likely malignant tumors in this age group are osteosarcoma, Ewing's sarcoma, fibrosarcoma and, possibly, chondrosarcoma. Most malignant tumors are metaphyseal. Based on location in the bone (Table 6–4), the most likely benign tumors are chondroblastoma and giant cell tumor. Most malignant tumors are metaphyseal. The geographic appearance implies a benign radiographic appearance. Thus, the working diagnosis would be chondroblastoma or, possibly, giant cell tumor if the lesion were benign, whereas it would be osteosarcoma or chondrosarcoma if the lesion were malignant, which is less likely. In this age group, metastatic disease is very unlikely, but low-grade infection may mimic a tumor, particularly if the patient is immunocompromised, as can be determined from the patient's history. Table 6–5 indicates the most useful studies for further workup.

B. ISOTOPE BONE SCANNING

Technetium (Tc)-99 radioisotope scans are used to assess the degree of osteoblastic activity of a given lesion

Table 6–2. Distribution of bone tumors by age (years).

Type of Tumor	0	10	20	30	40	50	60	70	80
Benign bone tumors									
Osteoid osteoma									
Osteoblastoma									
Osteofibrous dysplasia									
Enchodroma									
Periosteal chondroma									
Osteochondroma									
Chondroblastoma									
Chondromyxoid fibroma									
Fibrous cortical defect									
Nonossifying fibroma									
Fibrous dysplasia									
Solitary bone cyst									
Aneurysmal bone cyst									
Epidermoid cyst									
Giant cell tumor									
Hemangioma									
Malignant bone tumors									
Classic osteosarcoma									
Hemorrhagic osteosarcoma									
Parosteal osteosarcoma									
Periosteal osteosarcoma									
Secondary osetosarcoma									
Low-grade intramedullary osteosarcoma									
Irradiation-induced osteosarcoma									
Multicentric osteosarcoma									
Primary chondrosarcoma									
Secondary chondrosarcoma									
Clear cell chondrosarcoma									
Dedifferentiated chondosarcoma									
Mesenchymal chondosarcoma									
Ewing's sarcoma									
Lymphoma									
Multiple myeloma									
Solitary plasmacytoma									
Fibrosarcoma									
Malignant fibrous histiocytoma									
Adamantinoma									
Vascular sarcoma									
Chordoma									
Metastatic carcinoma									

Table 6–3. Aspects of physical exam that should be documented when evaluating a patient with a mass.[a]

1. **Skin color**
2. **Warmth**
3. **Location**
4. **Swelling.** Swelling, in addition to the primary mass effect, may reflect a more aggressive process.
5. **Neurovascular exam.** Changes may reflect a more aggressive process.
6. **Joint range of motion** of all joints in proximity to the region in question, above and below.
7. **Size.** A mass greater than 5 cm should raise the suspicion of malignancy.
8. **Tenderness.** Tenderness may reflect a more rapidly growing process.
9. **Firmness.** Malignant tumors tend to be firmer on examination than benign processes. This applies more to soft-tissue tumors than osseous ones.
10. **Lymph nodes.** Certain sarcomas (eg, rhabdomyosarcoma, synovial sarcoma, epithelioid, and clear cell sarcomas all have increased rates of lymph node involvement).

[a]*Note:* These findings assume the absence of trauma.

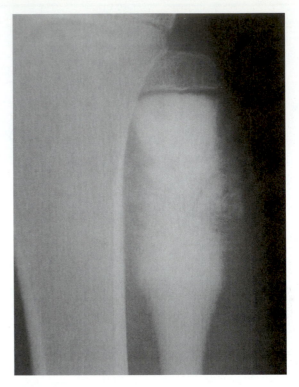

Figure 6–2. Radiograph of a proximal fibular osteosarcoma demonstrating the destructive, permeative nature of malignant bone tumors.

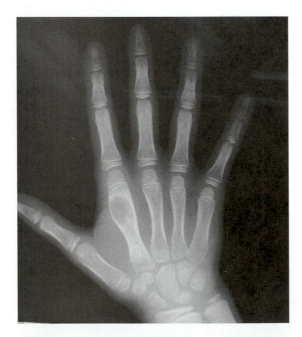

Figure 6–1. Radiograph of an enchondroma of the second metacarpal. Notice its geographic appearance.

of bone (Figure 6–4). In general they are quite sensitive, with a few exceptions, for active lesions of bone. Accordingly, technetium-99 scans are excellent screening tools for remote lesions (staging). The best indication for a bone scan is suspected multiple bony lesions, such as those commonly seen in metastatic carcinomas and lymphomas of bone. Isotope bone scanning is far simpler to perform, is less expensive, and requires less total body irradiation than skeletal surveys. It is common practice to use serial isotope scans to follow patients with suspected metastatic disease and at the same time evaluate the effectiveness of their systemic therapy program.

Isotope scanning is also used in the staging process of a primary sarcoma such as an osteosarcoma to make sure that the patient does not have an asymptomatic remote skeletal lesion. Technetium-99 scans are also useful in distinguishing blastic lesions of bone. Given that the study reflects metabolic activity, an enostosis (bone island) would not demonstrate significant increased activity compared with a blastic prostate metastasis. Inflammatory disease and trauma will also show increased activity. It is important to note, however, that multiple

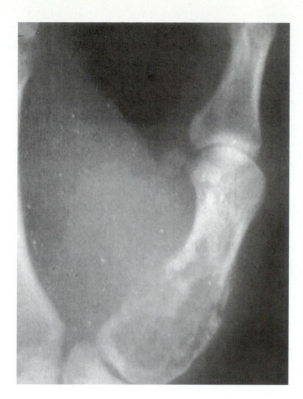

Figure 6–3. Radiograph of a giant cell tumor of the thumb. This is a typical moth-eaten appearance.

myeloma and metastatic squamous cell carcinoma may not demonstrate technetium uptake (ie, false-negative). Skeletal surveys are preferable for screening for additional sites of involvement in such cases.

C. COMPUTED TOMOGRAPHY AND MAGNETIC RESONANCE IMAGING

Computed tomography (CT) remains a standard imaging procedure for use in well-selected clinical situations. Perhaps the best indication for CT is for smaller lesions that involve cortical structures of bone or spine (Figure 6–5). In such cases, CT is superior to magnetic resonance imaging (MRI) because the resolution of cortical bone using MRI is inferior. CT scan of the lung is the modality of choice for evaluating the patient with a sarcoma for possible lung metastases. Abdominal CT scan is invaluable in surveying for a primary tumor in patients who present with a bone metastases. For tumors involving the pelvis and sacrum, CT can help to elucidate the extent of bone involvement (Figure 6–6). In cases involving a soft-tissue lesion, MRI is far superior to CT unless there is a heavily calcified process.

MRI has its greatest application in the evaluation of noncalcific soft-tissue lesions. The two most com-

monly used MRI variations are the T_1-weighted and T_2-weighted spin-echo imaging techniques (Figure 6–7). Unlike CT scanning, MRI allows for excellent imaging in the longitudinal planes as well as the axial plane. MRI can also demonstrate the normal anatomy of soft structures, including nerves and vessels, thereby nearly eliminating the need for arteriography and myelograms.

Laboratory Studies

A. BIOPSY

The biopsy should usually be the final staging procedure. Although the biopsy can distort the imaging studies, such as MRI, pathologic evaluation and interpretation may require information provided by the prior workup. Complications relating to the biopsy are not infrequent. Accordingly, careful preoperative planning is imperative. The imaging studies will aid the surgeon in selecting the best site for a tissue diagnosis. In most cases, the best diagnostic tissue will be found at the periphery of the tumor, where it interfaces with normal tissue. For example, in the case of a malignant bone tumor, soft-tissue invasion is usually evident outside the bone, and this area can be sampled without violating cortical bone and thus without causing a fracture at the biopsy site. If a medullary specimen is needed, a small round or oval hole should be cut to decrease the chance of fracture. If the medullary specimen is malignant, the cortical hole should be plugged with bone wax or bone cement to reduce soft-tissue contamination following the procedure.

Obtaining an adequate specimen is critical. A frozen section determines if appropriate tissue has been obtained. A few experienced tumor centers may make a definitive diagnosis based on a frozen section, allowing the surgeon to proceed with definitive operative treatment of the tumor. However, freezing artifact can cause overinterpretation of the material, so an aggressive resection should always be deferred until the permanent analysis is complete. Additional studies beyond conventional light microscopy, such as immunocytochemistries and cytogenetics, may also be necessary.

The placement of the biopsy site is a major consideration. If the surgeon is inexperienced and not familiar with surgical oncologic principles, a serious contamination of a vital structure such as the popliteal artery or sciatic nerve may occur. Such an error might necessitate an amputation instead of a limb-sparing procedure. To avoid this problem in the case of a suspected malignant condition, the surgeon who performs the biopsy should be the same surgeon who will perform the definitive operative procedure.

Table 6–4. Skeletal distribution of bone tumors, ranked from most common (1) to less common (5) sites.

Type of Tumor	Femur	Tibia	Foot or Ankle	Humerus	Radius	Ulna	Hand or Wrist	Scapula	Clavicle	Rib	Vertebra	Sacrum	Pelvis	Skull	Face
Benign bone tumors															
Osteoid osteoma	1	2		4			5				3				
Osteoblastoma	3	4		5							1				2
Osteofibrous dysplasia		1													
Chondroma	2		4	3		5	1								
Osteochondroma	1	3		2				5					4		
Chondroblastoma	1	3		2				5					4		
Chondromyxoid fibroma	3	1	2		5								4		
Fibrous cortical defect	2	1		3	4				5						
Nonossifying fibroma	2	1		3	4				5						
Solitary bone cyst	2	3		1		5							4		
Aneurysmal bone cyst	1	2		4							3		5		
Giant cell tumor	1	2		5	3							4			
Hemangioma	3	4		5							2			1	
Malignant bone tumors															
Classic osteosarcoma	1	2		3									4		
Hemorrhagic osteosarcoma	1	2		3							5		4		

Malignant bone tumors

Parosteal osteosarcoma	1	2		3	4		
Periosteal osteosarcoma	1	2	5	3	4		
Secondary osteosarcmoa	2	5		3		1	4
Low-grade intramedullary osteosarcoma	1	2					
Irradiation-induced osteosarcoma	1			2	3	5	4
Primary chondrosarcoma	1			4	3	5	2
Secondary chondrosarcoma	2			3	4	5	1
Dedifferentiated chondrosarcoma	1			3	4	5	2
Mesenchymal chondrosarcoma	5						
Ewing's sarcoma	1			3	5	3	2	1	4
Lymphoma	1			4	5	3	2
Myeloma	4			5	2	1	3
Fibrosarcoma	1	2		4		3	5
Malignant fibrous histiocytoma	1	3		5			
Adamantinoma	3	1		4	2		
Vascular sarcoma		4		3	5	1	2	4
Chordoma						3	1	2
Metastatic carcinoma	2			5	4	1	3

293

Table 6–5. Bone tumors: Imaging characteristics, location in a long bone, and beneficial studies, ranked from most common or most beneficial (1) to less common or less beneficial (3).

Type of Tumor	Imaging Characteristics			Location in a Long Bone					Beneficial Studies				
	Geo-graphic	Moth-Eaten	Permeative	Epiphyseal	Meta-physeal	Metadi-aphyseal	Diaphyseal	Surface	Plain Radiograph	CT Scan	MRI	Isotope Bone Scan	Blood Studies
Benign bone tumors													
Osteoid osteoma	1				1	2	3		1	2		3	
Osteoblastoma	2	1			2	1	3		1	2		3	
Osteofibrous dysplasia		1				2	1		1	2		3	
Chondroma	1				3	1	2		1	2		3	
Osteochondroma	1				2			1	1	2			
Chondroblastoma	1	2		1	2				1	2			
Chondromyxoid fibroma	1	2			1	2			1	2		3	
Fibrous cortical defect	1				1	2			1				
Nonossifying fibroma	1	2			1	2			1	2			
Solitary bone cyst	1				1	2	3		1				
Aneurysmal bone cyst	3	2	1		1	2		3	1	2	3		
Giant cell tumor	3	1	2	1	2				1	2			3
Hemangioma	2	1			3	1	2		1				
Malignant bone tumors													
Classic osteosarcoma	3	1	2		1	2	3		1	2	2	3	
Hemorrhagic osteosarcoma		1	2		1	2			1		2		3
Parosteal osteosarcoma	2	1			2	3		1	2	1			

Periosteal osteosarcoma	2	1			3	2		1	2	1	2	1	
Secondary osteosarcoma	1	1	2		1	2	3		2	1	2	1	3
Low-grade intramedullary osteosarcoma	1				1	2			1	2		2	3
Irradiation-induced osteosarcoma	1	1	2		1	2	3		1	1	1	1	3
Primary chondrosarcoma	2	1	1	3	1	2			2	1	2	1	3
Secondary chondrosarcoma	2	1	1		2	3		1	2	1	2	1	
Dedifferentiated chondrosarcoma	1	1	2		1	2	3		2	3	2	3	1
Mesenchymal chondrosarcoma	1	1	2		1	2			2	3	3	3	1
Ewing's sarcoma	2	2	1		1	2	3		2	3	2	1	3
Lymphoma	2	2	1		3	1	2		3	1	3	1	2
Myeloma	2	2	2		1	3	2		1	3	1	3	3
Fibrosarcoma	1	1	2		1	2	3		2	1	2	1	1
Malignant fibrous histiocytoma	1	1	2		1	2	3		2	2	2	1	1
Adamantinoma	2	1	1		3	2	1		1	2	2	3	3
Vascular sarcoma	2	1	3		1	2	3		1	1	1	2	3
Chordoma	2	1	1		1	1	2		3	2	3	2	1
Metastatic carcinoma	3	1	2		1	2	3		2	3	2	3	1

Table 6–6. Distribution of soft tissue tumors by age (years).

Type of Tumor	0	10	20	30	40	50	60	70	80
Benign soft tissue tumors									
Desmoid tumor		█							
Intramuscular lipoma			█	█	█	█	█		
Spindle cell lipoma					█	█	█		
Angiolipoma			█	█					
Diffuse lipomatosis	█	█	█						
Benign lipoblastoma	█	█		█					
Hibernoma			█	█					
Capillary hemangioma	█								
Cavernous hemangioma		█	█	█					
Arteriovenous hemangioma		█	█	█					
Epithelioid hemangioma			█	█					
Pyogenic granuloma		█	█	█	█	█	█		
Lymphangioma		█	█	█					
Glomus tumor			█	█					
Benign hemangiopericytoma			█	█					
Neurilemoma			█	█	█	█			
Solitary neurofibroma			█	█					
Neurofibromatosis		█	█	█	█				
Intramuscular myxoma					█	█	█	█	
Malignant soft tissue tumors									
Pleomorphic MFH						█	█	█	
Myxoid MFH						█	█	█	
Giant Cell MFH						█	█		
Angiomatoid MFH			█	█	█				
Dermatofibrosarcoma protuberans				█	█				
Fibrosarcoma				█	█	█			
Leiomyosarcoma				█	█	█	█		
Well-differentiated liposarcoma					█	█			
Myxoid liposarcoma				█	█	█			
Round cell and pleomorphic liposarcoma					█	█	█		
Embryonal rhabdomyosarcoma	█	█							
Alveolar rhabdomyosarcoma		█	█						
Pleomorphic rhabdomyosarcoma				█	█	█	█	█	
Synovial sarcoma		█	█	█					
Solitary malignant schwannoma									
Multiple malignant schwannoma									
Angiosarcoma									
Alveolar soft part sarcoma		█	█	█					
Epithelioid sarcoma			█	█					
Clear cell sarcoma			█	█					

MFH = Malignant fibrous histiocytoma.

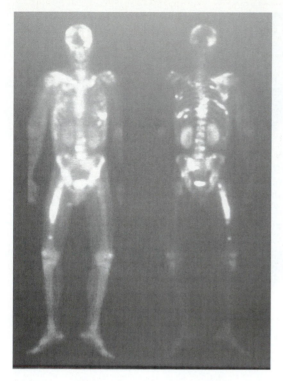

Figure 6–4. Technetium-99 scan demonstrating extensive osteoblastic activity in a patient with metastatic adenocarcinoma.

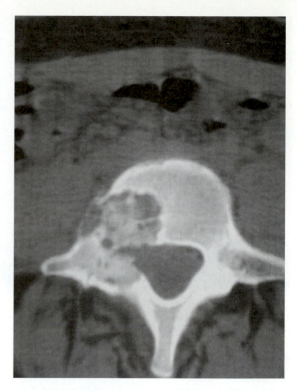

Figure 6–5. CT scan of an osteoblastoma arising from the right pedicle of a lumbar vertebral body.

Transverse incisions should be avoided because removing the entire biopsy site with the widely resected subjacent tumor mass is difficult. Adequate hemostasis is mandatory to avoid formation of a contaminating hematoma. A drain may be helpful, but frequently unnecessary. If a drain is used it must be placed in line with the incision.

Needle biopsies, either core or fine needle, can be used by experienced tumor centers, especially for lesions that are easily diagnosed, such as metastatic carcinomas or round cell tumors. Because the subtype of sarcoma is proving to be very important, architecture of the tumor is generally needed. This requires a core biopsy rather than a fine-needle aspirate. Core biopsies also allow the surgeon to sample various areas of the tumor to avoid sampling error in a heterogeneous tumor. In the case of a deep pelvic lesion or a spinal lesion, a CT-guided needle biopsy is ideal because it avoids excessive multicompartmental contamination.

In general excisional biopsies are discouraged unless the lesion is particularly small (< 2–3 cm) or in an area where a cuff of healthy, uninvolved tissue of at least 1

cm can be removed as well. This would hopefully avoid a second procedure to remove the entire biopsy site if the lesion turns out to be malignant.

B. CULTURES AND SPECIAL STUDIES

The damage of biopsy specimens after retrieval can make it impossible to perform special studies such as immunohistochemistry, cytogenetics, flow cytometry, and electron microscopy. For this reason, the biopsy surgeon should consult with the pathologist before specimens are retrieved and handled. Furthermore, many current studies require fresh tissue (no formalin). It is also a good habit to obtain cultures for bacterial culture (anaerobic and aerobic) as well as fungal and acid-fast bacteria if clinical suspicion warrants.

Molecular diagnostics is on the verge of revolutionizing sarcoma diagnostics. Specific translocations have been found in a variety of tumors (Table 6–7). Furthermore, therapeutics are beginning to be designed against specific molecular defects in malignancies. Gastrointestinal stromal tumor (GIST) a malignant mesenchymal tumor arising from the GI tract, omentum, and

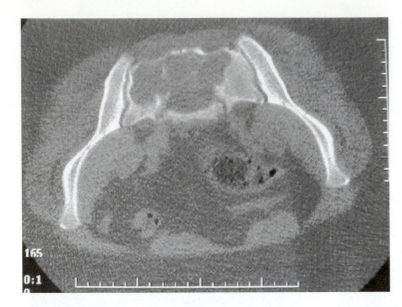

Figure 6–6. Pelvic CT demonstrating the bony destruction of the sacrum caused by a giant cell tumor.

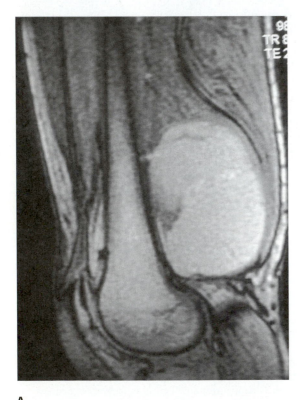

A

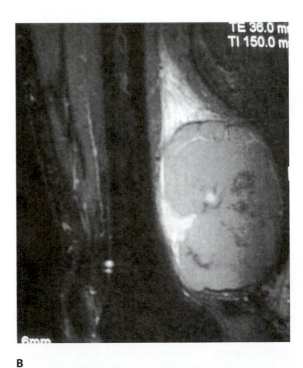

B

Figure 6–7. Synovial sarcoma involving the popliteal fossa. (**A**) T_1-weighted. (**B**) T_2-weighted.

Table 6–7. Common translocations seen in sarcomas.

Ewing's/primitive neuroectodermal tumor: t(11;22) (q24; q12), (t21; 22) (q22; q12), (t7; 22) (p22; q12)

Myxoid chondrosarcoma: t(9; 22) (q22; q12)

Myxoid & round cell liposarcoma: t12; 16) (q12; p11)

Synovial sarcoma: t(X; 18) (p11; q11)

Alveolar rhabdomyosarcoma: t2; 13) (q35; q14), t(1; 13) (p36; q14)

Alveolar soft parts sarcoma: t(X; 17) (p11.2; q25)

Desmoplastic small round cell tumor: t(11; 22) (p13; q12)

Congenital fibrosarcoma: t(12; 15)

---

mesentery has been shown to overexpress a mutant form of c-*kit*. The *KIT* gene encodes a tyrosine kinase receptor for the growth factor named stem cell factor or mast cell growth factor. Therapy directed against c-*kit* is having an early and remarkable effect on the previously difficult to treat malignancy. Similar pathways are being elicited in other sarcomas.

Staging Systems

After the appropriate studies have been completed, staging begins. Staging refers to an assessment of the grade of the tumor and the extent to which the disease has spread. There are several staging systems, but all have the purpose of helping the physician plan a logical treatment program and establish a prognosis for the patient. The two major systems are discussed here.

A. SYSTEM OF THE AMERICAN JOINT COMMISSION OF CANCER

The American Joint Commission of Cancer (AJCC) system is used by most surgical oncologists when dealing with soft-tissue sarcomas. It has a four-point scale for classifying tumors as grade 1, 2, 3, or 4 on the basis of their histologic appearance. A grade 1 or grade 2 tumor in the AJCC system is equivalent to a stage I tumor in the Enneking system. A grade 3 or 4 is equivalent to an Enneking stage II.

B. SYSTEM OF THE AMERICAN MUSCULOSKELETAL TUMOR SOCIETY (ENNEKING SYSTEM)

The Enneking system, which addresses the unique problems related to sarcomas of the extremities and applies to tumors of the bone as well as those of soft tissue, is generally preferred by orthopedic oncologists. The Enneking system has a three-point scale for classifying tumors as stage I, II, or III on the basis of their histologic and biologic appearance and their likelihood of metastasizing to regional lymph nodes or distant sites

such as the lung. Stage I refers to low-grade sarcomas with less than 25% chance of metastasis. Stage II refers to high-grade sarcomas with more than 25% chance of metastasis. Stage III is for either low-grade or high-grade tumors that have metastasized to a distant site, such as a lymph node, lung, or other distant organ system.

The Enneking system further classifies tumors on the basis of whether they are intracompartmental (type A) or extracompartmental (type B) in nature. Type A tumors are constrained by anatomic boundaries such as muscle fascial planes and stand a better chance for local control of tumor growth with surgical removal than type B tumors do. A lesion contained in a single muscle belly or a bone lesion that has not broken out into the surrounding soft tissue would be classified as a type A tumor. A lesion in the popliteal space, axilla, pelvis, or midportion of the hand or foot would be classified as a type B tumor. Although compartmentalization of a tumor is an important concept, studies have shown that the size of the tumor rather than whether it is contained within a compartment is more prognostic. Larger tumors, greater than 5 cm, do less well.

A low-grade fibrosarcoma located inside the fascial plane of the biceps muscle and having no evidence of metastasis would be classified as a stage I-A tumor. A typical malignant osteosarcoma of the distal femur with breakthrough into the surrounding muscle as determined by MRI would be classified as a stage II-B lesion. If CT scanning revealed metastatic involvement of the lung, the osteosarcoma would then be classified as a stage III-B lesion.

Enneking WF: A system of staging musculoskeletal neoplasms. Clin Orthop 1985;204:9.

Mankin HJ et al: The hazards of the biopsy, revisited. J Bone Joint Surg Am 1996;78:656. [PMID 8642021]

Miettinen M et al: Gastrointestinal stromal tumors—Definition, clinical, histological, immunohistochemical, and molecular genetic features and differential diagnosis. Virchows Arch 2001;438(1):1. [PMID: 11688571]

Moley JF et al: Soft-tissue sarcomas. Surg Clin North Am 2000; 80(2):687. [PMID: 10836012]

Oliveira AM et al: Grading in soft tissue tumors: Principles and problems. Skeletal Radiol 2001;30(10):543. [PMID: 11685477]

Simon MA et al: Diagnostic strategy for bone & soft tissue tumors. J Bone Joint Surg Am 1993;75:622. [PMID: 8478392]

Skrzynski MC et al: Diagnostic accuracy and charge savings of outpatient care needle biopsy compared with open biopsy of musculoskeletal tumors. J Bone Joint Surg Am 1996;78:644. [PMID: 8642019]

Zahm SH et al: The epidemiology of soft tissue sarcoma. Semin Oncol 1997;24(5):504. [PMID: 9344316]

■ DIAGNOSIS & TREATMENT OF TUMORS

BENIGN BONE TUMORS

Benign bone tumors have certain characteristics that favor their diagnosis over malignant conditions. If the condition is benign, the patient is frequently asymptomatic and the radiograph usually shows a well-defined geographic lesion with sclerotic reactive margins that suggest a long-standing process associated with slow growth potential. In contrast, if the condition is malignant, the patient usually complains of pain and the radiograph commonly shows a more permeative lesion with lytic destruction and poorly defined margins that suggest rapid progression. In many cases, further studies such as MRI or bone isotope studies are not necessary for a typical benign tumor, such as fibrous dysplasia, enchondroma, or nonossifying fibroma. A system of staging exists for benign bone tumors. Stage 1 lesions are considered latent. They generally are asymptomatic but not always. Although they can progress, they usually resolve. Initially, these lesions should be observed. Stage 2 lesions are considered active. They tend not to resolve spontaneously and are less well demarcated than stage 1 lesions. Frequently they require surgical intervention with aggressive treatment. Recurrence is not infrequent. Stage 3, or aggressive lesions, demonstrate extensive destruction. Treatment often requires wide, en bloc resection.

The more common types of benign bone tumor seen by the practicing orthopedic surgeon are discussed in this section.

Benign Osteoid-Forming Tumors

A. Osteoid Osteoma

The most common benign osteoid-forming tumor is the osteoid osteoma, accounting for 10% of all benign bone tumors. It is more common in males than in females, with a peak incidence in the second decade of life. The proximal femur is the most common site. Dull aching pain is the most frequent symptom. Symptoms are relieved with nonsteroidal anti-inflammatory drugs secondary to a high concentration of prostaglandins in the nidus. Osteoid osteoma may have a unique pathogenic nerve supply as well, a unique finding among bone tumors.

The characteristic radiographic feature of the osteoid osteoma is the central lytic nidus that measures up to 1 cm in diameter. In the common cortical lesion (Figure 6–8), an extensive reactive sclerosis is evident, creating a fusiform bulge on the bone surface. However, if the nidus is more centrally located in metaphyseal bone, less sclerosis is seen and the radiographic appearance is less diagnostic. If the nidus is close to a joint or actually in the joint, as in the case of a femoral neck lesion, inflammatory synovitis will result and suggest the diagnosis of a pyarthrosis or rheumatoid disease. Technetium bone scans are invariably positive. A CT scan is helpful to better anatomically locate the lesion in preoperative planning.

In the spine, the typical location for an osteoid osteoma is in the posterior elements, such as the lamina or pedicle. The lumbar spine is most commonly involved, whereas the dorsal spine is the second most commonly involved. A secondary scoliosis may develop, with the convexity toward the lesion. Furthermore, if the nidus is in proximity to a nerve root, root irritation can develop. In the lumbar spine this can present as sciatica and suggest the diagnosis of a herniated disk.

Previously, some investigators believed that the osteoid osteoma was an inflammatory process such as a Brodie's abscess, which has a similar clinical and radiographic appearance. Currently, it is accepted that osteoid osteoma is a true osteoid-forming neoplasm and is absent of lymphocytes or plasma cells. Histologically, the nidus will show aggressive but benign woven bone formation, with large numbers of osteoblasts and osteoclasts in a vascular fibrous stroma. No chondroid areas will be seen.

Most cases of osteoid osteoma are stage 1 lesions and can be treated symptomatically with aspirin or nonsteroidal anti-inflammatory agents. If the patient fails such treatment, surgical intervention is warranted. If surgery is undertaken, it is important to eradicate the entire symptomatic nidus. Removal of a large amount of the surrounding sclerotic bone should be avoided because it can severely weaken the bone and may result in a pathologic fracture. If the lesion is in cortical bone, adequate exposure is required so the surgeon can visualize the bulging cortex. Intralesional resection via the "burr-down" technique is generally preferred over en bloc resection. The nidus can be identified visually by the hyperemic pink color in the reactive bone adjacent to it. Simple curettage of the nidus followed by high-speed burring to advance the margin another 2–3 mm is all that is necessary. If the lesion is not visible on the surface, as in the case of a medullary lesion, then radiographic markers should be placed intraoperatively prior to placing the round cortical window. Alternatively, percutaneous radiofrequency ablation is another, less invasive method of treating osteoid osteoma. This method may prove to be the modality of choice in the future.

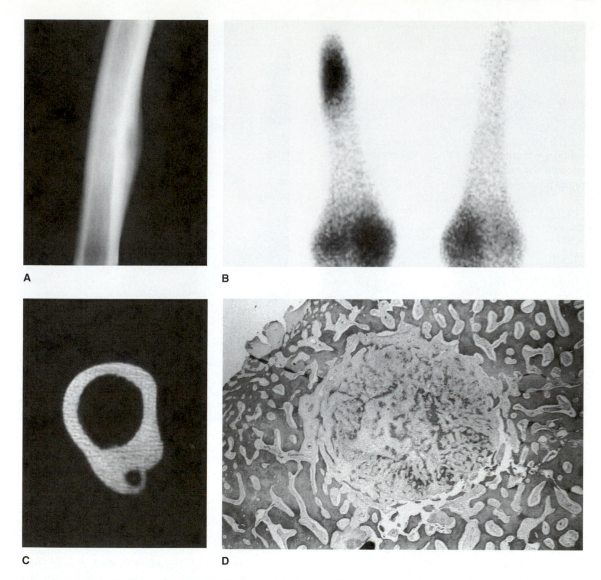

Figure 6–8. Radiograph (**A**), isotope bone scan (**B**), CT scan (**C**), and photomicrograph (**D**) of an osteoid osteoma in the femur of a 19-year-old man.

B. OSTEOBLASTOMA

Osteoblastoma is a large osteoid osteoma that demonstrates a propensity for the posterior elements of the spine. They are found more commonly in males than in females and occur in the same age group as osteoid osteomas. Osteoblastomas are less common than osteoid osteomas, accounting for 1% of all bone tumors. A few will be found in the metaphyses of long bone (raising suspicion about a possible osteosarcoma), and a few will be seen in the ankle and wrist areas. These lesions are usually stage 1–2 lesions.

Radiographically, the osteoblastoma has a more lytic and destructive appearance than the osteoid osteoma. Its nidus, which is greater than 1–2 cm, has a less sclerotic reactive bone at the periphery and may take on the appearance of an aneurysmal bone cyst. Histologically, the nidus of the osteoblastoma is nearly identical to that of the osteoid osteoma and shows excessive osteoblastic activity and osteoid formation with numerous giant cells in a vascular fibrous stroma.

In the spine area, the effects of osteoblastoma are similar to those of osteoid osteoma, with pressure on

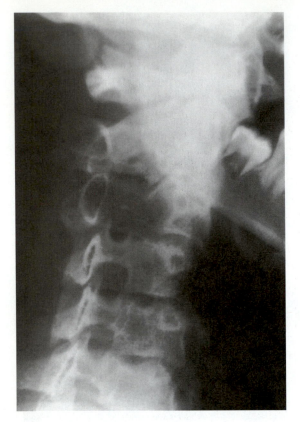

Figure 6–9. Radiograph of osteoblastoma in the pedicle area of the C3 vertebra of a 14-year-old boy.

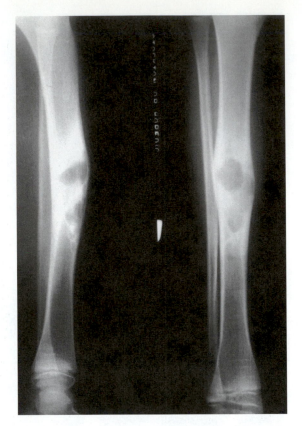

Figure 6–10. Radiograph of osteofibrous dysplasia in the tibia of an 8-year-old boy.

nerve roots causing pain down the leg or arm (Figure 6–9). In the thoracic area, a large lesion could result in cord compromise.

In patients with osteoblastomas, treatment usually consists of a vigorous curettement of the lesion, which may require a bone graft if instability results. Radiofrequency ablation may also prove useful in the management of this lesion.

C. OSTEOFIBROUS DYSPLASIA

Osteofibrous dysplasia is a rare condition that is seen almost exclusively in the tibia of children younger than 10 years, is more common in boys than in girls, and is usually asymptomatic. It commonly affects the diaphysis and results in anterior cortical bowing. Osteofibrous dysplasia can occur in the fibula and even more rarely can be seen bilaterally. It is most likely a hamartomatous process and tends to involute spontaneously with skeletal maturity.

In osteofibrous dysplasia (Figure 6–10), the lytic changes seen in the anterior tibial cortex are surrounded by sclerotic margins, thus creating a soap-bubbly appearance similar to the radiographic picture of both fibrous dysplasia and adamantinoma. Histologically, the lytic lesion shows a benign trabecular "alphabet-soup" pattern in a fibrous stroma. The histologic findings are similar to those in fibrous dysplasia, although the lesions of fibrous dysplasia lack the prominent surface layer of osteoblasts seen in osteofibrous dysplasia. These lesions are stage 1–2.

In a recent report of experience with 35 cases of osteofibrous dysplasia, investigators indicated that early attempts at surgical curettement and grafting of the lesions resulted in a high failure rate because of recurrence. For this reason, they suggested waiting until patients reach the age of 15 years and their disease arrests spontaneously before proceeding with a definitive debridement and bone grafting.

Benign Chondroid-Forming Tumors

A. ENCHONDROMA

Enchondroma refers to a centrally located chondroma of bone. These tumors are relatively common lesions, accounting for greater than 10% of benign bone tumors. In 50% of cases, the tumor is found in the small tubular bone of the hands and feet. It arises in growing bones as a hamartomatous process but is frequently asymptomatic and may avoid detection until the patient reaches adulthood, at which time the lesion may be discovered in association with a pathologic fracture or as an incidental finding on a routine radiographic examination.

Radiographs of enchondromas show geographic lysis with sharp margination and central calcification (Figure 6–11). In the case of an enchondroma of the hand, the cortex is frequently thinned out with slight dilatation. In contrast, with involvement of the large long bones, the lesion is centrally located with minimal evidence of cortical erosion or dilatation. Enchondromas are either stage 1 or 2 lesions.

Multiple enchondromatosis, or Ollier's disease (Figure 6–12), is a rare nonfamilial dysplasia that is typically seen on one-half of the body and appears similar to fibrous dysplasia. This condition can be quite extensive with significant involvement of metaphyseal areas resulting in bowing and shortening of the long bones. Such dramatic changes are rarely seen in cases of a solitary enchondroma. In patients with Maffucci's syndrome, enchondromatosis is seen in association with multiple soft-tissue hemangiomas.

A large solitary enchondroma in a large bone will convert to a low-grade chondrosarcoma in fewer than 5% of cases, and the conversion will take place during adulthood. A solitary enchondroma on the hand will rarely convert to a chondrosarcoma. A secondary chondrosarcoma is enchondromatosis can arise in up to 20% of cases and may be related to inactivation of particular tumor suppressor genes.

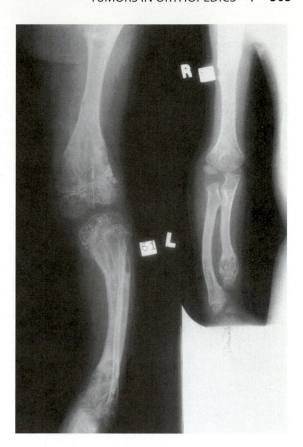

Figure 6–12. Radiograph of Ollier's disease of the upper and lower extremities.

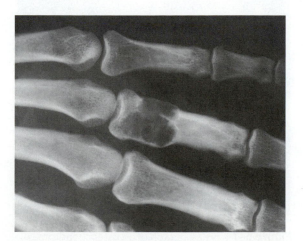

Figure 6–11. Radiograph of an enchondroma of the proximal phalanx of the ring finger.

There is no need to treat an asymptomatic patient with a solitary enchondroma of the hand or foot. If the patient has a pathologic fracture, it is best to allow the fracture to heal and then at a later date to perform a simple curettage and bone grafting procedure, which usually results in good function and a low chance of recurrence. Patients with Ollier's or Maffucci's disease must be followed carefully because of the increased risk of malignant degeneration.

B. PERIOSTEAL CHONDROMA

A benign chondroma seen on the surface of a bone is called a periosteal chondroma. Patients usually have more than one lesion, and the most common location is on the proximal humeral metaphysis. Radiographically, they often have a thin shell of bone and appear to lie on the cortical surface (Figure 6–13). These lesions are stage 1–2. Periosteal chondromas can grow to a sizable mass, but anything larger than 4 cm would suggest a peripheral primary chondrosarcoma.

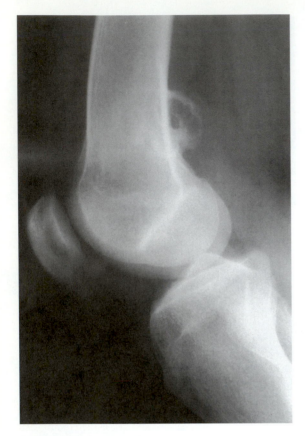

Figure 6–13. Radiograph of a periosteal chondroma of the distal femur.

Management of periosteal chondromas generally consists of observing the lesion at intervals to make sure that it does not continue growing as the patient reaches adulthood. In cases in which simple local resection without bone graft is indicated, the procedure is associated with a low recurrence rate.

C. OSTEOCHONDROMA

The nonossifying fibroma of bone is the most common benign tumor of bone, and the solitary osteochondroma is the second most common. Like the enchondroma, the osteochondroma is a developmental, or hamartomatous, process that arises from a defect in the outer edge of the growth plate on the metaphyseal side and that results in an exostosis that always points away from the joint of origin as the lesion moves away from the growth plate during the growing years.

The bony base of an osteochondroma is in direct communication with the medullary canal of the bone from which it arises. These lesions can be either pedunculated, as is commonly seen around the knee, or sessile, as is typically seen in the proximal humerus. There must be an associated cartilaginous cap on the bony base in order to make the diagnosis of osteochondroma (Figure 6–14). This cap will have the histologic features of a normal growth plate during the growing years. However, osteochondroma growth plate activity will subside at the same time as the activity in the larger plate from which the osteochondroma arose.

A familial form of osteochondroma, called multiple hereditary exostoses (MHE), is an autosomal-dominant disorder that is one tenth as common as solitary osteochondroma. Three genetic loci have been determined to be involved with MHE involving the EXT gene. This condition can vary from quite mild to extensive involvement with symmetric limb shortening. Forearm involvement can be quite deforming. The metaphyseal portions of long bones are deformed and widened (Figures 6–15 and 6–16). The histologic findings in multi-

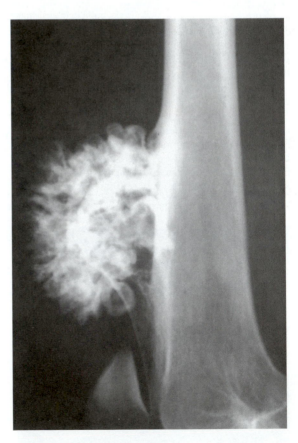

Figure 6–14. Radiograph of an osteochondroma of the distal femur.

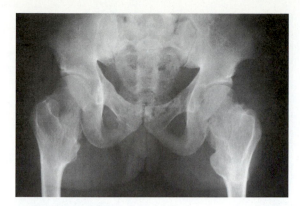

Figure 6–15. Radiograph of multiple exostoses of both hips.

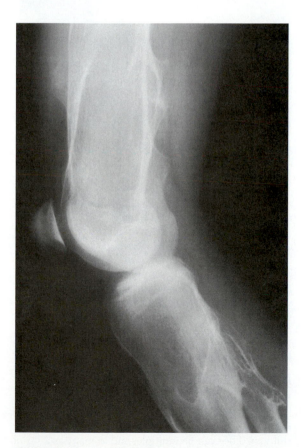

Figure 6–16. Radiograph of multiple exostoses in the knee.

ple exostoses are similar to those in solitary osteochondroma.

Conversion of solitary osteochondroma to chondrosarcoma occurs only during adulthood. The overall rate of conversion for all types of solitary lesions is quite rare. In MHE, there is approximately a 1% chance of malignant conversion to secondary chondrosarcoma in the cartilaginous cap, especially in the larger, more proximal lesions.

Osteochondromas are stage 1 lesions. Most children and adults with a solitary osteochondroma are asymptomatic and therefore do not require surgical treatment. In some cases the lesion may be palpable and irritating. Surgical removal is appropriate in these cases to address the symptoms only and not as a prophylaxis for chondrosarcomatous degeneration. In MHE symptomatic lesions are addressed surgically as needed. Corrective osteotomy is occasionally required because of angulatory deformity in the lower extremity. In adults with either a solitary osteochondroma or with multiple exostoses, if a previously quiescent lesion begins to enlarge, it should be removed. The surgical margin should be wide enough to include the entire cartilaginous cap as this is where malignant degeneration can occur.

D. CHONDROBLASTOMA

The term *chondroblastoma* suggests a benign cartilage-forming tumor, but in fact this epiphyseal lesion of childhood has a histologic appearance that is more typical of the benign metaphyseal-epiphyseal giant cell tumor of young adulthood. The chondroblastoma is about one fifth as common as the giant cell tumor. It differs from other bone tumors in that it is almost always associated with epiphyseal or apophyseal bone. The majority of cases arise in the second decade of life. Males are affected more often than females. The most common location is the outer portion of the proximal humeral epiphysis, but other common locations are the distal femoral and proximal tibial epiphyseal areas. Because of its proximity to a joint, chondroblastoma can present with a symptomatic joint effusion.

In cases of chondroblastoma, the radiograph demonstrates a lytic tumor with a sharp sclerotic margin and central stippled or flocculated calcification occurring in the chondroid portion of the tumor (Figure 6–17). As the growth plate closes, the tumor can expand gradually into the metaphyseal area and sometimes becomes quite aneurysmal, as in the case of a giant cell tumor. The chondroblastoma has the histologic appearance of a giant cell tumor, with numerous macrophages seen usually in areas of hemorrhage. The stromal cells of the chondroblastoma are polyhedral, like those of a giant cell tumor, but with associated halos that give the chondroblastoma a "chicken wire"

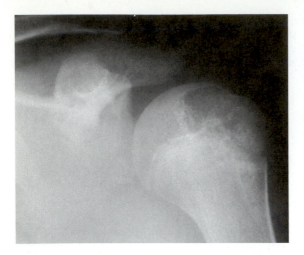

Figure 6–17. Radiograph of a chondroblastoma in the proximal humeral epiphysis of a 15-year-old boy.

appearance. Although chondroid metaplasia in the chondroblastoma is not easy to find, it must be present to firmly establish the diagnosis. Most chondroblastomas are stage 2 lesions but some can be stage 3.

The spontaneous conversion of chondroblastoma to a malignant tumor is extremely rare. However, as with the case of giant cell tumors, conversion to sarcoma can occur following radiation treatment. Even though the chondroblastoma is considered benign, it has been reported to metastasize to the lung on rare occasions. Nevertheless, it carries an excellent prognosis.

Treatment for chondroblastoma consists of aggressive intralesional resection with curettage; bone graft or bone cement (polymethyl methacrylate) may be used to reconstruct the defect. It has been our experience that this will suffice with local recurrence less than 10%. Some authors, however, recommend more aggressive marginal or wide resection.

E. CHONDROMYXOID FIBROMA

This very rare tumor generally affects males in the second or third decade of life. The most common location of the tumor is the proximal tibial metaphysis, followed by the distal femur and the first ray of the foot. The tumor is slow-growing and accompanied by mild pain symptoms.

Radiographs of chondromyxoid fibroma show a lytic tumor with sharp sclerotic margins and a pseudoloculated pattern resembling that of a bone cyst. The tumor is eccentrically located in metaphyseal bone with a slightly dilated and thinned out cortex similar to that shown (Figure 6–18). Histologic findings include a strange but specific mixture of fibrous, myxomatous,

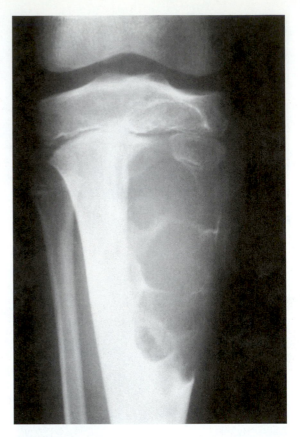

Figure 6–18. Radiograph of a chondromyxoid fibroma in the proximal tibia of an 11-year-old boy.

and chondroid tissues, which could mistakenly suggest the diagnosis of a chondrosarcoma. The findings also commonly include giant cells, which might suggest the diagnosis of a chondroblastoma seen in epiphyseal bone. This stage 2 lesion is quite active locally, especially in children. With simple curettement and bone grafting, the recurrence rate can approach 25%. Aggressive margin expansion should be performed. The conversion of chondromyxoid fibroma to chondrosarcoma is extremely rare.

Benign Fibrous Tumors of Bone

A. FIBROUS CORTICAL DEFECT

Fibrous cortical defects, or cortical desmoids, are small hamartomatous fibromas seen almost exclusively in the metaphyseal areas of the lower extremities of growing children. They can be multiple, and as many as 25% of normal children will demonstrate these asymptomatic lesions at 5 years of age. The lesions tend to disappear as the result of bone remodeling before skeletal maturity. If excessive stress is placed across the lesions, they can become symptomatic and can also cause findings of increased activity on an isotope bone scan.

In the case of fibrous cortical defects, microscopic studies show benign appearing fibroblasts with an occasional area of histiocytes, foam cells, and benign giant cells. The radiographic appearance is so characteristic of this entity (Figure 6–19) that a biopsy is usually not necessary. These are stage 1 lesions and can generally be observed.

B. Nonossifying Fibroma

Just as the osteoblastoma is considered a larger or more extensive form of osteoid osteoma, the nonossifying fibroma is considered a larger form of the fibrous cortical defect. It is typically seen in the lower extremity of children. Because of its size it may not entirely resolve by skeletal maturity and this can persist into adult life. If the lesion is quite large, approaching 50% of the diameter of the bone, pathologic fracture may ensue. The fracture-healing process may facilitate resolution of the lesions. Careful consideration to fracture prophylaxis should be reserved for large lesions only in children older than age 10. Nonossifying fibromas are stage 1 lesions, and neither they norfibrous cortical defects require biopsy as their radiographic appearance is so characteristic.

With nonossifying fibroma, multiple lesions may take on the appearance of fibrous dysplasia and can be associated with "café au lait" skin defects. Large lesions in the proximal tibia can assume the appearance of a chondromyxoid fibroma (Figure 6–20). The lesions have a well-defined sclerotic margin and a pseudomultiloculated lytic center that gives them a soap-bubbly radiographic appearance. Histologically, they appear identical to fibrous cortical defects and are character-

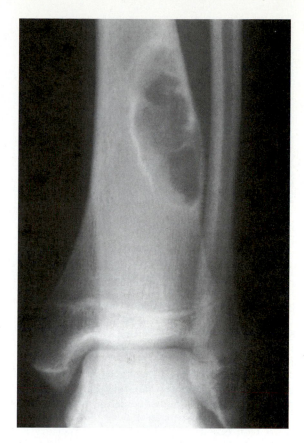

Figure 6–20. Radiograph of a nonossifying fibroma of the distal tibia.

ized by benign fibrous tissue speckled with areas of histiocytes, foam cells, and giant cells. As the lesion involutes in adulthood and the number of giant cells and histiocytes diminishes, large areas of cholesterol deposits become evident, which may suggest the diagnosis of a xanthofibroma or xanthoma of bone. Nonossifying fibromas are clearly separated from fibrous dysplasia by the absence of the metaplastic osteoid formation in the fibrous stroma.

C. Fibrous Dysplasia

Fibrous dysplasia can present in a variety of ways: monostotic, polyostotic, and with or without associated syndromes (Figure 6–21). Most cases are diagnosed within the first three decades and have a distinct female predilection. The monostotic presentation is more common than polyostotic. This condition is a dysplastic anomaly of bone-forming mesenchymal tissue with an inability to produce mature lamellar bone. Accordingly, the bone is arrested in the woven state with a resultant proliferation of spindle cell fibroblasts. In the

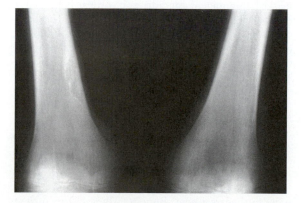

Figure 6–19. Radiograph of a metaphyseal fibrous defect in a 15-year-old boy.

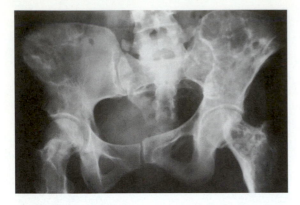

Figure 6–21. Radiograph of polyostotic fibrous dysplasia of the pelvis.

polyostotic form it tends to involve one side of the body rather than bilaterally. Nevertheless, it can involve any bone of the body. The most common location is the proximal femur, where it results in the so-called shepherd's crook deformity. Other areas frequently involved include the tibia, pelvis, humerus, radius, and ribs.

In addition to bony involvement patients can demonstrate café au lait skin pigmentation. These patches usually have a rough border, in contrast to the smooth border of those seen in neurofibromatosis. Patients with fibrous dysplasia may have associated endocrine problems. For example, 5% of patients with the polyostotic form of fibrous dysplasia will also exhibit precocious puberty (Albright McCune syndrome). Other associated endocrine abnormalities include hyperthyroidism, acromegaly, Cushing's disease, and hypophosphatemic osteomalacia. Polyostotic fibrous dysplasia with soft-tissue myxomas is known as Mazabrand's syndrome. Fibrous dysplasia can also involve the skull and jaw bones, mimicking ossifying fibroma of jaw bone.

In fibrous dyplasia, microscopic findings include an alphabet-soup pattern of metaplastic woven bone scattered through a benign fibrous tissue stroma. This woven stroma has an absence of osteoblastic rimming. Foam cells, giant cells, and cholesterol deposits can be seen. Large cystic areas and even areas of cartilage formation are commonly present.

Recent research has potentially implicated a mutation in the signal transducing G-proteins, interrupting cellular communication at the transmembrane cell surface receptor-intracellular signal transduction pathway. The c-fas oncoprotein may be involved as well.

Fibrous dysplasia tends to be active during the growing years then burns out in adult life. Fewer than 1 % of lesions will convert to osteosarcoma, fibrosarcoma, or even chondrosarcoma. If conversion does occur, it almost always happens during adulthood. Generally this disease is either stage 1 or 2.

In pediatric patients with active disease, curettage and grafting should be avoided because of high recurrence rates. The goals in treating pediatric patients should be the prevention and treatment of deformity, especially in the lower extremity. Most cases should become quiescent with skeletal maturity. If not, the best surgical treatment in adults consists of rigid fixation with an intramedullary implant with strut grafting as needed. The best surgical treatment in adults consists of the use of long autogenous fibular struts combined with autogenous cancellous bone graft. This treatment has a higher success rate in the adult group than in the pediatric group. Medical management with bisphosphonates has been shown to be of benefit in some cases. Irradiation is contraindicated because it may lead to irradiation-induced sarcoma at a later date.

Cystic Lesions of Bone

A. Simple Bone Cyst

Simple bone cysts are a common pseudotumor of bone and the most frequent cause of pathologic fractures in children. Bone cysts typically affect patients between 5 and 15 years of age and occur more often in boys than in girls. They are found in the proximal humerus in 50% of cases and in the upper femur in 25%. Patients are asymptomatic until a pathologic fracture occurs. Fractures seem to arise from the central metaphyseal side of an epiphyseal or apophyseal growth plate. The cystic process continues to grow away from the physis. When it remains in contact with the physis it is termed "active." When it separates it is termed "inactive."

Radiographs typically show a solitary cyst that is centrally located in the metaphyseal area and has marked thinning of the adjacent cortical bone and a pseudoloculated appearance (Figure 6–22). The bone cyst is filled with a clear serous fluid, and there is increased pressure during the active phase. The fact that this pressure gradually decreases as the cyst becomes inactive suggests a hydrodynamic mechanism.

The cyst cavity is lined with a fibrinous membrane that contains giant cells, foam cells, and a slight osteoid formation and is similar to the fibrous tissues seen in other fibrous bone lesions, including fibrous dysplasia. The periosteal covering in the area of a cyst is normal, and thus the pathologic fractures heal normally and in most cases do not require surgery. Unfortunately, the cyst will usually persist after fracture union and will require further treatment. Bone-resorbing factors such as matrix metalloproteinases, prostaglandins, interleukin-

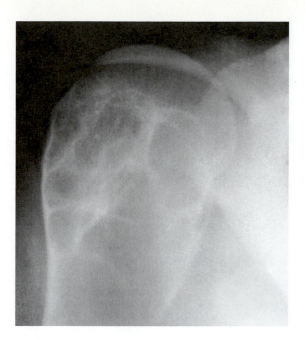

Figure 6–22. Radiograph of a solitary bone cyst on the proximal humerus of a 13-year-old boy.

1, interleukin-6, tumor necrosis factor-alpha and oxygen free radicals, have been demonstrated in the cyst fluid. Elevated nitrate and nitrite levels have also been noted to be higher in the cyst fluid than in serum.

Before the mid-1970s, the standard treatment for a solitary bone cyst was aggressive curettement or even resection followed by bone grafting. In patients with active disease, the recurrence rate was 30–50%, and repeated grafting was frequently necessary. In patients with inactive disease, particularly those older than 15 years, the surgical results were much better and the recurrence rate was lower. Unicameral bone cysts are generally considered stage 1 lesions, but occasionally they may be stage 2. Currently, treatment is a function of location. In weight-bearing bones, such as the proximal femur, lesions should be treated aggressively. Initial management usually involves aspiration/injection with either bone marrow or corticosteroid. The injections are carried out with bone biopsy needles and are repeated three to five times at intervals of 2–3 months, depending on the radiographic response. The best results are when the patient is between 5 and 15 years old, at which time the disease is active and macrophage activity is greatest in the cyst lining. Curettage and bone grafting may also be an effective modality.

Physicians should note that sarcomas can take on the radiographic appearance of a solitary bone cyst. For this reason, if needle aspiration does not reveal cystic fluid or if it is impossible to inject contrast material and obtain radiologic confirmation of the diagnosis, an open biopsy is indicated to rule out sarcoma.

B. Aneurysmal Bone Cyst

Aneurysmal bone cyst is a hemorrhagic lesion with many characteristics of a giant cell tumor but occurs only half as frequently. Although 75% of the cases of aneurysmal bone cyst occur in patients 10–20 years old, giant cell tumor is rare in patients younger than 20 years of age. Both aneurysmal bone cyst and giant cell tumor are more common in females than in males. The femur is the most frequently affected site, followed by the tibia, pelvis, and spine. In the spine, two thirds of aneurysmal bone cysts will arise from posterior elements and one third will arise from the vertebral body, whereas most giant cell tumors arise from the vertebral body.

Initially, the aneurysmal bone cyst appears on radiograph as an aggressive osteolytic lesion with extensive permeative cortical destruction that gives the impression of a malignant process such as Ewing's sarcoma or hemorrhagic osteosarcoma. Next, a large aneurysmal bulge will occur outside the bone, with a thin reactive shell of bone forming at the outer edge. Less soap-bubbly pseudoseptation is seen in an aneurysmal bone cyst than in a solitary cyst (Figure 6–23).

At the time of biopsy, the aneurysmal bone lesion will demonstrate large hemorrhagic cysts, but bleeding is modest. The hemorrhagic cysts are broken up by thick spongy fibrous septa that histologically contain great numbers of large giant cells and have thin osteoid

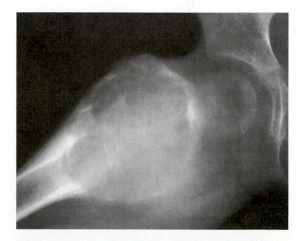

Figure 6–23. Radiograph of an aneurysmal bone cyst on the proximal femur of a 5-year-old boy.

seams. Even if a few mitotic figures are seen, the diagnosis of a benign lesion can remain. A carefully placed biopsy with multiple samples is needed to rule out other well-known skeletal tumors that may demonstrate an aneurysmal component. These include giant cell tumor, chondromyxoid fibroma, and malignant hemorrhagic osteosarcoma. Some authors believe that there is no such entity as the aneurysmal bone cyst and feel that it is merely a morphologic variant of some other underlying neoplastic process. Like the solitary bone cyst, this cyst may have a hydraulic pressure origin that is secondary to hemorrhage and could be traumatically induced. However, it is important to point out that abnormal cytogenic findings have been noted in aneurysmal bone cysts, which may suggest a distinct cellular pathogenetic etiology. Aneurysmal bone cyst is either a stage 2 or 3 lesion and frequently symptomatic.

If an aneurysmal cyst is left untreated, it may involute spontaneously during which time it will develop a heavy shell of reactive bone at the periphery. This involutional process can be hastened by surgical curettage and bone grafting. Radiation is no longer recommended. Another option for treating extremely large lesions is repeated embolization to reduce the rate of hemorrhagic expansion.

C. Epidermoid Cyst

The least common bone cyst is the epidermoid bone cyst. This lesion is found either in the distal phalanx or in the skull. No other bone is affected. In the case of the phalanx, the cyst is usually the result of nail bed epithelium being driven into the subjacent distal phalanx by a crushing blow. The ectopic squamous epithelium produces a keratinized cavity that is filled with clear fluid and creates a surface erosion with a sclerotic reactive base (Figure 6–24). The bulbous cyst seen at the fingertip will transilluminate with flashlight examination. Other conditions that might have a similar appearance are the glomus tumor and the enchondroma.

The epidermoid cyst is treated with a simple curettement and, in some cases, a bone graft.

Giant Cell Tumor of Bone

Numerous types of tumors contain giant cells but are not true benign giant cell tumors. Most of the variants are seen in children and include aneurysmal bone cyst, chondroblastoma, simple bone cyst, osteoid osteoma, and osteoblastoma. The hemorrhagic osteosarcoma is the most malignant of the variants, and it is difficult to distinguish from an aggressive benign giant cell tumor. The giant cell reparative granuloma is a benign variant seen in jaw bones or hand bones and has more spindle cells than a classic giant cell tumor does. The brown tumor of hyperparathyroidism is a nonneoplastic vari-

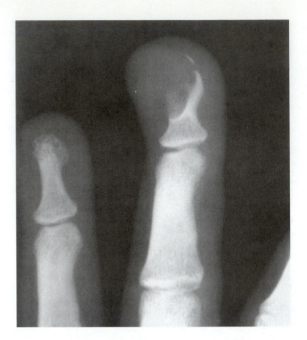

Figure 6–24. Radiograph of an epidermoid cyst in the distal phalanx.

ant seen in both primary and secondary hyperparathyroidism. Only after all of the variant conditions are excluded can the diagnosis of benign giant cell tumor be made.

Between 5 and 10% of all benign bone tumors are true giant cell tumors, occurring most frequently in the third decade of life. They are more frequently found in females than in males. In about half of the cases, the tumor is found about the knee. The next most common locations are the distal radius and sacrum. The tumor is usually painful for several months prior to diagnosis and can cause a pathologic fracture. It can also cause a painful effusion because of its juxtaposition to a major joint. Giant cell tumors may present as either stage 2 or stage 3 disease and less frequently as stage 1. On radiograph, the lesion appears lytic in nature and is located in the epiphyseal-metaphyseal end of a long bone (Figure 6–25). The lesion grows toward the joint surface and frequently comes into contact with articular cartilage but rarely breaks into the joint.

Like the chondroblastoma, the benign giant cell tumor has a 1–2% chance of metastasizing to the lung. Recurrent tumors have a 6% chance. Accordingly, pulmonary staging is an important component in the initial evaluation and follow-up of giant cell tumor of bone. The prognosis for survival with this complication is favorable, and the tumors may resolve spontaneously. The benign giant cell tumor can later convert to a ma-

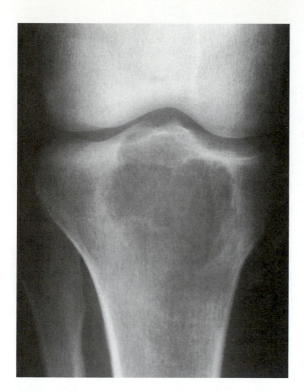

Figure 6–25. Radiograph of a giant cell tumor on the proximal tibia of a 22-year-old woman.

multiple recurrent tumors, intensive soft-tissue involvement, or massively destructive cases. Embolization may also prove palliative or curative in unresectable cases. For advanced, multiply recurrent, or aggressive metastatic cases, investigators are developing experimental medical protocols. Close follow-up for locally recurrent disease and pulmonary involvement is critical. Surveillance should include a plain chest radiograph every 6–12 months for the first 2–3 years at least.

Hemangioma

Hemangioma of bone is a hamartomatous process that occurs more frequently in females than in males. It is most commonly found in vertebral bodies (Figure 6–26). It is found only rarely in the diaphysis of long bone. Hemangiomas of bone can be associated with hemangiomas of soft tissue. The spinal lesion is usually discovered as an incidental radiographic finding and demonstrates a characteristic vertically oriented honey-

lignant condition such as an osteosarcoma or malignant fibrous histiocytoma. It is generally believed that this is secondary to treatment. A conversion rate of 15–20% has been reported in patients who were treated previously with more than 3000 cGy of radiation, with conversion occurring 3 or more years after treatment. The conversion rate in patients who have not received radiation therapy is less than 5%. This has come into question with newer radiation therapy modalities.

Until recent years, the standard treatment for giant cell tumor was curettage and bone grafting. The recurrence rate with this treatment has been reported as up to more than 50%. Follow-up treatment consisted of an aggressive resection of the recurrent lesion and reconstruction with a large osteoarticular allograft, endoprosthesis, or an excisional arthrodesis. Currently, most surgeons will elect an aggressive curettage, followed by the use of adjuvant phenol, hydrogen peroxide, or liquid nitrogen and by the subsequent packing of the defect with bone cement. With this new approach, the recurrence rate is between 10–25%. When giant cell tumor infrequently involves an expendable bone such as the proximal fibula or ilium, it should be primarily resected. En bloc resection continues to be used to treat

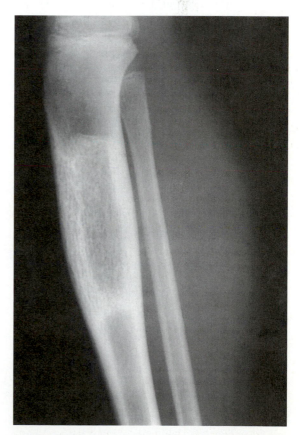

Figure 6–26. Radiograph of a hemangioma of the tibia in a 14-year-old boy.

combed or moth-eaten appearance. On rare occasions, a lesion can cause cord compression that may require surgical resection. In such cases, preoperative angiography is critical in evaluating the vascular blood supply to the spinal cord. Alternatively an attempt at arterial embolization may prove successful and is less aggressive.

Gorham's disease is characterized by massive osteolysis in children or young adults and is usually associated with the presence of benign cavernous hemangiomas or lymphangiomas of bone. This strange condition usually affects a particular area (such as the spine or the hip) but can involve multiple bones of that area and tends to resolve spontaneously.

Baruffi MR et al: Aneurysmal bone cyst with chromosomal changes involving 7q and 16p. Cancer Genet Cytogenet 2001;129 (2):177. [PMID: 11566352]

Bottner F et al: Cyclooxygenase-2 inhibitor for pain management in osteoid osteoma. Clin Orthop 2001;(393):258. [PMID: 11764357]

Boutou-Bredaki S et al: Prognosis of giant cell tumor of bone. Histopathological analysis of 15 cases and review of the literature. Adv Clin Path 2001;5(3):71. [PMID: 11753878]

Bovee JV et al: Malignant progression in multiple enchondromatosis (Ollier's disease): An autopsy-based molecular genetic study. Hum Pathol 2000;31(10):1299. [PMID: 11070122]

Cheung P et al: Etiological point mutations in the hereditary multiple exostoses gene EXT1: A functional analysis of heparan sulfate polymerase activity. Am J Hum Genet 2001; 69(1): 55. [PMID: 11391482]

Flemming DJ et al: Primary tumors of the spine. Semin Musculoskelet Radiol 2000;4(3):299. [PMID: 11371321]

Gallazzi MB et al: Percutaneous radio-frequency ablation of osteoid osteoma: Technique and preliminary results. Radiol Med (Torino) 2001;102(5-6):329. [PMID: 11779979]

Kivioja A et al: Chondrosarcoma in a family with multiple hereditary exostoses. J Bone Joint Surg Br 2000;82(2):261. [PMID: 10755438]

Komiya S et al: Increased concentrations of nitrate and nitrite in the cyst fluid suggesting increased nitric oxide synthesis in solitary bone cysts. J Orthop Res 2000;18(2):281. [PMID: 10815830]

Lindner NJ et al: Percutaneous radiofrequency ablation in osteoid osteoma. J Bone Joint Surg Br 2001;83(3):391. [PMID: 11341426]

Maki M et al: Comparative study of fibrous dysplasia and osteofibrous dysplasia: Histopathological, immunohistochemical, argyrophilic nucleolar organizer region and DNA ploidy analysis. Pathol Int 2001;51(8):603. [PMID: 11564214]

Marie PJ: Cellular and molecular basis of fibrous dysplasia. Histol Histopathol 2001;16(3):981. [PMID: 11510989]

Nakase T et al: Involvement of BMP-2 signaling in a cartilage cap in osteochondroma. J Orthop Res 2001; 19(6):1085. [PMID: 11781009]

Ramappa AJ et al: Chondroblastoma of bone. J Bone Joint Surg Am 2000;82-A(8):1140. [PMID: 10954104]

Randall RL et al: Aggressive aneurysmal bone cyst of the proximal humerus. Clin Orthop 2000;(370):212. [PMID: 10660716]

Robinson P et al: Periosteal chondroid tumors: Radiologic evaluation with pathologic correlation. Am J Roentgenol 2001; 177(5):1183. [PMID: 11641198]

Safar A et al: Recurrent anomalies of 6q25 in chondromyxoid fibroma. Hum Pathol 2000;31(3):306. [PMID: 10746672]

Soder S et al: Cell biology and matrix biochemistry of chondromyxoid fibroma. Am J Clin Pathol 2001;116(2):271. [PMID: 11488075]

Yanagawa T et al: The natural history of disappearing bone tumours and tumour-like conditions. Clin Radiol 2001;56(11): 877. [PMID: 11603890]

MALIGNANT BONE TUMORS

Osteoid-Forming Sarcomas

Aside form multiple myeloma, osteosarcoma of bone is the most common primary malignant tumor of bone constituting 20% of all primary malignancies of bone. In the United States, between 500 and 1000 new cases are diagnosed each year. The global incidence is felt to be between 1 and 3 per million people annually. There are currently many subtypes of osteoid-forming sarcomas, ranging from the extremely low grade variants such as the parosteal osteosarcoma to the extremely high grade variants such as osteosarcoma secondary to Paget's disease. This discussion begins with the more common, central form of sarcoma that is seen in children and known as classic osteosarcoma.

A. CLASSIC OSTEOSARCOMA

The classic form of osteosarcoma is typically seen in patients in their second or third decade, with a peak in the adolescent growth spurt. It occurs more frequently in males than in females and is found in the metaphyseal areas of long bones, with 50% of lesions seen about the knee joint (Figures 6–27 and 6–28). The distal femur is the most common site, followed by the proximal tibia and then the proximal humerus. It is rare to see osteosarcoma in small bones of the feet or hands or in the spine. When seen in the foot, it will occur in the larger bones of the hind foot. The prognosis is more favorable for a tumor in a small bone than for one in a large bone.

Most patients with classic osteosarcoma have symptoms of pain before a tumor mass is noticeable. A mass near a major joint may exist for several weeks or even as long as 4 months before a diagnosis is made. Dilated veins may be seen in the overlying skin. The radiographic findings will include permeated lytic destruction of metaphyseal bone, with eventual cortical breakthrough into the subperiosteal space and subsequent formation of "Codman's reactive triangle" at the diaphyseal end of the tumor. As the tumor continues to push its way into the extracortical soft tissue, a typical sunburst pattern of chaotic neoplastic bone may be seen outside the involved bone.

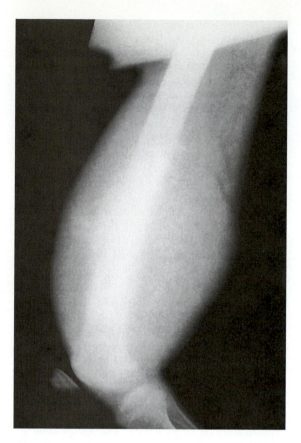

Figure 6–27. Osteosarcoma of the distal femur of a 15-year-old female patient. Notice the sunburst appearance.

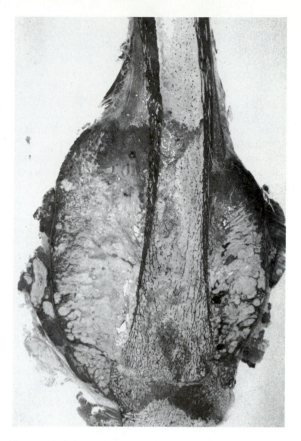

Figure 6–28. Gross surgical specimen from Figure 6–27. Notice the sharp upper medullary margin located about the same level as the extracortical mass. The tumor has not invaded the growth plate.

In less than 2–25% of cases, an additional lesion may be found at a higher level in the femur. Such a "skip" lesion may portend a worse probability of survival and should be considered a true metastatic focus (stage III [Enneking], stage IV [AJCC]). About 50% of osteosarcomas are of the more typical osteoblastic type, followed by chondroblastic, with a small percentage of them being fibroblastic. Whether the subtype portends a better or worse prognosis is controversial. Confounding variables such as multidrug resistance (*p*-glycoprotein expression) may be differentially expressed in different subtypes. *P*-glycoprotein overexpression has itself been found to bear a substantial relationship on clinical outcome.

Staging of osteosarcoma must include an MRI of the involved extremity (Figure 6–29). This technique offers excellent contrast of the extracortical portion of the tumor and at the same time gives good intramedullary contrast of the high-signal tumor next to a low-signal fatty marrow. The periphery of the tumor can readily be appreciated and represents the most anaplastic and rapidly growing part of the tumor. This region is the best tissue for a biopsy because it is easy to reach, soft enough for a diagnostic frozen section, and representative of the most aggressive portion of the tumor. Furthermore, the MRI provides the necessary anatomic data to determine the level of transection through the femur for a safe margin and to determine whether a limb-sparing procedure is feasible.

Before the advent of adjuvant multidrug chemotherapy, the treatment for osteosarcoma was radical amputation. Eighty percent of these patients proceeded to die from disseminated pulmonary disease. Today, with the combination of chemotherapy and surgical treatment, the prognosis for 5-year survival approaches 70%.

The drugs commonly used today include high-dose methotrexate, doxorubicin, cisplatin, and ifosfamide. They are administered intravenously in cyclic intervals

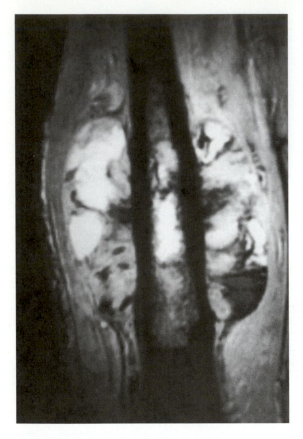

Figure 6–29. Fat-subtraction (STIR) MRI of a femoral osteosarcoma.

of 3–4 weeks for approximately 11–15 weeks prior to surgery. Surveillance imaging studies are performed during this period to assess possible reduction in tumor volume. Tumor necrosis secondary to neoadjuvant chemotherapy, determined at the time of tumor resection, is an important prognostic factor. Patients with greater than 90% tumor necrosis have a significantly improved 5-year survival rate, approaching 85%. Approximately half of patients will demonstrate this response to current chemotherapy regimens. Furthermore, the postoperative drug regimen can be adjusted based upon this evaluation.

In extremity osteosarcoma, limb-sparing surgery, with wide resection of the tumor, is the standard approach. Amputation is reserved for the exceptional or recurrent case. In less than 10% of cases, amputation is performed at a level about 5 cm above the upper pole of the tumor. Limb salvage techniques continue to evolve with reconstruction options including large prostheses, structural allografts, and composites reconstructions.

Endoprosthetics are composed of modular components in various lengths, linked together with taper fittings (Figure 6–30 and 6–31). The intramedullary stems are of various diameters and lengths and are usually cemented. The immediate functional results are excellent, with minimal early complications. However, subsequent loosening at 5–10 years has been shown to occur in as many as 15–30% of cases. Another limb-sparing procedure consists of the use of an osteoarticular allograft alone or in combination with a prosthesis. The major drawback with large bone allografts is a 10–15% chance of infection, nonunion, or stress fracture, especially in the immunosuppressed patient receiving chemotherapy. The use of an excisional arthrodesis was more popular in the past but is rarely elected today because patients have better function with a mobile joint.

Prior to the introduction of chemotherapy, the finding of a pulmonary metastasis portended a very poor prognosis. Today, however, in larger tumor centers where aggressive surgical approaches with multiple thoracotomies and continued chemotherapy are used, the 5-year survival rate is approximately 30%.

Molecular oncologic evaluation of osteosarcoma specimens is beginning to elucidate factors involved in its pathogenesis. The p53 suppressor genes have an increased mutation rate in osteosarcoma. However, wild type *TP53* and *MDM2* assays in and of themselves have not been shown to be of prognostic value. Loss of heterozygosity of the Rb gene has been shown to be a predictive feature of osteosarcoma. The *F33* isoform has also demonstrated a strong correlation with osteosarcoma disease progression. ErbB-2 (Her-2/*neu*), a protooncogene and transforming growth factor beta, isoform 3 expression has also been correlated with a worse prognosis in osteosarcoma patients. Controversy surrounds the significance of cytoplasmic versus membranous staining in Her-2/neu expression as relates to prognosis in osteosarcoma.

B. HEMORRHAGIC OR TELANGIECTATIC OSTEOSARCOMA

Telangiectatic osteosarcoma is an extremely lytic and destructive variant of classic osteosarcoma and is seen in the same age group and location. Its radiographic appearance is similar to that of an aneurysmal bone cyst, thereby making the diagnosis difficult (Figure 6–32). The pathologic specimen is hemorrhagic, with microscopic evaluation demonstrating the presence of malignant-appearing stromal cells with giant cells.

Because hemorrhagic osteosarcoma is a high-grade, purely lytic tumor, the incidence of pathologic fracture in the early course of the disease is high. If significant contamination of the adjacent neurovascular structures results, a pathologic fracture may necessitate amputation rather than limb salvage (Figure 6–33). This must be carefully evaluated with a preoperative MRI. Ac-

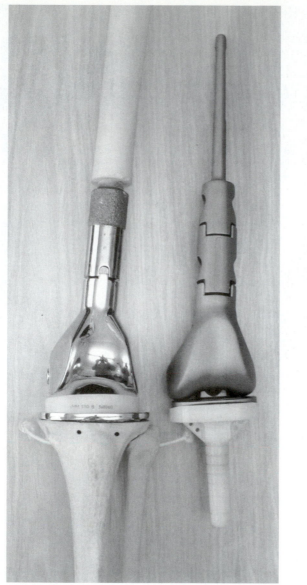

A

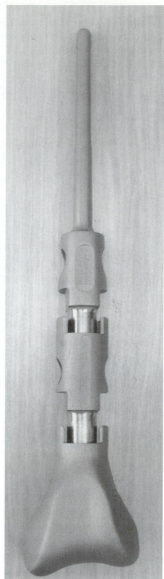

B

Figure 6–30. **A.** Two examples of distal femoral replacement systems. **B.** Modularity of system allows different size intercalary body segments.

cordingly, in cases with significant risk for fracture during the preoperative treatment regiment, it may be appropriate to immobilize the involved extremity or proceed with limb-sparing surgery earlier than usual. Prior to the advent of aggressive multidrug chemotherapy, the prognosis for patients with hemorrhagic osteosarcoma was extremely poor. At present, however, it is the same as the prognosis for patients who have classic osteosarcoma and is treated with similar protocols.

C. PAROSTEAL OSTEOSARCOMA

Parosteal osteosarcoma is a low-grade variant arising in an exophytic pattern from the cortical surface of bone. There is no medullary involvement. It is low-grade with

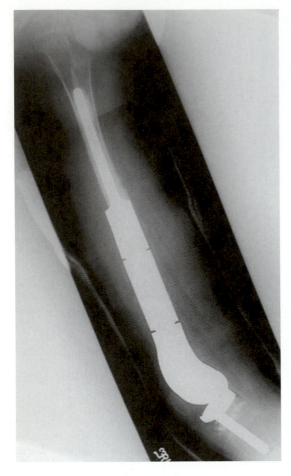

Figure 6–31. Lateral radiograph of distal femoral replacement system in skeletally immature patient. Expansion with larger intercalary body is possible.

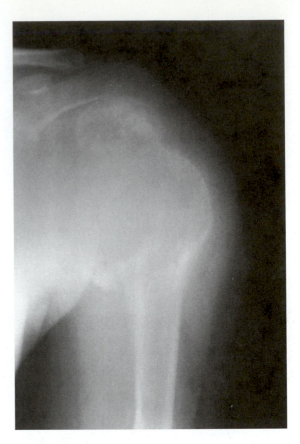

Figure 6–32. Radiograph of hemorrhagic osteosarcoma in a 6-year-old girl.

a 5-year survival rate in excess of 90% and a 10-year survival rate of 80%. It accounts for 3–4% of all osteosarcomas.

The tumor is composed of a spindle-cell fibroblastic component with well-developed bone trabeculae. There also may be areas of cartilage present. Osteoblasts are well differentiated, and few mitotic figures are present.

Parosteal osteosarcoma is more common in females than in males and affects a slightly older age group than classic osteosarcoma (see Table 6–2). It is a slow-growing tumor with minimal symptoms initially. It is metaphyseal in origin, with the vast majority of cases involving the posterior aspect of the distal femur (Figure 6–34).

Because the parosteal osteosarcoma is low-grade, it does not respond well to either chemotherapy or radiation therapy. Therefore, the only treatment is wide sur-

gical resection. Usually this requires distal femoral removal but in smaller cases side resection of the posterior cortex and tumor only may be feasible, sparing the knee joint. Nevertheless, a negative tumor margin is imperative. Otherwise, recurrence is likely. Recurrence may occur as late as 5–10 years because of the tumor's slow growth.

On occasion, low-grade parosteal osteosarcoma can dedifferentiate into a high-grade sarcoma. Such a lesion carries a similar prognosis to classic osteosarcoma.

D. PERIOSTEAL OSTEOSARCOMA

Periosteal osteosarcoma is another surface osteosarcoma of low to intermediate grade. This lesion represents less than 2% of all osteosarcomas. It arises beneath the periosteum, elevating it and inducing vigorous neo-osteogenesis with a predominant chondroblastic differentiation. It is slightly more common in females, with a peak incidence in the second decade of life. It almost exclusively arises in the long bone. The lesion can mimic an

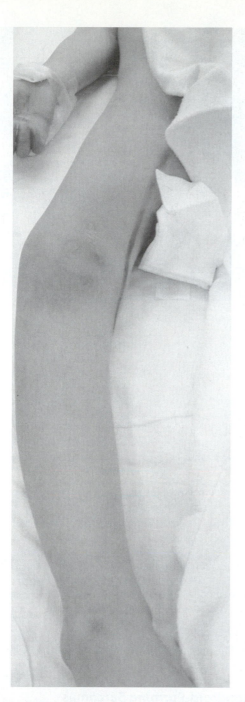

Figure 6–33. Clinical photograph of patient that sustained a pathologic fracture through a distal femur osteosarcoma contaminating the neurovascular structures precluding limb salvage.

aneurysmal bone cyst or periosteal chondroma radiographically (Figure 6–35).

Because of its low to intermediate grade, periosteal osteosarcoma is generally not treated with chemotherapy but may be in more advanced cases. Wide surgical resection is the modality of choice. Because periosteal osteosarcoma is a low-grade tumor, it carries a better prognosis than the classic osteosarcoma. Approximately 25% of patients will succumb to metastatic disease within 2–3 years. The surgical treatment is usually a limb-sparing procedure, and because the tumor is more diaphyseal in location, the adjacent joints may often be spared.

E. Secondary Osteosarcoma

Osteosarcoma can arise from benign disease through a process that may involve a second mutation and usually occurs at a later age (Table 6–2). Among the benign conditions that can result in secondary osteosarcoma are Paget's disease, osteoblastoma, fibrous dysplasia, benign giant cell tumor, bone infarction, and chronic osteomyelitis.

The classic example of a secondary osteosarcoma is seen in a small percentage of patients with Paget's disease. Pagetic osteosarcomas, which represent about 3% of all osteosarcomas, are the most common osteosarcomas in the older age group. The most frequent location for pagetic osteosarcoma is the humerus, followed next by the pelvis and femur. The typical patient has a long history (15–25 years) of dull, aching pain associated with the inflammation of Paget's disease before a new acute pain arises in an area of recent lytic destruction and the diagnosis of pagetic osteosarcoma is established (Figure 6–36). The prognosis for patients with pagetic osteosarcoma is extremely poor (5-year survival rate of approximately 8%). Because of the older age group involved, chemotherapy is usually not an option secondary to intolerance.

F. Low-Grade Intramedullary Osteosarcoma

Another rare and low-grade osseofibrous variant of osteosarcoma is the central or intramedullary form. Although this variant has a microscopic appearance similar to that of the parosteal osteosarcoma, it is usually located in metaphyseal bone about the knee joint in adults between 15 and 65 years of age. Males and females are equally affected. Radiographically, intramedullary osteosarcoma will create a sclerotic density in metaphyseal bone (Figure 6–37). Like the parosteal osteosarcoma, the low-grade intramedullary osteosarcoma carries an excellent prognosis and can be treated with local surgery alone.

G. Irradiation-Induced Osteosarcoma

Radiation-induced osteosarcoma may arise after any form of significant radiation exposure (in excess of 30

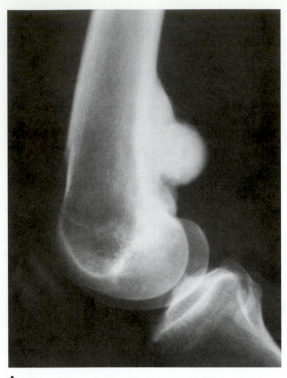

A

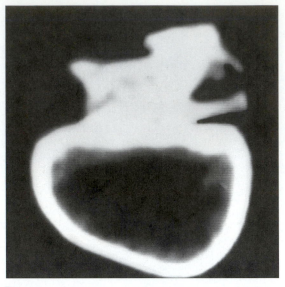

B

Figure 6–34. Radiograph (**A**) and CT scan (**B**) of a parosteal osteosarcoma of the distal femur in a 21-year-old woman.

Gy) (Figure 6–38). Onset is usually delayed an average of 15 years (range 3–55). Other irradiation-induced sarcomas, besides the osteosarcoma type, include irradiation-induced fibrosarcoma and malignant fibrohistiocytoma. All of these secondary sarcomas are invariably high grade and carry a poor prognosis for survival, with a very high rate of metastasis.

H. MULTICENTRIC OSTEOSARCOMA

Multicentric osteosarcoma has two clinical presentations: (1) synchronous—occurring in childhood and adolescents and (2) metachronous—occurring in adults. The synchronous type is a high-grade sclerosing intramedullary type, which is lethal. The adult form is less aggressive, with a lower histologic appearance, but prognosis remains grim (Figure 6–39).

I. SOFT-TISSUE OSTEOSARCOMA

Osteosarcoma can occur in muscle tissue outside bone and accounts for about 4% of all osteosarcomas (Figure 6–40). Soft-tissue osteosarcoma is rarely seen in patients younger than 40 years. The number of cases is

equal in males and females, and the tumor is usually seen in large muscle groups of the pelvis and thigh areas.

Soft-tissue osteosarcoma must be differentiated from the more common myositis ossificans. Although soft-tissue osteosarcoma shows heavy mineralization in the central area (see Figure 6–40), myositis ossificans has a zonal pattern of ossification, with the mature dense ossification concentrating at the periphery of the lesion.

The treatment of the soft-tissue form of osteosarcoma is the same as for the high-grade osseous form and includes a wide resection and adjuvant chemotherapy. The prognosis is worse with the soft-tissue form of osteosarcoma.

Chondroid-Forming Sarcomas

Chondroid-forming sarcomas re a heterogenous group of neoplasms consisting of a cartilage-based histology. A cornerstone to the diagnosis of chondrosarcoma is the absence of osteoid formation. If any osteoid is present with a malignant stroma, then the tumor is considered

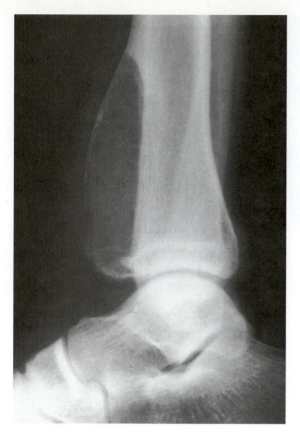

Figure 6–35. Radiograph of a periosteal osteosarcoma of the distal tibia in a 15-year-old boy.

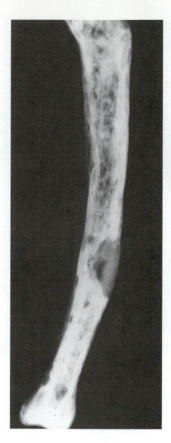

Figure 6–36. Radiograph of a pagetic osteosarcoma of the tibia.

an osteosarcoma with chondroblastic features. It is important to make the distinction because chondrosarcomas behave differently from osteosarcomas. However, this can be a difficult task. The surgeon must consider the age of the patient and carefully assess the radiographic and histologic features in order to confirm the diagnosis.

A. PRIMARY OR CENTRAL CONVENTIONAL CHONDROSARCOMA

The typical primary chondrosarcoma is a low-grade tumor seen in adults between 30 and 60 years of age. The tumor is found more frequently in men than in women. Minimal symptoms of pain may occur over a period of several years before a radiograph is obtained. The pelvis and femur are the most common locations, followed by the rib cage, proximal humerus, scapula, and upper tibia. Primary chondrosarcoma is extremely rare in small bones, including the hand and foot. The

metaphysis is the most common location in a long bone; however, a diaphyseal location is not unusual.

About 85% of central chondrosarcomas are low-grade lesions with a typical matrix calcification that can be described as flocculated. The high-grade lesions are rare, and radiographically they lose their typical lobulated and calcific pattern and take on the appearance of a more permeative high-grade tumor, such as a malignant fibrous histiocytoma. At the same time, histologically the high-grade chondrosarcomas loose their chondroid matrix pattern, which is replaced with that of a more aggressive spindle-cell tumor.

The radiologic feature that clearly separates this lesion from a benign enchondroma is the permeative lysis seen in the surrounding cortex (Figure 6–41). Because of the weakened cortex, the patient will usually complain of local pain not experienced with an enchondroma. Because most chondrosarcomas are low grade, they do not respond well to adjuvant irradiation or

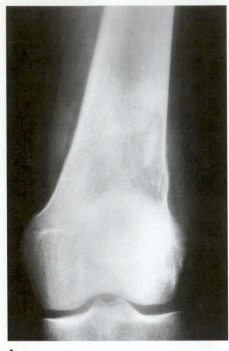

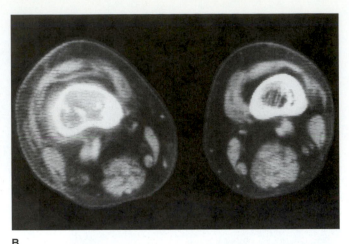

B

A

Figure 6–37. Radiograph (**A**) and CT scan (**B**) of a low-grade intramedullary osteosarcoma in the distal femur of a 65-year-old man.

chemotherapy. Therefore, aggressive surgical management is imperative. However, optimal surgical management is controversial. Although wide, en bloc resection is ideal from a margins standpoint, it can often produce considerable morbidity. On the contrary, aggressive intralesional resection (curettage) and margin expansion with an adjuvant therapy (eg, phenol or liquid nitrogen) can reduce morbidity and may provide equal local control. In fact, some authors have found that for grade 1 chondrosarcoma the margin of resection is not significant in terms of local recurrence or disease progression.

In general, the prognosis for low-grade central chondrosarcoma is very good, with a low rate of pulmonary metastasis if the primary lesion is widely resected. Nevertheless, recurrences can occur late, even over 15 years later.

For any intermediate- or high-grade chondrosarcoma, wide, en bloc resection is mandatory (Figure 6–42).

B. SECONDARY CHONDROSARCOMA

The vast majority of secondary chondrosarcomas arise from osteochondromas in patients afflicted with MHE. Patients with solitary osteochondromas do not generally form secondary chondrosarcomas in their lesions, making prophylactic removal unnecessary and unwarranted unless the solitary lesion is otherwise symptomatic. Even in patients with MHE the rate of malignant degeneration is less than 1% and generally does not occur in patients prior to skeletal maturity. However, patients with secondary chondrosarcoma tend to be younger than those with primary chondrosarcomas. The lesions tend to be slow growing with minimal to mild symptoms. The most common site is the pelvis, followed by the proximal femur, proximal humerus, and ribs. Plain radiographs demonstrate a flocculated calcific pattern (Figure 6–43). Anything thicker than 1–2 cm should raise suspicion of a secondary chondrosarcoma. The overall prognosis for patients with secondary or peripheral chondrosarcoma is even better than that for patients with primary or central chondrosarcoma. Surgical removal, without violation of the cartilage cap, is the only effective treatment modality.

C. DEDIFFERENTIATED CHONDROSARCOMA

Dedifferentiated chondrosarcoma is the most malignant variant of chondrosarcoma, accounting for between 5–10% of all chondrosarcomas. It is heralded by the transformation of areas of conventional chondrosarcoma into malignant fibrous histiocytoma or osteosar-

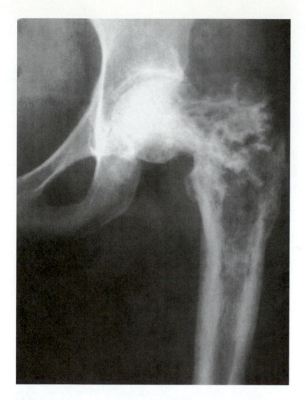

Figure 6–38. Radiograph of irradiation-induced osteosarcoma of the peritrochanteric area in a 35-year-old woman.

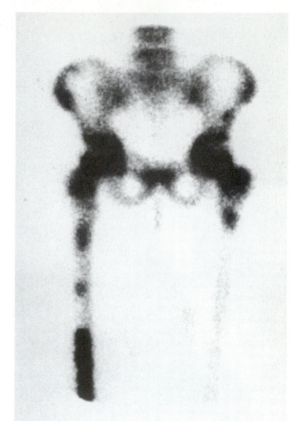

Figure 6–39. Isotope bone scan of multicentric osteosarcoma in an 8-year-old girl.

coma. Histologically, it is characterized by two distinct but neighboring areas of low- to intermediate-grade malignant chondroid tumor and heterogenous high-grade sarcoma. Dedifferentiated chondrosarcoma occurs in older patients, usually between 50 and 70 years of age. It is found in the same areas affected by central primary chondrosarcomas, including the pelvis, femur, and proximal humerus (Figure 6–44). Radiographs show areas of rarefication within the tumor with cortical attenuation. Pathologic fracture is not uncommon.

The prognosis in dedifferentiated chondrosarcoma is bleak, with the majority of patients developing and dying of metastatic disease within 1 year (historically 1-year survival rate approached 10%). Chemotherapy and radiation therapy are less effective than in a malignant fibrous histiocytoma or osteosarcoma that had arisen de novo. Surgical resection remains the mainstay of treatment, with adjuvant modalities employed in younger patients.

D. CLEAR CELL CHONDROSARCOMA

Clear cell chondrosarcoma is a rare low-grade variant of chondrosarcoma. Clear cell lesions occur more often in

males than in females and are usually seen in patients between the ages of 20 and 50 years. The vast majority of lesions are found in the femoral head (Figure 6–45). The radiographic appearance is one of a lytic tumor with sharp margination and a central matrix calcification, creating the appearance of a chondroblastoma. Although microscopic examination reveals the presence of some giant cells, as seen in a chondroblastoma, areas of low-grade chondrosarcoma are also evident in which no giant cells are seen. Even on gross examination, the clear cell chondrosarcoma does not look like a chondrosarcoma, and this explains why it is frequently mistaken for a chondroblastoma in younger adult patients. The tumor cells have abundant glycogen, giving them their characteristic clear cell phenotype. Although no significant genetic alteration have been found in clear cell chondrosarcoma, recent findings show that alkaline phosphatase activity may correlate with prognosis.

The treatment for clear cell chondrosarcoma is a wide excision and reconstruction. The prognosis with

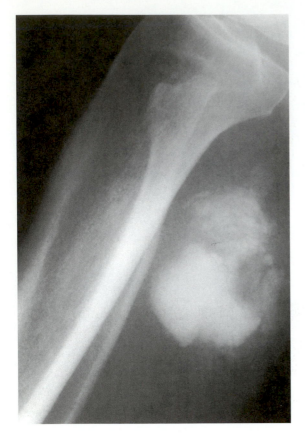

Figure 6–40. Radiograph of a soft-tissue osteosarcoma in the calf area of a 67-year-old man.

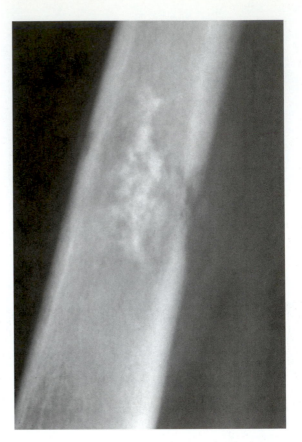

Figure 6–41. Radiograph of a low-grade primary chondrosarcoma in the distal femur of an 83-year-old man.

this type of treatment is good. In contrast, when lesions are mistaken for chondroblastomas and treatment consists of a simple curettement and bone grafting, the prognosis is poor and the recurrence rate is high.

E. MESENCHYMAL CHONDROSARCOMA

Another rare variant of chondrosarcoma is the mesenchymal chondrosarcoma. It is a highly cellular tumor composed of primitive mesenchymal cells with foci of cartilage differentiation. This tumor involves the soft tissue in one third of cases, occurs more frequently in females than in males, and is seen in young adults. The jaw is the most common location, followed by the spine and ribs, with very few cases noted in long bones.

Mesenchymal chondrosarcoma is a high-grade tumor with histologic features of low-grade chondrosarcoma. Heavily calcified areas, mixed with areas of malignant round cells, may give it the appearance of Ewing's sarcoma or hemangiopericytoma.

Treatment consists of resection, with a wide margin if possible, and adjuvant chemotherapy and radiation therapy. Despite aggressive treatment, the prognosis is very poor, with a high incidence of pulmonary metastasis.

Round Cell Sarcomas

This "group" of tumors is composed of distinct tumors that, other than their similar microscopic appearance using hematoxylin-eosin stain, are quite different. They behave and are treated in a variety of ways, given that each arises from a different cell type.

A. EWING'S FAMILY OF TUMORS

1. Ewing's sarcoma—Ewing's sarcoma is a well-known clinical entity that was originally described by James Ewing as a diffuse endothelioma of bone. Since the time of his description, many theories have evolved regarding the tumor's true histogenesis. Based on elec-

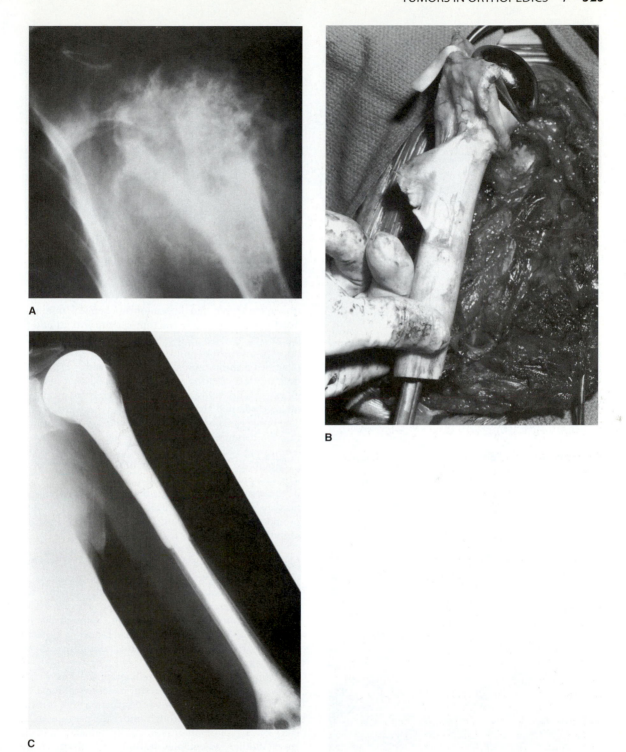

Figure 6–42. Preoperative radiograph of a large central chondrosarcoma in the proximal humerus of a 52-year-old woman (**A**), placement of a Neer prosthesis (**B**), and postoperative radiograph (**C**).

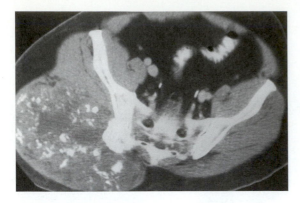

Figure 6–43. CT scan of a secondary peripheral chondrosarcoma in the ilium of a 56-year-old man with multiple exostoses.

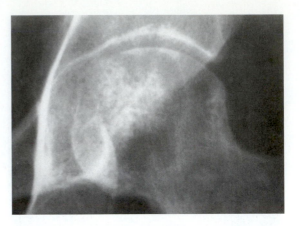

Figure 6–45. Radiograph of clear cell chondrosarcoma of the femoral head in a 25-year-old man.

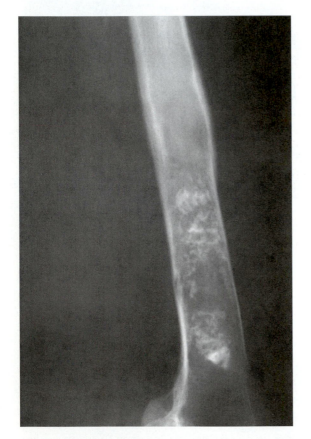

Figure 6–44. Radiograph of dedifferentiated chondrosarcoma in the distal femur of a 73-year-old woman.

tron microscopic and immunohistochemical findings, experts currently believe the tumor represents an undifferentiated member of the family of neural tumors distinct from neuroblastoma. Cytogenetic studies have identified a chromosomal abnormality with a reciprocal translocation in chromosomes 11 and 22 seen in 90% of cases. This translocation is also seen in primitive neuroectodermal tumor (PNET) and Askin's tumors. The breakpoints have been cloned and it is now known that the Ewing's sarcoma and *FLI1* genes are involved. The Ewing's sarcoma gene encodes a homologous sequence to the RNA binding site in RNA polymerase II. The FLI product is a transcription factor. Accordingly, in the resultant fusion protein the *FLI1* transcription factor is placed under control of the Ewing's sarcoma promoter. Two other translocations have also been described in Ewing's/PNET, t(21:22) and t(7:22).

In 90% of cases, Ewing's sarcoma is found in patients between 5 and 25 years of age. If the patient is younger than 5 years, the most likely diagnosis is metastatic neuroblastoma. Males are affected more frequently than females and carry a worse prognosis. The pelvis is the most common location, followed by the femur, tibia, humerus, and scapula. However, because Ewing's sarcoma is a myelogenous tumor, it can be found in any bone in the body.

Ewing's sarcoma appears radiographically as a central lytic tumor of the diaphyseal-metaphyseal bone. It creates extensive permeative destruction of cortical bone, and as it breaks through under the periosteum, it takes on a typical onionskin, multilaminated appearance. Another radiographic feature is the reactive hair-on-end appearance created by bone forming along the periosteal vessels that run perpendicularly between the cortex and the elevated periosteum (Figure 6–46).

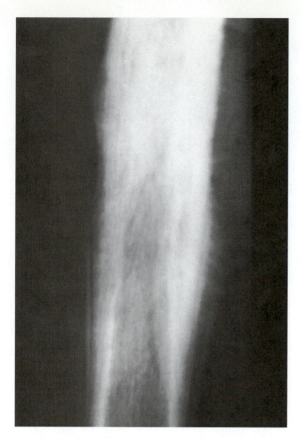

Figure 6–46. Radiograph of periosteal response in Ewing's sarcoma of the femur in a 15-year-old boy.

Ewing's sarcoma can frequently masquerade as osteomyelitis because it is a high-grade lesion with resultant areas of necrosis, liquefaction may occur that may be mistaken for pus. Furthermore, patients frequently present with systemic symptoms of low-grade intermittent fever, elevated white cell count and erythrocyte sedimentation rate.

Microscopically, small round like cells predominate in densely packed sheets. Formation of pseudorosettes may also be seen (in less than 20%). The rosette-like patterns are more frequently seen in PNET.

Ewing's sarcoma is an aggressive malignancy with a high local recurrence and metastatic rate. Patients with locally resectable disease treated with multidrug chemotherapy have a 5-year survival rate of approximately 70%. Unfortunately, 15–25% of patients will present with nonlocalized disease. For the patient who presents with advanced, metastatic disease, the 5-year survival rate is 30%. Resection of lung metastasis, if possible, does improve survival.

Ewing's sarcoma is a radiosensitive tumor. Historically, this has been a modality of choice employing 45–50 Gy over 5 weeks to treat local disease. Because of the not insignificant risk of secondary sarcomas, surgery has been investigated as the primary modality for local control. If the margins are contaminated, then local irradiation must still be used postoperatively. However, prospective well-controlled studies have not yet clearly established that surgery significantly improves survival without radiation.

2. Primitive neuroectodermal tumor—PNET is the less common relative to Ewing's sarcoma. Like Ewing's, this tumor demonstrates expression of neural markers by immunocytochemistry. PNET also exhibits the t(11:22) translocation with the resulting EWS/FI1-fusion protein. In fact, because of such similarities, it is generally agreed that PNET and Ewing's represent ends of a spectrum of disease.

By strict criteria, PNET is a rare tumor, representing approximately 10% of Ewing's-like tumors. The demographics are identical to those of Ewing's-like tumors. Treatment of PNET is similar to that of Ewing's; however, the survival rate is slightly less. Accordingly, some authors feel it should be distinguished from Ewing's.

B. Lymphoma

Lymphoblastic tumors are considered systemic neoplasms of the lymphatic organs, including the bone marrow, and they account for 7% of all malignant bone tumors. They can be roughly divided into Hodgkin's lymphomas and non-Hodgkin's lymphomas, both of which can affect bone. Of the two groups, the lymphomas associated with Hodgkin's disease carry a much better prognosis. When they are found in bone, they tend to be localized and have a considerable blastic response, especially when involving the vertebra.

There are two main types of non-Hodgkin's lymphomas. The type emphasized in this section is the primary lymphoma of bone, in which a localized lytic destruction occurs in a single bone, and the results of staging studies (including an isotope bone scan, a CT scan of the chest and abdomen, and marrow aspiration) all prove negative for other areas of involvement. The other type is the more generalized or systemic form of lymphoma, in which many lymphoid organs are involved, including the lymph nodes, liver, spleen, and bone. The prognosis is better for an isolated primary lymphoma of bone, but years later involvement may become generalized or systemic and carry a worse prognosis. This is similar to the case with plasma cell tumors, in which the findings in a patient can change from that of a solitary plasmacytoma with an excellent prognosis to that of the multiple myeloma form of the disease with a poor prognosis.

Primary lymphoma of bone, which was formerly called reticulum cell sarcoma of bone, accounts for about half of all lymphomas. To meet the criteria of being a primary bone lymphoma, there must be a 4–6-month interval from the onset of skeletal manifestations to the development of systemic disease. It occurs more frequently in males than in females, is usually found in patients over the age of 25 years, and affects the spine or pelvis in over 50% of the cases. In the extremities, the femur is the most commonly involved area, followed next by the humerus and the tibia. Multiple skeletal involvement occurs in 10–40% of cases.

Radiographic findings in primary lymphoma include extensive lytic permeation of cortical bone, with minimal sclerotic response in diaphyseal, metaphyseal, and epiphyseal locations (Figure 6–47). MRI studies demonstrate that the actual marrow involvement is frequently more extensive than the cortical disruption seen on simple radiographs suggests.

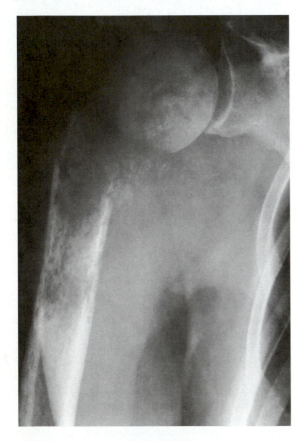

Figure 6–47. Radiograph of a lymphoma in the proximal humerus of a 64-year-old woman.

The most common histologic types of lymphoma of bone are the large cell or mixed small-large cell types. The cells tend to demonstrate little cytoplasmic structure. However, the nuclear pattern shows indented and folded nuclear patterns and a prominent pink-staining nucleolus, which may help to distinguish it histologically from Ewing's sarcoma. Immunohistochemical staining is often necessary to differentiate Ewing's sarcoma from the B-cell and T-cell subtypes of lymphoma. In the case of lymphomas, the glycogen stain is usually negative, but the reticulum stain is often positive.

In primary lymphoma of bone, as in Ewing's sarcoma, multidrug chemotherapy has greatly improved the 5-year survival rate, which now is about 70% for patients with either of these tumors. Like Ewing's sarcoma, primary lymphoma of bone is highly sensitive to local irradiation. If the primary lymphoma is localized, a wide resection and limb-salvage reconstruction may be carried out, thereby avoiding the need for local irradiation and possibly effect a cure. However, if the involvement is more extensive, as is commonly the case, then it will be necessary to use intralesional techniques such as cemented intramedullary nails or a long-stem prosthesis and subsequently use whole bone irradiation, similar to the management of metastatic carcinoma with pathologic fractures. In cases of extensive systemic involvement, bone marrow transplantation can be used.

C. PLASMA CELL TUMOR

A bone tumor composed of malignant monoclonal plasma cells is referred to as a myeloma or plasmacytoma. It is rare for a patient to have a solitary myeloma or plasmacytoma. Tumors are almost always found on multiple bony sites, in which case the term *multiple myeloma* is used.

1. Myeloma—Multiple myeloma, which is the most common primary tumor of bone, accounts for 45% of all malignant bone tumors. It is the second most common hematopoietic malignancy. 90% of cases are in patients older than 40 years. It accounts for 1% of all malignancies in Caucasians and 2% in African-Americans.

The disease is characterized by a triad of osteolytic "punched out" lesions (multifocal) (Figure 6–48) neoplastic proliferation of atypical plasma cells and a monoclonal gammopathy. Diagnostic criteria have been established for myeloma. Major criteria include plasmacytosis on biopsy of a lesion, marrow plasmacytosis, and an abnormal serum protein electrophoresis and light (Bence-Jones) proteinuria. It causes bony destruction similar to that caused by lymphomas, with most lesions occurring in the trunk, hip, and shoulder areas. Lesions are rarely found distal to the knee or elbow. About 3% of patients with myeloma have a sclerotic form of the disease, which appears to carry a better prognosis and is associated with peripheral neuropathy.

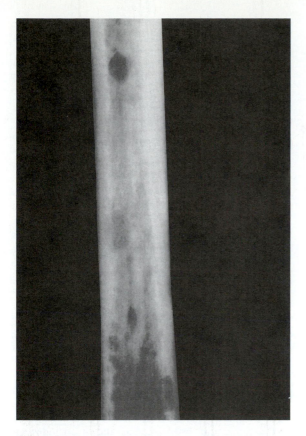

Figure 6–48. Radiograph of multiple myeloma in the femoral shaft of a 72-year-old man.

The serum, protein electrophoresis shows an elevated monoclonal immunoglobulin on either the a or y spike. Bence-Jones proteinuria is secondary to light-chain immunoglobulin spillover. Occasionally, electrophoresis of a urine sample will yield positive results, whereas that of a serum sample will yield negative results. In aggressive forms of myeloma, the extensive bone breakdown will cause hypercalcemia, which can lead to a semicomatose state and over a long period will result in nephrocalcinosis. Renal damage also results from protein plugging of the renal tubules and renal failure.

A marrow aspirate will usually demonstrate the abnormal plasma cells. These cells show an eccentrically placed nucleus in a well-structured eosinophilic cytoplasm. Although normal B-cell–derived plasma cells produce antibodies, the abnormal B-cell–derived plasma cells produce immunoglobulin that is ineffective, which helps explain the increased infection rate in patients with myelomas. Patients may also demonstrate extraosseous infiltrates, with the majority seen in the upper airway and oral cavity. Amyloidosis may be seen concurrently in 10–15% of cases. A quarter of these will have extensive cardiac involvement. In such cases the median survival is 4 months.

Plain radiographs show myeloma lesions to be sharply demarcated lytic lesions with minimal periostitis. Pathologic fixation is frequent. Bone scans have a high false-negative rate thought to be due to almost exclusive osteoclast activity.

Less than 2% of myeloma cases will demonstrate the POEMS syndrome: *P*olyneuropathy, *O*rganomegaly, *E*ndocrinopathy, *M*-component spike, *S*kin changes, *S*cleroses of bone.

Although treatment and prognosis have improved, myeloma remains a fatal disease, with more than 90% of patients dying within 2–3 years. Chemotherapy such as melphalan and cortisone may induce a transient remission in 50–70% of cases.

Local treatment of myeloma is similar to that of metastatic disease, with cemented intramedullary nails and prosthetic devices used after an intralesional debridement. The amount of bleeding at the surgical site is usually extensive, similar to that encountered with surgery for metastatic renal cell carcinoma and certain thyroid metastases. After surgery, the entire bone should be irradiated with 5500 cGy. Spinal lesions should be handled just like metastatic tumors, as discussed in a later section.

2. Solitary myeloma—Solitary lesions are rare (Figure 6–49). By definition there must be no marrow involvement. Seventy-five percent of these cases will have an entirely normal protein electrophoresis in serum (SPEP) and urine (UPEP). The remaining 25% may have mild abnormalities. Vertebral involvement is the most common site. Patients also tend to be younger. Unfortunately, 70% of these solitary cases develop multiple myeloma within 3 years. Until this happens, the treatment is only local, with a wide resection if possible or intralesional debridement and reconstruction followed by radiation therapy.

Fibrous Sarcomas of Bone

Malignant fibrous tumors of bone are clinically similar to the osteosarcoma, but they affect an older age group of patients and show a complete absence of tumor osteoid formation. The two major tumors in this category are the fibrosarcoma and the malignant fibrous histiocytoma.

A. FIBROSARCOMA OF BONE

Fibrosarcoma of bone is a malignant spindle-cell tumor seen in an older patient population with a peak incidence in the fourth decade. It is 10 times less frequent than osteosarcoma but tends to involve similar loca-

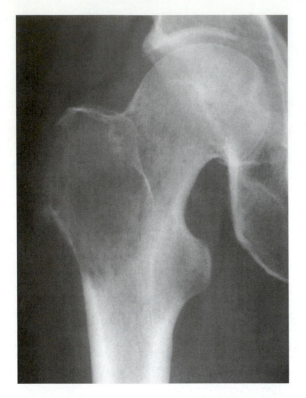

Figure 6–49. Radiograph of a solitary plasmacytoma in the proximal femur of a 46-year-old man.

tions. The most common site of fibrosarcoma is the distal femur, followed next in order by the proximal tibia, pelvis, proximal femur, and proximal humerus. It is rarely seen in the spine, hand, or foot.

On radiograph, fibrosarcomas appear to be almost purely osteolytic and permeative, similar to lymphomas. For this reason, they are painful and can lead to a pathologic fracture. Microscopically, myofibroblastic differentiation with osteoid formation or histiocytes permits distinction from fibroblastic osteosarcoma and malignant fibrous histiocytoma (MFH) of bone. The low-grade form is characterized by malignant-appearing fibroblasts that form a large amount of collagen fiber, giving the appearance of an aggressive desmoplastic fibroma. The high-grade form is characterized by a more anaplastic fibroblast with a higher index of mitotic activity and less collagen fiber formation. It is common to see a basket-woven or storiform pattern in the microscopic picture.

The prognosis and treatment are directly related to the histologic grade of the tumor. Low-grade fibrosarcoma has a better prognosis than osteosarcoma does, but it must be treated by means of an aggressive and wide resection to avoid local recurrence. Because the low-grade form has a low mitotic index, adjuvant chemotherapy and radiation therapy are of little help. High-grade fibrosarcoma has a prognosis and a rate of metastasis that are similar to those of osteosarcoma, and it is usually treated in a similar manner with a combination of surgery and, if the patient is young enough to tolerate the systemic toxicity adjuvant chemotherapy.

B. MALIGNANT FIBROUS HISTIOCYTOMA OF BONE

Prior to 1970, MFH was rarely diagnosed in bone but was commonly found in soft tissue. Now MFH is more common in bone than fibrosarcoma, but the two types of tumor run a similar clinical course. MFH of bone is seen in middle-age and older adults, is more common in males than in females, and affects the same bony sites as the fibrosarcoma and osteosarcoma.

MFH is a purely lytic tumor that shows aggressive permeation of metaphyseal-diaphyseal bone, similar to the findings in lymphoma (Figure 6–50). Lytic destruction is diffuse, with no evidence of a periosteal response to blastic repair. Microscopic analysis of MFH usually shows the tumor to be high grade and have highly anaplastic fibroblasts mixed with malignant histiocytes and a few giant cells in a typical storiform pattern.

Because the MFH is closely related to the high-grade fibrosarcoma, it carries a poor prognosis, with high rates of local recurrence and metastasis. The treatment program is therefore similar to that for high-grade fibrosarcoma and osteosarcoma, and it includes an aggressive wide resection and the use of adjuvant chemotherapy.

Adamantinoma of Bone

Adamantinomas account for only 0.33% of all malignant bone tumors; occur with equal frequency in males and females, usually during the second and third decades of life; are found in the tibia in 90% of cases; and are usually diaphyseal in location, frequently starting in the anterior cortex. The cause of adamantinoma remains unknown, although angioblastic synovial cells and epithelial cells have been considered in the past. Recent investigations, including immunohistochemistry and electron microscopic studies, lend support to the hypothesis of an epithelial origin, which goes along with the histologic appearance of a basal cell carcinoma and might explain the common site of origin subcutaneously in the anterior tibial cortex. The name *adamantinoma* was given to the tibial lesion because its histologic appearance is similar to that of the adamantinoma of jaw bone (ameloblastoma), but the two entities have no other relationship clinically.

In patients with adamantinoma, the radiograph shows a benign tumor with a lytic central core that is

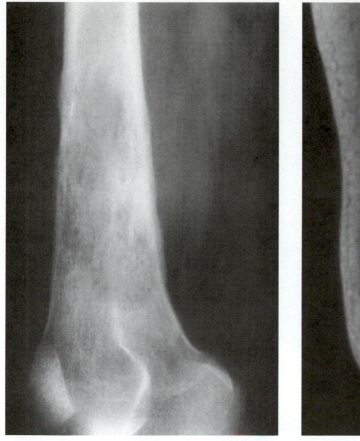

A

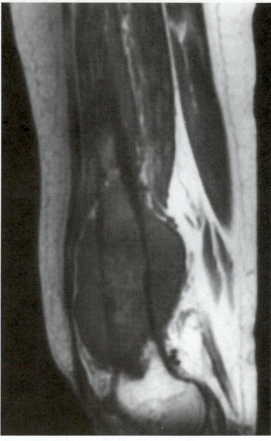

B

Figure 6–50. Radiograph (**A**) and T$_1$-weighted MRI (**B**) of malignant fibrous histiocytoma in the distal femur of a 50-year-old woman.

surrounded by reactive sclerotic bone which typically bulges the anterior cortex and thus takes on the appearance of either fibrous dysplasia or osteofibrous dysplasia (Figure 6–51). One consideration in the differential diagnosis is that osteofibrous dysplasia is painless, whereas pain is a frequent symptom in adamantinoma. Another is that fibrous lesions of bone will stop growing at bone maturity, whereas the adamantinoma will continue on into adult life, at which point a biopsy of the progressive lytic portion of the disease should be performed. There have been cases of osteofibrous dysplasia combined with small areas of adamantinoma scattered in the benign osseofibrous tissue. Adamantinoma has also occasionally been found in both the tibia and fibula, so the physician should look for multiple sites.

Microscopic findings include nests or cords of epithelial or angioid tissue growing in a fibrous tissue stroma, and this can give adamantinoma the appearance of a low-grade angiosarcoma or a metastatic carcinoma.

Adamantinoma grows extremely slowly, over many years, but will on occasion metastasize to regional lymph nodes and the lung. For this reason, it should be treated by a wide resection, which in most cases will be a segmental diaphyseal resection followed by an allograft reconstruction over an intramedullary nail. Because of the low-grade nature of this tumor, adjuvant irradiation or chemotherapy is rarely indicated. Even if pulmonary metastases occur, they can be resected and there will be a fairly good prognosis for survival.

Vascular Sarcomas of Bone

Vascular sarcomas are relatively rare. They include the hemangioendothelioma, angiosarcoma, and heman-

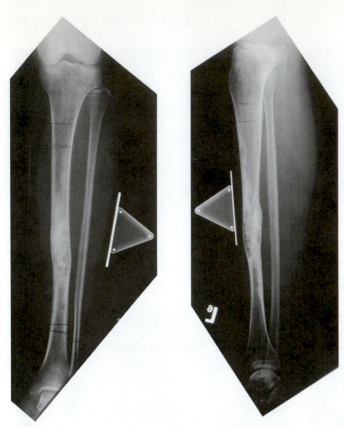

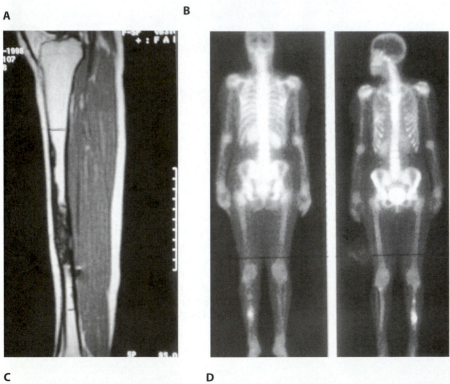

Figure 6–51. Adamantinoma of the tibia. Initial anteroposterior radiograph (**A**), lateral radiograph (**B**), bone scan (**C**), MRI (**D**).

A

B

C

D

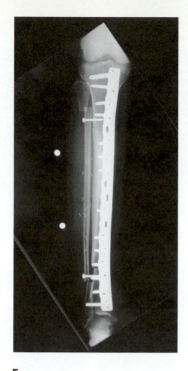

E

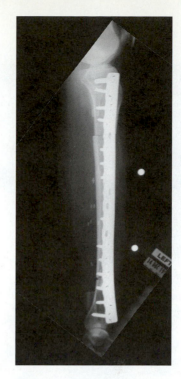

F

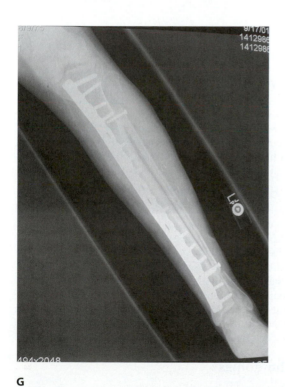

G

H

Figure 6–51. Immediate postoperative after resection with intercalary allograft reconstruction and vascularized fibula transport anteroposterior radiograph (**E**), lateral radiograph. 3 years postoperative (**F**) anteroposterior radiograph (**G**), lateral radiograph (**H**).

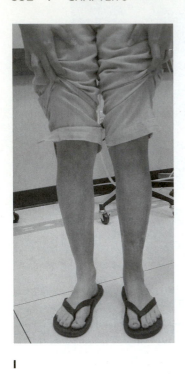 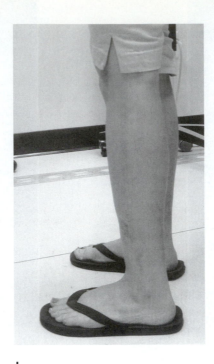 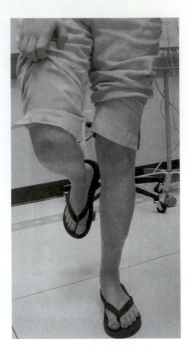

I   J   K

Figure 6–51. (**I–K**) Clinical photos 3 years postoperative.

giopericytoma of bone. The terms *hemangioendothe-lioma* and *angiosarcoma* are frequently used synony-mously; however, the first term refers to a low-grade tumor, and the second term usually suggests a higher grade lesion with a poorer prognosis. The vascular sar-comas have two different cell line origins: endothelial cells for the hemangioendotheliomas, in contrast to he-mangiopericytes for the hemangiopericytomas.

A. HEMANGIOENDOTHELIOMA

The hemangioendothelioma, which is more common in males than in females, is seen in a wide range of ages between the second and seventh decades. The femur, pelvis, spine, and ribs are the usual sites of origin, and the diaphyses and metaphyses of the long bones are also involved. One third of cases will be multicentric, usu-ally in the same bone or limb.

Radiographically, the lesion appears lytic, with sur-rounding sclerotic bone. The more anaplastic the dis-ease process is, the less reactive will the bone be. The clinical picture varies widely, depending on the histo-logic grade of the tumor. The low-grade lesions look like benign hemangiomas, are slow-growing, and carry an excellent prognosis. The high-grade lesions are fast-growing lytic lesions with a poor prognosis.

Treatment depends on the histologic grade. The low-grade lesions do well with simple curettement and bone graft, but the high-grade lesions require a more aggressive wide resection and reconstruction. Adjuvant chemotherapy and radiation therapy can be considered for high-grade lesions, especially in patients with multi-focal disease.

B. HEMANGIOPERICYTOMA

The hemangiopericytoma is an extremely rare form of vascular sarcoma that also has a wide spectrum of clini-cal presentations, depending on the histologic grading. This tumor is the malignant counterpart of the glomus tumor, which is discussed later in the section on soft-tissue tumors. The hemangiopericytoma is a round cell tumor located outside the endothelial membrane of the vascular channel. This can be demonstrated clearly by a silver staining of the reticulum fibers lying between the inner endothelial cells and the outer hemangiopericytes.

Chordomas

Chordoma of bone is rare and accounts for 4% of ma-lignant bone tumors. It takes its origin from the primi-tive notochord and has the clinical appearance of a chondrosarcoma. Chordomas affect males more frequently than females and are seen in patients between the ages of 30 and 80 years. Although 50% of the tumors are sacrococcygeal in origin, 37% arise in the sphenoccipital area and the remainder arise from vertebral bodies of the cervical or lumbar spine. The cranial lesions are seen in a younger age group and carry a poor prognosis because of the dangerous location next to the brain, where surgical removal is difficult.

On radiograph, the chordoma appears as a centrally located lytic process that has minimal sclerotic response at the periphery and may show slight matrix calcification, as in a chondrosarcoma. If the sacrum is involved, the lesion is seen usually in the lower three sacral segments and presents as an extracortical lobulated mass both in front and behind the sacrum. Because of the slow tumor growth, pain may not occur early, but constipation can be an early symptom that results from pressure on the rectum. Because the true anatomic borders are not readily defined by routine radiography, it is best to image this tumor with CT or MRI (Figure 6–52). Microscopically, nests or cords of cells, sprinkled in a sea of mucinous tissue give an appearance similar to low-grade chondrosarcoma. In most cases, large vacuolated cells appear like a signet ring and are referred to as physaliferous cells.

Treatment for the sacral lesions is an aggressive wide resection, which can be difficult because of excessive bleeding. Significant neurogenic bowel and bladder deficits can result. At the present time, it is common to use adjuvant radiation therapy to help reduce the chance of postoperative recurrence. Recent studies recommend using up to 5000 cGy preoperatively, followed with a boost of 1500 cGy postoperatively. If the surgeon is successful in obtaining clean margins, the local recurrence rate is about 30%. With contaminated margins, the recurrence rate climbs to 65%. Recurrence 10–15 years following surgery is common. Because of the low-grade characteristics of the chordoma, it is rare to see a pulmonary metastasis, even after a local recurrence following an inadequate local surgical resection.

Anthouli-Anagnostopoulou FA et al: Juxtacortical osteosarcoma. A distinct malignant bone neoplasm. Adv Clin Path 2000;4(3): 127. [PMID: 11080792]

Bacci G et al: Neoadjuvant chemotherapy for osteosarcoma of the extremity: Long-term results of the Rizzoli's 4th protocol. Eur J Cancer 2001;37(16):2030. [PMID: 11597381]

Bacci G et al: Histologic response of high-grade nonmetastatic osteosarcoma of the extremity to chemotherapy. Clin Orthop 2001;(386):186. [PMID: 11347833]

Bacci G et al: Telangiectatic osteosarcoma of the extremity: Neoadjuvant chemotherapy in 24 cases. Acta Orthop Scand 2001; 72(2):167 [PMID: 11372948]

Berend KR et al: Adjuvant chemotherapy for osteosarcoma may not increase survival after neoadjuvant chemotherapy and surgical resection. J Surg Oncol 2001;78(3):162. [PMID: 11745799]

Bruns J et al: Chondrosarcoma of bone: An oncological and functional follow-up study. Ann Oncol 2001;12(6):859. [PMID: 11484965]

Crapanzano JP et al: Chordoma: A cytologic study with histologic and radiologic correlation. Cancer 200125;93(1):40. [PMID: 11241265]

Ewing J: Diffuse endothelioma of bone, Proc NY Pathol Soc 1921; 21:17.

Gokgoz N et al: Comparison of p53 mutations in patients with localized osteosarcoma and metastatic osteosarcoma. Cancer 200115;92(8):2181. [PMID: 11596036]

Hoang MP et al: Mesenchymal Chondrosarcoma: A small cell neoplasm with polyphenotypic differentiation. Int J Surg Pathol 2000;8(4):291. [PMID: 11494006]

Kanamori M et al: Extra copies of chromosomes 7, 8, 12, 19, and 21 are recurrent in adamantinoma. J Mol Diagn 2001;3(1): 16. [PMID: 11227067]

Kaste SC et al: Thallium bone imaging as an indicator of response and outcome in nonmetastatic primary extremity osteosarcoma. Pediatr Radiol 2001; 31(4):251. [PMID: 11321742]

Kilpatrick SE et al: Clinicopathologic analysis of HER-2/neu immunoexpression among various histologic subtypes and grades of osteosarcoma. Mod Pathol 2001;14(12):1277. [PMID: 11743051]

Lewis VO et al: Parosteal osteosarcoma of the posterior aspect of the distal part of the femur. Oncological and functional results following a new resection technique. J Bone Joint Surg Am 2000;82-A(8):1083. [PMID: 10954096]

Maitra A et al: Aberrant expression of tumor suppressor proteins in the Ewing family of tumors. Arch Pathol Lab Med 2001; 125(9):1207. [PMID: 11520274]

Mandahl N et al: Cytogenetic aberrations and their prognostic impact in chondrosarcoma. Genes Chromosomes Cancer 2002; 33(2):188. [PMID: 11793445]

Oberlin O et al: Study of the French Society of Paediatric Oncology (EW88 study). Br J Cancer 2001;85(11):1646 [PMID: 11742482]

Ogose A et al: Elevation of serum alkaline phosphatase in clear cell chondrosarcoma of bone. Anticancer Res 2001;21(1B):649. [PMID: 11299821]

Park YK et al: Overexpression of p53 and absent genetic mutation in clear cell chondrosarcoma. Int J Oncol 2001;19(2):353. [PMID: 11445851]

Pring ME et al: Chondrosarcoma of the pelvis. A review of sixty-four cases. J Bone Joint Surg Am 2001;83-A(11):1630. [PMID: 11701784]

Rizzo M et al: Chondrosarcoma of bone: Analysis of 108 cases and evaluation for predictors of outcome. Clin Orthop 2001; (391):224. [PMID: 11603673]

Roland Durr H et al: Multiple myeloma: Surgery of the spine: Retrospective analysis of 27 patients. Spine 2002;27(3):320. [PMID: 11805699]

Scully SP et al: Pathologic fracture in osteosarcoma: Prognostic importance and treatment implications. J Bone Joint Surg Am 2002;84-A(1):49. [PMID: 11792779]

Sluga M et al: The role of surgery and resection margins in the treatment of Ewing's sarcoma. Clin Orthop 2001;(392):394. [PMID: 11716413]

Smith SE et al: Primary musculoskeletal tumors of fibrous origin. Semin Musculoskelet Radiol 2000;4(1):73. [PMID: 11061693]

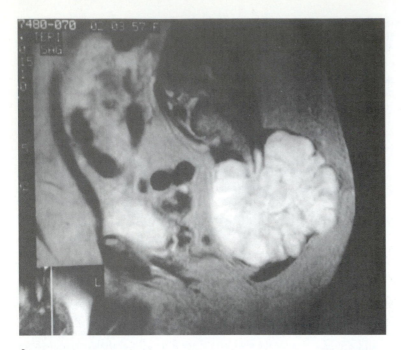

A

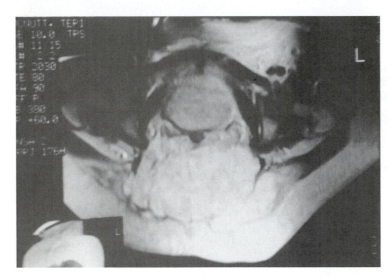

B

Figure 6–52. Sacral chordoma in middle-aged woman: T_2 sagittal image (**A**), T_2 transverse image (**B**).

Tallini G et al: Correlation between clinicopathological features and karyotype in 100 cartilaginous and chordoid tumours. A report from the Chromosomes and Morphology (CHAMP) Collaborative Study Group. J Pathol 2002;196(2):194. [PMID: 11793371]

Weisstein JS et al: Detection of c-fos expression in benign and malignant musculoskeletal lesions. J Orthop Res 2001;19(3):339. [PMID: 11398843]

Zhou H et al: Her-2/neu staining in osteosarcoma: Association with increased risk of metastasis. Sarcoma 2001;5(S1):9.

BENIGN SOFT-TISSUE TUMORS

"Soft tissue" can be defined as nonepithelial, extraskeletal mesenchymal exclusive of the reticuloendothelial system and glia. This would include fat, fibrous tissue, muscle, and the relating neurovascular structures.

Benign soft-tissue tumors, by definition, represent a differentiated neoplastic process with a limited capacity for autonomous growth. They generally demonstrate a marginal capacity to invade locally with infrequent local recurrence. Because of the extensive numbers of benign soft-tissue tumors, discussion will be limited to the more common entities.

Lipomas

The lipoma is by far the most common soft-tissue tumor and has a large number of variants. Some examples include the superficial subcutaneous lipoma; the intramuscular lipoma; the spindle-cell lipoma; the angiolipoma; the benign lipoblastoma; and the lipomas of tendon sheaths, nerves, synovium, periosteum, and the lumbosacral area.

A. SUPERFICIAL SUBCUTANEOUS LIPOMA

The most frequently seen type of lipoma is the superficial subcutaneous type, which can be solitary or multiple. Subcutaneous lipomas occur with equal frequency in men and women and seem to arise spontaneously during the fifth and sixth decade of life. The most common locations are the back, shoulder, and neck.

On palpation this tumor is soft and ballotable. Although it is found more commonly in obese patients, the size of the lipoma does not correlate with the weight of the patient. Lipomas do not reduce in volume with weight loss. They generally grow to a limited size and sarcomatous degeneration does not occur.

Surgical treatment is usually cosmetic in nature, and the recurrence rate is less than 5%.

B. INTRAMUSCULAR LIPOMA

The deep intramuscular lipoma is seen in adults between the ages of 30 and 60 years, affects men more frequently than women, and is commonly found in the large muscles of the extremities. The lesions are slow-growing and painless. The intramuscular lipoma has a characteristic radiolucency that contrasts with the surrounding muscle (Figure 6–53). On MRI this tumor demonstrates a uniform high-signal image on the T_1-weighted spin-echo sequence. On gross examination, the tumor can appear quite infiltrative in surrounding muscle and has a faint yellow color on sectioning. Histologic studies show that the intramuscular lipoma, like the subcutaneous lipoma, is composed of benign lipocytes with small pyknotic nuclei that are difficult to see on the surface of the large fat-laden cell. When samples are taken for biopsy purposes, the pathologist must take care to rule out a low-grade, well-differentiated liposarcoma that can coexist with a benign lipoma. On

rare occasions, a lipoma can have chondroid or osseous hamartomatous elements that have caused it to be classified as a mesenchymoma in the past. In other cases, evidence of hemorrhage or necrosis can be found in a lipoma and will create low-signal changes on the MRI that are similar to the changes seen in liposarcoma.

A marginal surgical excision is indicated for treatment of intramuscular lipoma. Local recurrence rates of 15–60% have been reported.

C. SPINDLE-CELL LIPOMA

The spindle-cell lipoma is seen typically in the posterior neck and shoulder area in men between the ages of 45 and 64 years. On gross examination, the spindle-cell lipoma has the appearance of an ordinary lipoma but with areas of gray-white gelatinous foci streaking through it. Microscopic examination of these areas reveals the presence of benign fibroblasts. Thus, with imaging studies, dense areas are scattered throughout the normal radiolucent areas of a lipoma. On MRI, findings generally consist of a low-signal streaking through the typical high-signal pattern of a benign lipoma.

The treatment for this lesion is a simple marginal resection, and the chance for local recurrence is minimal.

D. ANGIOLIPOMA

The angiolipoma (Figure 6–54) is a subcutaneous lesion that is seen in young adults, usually on the forearm. Multiple lesions are frequently present and are usually painful because of their vascularity. Grossly, the lobular lipoma will demonstrate vascular channels.

Treatment of angiolipoma consists of marginal excision.

E. DIFFUSE LIPOMATOSIS

An extremely rare variant of the lipoma is diffuse lipomatosis, which is characterized by the presence of multiple superficial and deep lipomas that involve one entire extremity or the trunk and usually have their onset during the first 2 years of life. Histologically, an individual lesion in a patient with diffuse lipomatosis looks no different from a typical solitary lipoma. An involved limb may become massive in size, sometimes making it impossible to surgically remove the fatty tumors. If this is the case, amputation may be indicated.

F. LUMBOSACRAL LIPOMA

This lipoma occurs in the lumbosacral area posterior to a spina bifida defect. It is frequently associated with both intradural and extradural lipomas and thus can result in neurologic deficits. Although lumbosacral lipoma is generally considered a pediatric tumor, it can be seen in adults (Figure 6–55).

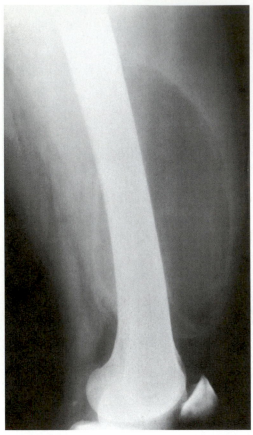

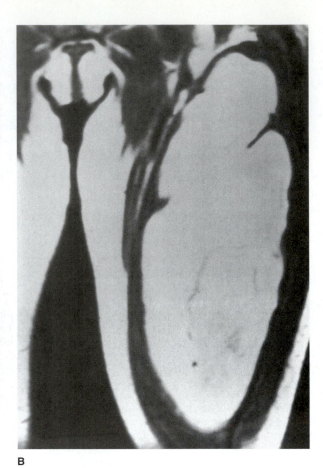

A   B

Figure 6–53. Radiograph (**A**) and coronal view T$_1$-weighted MRI (**B**) of an intramuscular lipoma in the quadriceps muscle of a 72-year-old man.

Surgical treatment consists of a marginal resection of the entire lipoma, including the portion arising from the vertebral canal and lumbosacral roots.

G. BENIGN LIPOBLASTOMA AND DIFFUSE LIPOBLASTOMATOSIS

These types of lipoma are seen in the extremities of infants. The lesions can be solitary or multiple and can be superficial or deep in muscle tissue. They demonstrate cellular immaturity, with lipoblasts similar to the myxoid form of liposarcoma. Even with the cellular aggressiveness of the lesions, the prognosis is excellent following simple surgical resection.

H. HIBERNOMA

This rare lipoma is usually seen in young adults, commonly occurs in the scapular and interscapular regions, is painless and slow-growing, and ranges between 10 and 15 cm in diameter. The hibernoma is composed of finely granular or vacuolated cells characteristic of brown fat and contains a considerable amount of glycogen. The treatment is marginal surgical resection with a low potential for recurrence.

Benign Vascular Tumors

Benign vascular proliferative tumors are the second most common benign tumor after lipomas. Three types of vascular tumors are discussed: hemangiomas, lymphangiomas, and glomus tumors.

Like lipomas, angiomas occur in a wide variety of clinical conditions seen more often in females than in males. The most common type of angioma is the hemangioma, which can be a superficial cutaneous lesions or a deep and intramuscular one. The lymphatic counterpart of the hemangioma is known as the lymphan-

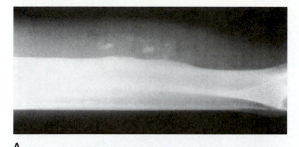

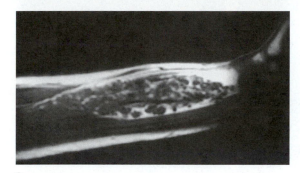

Figure 6–54. Radiograph (**A**) and T$_1$-weighted MRI (**B**) of a soft-tissue angiolipoma in the volar aspect of the forearm of a 27-year-old woman.

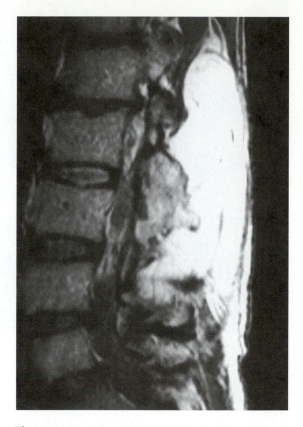

Figure 6–55. T$_1$-weighted MRI of a lumbosacral lipoma.

gioma or hygroma. In most cases, the lesion is solitary or localized. If it is extensive and involves an entire limb, the term *angiomatosis* is used. Because most hemangiomas and lymphangiomas are congenital in origin, the term *hamartomatous* or *arteriovenous malformation* will be applied in their classification. Hemangiomas and lymphangiomas arise from developmental dysplasias of the endothelial tube, whereas glomus tumors and hemangiocytomas arise from hemangiopericytes, which are cells that lie outside the endothelial tube. Most vascular anomalies arise sporadically, but some familial, autosomal-dominant inheritance patterns have also been described. Genetic analyses of these families has identified specific gene mutations supporting the genomic role in the regulation of angiogenesis.

A. HEMANGIOMA

Hemangiomas are the most frequently seen tumors of childhood and account for 7% of all benign tumors.

1. Solitary capillary hemangioma—The most common type of hemangioma is the solitary capillary type, which appears as an elevated red to purple cutaneous lesion on the head or neck. The lesion occurs during the first few weeks after birth, grows rapidly over a period

of several months, and regresses over a 7-year period in 75–90% of cases.

Because of the spontaneous regression, no treatment is needed in most cases. In the past, treatment has consisted of cryosurgery, sclerotherapy, or irradiation, but frequently this treatment was worse than the disease itself. Recently, lasers have been used with good preliminary results. This may prove to be the treatment of choice in selected cases.

2. Cavernous hemangioma—The cavernous hemangioma is larger and less common than the capillary hemangioma. The enlarged vascular spaces of the cavernous lesion give it the appearance of a cluster of purple grapes. It lies deep in the extremity, with common involvement of muscles and even the synovial membrane of the joints.

Imaging may be characteristic (Figure 6–56). In some patients with deep intramuscular forms of hemangioma, the skin shows no abnormalities and no phleboliths are apparent on radiograph. With MRI, deep intramuscular hemangiomas can be easily detected

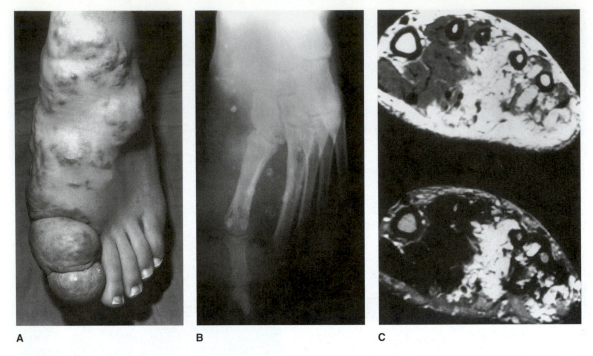

A **B** **C**

Figure 6–56. Clinical appearance (**A**) and radiographic appearance (**B**) of a cavernous hemangioma in the foot of one patient, and T_1-weighted and T_2-weighted MRIs (**C**) of a cavernous hemangioma in the foot of another patient.

by the characteristic mixed-signal serpiginous pattern seen in the T_1-weighted image.

The muscle lesions are usually asymptomatic until intralesional hemorrhage occurs either spontaneously or after a minor injury. The pain symptoms are usually short-lived but recur infrequently. In some patients, the pain is more severe and is associated with muscle contracture and joint deformity. These patients may require surgical resection of the scarred-down lesion to allow for better joint function and to reduce the pain. In rare cases of multiple hemangiomas involving the entire limb, amputation may be indicated. Vascular embolization of the feeder vessels has been attempted but may lead to a significant compartment syndrome, with severe contractures or with loss of muscle strength and limitation of joint movement.

3. Arteriovenous hemangioma—This type of hemangioma is seen in young patients, usually in the head, neck, or lower extremity. It is associated with significant arteriovenous shunting in the tumor, which creates increased perfusion of the tumor. This results in increased local temperature, pain, and continuous thrill or bruit over the mass. In the extremity, it also results in an overgrowth of the limb.

If shunting is excessive, surgical removal of the hemangioma may be necessary to prevent increased pulse pressure from leading to high-output heart failure. Arteriograms are helpful in determining the degree of shunting prior to treatment. Embolization or surgical ligation of feeder vessels is frequently not a successful form of treatment.

4. Epithelioid hemangioma (Kimura's disease)—This cutaneous hemangioma is found on the head or neck in women between 20 and 40 years old. It is associated with inflammatory changes and eosinophilia, and it sometime ulcerates. Its name is derived from the epithelial appearance of the endothelia-lined capillary structures.

5. Pyogenic granuloma—The pyogenic granuloma is a polypoid capillary hemangioma that affects the skin or mucosal surfaces of males and females in all age groups. It may be associated with trauma and is found about the mouth, gingivae, or fingers. The lesions have a purple-red color, bleed easily, and ulcerate.

B. LYMPHANGIOMA

The lymphangioma is nothing more than an angioma composed of lymphatic endothelial tubes that are filled with lymphatic fluid, rather than being filled with blood, as the hemangioma is. Lymphangiomas can be localized, as occurs with the cystic hygroma, and are usually seen about the head, neck, or axilla of young boys and girls. As with hemangiomas, the larger lymphomas are cavernous lesions seen in older patients with deeper involvement. In both lymphangioma and hemangioma, because of increased regional perfusion, bony overgrowth can occur (Figure 6–57).

C. GLOMUS TUMOR

The glomus tumor arises from the hemangiopericyte, which is a cell that is seen at the periphery of the capillary vascular network and is normally involved with the regulation of blood flow through the capillary system. Microscopic examination of the tumor reveals large vas-

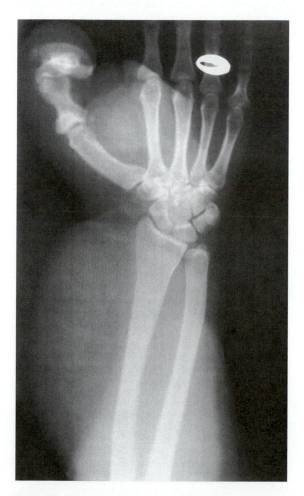

Figure 6–57. Radiograph of a lymphangioma in the forearm and hand of a 23-year-old woman.

cular spaces surrounded by a homogeneous field of round epithelioid hemangiopericytes, with no evidence of mitotic activity.

The glomus tumor is a pink lesion that measures less than 1 cm in diameter. It represents 1.6% of all soft-tissue tumors and occurs with equal frequency in men and women, usually between the ages of 20 and 40 years. Although the tumor is found most commonly in the subungual area of a digit, where it is readily visible, it also occurs subcutaneously on the hand, wrist, forearm, or foot, where it may be invisible and thus difficult to diagnose until localized lancinating pain leads to a surgical exploration. After the lesion is surgically removed, the pain subsides and recurrence is unlikely.

Extra-Abdominal Desmoid Tumors (Aggressive Fibromatosis)

In comparison with the infantile fibrous lesions mentioned earlier, the desmoid tumor is seen in older children and young adults up through 40 years of age. Whereas abdominal desmoids are seen in the abdominal wall of women following pregnancy, the extra-abdominal desmoids usually occur in men and are more common in proximal areas about the shoulder and buttock, followed next by the posterior thigh, popliteal area, arm, and forearm. In most cases, it presents as a solitary tumor. Multicentric involvement is seen at times, however, and can be associated with Gardner's syndrome, which is characterized by polyposis of the large bowel and by craniofacial osteomas. In patients with familial adenomatous polyposis (FAP), an inherited disease due to mutations in the APC gene, desmoids are a significant source of morbidity and mortality. The APC gene, located on chromosome 5, encodes for a 300-kDa protein, in which a germline mutation is an early event in tumor formation.

Desmoids are deep-seated tumors that arise from muscle fascial planes and infiltrate extensively into adjacent muscle tissue, tendons, joint capsules, and even bone. Compared with malignant fibrosarcomas, desmoids are poorly marginated and for this reason are difficult to resect surgically. Desmoids can engulf surrounding vessels and nerves, whereas fibrosarcomas will usually push these structures aside. A desmoid may cause local pain and grow quite rapidly, suggesting a malignant tumor. The desmoid tends to grow more longitudinally along muscle planes to a considerable size, frequently resulting in restricted joint motion about the shoulder, hip, or knee. Because the local aggressiveness of desmoids is so similar to that of malignant fibrosarcomas or malignant fibrous histiocytomas, some experts feel that the desmoid may be a low-grade fibrosarcoma that has lost its potential to metastasize; however, molecular analyses may suggest otherwise.

On gross examination, a desmoid tumor is firm and heavily collagenized. Microscopically, it has a low mitotic index, similar to that of a plantar or palmar fibromatosis. Radiographically, a desmoid is noncalcified and appears dense in comparison with normal muscle. It is easily seen in soft window CT scanning. More exact presurgical imaging can be obtained with MRI (Figure 6–58). As with an abdominal desmoid, an extra-abdominal desmoid physical injury may play a role in the activation of a preexisting oncogene located in the damaged fibroblast.

Desmoids are usually treated surgically with an aggressive wide resection similar to that used in treating a primary sarcoma. Even following a clean resection of the desmoid, the recurrence rate may approach 50%. For this reason, it is common to administer 50 Gy of radiation to the surgical site starting 2 weeks postoperatively. With radiation therapy, the recurrence rate decreases to 15%. In rare cases an amputation may be necessary after multiple recurrences. A few cases of spontaneous involution of desmoid tumors have been reported after 40 years of age.

Based on clinical and experimental evidence, estrogen may play a role in the development of desmoid tumors. Accordingly, agents such as tamoxifen are being utilized in some centers because of their antiestrogen effects. Nonsteroidal anti-inflammatories have also been implemented in attempts to treat aggressive cases. In selected patients with progressive disease, low-dose vinblastine and methotrexate chemotherapy may be used.

Benign Tumors of Peripheral Nerves

Benign tumors of peripheral nerve sheaths are common and take their origin from Schwann cells, which normally produces myelin and collagen fiber.

A. NEURILEMOMA

The neurilemoma (neurinoma or benign schwannoma) is the least common of the benign tumors of peripheral nerve sheaths. It usually affects individuals between the ages of 20 and 50 years and occurs with equal frequency in men and women. It has a predilection for spinal roots and for superficial nerves on the flexor surfaces of both upper and lower extremities. In most cases, the lesion is solitary, but multiple lesions are occasionally seen in von Recklinghausen's disease. The neurinoma is slow-growing and rarely causes pain or a neurologic deficit.

Unlike the neurofibroma, which has a fusiform appearance, the neurilemoma is round (Figure 6–59). Microscopic studies reveal the presence of a characteristic Verocay body, which consists of palisading Schwann cells and is found in the fibrotic Antoni A substance of the tumor. Other areas will reveal a more mucinous Antoni B substance. Neurilemomas may occur in an axial fashion involving spinal roots, often presenting as a dumbbell-shaped extradural defect (Figure 6–60). In comparison with the less restricted peripheral lesions, the nerve root lesions are more apt to cause pain associated with neurologic deficiency because of their bony constriction.

In some cases, simple excision of the neurilemoma is clinically indicated. This often can be performed without serious damage to the nerve. If the patient is asymptomatic, observation is appropriate because there is little chance for malignant degeneration.

B. SOLITARY NEUROFIBROMA

The solitary neurofibroma is a fusiform fibrotic tumor arising centrally from a smaller peripheral nerve (Figure 6–61). The tumor is seen with equal frequency in men and women, usually between the ages of 20 and 30 years.

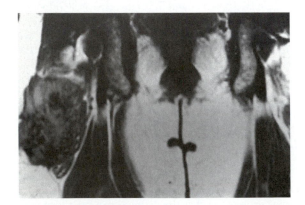

Figure 6–58. T$_1$-weighted MRI of a desmoid tumor in the gluteal area of a 45-year-old woman.

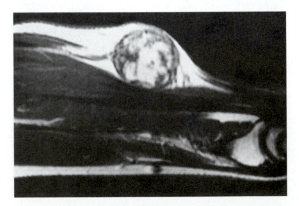

Figure 6–59. T$_1$-weighted MRI of a neurilemoma of the ulnar nerve in a 69-year-old man.

It is 10 times more common than the multiple form seen in von Recklinghausen's disease, is usually smaller, and carries less chance of malignant degeneration. Microscopic examination of the solitary neurofibroma shows interlacing bundles of elongated spindle cells with benign-appearing nuclei and occasionally with areas resembling the Antoni A tissue seen in the neurilemoma.

Treatment of the solitary neurofibroma consists of simple excision.

C. NEUROFIBROMATOSIS (VON RECKLINGHAUSEN'S DISEASE)

This is a familial dysplasia, inherited as an autosomal-dominant trait, with an incidence of about 1 in every 3000 live births. The disease usually begins during the first few years of life with the emergence of small café au lait spots. Over time, these lesions grow in number and size. Unlike the lesions seen in fibrous dysplasia, the lesions in von Recklinghausen's disease do not have rough edges. If a patient has more than six lesions that have smooth edges and are greater than 1.5 cm in diameter, the diagnosis of von Recklinghausen's disease is certain.

Later in life, the patient develops multiple neurofibromas, each of which appears as a soft cutaneous nodule (Figure 6–62). This pedunculated skin lesion,

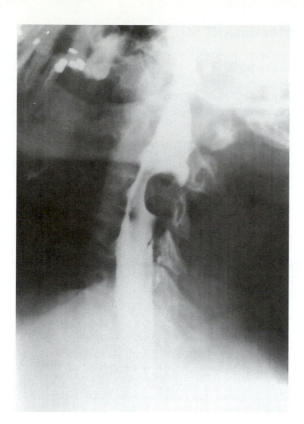

Figure 6–60. Myelogram of a neurilemoma in the cervical spine.

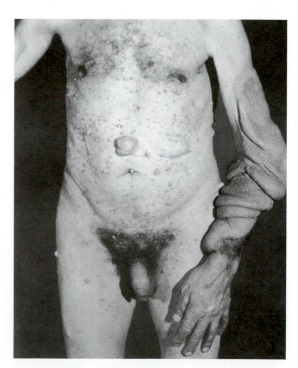

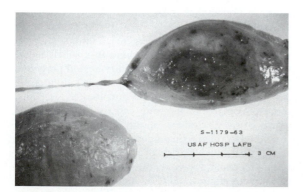

Figure 6–61. Photographic appearance of a solitary neurofibroma.

Figure 6–62. Cutaneous manifestations of neurofibromatosis.

which is called fibroma molluscum, can be large and pendulous. More pathognomonic of the disease is the plexiform neurofibroma, which appears in larger nerves and can involve an entire extremity (see Figure 6–62). When the overlying skin of an extremity is loose and hyperpigmented the condition is called elephantiasis neuromatosa, or "elephant man syndrome." (It is now thought that John Merrick, the "Elephant Man," was actually affected by Proteus syndrome.) Among the bony changes that can be seen in von Recklinghausen's disease are angular scoliosis, spinal meningocele, scalloping of the vertebra, pseudarthrosis of the tibia, and osteolytic lesions in bone.

A major threat to the patient's life is that a malignant schwannoma will develop from one of the large and deep neurofibromas. This occurs at a later age in 3–5% of patients.

Intramuscular Myxomas

The intramuscular myxoma is a rare tumor that is seen in patients past 40 years of age affecting the large muscles about the thighs, shoulders, buttocks, and arms. It is a slow-growing well-marginated tumor that has the gelatinous physical quality of a ganglion cyst or myxoid liposarcoma. The intramuscular myxoma causes no pain and can grow to greater than 15 cm in diameter. Although it appears radiolucent on CT scan, MRI demonstrates an intermediate signal on the T_1-weighted image and an extremely high signal on the T_2-weighted image. Multiple myxomas have been associated with polyostotic fibrous dysplasia.

The intramuscular myxoma can be resected marginally. After this procedure, the recurrence rate is extremely low.

Azzarelli A et al: Low-dose chemotherapy with methotrexate and vinblastine for patients with advanced aggressive fibromatosis. Cancer 2001;92(5):1259. [PMID: 11571741]

Bertario L et al: Genotype and phenotype factors as determinants of desmoid tumors in patients with familial adenomatous polyposis. Int J Cancer 2001;95(2):102. [PMID: 11241320]

Chun YS et al: Lipoblastoma. J Pediatr Surg 2001;36(6):905. [PMID: 11381423]

Kang HJ et al: Schwannomas of the upper extremity. J Hand Surg [Br] 2000;25(6):604. [PMID: 11106529]

Richards KA et al: The pulsed dye laser for cutaneous vascular and nonvascular lesions. Semin Cutan Med Surg 2000;19(4):276. [PMID: 11149608]

Shields CJ et al: Desmoid tumours. Eur J Surg Oncol 2001;27(8):701. [PMID: 11735163]

Sorensen SA et al: Long-term follow-up of von Recklinghausen neurofibromatosis: Survival and malignant neoplasms. N Engl J Med 1986;314:1010. [PMID: 3083258]

Vikkula M et al: Molecular genetics of vascular malformations. Matrix Biol 2001;20(5-6):327. [PMID: 11566267]

MALIGNANT SOFT-TISSUE TUMORS

Sarcomas are capable of invasive, locally destructive growth with a tendency to recur and to metastasize. All sarcomas do not behave the same, however. Some sarcomas such as dermatofibrosarcoma protuberans rarely metastasize. Malignant fibrous histiocytoma, in contrast, does so with alacrity.

A. FIBROHISTIOCYTIC TUMORS

The most common soft-tissue sarcomas seen in adults is malignant fibrous histiocytoma (MFH) (Figure 6–63). Strangely, although more frequently encountered than other adult soft-tissue sarcomas, the cell type(s) of origin remain unclear. Current debate is centered on whether MFH is a distinct entity or a diverse group of sarcomas that on histologic evaluation appear similar. At present, four main subtypes of MFH are accepted: (1) storiform-pleomorphic, (2) myxoid, (3) giant cell, and (4) inflammatory. Angiomatoid fibrous histiocytoma, a low-grade lesion seen in children is now considered a benign entity.

1. Storiform pleomorphic—Storiform pleomorphic is the most common subtype of MFH. It occurs more frequently in men than in women, primarily affecting individuals between the ages of 50 and 70 years. Usually it is a deep lesion found in the large muscles about the thigh, hip, and retroperitoneal areas. The tumor may be asymptomatic.

On gross examination, the tumor appears multinodular and may demonstrate several separate satellite lesions in the same muscle belly, especially at the superior and interior poles. It may be necrotic and ranges in color from dirty gray to a reddish tan. Microscopy demonstrates that it is composed of malignant fibroblasts mixed with anaplastic and pleomorphic histiocytes.

The prognosis and treatment vary, depending on the size and location of the tumor. The overall local recurrence potential is 45%, with a 40% incidence of metastasis to the lung and with a 10% incidence of regional lymph node involvement. Tumors that are under 5 cm in diameter and found in a subcutaneous location in the distal body parts carry a good prognosis, with a 5-year survival rate of 80%, whereas tumors that are 5 cm or more in diameter and located deep in a more proximal muscle group carry a poor prognosis, with a 5-year survival rate of only 55%.

Although the treatment depends on the clinical situation, it generally consists of an aggressive, wide resection after careful preoperative staging, including an MRI of the primary and CT scan of the chest. Amputation is rare, with limb salvage possible in the majority of cases.

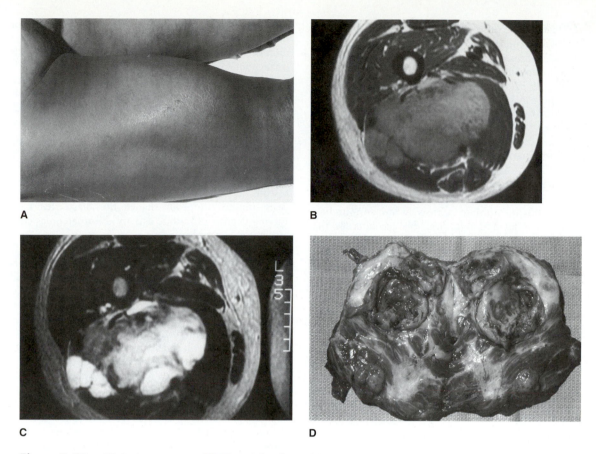

Figure 6–63. Clinical appearance (**A**), T$_1$-weighted MRI (**B**), T$_2$-weighted MRI (**C**), and resected surgical specimen (**D**) of a large pleomorphic malignant fibrous histiocytoma in the posterior thigh of a 55-year-old man.

The use of adjuvant radiation therapy is important in reducing the local recurrence rate. Most clinicians administer 55 Gy to a wide area, followed by a boost to 65 Gy aimed at the surgical site. An attempt is made to leave a longitudinal strip of tissue out of the field of radiation to reduce the chance of postirradiation edema distal to the treatment site. Some centers advocate preoperative and postoperative radiation with 50 Gy given before resection and about 15 Gy postoperatively. Some institutions employ preoperative radiation exclusively. Local recurrence rates are generally between 5–25%.

The use of adjuvant chemotherapy is more controversial. Because there are limited data to suggest that chemotherapy results in a significant improvement in survival and because most patients are older individuals who cannot tolerate the high-dose protocols, medical oncologists are divided on whether to advocate the use of chemotherapeutic agents in the treatment of MFH.

2. Myxoid—The myxoid type is the second most common type of MFH and is seen in the same age group of patients and the same locations as the pleomorphic type. On gross examination, myxoid MFH has a multinodular and translucent or gelatinous appearance similar to the appearance of a myxoid liposarcoma or a benign myxoma of muscle. Because of its gelatinous nature, myxoid MFH has a greater chance for local contamination and thus has a higher local recurrence rate than pleomorphic MFH. However, the metastasis rate in cases of myxoid MFH is about 25%.

3. Giant cell—The giant cell type of MFH also affects older patients and is seen in large muscle groups, but it is hemorrhagic in nature and carries a 50% chance of pulmonary metastasis.

4. Inflammatory—The inflammatory type of MFH affects the older age groups, is more common in the retroperitoneal areas, and has a 50% metastasis rate.

B. Dermatofibrosarcoma Protuberans

This low- to intermediate-grade fibrohistiocytic tumor is unique because of its nodular cutaneous location. It is seen more commonly in males than females and occurs in young or middle-aged adults. It is typically located about the trunk and proximal extremities. Antecedent trauma is recorded in 10–20% of cases. Dermatofibrosarcoma protuberans begins as a painless subcutaneous nodule or nodules and slowly develops into an elevated multinodular plaque (Figure 6–64). Microscopic examination of the lesion reveals the same storiform or basket-weave pattern of a benign or malignant fibrous histiocytoma but with a very low mitotic index. The pattern tends to infiltrate extensively into surrounding subcutaneous fat and skin, and this accounts for the high local recurrence rate, which is sometimes reported to approach 50%.

Characteristic cytogenetic abnormalities have been described with characteristic features such as reciprocal t(17;22)(q22;q13) or, more commonly, supernumerary ring chromosomes containing sequences from chromosomes 17 and 22.

Surgical treatment, consisting of an aggressive resection, is associated with a lower recurrence rate of 20%. Because of the low mitotic index, radiation therapy is not usually indicated and the chance of pulmonary metastasis is only 1%.

C. Fibrosarcoma

Fifty years ago, fibrosarcoma was considered the most common of the soft-tissue sarcomas, secondary to imprecise pathologic classification of MFH, certain liposarcomas, rhabdomyosarcoma, leiomyosarcomas, and malignant peripheral nerve sheath tumors. Currently, fibrosarcoma is considered one of the least common soft-tissue sarcomas. The diagnosis is reserved for those tumors in which the histology demonstrates a uniform fasciculated growth pattern of spindle cells (malignant fibroblasts). It is clinically similar to MFH, occurs with nearly equal frequency in men and women, is found in patients between 30 and 55 years of age, is sometimes slow-growing and painless, and tends to affect deep fascial structures of muscle about the knee and thigh, followed next by the forearm and leg.

On gross examination, fibrosarcoma appears as a firm and lobulated lesion that has a yellowish white to tan color. The lesion may demonstrate a few calcific or osseous deposits on radiographic exam. Microscopy reveals spindle, uniformly shaped fibroblasts that have varying degrees of mitotic activity. Fibrosarcomas contain no malignant histiocytes.

The treatment and prognosis depend on the grade of tumor in a particular patient. Low-grade fibrosarcoma is nearly the same tumor as a benign desmoid tumor and has an extremely low rate of metastasis. However, high-grade fibrosarcoma requires an aggressive wide surgical resection, along with radiation therapy, and has a pulmonary metastasis rate of 50–60%. Lymph node involvement is rare. The use of chemotherapy is considered controversial in patients with fibrosarcoma, as it is in patients with MFH.

D. Liposarcomas

Liposarcoma is the second most common soft-tissue sarcoma after MFH. Like MFH, liposarcoma is a tumor of older patients and can be large and deep-seated. Four types of liposarcoma are discussed in the following sections. The well-differentiated type and the myxoid type are associated with a low chance for lung metastasis, whereas the round cell and the pleomorphic types tend to behave in a more aggressive fashion.

1. Well-differentiated liposarcoma—This very low grade tumor affects individuals who are 40–60 years old and occurs more frequently in men than in women. It grows extremely slowly and reaches a large size without causing pain. The deep-seated tumor is found in the retroperitoneum, buttock, or thigh. In some cases of well-differentiated liposarcoma, findings will include inflammation and sclerosis.

On gross examination, this tumor has a fatty lobulated appearance similar to a benign lipoma. Even under the microscope, many large areas of the tumor will appear benign. However, with proper sampling, the pathologist will find a few areas of lipoblast activity to suggest the diagnosis of a liposarcoma. MRI findings are sometimes difficult to distinguish from a large, deep lipoma (Figure 6–65).

In cases of well-differentiated liposarcoma, a conservative, wide resection is performed to avoid local recur-

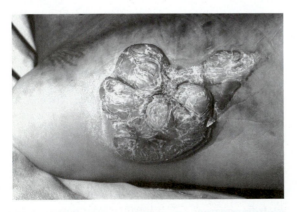

Figure 6–64. Clinical appearance of dermatofibrosarcoma protuberans on the bottom of the heel of a 30-year-old man.

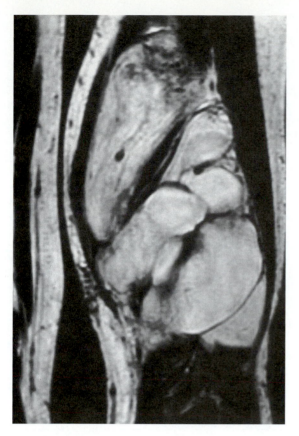

Figure 6–65. T$_1$-weighted MRI of a well-differentiated liposarcoma in the thigh of a 63-year-old man.

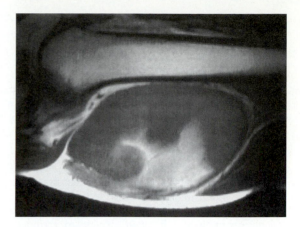

Figure 6–66. Sagittal view T$_1$-weighted MRI of a myxoid liposarcoma in the thigh of a 32-year-old man.

rence. Adjuvant radiation therapy is not helpful, and chemotherapy is never used. The chance of metastatic disease is very low, and the prognosis for survival is excellent.

2. Myxoid liposarcoma—Myxoid liposarcoma is the most common fat sarcoma, accounting for 40–50% of all liposarcomas. The myxoid type is low to intermediate grade and is seen in older patients. The clinical presentation is similar to the well-differentiated liposarcoma.

Gross examination of a myxoid liposarcoma reveals a lobulated pattern with some areas that appear similar to those of a lipoma but with other myxomatous areas. Microscopic examination shows myxoid tissue with areas of signet ring lipoblasts. It is common to find a delicate pattern of capillaries running through the myxoid areas. MRI frequently demonstrates a heterogeneous high- and low-signal pattern that is typical of myxoid liposarcoma but is not present in cases of benign lipoma (Figure 6–66).

Characteristic translocations have also been seen in myxoid liposarcoma. The predominant type is t(12;16)(q13;p11) however t(12;22)(q13;q12) has also been described.

Multifocal myxoid liposarcoma has also been described. Consideration for additional advanced axial imaging should be entertained with this histologic subtype.

Although myxoid liposarcoma carries a very good prognosis, the tumor should be removed with wide margins, and adjuvant radiation therapy should be given. Chemotherapy is not indicated.

3. Round cell and pleomorphic liposarcoma— These high-grade liposarcomas are seen in the same locations and age group as the well-differentiated and myxoid subtypes. But unlike the latter, the round cell and pleomorphic types are fast-growing tumors that may be painful.

In cases of round cell or pleomorphic liposarcoma, the lesion does not have a fatty appearance on gross examination but instead looks more like an MFH or a fibrosarcoma. Moreover, on MRI, the lesion appears more like an MFH, with a low-signal pattern in the T$_1$-weighted image and a high-signal pattern in the T$_2$-weighted image. Microscopically, the round cell type of liposarcoma shows areas of uniformly shaped round cells similar to those found in Ewing's sarcoma or lymphoma and also shows areas of myxoid tissue. In the pleomorphic type of liposarcoma, large and bizarre giant cells occur similar to those found in the pleomorphic type of MFH and rhabdomyosarcoma.

In round cell and pleomorphic liposarcoma, there is an early and high rate of pulmonary metastasis. Accordingly, the prognosis for survival is poor. Thus, the treatment should include aggressive resection, adjuvant radiation therapy as necessary, and chemotherapy in selected patients.

E. Rhabdomyosarcomas

Rhabdomyosarcomas account for 20% of all soft-tissue sarcomas. The embryonal and alveolar types of rhabdomyosarcoma affect pediatric patients, and the rarer pleomorphic type affects adults.

1. Embryonal rhabdomyosarcoma—The embryonal type is seen in patients from birth to 15 years of age and is encountered more frequently in boys than in girls. It is most common in the head and neck area. The so-called botryoid form is seen as a cluster of grapes under mucous membranes in the vagina, bladder, or retroperitoneal area. Histologically, it is a round cell tumor like Ewing's sarcoma, but some rhabdomyoblasts with cross striations are present in a few area.

Embryonal rhabdomyosarcoma is treated with local surgical resection plus preoperative and postoperative chemotherapy consisting of vincristine, dactinomycin, cyclophosphamide, and doxorubicin given in cyclic courses during a 2-year span. If the surgical margins are contaminated, local radiation therapy is used. With this program, the 5-year survival rate is 80%. Prior to the advent of chemotherapy, it was only 10%.

2. Alveolar rhabdomyosarcoma—This type of rhabdomyosarcoma affects individuals between the ages of 10 and 25 years and is found more commonly in males than in females. Besides affecting the head and neck, it can be seen in the extremities, especially the thigh and calf. Microscopic examination of the lesion reveals a typical alveolar pattern of round cells, with fewer rhabdomyoblasts seen in this type of rhabdomyosarcoma than in the embryonal type. This type of rhabdomyosarcoma is associated with the fusion genes PAX3-FKHR and PAX7-FKHR. Although not definitive, the presence of the translocation t(2;13)/PAX3-FKHR may be an adverse prognostic factor, with molecular screening being implemented in the future. Currently, he treatment is the same as for the embryonal type, but the prognosis is a bit worse.

3. Pleomorphic rhabdomyosarcoma—In the 1940s, pleomorphic rhabdomyosarcoma was a popular histologic diagnosis and MFH was a rare one. Based on today's criteria, most of the old cases classified as pleomorphic rhabdomyosarcoma would now be classified as MFH. Currently, the pleomorphic type of rhabdomyosarcoma is the rarest type.

Pleomorphic rhabdomyosarcoma is a high-grade tumor that affects middle-aged and older adults and is seen most commonly in the large muscle groups of the proximal extremities, usually the lower extremities. Microscopic examination of the tumor reveals large, atypical giant cells, along with racket- or tad-pole-shaped malignant rhabdomyoblasts that stain positive for glycogen, actin, and myosin. The tumor carries a poor prognosis and is associated with a high rate of metastasis to the lung. The treatment for pleomorphic rhabdomyosarcoma is similar to that for MFH and consists of a wide local resection and adjuvant radiation therapy. Chemotherapy is rarely indicated.

F. Leiomyosarcoma

Leiomyosarcoma is a very rare soft-tissue tumor whose cell type of origin is smooth muscle. It is seen in the middle-aged adult and is much more common in women than in men. Its usual locations, in order of frequency are retroperitoneal, intra-abdominal, cutaneous, and subcutaneous. In some cases, the lesion has a venous wall origin and is found in the vena cava or large vessels of the leg. On microscopic examination, leiomyosarcoma can demonstrate a palisading, orderly fascicular pattern similar to a malignant schwannoma. A specific immunohistochemical staining for actin may be helpful in the differential diagnosis.

The prognosis and the treatment for leiomyosarcoma are similar to those for fibrosarcoma. However, leiomyosarcomas of venous wall origin have a worse prognosis because they are difficult to resect and have a high rate of pulmonary metastasis.

G. Synovial Sarcomas

Synovial sarcoma (Figure 6–67) is the fourth most common soft-tissue sarcoma. It is seen in young adults between 15 and 35 years of age and affects males slightly more than females. The name of this tumor suggests a synovial cell origin, but only 10% of synovial sarcomas are found in a major joint. Nevertheless, they frequently arise from juxta-articular structures, especially around the knee, and can also arise from tendon sheaths, bursal sacs, fascial planes, and deep muscles. Synovial sarcomas can be seen about the shoulder, arm, elbow, and wrist and are the most common soft-tissue sarcoma in the foot.

Synovial sarcomas initially grow slowly and cause pain in about half of the affected patients. The tumors may appear after an injury, and because dystrophic calcification or even heterotopic bone formation is seen in half of the cases, the tumors are assumed to be a benign process for 2–4 years before a diagnostic biopsy is performed.

Microscopic examination of the tumor shows a typical biphasic pattern composed of epithelium-like cells that form nests, clefts, or tubular structures surrounded by malignant fibroblastic spindle cells. The epithelium-like cells produce a mucinous material that has suggested a synovial cell origin, although this origin is un-

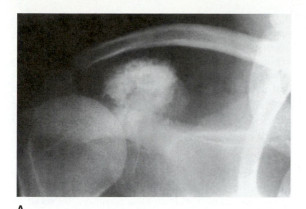

A

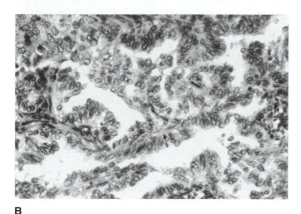

B

Figure 6–67. Radiograph (**A**) and microscopic appearance (**B**) of a synovial sarcoma in the shoulder of a 20-year-old woman.

likely. A monophasic form of synovial sarcoma has been described and is reported to consist of a dominant fibroblastic or epithelial cell pattern. If the lesion shows no biphasic component, however, it is difficult to confirm the diagnosis of synovial sarcoma.

Molecular characterization of this tumor has revealed a particular translocation, t(X;18) representing the fusion of SYT (at 18q11) with either SSX1 or SSX2 (both at Xp11). Both SYT and SSX appear to be transcription regulation factors whose fusion product is seen in the majority of synovial sarcomas.

Despite the slow growth of synovial sarcoma, the 5-year and 10-year survival rates are only 50% and 25%, respectively. In cases in which the tumors are heavily calcified, the 5-year survival rate is 80%. Because of the poor prognosis, the treatment plan should include aggressive wide resection, along with both radiation therapy and chemotherapy. Lymph node involvement is seen in 20% of affected patients and

might require a surgical excision followed by local radiation therapy.

H. Malignant Peripheral Nerve Sheath Tumor

A malignant peripheral nerve sheath tumor can arise from a pre-existing benign solitary neurofibroma but more frequently arises from the multiple lesions of neurofibromatosis type 1. In both cases, the tumor mass is usually larger than 5 cm in diameter and may arise from a large deep neurogenic structure such as the sciatic nerve (Figure 6–68) or one of the spinal roots. Smaller nerves, even cutaneous branches, however, can give rise to these sarcomas. Malignant degeneration from a solitary neurofibroma usually occurs after age 40 years with a 5-year survival rate of 75%. In contrast, patients whose schwannoma arose from the lesions of neurofibromatosis type 1 are generally younger and have a 5-year survival rate of 30%. Surgical treatment consists

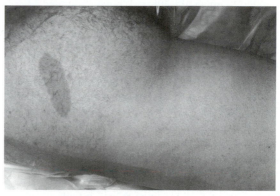

A

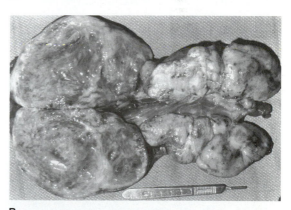

B

Figure 6–68. Clinical appearance of a café au lait defect in the skin overlying a malignant schwannoma in the buttock area of a 42-year-old man (**A**), and gross appearance of the tumor in resected sciatic nerve (**B**).

of a wide resection if possible. Adjuvant radiation and chemotherapy are used in selected cases.

I. MALIGNANT VASCULAR TUMORS

l. Kaposi's sarcoma—Of the malignant vascular tumors, Kaposi's sarcoma is the most common with four specific subtypes: (1) chronic, (2) lymphadenopathic, (3) transplant-associated, (4) AIDS-related. It is found directly beneath the skin, generally in the lower extremity of adults, is seen more often in men than in women, and is endemic in central Africa. The cutaneous lesions seen frequently in the foot and ankle area are purplish in color and are nodular (Figure 6–69). Microscopic examination of Kaposi's sarcoma shows an aggressive vascular pattern with rare mitosis. However, over a period of many years, the tumor will progress into a full-blown angiosarcoma or fibrosarcoma. It is associated with acquired immunodeficiency syndrome (AIDS) and other immunosuppressive disorders and can also be seen with lymphomas and multiple myeloma. Although the behavior of Kaposi's sarcoma is a function of the immunologic status of the patient and other variables, the overall mortality rate is 10–20%.

2. Angiosarcoma—Soft-tissue angiosarcoma is rare, accounting for less than 1% of all sarcomas. Although angiosarcomas are usually cutaneous lesions and tend to affect men more than women, they sometimes take the form of a deep tumor and they are typically seen in the upper extremities of women who have chronic lymphedema following radical breast surgery and radiation therapy. Histologic examination of angiosarcoma shows anaplastic endothelial cells surrounded by reticulum fiber. Prognosis for the older patient is poor. Smaller lesions in younger patients have a distinctively better outcome. The treatment is wide resection, sometimes with radiation therapy.

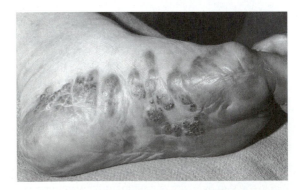

Figure 6–69. Clinical appearance of Kaposi's sarcoma of the foot.

3. Hemangiopericytoma—This rare perivascular tumor arises from pericytes. Pericytes are highly arborized perivascular cells that line capillaries and venules. The lesion affects male and female adults with equal frequency, is usually found deep in muscle bellies, and is generally located in the thigh or retroperitoneal area of the pelvis. Microscopic examination of the malignant hemangiopericytoma reveals tightly packed cells with round nuclei with moderate amounts of cytoplasm with poorly defined borders. The bifurcating sinusoidal vessels have a typical "staghorn" appearance. Cytogenetic analysis has revealed multiple chromosome translocations including t(12:19) and t(13:22). Treatment consists of a wide surgical resection, followed by local radiation therapy. Some authors recommend preoperative embolization or afferent vessel ligation (or both) intraoperatively.

MISCELLANEOUS SOFT-TISSUE SARCOMAS

The remaining soft-tissue sarcomas are rare and only a brief description of their clinical patterns will be summarized.

A. SOFT-TISSUE CHONDROSARCOMA

There are three types of soft-tissue chondrosarcomas.

1. Myxoid chondrosarcoma—The myxoid chondrosarcoma is sometimes referred to as a chordoid sarcoma because it looks like a chordoma. It is a slow-growing tumor that is seen in adults, usually in deep structure of the leg. It has a myxoid appearance, does not calcify, and is low-grade. Like the chordoma, the myxoid chondrosarcoma responds only to surgical removal.

2. Mesenchymal chondrosarcoma—This tumor affects individuals between 15 and 40 years of age, is found deep in the lower extremity and neck areas, is fast-growing, and carries a poor prognosis because of the high risk of pulmonary metastasis. Calcification may be seen on radiograph, and microscopic examination reveals round cells scattered in a chondroid matrix. Treatment consists of a wide resection in conjunction with chemotherapy and radiation therapy.

3. Synovial chondrosarcoma—The conversion of a synovial chondromatosis to a malignant synovial chondrosarcoma is an extremely rare phenomenon. It can occur with lesions of the hip or knee region in older adults.

B. EWING'S SARCOMA

Extraskeletal Ewing's sarcoma can be found in individuals between the ages of 10 and 30 years and is usually located in the paravertebral area, thorax, or deep muscle area of the lower extremity. It is a fast-growing tumor with minimal pain symptoms. It carries the same prognosis as its counterpart in bone and is treated with the same combination of surgery, chemotherapy, and radiation therapy.

C. ALVEOLAR SOFT PART SARCOMA

This round cell sarcoma affects more females than males, is usually found in patients between the ages of 15 and 35 years, and arises in the deep muscle tissue of the lower extremity, usually the thigh. Alveolar soft part sarcoma is a slow-growing tumor but carries a poor prognosis because of early pulmonary metastasis. The tumor has increased vascularity and is thought to originate from a neurogenic stem cell. It derives its name from its alveolar pattern, which is seen on microscopic examination and can cause this tumor to be mistaken for an alveolar form of rhabdomyosarcoma. A cytogenetic, unbalanced abnormality, t(x;17)(p11.2;q25) has been described. Treatment of alveolar soft part sarcoma consists of a wide surgical resection plus radiation therapy and chemotherapy.

D. EPITHELIOID SARCOMA

Although this superficial skin lesion is seen most commonly in the palm of the hand, it can also be found on the dorsum of the forearm or on the plantar aspect of the foot. It is a slow-growing tumor that affects patients between the ages of 20 and 30 years, causes minimal pain symptoms, and is associated with ulceration.

Because epithelioid sarcoma has a whitish color that under the microscope demonstrates cords of epithelium-like cells, it can be mistaken for a synovial sarcoma. Moreover, because of its firm multilobulated presentation, the epithelioid sarcoma may be mistaken for a plantar of palmar fibromatosis (Figure 6–70).

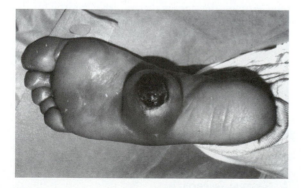

Figure 6–70. Clinical appearance of epithelioid sarcoma on the plantar aspect of the foot of a 36-year-old man.

Epithelioid sarcoma spreads as a lumpy nodularity along tendon sheaths or fascial planes and frequently involves local lymph nodes. Local surgical resection is followed by a high local recurrence rate, and a late pulmonary metastasis is common. For this reason, early treatment should consist of an aggressive wide surgical resection.

E. CLEAR CELL SARCOMA

The clear cell sarcoma is thought to be a deep, noncutaneous variant of the well-known cutaneous melanoma. It is extremely rare, affects women more often than men, and commonly occurs between the ages of 20 and 40 years. It arises in tendon sheaths and fascial planes, most frequently in the foot and ankle but also in the knee and arm. Clear cell sarcoma starts slowly as a painless lump and has a high potential to spread to local lymph nodes. The lesion in many cases will demonstrate evidence of melanin and melanosomes and may be of neural crest origin. The microscopic clear cell appearance can cause this sarcoma to be confused with epithelioid sarcoma and synovial sarcoma.

The prognosis is poor because of a high rate of pulmonary metastasis. This tumor may spread via lymphatics as well. Treatment consists of early aggressive wide resection and may include chemotherapy and local radiation therapy.

Ahmad SA et al: Extraosseous osteosarcoma: Response to treatment and long-term outcome. J Clin Oncol 2002;20(2):521. [PMID: 11786582]

Anderson J et al: Detection of the PAX3-FKHR fusion gene in paediatric rhabdomyosarcoma: A reproducible predictor of outcome? Br J Cancer 2001;85(6):831. [PMID: 11556833]

Antonescu CR et al: Monoclonality of multifocal myxoid liposarcoma: Confirmation by analysis of TLS-CHOP or EWS-CHOP rearrangements. Clin Cancer Res 2000;6:2788. [PMID: 10914725]

Bowne WB et al: Dermatofibrosarcoma protuberans: A clinicopathologic analysis of patients treated and followed at a single institution. Cancer 2000;88(12):2711. [PMID: 10870053]

Cormier JN et al: Concurrent ifosfamide-based chemotherapy and irradiation. Analysis of treatment-related toxicity in 43 patients with sarcoma. Cancer 2001;92(6):1550. [PMID: 11745234]

Dei Tos AP: Liposarcoma: New entities and evolving concepts. Ann Diagn Pathol 2000;4(4):252. [PMID: 10982304]

dos Santos NR et al: Molecular mechanisms underlying human synovial sarcoma development. Genes Chromosomes Cancer 2001;30(1):1. [PMID: 11107170]

Gibbs J et al: Malignant fibrous histiocytoma: An institutional review. Cancer Invest 2001;19(1):23. [PMID: 11291552]

Hayes-Jordan AA et al: Nonrhabdomyosarcoma soft tissue sarcomas in children: Is age at diagnosis an important variable? J Pediatr Surg 2000;35(6):948-53; discussion 953. [PMID: 10873042]

Ladanyi M: Fusions of the SYT and SSX genes in synovial sarcoma. Oncogene 2001;20(40):5755. [PMID: 11607825]

Meis-Kindblom JM et al: Cytogenetic and molecular genetic analyses of liposarcoma and its soft tissue simulators: Recognition of new variants and differential diagnosis. Virchows Arch 2001;439(2):141. [PMID: 11561754]

Nishio J et al: Supernumerary ring chromosomes in dermatofibrosarcoma protuberans may contain sequences from 8q11.2-qter and 17q21-qter: A combined cytogenetic and comparative genomic hybridization study. Cancer Genet Cytogenet 2001;129(2):102. [PMID: 11566338]

Orvieto E et al: Myxoid and round cell liposarcoma: A spectrum of myxoid adipocytic neoplasia. Semin Diagn Pathol 2001;18:267. [PMID 11757867]

Spillane AJ et al: Synovial sarcoma: A clinicopathologic, staging, and prognostic assessment. J Clin Oncol 200015;18(22):3794. [PMID: 11078492]

MANAGEMENT OF CARCINOMA METASTASIZED TO BONE

Incidence & Natural History of Metastases

A. COMMON METASTATIC CARCINOMAS AND AREAS OF SKELETAL INVOLVEMENT

Metastatic involvement of the musculoskeletal system is one of the most significant clinical issues facing orthopedic oncologists. The number of patients with metastasis to the skeletal system from a carcinoma is 15 times greater than the number of patients with primary bone tumors of all types. Approximately one third of all diagnosed adenocarcinomas will include skeletal metastases resulting in about 300,000 cases per year. Furthermore, 70% of patients with advanced, terminal carcinoma will demonstrate bone metastases at autopsy. The carcinomas that commonly metastasize to bone are prostate, breast, kidney, thyroid, and lung carcinomas. One study showed that nearly 90% of patients with these types of carcinoma had bone metastases. Among the carcinomas that less commonly metastasize to bone are cancers of the skin, oral cavity, esophagus, cervix, stomach, and colon.

The spine is the most frequent area of bone metastasis. Other common skeletal sites include the pelvis, femur, rib, proximal humerus, and skull, in that order. Metastatic lesions are rarely found distal to the elbow or knee. If lesions are found in these areas, the lung is the most common source. Solitary bone lesions comprise only approximately 10% of cases of bone metastasis.

B. CLINICAL COURSE OF METASTASES

The mechanism of metastases is accounted for in a modified "seed/soil" theorem. Less then one in 10 thousand neoplastic cells that escape into the circulation from the primary site are able to set up a metastatic focus. This is a complex multistep process by which the cell must first break free. This is a function of *degradative* enzymes such as collagenases, hydrolases, cathepsin D, and proteases. Once the cell invades the vascular channel it circulates through the body. It is theorized that the cell is protected by a fibrin platelet clot. However, clinical trials with heparin have not shown a significant change in metastatic outcome. Local factors such as integrins are instrumental in attracting the circulating metastatic cell to a particular remote tissue site. Once within the new tissue, the metastatic cell releases factors such as tumor angiogenesis factor inducing neovascularization, which in turn facilitates growth of the metastatic focus.

Patients with advanced metastatic disease frequently experience dysfunction of their hematopoietic and calcium homeostases systems. Patients may develop a normochromic, normocytic anemia with leukocytosis. In response to the anemia, the increased production of immature cells is noted on the peripheral blood smear. This is termed "leukoerythroblastic" reaction. Hypercalcemia may result in up to 30% of cases with extensive metastases. This is most frequently seen in myeloma, breast cancer and non-small–cell lung cancer.

Blastic metastases are frequently painless and are associated with a lower incidence of pathologic fracture because the bone is not as severely weakened (Figures 6–71 and 6–72). Not all tumors that metastasize from the prostate to the bone are blastic in nature. The lytic variants are painful and can cause pathologic fractures.

Most tumors that metastasize from the breast to the bone are blastic, but some demonstrate mixtures of blastic and lytic areas in the same bone. By taking serial radiographs and noting the appearance of bone metastases, it is possible to follow the progress of treatment consisting of systemic therapy with hormones or chemotherapeutic agents plus local radiation therapy. A favorable response may show a gradual conversion from a lytic to a blastic appearance as the pain decreases.

Bone destruction in lytic lesions is a response by native osteoclasts to the tumor. Neovascularity is common. Among the tumors that are characteristic for this hemorrhagic response are thyroid carcinomas (Figure 6–73), renal cell (Figure 6–74), and multiple myeloma. Before a surgical intervention, it is beneficial to perform a prophylactic embolization of the area to reduce perioperative bleeding. If a lesion is unexpectedly found to be aneurysmal at the time of surgical exploration, it is best to debulk the friable tumor mass rapidly down to normal bone and then pack the area until it can be stabilized with bone cement.

Diagnosis

A. GENERAL APPROACH

A methodical approach is mandatory in the workup of a patient with presumed metastatic disease to bone in order to locate the primary tumor. A thorough biopsy and

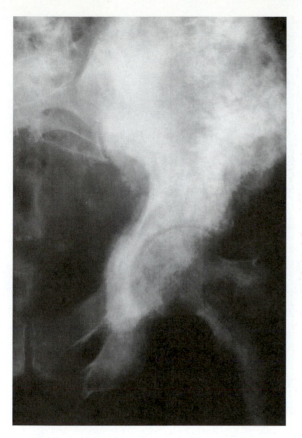

Figure 6–71. Radiograph of a blastic carcinoma that metastasized from the prostate to the pelvis in an 85-year-old man.

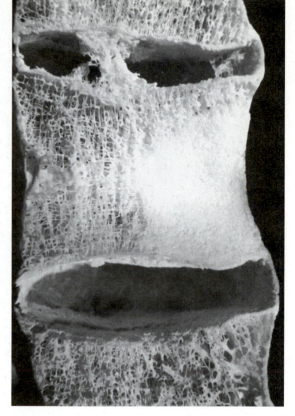

Figure 6–72. Skeletal specimen of a blastic carcinoma that metastasized from the prostate to the lumbar spine.

physical examination must be completed prior to laboratory and radiographic analysis. Eight percent of patients may have their primary carcinoma detected on physical exam. Lab analysis should include complete blood count, erythrocyte sedimentation rate, renal and liver panels, alkaline phosphate, and serum protein electrophoresis.

Radiographic examination should follow with a plain chest radiograph and radiographs of known involved bones. Approximately 45% of primaries will be detected in the lung on the chest radiograph. The workup should also include a staging bone scan. If this is negative, myeloma should be suspected. Furthermore, a lesion at a more convenient biopsy site may be found. Bone scan is also more sensitive than plain radiographs in detecting early lesions. CT scans of the chest, abdomen, and pelvis should be performed. Lung CT can detect up to 15% of primaries missed on the plain radiograph.

These studies in conjunction with a well-planned biopsy will detect the majority of cases. Routine radio-

graphic screening studies in search of early metastatic disease are not very helpful (Figure 6–75). Lytic changes become evident on routine radiographs only when cortical destruction approaches 30–50% (Figure 6–76).

Treatment & Prognosis

A. Nonsurgical Treatment

Nonsurgical management of metastatic carcinoma to bone includes observation, radiation treatment, and hormonal/cytotoxic chemotherapy. Radiation is reserved for palliative management. Each patient must be carefully evaluated as a candidate for radiation therapy. The histologic type of disease, extent of disease, prognosis, marrow reserve, and overall constitution must be assessed.

After sustaining a pathologic fracture secondary to metastatic carcinoma, the average survival time is 19 months. Each histologic type has varying lengths of sur-

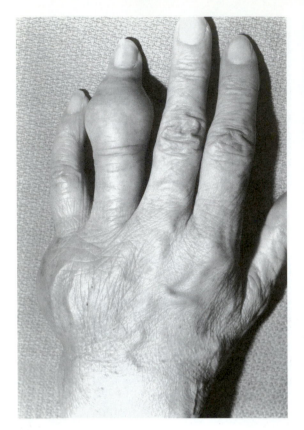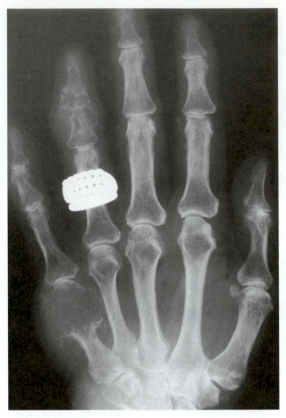

Figure 6–73. Clinical appearance (**A**) and radiographic appearance (**B**) of aneurysmal lesions in a case of carcinoma that metastasized from the thyroid to the hand.

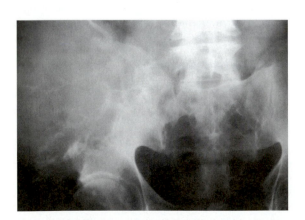

Figure 6–74. Radiograph of a metastatic hypernephroma in the ilium.

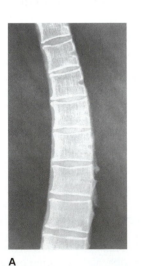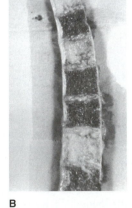

A   B

Figure 6–75. Radiograph (**A**) and gross appearance (**B**) of bone in a case of carcinoma that metastasized from the lung to the spine.

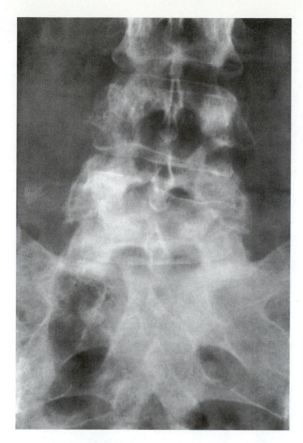

Figure 6–76. Radiograph of the spine of a 45-year-old woman whose cancer had metastasized from the breast.

vival: (Prostate 29 months, breast 23 months, renal 12 months, lung 4 months). Furthermore, each type of carcinoma exhibits varying radiosensitivity. Prostate and lymphoreticular types demonstrate excellent sensitivity. Breast is intermediate, and renal and gastrointestinal are poor. When used, appropriately 90% of patients gain at least minimal relief, with up to two thirds obtaining complete relief. Seventy percent of patients who are ambulatory retain this function after radiation therapy to the lower extremities. Systemic radioisotopes may also be used. Strontium-89 mimics calcium distribution in the body and has shown promise in clinical applications.

When a patient has sustained a true pathologic fixation (rather than an impending lesion) surgical stabilization is usually indicated with subsequent radiation therapy. Because of poor bone quality, augmentation of fixation with bone cement may be necessary.

Hormonal therapy has an important role in the management of metastatic breast and prostate cancer. Fortunately, these agents are easy to administer and have few side effects.

For breast cancer, medical hormonal manipulation can be done by use of antiestrogens, progestins, luteinizing hormone-releasing hormone or adrenal suppressing agents. Tamoxifen is effective in 30% of all breast cancer cases but increases to 50–75% of cases when the tumor is known to be estrogen receptor-, progesterone receptor-positive. Surgical ablation (oophorectomy) may also have a role in certain cases.

For prostate cancer, reduction in testosterone levels via bilateral orchiectomy or administration of estrogens or antiandrogens may produce dramatic results in certain cases. Estrogens are no longer used as a first agent because of the risk of cardiovascular complication.

Cytotoxic chemotherapy is used in adenocarcinoma treatment quite extensively. In older patients with advanced disease, however, the side effects of the drugs may be too severe.

B. SURGICAL TREATMENT

The goals for surgical intervention in the patient with metastatic carcinoma to bone are relief of pain; prevention of impending pathologic fixations; stabilization of true fixations; enhancement of mobility, function, and quality of life; and perhaps improvement of survival. It is generally agreed that a patient must have a life expectancy of at least 6 weeks to warrant operative intervention. Special considerations to surgical management include noting that bone quality is attenuated and healing will be delayed if even possible. Cancer patients, irrespective of their age, may have increased difficulty protecting their fixation device/prothesis secondary to systemic debilitation. Accordingly, rigid fixation, with polymethylmethacrylate (PMMA) augmentation as needed, is mandatory.

1. Hip—Seventy-five percent of all surgery for cancer that has metastasized to bone is performed in the hip area (Figure 6–77). Prior to 1970, surgeons attempted to stabilize these fractures with conventional hip nails or Austin-Moore prostheses, but results were poor because of deficient local bone stock. After 1970, with the advent of bone cement as an adjuvant form of therapy, these same devices could be used, with improved results in most cases, along with local radiation therapy starting 2 weeks after the surgery. This technique allowed for early ambulation with less pain. However, as time passed and survival times increased, more failures were noted after 1–2 years with the hip nail and cement technique. For this reason, most surgeons currently use a cemented bipolar hemiarthroplasty for the femoral neck fractures and a longer stem calcar replacement hemiarthroplasty for the intertrochanteric fractures. Be-

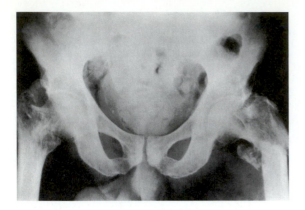

Figure 6–77. Radiograph of the pathologic fractures of both hips in a 55-year-old man with lung carcinoma.

fore these procedures are performed, it is wise to evaluate the entire shaft of the femur and the supra-acetabular area for other lytic lesions that might require a longer stem femoral component for the shaft or a modified cemented acetabular component with a total hip replacement for acetabular lesions.

In many cases, the diagnosis of metastasis to the proximal femur will be made before a fracture occurs. In these cases, it is the responsibility of the orthopedic surgeon to decide whether the patient should receive some form of internal stabilization prior to radiation therapy. A CT scan of the involved area will help make this decision. Criteria for the performance of a prophylactic stabilization procedure include the following: (1) 50% cortical lysis, (2) a femoral lesion greater than 2.5 cm in diameter, (3) an avulsion fracture of the lesser trochanter, and (4) persistent pain in the hip area 4 weeks following the completion of radiation therapy. It is important to point out that these criteria are not perfect, and large errors arise in estimation of the load-bearing capacity of the bone.

2. Supra-acetabular area—In the case of a small supra-acetabular lesion with intact cortical bone, a cemented cup with a total hip system is generally most appropriate. Augmentation of the fully cemented reconstruction with threaded Steinmann pins or similar anchoring screws may be necessary in advanced cases (Figure 6–78). The principles of treatment are always the same, irrespective of the extent of disease: aggressive intralesional curettage of the area back to healthy bone,

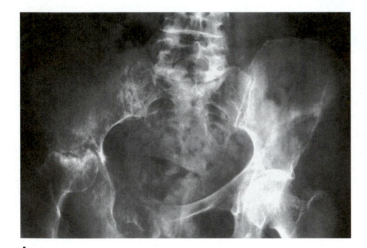

A

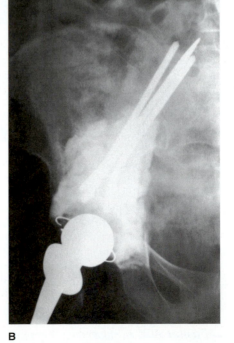

B

Figure 6–78. Preoperative (**A**) and postoperative (**B**) radiographs of the pelvis of a 73-year-old woman whose cancer had metastasized from the breast.

followed by the placement of large (³⁄₁₆-in., or 4.76-mm) threaded Steinmann pins into the sacroiliac area. The pins are placed with an initial foundation batch of cement, leaving them exposed for a second batch of cement, on top of which the cup is placed. A routine femoral component is then cemented.

3. Femoral shaft—Diaphyseal lesions that affect the femur but spare the peritrochanteric area are best handled with some form of intramedullary nail (Figure 6–79). Fixation of the entire femur, including the peritrochanteric area, with a reconstruction type nail is preferable in the event the disease progresses within the bone. Current intramedullary fixation devices often do not need cement augmentation. However, in cases of severe bone deficiency, PMMA introduction either directly into the defect or indirectly at the nail insertion site, is preferable.

4. Humerus—The principle for the management of metastatic disease to the humerus is no different from that for the femur. In the case of diaphyseal lesions, surgeons will either use a conventional intramedullary rod or they will plate the lesion. PMMA may be used with either technique.

In the case of the proximal humerus involving a large amount of the humeral head and neck, it is frequently necessary to cement a long-stem prosthesis (Figure 6–80). Just as with the proximal femur, in the proximal humerus there is no need to widely resect the tumor, and the rotator cuff is usually left intact.

5. Spine—In most cases of metastasis to the spine, the patient's pain can be managed adequately with local radiation therapy and medication. However, in cases of mechanical collapse associated with bony protrusion into the vertebral canal and cord compromise, surgical decompression and stabilization are frequently indicated. In the past, most of these problems were treated with posterior decompression by laminectomy alone. The results were poor because the spine was further destabilized, which resulted in increased kyphosis and anterior cord compression. With advances in the area of spinal instrumentation, the treatment has shifted toward a more aggressive anterior decompression and stabilization if the patient's general condition will allow. Even in cases in which the patient's general health will not tolerate the larger anterior approach, a less aggressive alternative might include posterior decompression supplemented by posterior spinal fixation.

The midthoracic spine is the most common area for paraplegia secondary to metastasis because of the narrow vertebral canal at this level of the spine. The ideal surgical approach to the problem in a patient with a reasonable prognosis consists of an anterior thoracotomy and anterior decompression by vertebrectomy, followed by anterior stabilization. As an alternative approach in a patient with a worse prognosis and a circumferential cord compression, a posterior decompression stabilization can be considered (Figure 6–81).

The second most common site for cord compression is the thoracolumbar region. The anterior reconstruction is the same in the thoracolumbar area as in the midthoracic area. A posterior stabilization may be advisable, especially in cases in which the prognosis is good.

The cervical spine is the least likely area for surgical treatment, mainly because the vertebral canal is wide at this level and cord compromise is uncommon. If surgery is needed, an ideal reconstruction is an anterior decompression and stabilization.

Radiation therapy is required postoperatively with all of these reconstructions. The use of bone graft is therefore undesirable because of inhibited osteoblastic healing.

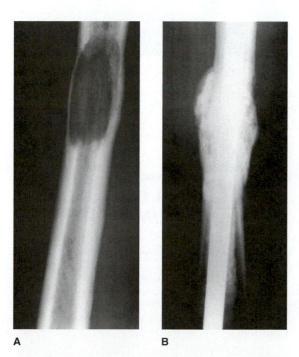

A   B

Figure 6–79. Preoperative (**A**) and postoperative (**B**) radiographs of the midshaft of the femur of a patient whose treatment involved fixation with a cemented intramedullary nail.

Beauchamp CP: Errors and pitfalls in the diagnosis and treatment of metastatic bone disease. Orthop Clin North Am 2000;31 (4):675. [PMID: 11043105]

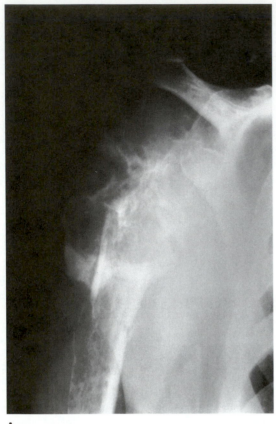

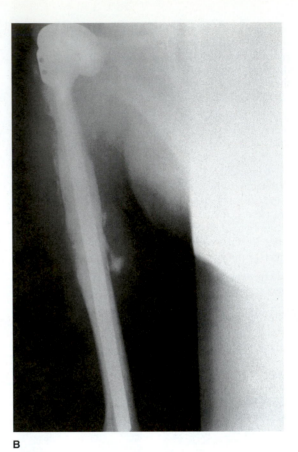

A

B

Figure 6–80. Preoperative (**A**) and postoperative (**B**) radiographs of the proximal humerus of a patient whose treatment involved the use of a cemented long-stem Neer prosthesis.

Hipp JA et al: Predicting pathologic fracture risk in the management of metastatic bone defects. Clin Orthop 1995;312:120. [PMID: 7634597]

Hortobagyi GN et al: Efficacy of pamidronate in reducing skeletal complications in patients with breast cancer & lytic bone metastases. N Engl. J Med 1996;24:1785. [PMID: 8965890]

Mirels H: Metastatic disease in long bones. A proposed scoring system for diagnosing impending pathologic fractures. Clin Orthop 1989;(249):256. [PMID: 2684463]

Mundy GR: Mechanisms of bone metastasis. Cancer 1997;80S:1546. [PMID: 9362421]

Rougraff BT et al: Skeletal metastases of unknown origin: A prospective study of a diagnostic strategy. J Bone Joint Surg 1993;75A:1276. [PMID: 8408149]

Wedin R: Surgical treatment for pathologic fracture. Acta Orthop Scand Suppl 2001;72(302):2p. [PMID: 11582636]

Wedin R et al: Surgical treatment for skeletal breast cancer metastases: A population-based study of 641 patients. Cancer 2001;92(2):257. [PMID: 11466677]

■ DIFFERENTIAL DIAGNOSIS OF PSEUDOTUMOROUS CONDITIONS

In addition to benign, malignant and metastatic neoplasms, a group of pseudotumors masquerade as bone and soft-tissue tumors. These lesions actually appear with greater frequency than either primary bone or soft-tissue tumors.

Stress-Reactive Lesions

The most common pseudotumors are those related to either bone or soft-tissue injury.

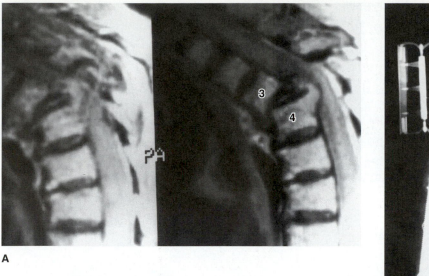

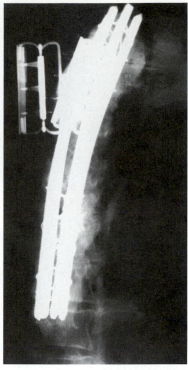

Figure 6–81. Preoperative T$_1$-weighted MRI (**A**) and postoperative radiograph (**B**) of the spine of a patient whose treatment involved use of posterior rods and sublaminal wires for stabilization.

A. Stress Fracture of Bone

Stress fractures are common in young athletic individuals and can produce radiographic features that might suggest the diagnosis of a bone-forming sarcoma or Ewing's sarcoma. It is important to obtain a careful history from the patient regarding his or her physical activity both at work and at play. There will be no history of a single injury if the bone symptoms are due to repetitive impact loading stress such as occurs with working out for cross-country running. The stress fracture will usually occur several weeks after a sudden increase of physical activity for which the patient is not properly conditioned. This is a common situation in the military, particularly during initial training.

Stress fractures are commonly located in the metaphyseal-diaphyseal areas of long weight-bearing bones. Early radiographs frequently appear normal before periosteal new bone begins to form. The most sensitive early diagnostic tool is a bone scan, which can appear hot or abnormal in the case of stress fractures, neoplasms, and infections. The MRI is sensitive to early fluid shifts in the periosteum overlying a stress fracture, but it is also sensitive to neoplastic and infectious conditions. One of the best methods to help rule out tumors and infection is to simply stop all physical stress to the injured bone for a period of 4 weeks. In patients with stress fracture, the pain should resolve spontaneously during this period, and a follow-up radiograph taken after this period will reveal a typical fusiform circumferential periosteal callous formation. In patients with a tumor or infection, the pain will persist, and the radiographic signs of permeative osteolysis will predominate, in which case a biopsy and culture are indicated.

At times, the clinical picture of a stress fracture will be confused by the preexistence of a benign stress raiser, such as a nonossifying fibroma or fibrous cortical defect (Figure 6–82).

In older patients, especially in postmenopausal women, stress fractures can occur with minimal physical activity. The circumstances under which the fracture occurred might not come out in a routine history. A common location of osteoporotic stress fractures is in the sacrum (Figure 6–83).

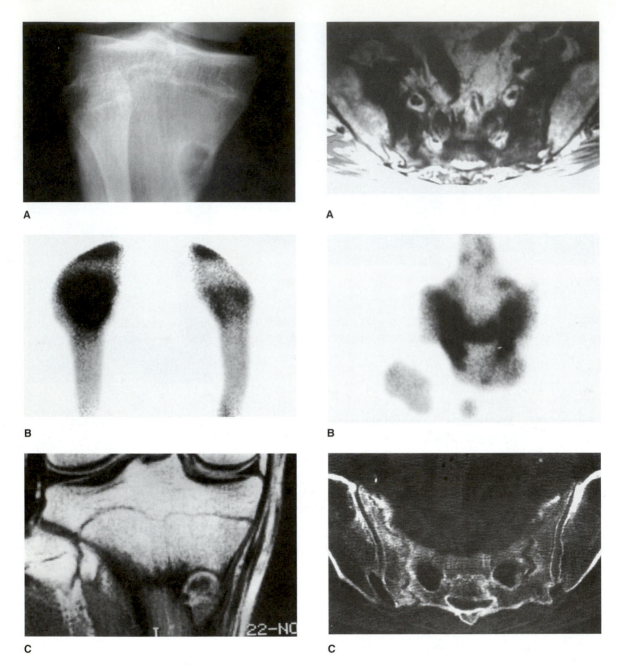

Figure 6–82. Radiograph (**A**), isotope bone scan (**B**), and T$_1$-weighted MRI (**C**) of the proximal tibia in a 16-year-old boy with a stress fracture.

Figure 6–83. T$_1$-weighted MRI (**A**), isotope bone scan (**B**), and CT scan (**C**) of the sacrum in a 71-year-old woman with stress fracture.

B. Myositis Ossificans

Another common stress-reactive pseudotumor seen in the extremity is myositis ossificans. This occurs most frequently in the lower extremity in young men. The quadriceps muscle is commonly involved because of direct blows or tearing injury to this muscle. The pseudotumor mass may not arise for several months after the injury and may not be related to a specific injury. In older, more sedentary patients, there may be no history of stress injury.

Early radiographs may not reveal soft-tissue calcification. With maturation, ossification will occur in the traumatized muscle fascial planes, and this may suggest the diagnosis of a synovial sarcoma or other calcifying sarcoma. If the myositis pseudotumor is attached to the subjacent bone it can mimic a parosteal osteosarcoma (Figure 6–84).

Infectious Diseases

Bacterial, viral, tuberculous, or fungal infections of the bone or soft tissue can frequently mimic a neoplastic process. This is particularly the case with infections that are not highly virulent, do not create systemic symptoms or a febrile response, and do not cause a large alteration in acute-phase reactant laboratory work. If a tender mass is present on examination and a bone or soft-tissue tumor is suggested by imaging studies, a biopsy may be indicated and should include a tissue culture in order to make the correct diagnosis. Inflammatory pseudotumors can be seen in any age group but are more common in children and frequently affect the lower extremity.

A. Bacterial Infection

Bacterial infections of bone can take on the appearance of a round cell tumor such as Ewing's sarcoma in children or lymphoma in adults (Figure 6–85). In contrast, tuberculous and fungal infections are less inflammatory and thus have more localized, well-marginated lesions that take on the imaging appearance of a benign tumor.

B. Tuberculous or Fungal Infection

A tuberculous or fungal infection of the spine or extremity can present as a pseudotumor in children or

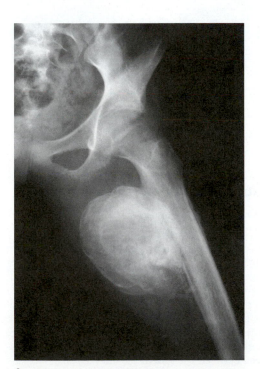

A

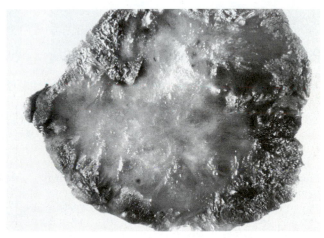

B

Figure 6–84. Radiograph (**A**) and gross appearance of a resected specimen (**B**) of myositis ossificans in the adductor muscles of a 12-year-old girl.

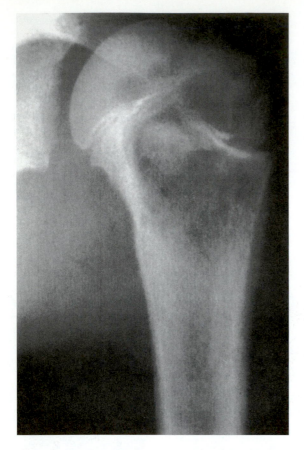

Figure 6–85. Radiograph of acute osteomyelitis due to *Staphylococcus aureus* in the proximal humerus of a 13-year-old boy.

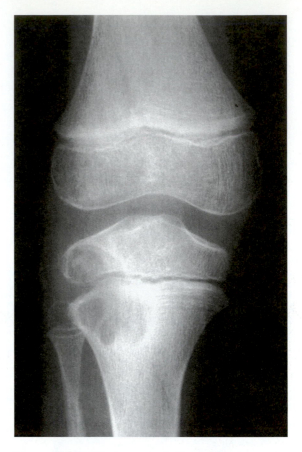

Figure 6–86. Radiograph of tuberculous osteomyelitis in the proximal tibia of a 10-year-old girl.

young adults, especially in Asian or Mexican patients (Figure 6–86). The incidence of tuberculous and fungal infections, which are low-grade infections that typically have an insidious onset, has also increased in patients with AIDS.

C. CAFFEY'S DISEASE

Caffey's disease can mimic a neoplastic process. It is an idiopathic form of periostitis that is seen in infants under 6 months of age and affects the extremities, shoulder girdle, and mandible (Figure 6–87). It may have a viral origin and is currently much rarer than it was 30 years ago. The bony changes are osteoblastic in nature and could suggest the diagnosis of an osteosarcoma, which is rare in infants. Caffey's disease is self-limiting and usually clears spontaneously without disability.

Metabolic Disorder

A. BROWN TUMOR OF PRIMARY HYPERPARATHYROIDISM

Brown tumor is the most common metabolic disorder that mimics a neoplastic process in bone. The lytic giant cell lesions occur symmetrically in metaphyseal-epiphyseal bone as the result of increased parathyroid hormone production by a solitary parathyroid adenoma, by hyperplastic parathyroid glands, or by a solitary parathyroid carcinoma. Brown tumors occur three times more often in females than in males and are usually seen between the ages of 15 and 70 years. They are most common in the ends of the long bone, followed next in frequency in the pelvis, long bone diaphysis, maxillary bone, cranium, rib, and hand. Brown tumors

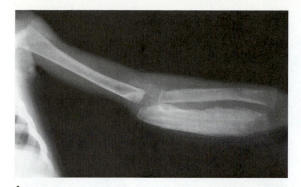

A

B

Figure 6–87. Preoperative (**A**) and postoperative (**B**) radiographs of Caffey's disease in the upper extremity and shoulder of a 5-month-old infant.

are rarely seen in the spine. Symptoms of pain are related to the local bone destruction, but widespread pain may result from generalized osteomalacia. The hyperparathyroid condition can lead to weight loss, psychologic disorders, gastrointestinal disorders, renal stones, polyuria, and polydipsia.

The radiographic features of the brown tumor in bone include a round lytic area that may be multicentric and may suggest the diagnosis of metastatic carcinoma, multiple myeloma, or histiocytic lymphoma (Figure 6–88). In the case of a solitary lesion, it may suggest the diagnosis of a nonossifying fibroma, fibrous dysplasia, giant cell tumor, or aneurysmal bone cyst. At the time of biopsy, the brown tumor will have the reddish brown appearance of a giant cell tumor. Microscopically, it will look like a giant cell tumor except that the background stromal cells will be more fibroblastic and the bone trabeculae will demonstrate abnormally

thick and poorly mineralized osteoid seams. Because of the marked similarity between the brown tumor and the giant cell tumor, clinicians should routinely order an analysis of serum calcium, phosphorus, and alkaline phosphatase levels in all patients with bone lesions that produce giant cells.

In patients with brown tumors, the treatment consists of removing the source of the excessive parathyroid hormone. After this, the bony defects will usually heal spontaneously. Bone grafting is rarely required. Although the secondary hyperparathyroidism seen in renal failure patients does not usually develop into brown tumors, it does produce pseudotumorous calcification in soft tissue, a condition similar to tumoral calcinosis, which is discussed later in this section.

B. PAGET'S DISEASE

Paget's disease is frequently included in discussions of metabolic bone disorders although the demonstration of cytoplasmic and nuclear inclusion bodies in osteoclasts of pagetic bone similar to paramyxovirus infections may suggest a viral origin. Most clinicians are familiar with the late changes in Paget's disease, which include the bowing of long bones and the finding of dense blastic changes on radiographic examination. However, many are unfamiliar with the early lytic phase of Paget's disease, when the radiographic findings are more suggestive of metastatic carcinoma, histiocytic lymphoma, primary sarcoma, or even primary hyperparathyroidism (Figure 6–89).

C. GAUCHER'S DISEASE

Gaucher's disease is a rare familial disorder in which accumulation of glucocerebroside causes enlargement of the liver, spleen, and marrow tissues. The marrow infiltration in children and young adults causes a gradual loss of bone that can mimic a neoplastic condition. The most common areas involved include the distal femur, tibia, humerus, vertebral column, skull, and mandible. Isolated focal destructive changed with endosteal scalloping and moth-eaten patterns may suggest the diagnosis of metastatic disease, myelomatosis, primary sarcoma, or fibrous dysplasia (Figure 6–90).

Hemorrhagic Conditions

A. PSEUDOTUMOR OF HEMOPHILIA

A hematoma in the soft tissue or bone under the periosteum may be difficult to distinguish from a tumor. Hematoma formation is frequently precipitated by some form of trauma, and the bones most commonly involved are the femur, pelvis, tibia, and small bones of

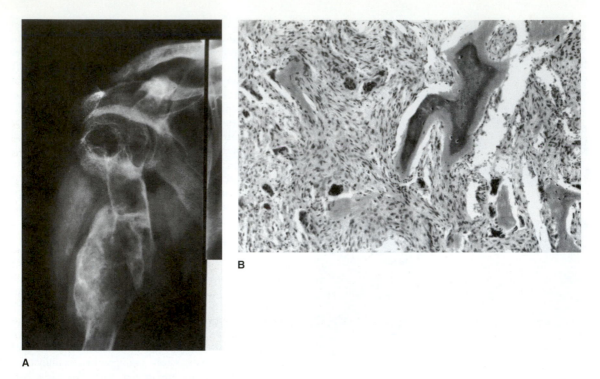

B

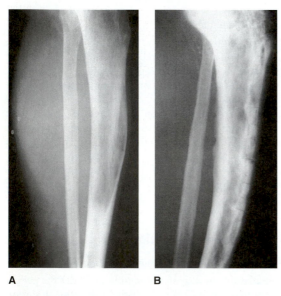

A

Figure 6–88. Radiograph (**A**) and photomicrograph (**B**) of a brown tumor of hyperparathyroidism in the proximal humerus of a 40-year-old woman.

A   **B**

Figure 6–89. Early and late radiographs of Paget's disease of the tibia, taken when the male patient was 45 years old (**A**) and when he was 65 years old (**B**).

the hand. It is rare to see multiple lesions. The bony lesions can be central or eccentric. The finding of lytic destruction followed by sclerotic reaction at the periphery may mimic the radiographic picture of an aneurysmal bone cyst or a giant cell tumor. In the hand bones, the osseous pseudotumors take on the appearance of a giant cell reparative granuloma or an osteoblastoma. The subperiosteal lesions bulge into the surrounding soft tissue and show reactive periosteal new bone formation and subjacent cortical erosion that may mimic Ewing's sarcoma or hemorrhagic osteosarcoma (Figure 6–91).

B. INTRAMUSCULAR HEMATOMA

Another hemorrhagic disorder that can produce a pseudotumor of soft tissue is the intramuscular hematoma. This is similar to the soft-tissue pseudotumor of hemophilia but without a bleeding abnormality. Intramuscular hematomas are almost always related to blunt trauma, but they occasionally result from a traction injury that may subsequently produce myositis ossificans. There may be no superficial signs of bruising in the overlying skin, and sometimes the hematoma

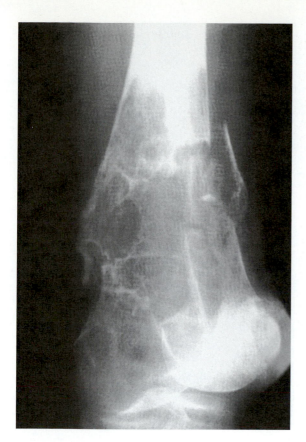

Figure 6–90. Radiograph of a pathologic fracture secondary to Gaucher's disease involving the distal femur in a 29-year-old man.

will grow in size at a later date, even as long as several years after the initial injury. The radiographic examination is of little help because no calcification or bony abnormality is evident. The MRI is the best imaging study, but unfortunately, the appearance of an intramuscular hematoma on MRI can mimic that of a deep soft-tissue sarcoma such as a malignant fibrous histiocytoma (Figure 6–92).

Ectopic Calcification

Ectopic calcification in soft tissue has many causes, most of which are related to chronic degenerative disorders in collagenous structures such as tendons or ligaments about a joint. However, in cases in which the dystrophic calcification is associated with a soft-tissue

mass, the clinician must rule out the diagnosis of a soft-tissue sarcoma such as synovial sarcoma.

A. TUMORAL CALCINOSIS

Tumoral calcinosis is seen about the hip, shoulder, and elbow and is characterized by extensive calcium phosphate deposition in a benign fibrous mass. It is an idiopathic condition that affects patients between the ages of 10 and 30 years and occurs more frequently in males than in females. Multiple lesions occur, and the lesions cause minimal pain and tenderness.

In cases of tumoral calcinosis, the extensive central fluffy calcification might suggest the diagnosis of a synovial sarcoma, soft-tissue chondrosarcoma, or tuberculosis (Figure 6–93). At biopsy, a chalky white paste will exude from a sponge-like fibrous mass. Microscopic findings include extensive amorphous calcium phosphate deposits in a fibrous stroma speckled with macrophages and inflammatory cells. If the pseudotumor is not completely removed, a recurrence is very likely.

A similar condition is seen in patients with renal osteodystrophy with secondary hyperparathyroidism, and the mechanism for the deposition in this case is a high level of calcium phosphorus production.

B. COMPARTMENT SYNDROME

The ischemic calcification and even ossification that occur in traumatic compartment syndromes in the lower extremity can often mimic a tumor. The initial injury is usually a crushing type that causes increased compartment pressure from muscle swelling. This pressure eventually leads to ischemic necrosis of the compartment muscle, which several years later will become calcific or even ossified. Because the muscle appears firm and calcified on radiographic examination, the clinician may not relate the finding to an old injury and may suspect a calcifying sarcoma such as synovial sarcoma. The most common place for this pseudotumor will be in one of the muscle compartments of the leg, and it will cause stiffness and muscle weakness at the ankle and foot area (Figure 6–94). This process can mimic soft-tissue calcifications secondary to a neoplastic process (Figure 6–95).

Dysplastic Disorders

Many developmental or dysplastic conditions can create bony abnormalities, which, on radiographic examination, can mimic a bone tumor. These are usually focal defects in enchondral bone formation that result from a failure to remodel primary woven bone forming at the metaphyseal end of the physis.

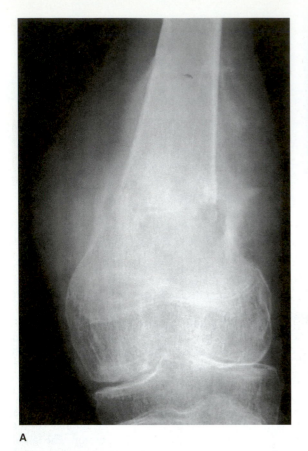

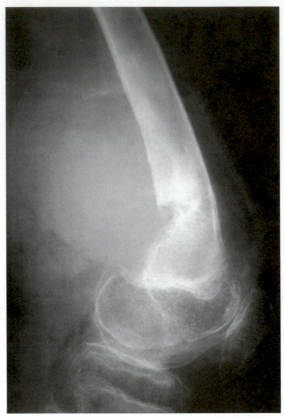

A   **B**

Figure 6–91.   Anteroposterior (**A**) and lateral (**B**) radiographs of a pseudotumor of hemophilia in the distal femur of a 14-year-old boy.

A. OSTEOMA

Osteoma commonly occurs in the skull or maxilla and is composed of dense unorganized woven bone seen just beneath the cortex. There is no lytic component in or around the dense bone, and no symptoms are associated with the presence of osteomas. Because the lesions are commonly seen in the metaphyseal areas about the knee, the clinician may become concerned about the diagnosis of an early osteosarcoma. However, the lack of periosteal response and minimal uptake on an isotope bone scan will help rule out sarcoma (Figure 6–96). In such cases, there should be no concern about future problems from the lesion and usually no intervention is necessary.

B. BONE ISLAND

The bone island is an even more sharply marginated dysplastic process than the osteoma. It is most commonly located in the pelvis. It can mimic a blastic metastatic lesion in patients with prostate cancer. However, with a bone island, as with an osteoma, the bone scan will show minimal and very focal activity, and the CT scan and MRI will show no reaction in the surrounding marrow. Figure 6–97 shows the findings of a bone island through the pelvis of a 35-year-old man.

Bone Infarcts

The two types of bone infarcts that can mimic bone tumors are the metaphyseal type and the epiphyseal type. They can be idiopathic in origin or secondary to increased alcohol consumption or corticosteroid use.

A. METAPHYSEAL BONE INFARCT

The most common bone infarct is in the metaphyseal region, which is typically seen about the knee, hip, and shoulder in adults. Radiographically, the infarct can mimic a low-grade cartilaginous tumor such as an enchondroma. An infarct presents with a sclerotic honey-

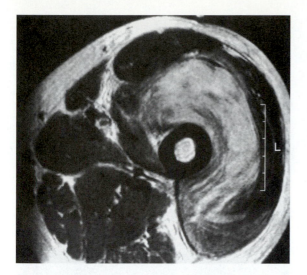

Figure 6–92. Axial view T$_2$-weighted MRI of a hematoma in the quadriceps muscles of a 46-year-old man.

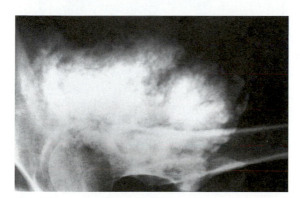

A

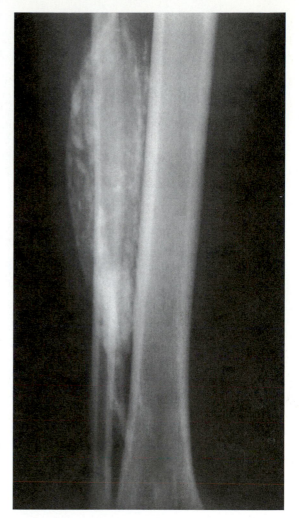

Figure 6–94. Radiograph of an old compartment syndrome in the flexor hallucis longus.

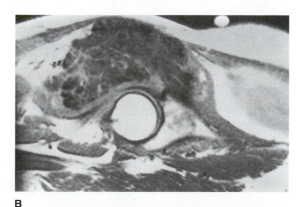

B

Figure 6–93. Radiograph (**A**) and T$_1$-weighted MRI (**B**) of tumoral calcinosis in the hip of a 54-year-old woman.

combed pattern (Figure 6–98), whereas a cartilaginous lesion presents with central flocculated calcification (Figure 6–99).

B. EPIPHYSEAL BONE INFARCT

Although epiphyseal bone infarcts have the same etiology as those in the metaphysis, these are most commonly found in the femoral condyles and the proximal femoral and humeral epiphyses. In these locations, the lytic change seen in the epiphyseal bone can mimic a chondroblastoma. The differential diagnosis can be difficult before the appearance of a crescent sign or other radiographic signs of subchondral collapse that usually rule out the chondroblastoma (Figure 6–100).

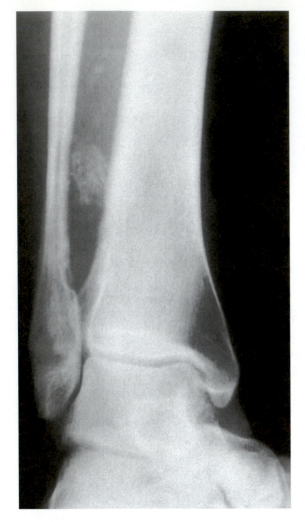

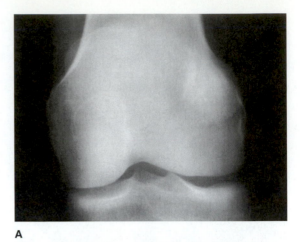

A

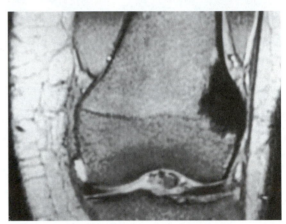

B

Figure 6–96. Radiograph (**A**) and T$_2$-weighted MRI (**B**) of a dysplastic process in the distal femur of a 64-year-old woman.

Figure 6–95. Radiograph of calcification in synovial sarcoma of the leg.

Histiocytic Disorders

A. LANGHERHANS' CELL HISTIOCYTOSIS

Sometimes inappropriately called histiocytosis X, Langerhans' cell histiocytosis can present in a variety of ways. Previously considered distinct diseases, including eosinophilic granuloma, Hand-Schüller-Christian disease, and Letterer-Siwe disease, are now considered part of the same spectrum of histiocytosis presentation. Of these, the localized granulomatous form, which is called eosinophilic granuloma or Langerhans' cell granulomatosis, is the one that mimics a tumor radiographi-

cally. Eosinophilic granuloma is seen twice as often in boys as in girls and commonly occurs between the ages of 5 and 15 years. It is usually monostotic but in 10% of cases involves two or three separate areas. It is a histiocytic process of unknown cause but may have a viral origin. It causes local inflammatory pain and may result in low-grade fever associated with an elevated sedimentation rate. Although the most common location of eosinophilic granuloma is the skull, it is also seen in the rib, pelvis, maxilla, vertebral body (vertebra plana), clavicle, and scapula, listed in the order of frequency. Besides affecting flat bones, it can arise in the diaphysis

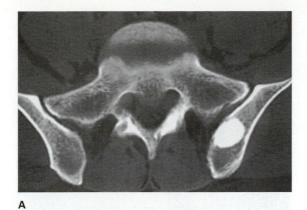

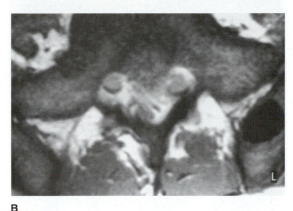

Figure 6–97. CT scan (**A**) and T_2-weighted MRI (**B**) of a bone island through the pelvis of a 35-year-old man.

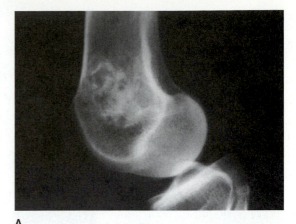

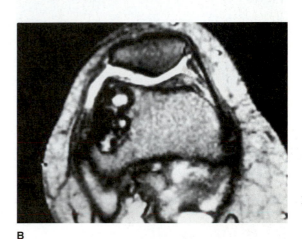

Figure 6–98. Radiograph (**A**) and T_1-weighted MRI (**B**) of a metaphyseal infarct in the distal femur of a 52-year-old woman.

of long bones, followed next by the metaphysis, and is least common in the epiphysis.

Eosinophilic granuloma can be extremely permeative and destructive, especially in long bones (Figure 6–101) and vertebrae (Figure 6–102), thereby mimicking a more aggressive process, such as Ewing's sarcoma, metastatic neuroblastoma, or osteomyelitis. It can also produce an "onionskin" periostitis of the type seen in Ewing's sarcoma. The lesion has a more aggressive pattern in younger children and later becomes more focal and granulomatous. Microscopic findings include large pale-staining histiocytes speckled with small bright-staining eosinophils and an occasional giant cell.

Eosinophilic granulomas tend to involute spontaneously without treatment, and therefore treatment should be conservative. Simple curettement and corticosteroid injections have proven beneficial. In difficult areas such as the spine or pelvis, low-dose radiation treatment (10 Gy) can be considered. In more disseminated cases that do not respond to simple treatment, low-dose chemotherapy is appropriate.

B. Pigmented Villonodular Synovitis

Although this form of synovitis can mimic a histiocytic tumor, it is thought to be a nonneoplastic condition involving histiocytic proliferation. It occurs in the subsynovial tissue about major joints of the lower extremity in patients between the ages of 20 and 40 years. The knee joint is the most common site of involvement, followed next by the hip, ankle, and foot. Involvement of the upper extremity is rare.

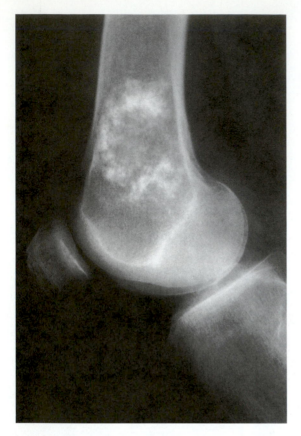

Figure 6–99. Radiograph of a large enchondroma in the distal femur.

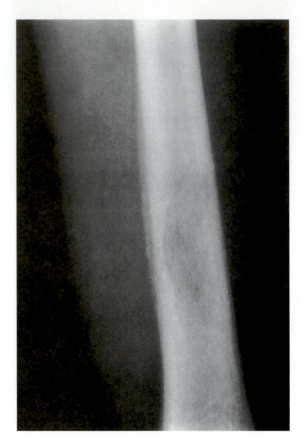

Figure 6–101. Radiograph of an eosinophilic granuloma of the humerus in a 12-year-old boy.

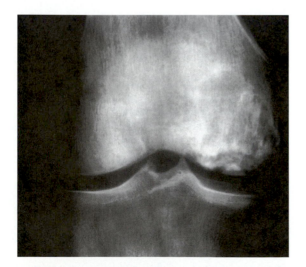

Figure 6–100. Radiograph of an epiphyseal infarct in the femoral condyle of a 45-year-old woman.

The histopathology of pigmented villonodular synovitis is similar to that of a giant cell tumor of the tendon sheath, which presents with soft-tissue tumors about the ankle and on the fingers of the hand. The usual situation involves spontaneous swelling of one knee secondary to synovial hypertrophy. The swelling can grow gradually to a massive amount and be associated with intermittent hemarthroses. The inflamed synovium can cause juxta-articular erosion into bone at the point of attachment of the joint capsule, as is seen in any chronic proliferative synovitis, including hemophilia and coccidioidomycosis.

In fewer than 10% of cases, pigmented villonodular synovitis is more localized and presents as a focal soft-tissue mass high in the suprapatellar pouch or in the popliteal space, and no generalized swelling of the knee occurs. In these cases, the mass can mimic a soft-tissue sarcoma such as a synovial sarcoma (Figure 6–103). Cortical erosion with secondary bony changes can also be appreciated frequently (Figure 6–104).

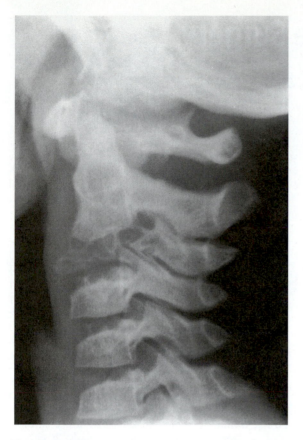

Figure 6–102. Radiograph of an eosinophilic granuloma in the body of the C3 vertebra in a 5-year-old girl.

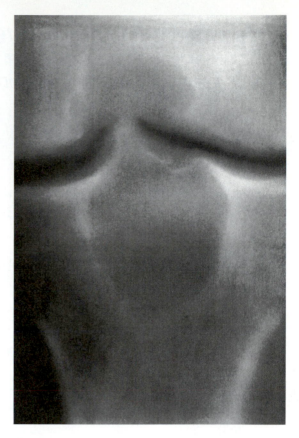

Figure 6–104. Laminagram of pigmented villonodular synovitis in the proximal tibia of a young man.

Mankin HJ et al: Gaucher disease. New approaches to an ancient disease. J Bone Joint Surg Am 2001;83-A(5):748. [PMID: 11379747]

Roodman GD: Studies in Paget's disease and their relevance to oncology. Semin Oncol 2001;28(4 Suppl 11):15. [PMID: 11544571]

Shidham V et al: Evaluation of crystals in formalin-fixed, paraffin-embedded tissue sections for the differential diagnosis of pseudogout, gout, and tumoral calcinosis. Mod Pathol 2001;14(8):806. [PMID: 11504841]

Zelger B: Langerhans cell histiocytosis: A reactive or neoplastic disorder? Med Pediatr Oncol 2001;37(6):543. [PMID: 11745894]

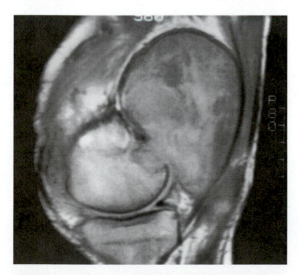

Figure 6–103. T_1-weighted MRI of pigmented villonodular synovitis in the popliteal space of a 50-year-old man.

Adult Reconstructive Surgery

7

Robert S. Namba, MD, Harry B. Skinner, MD, & Ranjan Gupta, MD

Adult reconstructive surgery in orthopedics has rapidly evolved over the past 30 years. Prior to the successful development of "low-friction" arthroplasty of the hip in the late 1960s, reconstructive options for the hip and the knee were limited. Reconstructive procedures with high success rates are now available for a variety of disorders, from marked degenerative hip disease to rotator cuff tears of the shoulder. Research done in the last 30 years has increased the understanding of major joint function and contributed to the success of reconstructive surgical procedures in almost all cases, and there is now a tremendous demand for these procedures. In 1997, total knee arthroplasty and total hip arthroplasty procedures numbered 338,000 and 289,000, respectively. This was the result of their great success in returning patients to active lifestyles. Millions of Americans are now benefiting from these procedures for extended periods. Because their cumulative procedure failure rate is approximately 1% per year, 10 years after their operation, patients have about a 90% chance of still having a successful, well-functioning joint replacement.

Statistics from American Academy of Orthopedic Surgeons. Arthroplasty and Total joint Replacement Procedures in the United States 1990 to 1997. http://www.aaos.org/wordhtml/press/arthropl.htm

ARTHRITIS & RELATED CONDITIONS

Evaluation of Arthritis

To appropriately treat arthritic conditions of the joints, an understanding of the disease process is essential. This begins with accurate diagnosis and a history of the progression of the disease, so that the future progression can be predicted and appropriate decisions regarding treatment can be made. The physician must evaluate the possibility of traumatic, inflammatory, developmental, idiopathic, and metabolic causes of the arthritis (Table 7–1). Evaluation of the history, physical examination, and laboratory data is helpful in arriving at a diagnosis.

A. HISTORY

Clearly the history is important in defining the disease process. The time course, including duration and behavior of symptoms since onset, is a key factor. Gradual rather than acute onset implies a nontraumatic cause. Swelling in the joints is an important sign, as is the distribution of joints if more than one is involved. The degree of interference with activities indicates the seriousness of the disorder.

The presence and extent of pain are valuable pieces of information. Constant pain, night and day, implies infection, cancer, or a functional disorder. Pain only with activity such as walking, standing, or running suggests joint loading. Pain that awakens the patient is considered severe and requires evaluation. Location helps distinguish referred pain from joint pain.

Knowledge of the age distribution of the various arthritic disorders can be very helpful to the student in diagnosing the disease. A hip disorder in the younger patient is unlikely to be osteoarthritis unless a predisposing condition is present, such as trauma. A more likely diagnosis is osteonecrosis. Similarly, a chronic condition of the knee in the 45-year-old man is likely to be a degenerative meniscus tear, unless the patient had a meniscectomy in his early 20s. This concept can be extended to all age groups for the common disorders of the hip and knee (Figures 7–1 and 7–2). Further, a history of one of these disorders at an earlier age predisposes a patient to earlier osteoarthrosis.

Hip pain is felt typically in the groin or in the lateral aspect of the hip or anterior thigh but seldom in the buttock. Pain arising from the spine may be appreciated in the buttock and less often in the groin and anterior thigh. Acetabular pain or femoral head pain is frequently felt in the groin. Proximal femur pain is usually appreciated in the anteroproximal thigh.

Knee pain is frequently anterior (patellofemoral), medial (medial compartment), or lateral (lateral compartment). It may also be poorly localized by the patient. Pain in the back of the knee may result from a popliteal cyst (Baker's cyst) or a torn meniscus. A swollen knee may be painful because of pressure. Pain with any motion may indicate a septic joint or possibly a gouty joint. Arthritic pain in the elbow and shoulder is less clearly defined by patients, and in such cases the physical examination is important. Shoulder pain may

370

Table 7–1. Causes of arthritic conditions.

Traumatic causes	Traumatic arthritis, osteonecrosis (posttraumatic)
Inflammatory causes	Infectious arthritis, gout, pseudogout, rheumatoid arthritis, systemic lupus erythematosus, ankylosing spondylitis, juvenile rheumatoid arthritis, Reiter's syndrome
Developmental causes	Developmental dysplasia of the hip, hemophilic arthritis, following slipped capital fermoral epiphysis, following Legg-Calvé-Perthes disease
Idiopathic causes	Osteoarthritis, osteonecrosis
Metabolic causes	Gout, calcium pyrophosphate deposition disease, ochronosis, Gaucher's disease

be caused by cervical, cardiac, or even diaphragmatic disorders.

B. Physical Examination

1. Hip—The physical examination of the hip is important to verify that the reported pain arises from the hip joint and to determine the severity of the pain. It is also useful to document range of motion (ROM), gait, leg length-discrepancy, and muscle weakness. Pain arising from the hip is typically elicited at the extremes of ROM. Active straight leg raising or resisted straight leg raising may produce pain (Figure 7–3). Log rolling (internal and external rotation of the hip in extension) will usually elicit hip pain if pain is severe. Frequently, internal rotation of the hip in flexion will be limited; this condition is one of the first signs of osteoarthritis (OA) of the hip. Abduction of the hip against gravity loads the hip and may produce hip pain of arthritis, but will not do so if pain in the buttock or thigh is referred from the spine. Increased loading may be achieved by applying resistance to abduction. In the young patient

with groin pain, provocative maneuvers can be used to diagnose labral tears. Flexion of the hip with external rotation (ER) and abduction (ABD) is followed by extension, adduction (ADD) and internal rotation (IR). Clicking or catching is observed in patients with anterior labral tears. Posterior tears of the labrum are identified by moving the hip from extension, ABD, and ER, to flexion, ADD, and IR.

The ROM in flexion, extension (flexion contracture), abduction, adduction, and internal and external rotation is measured. Decreased internal rotation is an early finding in osteoarthritis.

2. Knee—The physical examination of the knee localizes the pain to the knee and to the specific involved compartment. Range of motion of the hip should be evaluated to rule out referred hip pain. Ligamentous

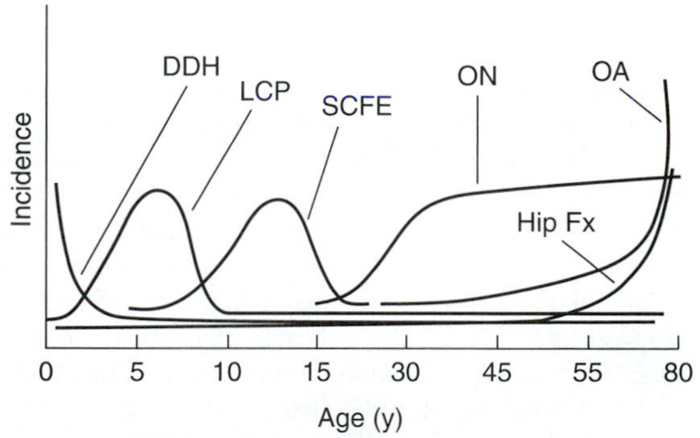

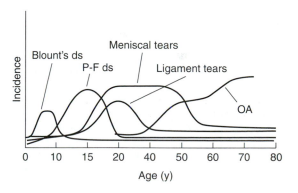

Figure 7–2. The age distribution of knee disorders is given schematically as a function of age. Blount's ds = tibia vara; P-F ds = patellofemoral arthralgia; and OA = osteoarthrosis. Meniscal tears can be either medial or lateral and are traumatic in the younger age group and degenerative in the older age group. Osteoarthrosis shows an earlier onset with the knee than with the hip, because there is an incidence of medial gonarthrosis in the 40s and 50s because of medial meniscectomy in the late teens and early 20s.

Figure 7–1. The age distribution of hip disorders is given in a schematic representation. DDH = developmental dysplasia of the hip; LCP = Legg-Calvé-Perthes disease; SCFE = slipped capital femoral epiphysis; ON = osteonecrosis; OA = osteoarthrosis; and Hip Fx = hip fracture.

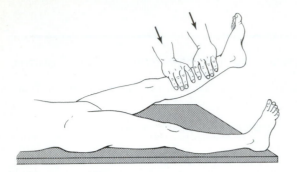

Figure 7–3. Resisted straight leg-raising test. The examiner asks the patient to actively raise the straight leg to about 30 degrees. This will produce hip pain in severe arthritis. If no pain is produced, the examiner applies pressure to the thigh, which the patient resists. This increased joint loading uncovers mild to moderate hip pain.

stability is discerned in the mediolateral and anteroposterior planes (see Chapter 4). Instability is not common in osteoarthritis but is often seen in rheumatoid arthritis. Alignment of the knee (varus or valgus) while standing is measured. Varus and valgus alignment have been found to increase the odds of progression of osteoarthritis (OA) fourfold and fivefold, respectively, in 18 months. Range of motion of the knee is measured, and any flexion contracture or extensor lag is noted. Flexion contracture is an inability to come to full extension passively, whereas an extensor lag indicates an inability to actively extend the knee as far as it will extend passively. The contracture is common in advanced OA, whereas the lag is generally a quadriceps muscle or tendon problem. The medial and lateral compartments are loaded during flexion and extension with varus and valgus stress, respectively, to elicit pain arising from arthritis in each compartment. The patellofemoral joint may be assessed for pain and bone-on-bone crepitance by flexion and extension with pressure on the patella. The presence of fluid, synovitis, and erythema is also important.

3. Shoulder—After the cervical spine has been ruled out as the source of pain, examination of the shoulder begins with visual inspection for obvious asymmetry of bone and muscle contours. Palpation of muscle tone and of the clavicle, as well as the acromioclavicular and sternoclavicular joints, follows. Tenderness over the anterolateral humeral head is often found with rotator cuff disorders. Tendinitis of the long head of the biceps is easily demonstrated by palpation of the tendon over the anteromedial humeral head. Active ROM is then assessed in flexion and abduction. External rotation is

reproducibly measured by keeping the elbow on the waist and rotating the hand away from the body. Internal rotation is best recorded by measuring how high the thumb can be positioned along the spine. Most individuals can position the thumb to the midthoracic area (eg, T6 or T7). When internal rotation is limited, the thumb may only be elevated to L5. If active ROM is at all limited, passive ROM should be assessed. Strength of the upper extremity muscle is then evaluated along with sensation and deep tendon reflexes. Decreased strength in external rotation with the elbow at the side indicates significant rotator cuff weakness. Provocative tests can help evaluate the cause of pain, particularly with instability. The apprehension test is positive, indicating anterior instability, when abduction, extension, and external rotation of the shoulder elicit anxiety or discomfort. Impingement signs are present with rotator cuff disorders and produce pain with passive flexion or internal rotation of the flexed and adducted arm.

4. Elbow—Inspection of the elbow includes measurement of the "carrying angle," the normal 5–7 degrees angle of valgus inclination between the humerus and forearm. Scars and obvious deformities are noted, as well as swelling or masses. Bony prominences are palpated, including the mediolateral epicondyles, radial head, and olecranon. Active and passive motion is recorded for both flexion and extension and pronation and supination. Tenderness over the lateral epicondyle exacerbated by resisted wrist dorsiflexion is often seen in lateral epicondylitis (tennis elbow). Tenderness over the medial epicondyle with pain elicited by resisted wrist flexion is seen in medial epicondylitis. Limitation of flexion and extension is seen with arthritis and posttraumatic stiffness.

C. IMAGING STUDIES

Radiologic data, synovial fluid analysis, and blood testing may be beneficial in confirming the diagnosis of arthritis. The most fundamental radiographic data can be provided by a plain x-ray film with a minimum of two views. Evaluation of joint pain includes ruling out fracture, joint space narrowing, osteophyte formation, or osteopenia. Views of the hip include a modified anteroposterior view of the pelvis (which clips the iliac wings to show the proximal femora) and a lateral view of the affected hip (either "frog," an anteroposterior view with the hip externally rotated and abducted, or a true lateral view). Views of the knee should include a 10 degrees down-angled beam posteroanterior radiograph of the bent knee (30–45 degrees of flexion) taken while the patient is standing, a lateral view, and a tangential patellar view (Merchant view, 45 degrees of flexion) (Table 7–2). Views of the shoulder should include anteroposterior, axillary, and lateral views of the

Table 7–2. Radiographic findings in arthritis.

Disease State	Findings in Hip or Knee
Osteoarthritis	Joint space narrowing, subchondral sclerosis, osteophytes, subchondral cysts Hip: Superior or medial narrowing Knee: Early narrowing on Rosenberg views; flattening of femoral condyles
Rheumatoid arthritis or sytemic lupus erythematosus	Uniform joint narrowing, erosion near joint capsule
Ankylosing spondylitis	Osteopenia, osteophytes, ankylosis of sacroiliac joints
Gout	Tophi, erosions
Calcium pyrophosphate deposition disease	Calcification of menisci and hyaline cartilage
Osteonecrosis	Crescent sign, spotty calcification
Gaucher's disease	"Erlenmeyer flask" appearance, distal femora
Neuropathic joint	Four *D*s: destruction, debris, dislocation, densification (sclerosis, hypertrophy)
Hemophilic arthropathy	Epiphyseal widening, sclerosis, cysts, joint space narrowing

scapula. Supraspinatus outlet views may be helpful in revealing acromial bone spurs, which produce impingement. The elbow usually can be visualized with anteroposterior and lateral radiographs.

D. LABORATORY FINDINGS

Basic blood testing should include a complete blood count and sedimentation rate. These are indicated in a suspected septic process or in the evaluation of a painful joint replacement. A normal white cell count may be helpful in the diagnosis of gout, especially in an inflamed joint other than the first metatarsophalangeal joint.

Synovial fluid analysis is indicated at any time to rule out infection, and it may also be quite helpful in the diagnosis of other arthritides. Table 8–2 shows the significance of yellow and clear synovial fluid. Aspiration of synovial fluid may reveal hemorrhagic fluid. If this is the result of a traumatic tap, it should be so noted and the fluid should be sent for analysis. If the fluid is grossly hemorrhagic, several diagnoses must be entertained, including hemophilia, neuropathic arthropathy, pigmented villonodular synovitis, hemangioma, or trauma. A finding of fat floating on the bloody fluid in the setting of a traumatic injury suggests the presence of an intra-articular fracture.

The combined history, physical examination, and appropriate laboratory studies should narrow the diagnoses to a relative few, if not the definitive one. It is helpful to consider diagnoses in categories, which, despite some overlap, provide a framework for further workup. Many of these arthritic conditions are described in the following pages.

Sharma L et al: The role of knee alignment in disease progression and functional decline in knee osteoarthritis. JAMA 2001; 286:188.

Solomon DH et al: Does this patient have a torn meniscus or ligament of the knee? Value of physical exam of the knee. JAMA 2001; 286:1610

1. Noninflammatory Arthritis

The term **osteoarthritis** is a misnomer, because inflammation is not the primary pathologic process observed in this form of articular joint disruption. More accurately described as degenerative joint disease, the disease represents a final common pathway of injury to articular cartilage. Although the true nature and cause of osteoarthritis are unclear, radiographic findings and gross and microscopic pathologic features are fairly typical in most cases.

Categorization of primary and secondary forms of osteoarthritis, though still useful, has become blurred. A designation of primary or idiopathic osteoarthritis has been made when no identifiable predisposing conditions could be recognized. Osteoarthritis is considered secondary when an underlying cause such as trauma, previous deformity, or systemic disorder exists. Although many cases of hip osteoarthritis were considered idiopathic when the end-stage changes were observed, careful analysis has indicated predisposing conditions such as slipped capital femoral epiphysis and mild forms of acetabular dysplasia in many cases.

The joints most commonly involved include the hip; knee; distal interphalangeal, proximal interphalangeal, and first carpometacarpal joints of the hand; and cervical, thoracic, and lumbar spine.

Primary Osteoarthritis

A. EPIDEMIOLOGIC FEATURES

Osteoarthritis is a widespread joint disorder in the United States, significantly affecting approximately 40 million people. Though autopsy studies show degenerative changes of weight-bearing joints in 90% of people older than 40 years, clinical symptoms are usually not present. The prevalence and severity of osteoarthritis increase with age.

When all ages are considered, men and women are equally affected. Under age 45, the disease is more prevalent in men; over age 55, women are more commonly afflicted. The pattern of joint involvement commonly includes the joints of the hands and knees in women and the hip joints in men.

The incidence of hip osteoarthritis is higher in European and American white males than in Chinese, South African blacks, and East Indian persons. Primary hip osteoarthritis in Japanese persons is rare, but secondary osteoarthritis is common because of developmental dysplasia of the hip.

There is evidence that some distinct forms of osteoarthritis may be inherited as a dominant trait with a mendelian pattern. These include a primary generalized osteoarthritis in which Heberden's nodes and Bouchard's nodes are a prominent feature and symmetric and uniform loss of articular cartilage of the knee and hip joints is evident. Other types of inherited osteoarthritis include familial chondrocalcinosis (with deposition of calcium pyrophosphate dihydrate crystals in cartilage), Stickler syndrome (characterized by vitreoretinal degeneration), hydroxyapatite deposition disease, and multiple epiphyseal dysplasias. Certain inherited forms are caused by mutations in the gene for cartilage-specific type II procollagen.

B. Pathologic Features

Early features of osteoarthritis include focal swelling and softening of the cartilage matrix. Mild loss of metachromatic staining ability represents loss of proteoglycans in the extracellular matrix. Surface irregularities in the form of fibrillation occur. Diffuse hypercellularity of the chondrocytes can be seen. The tidemark, an interface plane between hyaline cartilage and the zone of calcified cartilage, is thin and wavy early in osteoarthritis.

Later features of osteoarthritis include progressive loss of proteoglycans manifesting as reduction in safranin-O staining. Fibrillations in the surface deepen into fissures and later into deeper clefts. Chondrocyte cloning is seen and also reduplication of the tidemark, with discontinuous parallel lines indicating progression of calcification of the basal portion of the articular cartilage. Regions of eburnated bone represent complete loss of cartilage.

New bone formation occurs in a subchondral location as well as at margins of the articular cartilage. Areas of rarefaction of bone below eburnation are represented by "cysts" on radiographs and on gross inspection.

C. Laboratory Findings

Specific diagnostic tests for osteoarthritis are currently not available. Routine blood tests, urinalysis, and even synovial fluid analysis do not provide useful information, except for exclusion of inflammatory or infectious arthritis. Recent experimental work on identification of markers of cartilage degradation in osteoarthritis may provide diagnostic tests in the future. These include sensitive and specific assays for synovial fluid cytokines, proteinases and their inhibitors, matrix components and their fragments, and serum antibodies to cartilage collagen, and identification of proteoglycan subpopulations.

D. Imaging Studies

Typical radiographic features indicate late pathologic changes in osteoarthritis. Specifically, narrowing of the joint space, subchondral sclerosis, bony cysts, and marginal osteophytes are seen. End-stage disease is complicated by bony erosions, subluxation, loose bodies, and deformity.

Heberden's nodes are commonly seen in primary osteoarthritis, represented by bony and cartilaginous enlargement of the distal interphalangeal joints of the fingers. Similar enlargements of the proximal interphalangeal joints of the fingers are called **Bouchard's nodes.**

Secondary Osteoarthritis

The term **secondary osteoarthritis** is applied when an underlying recognizable local or systemic factor exists. These include conditions leading to joint deformity or destruction of cartilage, followed by signs and symptoms typically seen with primary osteoarthritis. Examples of preexisting conditions leading to secondary osteoarthritic changes in joints include acute and chronic trauma, Legg-Calvé-Perthes disease, developmental dysplasia of the hip, rheumatoid arthritis, bleeding dyscrasias, achondroplasia, infection, crystal deposition disease, neuropathic disorders, overuse of intra-articular steroids, and multiple epiphyseal dysplasias. Radiographic features of secondary osteoarthritis reflect the underlying pathologic changes plus the changes resulting from the primary osteoarthritis.

Bjell A: Cartilage matrix in hereditary pyrophosphate arthropathy. J Rheumatol 1981;8:959.

Hoaglund FT, Steinbach LS: Primary osteoarthritis of the hip: Etiology and epidemiology. J Am Acad Orthop Surg 2001;9(5): 320.

Kellgren JH et al: Genetic factors in generalized osteoarthrosis. Ann Rheum Dis 1963;22:237.

Knowlton RG et al: Genetic linkage analysis of hereditary arthro-ophthalmopathy and the type II procollagen gene. Am J Hum Genet 1989;65:681.

Lawrence RC et al: Estimates of the prevalence of arthritis and selected musculoskeletal disorders in the United States. Arthritis Rheum 1999;42(2):396.

Lowman EW: Osteoarthritis. JAMA 1955;157:487.

Marcos JC et al: Idiopathic familial chondrocalcinosis due to apatite crystal deposition. Am J Med 1981;71:557.

Mukhopadhaya B, Barooah B: Osteoarthritis of hip in Indians. Indian J Orthop 1975;1:55.

Palotie A et al: Predisposition to familial osteoarthrosis linked to type II collagen gene. Lancet 1989;1:924.

Reginato AJ: Articular chondrocalcinosis in the Chiloe islanders. Arthritis Rheum 1976;19:396.

Solomon L et al: Rheumatic disorders in the southern African Negro. S Afr Med J 1975;49: 1737.

Spranger J: The epiphyseal dysplasias. Clin Orthop 1975; 114:46.

Stickler GB et al: Hereditary progressive arthro-ophthalmopathy. Mayo Clin Proc 1965;40:433.

2. Inflammatory Arthritis

Rheumatoid Arthritis

A chronic systemic inflammatory disorder, rheumatoid arthritis is a crippling disease affecting approximately 1% of the population in the United States. Although similar synovial histopathologic and joint abnormalities are identifiable in all patients, the articular and systemic manifestations, outcomes, and differences in genetic makeup and serologic findings vary widely in individual patients. The cause is unknown, though the disease probably occurs in response to a pathogenic agent in a genetically predisposed host. Possible triggering factors include bacterial, mycoplasmal, or viral infections, as well as endogenous antigens in the form of rheumatoid factor, collagens, and mucopolysaccharides.

Joint involvement is typically symmetric, affecting the wrist, metacarpal, phalangeal, proximal, interphalangeal elbow, shoulder, cervical spine, hip, knee, and ankle joints. The distal interphalangeal joints are typically spared. Extra-articular manifestations include vasculitis, pericarditis, skin nodules, pulmonary fibrosis, pneumonitis, and scleritis. The triad of arthritis, lymphadenopathy, and splenomegaly is known as **Felty's syndrome** and is associated with anemia, thrombocytopenia, and neutropenia.

A. Epidemiologic Features

Rheumatoid arthritis occurs two to four times more often in women than men. The disease occurs in all age groups, but increases in incidence with advancing age, with a peak between the fourth and sixth decades.

Evidence for a genetic basis is provided by the association of rheumatoid arthritis with a certain haplotype of class II gene products of the major histocompatibility complex. Seventy-five percent of patients with rheumatoid arthritis carry circulating rheumatoid factors, which are autoantibodies against portions of the IgG antibody. In rheumatoid factor-positive patients, there is a high incidence of HLA-DR4, except in black patients. Only a minority of individuals with HLA-DR4 develop rheumatoid arthritis, however. (See Chapter 13, especially Tables 13–4 and 13–5.)

B. Pathologic Features

Early rheumatoid synovitis consists of a local inflammatory response with accumulation of mononuclear cells. The antigen-presenting cell (macrophage) activates T lymphocytes, resulting in cytokine production, B-cell proliferation, and antibody formation. Chronic inflammation results in formation of a pannus, a thickened synovium filled with activated T and B lymphocytes and plasma cells, as well as fibroblastic and macrophagic types of synovial cells. Joint destruction begins with exposed bone at the margins of articular cartilage denuded of hyaline cartilage. Eventually, the cartilage itself is destroyed by inflammatory by-products of the pannus.

The synovial fluid, in contrast to the mononuclear cell infiltrate seen in the synovial membrane, has neutrophils forming 75–85% of the cells.

Rheumatoid factors are antibodies specific to antigens on the Fc fragment of IgG. The antibodies include IgM, IgG, IgA, and IgE classes, but the IgM rheumatoid factor is typically measured. Rheumatoid factor may be a triggering factor for rheumatoid arthritis and may contribute to the chronic nature of the disease. Rheumatoid factor is also frequently found in patients with other inflammatory diseases, however, as well as in 1–5% of normal patients.

C. Laboratory Findings

No specific laboratory test exists for rheumatoid arthritis, but a series of test results help in the diagnosis. A high titer of rheumatoid factor (> 1:160) is the most significant diagnostic finding. Anemia is moderate, and leukocyte counts are normal or mildly elevated. Acute-phase reactants reflect the degree of inflammation nonspecifically and are often elevated in rheumatoid arthritis. These include the erythrocyte sedimentation rate and levels of C-reactive protein and serum immune complexes. Antinuclear antibodies are often positive in patients with severe rheumatoid arthritis (up to 37% in one study) but are not specific for the disease.

D. Imaging Studies

Early radiographic changes in rheumatoid arthritis include swelling of the small peripheral joints and marginal bony erosions. Joint space narrowing occurs later and is uniform, unlike the focal narrowing seen in osteoarthritis. Regional osteoporosis occurs, unlike the sclerosis seen in osteoarthritis. Advanced changes include bone resorption, deformity, dislocation, and fragmentation of affected joints. Protrusio acetabuli may be seen in the hips, and ulnar subluxation is common in the metacarpophalangeal joints.

Cush JJ, Lipsky PE: The immunopathogenesis of rheumatoid arthritis: The role of cytokines in chronic inflammation. Clin Aspects Autoimmun 1987;1:2.

Saulsbury FT: Prevalence of IgM, IgA, and IgG rheumatoid factors in juvenile rheumatoid arthritis. Clin Exp Rheum 1990;8:513.

Sutton B et al: The structure and origin of rheumatoid factors. Immunol Today. 2001; 21: 177.Winchester RG: Genetic aspects of rheumatoid arthritis. Springer Semin Immunopathol 1981;4:89.

Zvaifler NJ: Etiology and pathogenesis of rheumatoid arthritis. In: McCarty DJ, ed: *Arthritis and Allied Conditions.* Philadelphia: Lea & Febiger, 1989.

Ankylosing Spondylitis

A seronegative (negative rheumatoid factor) inflammatory arthritis, ankylosing spondylitis consists of bilateral sacroiliitis with or without associated spondylitis and uveitis. An insidious disease, the diagnosis is often delayed because of vagueness of the early symptom of low back pain. Diagnostic clinical criteria include low back pain, limited lumbar spine motion, decreased chest expansion, and sacroiliitis.

Joint involvement is primarily axial, including all portions of the spine, sacroiliac joint, and hip joints. Extraskeletal involvement includes dilatation of the aorta, anterior uveitis, and restrictive lung disease secondary to restriction of thoracic cage mobility.

A. Epidemiologic Features

The association of HLA-B27 and ankylosing spondylitis is strong, with 90% of patients testing positive for this haplotype; however, only 2% of HLA-B27-positive patients develop ankylosing spondylitis. First-degree family members of a patient who has ankylosing spondylitis and is positive for HLA-B27 have a 20% risk of developing the disease. Clinical and experimental evidence shows that *Klebsiella* infection may be a triggering factor for arthritis in patients positive for HLA-B27.

B. Laboratory Findings

During the active phase of the disease, the erythrocyte sedimentation rate is increased. Testing for rheumatoid factor and antinuclear antibodies is negative.

C. Imaging Studies

Early in the course of ankylosing spondylitis, the sacroiliac joints may be widened, reflecting bony erosions of the iliac side of the joint. Later, the inflamed cartilage is replaced by ossification, resulting in ankylosis of the bilateral sacroiliac joints. Vertebrae of the thoracolumbar spine are "squared off," with bridging syndesmophytes, forming a "bamboo spine." Ankylosis of peripheral joints may be seen. Magnetic resonance imaging may provide sensitive and specific radiographic evidence of sacroiliitis.

Ebringer RW et al: Sequential studies in ankylosing spondylitis: Association of *Klebsiella pneumoniae* with active disease. Ann Rheum Dis 1978;37:146.

Geczy AF et al: A factor in *Klebsiella* filtrates specifically modifies an HLA-B27 associated cell-surface component. Nature 1980;283:782.

Luong AA, Salonen DC: Imaging of the seronegative spondyloarthropathies. Curr Rheumatol Rep 2000; 2(4):288.

Moll JMH, Wright V: New York clinical criteria for ankylosing spondylitis: A statistical evaluation. Ann Rheum Dis 1973; 32:354.

Van der Linden S et al: The risk of developing ankylosing spondylitis in HLA-B27 positive individuals: A family and population study. Br J Rheum 1983;22 (Suppl):18.

Psoriatic Arthritis

A seronegative inflammatory arthritis associated with psoriasis, psoriatic arthritis was long considered a variant of rheumatoid arthritis. The discovery of rheumatoid factor led to the division of inflammatory arthritides into seropositive and seronegative diseases, separating psoriatic arthritis from rheumatoid arthritis.

Though psoriatic arthritis is characterized by a relatively benign course in most patients, up to 20% develop severe joint involvement. The distal interphalangeal joints of the fingers are commonly affected, but several patterns of peripheral arthritis exist, including an asymmetric oligoarthritis, a symmetric polyarthritis (similar to rheumatoid arthritis), arthritis mutilans (a destructive, deforming type of arthritis), and a spondyloarthropathy (similar to ankylosing spondylitis, with sacroiliac joint involvement).

In addition to the dry erythematous papular skin lesions, nail changes are found. These include pitting, grooves, subungual hyperkeratosis, and destruction.

A. Epidemiologic Features

One third of patients with psoriasis have arthritis, with joint symptoms delayed as long as 20 years after onset of skin lesions. Both sexes are affected equally.

B. Laboratory Findings

There are no specific laboratory tests for psoriatic arthritis. Nonspecific inflammatory markers may be elevated, including the erythrocyte sedimentation rate. Rheumatoid factor is usually negative but is present in up to 10% of patients.

C. Imaging Studies

Coexistence of erosive changes and bone formation is seen in peripheral joints, with absence of periarticular osteoporosis. Gross destruction of phalangeal joints ("pencil-in-cup" appearance) and lysis of terminal phalanges are seen. Bilateral sacroiliac joint ankylosis and syndesmophytes of the spine are seen, as in ankylosing spondylitis.

Gladman DD et al: HLA antigens in psoriatic arthritis. J Rheum 1986;13:586.

Hohler T, Marker-Hermann E: Psoriatic arthritis: Clinical aspects, genetics, and the role of T cells. Curr Opin Rheumatol 2001;13(4):273.

Mader R, Gladman D: Psoriatic arthritis: Making the diagnosis and treating early. J Musculoskel Med 1993;10:18.

Juvenile Rheumatoid Arthritis

Juvenile rheumatoid arthritis is an inflammatory arthritic syndrome with a variety of symptoms. Early diagnosis is often difficult. Criteria for juvenile rheumatoid arthritis include distinction of mode of onset as systemic, polyarticular, or pauciarticular. Systemic onset (also known as **Still's disease**) occurs in 20% of patients and is characterized by high fever, rash, lymphadenopathy, splenomegaly, carditis, and varying degrees of arthritis. Polyarticular onset occurs in 30–40% of patients, and is notable for fewer systemic symptoms, low-grade fever, and synovitis of four or more joints. Pauciarticular onset develops in 40–50% of patients and involves one to four joints; there are no systemic signs, but there is an increased incidence of iridocyclitis. Iridocyclitis is an insidious complication that requires early ophthalmologic slit lamp evaluation, if juvenile rheumatoid arthritis is suspected, to prevent blindness.

A. EPIDEMIOLOGIC FEATURES

The two peak ages of onset are between 1 and 3 years and between 8 and 12 years. Females are affected twice as often as males.

B. LABORATORY FINDINGS

Leukocytosis up to 30,000/mL is seen with systemic-onset juvenile rheumatoid arthritis, with mild elevations in polyarticular-onset disease and normal values in pauciarticular-onset disease. White blood cell counts in synovial fluid range from 150 to 50,000/mL. The erythrocyte sedimentation rate is elevated, as are other acute-phase reactants.

Rheumatoid factor is typically negative in juvenile rheumatoid arthritis. As many as 50% of patients have positive antinuclear antibodies, a finding correlated with iridocyclitis and pauciarticular-onset disease.

C. IMAGING STUDIES

Soft-tissue swelling and premature closure of physes may be seen early, as well as juxta-articular osteopenia.

Erosive changes are seen late and resemble those of rheumatoid arthritis.

Falcini F, Cimaz R: Juvenile rheumatoid arthritis. Curr. Opin. Rheumatol. 2000; 12(5): 415.

Schaller JG: The association of antinuclear antibodies with the chronic iridocyclitis of juvenile rheumatoid arthritis. Arthritis Rheum 1974;17:409.

Systemic Lupus Erythematosus

Systemic lupus erythematosus is a chronic inflammatory disease that may affect multiple organ systems. It is an autoimmune disorder in which autoantibodies are formed. The large variety of clinical appearances and laboratory findings may mimic many disorders. The diagnosis is based on the presence of 4 of the following 11 criteria: (1) malar rash; (2) discoid rash; (3) photosensitivity; (4) oral ulcers; (5) arthritis; (6) serositis; (7) renal disorders (proteinuria or casts); (8) neurologic disorders (seizures or psychosis); (9) hematologic disorders (hemolytic anemia, leukopenia, lymphopenia, thrombocytopenia); (10) immunologic disorders (positive lupus erythematosus (LE) cell preparation, anti-DNA antibody, anti-Sm antibody, false-positive serologic test for syphilis); and (11) abnormal titer of antinuclear antibody.

A. EPIDEMIOLOGIC FEATURES

Females are affected eight times as often as males. An increased risk for systemic lupus erythematosus has been noted for Asians and Polynesians over whites in Hawaii. Black females are also associated with an increased risk over white females. Genetic susceptibility has been demonstrated with increased frequency (5%) among relatives of patients with the disease. An inherited complement deficiency is inferred from the absence, or near absence, of individual complement components, the most common being C2.

B. LABORATORY FINDINGS

Antinuclear antibody determination is the most helpful screening test for systemic lupus erythematosus. The LE cell preparation was the first immunologic test for systemic lupus erythematosus, but it is laborious, insensitive, and difficult to interpret. In patients with untreated active disease, 98% have positive antinuclear antibody tests. The higher the titer of antinuclear antibodies, the more likely is the diagnosis of systemic lupus erythematosus or related rheumatic syndrome. A low value for the antinuclear antibody test is 1:320; values greater than 1:5120 are considered high.

If antinuclear antibody levels are positive, more specific tests may be performed, including testing for anti-DNA antibodies, antibodies to extractable nuclear antigens, and complement levels. High titers of antibodies to double-stranded DNA are highly suggestive for systemic lupus erythematosus. Low complement levels (C3, C4, and total hemolytic complement levels) are found in the disease but are also seen in related illnesses.

Anemia, leukopenia, and thrombocytopenia are seen, as well as elevations in the erythrocyte sedimentation rate. Renal function tests and muscle and liver enzyme tests are often abnormal, reflecting multiple organ system involvement.

C. Imaging Studies

The radiographic features of arthritis in systemic lupus erythematosus are similar to those of rheumatoid arthritis. Much of the joint pain may be related to osteonecrosis, particularly of the femoral and humeral heads.

Agnello V: Association of systemic lupus erythematosus and systemic lupus erythematosus-like syndromes with hereditary and acquired complement deficient states. Arthritis Rheum 1978;21:S146.

Block SR et al: Immunologic observations on 9 sets of twins either concordant or discordant for systemic lupus erythematosus. Arthritis Rheum 1976;19:545.

Kaine JL, Kahl LE: Which laboratory tests are useful in diagnosing SLE? J Musculoskel Med 1992;9:15.

Serdula MK, Rhoads GG: Frequency of systemic lupus erythematosus in different ethnic groups in Hawaii. Arthritis Rheum 1979;22:328.

Tan EM et al: Revised criteria for classification of systemic lupus erythematosus: ARA subcommittee. Arthritis Rheum 1982; 25:1271.

Arthritis Associated with Inflammatory Bowel Disease

Peripheral arthritis and spondylitis are associated with ulcerative colitis and Crohn's disease. Joint involvement is typically monarticular or oligoarticular and often parallels the activity of the bowel disease. The arthritis is frequently migratory and is self-limiting in most cases, with only 10% of patients having chronic arthritis. The joints most commonly affected are the knees, hips, and ankles, in order of prevalence. Spondylitis associated with inflammatory bowel disease occurs in two forms. One is very similar to ankylosing spondylitis, including the increased incidence of the HLA-B27 haplotype. The other form has no identifiable genetic predisposition.

A. Epidemiologic Features

Up to 25% of patients with inflammatory bowel disease develop arthritis. There is no difference between the sexes in incidence.

B. Laboratory Findings

There is no specific diagnostic test. Synovial fluid analysis reveals an inflammatory process, with leukocyte counts of 4000–50,000/mL.

C. Imaging Studies

Peripheral arthritis is nonerosive, with juxta-articular osteopenia and joint space narrowing. Spondylitis associated with inflammatory bowel disease resembles ankylosing spondylitis.

Enlow RW et al: The spondylitis of inflammatory bowel disease. Arthritis Rheum 1980;23: 1359.

Morris RI et al: HLA-B27, a useful discriminator in the arthropathy of inflammatory bowel disease. N Engl J Med 1974;290: 1117.

Wollheim FA: Enteropathic arthritis: How do the joints talk with the gut? Curr Opin Rheumatol 2001:13(4):305.

Reiter's Syndrome

The classic triad of conjunctivitis, urethritis, and peripheral arthritis is known as **Reiter's syndrome. Reactive arthritis** is becoming accepted as a more precise term, because the initiating condition may be enteritis as well as a sexually transmitted disease. The peripheral arthritis is polyarticular and asymmetric, with knees, ankles, and foot joints most commonly affected.

A. Epidemiologic Features

Nongonococcal urethritis caused by *Chlamydia* or *Ureaplasma* accounts for the precipitating event in about 40% of cases. Patients who test positive for HLA-B27 are predisposed to developing arthritis after contracting nongonococcal urethritis. A reactive arthritis following enteric infection with *Salmonella, Shigella, Yersinia,* and *Campylobacter* has also been noted. For enteric infections with *Shigella,* the risk of developing arthritis in individuals positive for HLA-B27 is close to 20%.

B. Laboratory Findings

There are no specific diagnostic tests for Reiter's syndrome. Anemia, leukocytosis, and thrombocytosis occur, and the erythrocyte sedimentation rate is often elevated.

C. Imaging Studies

The radiographic features of Reiter's syndrome are similar to those of ankylosing spondylitis, with calcifications of ligamentous insertions and ankylosing of joints. The sacroiliitis is unilateral, unlike in ankylosing spondylitis.

Caelin A, Fries JF: An "experimental" epidemic of Reiter's syndrome revisited: Follow-up evidence on genetic and environmental factors. Ann Intern Med 1976;85:563.

Ford DK: Reiter's syndrome: Reactive arthritis. In McCarty DJ, ed: *Arthritis and Allied Conditions.* Philadelphia: Lea and Febiger, 1989.

Grayston JT, Wan SP: New knowledge of chlamydiae and the diseases they cause. J Infect Dis 1975;132:87.

Shepard MC: Current status of *Ureaplasma urealyticum* in nongonococcal urethritis. J Clin Sci 1980;1:198.

3. Metabolic Arthropathy

Gout

Deposition of monosodium urate crystals in the joints produces gout. Although most patients with gout have hyperuricemia, few patients with hyperuricemia develop gout. The causes of hyperuricemia include disorders resulting in overproduction or undersecretion of uric acid or a combination of these two abnormalities. Examples of uric acid overproduction include enzymatic mutations, leukemias, hemoglobinopathies, and excessive purine intake.

The first attack involves sudden onset of painful arthritis, most often in the first metatarsophalangeal joint, but also in the ankle, knee, wrist, finger, and elbow. The intensity of the pain is comparable to that from a septic joint, and differentiation is necessary as the treatment is different. Coexistence of a septic joint is unusual but possible. Rapid resolution with colchicine or indomethacin is seen. Chronic gouty arthritis is notable for tophaceous deposits, joint deformity, constant pain, and swelling. Definitive diagnosis is made upon demonstration of intracellular monosodium urate crystals in synovial cell leukocytes.

A. EPIDEMIOLOGIC FEATURES

Primary gout has hereditary features, with a familial incidence of 6–18%. It is likely that the serum urate concentration is controlled by multiple genes.

B. LABORATORY FINDINGS

The key diagnostic test is detection of monosodium urate crystals in white blood cells in synovial fluid. Negative birefringence of the needle-shaped crystals is seen by their yellow coloration on polarized light microscopy.

Hyperuricemia is usually seen, but up to one-fourth of gout patients may have normal uric acid levels. Uric acid levels are elevated when they exceed 7 mg/dL. An elevated white blood cell count and sedimentation rate can be seen in acute gout, and thus these tests cannot be used to differentiate between the two processes. Aspirates should be sent for culture to rule out coexisting infection.

C. IMAGING STUDIES

Tophi may be seen when they are calcified. Soft-tissue swelling is seen, as well as erosions. Chronic changes consist of extensive bone loss, joint narrowing, and joint deformity.

Abubaker MY et al: The management of gout. N Engl J Med 1996; 334:445.

Agudelo CA, Wise CM: Gout: Diagnosis, pathogenesis, and clinical manifestations. Curr Opin Rheumatol 2001;13(3):234.

Emmerson BT: Coexistence of acute gout and septic arthritis. Arthritis Rheum 2000;43:S189.

Kelley WN et al: Gout and related disorders of purine metabolism. In Kelly WN et al, eds: *Textbook of Rheumatology.* Philadelphia: WB Saunders, 1989.

Levinson DJ: Clinical gout and the pathogenesis of hyperuricemia. In McCarty DJ, ed: *Arthritis and Allied Conditions.* Philadelphia: Lea & Febiger, 1989.

Calcium Pyrophosphate Crystal Deposition Disease

This goutlike syndrome is also known as pseudogout or chondrocalcinosis. Crystals of calcium pyrophosphate dihydrate are deposited in a joint, most commonly the knee and not the first metatarsophalangeal joint, as in gout. The diagnosis is made by demonstration of the crystals in tissue or synovial fluid and by the presence of characteristic radiographic findings.

Aging and trauma have been associated with this disorder, as well as conditions such as hyperparathyroidism, gout, hemochromatosis, hypophosphatasia, and hypothyroidism.

A. EPIDEMIOLOGIC FEATURES

Hereditary forms of calcium pyrophosphate dihydrate deposition disease have been reported, with transmission as an autosomal trait. Idiopathic cases have not been rigorously examined for genetic factors or association with other diseases.

B. PATHOLOGIC FEATURES

Calcification of multiple joint structures occurs, including hyaline cartilage and capsules, with heaviest deposition in fibrocartilaginous structures such as the menisci. The crystals are more difficult to see than urate crystals but have weak positive birefringence.

C. IMAGING STUDIES

Calcification of menisci and hyaline cartilage is seen as punctate or linear radiodensities, which delineate these normally radiolucent structures. Bursas, ligaments, and tendons may have calcifications as well. Bony signs include subchondral cyst formation, signs of carpal instability, sacroiliac joint erosions with vacuum phenomenon, and "crowning" of the odontoid process.

Kohn NN et al: The significance of calcium phosphate crystals in the synovial fluid of arthritis patients: The "pseudogout syndrome." II. Identification of crystals. Ann Intern Med 1982;56:738.

McCarty DJ et al: The significance of calcium phosphate crystals in the synovial fluid of arthritis patients: The "pseudogout syndrome." I. Clinical aspects. Ann Intern Med 1962;56:711.

Resnick D: Rheumatoid arthritis and pseudorheumatoid arthritis in calcium pyrophosphate dihydrate crystal deposition disease. Radiology 1981;140:615.

Rosenthal AK: Calcium crystal-associated arthritides. Curr Opin Rheumatol 1998;10(3):273.

Ochronosis

A hereditary deficiency in the enzyme homogentisic acid oxidase is present in the disease known as **alkaptonuria.** The presence of unmetabolized homogentisic acid results in a brownish black color of the urine (thus the name of the disease). The term **ochronosis** describes the clinical condition of homogentisic acid deposited in connective tissues, manifested by bluish black pigmentation of the skin, ear, and sclera, and in cartilage.

The diagnosis is made when the triad of dark urine, degenerative arthritis, and abnormal pigmentation is present. Freshly passed urine is normal in color but turns dark when oxidized. Spondylosis is common, with knee, shoulder, and hip joint involvement also seen.

A. EPIDEMIOLOGIC FEATURES

Transmission of alkaptonuria is by a recessive autosomal gene.

B. IMAGING STUDIES

Spondylosis is seen, with calcification of intervertebral disks with few osteophytes. Joint involvement is similar in appearance to that of osteoarthritis, except for protrusio acetabuli.

Schumacher HR, Holdsworth DE: Ochronotic arthropathy: Clinicopathologic studies. Semin Arthritis Rheum 1977; 6:207.

4. Osteochondroses

Osteonecrosis of the Femoral Head

A variety of conditions and diseases are associated with femoral head osteonecrosis, but the pathogenesis is unknown in most cases. Direct injury to the blood supply of the femoral head is implicated in traumatic causes of avascular necrosis such as subcapital femoral neck fracture and dislocation of the hip. The disorder is bilateral in more than 60% of cases and affects other bones in about 15% of cases. The leading nontraumatic causes of osteonecrosis of the femoral head include alcoholism, idiopathic causes, and systemic steroid treatment. The mechanism by which steroids cause osteonecrosis may be by adipogenesis, because the effects may be reduced, at least in an animal model, by using lovastatin.

Other associated conditions include hemoglobinopathies, Gaucher's disease, caisson disease, hyperlipidemia tobacco use, hypercoagulable states, irradiation, and diseases of bone marrow infiltration such as leukemia and lymphoma.

A. PATHOLOGIC FEATURES

Regardless of underlying causes, the early lesions in femoral head osteonecrosis include necrosis of marrow and trabecular bone, usually in a wedge-shaped area in the region of the anterolateral superior femoral head. The overlying articular cartilage is largely unaffected because it is normally avascular, obtaining nutrition from the synovial fluid. The deep calcified layer of cartilage, however, does derive nutrition from epiphyseal vessels and also undergoes necrosis. Histologically, necrotic marrow and absence of osteocytes in lacunae are seen.

Leukocytes and mononuclear cells collect around necrotic and fibrovascular tissue and eventually replace necrotic marrow. Osteoclasts resorb dead trabeculae, and osteoblasts then attempt to repair the damaged tissue; during attempted repair, the necrotic trabeculae are susceptible to fatigue fracture. Grossly, a subchondral fracture forms, with deformation of overlying hyaline cartilage. With time, fragmentation of articular cartilage ensues, resulting in degenerative arthritis.

B. IMAGING STUDIES

Ficat has created a classification based on the plain radiographic appearance of femoral head osteonecrosis in progressive stages. Stage I represents normal or minimal changes (mild osteopenia or sclerotic regions) in an asymptomatic hip. In stage II, subchondral sclerosis and osteopenia are evident, often in a well-demarcated wedge in the anterolateral femoral head seen best with radiographs taken with the patient in the frogleg position from the lateral views. Stage III is heralded by collapse of subchondral bone; this is known as the crescent sign and is pathognomonic for femoral head osteonecrosis. Femoral head flattening is often seen, but the joint space is preserved. Stage IV consists of advanced degenerative arthritic changes, with loss of joint space and bony changes in the acetabulum.

A more recent classification system devised by Steinberg has become popular. It is based on extent of head involvement as determined by MRI. This system, called the University of Pennsylvania System, has seven stages from normal (stage 0) to stage VI in which advanced degenerative changes are evident. Stages I to V are divided into three subcategories of mild moderate and severe. Stage III of the Steinberg system corresponds to stage III of the Ficat system.

Cui Q et al: The Otto Aufranc Award: Lovastatin prevents steroid-induced adipogenesis and osteonecrosis. Clin Orthop 1997; 344:8.

Ficat RP: Idiopathic bone necrosis of the femoral head: Early diagnosis and treatment. J Bone Joint Surg Br 1985;67:3.

Lavernia CJ et al: Osteonecrosis of the femoral head. J Am Acad Orthop Surg 1999;7:250.

Steinberg ME et al: A quantitative system for staging avascular necrosis. J Bone Joint Surg 1995;77B:34.

5. Other Disorders Associated with Arthritis

Hemophilia

Hemophilia A is a heritable bleeding disorder produced by deficiency of factor VIII. Hemophilia B is a disease caused by lack of clotting factor IX. Both hemophilia A (classic hemophilia) and hemophilia B (Christmas disease) are sex-linked recessive disorders, though 30% of patients may have no family history of the disease. Hemophilic arthropathy primarily involves the knee joint, with the elbow and ankle joints affected less frequently.

A. PATHOLOGIC FEATURES

Recurrent hemarthrosis produces deposits of hemosiderin and synovitis. In the acute phase, hypertrophy of synovium occurs, causing a higher risk of repeated bleeding. A pannus may form, as in rheumatoid arthritis, with underlying cartilage destruction. With time, synovial fibrosis occurs, resulting in joint stiffness.

B. IMAGING STUDIES

Soft-tissue swelling is seen early and is associated with hemarthroses. Later stages include widening of epiphyseal regions caused by overgrowth from increased vascularity. Skeletal changes are manifested as subchondral sclerosis and cyst formation early, with later loss of cartilage and secondary osteophyte formation. Squaring of the patella is seen, possibly resulting from overgrowth.

Luck JV, Kasper CK: Surgical management of advanced hemophilic arthropathy. Clin Orthop 1989;242:60.

Gaucher's Disease

A rare familial disorder, Gaucher's disease is an inborn error of metabolism caused by a deficiency of the lysosomal hydrolase enzyme β-glucocerebrosidase. Accumulation of glucosylceramidase in phagocytic cells of the reticuloendothelial cells occurs, including the liver, spleen, lymph nodes, and bone marrow.

The femur is the most commonly affected bone, but the vertebrae, ribs, sternum, and flat bones of the pelvis may also be affected. The manifestations of skeletal disease are the result of mechanical effects of infiltration of the abnormal cells, leading to erosion of cortices and interference with the normal vascular supply. Expansion of bone and areas of osteolysis predispose affected bones to pathologic fracture, and vascular interruption leads to avascular necrosis of the femoral hip.

A. EPIDEMIOLOGIC FEATURES

Inherited in an autosomal recessive manner, Gaucher's disease is the most common inherited disorder of lipid metabolism. The disease is especially common in the Ashkenazi Jewish community.

B. PATHOLOGIC FEATURES

Histologic examination of involved reticuloendothelial tissues demonstrates foam cells, which are large lipid-laden macrophages.

C. IMAGING STUDIES

Early stages of skeletal involvement in Gaucher's disease include diffuse osteoporosis and medullary expansion. The distal femur may expand to form a characteristic "Erlenmeyer flask deformity." Localized erosions and sclerotic areas are seen. Osteonecrosis may be seen in the femoral head, humeral head, and distal femur. Secondary degenerative changes follow collapse of necrotic articular bone.

Amstutz HC, Carey EJ: Skeletal manifestations and treatment of Gaucher's disease. J Bone Joint Surg Am 1966;48:670.

Goldblatt J et al: The orthopaedic aspects of Gaucher's disease. Clin Orthop 1978;137:208.

Hip Labral Tears

The hip has a cartilaginous extension of the bony acetabulum called the labrum that deepens the acetabulum and stabilizes the hip. Labral tears have recently been rediscovered as a source of pain and a cause of osteoarthrosis. This has partially occurred due to the relative ease of evaluating their presence and subsequently treating them. Arthroscopy can be used to remove the torn labrum, similar to torn menisci.

A. PATHOLOGIC FEATURES

The normal labrum is triangular in shape and variable in size from 1 to 10 mm in length. The pathologic labrum has been classified into types A and B, depending on whether the labrum is traumatic (triangular; A) or degenerative (thick and rounded; B) and three stages: (1) intrasubstance degeneration, (2) partial tear, (3) complete tear.

B. IMAGING STUDIES

Magnetic resonance imaging (MRI) arthrography is the test of choice for suspected labral tears. Contrast is seen going into the tear which is frequently in the weight bearing area of the acetabulum. computed tomographic (CT) arthrography and MRI are not as sensitive.

Plotz GM et al: Magnetic resonance arthrography of the acetabular labrum. J Bone Joint Surg Br 2000;82:426.

■ MEDICAL MANAGEMENT

Nonsteroidal Anti-Inflammatory Drugs

The use of nonsteroidal anti-inflammatory drugs (NSAIDs) in the management of osteoarthritis is widespread but controversial. Because only minimal inflammatory changes are present in joints with osteoarthritis, the use of acetaminophen has been advocated as a first-line drug. In a short-term study of patients treated for osteoarthritis, acetaminophen (4000 mg/d) was found to be as effective as ibuprofen (2400 mg/d).

The therapeutic effect of NSAIDs can be dramatic in the osteoarthritic patient, even with severe disease. The main problems with routine NSAID therapy are the gastrointestinal (GI) and renal complications and the inhibition of normal platelet function. Thus, alternative therapies should be carefully considered, and therapy should be closely monitored. Current NSAIDs work by altering prostaglandin synthesis through nonspecific inhibition of both cyclooxygenase isoforms 1 (COX-1) and 2 (COX-2). COX-1 inhibition can have deleterious effects on hemostasis and the GI tract.

Patients treated with NSAIDs have a three-times greater relative risk of developing GI complications than nonusers. In one study, NSAIDs were associated with acute hospital admissions of 30% of elderly patients. Patients at high risk for developing ulcers with use of NSAIDs are those with any of the following characteristics: age older than 65 years, history of prior ulcer disease, use of multiple dose or high-dose NSAIDs, or use of concomitant corticosteroids. The antiprostaglandin effects of NSAIDs can reduce renal blood flow, leading to acute and chronic renal insufficiency. Patients at risk for acute renal insufficiency because of NSAIDs are elderly patients, those with atherosclerotic cardiovascular disease, and those with preexisting renal impairment. The platelet effects of these drugs are variable, depending on the NSAID half-life, on whether the NSAID inhibits thromboxane A, and on whether that inhibition is reversible. Aspirin, for example, is permanent for the life of the platelet. Many patients report increased bruising as a result of taking these drugs.

The toxicities of currently available NSAIDs are compared in Table 7–3. Because the effects are not caused solely by the inhibitory effects on prostaglandin synthesis, the various chemical origins of these drugs may lead to slightly different clinical effects in different patients.

The chemical families of these drugs are noted in Table 7–4 with their half-lives and their dosing frequency. Dosing frequency is important because it has been shown that patient compliance with use of these drugs goes up with less frequent dosing, such as daily or twice daily.

Much anticipated has been the development of COX-2-selective NSAIDs, which have recently become available. Most of the side effects attributable to NSAIDs are caused by inhibition of COX-1, an isoform that is normally present ("constitutive") in renal and gastrointestinal tissues. COX-2-selective NSAIDs inhibit the isoenzyme that develops ("inducible") as a response to inflammation. By selectively inhibiting COX-2, the efficacy of NSAIDs is retained with much less side effects.

Though COX-2-selective NSAIDs are purportedly safe, they are not without side effects. Celecoxib did not exhibit statistically significant decreased rates of complicated upper GI events in a recent randomized controlled trial. Rofecoxib was shown to significantly decrease complicated upper GI events compared with conventional NSAIDs, but the rate of myocardial infarction was increased, possibly related to loss of the antiplatelet effect normally present in NSAIDs.

The choice of an appropriate NSAID should be based on the following factors: clotting problems, compliance of the patient, GI symptom history, renal function, drug cost, and the effect on the patient with previously used NSAIDs. Patients taking warfarin would probably be better treated with a drug having no platelet effect, that is COX-2-specific. Patients with a poor response to one type of NSAID may benefit from a trial with one from another chemical family. A patient with a history of poor drug compliance with other medications would benefit from daily dosing, whereas a patient already taking another drug three times daily would probably find tid, or three-times-daily, dosing more convenient. Obviously, a patient with renal disease should be treated with a drug having not only low renal toxicity, but also probably a short half-life to minimize the accumulation of the drug in the body because of lack of renal excretion. The COX-2-selective NSAIDs will not eliminate the need for the other drugs. The vast majority of patients tolerate the side effects of the older drugs, and the risk-benefit ratio for these drugs is quite favorable, especially for short courses of treatment.

The advent of the COX-2-specific NSAIDs has added to their safety as analgesics for acute pain because the COX-2 inhibitors block the pain, fever, and inflammatory response, while not affecting clotting. Thus,

Table 7–3. Toxicity profiles of currently available NSAIDs.

Generic Name	Proprietary Name	Gastrointestinal Toxicity	Renal Toxicity	Platelet Effects (d)[a]	Other Toxicity[b]
Diclofenac	Voltaren	Moderate	Moderate	1	Hepatitis
Etodolac	Lodine	Low[c]	Moderate	NA	—
Indomethacin	Indocin	High	Moderate	1	Headache
Nabumetone	Relafen	Low[c]	Moderate	NA	Hepatitis
Sulindac	Clinoril	Moderate	Low	1	Dermatitis
Tolmetin	Tolectin	Moderate	Moderate	2	—
Meclofenamate	Meclomen	Moderate	Moderate	1	Diarrhea
Piroxicam	Feldene	Moderate	Moderate	14	—
Fenoprofen	Nalfon	Moderate	Moderate	1	—
Flurbiprofen	Ansaid	Moderate	Moderate	1	—
Ibuprofen	Motrin	Moderate	Moderate	1	—
Ketoprofen	Orudis	Moderate	Moderate	2	—
Naproxen	Naprosyn	Moderate	Moderate	4	—
Oxaprozin	Daypro	Moderate	Moderate	NA	—
Ketorolacq	Toradol	High	Moderate	1	—
Salicylsalicylic acid[d]	Disalcid	None	None	None	—
Sodium salicylate[d]	—	None	None	None	—
Aspirin	—	High	Moderate	10	Tinnitus
Diflunisal[e]	Dolobid	Low	Low	None	—
Celecoxib	Celebrex	Low	Low	None	Sulfa allergies

[a]Average time to normal platelet function after discontinuation of drug.
[b]Other NSAIDs may have similar toxicity, but the effects are more prevalent with these agents.
[c]Simultaneous efficacy comparisons in inflammatory disease not available.
[d]No prostaglandin inhibition.
[e]Weak prostaglandin inhibitor.
NA = data not available.

their use in the perioperative setting has significantly increased.

Surgical intervention is generally indicated for patients who have failed conservative therapy with NSAIDs. For patients who are not surgical candidates, a long-term regimen of narcotic medication may be considered.

Batchlor EE, Paulus HE: Principles of drug therapy. In Moskowitz RW et al, eds: *Osteoarthritis: Diagnosis and Medical Surgical Management.* Philadelphia: WB Saunders, 1993.

Berger RG: Nonsteroidal anti-inflammatory drugs: Making the right choice. J Am Acad Orthop Surg 1994;2:255.

Bombardier C et al: Comparison of upper gastrointestinal toxicity of rofecoxib and naproxen in patients with rheumatoid arthritis. VIGOR Study Group. N Engl J Med 2000;343(21): 1520.

Bradley JD et al: Comparison of an anti-inflammatory dose of ibuprofen, an analgesic dose of ibuprofen, and acetaminophen in the treatment of patients with osteoarthritis of the knee. N Engl J Med 1991;325:87.

Gabriel SE et al: Risk for serious gastrointestinal complications related to use of nonsteroidal anti-inflammatory drugs. Ann Intern Med 1991; 115:787.

Hochberg MC et al: Guidelines for the medical management of osteoarthritis, I Osteoarthritis of the hip. Arthritis Rheum 1995;38:1535.

Hochberg MC et al: Guidelines for the medical management of osteoarthritis, II Osteoarthritis of the knee. Arthritis Rheum 1995;38:1541.

Hosie J et al: Meloxicam in osteoarthritis: A 6-month, double-blind comparison with diclofenac sodium. Br J Rheumatol 1996;35 (Suppl 1):39.

Silverstein FE et al: Gastrointestinal toxicity with celecoxib vs nonsteroidal anti-inflammatory drugs for osteoarthritis and rheumatoid arthritis: the CLASS study: A randomized controlled trial. Celecoxib long term arthritis safety study. JAMA 2000;284(10):1247.

Simon LS et al: Preliminary study of the safety and efficacy of SC-58635, a novel cyclooxygenase 2 inhibitor: Efficacy and safety in two placebo-controlled trials in osteoarthritis and rheumatoid arthritis, and studies of gastrointestinal and platelet effects. Arthritis Rheum 1998; 41:1591.

Disease-Modifying Agents in Rheumatoid Arthritis

Three new disease-modifying antirheumatic drugs (DMARD) are now available for the medical treatment of rheumatoid arthritis. Although the experience of these new agents is limited, the mechanisms of their actions may guide orthopedic surgeons with respect to their potential effect on the surgical procedures. Etaner-

Table 7–4. Dosage data of currently available NSAIDs.

Generic Name	Proprietary Name	Largest Unit Dose (mg)	Half-life (h)	Dosing Frequency[a]	Family
Diclofenac	Voltaren	75	2	bid	Acetic acid
Etodolac	Lodine	300	6	qid	"
Indomethacin	Indocin	50	4	tid	"
Nabumetone	Relafen	500	20–30	2 qd	"
Sulindac	Clinoril	200	8–14	bid	"
Tolmetin	Tolectin	400	1–2	tid	"
Meclofenamate	Meclomen	100	2	tid	Fenamates
Piroxicam	Feldene	20	30–86	qd	Oxicams
Fenoprofen	Nalfon	600	2–3	qid	Proprionates
Flurbiprofen	Ansaid	100	6	tid	"
Ibuprofen	Motrin	800	2	qid	"
Ketoprofen	Orudis	75	3	tid	"
Naproxen	Naprosyn	500	14	bid	"
Oxaprozin	Daypro	600	40–50	2 qd	"
Ketorolac	Toradol	10	5	qid	Pyrrolo-pyrrole
Salicylsalicylic acid	Disalcid	750	1	qid	Salicylates
Sodium salicylate	—	650	0.5	q4h	"
Aspirin	—	325	0.25	2q4h	"
Diffunisal	Dolobid	500	10	bid	"
Celeboxib	Celebrex	200	11	bid	Sulfonamide

[a]Dosage required for treatment of inflammation.
bid = twice a day; qd = each day; q4h = every 4 hours; qid = four times a day; tid = three times a day.

cept is an artificially bioengineered molecule that binds to the receptor of TNF (tumor necrosis factor), preventing activation of the inflammatory cascade. Infliximab, is a chimeric antibody which also targets TNF. Both of these drugs will probably have little effect on healing and probably can be continued up to any surgical procedure. Leflunomide inhibits an enzyme, decreasing levels of pyrimidine nucleotides, inhibiting clonal expansion of T cells in rheumatoid arthritis. This DMARD should probably be discontinued one week prior to surgery, similar to methotrexate.

Kremer JM: Rational use of new and existing disease-modifying agents in rheumatoid arthritis. Ann Intern Med 2001;134: 695.

OTHER THERAPIES

Nutritional Supplements

The nutritional supplements glucosamine sulfate and chondroitin sulfate have become popular as nonprescription products for arthritis therapy. This popularity arises from the concept that these products may serve as substrate for the reparative processes in cartilage. Glucosamine sulfate is found as an intermediate product in mucopolysaccharide synthesis, and an elevated urinary excretion is seen in patients with osteoarthritis and rheumatoid arthritis. Oral administration of glucosamine sulfate was compared with analgesic doses of ibuprofen in a 4-week trial in patients with osteoarthritis of the knee. Ibuprofen was found to provide pain relief more quickly, but the response rates were similar at 4 weeks.

Chondroitin sulfate is another glycosaminoglycan present in articular cartilage; its oral administration in one study resulted in no change in serum levels. In another study, patients with osteoarthritis of the hip and knee used fewer NSAIDs when given chondroitin sulfate compared with a placebo control group. Although glucosamine sulfate and chondroitin sulfate are unproven therapies at this time, their use may provide safe and effective symptomatic relief in some patients with osteoarthritis. Recent reports indicate improved symptoms of osteoarthritis with oral glucosamine and chondroitin sulfate, but the mechanisms of action are unknown.

Brief AA et al: Use of glucosamine and chondroitin sulfate in the management of osteoarthritis. J Am Acad Orthop Surg 2001; 9:71.

Houpt JB et al: Effect of glucosamine hydrochloride (GHCl) in the treatment of pain of osteoarthritis of the knee. J Rheumatol 1998;25 (supplement 52):8.

Hughes RA, Carr AJ: A randomized double-blind placebo-controlled trail of glucosamine to control pain in osteoarthritis of the knee. Arthritis Rheum 2000;43(9(Suppl)):S384.

Leffter CT et al: Glucosamine, chondroitin, and manganese ascorbate for degenerative joint disease of the knee or low back: A randomized, double-blind, placebo-controlled pilot study. Mil Med 1999;164(2):85.

Mazieres B et al: Chondroitin sulfate in the treatment of gonarthrosis and coxarthrosis. Five-month results of a multicenter double-blind controlled prospective study using placebo. Rev Rhum Mal Osteoartic 1992;59:466.

McAlindon TE et al: Glucosamine and chondroitin for treatment of osteoarthritis: A systemic quality assessment and meta-analysis. JAMA 2000; 283:1469.

Muller-Fabender H et al: Glucosamine sulfate compared to ibuprofen in osteoarthritis of the knee. Osteoarthritis Cartilage 1994;2:61.

Reginster JY et al: Long term effects of glucosamine sulphate on osteoarthritis progression: A randomized, placebo-controlled clinical trial. Lancet 2001;357:251.

Rindone JP et al: Randomized, controlled trial of glucosamine for treating osteoarthritis of the knee. West J Med 2000;172 (2):91.

Injections

One of the mainstays of the treatment of osteoarthrosis and rheumatoid arthritis is the cortisone injection. These can be used for joints, bursae, and trigger points. Generally, shoulders, elbows, wrists, finger joints, knees, ankles and joints of the foot can be given in the office without radiographic control. Hips and some joints of the foot and hand are best done with radiographic control to ensure location of the injection. The injections can be therapeutic with steroids or diagnostic with local anesthetic. For example, differentiation between the amount of a patient's pain coming from the back and the proportion coming from the hip can be ascertained with a lidocaine injection into the hip. This will reliably inform the patient as to the realistic expectations of pain relief after a hip replacement. Similarly, an ankle injection will predict pain relief after ankle fusion. Recently, intra-articular administration of hyaluronic acid has become available for treatment of osteoarthritis of the knee with products of different molecular weight currently available. The treatment protocols for these drugs call for weekly injections for 3–5 weeks to obtain a therapeutic effect.

Hyaluronic acid is a long-chain polysaccharide responsible for the viscoelastic properties of synovial joint fluid. In pathologic states, such as osteoarthritis and rheumatoid arthritis, both the concentration and molecular size of hyaluronic acid is diminished. In animal experimental models, there is evidence that hyaluronic injections may retard progression of osteoarthritis. Serial injections of hyaluronic acid in patients with osteoarthritic knees have been reported to reduce pain for up to 10 months, but the mechanism of action is unknown. Because of the short half-life of hyaluronic acid, it is unlikely that the injections significantly boost lubrication of arthritic joints. Rather than being a disease-modifying therapy, the injectable hyaluronic acid products should be considered long-acting, pain-relieving drugs.

Adams ME et al: The role of viscosupplementation with hylan G-F 20 (Synvisc) in the treatment of osteoarthritis of the knee: A Canadian multicenter trial comparing hylan G-F 20 alone, hylan G-F 20 with nonsteroidal anti-inflammatory drugs (NSAIDs) and NSAIDs alone. Osteoarthritis Cartilage 1995; 3(4):213.

Altman RD, Moskowitz R: Intraarticular sodium hyaluronate (Hyalgan) in the treatment of patients with osteoarthritis of the knee: A randomized clinical trial. Hyalgan Study Group. J Rheumatol 1998;25(11):2203.

Marshall KW et al: Amelioration of disease severity by intraarticular hylan therapy in bilateral canine osteoarthritis. J Orthop Res 2000;18(3):416.

Watterson JR, Esdaile JM: Viscosupplementation: Therapeutic mechanisms and clinical potential in osteoarthritis of the knee. J Am Acad Orthop Surg 2000;8:277.

Orthotic Treatment

The use of orthotics can ameliorate the symptoms of osteoarthrosis in the knee, the ankle, and possibly the elbow, but other joints are not really amenable to this treatment. The medial compartment of the knee is more commonly affected than the lateral, leading to, or resulting from varus deformity. Thus this disorder lends itself to orthotic treatment to remove the deformity. Heel wedges and valgus braces can be helpful in relieving the pain and improving the ambulatory function of patients with medial gonarthrosis. Similarly, orthotics to control varus and valgus forces at the ankle can be very helpful for ankle arthrosis.

Draper ERC et al: Improvement of function after valgus bracing of the knee. J Bone Joint Surg Br 2000;82:1001.

Pollo FE: Bracing and heel wedging for unicompartmental osteoarthritis of the knee. Am J Knee Surg 1998;11:47.

■ SURGICAL MANAGEMENT

PROCEDURES FOR JOINT PRESERVATION

A joint can potentially deteriorate for the following reasons: (1) trauma, which may distort the joint so that abnormal loads are applied; (2) hemophilia, which forces the joint to dispose of blood on multiple occasions, causing synovitis; (3) rheumatoid arthritis, which causes a proliferation of the synovium, which may destroy the hyaline joint cartilage; and (4) osteonecrosis, which may result in fatigue fractures and collapse of the joint, with subsequent incongruity or (5) rotator cuff tear, leading possibly to cuff arthropathy. Certain procedures can slow progression of the deterioration and prolong the useful service of the joint. These include synovectomy, core decompression, osteotomy, and rotator cuff repair.

Rotator Cuff Repair

Chronic rotator cuff tears of the shoulder can lead to a degenerative condition called **cuff arthropathy.** The rotator cuff functions to counter the upward shear force on the articular cartilage exerted by the unopposed deltoid musculature. By repairing a torn rotator cuff, kinematic balance can be restored, preventing degeneration of the glenohumeral joint. Rotator cuff tears are repaired by mobilizing the rotator cuff and debriding the degenerated margins. These freshened edges are then sutured into bone at their insertion to restore function of the rotator cuff muscles. Removal of acromial spurs and excision of the coracoacromial ligament are also performed at the time of repair.

Synovectomy

Synovectomy is a treatment that may prolong the life of the hyaline joint surface through removal of proliferative synovitis, which damages cartilage. Synovectomy is indicated for chronic but not acute synovitis. Chronic synovitis is a clinical entity characterized by proliferation of the synovium and may be monarticular, as in pigmented villonodular synovitis, or polyarticular, as in rheumatoid arthritis or hemophilia. The term **synovitis** is relatively nonspecific, and the disorder is usually the result of a reaction to joint irritation.

A. INDICATIONS AND CONTRAINDICATIONS

The most common indication for synovectomy is rheumatoid arthritis, but the procedure may be beneficial in many other conditions, such as synovial osteochondromatosis, pigmented villonodular synovitis, and hemophilia, and occasionally following chronic or acute infection.

More specific indications for synovectomy include the following conditions:

(1) synovitis with disease limited to the synovial membrane with little or no involvement of the other structures of the joint;

(2) recurrent hemarthroses in conditions such as pigmented villonodular synovitis or hemophilia;

(3) imminent destruction of the joint by lysosomal enzymes derived from white blood cells that may be liberated from infection; and

(4) failure of an adequate trial of conservative management.

Contraindications include reduced ROM, significant degenerative arthrosis of the involved joint or other joint, or cartilage involvement.

B. TECHNIQUE

Synovectomy is most commonly performed on the knee and also often on the elbow, ankle, and wrist. Three main techniques are available: open synovectomy, synovectomy with use of the arthroscope, and radiation synovectomy.

1. Open synovectomy—Open synovectomy is becoming less common because of pain that causes difficulty in obtaining full motion following surgery. Continuous passive motion may be beneficial in these cases. Open synovectomy may be necessary in cases of pigmented villonodular synovitis or synovial osteochondromatosis, although these diseases may also be treated by arthroscopy, which permits noninvasive complete removal of the synovium in many cases.

2. Synovectomy with use of arthroscope—Synovectomy with use of the arthroscope may be tedious, especially in large joints such as the knee, because complete treatment requires removal of the entire synovium in many cases.

A recent study of pigmented villonodular synovitis of the knee treated by total and partial arthroscopic synovectomy demonstrated that total synovectomy resulted in a low recurrence rate, whereas partial synovectomy resulted in symptomatic and functional improvement but a fairly high recurrence rate. Arthroscopic synovectomy was recommended only for localized lesions.

3. Radiation synovectomy—Radiation synovectomy is a technique that is becoming much more popular. It has been used in knee joints affected by rheumatoid arthritis. An injection of dysprosium-165-ferric hydroxide macroaggregates is given and leads to improvement in a significant percentage of patients. Proliferation of synovium decreases following this procedure, and there is less pain, blood loss, and expense than with more invasive procedures.

A similar technique has been used in the knee joint in hemophiliacs. Phosphorus-32 chromic phosphate colloid is used and can be given on an outpatient basis. This is a safer technique for health care personnel, who have less contact with the blood of the hemophiliac patients, many of whom have become HIV-positive through contaminated blood factor replacement.

Cartilage Transplant Techniques

Defects of hyaline cartilage have long been considered permanent injuries, and the irrevocable sequelae have been gradual deterioration of the architecture of the tissue. The treatment of cartilaginous diseases and injuries has been limited by the slow and poorly understood metabolism of articular chondrocytes. Recent development of cartilage repair procedures pertain only to focal defects of full-thickness cartilage loss. Such injuries occur typically in young patients during athletic activities or in patients with osteochondritis dissecans.

Because cartilaginous tissues are avascular, prior surgical treatment has consisted of chondroplasty, where underlying subchondral bone is either drilled, burred, or microfractured to produce bleeding and an inflammatory response. Although multiple growth factors may be released with bleeding, the ensuing repair tissue is essentially fibrous scar tissue with inferior load-bearing capabilities compared with hyaline articular cartilage. As a result, the repair tissue eventually degrades leaving the defect little better than if left alone.

Much enthusiasm has followed the procedure described by Brittberg and colleagues, in which viable articular chondrocytes are harvested from a patient with a focal cartilaginous defect and cultured in a laboratory. The population of chondrocytes is expanded and placed back in the patient at the site of the cartilage injury. The cells are held in place with a flap of periosteum sutured to surrounding healthy cartilage. Although encouraging early clinical results have been reported with this method, similar results have been shown using only the flap of periosteum. Further, the procedure using cells failed to demonstrate reconstitution of normal hyaline cartilage in a canine model experiment.

Another method of dealing with focal defects of cartilage includes transplantation of small plugs of mature cartilage and bone. Small cylinders of cartilage and bone are removed from non-weight–bearing portions of cartilage and transplanted into focal femoral defects. Although encouraging short-term results have been reported, whether the reconstructed cartilage endures remains to be seen.

In contrast, osteoarthritis is a more prevalent affliction of cartilage, affecting more than 40 million patients in the United States. The early pathologic observations of osteoarthritis indicate structural degradation of the superficial layers of the cartilage architecture. Meaningful spontaneous repair of injuries limited to cartilage has not been observed clinically, but a variety of experimental evidence suggests a latent ability to effect some degree of healing after injury and possibly in osteoarthritis. These suppositions include observation of increased DNA synthesis and proteoglycan synthesis in chondrocytes during intermediate stages of osteoarthritis. The procedures described above for cartilage repair do not apply for osteoarthritic involvement of any significant portions of a joint.

Brittberg M et al: Treatment of deep cartilage defects in the knee with autologous chondrocyte implantation. N Engl J Med 1994;331:889.

Hangody L et al: Mosaicplasty for the treatment of articular defects of the knee and ankle. Clin Orthop 2001; 391 Suppl:S328.

Rodrigo JJ et al: Improvement of full-thickness chondral defect healing in the human knee after debridement and microfracture using continuous passive motion. Am J Knee Surg 1994; 7:109.

Core Decompression with or Without Structural Bone Grafting

A. INDICATIONS AND CONTRAINDICATIONS

Core decompression with or without bone grafting is a surgical treatment primarily used for the femoral head because the hip is the joint most commonly affected by osteonecrosis. The knee and the shoulder may also be affected. Osteonecrosis results from loss of blood supply to the bone and is associated with a variety of conditions. Under repetitive stress, microfractures occur, are not repaired, and eventually lead to collapse of the necrotic bone and disruption of the joint surface.

The treatment of osteonecrosis is controversial because the outcome is frequently unsatisfactory. Spontaneous repair of the osteonecrotic lesion may occur but is an exception to the usual natural history of osteonecrosis. Core decompression, core decompression with electrical stimulation and bone grafting, and core decompression with structural bone grafting are considered acceptable forms of treatment for this disorder. Another treatment involves use of a free vascularized fibula transplant after core decompression.

B. TECHNIQUE

The goal of core decompression is to alleviate hypertension in the bone caused by obstructed venous egress from the affected area. The theory is that drilling a hole in an involved bony area will diminish pressure and permit the ingrowth of new blood vessels, which will allow repair of the avascular bone and prevent joint destruction. Corticocancellous bone grafting has been considered an alternative to simple core decompression, as there is some evidence that this would place the femoral head at less risk of collapse in the postoperative period before new bone formation can occur. Core decompression or structural bone grafting is indicated in early osteonecrosis prior to collapse of the femoral head (Ficat stage I or II).

Core decompression is usually performed on the hip but may also be done on the knee or the shoulder. A lateral approach is used for the hip, and a pin is placed into the osteonecrotic area under fluoroscopic control. A reamer or core device is then passed over the pin to achieve decompression, and a sample of bone may be obtained for pathologic analysis. If structural bone grafting is to be performed, the graft may be placed over the pin (allograft or autograft fibula). Again, placement is performed under direct radiograph control.

The results of core decompression have been mixed, but this may be the result of poor technique, lack of standardization of staging, and factors causing the osteonecrosis. The major complication of the procedure in the hip is torsional failure resulting from the stress concentration site in the lateral aspect of the cortex. Reports of structural bone grafting by some investigators are highly favorable, with a high percentage of asymptomatic hips showing no evidence of progression of necrosis or collapse. One series has reported a relatively high rate of postoperative or intraoperative fracture (4 of 31 cases).

Osteotomy

Osteotomy is a treatment that should be considered part of the armamentarium of the orthopedic surgeon in the treatment of biomechanical disorders of the knee and the hip. Osteotomy of the hip for osteoarthritis is less frequently performed than osteotomy of the knee. Abnormal distribution of load may be alleviated by osteotomy. Femoral head coverage may be improved with osteotomy of the pelvis, orientation of the femoral head may be improved with osteotomy of the proximal femur, and realignment of the load on the medial and lateral condyles of the tibia may be improved with osteotomy of the femur and the tibia. The most common procedure is high tibial osteotomy, sometimes referred to as **Coventry osteotomy,** which corrects varus deformity of the knee by removal of a wedge of bone from the lateral side of the tibia. Other osteotomies are performed for residual deformity for fracture. These are tailored to the particular problem presented by the patient. Either intra-articular (ie, condylar osteotomy of the medial compartment [Figure 7–4]) or extra-articular osteotomies can be done to correct deformity.

A. HIGH TIBIAL OSTEOTOMY

Alleviation of abnormal stress through high tibial osteotomy will prevent osteoarthrosis or, alternatively, reduce pain caused by unicompartmental gonarthrosis. The procedure is indicated in relatively young patients who have unicompartmental degeneration with relative sparing of the patellofemoral joint. The knee should have a good ROM, preferably with no flexion contrac-

ture. The knee must be stable, with no demonstrated medial or lateral subluxation. The ideal patients are younger than 65 years, are not obese, and wish to continue an active lifestyle, including activities such as skiing or tennis. These activities are contraindicated in total joint replacement or unicompartmental replacement. Evaluation of the uninvolved compartment (either medial or lateral) may be accomplished by arthroscopy or with a technetium bone scan. A cold scan of the uninvolved compartment indicates relative normalcy. The normal anatomic axis of 5–7 degrees (angle between the shaft of the femur and the shaft of the tibia) on the standing anteroposterior film must usually be overcorrected to 10 degrees. High tibial osteotomy is usually indicated for patients with medial gonarthrosis, although it can be performed in patients with a valgus angulation of less than 12 degrees. If the angle is outside of this range, the patient may be a candidate for distal femoral supracondylar osteotomy. A high tibial osteotomy that will result in a joint line that is not parallel to the ground indicates that the osteotomy should probably be performed through the distal femur.

Proximal tibial osteotomy is performed through a lateral "hockey stick" incision or a straight lateral incision. Exposure of the lateral, anterior, and posterior aspects of the tibia is made, and a closing wedge osteotomy is performed. The proximal portion of this osteotomy is made parallel to the joint surface under image intensifier control (Figure 7–5). With the help of guidepins, the appropriate distal cut is made, as determined from preoperative standing radiographs, to provide the necessary correction, which in the average case is approximately 1 mm per degree of correction as measured on the lateral cortex. This technique should only be used to double-check previous calculations, however. Resection of the fibular head or the proximal tibiofibular joint allows correction of the valgus angle. Fixation can reliably be obtained with staples, and other commercial fixation devices are available. Care must be taken to avoid damage to the peroneal nerve. Other problems that may be encountered include fracture of the proximal fragment or avascular necrosis of this fragment, which may occur if care is not exercised in performing the procedure.

The results of high tibial osteotomy are not as predictable as unicompartmental knee replacement or total knee replacement. Although pain is relieved in a high percentage of patients, this relief will deteriorate over time. Clinical reports indicate that about 65–85% of patients have a good result after 5 years. Results of series vary because of the differences in patient population, surgical technique, and preexisting pathologic factors. The procedure should be considered in a patient who wants to maintain a more active lifestyle and

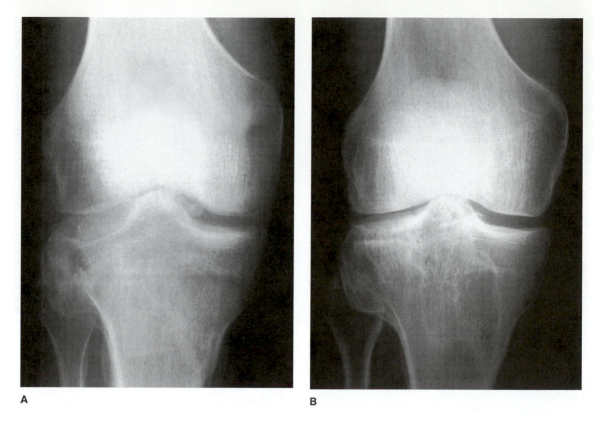

A   B

Figure 7–4. An intra-articular osteotomy can be of benefit in tibial plateau fractures. **A:** Preoperative radiograph of an intracondylar fracture of the tibial plateau. **B:** Postoperative view after osteotomy of the medial tibial condyle.

would be willing to accept the possibility of some pain or loss of pain relief over time.

Lateral gonarthrosis from genu valgum is a relatively frequent result of lateral tibial plateau fractures, although rheumatoid arthritis, rickets, and renal osteodystrophy may also produce this disorder. There has been limited success in using varus tibial osteotomy in treating genu valgum because the procedure frequently produces a joint line that is not parallel to the ground, resulting in medial subluxation of the femur. Several reports of distal femoral osteotomy for genu valgum have demonstrated that this is a viable alternative for treating painful lateral gonarthrosis.

B. Osteotomy of the Hip

Certain unusual conditions of the hip can be treated with osteotomy to prevent or retard coxarthrosis. These include osteochondritis dissecans and other traumatic conditions that produce localized damage to the surface of the hip. Various biomechanical theories have been proposed regarding the benefit of osteotomy of the

pelvis and hip in decreasing the load on the hip. Although the theoretical arguments may be correct, in practical terms there are two reasons for performing this procedure: (1) a normal viable cartilage surface is moved to the weight-bearing area where previously there was degenerated, thinned articular cartilage; and (2) the biomechanical loads on the joints that cause pain have been reduced. These can be reduced either through alteration of moment arms for muscles or, alternatively, by releasing or weakening the muscles. Significantly lengthening or shortening a muscle will reduce the force it can apply across a joint. In hip disorders, disease on one side of the hip joint cannot be addressed by an operation on the other side. For example, though it is tempting to use femoral osteotomy to treat acetabular dysplasia, only temporary relief may be obtained.

1. Treatment for acetabular dysplasia—Acetabular dysplasia may be defined by the center edge angle. The normal center edge angle is 25–45 degrees; an angle of

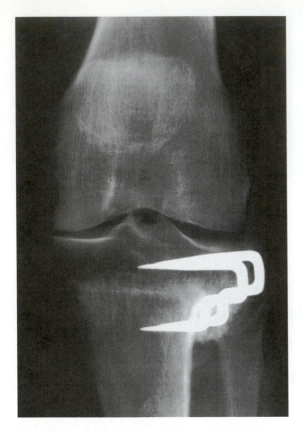

Figure 7–5. High tibial osteotomy, showing staples holding the osteotomy in place.

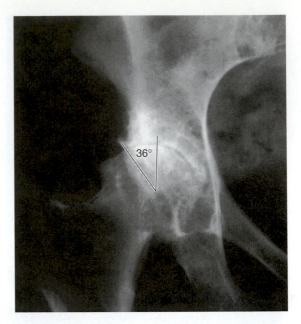

Figure 7–6. Anteroposterior pelvis film demonstrating the center edge angle.

less than 20 degrees is definitely considered dysplastic (Figure 7–6). The anterior center edge angle can also demonstrate an acetabulum that is too open anteriorly; an angle of 17–20 degrees is considered the lower limit on the falso profile view. In individuals with a mature skeleton, limited pelvic osteotomies such as the Salter innominate or shelf procedure are not appropriate. These measurements are probably best considered in a three-dimensional view with CT.

To significantly improve coverage and hip biomechanics, an acetabular-reorienting procedure that also permits medialization is ideal. The Wagner spherical osteotomy permits complete redirection of the acetabulum but does not permit medialization and is technically demanding. A triple osteotomy is useful in positioning the acetabulum but causes severe pelvic instability. The periacetabular osteotomy described by Ganz permits acetabular redirection and medialization but preserves the posterior column, minimizing instability.

2. Treatment of femoral disorders—Osteotomy of the femur can safely and reliably be performed in the intertrochanteric region, with the expectation of union. Osteotomy of the femoral neck is likely to compromise the blood supply to the femoral head. Intertrochanteric osteotomies of the femur of various types have been described. The goal of osteotomy is removal of degenerated articular cartilage from the weight-bearing dome and replacement of it with more viable cartilage. This may involve any of the three degrees of freedom: varus and valgus angle, internal and external rotation, and flexion and extension. It is necessary when planning these procedures to be sure that the osteotomy will provide an adequate ROM for the patient. These osteotomies have usefulness in very specific cases for osteoarthrosis, but their usefulness for osteonecrosis has been found to be extremely limited in the United States.

Bonfiglio M, Voke EM: Aseptic necrosis of the femoral head and nonunion of the femoral neck: Effect of treatment by drilling and bone-grafting (Phemister technique). J Bone Joint Surg Am 1968;50:48.

Buckley PD et al: Structural bone-grafting for early atraumatic avascular necrosis of the femoral head. J Bone Joint Surg Am 1991;73:1357.

Coventry MB: Osteotomy about the knee for degenerative and rheumatoid arthritis: Indications, operative technique, and results. J Bone Joint Surg Am 1973;55:23.

Crockarell JR et al: The anterior center-edge angle: a cadaver study. J Bone Joint Surg Br 2000:82.532

Edgerton BC et al: Distal femoral varus osteotomy for painful genu valgum: A five-to-11-year follow-up study. Clin Orthop 1993;288:263.

Fairbank AC et al: Long-term results of core decompression for ischaemic necrosis of the femoral head. J Bone Joint Surg Br 1995;77:42.

Haddad FS et al: CT evaluation of periacetabular osteotomies. J Bone Joint Surg Br 2000:82;526.

Mont MA et al: Core decompression versus nonoperative management for osteonecrosis of the hip. Clin Orthop 1996; 324:169.

Morita S et al: Long-term results of valgus-extension femoral osteotomy for advanced osteoarthritis of the hip. J Bone Joint Surg Br 2000:82:824.

Ogilvie-Harris DJ et al: Pigmented villonodular synovitis of the knee: The results of total arthroscopic synovectomy, partial arthroscopic synovectomy, and arthroscopic local excision. J Bone Joint Surg Am 1992;74:119.

Ohashi H et al: Factors influencing the outcome of Chiari pelvic osteotomy: A long-term follow-up. J Bone Joint Surg Br 2000:82;517.

Shoji H, Insall J: High tibial osteotomy for osteoarthritis of the knee with valgus deformity. J Bone Joint Surg Am 1973; 55:963.

Sledge CB et al: Synovectomy of the rheumatoid knee using intra-articular injection of Dysprosium-165-ferric hydroxide macroaggregates. J Bone Joint Surg Am 1987;69:970.

Urbaniak JR, Harvey EJ: Revascularization of the femoral head in osteonecrosis. J Am Acad Orthop Surg 1998;6(1):44.

JOINT SALVAGE PROCEDURES

1. Arthrodesis

Arthrodesis is the creation of a bony union across a joint. The creation of a fibrous union across a joint with no motion is ankylosis. With bony union across a joint, motion of one bone on another is eliminated, relieving pain caused by arthritis. Although ankylosis may prevent observable motion, micromotion may be associated with significant pain. Ankylosis or arthrodesis may occur spontaneously, as in infection or ankylosing spondylitis, or may be surgically produced. The functional results of spontaneous arthrodesis are not ideal, because the patient will typically hold the joint in the position that causes minimum pain, which frequently is an inappropriate angle for function. Although surgical arthrodesis can be created in almost any joint, including the spine, the most common joints fused are the ankle, knee, shoulder, and hip. The technique used in any of the joints follows the same general pattern. The articular surfaces are denuded of remaining hyaline cartilage and are then placed together in the optimal position of function after shaping to achieve maximum contact between the two opposing surfaces. Bone grafting is frequently used, and some form of fixation, either internal (plates, rods, or screws) or external (external fixators or a cast), is used to immobilize the arthrodesis site in the optimal position (Table 7–5). After adequate healing, the rehabilitation process is begun. Multiple techniques of arthrodesis have been described for each joint.

Ankle Arthrodesis

Arthrodesis of the tibiotalar joint has generally been considered by the orthopedic community to be a good operation for treatment of tibiotalar arthrosis. A well-done ankle arthrodesis results in freedom from pain and nearly normal walking ability. Perhaps the main reason that the ankle arthrodesis is regarded so highly, how-

Table 7–5. Optimal position of joints after arthrodesis.

Joint	Angle	Length	Other Consideration
Ankle	0° dorsiflexion 0–5° valgus of hindfoot 5–10° external rotation	Slight shortening	Talus displaced posteriorly.
Knee	15° flexion 5–8° flexion	Slight shortening	—
Shoulder	20–30° flexion 20–40° abduction (lateral border of scapula) 25–40° internal rotation	—	Patient's hand should be able to touch the head and face.
Hip	25° flexion 0–5° abduction (measured between the shaft and a line through the ischia) 0–5° external rotation	Slight shortening	Do *not* destroy abductor mechanism.

ever, is that other options, such as total ankle replacement, have been less viable.

The indications for ankle arthrodesis are

(1) degenerative arthrosis,

(2) rheumatoid arthritis,

(3) posttraumatic arthritis,

(4) avascular necrosis of the talus,

(5) neurologic disease resulting in an unstable ankle, and

(6) neuropathic ankle joint.

The relative contraindications include degenerative joint disease in the subtalar and midtarsal joints.

The ankle arthrodesis can be performed through an anterior, lateral, or medial approach, and even posterior approaches have been described. Recently, arthroscopic techniques have been employed. The most common techniques are probably external fixation or internal screw fixation to achieve compression. Preparation of the ankle for arthrodesis is performed as mentioned earlier. Positioning of the ankle is important, with the talus in a neutral position or at an angle of 5 degrees of dorsiflexion. The midtarsal joints have a greater ROM in plantar flexion than in dorsiflexion, resulting in a more flexible foot. The talus is also displaced slightly posteriorly to make it easier for the patient to roll the foot over at the completion of the stance phase. A varus position is to be avoided because this restricts mobility at the midtarsal joints.

Kitaoka HB, Patzer GL: Arthrodesis for the treatment of arthrosis of the ankle and osteonecrosis of the talus. J Bone Joint Surg 1998;80:370.

Scranton PE: An overview of ankle arthrodesis. Clin Orthop 1991;268:96.

Knee Arthrodesis

Knee arthrodesis is seldom done for primary problems and is generally done as the last resort for other problems. Indications for the procedure include infection, such as tuberculosis, neuropathic joint secondary to syphilis or diabetes, and loss of quadriceps function. The latter is a relative indication for arthrodesis, because joint mobility can be maintained without quadriceps function, and joint stability can be obtained through the use of orthosis, which locks the joint in the fully extended position but which can be unlocked for sitting. Although knee arthrodesis is usually successful and provides pain-free weight bearing, it is associated with other problems, especially in tall people. Sitting in airplanes, movie theaters, and even automobiles may be difficult. The most common indication for knee

arthrodesis at the present time is failed total knee arthroplasty, usually because of infection. In a patient who wishes to maintain an active lifestyle, such as hunting on rough ground or performing manual labor, a knee arthrodesis is a viable alternative. The relative contraindications include bilateral disease or a problem such as an above-knee amputation of the other leg. In such a case, it would be extremely difficult for a person to arise from a chair with an arthrodesis on the contralateral side.

The technique of arthrodesis varies with the problem being treated. After infection, particularly when it is associated with total knee replacement, bone loss is often moderate to severe. Cancellous bone from the distal femur and proximal tibia may be nearly nonexistent, and external fixation may be necessary to obtain adequate immobilization for arthrodesis. For less severe cases, intramedullary rod fixation may be indicated, particularly if the infection is under control. Similarly, use of double plates at 90 degrees is a viable method of immobilization. Frequently, iliac crest bone grafting is necessary to stimulate healing. Although bone loss often makes it necessary to shorten the extremity, some shortening (2–3 cm) is desirable to prevent a circumduction gait after fusion. The knee should be positioned at 10–15 degrees of flexion and at the normal valgus alignment of 5–8 degrees, if possible.

Donley BG et al: Arthrodesis of the knee with an intramedullary nail. J Bone Joint Surg Am 1991;73:907.

Nichols SJ et al: Arthrodesis with dual plates after failed total knee arthroplasty. J Bone Joint Surg Am 1991;73:1020.

Papilion JD et al: Arthroscopic assisted arthrodesis of the knee. Arthroscopy 1991;7:237.

Elbow Arthrodesis

Elbow arthrodesis is an uncommon procedure. Loss of elbow motion may be particularly disabling. Thus, the indications for arthrodesis are few, and few are performed because fusion causes severe functional limitations. To perform activities of daily living, a flexion arc of 100 degrees from 30 degrees of extension to 130 degrees of flexion is required. A range of 100 degrees for pronation and supination is also required. Painful arthrosis in a patient who is willing to accept the trade-off between stability and loss of motion is the indication for arthrodesis. Infectious processes, such as tuberculosis or fungus, are also indications for arthrodesis.

Several techniques have been described, but the relative rarity of the operation has prevented recommendation of one particular method. A recent report recommends screw fixation. Resection of the radial head may be necessary to allow for pronation and supination. The position of fusion is 90 degrees.

Irvine GB, Gregg PJ: A method of elbow arthrodesis: Brief report. J Bone Joint Surg Br 1989;71:145.

Morrey BF et al: A biomechanical study of normal elbow motion. J Bone Joint Surg Am 1981;62:872.

Shoulder Arthrodesis

Paralysis of the deltoid muscle and sepsis after an arthroplasty are possible indications for shoulder arthrodesis. Obtaining fusion may be a relatively difficult process because of the very long lever arm on the shoulder joint. This is accentuated by the position of fusion, which places the arm in abduction. Before the advent of comprehensive internal fixation devices, intra-articular and extra-articular arthrodeses were performed to provide a reasonable probability of obtaining fusion.

The AO technique (Arbeitsgemeinschaft für Osteosynthese technique) is the most promising because it provides rigid internal fixation and the potential for immobilization without postoperative external immobilization. The patient is placed in the lateral decubitus position. The incision is made over the spine of the scapula, over the acromion, and down the lateral aspect of the humerus. The surface of the glenohumeral joint and the undersurface of the acromion are cleaned of residual cartilage and cortical bone to provide as much contact as possible with the arm in the appropriate position (see Table 7–5). A broad bone plate or pelvic reconstruction plate is then used to fix the humerus to the scapula. The bone plate is fixed to the spine of the scapula and the shaft of the humerus and is bent into the appropriate position. Additional fixation may be obtained by placing another plate posteriorly. Bone grafting may be necessary for defects. Rigid fixation must be obtained. After surgery, a soft dressing is used until pain is controlled. A shoulder spica cast is preferred for immobilization by some surgeons. Exercises are begun to gently obtain scapular motion if no cast is used.

A modification of the AO technique that uses an external fixator to neutralize forces on interfragmentary screws has been reported to have good results.

Functional results are varied and depend on the position of fusion. Overhead work or work with the arm abducted is not possible. Excessive internal and external rotation must be avoided.

Johnson CA et al: External fixation shoulder arthrodesis. Clin Orthop 1986;211:219.

Muller ME et al: *Manual of Internal Fixation.* Berlin: Springer Verlag, 1970.

Richards RR et al: Shoulder arthrodesis using a pelvic-reconstruction plate. J Bone Joint Surg Am 1988;70;416.

Riggins RS: Shoulder fusion without external fixation: A preliminary report. J Bone Joint Surg Am 1976;58:1007.

Hip Arthrodesis

Arthrodesis of the hip, as of other joints, produces a relatively pain-free, stable joint that allows the patient to perform heavy labor. The disadvantage of hip arthrodesis in a young person who performs heavy labor is that over a period of time, degenerative disk disease of the lumbar spine and degenerative arthrosis of the ipsilateral knee frequently occur, even with optimal position of the arthrodesis. In fact, an indication for converting a hip fusion to a total hip arthroplasty is incapacitating back or knee pain.

The most obvious indication for arthrodesis of the hip is tuberculosis. Chronic osteomyelitis is a relative indication. Contraindications to arthrodesis include limited motion of the ipsilateral knee or degenerative arthrosis of the ipsilateral knee, as well as significant degenerative lumbar spine disease and arthrosis of the contralateral hip. Perhaps the biggest problem in performing a hip arthrodesis in a patient with adequate indications is obtaining agreement from the patient. Because joint replacement offers mobility, early rehabilitation, and a less extensive operation, patients are reluctant to consider the potential problems of hip arthrodesis. This is particularly true when total hip arthroplasty is performed in professional athletes, permitting some of them to continue in sports. Because of these factors, hip arthrodesis has become a relatively uncommon operation.

Multiple techniques have been described for performing hip arthrodesis. Truly rigid fixation is difficult to achieve, and cast immobilization after surgery is usually needed. During the fusion procedure, care should be taken to preserve the abductors, so that future reconstructive procedures may be performed if desired. The crucial aspect of the operation is fusing the hip in the appropriate position. The optimal position is slight flexion (25 degrees) from the normal position of the pelvis and spine, slight external rotation (5 degrees), and neutral abduction and adduction. Previously, the hip was placed in abduction, producing a very abnormal gait with additional stress on the lumbar spine. A position of neutral to slight abduction minimizes this problem because the body's center of gravity when the patient is in a one-legged stance is moved closer to the foot. Too much flexion makes both walking and lying in bed difficult, and too little flexion makes sitting difficult. Too much external rotation forces the knee joint to move in a plane oblique from that defined by the collateral and cruciate ligaments.

Blasier RB, Holmes JR: Intraoperative positioning for arthrodesis of the hip with the double bean bag technique. J Bone Joint Surg Am 1990;72:766.

Callaghan JJ et al: Hip arthrodesis: A long-term follow-up. J Bone Joint Surg Am 1984; 67:1328.

2. Resection Arthroplasty

Resection arthroplasty, or excisional arthroplasty, is a procedure that has been primarily applied to the hip, the elbow, and, more recently, the knee. Resection arthroplasty, or a modification called **fascial arthroplasty,** was a procedure used in the elbow for many years. Resection arthroplasty of the hip is also called **Girdlestone pseudoarthrosis** and dates back to 1923. Resection arthroplasty of the knee is a relatively new procedure that has been used when infection compromises total knee replacement. Similarly, Girdlestone pseudoarthrosis has been performed with increasing frequency as an intervening, sometimes permanent treatment for infection following total hip arthroplasty.

Hip Arthroplasty

Resection arthroplasty of the hip produces a relatively pain-free joint with reasonably good motion. It is indicated as a primary procedure when ankylosis has caused the hip to be placed in an unsuitable position; such patients would otherwise be at high risk for dislocation or infection with a total hip arthroplasty. Spinal cord injury, head injury, and, perhaps, severe Parkinson's disease would be diagnoses that might warrant primary resection arthroplasty. Disadvantages of the procedure result from lack of mechanical continuity between the femur and the pelvis; this causes an abnormal gait and the need for support with a cane or other device, and shortening occurs with each step. Patients who have previously had infection following total hip replacement usually have the most stable hip joints because dense scar tissue has formed. The procedure can be very helpful in reambulating wheelchair-bound patients in whom peroneal care is very difficult.

For infection compromising total hip replacement, resection arthroplasty is accomplished by removing all of the cement, the prosthesis, any necrotic bone, and the soft tissue. In primary resection arthroplasty, the procedure is more of a reconstructive procedure in which the femoral head and neck are removed flush with the intertrochanteric line and the capsule is reconstructed to help provide some stability of the hip. Traction with a pin in the tibia is frequently used for variable periods to maintain leg length.

Knee Arthroplasty

Resection arthroplasty of the knee has a much less satisfactory functional result. After removal of an infected knee prosthesis, there is usually significant bone loss and the knee is quite unstable. Bracing improves the condition only modestly, and the patient still requires crutches or a walker to ambulate.

Elbow Arthroplasty

Resection arthroplasty or fascial arthroplasty of the elbow is one means of managing ankylosis after trauma or infection. Resection arthroplasty may be performed for failure of total elbow arthroplasty resulting from sepsis. Resection arthroplasty in the rheumatoid arthritis patient should be discouraged because one of the problems associated with the procedure is instability. The rheumatoid patient frequently is dependent upon the upper extremity to ambulate with walking aids. Interpositional arthroplasty, using fascia or split-thickness skin grafts, was thought to reduce resorption of bone, but the additional benefit of the interpositional tissue is doubtful. Although resection arthroplasty frequently relieves pain, instability is a major problem, and bracing is required in most cases. With the availability of elbow arthroplasty, this procedure is rarely performed.

Milgram JW, Rana NA: Resection arthroplasty for septic arthritis of the hip in ambulatory and nonambulatory adult patients. Clin Orthop 1991;272:181.

Thornhill TS et al: Alternatives to arthrodesis for failed total knee arthroplasty. Clin Orthop 1982;170:131.

JOINT REPLACEMENT PROCEDURES

1. Hemiarthroplasty

Hemiarthroplasty is the replacement of only one side of a diarthrodial joint. The procedure is indicated for displaced fractures of the femoral neck or four-part fractures of the humeral head, but there are other indications in adult reconstructive surgery. In both the shoulder and the hip, osteonecrosis may result in collapse of the humeral or femoral articulating surface, with sparing of the glenoid or acetabulum. In the hip, nonunion of the femoral neck after open reduction and internal fixation may also be an indication for endoprosthetic replacement. In either joint, pathologic fracture or tumor may be an indication. Contraindications include active infection, rheumatoid arthritis, and possibly the patient's age. Endoprosthetic replacement in a young individual is certain to result, with time, in destruction of the articular surface of the acetabulum. This may, however, take many years, and the patient may have a serviceable joint in the intervening period.

The choice of prosthesis depends on factors such as life expectancy, cost, and physiologic demand. For the shoulder, a cemented prosthesis should probably be modular to permit conversion to total shoulder replacement at a later date without removal of the stem, should that become necessary. Similar concerns for the hip apply. The femoral head can be replaced with a unipolar or bipolar prosthesis. The bipolar prosthesis allows motion to occur between the acetabulum and the prosthesis, as well as between the prosthesis and the articulating surface of the metal femoral head. This articulation is metal or ceramic on plastic and is certain to produce debris from wear that may be detrimental to the durability of the hip prosthesis. Selection of a monopolar prosthesis, however, must not compromise conversion of the hemiarthroplasty to a total hip arthroplasty, should this become necessary.

The operative technique is quite similar to that of total joint replacement for each joint. The main difference in the hip is that the capsule is usually repaired after hemiarthroplasty. A posterolateral approach is most commonly used in the hip, although an anterolateral approach may be preferred in a patient with associated mental problems that may limit postoperative cooperation. If the posterolateral approach is used in such patients, a knee immobilizer may be necessary to prevent hip flexion that might lead to dislocation.

2. Total Joint Arthroplasty

Joint replacement surgery became a viable treatment for arthritic afflictions of joints when the low-friction hip arthroplasty was developed by Sir John Charnley in the 1960s. This procedure consisted of the articulation of a metal femoral head on an ultrahigh-molecular-weight polyethylene (UHMWPE) acetabular component, with both components fixed in place with acrylic cement (polymethylmethacrylate [PMMA]). The long-term results have been quite satisfactory, and the concept has been applied to other joints with variable success. The knee replacement, shoulder replacement, and elbow replacement have evolved to the point that satisfactory results are routine when the indications for surgery are appropriate. Other arthroplasties such as the ankle, wrist, and first metatarsophalangeal joint have been less successful. In fairness, the application of technology to these joints has not been at the level applied to other joints. Success of all arthroplasties is dependent on the skill of the surgeon, the surgeon's understanding of the basic biomechanics underlying the joint function, the design of the prosthesis, and the technical equipment used to insert the prosthesis.

The design of the prosthesis is an evolutionary process that has been dependent on laboratory and clinical experience. Hip replacement surgery is performed often and is highly successful. Less frequently performed arthroplasties, such as elbow replacement, have been associated with less clinical and laboratory experience.

Total Hip Arthroplasty

The original Charnley total hip arthroplasty was a stainless steel femoral prosthesis with a small collar, a rectangular cross section, and a 22-mm femoral head. The

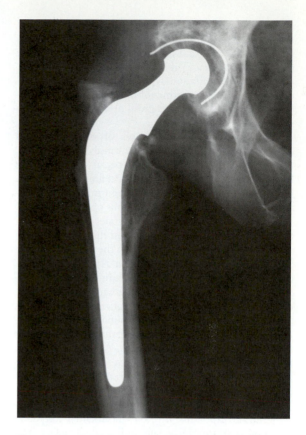

Figure 7–7. Radiograph of a Charnley arthroplasty.

acetabular component was a UHMWPE cup (Figure 7–7). Both components were cemented into place with acrylic bone cement. Since then, an entire industry has evolved to produce new designs for hip components, including different head sizes (22, 25, 25.4, 28, 32, and 35 mm), different femoral component lengths (ranging from 110 mm to 160 mm for standard prostheses), different cross sections (square, round, oval, I-beam), a porous coating for bone ingrowth attachment, and metal backing for the acetabulum (cemented or porous coated). The two generic designs that have evolved from experience with bone attachment technique are the porous ingrowth and cement fixation prostheses.

A. INDICATIONS

The indications for hip arthroplasty are incapacitating arthritis of the hip combined with appropriate physical and roentgenographic findings. The historical data that justify consideration of hip replacement surgery include pain requiring medication stronger than aspirin, inability to walk more than a few blocks without stopping, pain following activity, pain that wakes the patient at night, difficulty with shoes and socks or foot care such as cutting nails, and difficulty in climbing stairs. It is good practice to use a clinical rating score to evaluate these historical data (Table 7–6).

Physical examination typically demonstrates a limited ROM, pain at extremes of motion, a positive Trendelenburg test, a limp, and groin or anterior thigh pain with active straight leg raising.

Radiographs demonstrate loss of joint space and other findings consistent with the cause of the disorder. Noteworthy features requiring special considerations for surgery are dysplasia of the acetabulum, protrusio acetabuli, and proximal femoral deformity or the presence of metal implants from previous operations.

After consideration of the lifestyle requirements of the patient, the surgeon may suggest this procedure as a means of alleviating pain, which is the main indication for hip replacement surgery. Other reconstructive procedures should be considered, including arthrodesis, osteotomy, and hemiarthroplasty. When selecting a procedure, one should consider the patient's goals in terms of work and leisure activity. A young person who performs heavy labor and has unilateral traumatic arthritis may be best served by arthrodesis. A 50-year-old bank executive who does not ski, play tennis, or ride horses but does swim and bicycle will probably have best results with hip arthroplasty.

A choice must be made between cemented and uncemented arthroplasty, with the uncemented acetabular component nearly universally indicated. Its advantages include a consistently pain-free result, long-lasting fixation, and modularity to permit latitude in selecting head size and acetabular polyethylene component offset designs. Its disadvantages include the need for metal backing of the polyethylene liner, which may increase wear, and the possibility of dissociation of the plastic component from the metal. A cemented acetabular component manufactured from UHMWPE is usually reserved for an individual with a life expectancy of 10 years or less. The indications for an uncemented femoral component vary with the surgeon but usually depend on the age of the patient, with younger patients most likely to benefit from the porous-coated prosthesis.

B. SURGICAL TECHNIQUE

Certain aspects of hip replacement surgery apply to all arthroplasty techniques, including cement technique and bone surface preparation.

1. Posterolateral approach—The most common approach for total hip arthroplasty is the posterolateral approach. After administration of anesthesia and placement of a thromboembolic stocking and intermittent compression stocking on the unaffected limb, the patient is rolled into the lateral decubitus position, with

the affected side superior. Draping should leave the entire leg free and extending above the iliac crest. Kidney rests are used to support the pelvis at the pubis and the sacrum, and bony prominences should be protected. The incision is outlined on the skin before the skin is completely covered with an adhesive drape. By flexing the hip to 45 degrees, the incision can be made in line with the femur from approximately 10 cm proximal to the tip of the trochanter to 10 cm distal to the tip of the trochanter. Alternatively, with the hip in the extended position, the incision is made from 10 cm distal to the tip of the trochanter extending proximally along the line of the trochanter and then curving posteriorly at about a 45 degrees angle for another 10 cm. The incision is deepened to show the fascia lata and the gluteus maximus. An incision is made in the fascia lata directly lateral and this is extended proximally into the gluteus maximus, which is split in line with its fibers. A Charnley retractor is placed, and fat overlying the external rotators is removed. After putting the femur into internal rotation, the external rotators (piriformis, gemelli, obturator internus, and quadratus femoris) are tagged with sutures for reattachment and removed from their attachments at the trochanter. The gluteus minimus is separated from the capsule and preserved and protected, and a capsulectomy is performed. Alternatively, portions of the posterior capsule can be reflected for later reattachment. If the patient is not paralyzed with nondepolarizing muscle relaxant agents, excision of the capsule with electrocautery will signal whether the sciatic nerve is particularly closely applied to the posterior of the acetabulum. The sciatic nerve must be identified and protected throughout the procedure if there is electrical transmission. Internal rotation of the flexed hip dislocates the hip, and the femoral head is delivered into the operative field. Using an appropriate template, the femoral head is resected with an oscillating saw. The femur is then externally rotated, and Taylor retractors are placed anteriorly and posteriorly to permit visualization of the acetabulum. The acetabulum is medialized if appropriate when medial osteophytes are present. Anterior osteophytes, if present, are removed under direct visualization. Reaming of the acetabulum is performed until a good bed of bleeding subchondral bone is obtained; progressive reamers are usually used. At this point, techniques diverge based on whether a cemented or an uncemented cup is used.

If a cemented cup is used, multiple holes with a diameter of ¼ to ⅜ in. are drilled in the acetabulum to provide firm cement interdigitation. One of the commercially available techniques that prevents bottoming out of the acetabular cup should be used, so that the medial cement mantle will be adequate. The position of the cup is determined with trials, using the native acetabulum for guidance and radiograph if there is any

Table 7–6. Harris hip evaluation (modified).

I. Pain (44 possible)
  A. None or ignores it 44
  B. Slight, occasional, no compromise in activities 40
  C. Mild pain, no effect on average activities, rarely moderate pain with
     unusual activity may take aspirin 30
  D. Moderate pain, tolerable, but makes concessions to pain; some limitation of ordinary
     activity or work; may require occasional pain medicine stronger than aspirin 20
  E. Marked pain, serious limitation of activities 10
  F. Totally disabled, crippled, pain in bed, bedridden 0
II. Function (47 possible)
  A. Gait (33 possible)
    1. Limp
      a. None 11
      b. Slight 8
      c. Moderate 5
      d. Severe 0
    2. Support
      a. None 11
      b. Cane for long walks 7
      c. Cane most of the time 5
      d. One crutch 3
      e. Two canes 2
      f. Two crutches 0
      g. Not able to walk (specify reason) 0
    3. Distance walked
      a. Unlimited 11
      b. Six blocks 8
      c. Two or three blocks 5
      d. Indoors only 2
      e. Bed and chair 0
  B. Activities (14 possible)
    1. Stairs
      a. Normally without using a railing 4
      b. Normally using a railing 2
      c. In any manner 1
      d. Unable to do stairs 0
    2. Shoes and socks
      a. With ease 4
      b. With difficulty 2
      c. Unable 0
    3. Sitting
      a. Comfortably in ordinary chair 1 hour 5
      b. On a high chair for one-half hour 3
      c. Unable to sit comfortably in any chair 0
    4. Enter public transportation 1
  C. Range of Motion   R   L
    Flexion   ____ ____
    Flexion contracture ____ ____
    Abduction ____ ____
    Adduction ____ ____
    External rotation ____ ____
    Internal rotation ____ ____
  D. Location of pain
    Groin ____ ____
    Thigh ____ ____
    Buttock ____ ____

concern about positioning. The cup is cemented into place after the acetabular bone has been prepared with pulsable lavage, epinephrine-soaked sponges, and pressurization of the cement.

If an uncemented cup is to be used, reaming progresses to a diameter 1–2 mm smaller than the actual size of the cup to be implanted. The cup is impacted into place, ensuring appropriate positioning. Fixation is achieved with screws or pegs, as specified by the manufacturer. A trial plastic component is inserted, and attention is returned to the femur.

The hip is internally rotated, flexed to approximately 80 degrees, and adducted, so that the cut femoral neck is presented to the surgeon. Homan retractors may be used to help elevate the amputated femoral neck into the wound. A box chisel is then used to remove the femoral neck laterally. The canal is broached with a curet to provide an indication of the direction of the intramedullary canal. The femoral canal is then broached with increasing sizes of broaches, until all weak cancellous bone has been removed. The prosthesis size is determined, and a cement restrictor is placed 2 cm distal to the final position of the stem tip. The canal is prepared for cementing with pulsable lavage, medullary canal brushing, and sponges soaked with hydrogen peroxide or epinephrine. The cement is prepared and centrifuged, or vacuum mixed and inserted into the femoral canal with a cement gun. The cement is pressurized, and the prosthesis is inserted into appropriate anteversion (about 10 degrees) and held in position until the cement has cured. When the appropriate broach, as indicated by preoperative templating, has been reached, a trial femoral prosthesis is inserted, the neck length is checked, and the prosthesis is reduced into position. Range of motion is tested at 90 degrees of flexion and should be stable to 40–45 degrees of internal rotation. External rotation to 40 degrees in the fully extended position must be obtained without impingement on the femoral neck posteriorly. Proper myofascial tension is assessed by telescoping the hip at 45 degrees (approximately 3 or 4 mm). Proper leg length is usually achieved when the rectus femoris tightness (flexion of the knee with the hip extended) is similar to prior to surgery. A further check on leg lengths can be made by comparing the center of the femoral head preoperatively with the proximal tip of the trochanter to trochanter-prosthesis center distance with the prosthesis in place. Measuring devices have been designed to measure leg lengths, but up to a centimeter of discrepancy can still occur. An extended lip on the UHMWPE component may provide additional stability but may form a fulcrum on which the head may be levered out. The prosthesis trial is removed and the permanent polyethylene component is put into place in the acetabular metallic shell. The femoral canal is then prepared for cementing.

After the cement has hardened, a trial femoral head is used to put the hip through a second ROM. The optimal neck length is selected, and the appropriate prosthetic component is impacted into place. When combining modular components held together with a Morse-type taper, the manufacturers' components should not be mixed. It is mandatory that the surfaces be clean and dry. The bore in the femoral head is placed on the trunion and twisted and impacted into place with several sharp blows. The acetabulum is cleaned of debris, the femoral head is reduced, and the wound is closed. The external rotators are reattached with sutures placed through bone while the hip is in external rotation and abduction. The fascia is closed with interrupted sutures.

The design and insertion technique of the uncemented femoral components are quite variable and therefore will not be described here.

Abbreviated "mini" incisions for the posterolateral approach to the hip have been described. These generally utilize a small portion of the routine incision but are carefully placed to optimize visualization of the hip.

2. Lateral approach—The lateral approach to the hip is performed with a trochanteric osteotomy after the fascia of the tensor fascia lata and gluteus maximus have been entered. The patient may be in the supine position with a bump under the hip or in the lateral position. Prior to osteotomy, the trochanter is mobilized, and the trochanteric osteotomy is performed with an osteotome or a Gigli saw. The gluteus minimus is peeled off of the capsule as the trochanter is mobilized proximally. After capsulectomy, the femoral head is dislocated anteriorly. The procedure is essentially identical from this point on until the trochanter is reattached. Various modifications of trochanteric osteotomy techniques have been described. The abductor mechanism is extremely important in preserving the stability of the hip as well as the gait. Thus, extreme care must be taken to reattach the trochanter when the procedure is completed, so that reliable union is achieved. Even in the best of hands, approximately 1 in 20 trochanters fails to unite, although the number of people who have disability or pain from a fibrous union is much lower. If wires are to be used to reattach the trochanter, they should be biocompatible with the prosthetic component, and a minimum of three should be used to achieve adequate fixation.

3. Anterolateral approach (Watson-Jones approach)—The interval between the gluteus medius muscle and the tensor fascia lata is utilized proximally to gain access to the femoral neck and hip joint. The patient is in the supine position, with a bump under the buttock. The skin incision follows the shaft of the femur distally and curves slightly anteriorly proximally. The fascia is incised in line with the skin incision and proximally splits the interval between the tensor fascia lata and the gluteus medius. The tensor fascia lata is then retracted anteriorly, and the gluteus medius is retracted superiorly and laterally. Because the fibers of the gluteus medius and minimus tend to run anteriorly, particularly in the osteoarthritic hip with destruction and shortening, these fibers must be released to provide access to the hip joint. The hip is externally rotated. The anterior capsule is incised, and the hip joint can then be dislocated. Osteotomy of the femoral neck proceeds at the appropriate level. Capsulotomy is performed, retractors are placed to provide acetabular exposure, and hip replacement is performed. The femur during this procedure is externally rotated. Care must be taken in exposing the acetabulum to prevent damage to the femoral nerve and femoral muscles.

4. Other approaches—Other approaches have been used for hip replacement, some of which are successful according to the skill of the individual surgeon. Some approaches, including the direct lateral approach, may be fraught with problems such as abductor weakness after surgery, and the result may be disappointing to the patient as well as the surgeon.

C. IMPLANTS

There are two basic types of total hip replacement: cemented and uncemented. The bearing surfaces for both are the same, either cobalt chromium alloy or ceramic (alumina or zirconia), articulating with a UHMWPE bearing surface. The femoral stem replacement may be cobalt chromium or titanium alloy, either of which is also used for the metal backing of the acetabulum. Cobalt chromium alloy is associated with much less stress on the bone-cement interface because of its higher modulus; this will prolong fixation. The femoral component should be designed to provide intrinsic torsional stability without having sharp edges that would create stress concentration sites in the bone cement. A matte surface should be created to allow some mechanical interlocking with the cement, although currently this is controversial, and some surgeons recommend a polished surface. Adequate offset is necessary to restore the mechanical advantage of the abductors.

The choice of material for the femoral head is a trade-off between cost and theoretical advantages. The harder, wettable surface of ceramic heads will theoretically result in less production of debris from wear and longer service of the hip replacement without loosening, but the cost is two to three times that of an equivalent-sized cobalt chromium (Co/Cr) head. Thus, in most individuals undergoing total hip arthroplasty, a cobalt chromium head is probably optimal. In younger patients, the increased cost of a ceramic head may be warranted. Femoral heads are available now in 22-, 26-, 28-, and 32-mm sizes. One clinical investigation of total hip replacements showed that 26- and 28-mm heads were associated with the least amount of linear and volumetric wear. A head of 22 mm may be necessary for patients with smaller acetabular sockets to provide adequate thickness of the polyethylene bearing surface. A minimum of 6 mm, preferably 8 mm or more, is suggested to lower the contact stress on the polyethylene and thereby reduce wear.

New bearing surfaces for the articulation of the hip joint are becoming popular. The possibilities include ceramic-on-ceramic, Co/Cr-on-Co/Cr, and ceramic or Co/Cr on radiation cross-linked polyethylene. The impetus for this change is the possibility of lower wear debris. These articulation couples will require long-term follow-up to determine if they will live up to their promise.

There is no evidence to justify use of a metal backing on the cemented acetabular component. Other design considerations to avoid are deep grooves that might evolve into cracks in the PMMA. The surface must be rough enough to allow the cup to bond to the cement through mechanical interlock.

Uncemented acetabular components have a spherical outer surface with at least one hole to permit the surgeon to determine if the prosthesis is fully impacted into place. The shell should have a minimum of 3 mm of metal to reduce the risk of fatigue failure. Cobalt chromium alloy or titanium alloy appears to be equally efficacious. The inner surface should lock the polyethylene in some fashion to reliably limit rotation and dissociation. The inner surface should be the mate of the polyethylene outer surface to reduce the chance of cold flow of the plastic as well as wear from relative motion. Recommended materials are listed in Table 7–7.

Design considerations for the uncemented femoral component are unclear at present. Use of porous coating, hydroxyapatite, or tricalcium phosphate coating has been driven by manufacturing concerns and prosthesis strength requirements rather than an understanding of the biologic principles of hip replacement. Two design factors are important: (1) If a prosthesis is excessively stiff in relation to the bone to which it is attached, proximal osteopenia may result from "stress shielding" or "stress bypassing" of the bone. (2) Stiffer prostheses also seem to be associated with more pain in the thigh. Therefore, strategies to reduce stiffness seem appropriate. Both of these factors are addressed by using titanium alloy as opposed to cobalt chromium alloy, but other factors may surface to affect this choice. Creating slots or grooves to reduce the torsional and bending stiffness also seems to be effective in reducing stiffness and resulting thigh pain.

Table 7–7. Preferred materials for total hip replacement.

Component	Material	Alternative Material
Uncemented femoral component	Titanium alloy	Cobalt chromium alloy
Cemented femoral component	Cobalt chromium alloy (forged)	Cast cobalt chromium alloy, titanium alloy
Femoral head	Cobalt chromium alloy	Zirconia, alumina
Cemented acetabulum bearing surface	Ultrahigh-molecular-weight polyethylene component (no metal backing)	—
Uncemented acetabulum bearing surface	Ultrahigh-molecular-weight polyethylene component	—
Acetabulum ingrowth surface	Titanium alloy, cobalt chromium alloy	

D. COMPLICATIONS

Any major surgery is associated with a certain incidence of complications, and this is certainly true for total hip arthroplasty. The surgeon must recognize these complications in a timely manner and treat them appropriately. The most common complications include deep venous thrombosis, fracture or perforation of the femoral shaft, infection, instability (dislocation), heterotopic bone formation, and nerve palsies.

1. Deep venous thrombosis—Although some morbidity results from deep venous thrombosis, the real risk is pulmonary embolism, which is occasionally fatal. The incidence of deep venous thrombosis is high, but the incidence of fatal pulmonary emboli fortunately is low, in the range of 0.3.%. The high incidence of deep venous thrombosis during hip replacement surgery has been related to femoral vein damage from manipulation or retraction, intraoperative or postoperative venous stasis caused by immobility and limb swelling, and a hypercoagulable state directly resulting from the surgical trauma to the patient. Certain factors have been recognized as predisposing the patient to higher risk for deep venous thrombosis, including a prior history of pulmonary embolus, estrogen treatment, preexisting cancer, older age of the patient, and length of the operative procedure, one factor that is under the surgeon's control.

Pharmacologic and mechanical measures have been used to reduce the risk of deep venous thrombosis. Some surgeons prefer surveillance through clinical or laboratory tests such as duplex scanning, venograms, and fibrinogen scans, followed by anticoagulation therapy in patients with clot formation. The National Institutes of Health Consensus Conference concluded that mechanical measures such as intermittent pneumatic compression provided adequate prophylaxis for patients who would be mobilized quickly, whereas anticoagulation therapy was recommended for those expected to undergo prolonged bed rest. Pharmacologic prophylaxis has included sodium warfarin, subcutaneous heparin, and aspirin. The efficacy of subcutaneous "minidose" heparin and aspirin is controversial. The first low-molecular-weight heparin (enoxaparin) is administered subcutaneously and was approved by the FDA for prophylaxis in total hip arthroplasty patients. This drug offers the benefit of twice-daily administration without the need for coagulation monitoring. Its indications have been extended to total knee replacement prophylaxis. Other similar low-molecular-weight heparin products have become available and may permit single daily dosing. These include such products as dalteparin sodium and tinzaparin sodium. These drugs offer higher factor Xa inhibition in relation to factor IIa inhibition than unfractionated heparin, which prevents clotting without affecting the activated partial thromboplastin time (PTT). Other chemotherapeutic agents include fondaparinux, a pentasaccharide that is a factor Xa inhibitor, also given by injection once daily. On the horizon are oral thrombin (IIa) inhibitors that may be more convenient for out patient use.

Because deep venous thrombosis can lead to a catastrophic outcome, preventative measures are indicated starting in the presurgical area. The patient should wear an antiembolic stocking on the unaffected extremity, and both extremities can be treated with intermittent pneumatic compression during the operative procedure. Following surgery, a low-molecular-weight heparin (enoxaparin or dalteparin) is the treatment of choice.

Patients who develop pulmonary embolus should receive routine treatment with heparin followed by warfarin.

2. Nerve palsies—Three degrees of nerve injury are recognized. In order of increasing severity, these are neuropraxia, in which conduction is disrupted; axonotmesis, in which the neuron is affected but not the myelin sheath; and neurotmesis, in which the nerve is completely disrupted, as in laceration. In total hip arthroplasty, the most common injuries are neuropraxia and axonotmesis. Neurotmesis is unlikely to occur, except when severe scar tissue predisposes the nerve to laceration. Early nerve recovery (days to weeks) indicates neuropraxia, while longer recovery (months) indicates axonotmesis.

Nerve palsies after total hip arthroplasty are relatively infrequent, but the incidence increases as the complexity of the surgical procedure increases. The sciatic nerve is most commonly involved, with the peroneal division of the sciatic nerve at the greatest risk (80% of cases). The femoral nerve is involved less frequently. An early study indicated an overall prevalence of 1.7%, with total hip arthroplasty for congenital hip dysplasia having a rate of 5.2% and for osteoarthrosis 1%, but a subsequent review suggested that the overall rate of palsy has been reduced to about 1%. Revision surgery was associated with a rate of 3.2%. The type of injury most likely to produce nerve palsy is stretching or compression, although other mechanisms, such as ischemia, intraneural hemorrhage, dislocation of the femoral component, and cement extrusion have also been suggested as causes.

Nerve injury may be prevented by identifying high-risk cases, protecting the sciatic nerve from compression, and evaluating the sciatic nerve for possible stretching before the wound is closed. Stretching the sciatic nerve by as little as 2 cm increases the risk of palsy significantly. Palpation of the sciatic nerve for tautness with the hip and knee extended and with the hip flexed and knee extended (straight leg-raising test) indicates whether there is danger of stretching the sciatic nerve. Shortening the femoral neck is one means of addressing this problem. If any doubt exists as to whether stretching occurred, the patient should be placed in the hospital bed following operation with the hip extended and the knee flexed to relieve tension of the nerve, until the patient is awake and function of the nerve can be monitored.

Management of nerve palsy is generally conservative, with observation when the nerve is known to be in continuity and not stretched. Electromyograms and nerve conduction studies may be helpful but may not show changes until 3 weeks after injury. Recovery of some motor function in the hospital heralds a good prognosis, and if complete return is to occur, it will do so by 21 months, according to one study.

3. Vascular complications—Significant vascular complications are reported to occur in about 0.25% of total hip replacements. These may be caused by placement of retractors and acetabular screws and by damage to atherosclerotic vessels. Early recognition is important in these injuries.

4. Fracture or perforation—The typical fracture associated with total hip arthroplasty involves the femoral shaft, but other fractures do occur. Fatigue fractures of structures such as the pubic ramus may occur following increased activity after hip replacement has relieved pain. The intraoperative problem of fracture or perforation of the femur is relatively uncommon in primary arthroplasty. Perforation may occur in disorders such as sickle cell anemia and osteopetrosis or following previous internal fixation. These conditions may have resulted in sclerotic bone, which may direct the broach astray. Perforations are relatively easily managed by extending the prosthesis past the area of perforation. This distance is generally considered to be two femoral diameters for a perforation with a cemented arthroplasty, but longer distances may be necessary with uncemented arthroplasties, depending on the size of the perforation. An alternative is to use a structural allograft held in place with cerclage wires. In either case, cancellous bone grafting is prudent to facilitate healing.

After total hip arthroplasty, the stress state of the bone is definitely changed, and there is a stress concentration area at the tip of the prosthesis. Fractures in the periprosthetic area have become relatively common. These fractures are classified as type A, involving the greater or lesser trochanter; type B1, B2, B3, around or just below the stem, with the stem well fixed (B1), stem loose (B2), or poor bone stock in the proximal femur (B3); or type C, well below the stem. Type A fractures are treated nonoperatively unless the cause is osteolysis, which may predispose the femur to more serious injury. Type B and C fractures are generally treated surgically. Revision is usually the treatment of choice if the prosthesis demonstrates loosening on plain radiographs. Bone grafting is generally necessary with bone deficiencies and bicortical onlay grafting techniques may be necessary with poor bone stock. Open reduction and internal fixation may be indicated if the prosthesis is tight (types B1 and C), but generous bone grafting and careful observation are necessary to ensure healing. Fracture fixation devices applied in the vicinity of the femoral component may be tenuous and these devices must not compromise the integrity of the cement mantle or prosthesis.

5. Dislocation following total hip arthroplasty—The incidence of dislocation following total hip arthroplasty varies somewhat from series to series, but ranges from 1% to 8% and averages 2–2.5%. Several factors are associated with higher rates of dislocation, including female sex of the patient and nonunion of the trochanteric osteotomy, revision surgery, and use of the posterior approach. Dislocation after revision surgery in one series was 10% after the first revision and 26.7% after two or more revisions. An ununited trochanter after revision was associated with a 25% rate of dislocation.

Factors important in preventing dislocation are proper placement of components, adjustment of myofascial tension, component design, and patient compliance. Variables found to have no effect on the dislocation rate include the ROM of the hip and the femoral head size. A 32-mm head has a theoretic advantage over a 22-mm head because a neck of the same diameter would impinge earlier with a 22-mm head. At the time of surgery, the myofascial tension is tested by traction on the femur. Displacement of 1 cm or more suggests an increased probability of dislocation after surgery.

The risk of dislocation after total hip arthroplasty diminishes as time passes without dislocation. A first dislocation often occurs within 6 weeks following surgery and is frequently a result of patient noncompliance with postsurgical guidelines. For a first dislocation, closed reduction is used and careful assessment of the cause of dislocation should be made. If component position appears to be adequate, bracing for 3 months is recommended, along with careful explanation of hip dislocation precautions to the patient. Alternatively, removal of the acetabular component with replacement by a bipolar into the reamed acetabulum may be the best salvage procedure. Recurrent dislocation should be examined carefully for cause, with radiographs taken to evaluate the abduction and anteversion of the cup as well as the anteversion of the femoral head (Figure 7–8). Examination under fluoroscopy may reveal impingements, and push and pull films may reveal inadequate myofascial tension.

After careful evaluation of the cause(s) of dislocation, surgical correction may be undertaken. Possible solutions include reorienting the offset lip of the acetabulum, changing the anteversion or abduction of the acetabulum, changing the anteversion of the femoral component, or advancing the trochanter to tighten the muscle envelope. Failure of these methods may require the use of a constrained acetabulum to prevent dislocation. This treatment should be considered a "last resort," because the reduced ROM resulting from the design of these cups can predispose the patient to dislocation as a result of levering out of the cup from neck impingement. Long-term bracing is a possible solution for recurrent dislocation in a patient with limited goals for activity. Recurrent dislocation causes significant anxiety, which encourages patients to seek surgical correction. The recurrence rate in such patients is as high as 20% after surgical correction.

6. Leg-length discrepancy—During hip replacement surgery, an attempt is made to maintain the preoperative length of the affected leg, so that it is as long as the unaffected leg. This goal, however, is sometimes incompatible with (and therefore subservient to) myofascial tension in the ligamentously lax individual or may be a potential cause of damage to nerve or vascular structures. Hence, most surgeons advise their patients

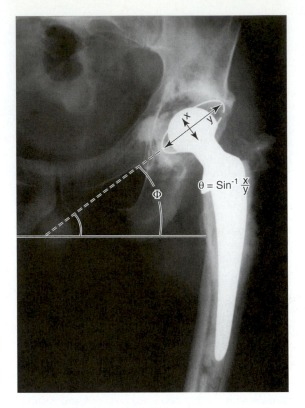

$$\theta = \text{Sin}^{-1} \frac{x}{y}$$

Figure 7–8. Approximate determination of the abduction-adduction angle and angle of anteversion of the cup. Exact measurement requires careful control of the direction of the x-ray beam.

that the leg may be longer or shorter than normal after operation.

7. Trochanteric nonunion—The rate of trochanteric nonunion after a primary total hip arthroplasty is about 5%. The percentage of patients who will develop symptoms from this complication is smaller. Usually, migration of less than 1 cm is not associated with functional symptoms or pain.

The rate of nonunion after revision surgery is much higher, as much as 40%, particularly if there has been nonunion following the primary procedure. Diminished function, as evidenced by weakness in abduction and a limp that cannot be compensated for with a cane, is an indication for an attempt at reattachment of the trochanter. The surfaces should be freshened and rigidly fixed together; bone grafting may be necessary. Subperiosteal release of the iliac wing muscles may be necessary to allow the trochanter to be reattached to the femur.

Pain after trochanteric nonunion may be the result of a painful pseudoarthrosis or, alternatively, to fixation wires that may form a painful bursa.

8. Heterotopic ossification—The incidence of significant heterotopic ossification after total hip arthroplasty is 5% or 10%, although it is present to a lesser degree in perhaps 80% of patients. Definite risk factors include previous heterotopic ossification, ankylosing spondylitis, diffuse idiopathic skeletal hyperostosis or spinal ostosis (Forestier's disease), unlimited hip motion preoperatively, head injury, and male sex of the patient. Other possible risk factors include trochanteric osteotomy, interoperative fracture, bone grafting, or localized muscle damage or hematoma.

Heterotopic bone is classified by either the Brooker or the Mayo classification (Table 7–8). Patients identified as being at risk for heterotopic ossification should undergo prophylactic treatment, careful surgical treatment, wound drainage, and irrigation of the wound prior to closing. In patients at risk, low-dose radiation, 6–8 cGy in the first 3 days after surgery, will prevent grade 3 or 4 heterotopic ossification. Indomethacin has been demonstrated to be effective, although it may be poorly tolerated by some patients. Early studies indicate that the bone inhibition is a COX-1 function, suggesting that COX-2 inhibitors may not prevent heterotopic bone. Diphosphonates are not effective in prevention of heterotopic ossification and should not be used. Indomethacin may not be optimal for prophylaxis in uncemented total hip arthroplasty, because ingrowth may be retarded. Irradiation may cause problems if ingrowth components are not appropriately shielded.

If heterotopic ossification causes symptoms (pain, decreased ROM), surgical excision may be considered after the ossification is fully mature. Irradiation and

Table 7–8. Heterotopic bone classification systems.

Stage	Mayo Classification	Brooker Classification
I	5 mm or less	Islands of bone
II	< 50% bridging laterally	Bone spurs 1 cm or greater gap
III	> 50% bridging laterally	Bone spurs less than 1 cm
IV	Apparent ankylosis	Apparent ankylosis

Reprinted, with permission, from Brooker AF et al: Ectopic ossification following total hip replacement. J Bone Joint Surg Am 1973;55:1629; and Morrey BF, Adams RA, Cabanela ME: Comparison of heterotopic bone after anterolateral, transtrochanteric, and posterior approaches for total hip arthroplasty. Clin Orthop 1984;188:160.

nonsteroidal anti-inflammatory medication are recommended postoperatively to prevent recurrence.

9. Infection—Prevention of infection after total hip arthroplasty is important because of the grave consequences. Frequently, the only way to treat an infected total hip arthroplasty is to remove the components and control the infection with antibiotics. Reinsertion of the components will then be required 1½–6 months later.

A recent innovation in the treatment of infected total hips and knees is the PROSTALAC technique. The prostheses are removed, sterilized, and reinserted as press-fit components with a layer of antibiotic-impregnated bone cement covering all surfaces except the bearing surface. This procedure is performed at the initial, meticulous debridement, to provide a spacer for subsequent, definitive joint replacement.

Prevention is much more desirable than subsequent treatment of infection. Total joint arthroplasty implants are such large foreign bodies that all reasonable prophylactic measures should be employed. Laminar flow and ultraviolet lights are used in operating rooms to reduce the number of viable particles per volume of air in the room. Because bacteria are shed from people, keeping the number of people in an operating room to a minimum and reducing the exposed skin area may be beneficial. Antimicrobial therapy may be the single most important prophylaxis against infection. Good surgical technique and minimal operating times also contribute to lowering of infection rates. Infections occurring 6 weeks to 3 months after surgery probably originate from intraoperative contamination. Careful surveillance in this period for signs of infection, including pain, elevated white blood cell count, fever, and wound drainage, allows for early identification of deep wound infection, and early debridement is then indicated to eradicate the infection. Similarly, large hematomas should be debrided because they may cause chronic drainage and constitute a culture media for infectious agents. A recent report indicates that prophylactic antibiotics given in the period before and immediately after significant dental procedures may be beneficial in preventing hematogenous infection of total joints, despite recent recommendations that routine prophylaxis 2 years after joint arthroplasty is not necessary.

Amoxicillin, 3 g taken 1 h before and 1.5 g taken 6 h after a dental procedure, is recommended to reduce the risk of hematogenous infection. For penicillin-allergic patients, erythromycin, 1 g before and 500 mg after the procedure, is recommended.

Barrack RL, Harris WH: The value of aspiration of the hip joint before revision total hip arthroplasty. J Bone Joint Surg Am 1993;75:66.

Callaghan JJ et al: Charnley total hip arthroplasty with cement: Minimum twenty-five year follow-up. J Bone Joint Surg Am 2000;82:487.

Coventry MB: Late dislocations in patients with Charnley total hip arthroplasty. J Bone Joint Surg Am 1985; 67:832.

Daly P, Morrey BF: Operative correction of an unstable total hip arthroplasty. J Bone Joint Surg Am 1992; 74:1334.

DeHart MM and Riley LH: Nerve injuries in total hip arthroplasty. J Am Acad Orthop Surg 1999;7:101.

Dorr LD et al: Total hip arthroplasty with use of the Metasul metal-on-metal articulation: Four to seven year results. J Bone Joint Surg Am 2000;82:789.

Harris WH: Traumatic arthritis of the hip after dislocation and acetabular fractures: Treatment by mold arthroplasty. J Bone Joint Surg Am 1969;51:737.

Harris WH, Barrack RL: Contemporary algorithms for evaluation of the painful total hip replacement. Orthop Rev 1993; 22:531.

Huddleston HD: An accurate method for measuring leg length and hip offset in hip arthroplasty. Orthopedics 1997;20:331.

Khan MAA et al: Dislocation following total hip arthroplasty. J Bone Joint Surg Br 1981;63:214.

Lester DK, Helm M: Mini-incision posterior approach for hip arthroplasty. Orthop Traumatol 2001;4:245.

Lewinnek GE et al: Dislocations after total hip replacement arthroplasties. J Bone Joint Surg Am 1970;60:217.

Markolf KL et al: Mechanical stability of the greater trochanter following osteotomy and reattachment by wiring. Clin Orthop 1979;141:111.

McDonald DJ, Fitzgerald RH Jr: Two-stage reconstruction of a total hip arthroplasty because of infection. J Bone Joint Surg Am 1989;71:828.

Mont MA et al: Total hip replacement without cement for noninflammatory osteoarthrosis in patients who are less than forty-five years old. J Bone Joint Surg Am 1993;75:740.

Ritter MA: A treatment plan for the dislocated total hip arthroplasty: Treatment with an above-knee hip spica cast. Clin Orthop 1980;153:153.

Schmalzried TP et al: Update on nerve palsy associated with total hip replacement. Clin Orthop 1997;344:188.

Waldman BJ et al: Total knee arthroplasty infections associated with dental procedures. Clin Orthop 1997;343:164.

Revision Total Hip Arthroplasty (THA)

The clinical success of revision THA procedures has historically been greatly inferior to the results of primary hip arthroplasty procedures. Loosening rates from 13% to 44% of cemented femoral revision procedures were reported at follow-ups of less than 5 years.

Improved techniques of cementing femoral stems led to improved results with cemented femoral revision. Pressurization of cement delivered, in a doughy stage, with a cement gun, use of pulsatile lavage and an intramedullary plug permitted reproducible creation of adequate cement mantles. Only 14% of revised cemented femoral components were loose radiographically in one series after an average of 6 years. Other series indicate a revision rate of approximately 10% at 10 years, which is much improved from earlier series, but inferior to those obtained with primary cemented stems.

Estok DMD II, Harris WH: Long-term results of cemented femoral revision surgery using second-generation techniques: An average 11.7 years follow-up evaluation. Clin Orthop 1994;299:190.

Katz RP et al: Cemented revision total hip arthroplasty using contemporary techniques: A minimum ten-year follow-up study. J Arthroplasty 1994;9:103.

Kavanagh BF et al: Revision total hip arthroplasty. J Bone Joint Surg 1985;67:517.

Pellicci PM et al: Revision total hip arthroplasty. Clin Orthop 1982;170:34.

Rubash HE, Harris WH: Revision of nonseptic, loose, cemented femoral components using modern cementing techniques. J Arthroplasty 1988;3:241.

Cementless reconstructions of failed femoral components were developed in response to the early high rates of failure with cemented revision procedures. However, early cementless revision series were generally unsuccessful, with failure rates of 4–10% at follow-ups less than 4 years. The use of proximally porous coated stems with inadequate stabilization, in the setting of deficient femoral bone stock led to unreliable bone ingrowth fixation. More recently, encouraging reports have been obtained with modular proximally coated stems, such as the S-ROM (Johnson and Johnson, Raynham, Massachusetts) prosthesis and extensively porous coated stems, such as the AML and Solution (Depuy, Warsaw, Indiana). Re-revision rates from 1.5% to 6% have been achieved with use of these types of cementless femoral component at follow-ups from 5 to 8.4 years.

Gustilo RB, Pasternak HS: Revision total hip arthroplasty with titanium ingrowth prosthesis and bone grafting for failed cemented femoral component loosening. Clin Orthop 1988;235:111.

Harris WH et al: Results of cementless revisions of total hip arthroplasties using the Harris-Galante prosthesis. Clin Orthop 1988;235:120.

Hedley AK et al: Revision of failed total hip arthroplasties with uncemented porous-coated anatomic components. Clin Orthop 1988;235:75.

Lawrence JM et al: Revision total hip arthroplasty: Long term results with cement. Orthop Clin North Am 1993;24:635.

McCarthy JC et al: Revision of the deficient femur with a modular femoral component. Orthop Trans 1993;17:966.

Paprosky WG et al: Cementless femoral revision in the presence of severe proximal bone loss using diaphyseal fixation. Orthop Trans 1993; 17:965.

In the situation where inadequate femoral bone stock exists, the use of allograft bone has been advocated. For extended loss of proximal femoral bone stock, cementing a smooth tapered femoral stem in a bed of impacted particulate allogenic bone has been reported to produce promising short-term clinical results. When deficiency of proximal bone stock is severe, use of structural femoral allografts may be required, and short-term reports suggest good clinical results.

Gie GA et al: Impacted cancellous allografts and cement for revision total hip replacement. J Bone Joint Surg 1993;75:14.

Gross AE et al: Proximal femoral allografts for reconstruction of bone stock in revision arthroplasty of the hip. Clin Orthop 1995;319:151.

Similar to early experience with cemented revisions of the femoral component, acetabular revision with cement was generally unsuccessful. Because of the difficulty of interdigitating cement into a sclerotic and often deficient acetabular bone stock, failure rates of loosening were reported from 53% to 93% at follow-ups from only 2–4.5 years.

Kavanagh BF et al: Charnley total hip arthroplasty with cement: Fifteen-year results. J Bone Joint Surg 1985;71:1496.

Snorrason F, Karrholm J: Early loosening of revision hip arthroplasty: A roentgen stereophotogrammetric analysis. J Arthroplasty 1990;5:217.

The introduction of cementless porous-coated acetabular implants for revision of failed cemented cups greatly facilitated early clinical results. Large hemispherical cementless acetabular implants can accommodate most bone defects encountered after removal of failed cemented cups. Where an adequate press-fit cannot be obtained, adjuvant fixation of the implant with screws or spikes can provide adequate stability to permit bone ingrowth fixation. Re-revision rates have been reported to be from 0% to 1.6% with follow-up of 2–4 years (Engh, Harris, Hedley, Padgett).

Engh CA et al: Results of cementless revision for failed cemented total hip arthroplasty. Clin Orthop 1988;235:91.

Harris WH et al: Results of cementless revision of total hip arthroplasties using the Harris-Galante prosthesis. Clin Orthop 1988;235:120.

Hedley AK et al: Revision of failed total hip arthroplasties with uncemented porous-coated anatomic components. Clin Orthop 1988;235:75.

Padgett DE et al: Revision of the acetabular component without cement after total hip arthroplasty: Three- to six-year follow-up. J Bone Joint Surg 1993;75A:663.

Where inadequate bone stock of the acetabulum precludes reconstructions with conventional hemispherical implants, structural allografts fixed to the pelvis with screws can provide acceptable middle-term results. Other alternatives include the use of eccentric shaped cementless implants and cemented reconstructions with particulate allografting and antiprotrusio cages.

Berry DJ, Muller M: Revision arthroplasty using an antiprotrusio cage for massive acetabular bone deficiency. J Bone Joint Surg 1992;74:711.

Garbuz D et al: Revision of the acetabular component of a total hip arthroplasty with a massive structural allograft. J Bone Joint Surg 1996;78:693.

Peters CL, Curtain M, Samuelson KM: Acetabular revision with the Burch-Schnieder antiprotrusio cage and cancellous allograft bone. J Arthroplasty 1995;10:307.

Sutherland CJ: Early experience with eccentric acetabular components in revision total hip arthroplasty. Am J Orthop 1996; 25:284.

Total Knee Arthroplasty

A. INDICATIONS

As with other joints, the primary indication for total knee arthroplasty is pain. Absolute contraindications to total knee arthroplasty include active sepsis, absence of an extensor mechanism, and neuropathic joint. Relative contraindications include a patient's young age, heavy demand for activity, or a patient's unreliability.

When both hips and knees are involved with painful arthritis, the joint causing the most discomfort should be replaced first. If hips and knees are equally painful, hip arthroplasty should precede knee arthroplasty. Rehabilitation following total hip arthroplasty is easier and less affected by a painful knee than vice versa. Additionally, motion of the hip joint greatly facilitates surgery for the knee.

B. IMPLANTS

Early designs of total knee arthroplasty were developed in Europe and may be categorized as constrained or resurfacing. Constrained devices consisted of fixed hinges, and resurfacing devices relied upon ligaments for stability. Constrained devices predictably loosened, though they were used primarily in severe bone or ligamentous deficiency states. Early resurfacing implants were flat, roller pin-shaped implants or unicondylar devices that replaced only the medial or lateral compartment. Early knee replacements did not resurface the patellofemoral joints.

Contemporary total knee replacements represent a convergence of two major designs developed in the United States during the early 1970s: the total condylar and the duopatellar prostheses. The total condylar prosthesis had a femoral component made of Co/Cr and an all-polyethylene tibial component with a central peg. Excision of the posterior cruciate ligament was required because the entire surface of the tibial plateau was resurfaced. The patellar component was a dome-shaped polyethylene implant. All components were fixed with acrylic cement.

The Duocondylar knee replacement was the forerunner of the duopatellar prosthesis, and did not resurface the patellofemoral joint. Extension of the anterior flange of the Co/Cr femoral component provided an articulation surface for an all-polyethylene dome-shaped patellar component. The tibial component was originally designed with separate medial and lateral runners, allowing preservation of the central insertion of the posterior cruciate ligament. Later, the two components were joined together, but a cutout was made posteriorly to permit retention of the posterior cruciate ligament.

Retention of the posterior cruciate ligament permitted increased flexion over that with the total condylar design because the normal femoral rollback during knee flexion was retained. Shifting of the center of rotation posteriorly during knee flexion greatly improves the lever arm of the quadriceps mechanism. The ability to climb stairs was superior when the cruciate ligament was retained. Central to the design of a cruciate ligament-retaining prosthesis is avoidance of excessive constraint by the tibial surface to permit rollback.

To overcome limitations in flexion and stair climbing function, the total condylar prosthesis was modified with a cam mechanism (posterior-stabilized condylar prosthesis). The central cam design permits substitution of the function of the posterior cruciate ligament, providing a mechanical recreation of femoral rollback.

The differences in ROM and stair climbing function achieved with cruciate-retaining and posterior-stabilized knee replacements are now considered negligible. Arguments in favor of the posterior-stabilized implant include technical ease in reconstructing severely deformed knees and less shear force at the articular bearing because sliding is reduced. The arguments in favor of cruciate-retaining designs are reduction of bone-cement interface forces because of less constraint, improved stability in flexion, less removal of bone from the intercondylar region, and absence of patellofemoral impingement syndrome (formed by scar tissue in the intercondylar recess of the posterior stabilized femoral component).

Problems with high-contact, stress-inducing fatigue wear of the polyethylene surfaces has stimulated a new design concept in knee replacement. This design utilizes a polyethylene component that can move in relation to the tibial base plate. Thus, the surface of polyethylene in contact with the femoral component can be made to be more conforming because it can change positions during flexion and extension of the knee. Two types have evolved: the rotating platform, which only allows rotation of the polyethylene around an axis approximating the axis of the tibia, and variations on the

"meniscal bearing" knee. In this design, the individual medial and lateral poly components can rotate (tibial axis) and translate(AP direction), or the entire poly plateau can rotate and translate in the AP direction. The latter concept seems to better address the biomechanical aspects of the knee but results are early or limited on all designs.

C. SURGICAL TECHNIQUE

Total knee replacement surgery is greatly facilitated by use of a thigh tourniquet. Following exsanguination of the lower limb with an elastic wrap, the tourniquet is inflated to 250–300 mm Hg. An anterior midline skin incision is made, followed most commonly by a deep medial parapatellar approach. The lateral flap containing the patella is everted to allow exposure of the tibiofemoral joint. Remnants of menisci and anterior cruciate ligament are excised, with careful release of contracted soft tissue structures as needed.

Instrumentation systems guide the surgeon to create bone cuts with a saw that match the prosthetic fixation surface and reproduce anatomic alignment of the knee joint. Typically, in the coronal plane, the tibial plateau is cut horizontally to be at a right angle with the shaft of the tibia. The distal femur is usually cut at 5–7 degrees of valgus from the shaft of the femur. Such bone cuts provide a neutral mechanical alignment in the coronal plane such that a line can be drawn from the center of the femoral head, through the middle of the knee joint, and through the center of the ankle joint. In the sagittal plane, the femoral cut is at right angles to the femoral shaft but the tibial cut is made with 3–5 degrees of posterior slope. Slight external rotation of the femoral component allows symmetric tension of collateral ligaments during knee flexion and facilitates tracking of the patellar component.

Retention or sacrifice of the posterior cruciate ligament depends on the design of the implant used. When the cruciate ligament is sacrificed, bone from the intercondylar notch is removed to accommodate the box that houses the cam mechanism.

When the patellar surface is replaced, a saw is used to create a flat surface with symmetric bone thickness. Inadequate resection will predispose to subluxation because excessive extensor mechanism length will be used, and the lateral ligamentous structures will be relatively tightened. Many patellar components are 10 mm thick; thus, adequate resection must be almost 10 mm, within the limits of the anatomy of the patella. At least 10 mm and preferably 15 mm of patella (anteroposterior thickness) should remain. Patellar tracking is assessed by using trial components and ranging the knee from full extension to full flexion. In knees with valgus deformity, it is common to have lateral subluxation of the patella. In such cases, a careful lateral retinacular release that preserves the superior lateral geniculate vessels is performed. Positioning the patellar implant slightly medially on the patellar bone surface will also improve tracking.

After appropriate trials are used to confirm accurate sizes of the components as well as ligamentous stability, cementing is performed. Careful cleansing of the bone surfaces with pulsatile lavage facilitates interdigitation of "doughy"-stage methylmethacrylate cement. The prosthetic components must be seated in the correct orientation, and excess acrylic cement must be removed. Before closure of the knee, it is prudent to lavage fragments of bone and cement and release the tourniquet to obtain hemostasis. At surgery, little bleeding is seen in the flexed knee. Thus, many surgeons close the wound and maintain the knee in flexion for periods up to 24 h to decrease blood loss.

D. CLINICAL RESULTS

Long-term results of contemporary cemented total knee arthroplasty designs are excellent. Survivorship of the total condylar prosthesis has been calculated to be 90–95% at 15 years. Excellent functional results of posterior stabilized total knee replacements have also been reported, with a 12-year survival rate of 94% for functional prostheses. Similarly, excellent function and only a 1% rate of loosening of the tibial or femoral component was reported with a cruciate ligament-retaining knee replacement when followed up at 10–14 years.

E. COMPLICATIONS

Complications are infrequent with total knee arthroplasty but include many of the same problems encountered with total hip arthroplasty. Additional problems arise from wound healing, fracture, extensor mechanism problems, and stiffness of the knee.

1. Deep vein thrombosis—Deep venous thrombosis is common following knee arthroplasty, occurring in more than 50% of patients in one study. Further, 10–15% of patients will develop deep vein thrombosis in the contralateral leg after unilateral knee arthroplasty. The use of the tourniquet during surgery does not have a clear, detrimental effect on thrombus formation. The incidence of pulmonary embolism is lower than that reported in hip arthroplasty. This may be caused by the greater propensity to form calf thrombi after total knee arthroplasty; these thrombi may be less likely to cause emboli than thigh thrombi. Antithrombotic prophylactic measures include use of pulsatile compression stockings and administration of warfarin or low-molecular-weight heparin.

2. Wound problems—Wound problems can arise from incision-related issues and from patient-related risk factors. The skin incision should optimally be mid-line and longitudinal, and the skin should have minimal undermining. Preexisting skin incisions should be used when possible. Because wound healing is crucial to the success of the procedure, preoperative plastic surgery consultation may be beneficial if multiple scars, burns, or previous irradiation to the skin are present. Patient-related risk factors include chronic corticosteroid use, obesity, malnutrition, tobacco use, diabetes, and hypovolemia.

Treatment of wound problems depends on the type of problem. Drainage of serous material that does not clear in 5–7 days is an indication for open debridement. Hematoma formation (without drainage) is treated nonoperatively unless there are signs of impending skin necrosis or compromise of ROM. Small areas of superficial necrosis at the wound edge are treated with routine local wound care. Full-thickness soft-tissue necrosis places the joint space at high risk of infection and must be treated aggressively. Debridement with flap closure is frequently required. The medial gastrocnemius flap is useful, because the tissue necrosis is frequently medial.

Prevention of wound problems through careful planning, gentle handling of soft tissues, and patient education to minimize risk factors is preferable to subsequent treatment of the problems.

3. Nerve palsy—Nerve palsies are a rare complication of total knee arthroplasty. The peroneal nerve is believed to be at increased risk for injury from surgery performed on valgus knees with flexion contractures or other significant deformity, ischemia from stretching small vessels in the surrounding soft tissue, and compression resulting from a tight dressing or splint. The risk is reported to be about 0.6%.

4. Femoral fracture—Notching of the anterior femoral cortex may predispose to distal femoral fracture. A technical error, notching can be prevented by careful femoral sizing before use of the anterior distal femur cutting block and by avoidance of posterior displacement or extension of the cutting block. Use of an intramedullary stem extension is advised if notching occurs. Fracture of the medial or lateral condyle may occur, particularly in patients with poor bone stock, such as those with rheumatoid arthritis or osteoporosis or in patients with cruciate-sacrificing femoral components. Large intercondylar boxes in these prostheses can cause weakening of the distal femur. Prevention is the rule, facilitated by vigilance during exposure of a stiff knee. Useful techniques to avoid avulsion include a V turndown quadricepsplasty, quadriceps "snip," tibial tubercle osteotomy, and placement of a Steinmann pin in the tubercle to prevent excessive traction on the patellar tendon. Treatment of the disruption is similar to the treatment in a normal knee. The patellar tendon is attached to bone, and the repair is protected with a wire around the patella and the tibial tubercle, holding the patella at the correct length from the tibial tubercle.

Patellar complications include maltracking, loosening of the patellar component, fractures, and impingement. The patellofemoral forces are among the highest anywhere in the body, and avoidance of intraoperative technical errors may minimize patellar complications. Patellar tracking should be assessed intraoperatively during flexion and extension of the prosthetic knee. Lateral patellar subluxation or dislocation may be caused by internal rotation of the femoral or tibial component, as well as a tight lateral patellar retinaculum. Careful release of the lateral patellar retinaculum may correct maltracking. Subluxation can predispose to patellar component loosening, as can abnormal stress caused by uneven patellar bone resection. Excessive bone resection and avascularity, caused by damage to the superior lateral geniculate artery during lateral release, can predispose to fractures. When using a posterior stabilized prosthesis, maintaining the inferior pole of the patella within 10–30 mm of the joint line may prevent impingement syndrome, which is characterized by pain or clicking when peripatellar synovial scar tissue impinges against the intercondylar box of the femoral component during flexion and extension.

In some studies, patellar complications are the cause for as many as one half of the knee revisions performed. For this reason, some surgeons do not resurface the patella when the appearance is relatively normal. Because most patellofemoral replacement problems have been attributed to technical errors, inferior prosthetic design, and excessive loads, replacement will probably become more prevalent as these problems are resolved.

5. Extensor mechanism complications—Many of these problems can be prevented by careful surgical technique, because many of these arise from technical problems, such as quadriceps (or patellar) tendon rupture, patellofemoral instability, and patella fracture.

Intraoperative rupture of the patellar or quadriceps tendon at the time of arthroplasty can be repaired, but a repair complicates the postoperative ROM regimen, at least to some extent. The incidence ranges from 0.2% to 2.5%.

6. Knee stiffness—Knee stiffness is a common problem in the early postoperative period. Methods to reduce stiffness include physical therapy (active or active-assisted ROM) and continuous passive motion (CPM). The CPM machine moves the knee through a preset passive ROM This modality is generally accepted and even liked by patients but has not been shown to affect the final ROM or reduce hospital stay. An acceptable ROM is 90–95 degrees of flexion with less than 10 degrees of flexion contracture, but the activities of daily living, such as getting out of a chair or climbing stairs, should be painless. Postoperative stiffness would have generally subsided by 6–8 weeks after surgery, and improvement in ROM should occur for 1 year with most gain in the first 3 months. The preoperative ROM is an important indicator of the ROM to be expected postoperatively.

Prevention of significant flexion contracture at the time of surgery and in the early postoperative period is important, because improvement with manipulation is unrewarding. Manipulation with or without steroid injection can be beneficial in the first 3 months. Arthroscopic debridement may be necessary after intra-articular fibrosis has occurred. Decreases in ROM after initial gains should alert the surgeon to possible infection, reflex sympathetic dystrophy, or mechanical problems, such as loose components or interposed soft tissue.

Ayers DC et al: Common complications of total knee arthroplasty. J Bone Joint Surg Am 1997;79:278.

Barrack RL, Wolfe MW: Patellar resurfacing in total knee arthroplasty. J Am Acad Orthop Surg 2000;8:75.

Callaghan JJ et al: Cemented rotating-platform total knee replacement: A nine to twelve year follow-up study. J Bone Joint Surg Am 2000;82:705.

Callaghan JJ et al: Mobile-bearing knee replacement: Concepts and results. J Bone Joint Surg 2000;82:1020.

Figgi HF et al: The influence of tibial-patellofemoral location on function of the knee in patients with the posterior stabilized condylar knee prosthesis. J Bone Joint Surg Am 1986;68:1035.

Hahn SB et al: A modified Thompson quadricepsplasty for stiff knee. J Bone Joint Surg Br 2000;82:992.

Rinonapoli E et al: Long-term results and survivorship analysis of 89 total condylar knee prostheses. J Arthroplasty 1992;7:241.

Scuderi GR et al: Survivorship of cemented knee replacements. J Bone Joint Surg Br 1989;71:798.

Ververeli PA et al: Continuous passive motion after total knee arthroplasty: Analysis of cost and benefits. Clin Orthop 1995;321:208.

Total Shoulder Arthroplasty

A. INDICATIONS

The primary indication for shoulder arthroplasty is severe pain that has been unsuccessfully treated with nonsurgical management. The underlying causes for the loss of articular cartilage and the incongruent osseous surfaces of the glenohumeral joint are usually osteoarthritis, rheumatoid arthritis, posttraumatic arthritis, and dislocation arthropathy. The functional status of the soft tissues is vitally important because they provide a significant component of the joint stabilizing force through the concavity-compression mechanism. Replacement of the glenoid may be performed if and only if the rotator cuff is intact or is reparable at the time of surgery. Although still controversial, most surgeons agree that a shoulder hemiarthroplasty is performed for patients with rotator cuff arthropathy and osteonecrosis. If rheumatoid arthritis has caused profound bony erosion of the glenoid, hemiarthroplasty may be the only viable option as the glenoid may not support a prosthetic component. Contraindications to shoulder arthroplasty include active sepsis, neuropathic arthropathy, and the absence of a functional deltoid.

B. SURGICAL TECHNIQUE

A deltopectoral surgical approach is performed, with careful retraction of the conjoined tendon medially to avoid injury to the musculocutaneous nerve. Although some suggest releasing the subscapularis tendon 1 cm lateral to its humeral insertion because it may facilitate later repair, most currently recommend to detach the subscapularis directly off the humeral insertion. Attachment of the subscapularis to the edge of the humeral osteotomy lengthens the muscle-tendon unit so that a coronal Z-plasty is not required to improve external rotation of the glenohumeral joint. Palpation of the axillary nerve medially along the inferior border of the subscapularis is recommended to avoid injury to this vital nerve. A capsulotomy is then performed from the humeral attachment, and the humeral head is delivered out of the wound, with extension and external rotation of the arm. The humeral head is carefully resected to protect the rotator cuff insertion, and the humeral component is placed in 30–35 degrees of retroversion. Preparation of the humeral intramedullary canal is followed by insertion of a trial stemmed humeral component. After the appropriate thickness of the humeral head and stem is determined, the trial humeral head component is removed and the stem is left in place to tamponade the intramedullary bleeding and to provide strength to the humerus during glenoid preparation. Posterior displacement of the proximal humerus is performed using a humeral head retractor, such as a Fukuda retractor, for exposure of the glenoid vault. Minimal bone is removed from the glenoid bone with a motorized burr to preserve cortical bone for support of the glenoid component. Long-term follow-up studies have shown that both bone grafting of deficient glenoid bone and building up defects with cement are not routinely recommended. With posterior glenoid wear, bone is removed form the glenoid anteriorly to match the posterior aspect of the glenoid. A keel or drill holes for peg insertion are made for cemented applications. Currently, the FDA has not approved any noncemented glenoid components. The humeral component is then implanted with or without cement, depending on surgeon preference and quality of bone stock. The closure must include a robust repair of the subscapularis tendon so that physical therapy may be initiated in the immediate postoperative period.

C. IMPLANTS

Early total shoulder arthroplasties were designed with constrained articulations between the humeral and glenoid components. Predictably, glenoid loosening and implant failures were commonplace, leading to development of unconstrained designs. Currently, nonconstrained resurfacing devices are primarily used with stemmed metal humeral components. Options include modular head and neck assemblies as well as a porous coating for cementless implantation. Although most commonly used glenoid components are made of high-density polyethylene, some designs of metal backing with porous coating and screw fixation for cementless applications are being explored.

D. CLINICAL RESULTS

Shoulder arthroplasty has made significant progress, similar to the advances in hip and knee arthroplasty. The current "third-generation" prosthetic designs incorporate variable offset and inclination, anatomic humeral heads, precision instruments, and variable glenoid curvature in their designs. Pain relief is reliably achieved with shoulder arthroplasty in more than 90–95% of patients. Pain relief obtained from hemiarthroplasties is equivalent to total shoulder replacement in selected patients under 50 years of age.

Functional results are variable, however, depending largely on the underlying cause. A recent study by Matsen and colleagues demonstrated that the overall well-being of the patient prior to surgery strongly correlates with the final functional outcome. A ROM three quarters to four fifths of normal can be expected in patients treated for osteoarthritis or osteonecrosis. For rheumatoid arthritis, one half to two thirds of normal motion is usually obtained. For patients with cuff tear arthropathy, the ROM achieved may be only one third to one half of normal.

The major complication associated with total shoulder arthroplasty involves loosening of the glenoid component; instability and late rotator cuff tears are next in frequency. Less common complications are humeral component loosening, sepsis, nerve injury, and humeral fractures. The incidence of shoulder arthroplasty infection is < 0.5% and is usually attributed to the abundant blood supply and surrounding musculature of the joint.

Radiolucent lines have been observed around the glenoid component in 30–90% of cases in most published series, but the rate of definite and probable radiographic loosening is between 0–11%. Despite this, the revision rate for glenoid loosening is about 6% at 12 years. A higher failure rate caused by glenoid component loosening is associated with deficiency of the rotator cuff. Superior migration of the humeral articulation leads to eccentric loading and a rocking-horse effect on the glenoid component and loosening. Most surgeons currently perform hemiarthroplasty for rotator cuff tear arthropathy. In certain cases of cuff tear arthropathy or of significant medial glenoid erosion, one may use of a large-diameter humeral head or bipolar hemiarthroplasty to lateralize the joint center, thereby facilitating the mechanical advantage of the deltoid.

Bonsell S et al: The relationship of age, gender, and degenerative changes observed on radiographs of the shoulder in asymptomatic individuals. J Bone Joint Surg Br 2000; 82:1135.

Gartsman GM et al: Shoulder arthroplasty with or without resurfacing of the glenoid in patients who have osteoarthritis. J Bone Joint Surg Am 2000; 82:26.

Godeneche A et al: Prosthetic replacement in the treatment of osteoarthritis of the shoulder: Early results of 268 cases. J Shoulder Elbow Surg 2002;11:11.

Green A, Norris TR: Shoulder arthroplasty for advanced glenohumeral arthritis after anterior instability repair. J Shoulder Elbow Surg 2001;10:539.

Hill JM, Norris TR: Long-term results of total shoulder arthroplasty following bone grafting of the glenoid. J Bone Joint Surg Am 2001; 83:877.

Matsen FA et al: Correlates with comfort and function after total shoulder arthroplasty for degenerative joint disease. J Shoulder Elbow Surg 2000; 9:465.

Sperling JW et al: Neer hemiarthroplasty and Neer total shoulder arthroplasty in patients 50 years old or less. Long term results. J Bone Joint Surg Am 1998;80:464.

Total Elbow Arthroplasty

A. INDICATIONS

Although total elbow arthroplasty (TEA) may be an appropriate method of restoring joint function and stability, the primary goal of TEA is pain relief. With increased surgical experience, improvement of prosthetic designs, and evolving biomechanical knowledge, the indications for TEA have broadened to include the following, in order of frequency:

(1) rheumatoid arthritis (RA),

(2) posttraumatic arthritis,

(3) juvenile rheumatoid arthritis (JRA),

(4) distal humeral nonunions and severe comminuted distal humeral fractures, especially in the elderly, and

(5) primary osteoarthritis.

The severity of the disease and the choice of prosthesis in all of these situations are critical to the final outcome. TEA achieves its best results in individuals who do not tax the functional design of the prosthesis and who do not expect to use their upper limb beyond the level of basic daily functional activities such as combing hair, eating, and drinking. Active sepsis is an absolute contraindi-

cation to total elbow arthroplasty. Relative contraindications for TEA include previously open wound associated with trauma around the elbow, a previous infection of the elbow associated with prior TEA, arthrodesis, paralysis of the biceps or triceps, severe joint capsule contracture, and poor patient compliance. Lifting limitations after TEA remain 2.25 kg for repetitive lifting and 4.5 kg for single-episode lifting. Thus, patient selection, compliance, and age become critical factors in determining the successful long-term outcome of prosthetic elbows.

B. SURGICAL TECHNIQUE

Attention to the soft tissue, including the triceps insertion, collateral ligaments and the ulnar nerve, is of vital importance when performing a TEA. Although the direct posterior approach is routinely recommended, especially early in the surgeon's learning curve, failures in total elbow arthroplasty have been attributed to this approach. After the flap of triceps muscle is turned down, the tissue may be devascularized and lead to overlying skin necrosis and weakness of the triceps muscle. If this approach is used, careful reattachment of the triceps insertion to the ulna is mandatory.

As maintenance of the collateral ligaments is of vital importance when a nonconstrained device is used, the Kocher posterolateral approach allows preservation of the ulnar collateral ligament. As this ligament provides the major restraint against valgus forces in the flexed elbow, it must be preserved when a nonconstrained device is used. The surgical plane is between the anconeus and extensor carpi ulnaris muscles distally and proximally between the triceps and brachioradialis muscles.

The Bryan posteromedial approach is routinely used for implantation of semiconstrained devices. The surgical plane is between the medial triceps and forearm flexors proximally and between the flexor carpi ulnaris and flexor carpi radialis distally. This approach allows direct visualization of the ulnar nerve and facilitates transposition of the nerve. Great care should be taken when encountering Sharpey's fibers during elevation of the triceps from its olecranon insertion to prevent discontinuity with the forearm fascia. Release of the medial collateral ligament is required in order to proceed with implantation.

C. IMPLANTS

Early total elbow arthroplasty designs included constrained devices, which predictably failed owing to early aseptic loosening. In response to these failures, devices with less constraint and those permitting more normal elbow kinematics were developed. The two currently available types of elbow implants include resurfacing nonconstrained devices and semiconstrained devices. The most popular semiconstrained devices are the Coonrad Morrey, Pritchard-Walker, and GSB III

(Gschwend Mach III) prostheses. These implants have a linked hinge that provides stability but less constraint than early designs. The "sloppy fit" of these hinges permits varus, valgus, and rotatory forces to the implant and fixation to be dissipated. The inherent stability of these designs permits application in cases of soft-tissue and bony insufficiency, but theoretically there is increased risk of loosening. Excision of the radial head is also recommended during implantation of semiconstrained total elbow arthroplasties. Nonconstrained devices are widely used outside the united States, and the most popular devices are the Souter-Strathclyde, Roper-Tuke, and the Kudo implants. These nonconstrained implants permit restoration of the center of rotation of the ulnotrochlear joint with a metal-on-polyethylene articulation. The humeral and ulnar components are not linked, minimizing stresses to the fixation of these components. As these implants lack intrinsic stability, they should not be used in cases of ligamentous instability or deficiency of supporting bone.

D. CLINICAL RESULTS

Ten-year follow-up studies for TEA are currently only available for two semiconstrained, linked devices, the Coonrad-Morrey and the GSB III designs, as well as for three nonconstrained devices, the Kudo, the Souter-Strathclyde, and the Roper-Tuke designs. Most of the experience using resurfacing devices in this country has been with the capitellocondylar design. Although no consistent 10-year studies exist for the capitellocondylar device, supporters of these implants report functional outcome of TEAs with nonconstrained devices comparable to those with semiconstrained device. Nevertheless, most of the reported past experiences suggest that high complication rates, particularly joint subluxations and dislocations are associated with the use of these devices. The currently available 10-year, long-term studies, as well as previous intermediate follow-up results, seem to suggest that the better semiconstrained designs may be associated with smaller numbers of revisions and aseptic loosening, and greater success in maintaining pain relief and joint stability compared with the best nonconstrained devices.

Common complications encountered following TEA include aseptic loosening and joint instability, ulnar neuropathy, and infections. Ulnar neuropathies do not tend to require additional procedures, usually manifesting as paraesthesias and rarely showing signs of motor weakness. Many cases resolve or ameliorate over time. Recently, Spinner and coworkers reported that 40% of the patients in their series with rheumatoid arthritis already had preoperative evidence of ulnar neuropathy and that TEA did not contribute significantly to postoperative ulnar nerve dysfunction. Aseptic loosening of the cement-stem interface, polyethylene bush-

ing wear (in semiconstrained devices), metallosis, and infections are major reasons for reoperation. Infections are the most serious complications among these indications and have the potential to develop further into devastating local and systemic complications.

Gambirasio R et al: Total elbow replacement for complex fractures of the distal humerus. An option for the elderly patient. J Bone Joint Surg Br 2001;83:974.

Gill DRJ, Morrey BF: The Coonrad-Morrey total elbow arthroplasty in patients who have rheumatoid arthritis: A ten to fifteen year follow-up study. J Bone Joint Surg Am 1998;80: 1327.

Hildebrand KA et al: Functional outcome of semiconstrained total elbow arthroplasty. J Bone Joint Surg Am 2000; 82:1379.

Mansat P, Morrey BF: Semiconstrained total elbow arthroplasty for ankylosed and stiff elbows. J Bone Joint Surg Am 2000; 82:1260.

Tanaka N et al: Kudo total elbow arthroplasty in patients with rheumatoid arthritis: A long term follow-up study. J Bone Joint Surg Am; 83:1506.

Ronzig P: Souter-Strathclyde total elbow arthroplasty: A long-term follow-up study. J Bone Joint Surg Br 2000; 82:1129.

Spinner RJ et al: Ulnar nerve function following total elbow arthroplasty: A prospective study comparing preoperative and postoperative clinical and electrophysiologic evaluation in patients with rheumatoid arthritis. J Hand Surg Am 2000; 25:360.

Yanni ON et al: The Roper-Tuke total elbow arthroplasty: Four- to 10- year results of an unconstrained prosthesis. J Bone Joint Surg Br; 82:705.

Total Ankle Arthroplasty

The total ankle arthroplasty has been under development for many years as a result of the success with total joint replacement of the knee and the hip. Initial designs met with modest short-term success and caused almost an abandonment of the procedure because of the comparison to ankle arthrodesis. The longevity of present total ankle joint replacements has been somewhat erratic for a variety of reasons. The articular surface that must be replaced is unlike any other joint and, thus, experience cannot be carried directly from the knee or the hip to the ankle. Joint loads and requirements are less well characterized, and surgical technique is less well developed and, therefore, less reliable. For these reasons, total ankle replacement remains a developmental procedure indicated for patients with low activity demand and the need for ankle motion.

Encouraging early reports with newer designs of total ankle arthroplasty have emerged and are being closely observed. Results from Scandinavia with the STAR prosthesis in short-term follow-up are promising. Total ankle replacement is desirable because of the drawbacks of ankle arthrodesis, which include a significant pseudoarthrosis rate of 10–20%, despite extended cast immobilization to achieve arthrodesis. Furthermore, extended arthrodesis results in osteopenia and diminished motion in the subtalar and midtarsal joints. The additional stress on these joints from the ankle arthrodesis predisposes them to degenerative changes over the long term, as is seen frequently above and below the arthrodesis in other joints such as the cervical spine, the lumbar spine, and the hip.

Kitaoka HB, Patzer GL: Clinical results of the Mayo total ankle arthroplasty. J Bone Joint Surg 1996;78:1658.

Pyevich MT et al: Total ankle arthroplasty: A unique design. Two to twelve-year follow-up. J Bone Joint Surg. 1998;80:1410.

Evaluation of Painful Total Joint Arthroplasty

A certain degree of adaptation and accommodation is possible in the normal joint, allowing it to last for a lifetime in most persons. After replacement of a diseased joint by a metal-and-plastic artificial joint, no remodeling or accommodation is possible. Loosening of the interface between bone and prosthesis is possible and, indeed, may be inevitable. In addition, during and subsequent to the implantation process, bacteria may find their way into a prosthetic joint, causing pain or loosening. Implantation of a new joint markedly alters the stress state in the bone, particularly with uncemented prostheses, and a certain amount of pain may result. The presence of the new joint is likely to markedly alleviate pain, and the patient's activity level may increase, resulting in bone remodeling around the prosthesis or at a remote site or even fatigue fractures. All of these problems may result in a painful arthroplasty. Evaluation is complicated by the presence of the artificial joint, which introduces several new variables when compared with a normal arthritic joint. The same process of evaluation is used as with an arthritic joint; a history is obtained, physical examination is performed, and laboratory data are obtained.

A. History

Referred pain from other sources must be ruled out, particularly with the shoulder and the hip, where referred pain from the lumbar and cervical spine may confuse the picture. A history of pain radiating into the shoulder with motion of the neck, for example, may be helpful in this process. Pain related to activity of the affected joint, as compared with pain all the time, is an important fact, with constant pain or night pain suggesting chronic infection. Pain in the hip or knee that occurs with the first few steps but then improves is likely to be caused by loosening of the prosthesis. This pain probably arises from a fibrous membrane between the prosthesis and bone, which, with weight bearing, compresses and provides better contact, thereby lessen-

ing the pain. A history of swelling, redness, fevers, or chills must be obtained.

B. Physical Examination

The same tests are performed as for an arthritic joint to evaluate the location, magnitude, and severity of pain.

C. Workup

1. Laboratory findings—Laboratory data may be helpful. The erythrocyte sedimentation rate (> 35–40 mm/h) or C-reactive protein (> 0.7) points toward an infected arthroplasty; with the knee, a lower rate does not rule out infected arthroplasty. A complete blood count is sometimes also helpful in demonstrating an elevated white blood cell count.

2. Arthrographic evaluation—Arthrographic evaluation may be helpful by showing dye penetration into the cement-bone interface, prosthesis-bone interface, or prosthesis-cement interface. The most important aspect of arthrographic evaluation is the fluid obtained for culture. Arthrographic evaluation is mainly indicated when infection is suspected, as there is a risk of contaminating the joint as well as the possibility of obtaining false-positive and false-negative cultures. Another important aspect of arthrographic evaluation is the pain response to injection of lidocaine into the joint. Alleviation of essentially all pain when weight bearing is attempted after injection localizes the problem to the affected joint.

Bone scans have little value immediately after surgery. Significant bone remodeling is present, which continues for several months. Bone scans may not be helpful until 6 months to 1 year after surgery. At that point, increased uptake indicates bone remodeling and loosening of the prosthesis.

3. Indium-labeled white blood cell scan—This nuclear medicine study uses the patient's polymorphonuclear leukocytes, which are labeled with radioactive indium and injected back into the patient. It may be quite beneficial in localizing acute infectious processes but is frequently not helpful in the evaluation of chronic infection.

4. Plain radiographs—Roentgenographic examination is the single most useful test in the evaluation of nonseptic loosening. Important signs are radiolucent lines adjacent to the prosthesis or cement, particularly if they are 2 mm or greater or are becoming enlarged on serial radiographs (Figure 7–9). Fracture of the cement and change in position of the component are indications of loosening.

Treatment of Infected Total Joint Arthroplasty

Definitive evidence of a septic total joint arthroplasty forecasts a poor prognosis for the patient. The infec-

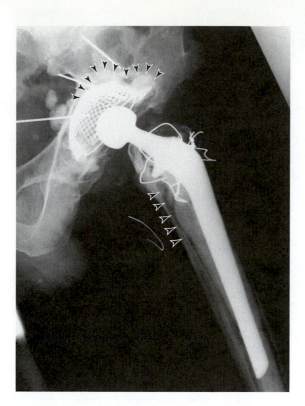

Figure 7–9. Radiograph of radiolucent lines around an acetabular component.

tious process is either acute or chronic, and the infection is either gram-negative or gram-positive. The components will either be tightly fixed to bone, or one or more of the components will be loose. In acute infection with tightly fixed components, most surgeons will debride the joint without removing the components and treat the infection locally and with systemic antibiotic therapy. A chronically infected or loose prosthesis is usually treated with removal of the prosthesis, local wound care, and systemic antimicrobial therapy. Therapy for an acutely infected, firmly fixed prosthesis varies according to surgeon preference.

There is general concurrence that thorough debridement of the joint, synovectomy, removal of necrotic material, and copious irrigation are necessary at the time of debridement. Because of the potential presence of glycocalyx, surfaces of the prosthesis that are available for inspection are scrubbed with Dakin's solution, which will dissolve the glycocalyx. Removable components are removed, and the undersurfaces are cleaned with Dakin's solution. New polyethylene components are inserted if available; if this is not possible, the old polyethylene prosthesis is scrubbed with Dakin's solution and rein-

serted. To prevent superinfection, the wound must be tightly closed. To help eradicate the existing infection, however, irrigation and drainage must be continued. One suitable method is that described by Jergesen and Jawetz, in which small volumes of antibiotic solution are instilled into the joint twice a day, the joint is sealed off for 3 h, followed by 9 h of suction (Figure 7–10). This protocol begins 24 h after surgery, during which time suction drainage is maintained. The installation-suction system is maintained for 10 days. At the end of the course of irrigation and instillation, a culture is aspirated from the joint after one antibiotic instillation. This system can also be used for osteomyelitis and routine joint infections. Antibiotics are continued for an appropriate period of time (usually 6 weeks) after the tubes are withdrawn.

In cases of loose prostheses, little alternative is available except to remove the prosthesis. A similar system of instillation and suction is then used, using the same protocol. If reimplantation is likely after infected total knee prosthesis, an antibiotic cement block is used to separate the bone ends and maintain a potential joint space. An alternative to the cement block is the PROSTALAC system as described in Section D9 Infection—Complications—Total Hip Arthroplasty. This technique has the benefit of maintaining quadriceps length and elasticity. In patients in whom reimplantation is planned, the erythrocyte sedimentation rate is followed monthly until it is normal without antibiotic therapy. In patients with rheumatoid arthritis or other disorders where the rate may be elevated, 6 months is an appropriate time to wait for possible recrudescence of the infection. At this point, either an aspiration arthrogram or a Craig needle biopsy is used to obtain specimens for culture. If these are negative, reimplantation surgery is planned.

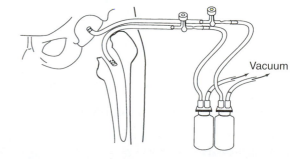

Figure 7–10. Schematic diagram of the Jergesen system of instillation of antibiotics. The antibiotics can be varied depending on the susceptibility of the infecting bacteria (fungus). The amount instilled is approximately 5 mL per tube plus the dead space from the valve to the joint.

Orthopedic Infections

8

Scott C. Wilson, MD

OVERVIEW

Introduction

Musculoskeletal infections are common; they can affect all parts of the musculoskeletal system; and they can be dangerous and even life threatening. Much has been learned in the last twenty years to effectively treat a wide range of musculoskeletal infections. Often a team including orthopedic surgeons, plastic surgeons, infectious disease specialists, as well as internists, nutritionists, and therapists must collaborate to orchestrate the multidisciplinary care that may be required to optimally treat these patients. This chapter will summarize the pathogenesis, diagnosis, and treatment of infections relevant to orthopedics. The management of osteomyelitis, septic arthritis, and soft tissue infections will be discussed and highlighted with clinical examples.

Because this subject is so important, other chapters in this book include discussions of special aspects of infection. Chapter 3 (Musculoskeletal Trauma Surgery), discusses appropriate management of open fractures, traumatic arthrotomies, and gun shot wounds to minimize the risk of infection. Chapter 5 (Disorders, Diseases, & Injuries of the Spine), describes the clinical identification and management of osteomyelitis of the spine, discitis, and epidural abscess. Chapter 7 (Adult Reconstructive Surgery), outlines the care of patients with prosthetic joint infections. Chapter 9 (Foot and Ankle Surgery), carefully details the management of diabetic foot ulcers and infections. Chapter 10 (Hand Surgery), discusses the treatment of paronychia, felons, chronic hand infections, human bites, and web space abscesses. Chapter 11 (Pediatric Orthopedic Surgery), reviews acute hematogenous osteomyelitis, septic arthritis especially of the hip joint, puncture wounds of the foot, skeletal tuberculosis, and spinal discitis.

Pathogenesis

A. GENERAL

All clinical infections must be thought of in terms of the attacking microbes and the host's defenses. Infections are more likely to occur if the organisms are more virulent and if the inoculum is larger. Bacteria can gain entry into the body from direct penetrating trauma, by hematogenous spread from adjacent or remote sites of infection, or during surgical exposures. This represents a wide spectrum of clinical possibilities ranging from fight bites to seeding from bacterial endocarditis to intraoperative breaks in sterile technique.

In acute osteomyelitis in children, the metaphysis is commonly involved. It is thought that the end vessels of the nutrient artery empty into much larger sinusoidal veins, causing a slow and turbulent flow of blood at this junction. These conditions predispose bacteria to migrate through adjacent gaps in the endothelium and adhere to the matrix. Also, low oxygen tension in this region may compromise phagocytic activity of white blood cells. Thrombosis due to infection results in a region of avascular necrosis that may lead to abscess formation. As pus accumulates and pressurizes, it can track through the cortex via the Haversian system and Volkmann's canals to collect beneath the periosteum. Subperiosteal abscesses may stimulate the formation of a periosteal involucrum. Once out of the cortex, pus can also track through soft tissues to the surface of the skin, forming a draining sinus.

The physis and joint capsule act as barriers to the flow of pus. However, secondary septic arthritis may occur if the infection begins in a region of bone within the confines of a joint capsule. This is why the hip joint is particularly susceptible to secondary infection arising from a spreading osteomyelitis of the femoral head or neck. Additionally, pus may track through the transphyseal vessels found in infants up to 6 months of age, causing secondary septic arthritis.

In hematogenous septic arthritis the synovial membrane lacks a basement membrane, facilitating the ingress of hematogenous bacteria into the joint space and resulting in an acute inflammatory reaction. The synovium becomes hyperemic and produces increased amounts of synovial fluid. Acute white blood cells infiltrate the joint space and the synovium hypertrophies. The cartilage may be eroded by the proteolytic enzymes released during phagocytosis. Cytokines and other inductive molecules produced by the leukocytes and synovial tissue recruit a further inflammatory response, which can eventually destroy all articular surfaces. Concurrent bone erosion usually begins in the periarticular folds of synovium at the junction of synovium and cartilage. Arthritis is the end result of articular bone and cartilage loss due to joint sepsis.

B. ORGANISMS

Although the musculoskeletal system may be infected by any infectious agent, the great majority of infections are bacterial. *Staphylococcus aureus, Streptococcus,* and *Haemophilus influenzae* are the most common causes of acute hematogenous osteomyelitis in children. The most common causes of septic arthritis are *Neisseria gonorrhoeae, Staphylococcus aureus,* and group A *Streptococcus.* Septic arthritis is less often caused by gram-negative organisms, including *Escherichia coli, Pseudomonas aeruginosa, Klebsiella, Enterobacter, Serratia, Proteus,* and *Salmonella.* Uncommon bacterial organisms include *Borrelia burgdorferi* (Lyme disease), *Mycobacterium tuberculosis, Brucella,* and the anaerobes *Clostridium* and *Bacteroides.* Unusual organisms that may preferentially infect immunocompromised patients include fungi (*Blastomyces, Cryptococcus, Histoplasma, Sporotrichum,* and *Coccidioidomycoses*), and atypical mycobacteria (*kansasii, avium-intracellulare, fortuitum, triviale,* and *scrofulaceum*). There is even some evidence to suggest that Paget's disease is the manifestation of a slow virus infection of bone.

Table 8–1 is a listing of common conditions associated with specific bacterial species.

Antibiotic resistance is conferred in these circumstances by spontaneous mutation, transduction of resistance genes via plasmids, and conjugation.

Table 8–1. Bacterial species associate with common conditions.

Organism	Common Occurrence
Staphylococcus aureus	Most common organism in osteomyelitis, acute hematogenous osteomyelitis (90%), and infected metal implants.
Group B strep	Infants < 1 year old
Hemophilus influenza	Children 1–16 years old
Pseudomonas aeruginosa	Nosocomial, puncture wound through shoe
Pasteurella multocida	Animal bite
Eikenella corrodens	Human bite
Salmonella	Sickle cell disease
Anaerobes	Diabetic ulcers, fight bites
Candida albicans	Immunocompromised
Aspergillus	" "
Atypical mycobacteria	" "
Escherichia coli	Neonatal
Neisseria gonorrhoeae	Septic arthritis in young adult

Ahmed S, Ayoub EM: Poststreptococcal reactive arthritis. Pediatr Infect Dis J 2001;20:1081. [PMID: 11734716]

Bezwada HP et al: Haemophilus influenza infection complicating a total knee arthroplasty. Clin Orthop 2002;402:202.

Brook I: Joint and bone infections due to anaerobic bacteria in children. Pediatr Rehabil 2002;5:11. [PMID: 12396847]

Dubost JJ et al: No changes in the distribution of organisms responsible for septic arthritis over a 20 year period. Ann Rheum Dis 2002;61:267. [PMID: 11830437]

Eiffert H et al: Characterization of Borrelia burgdorferi strains in Lyme arthritis. Scand J Infect Dis 1998;30:265. [PMID: 9790135]

Geyik MF et al: Musculoskeletal involvement of brucellosis in different age groups: A study of 195 cases. Swiss Med Wkly 2002;132:98. [PMID: 11971204]

Gonzalez TB et al: Acute bacterial arthritis caused by group C streptococci. Semin Arthritis Rheum 2001;31:43. [PMID: 11503138]

McLemore MM, Stapleton FB: Atypical septic arthritis due to Neisseria meningitides. J Tenn Med Assoc 1984;77:149.

Press J et al: Leukocyte count in the synovial fluid of children with culture-proven brucellar arthritis. Clin Rheumatol 2002;21:191. [PMID: 12111621]

Shirtliff ME, Mader JT: Acute septic arthritis. Clin Microbiol Rev 2002;15:527. [PMID: 12364368]

Tachi M et al: Pathophysiology and treatment of streptococcal toxic shock syndrome. Scan J Plast Reconstr Surg 2002;36:305. [PMID: 12477090]

Valesova H et al: Long-term results in patients with Lyme arthritis following treatment with ceftriaxone. Infection 1996;24:98. [PMID: 8852482]

C. HOST FACTORS

Any host with compromised immunity and wound healing, or with an implanted synthetic or allograft material has an increased risk for musculoskeletal infection.

Nonspecific factors include the skin as a mechanical barrier. Local host factors include the adequacy of the vascular supply and the presence of tissue injury. Systemic host factors that compromise immunocompetence include nutritional wasting; comorbid diseases such as diabetes mellitus, chronic renal and liver disease, cancer, AIDS, and autoimmune connective tissue diseases; and usage of immunosuppressing medications such as corticosteroids.

Patients with chronic renal and liver disease, diabetes, cancer, AIDS, autoimmune connective tissue disease, and nutritional wasting and those on immunosuppressive medications are particularly susceptible to infection.

Nutritional depletion with negative nitrogen balance, weight loss, and tissue-wasting can easily develop in patients with severe musculoskeletal injuries, as well as in patients who suffer from cancer, gastrointestinal malabsorption syndromes, and other chronic medical conditions. The signs of gross long-standing malnutrition, including profound weight loss, pitting edema, and intercostal wasting, are easily identified, but the signs of acute malnutrition are less apparent and often go undetected. A patient with a major fracture has a 20–25% increase in energy expenditure, and one with multiple trauma or infection has a 30–55% increase. Liver and skeletal muscle glycogen stores can be depleted within 12 h during severe stress. Even with adequate stores of fat, visceral and skeletal muscle protein may not be spared because fat is not a readily available energy source during severe stress.

Therefore, patients who are malnourished have significantly higher infection rates after surgery than patients who have normal nutritional status.

Methods to detect malnutrition include the following (Table 8–2).

D. Foreign Material

Recent experimental studies indicate that all biomaterials commonly used for total joint arthroplasty increase the incidence of *S aureus* infections. In contrast, biomaterials appear to have no effect on *E coli* and *S epidermidis* infections except when polymethylmethacrylate is used, in which case the incidence rises markedly.

Adherence of bacteria to the surface of implants is promoted by a polysaccharide biofilm called glycocalyx that acts as a barrier against host defense mechanisms and antibiotics. In addition, this film makes culture of organisms difficult, even with the use of special techniques.

Mixing antibiotics such as vancomycin and gentamicin to methacrylate cement can lower the risk of infection from cemented metal joint replacements, presumably by killing surface bacteria before they can produce glycocalyx.

Implantation of small amounts of allograft bone and connective tissue may slightly increase the risk of postoperative infection, but massive osteoarticular allografts can dramatically elevate the risk (> 10%).

Synthetic suture materials such as nylon and polyglycolic acid are less likely to facilitate wound infection than natural suture materials such as silk and cotton. In this regard monofilaments are superior to braided sutures in preventing infection; and resorbable materials are superior to nonresorbable materials. Therefore synthetic resorbable monofilaments are preferred in wounds that are potentially susceptible to infection.

Prophylaxis

A. General

Transmission of bacterial and viral infections can easily occur in the clinic and hospital setting because health care workers are often in direct contact with patients. The risk of transmission can be reduced by using universal precautions that include hand washing before and after all patient or body fluid contact; and wearing gloves, masks, eye protection, and gowns when in contact with patients with known infections. Proper disposal of patients' waste, dressing materials, and surgical drains should be mandatory. Blades and needles (which should not be recapped) must be disposed of in a dedicated "sharps box." Inpatients with easily transmitted infections or infections caused by bacteria resistant to certain antibiotics should be isolated in private rooms, and movement of these patients should be limited to reduce possible contact with other patients or health care workers.

B. Antibiotics

The administration of prophylactic antibiotics immediately before surgery and intraoperatively for cases lasting longer than 3–4 h has become a uniformly accepted standard of practice. Generally a first-generation cephalosporin is used. Vancomycin, clindamycin, or ciprofloxacin are useful alternatives if the patient has a cephalosporin allergy or an anaphylactic response to penicillin that indicates a potential cross-reactivity. However, the administration of preoperative antibiotics should be withheld when intraoperative bacterial cultures are to be obtained because they will inhibit the in vitro growth of the cultured bacteria and reduce the ability to identify the causative organism(s).

C. Operating Room Sterility

Sterile technique in the operating room is extremely important. The operative site is thoroughly prepped with a variety of topical antiseptics including isopropyl alcohol, chlorhexidine soaps, and iodine-based scrubs and paints. Sterile drapes effectively isolate the operative site from the rest of the patient, and sterile gowns and gloves isolate the surgeons and assistants from the patient. Surgeons may use double gloves, space suits, adherent plastic drapes, pulsatile lavage, and laminar flow operating rooms with ultraviolet lights as additional techniques that may lower the risk of intraopera-

Table 8–2. Tests to measure nutritional depletion.

Serology	
Albumin	< 3.5 g/dL
Prealbumin	< 10 mg/dL
Total lymphocyte count	< 1500/μL
Transferrin	< 150 mg/dL
Other	
Anergy panel	Nonreactive
Weight loss	> 4.5 kg
Arm circumference	< 80% standard

tive contamination, which is approximately 1% for clean, elective orthopedic cases. Breaks in sterile technique should be dealt with immediately and aggressively even if the operative site has to be reprepped and redraped and the surgeons have to regown and reglove.

D. EXPOSURE TO BLOOD-BORNE PATHOGENS

Health care workers may be accidentally exposed to infection when poked by a needle or sharp wire, cut by a knife or a sharp bone fracture edge, or splashed in the eye. The primary concern is the possible transmission of hepatitis B virus (HBV), hepatitis C virus (HCV), and human immunodeficiency virus (HIV). The estimated risk of acquiring an infection by accidental blood transmission is 6–30% for HBV, 1.8% for HCV, and 0.3% for HIV. Logically, larger inoculations confer an increased risk of infection. If exposure with a potentially infected source occurs, the worker must wash the contact area with disinfectant and immediately report to the occupational health center to document the exposure. The viral status is determined in the exposed worker and the source patient by obtaining serologic tests for HBV, HCV, and HIV. HIV testing requires the source's informed written consent. (Rapid plasma reagent (RPR) for syphilis should also be checked.)

The threat of health care workers acquiring hepatitis B has been dramatically reduced in recent years because many health care institutions now require that their employees be immunized against HBV. Immunization status is confirmed if the concentration of hepatitis B serum antibody (anti-HBV) is ≥ 10 mIU/mL. However, if the worker is unvaccinated or a nonresponder to

the vaccine and the source is known to be positive for hepatitis B, the worker should receive hepatitis B immunoglobulin (HBIG) and a series of hepatitis B vaccinations.

Currently there is no vaccination against HCV and there is no recommended prophylactic therapy for workers exposed to HCV. However, new drugs are being developed to treat active HCV infections and effective prophylaxis may soon be developed. If the source is known to have HIV, the worker should immediately begin a 28-day course of double or triple antiretroviral therapy.

Workers with any viral exposures should be subsequently monitored with serologic tests for HIV, HBV, and HCV at 6 weeks, 3 months, 6 months, and 1 year after exposure. These guidelines are frequently updated, and specific treatment recommendations should be discussed with the institution's occupational health specialist (Table 8–3).

Diagnosis

A. RADIOLOGIC WORK-UP

1. Plain films—Plain radiographs are useful in establishing a diagnosis of osteomyelitis or chronic septic arthritis. Initially plain radiographs do not show any bony changes in early osteomyelitis. After 7–10 days an area of osteopenia may appear, heralding cancellous bone destruction. As the infection progresses, a periosteal reaction may be seen, and focal areas of cancellous and cortical bone destruction may become apparent. Chronic osteomyelitis is identified by more

Table 8–3. Testing and treatment of exposed persons, assuming source tests positive and exposed person tests negative.

Virus	Seroconversion (percutaneous exposure)[a]	Serologic Test of Exposed Person	Prophylaxis	Efficacy of Rx
Hepatitis B	6–30%	Virus antibody-positive	None, immunity intact	
		Virus antibody-negative	Hepatitis B immunoglobulin Hepatitis B vaccination series	90%
Hepatitis C	1.8% (0–7%)		None[b]	
HIV	0.3%[c]		Antiretroviral drugs for 4 weeks Two- or three-drug regimen[d]	81%

[a]Larger inoculations from increased exposure confer higher risk of seroconversion.
[b]Patient may benefit from early treatment if symptoms develop.
[c]0.09% risk of seroconversion from mucosal exposure.
[d]Three drugs recommended if large exposure or source has AIDS.

Adapted, with permission, from: Updated U.S. Public Health Service guidelines for the management of occupational exposures to HBV, HCV and HIV and recommendations for postexposure prophylaxis. MMWR 50(RR11):1–42, 2001. And from Guidelines for using retroviral agents among HIV infected adults and adolescents. Recommendations of the Panel on Clinical Practices for Treatment of HIV. MMWR 51(RR–7):1, 2002.

extensive bone destruction and the appearance of a re-active rim of bone called the involucrum, which en-velops a sclerotic focus of necrotic bone called the sequestrum. The sequestrum is often radiodense com-pared with the adjacent involucrum.

Plain radiographs are usually normal in early septic arthritis. Only later in the disease will radiographs show cartilage loss and periarticular bone erosion. These radi-ographic features are not specific for infection and may be present in other arthropathies such as rheumatoid arthritis (RA) and pigmented villonodular synovitis.

Soft-tissue infections are virtually invisible on plain radiographs except for an occasional suggestion of soft-tissue swelling. The striking exception is encountered with air-producing infections causing "gas gangrene." Air in the soft tissues is quite clearly identifiable on plain radiographs as discrete radiolucent areas, analo-gous to bowel gas in a plain radiograph of the ab-domen. Figure 8–1 is a radiograph of air in the calf of a patient with a life-threatening clostridial infection.

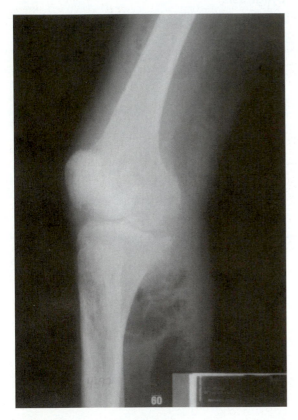

Figure 8–1. Plain radiograph of the knee, showing air in the soft tissues of the calf and thigh arising from a necrotizing clostridial infection.

2. Ultrasound—Ultrasound is useful at identifying a joint effusion and is particularly beneficial in the evalu-ation of pediatric patients with suspected infections of the hip joint. Ultrasound may also aid in the identifica-tion and aspiration of soft-tissue abscesses.

3. Radionuclide imaging—Radionuclide imaging is not routinely necessary to diagnose acute osteomyelitis and is often falsely negative in acute septic arthritis. This imaging modality is very sensitive but nonspecific in identifying bone disease. Commonly, infection cannot be distinguished from neoplasm, infarction, trauma, gout, stress fracture, postsurgical changes, adja-cent soft-tissue infection, neurotrophic joints (Charcot joint), or arthritis. However, in equivocal cases ra-dionuclide imaging may help to identify an infectious process before an invasive procedure is performed.

The most common imaging agents are technetium-99m and indium-111. Technetium-99m is adminis-tered intravenously. An early-phase scan is performed in 10–15 min. At this time most of the radioisotope is in equilibrium with the extracellular compartment and accumulates in areas of increased blood flow, such as areas associated with cellulitis. The late-phase scan is performed in 3 h, and the radioisotope is localized to the skeleton in both the organic matrix and the mineral phase of the bone.

Imaging with indium-111 requires collection of 80–90 mL of venous blood, separation of the leuko-cytes in the sample, and labeling the leukocytes with in-dium-111 in vitro. The indium-labeled leukocytes are then returned to the patient's bloodstream intra-venously, and scanning is done 18–24 h later.

Imaging with technetium99m methylene diphos-phonate is a highly sensitive technique and is useful in cases of suspected acute hematogenous osteomyelitis. In an extensive study of 280 children, the sensitivity of technetium-99m imaging in accurately detecting acute osteomyelitis was 89%, the specificity was 94%, and the overall accuracy was 92%. All soft-tissue infec-tions were correctly identified by this technique, and 37 studies were positive for septic arthritis, although 8 were falsely positive.

Although radionuclide imaging can be sensitive for chronic musculoskeletal infections, it is often nonspe-cific, and false-positive results may hinder diagnosis. Radionuclide imaging often cannot distinguish a chronic infection from aseptic loosening in patients with painful prosthetic joint replacements, and it is rarely necessary in establishing a diagnosis of septic arthritis.

4. Computed tomography—Computed tomography (CT) with sagittal and coronal reformatting is particu-larly useful in identifying sequestra in cases of chronic osteomyelitis. Routinely discrete sequestra are isolated from the viable bone and are more radiodense than the surrounding involucrum. Also, sagittal and coronal reformatting can be very useful in further assessing the mechanical integrity of the bone and in determining the extent of fracture healing even in the presence of metal fixation hardware.

CT will show expansion of a joint capsule and any evidence of bony destruction but is not specific for septic arthritis.

5. Magnetic resonance imaging—Magnetic resonance imaging (MRI) with T_2 and inversion recovery sequencing offers unparalleled visualization of bone marrow and soft-tissue inflammation associated with infection. Intravenous gadolinium concentrates in areas of increased vascularity and enhances regions of inflammation. Fluid collections are identified as dark signal voids where the gadolinium cannot penetrate due to the absence of vascular ingress. Thus, contrast MRI facilitates the identification of fluid collections within bones, joint spaces, and soft tissues that may represent abscesses and septic effusions.

Acute inflammation in bone and soft tissues is nonspecific. Acute inflammatory arthropathies may reveal synovial and adjacent soft-tissue inflammation, effusion, and periarticular bone inflammation especially at the synovial-cartilage junction. These findings may be identical with acute septic arthritis, gout, or other inflammatory arthropathies including neuropathic Charcot joints. Pigmented villonodular synovitis may have many of the same features although it can often be distinguished by areas of decreased signal uptake on T_2 images that represent areas of hemosiderin deposition.

As infection progresses in a joint, eroded cartilage and subchondral bone can be seen along with hypertrophic synovium and pronounced effusion. Periarticular erosion usually precedes erosion along weight-bearing surfaces. These changes are accompanied by generalized inflammation in the adjacent bone marrow and soft tissues, including bursas and tendon sheaths. Formation of abscesses, synovial cysts, and sinus tracts are particularly well visualized.

Keat A: Reactive arthritis or post-infective arthritis? Best Pract Res Clin Rheumatol 2002;16:507. [PMID: 12406424]

Roddy E, Jones AC: Reactive Arthritis associated with genital tract Group A streptococcal infection. J Infec 2002;45:208. [PMID: 12387782]

Sigal LH: Update on reactive arthritis. Bull Rheum Dis 2001;50:1. [PMID: 12386943]

B. IDENTIFICATION OF PATHOGENS

Whenever possible, antibiotic therapy must be delayed until deep cultures of the infection site are obtained. It is imperative to take appropriate cultures prior to antibiotic administration because antibiotics can often inhibit bacterial growth in vitro. If the cultures fail to grow, the clinician must choose antibiotics empirically. However well-informed the clinician may be, the selection of empiric antibiotics is a matter of guesswork, and treatment failure is more likely.

Deep cultures must be obtained percutaneously or intraoperatively using strict sterile technique. The overlying skin must be prepped with antiseptic to decrease the concentration of skin flora that might contaminate the culture sample. In addition to swabs of purulent fluid, bone and soft-tissue samples of the infected site should also be obtained. Additional tissue should be sent for histologic analysis because an acute suppurative infection can be distinguished from a chronic granulomatous infection, and an infection can be distinguished from an unsuspected neoplasm.

Superficial swabs of skin ulcers and draining sinus tracts usually identify colonizing bacteria rather than the pathogenic bacteria that must be eradicated. Therefore, avoid the practice of obtaining superficial cultures of deep-seated infections. Also, it is important to employ appropriate techniques for anaerobic cultures because these organisms can be difficult to isolate and may be responsible for a considerable amount of osteomyelitis. This is particularly true for diabetic patients with infected foot ulcers who have a high risk for mixed aerobic/anaerobic infections.

A Gram stain of the culture samples is not diagnostic by itself but may help to identify the organism. Therefore, the preliminary information gained from a Gram stain should be used to confirm clinical suspicions such as a staphylococcal osteomyelitis (positive cocci in clusters) or a gonococcal septic arthritis (gram-negative cocci in pairs). Blood cultures should also be obtained in patients who present with acute symptoms of bacteremia, such as fever, chills, and sweats.

Joint aspiration is usually necessary to identify the organisms responsible for septic arthritis, although blood cultures may also be helpful in acute cases. The synovial fluid from an infected joint is opaque, light yellow or light gray, and nonviscous. Cell analysis often reveals a WBC count of > 100,000 and > 90% PMNs (Table 8–4). Iatrogenic contamination of a sterile joint space may occur if the arthrocentesis needle passes through an overlying soft-tissue infection. Therefore, erythematous skin or indurated soft tissue should be avoided when choosing a site for arthrocentesis.

C. HISTOLOGY

Pathologic examination of a tissue sample can help to determine the presence of an infection, to histologically characterize the type and time frame of the infection, to

Table 8–4. Analysis of synovial fluid.

Analysis	Normal Results	Noninflammatory Effusion	Inflammatory Effusion	Septic Effusion
Gross Exam				
Volume	1–4 mL	Increased	Increased	Increased
Clarity	Transparent	Transparent	Transparent	Opaque
Color	Clear/pale yellow	Yellow	Yellow/white	Yellow/white/gray
Viscosity	High	High	Low	Low
Mucin clotting	Good	Good/fair	Fair/poor	Poor
Microscopic Exam				
Leukocytes	< 300	< 2000	2000–80,000	> 80,000
Neutrophils	< 25%	< 25%	25–75%	> 75%
Bacterial smear	Negative	Negative	Negative	Positive
Serum				
Glucose ratio	0.8–1.0	0.8–1.0	0.5–0.8	< 0.5
Protein g/dL	< 3	< 3	≤ 8	≤ 8
Culture	Negative	Negative	Negative	Positive

Normal synovial fluid is clear and viscous. Inflammation causes synovial fluid to become more cloudy as the concentration of white cells increases. Traditionally, newsprint can be read through a vial of noninfectious transudate but not through a vial of infectious exudate. The synovial fluid/serum glucose ratio will decrease and the synovial protein concentration will increase. Besides a positive bacterial smear the most helpful indicators of infection are a white blood cell count greater than 50,000 and a percentage of polymorphonuclear leukocytes exceeding 75%. Many acute bacterial infections will generate a white cell count of greater than 100,000 and > 90% PMNs.

identify the causative organism, and occasionally to distinguish an infection from an unsuspected neoplasm.

During revision arthroplasty, samples of periprosthetic tissue may be submitted for frozen section analysis. If less than 5 polymorphonuclear leukocytes occur per high-powered field, there is a low probability of residual infection. Extensive debridement and prosthetic removal should be considered rather than reimplantation of revision components if there are greater than 10 polymorphonuclear leukocytes per high-powered field.

Histologic study can distinguish between acute inflammatory responses characterized by the presence of polymorphonuclear leukocytes and chronic inflammatory responses characterized by plasma cells and lymphocytes. Granulomatous responses with central caseation help to establish the diagnosis of *Mycobacterium tuberculosis.* Noncaseating granulomas can occur with fungal and atypical mycobacterial infections.

Occasionally the inciting organisms can be identified as well. For example budding yeast forms of Blastomyces can be visualized with special stains or by using immunohistochemical markers.

This is particularly important because mycobacterial and fungal organisms are slow growing in vitro, and they may take 3–6 weeks to identify in culture.

Also, histologic analysis can distinguish an infection from an unsuspected tumor such as squamous cell carcinoma arising within a chronic infection or a tumor that radiographically may mimic an infection such as eosinophilic granuloma, Ewing's sarcoma, and lymphoma of bone.

Cucurull E and Espinoza LR: Gonococcal arthritis. Rheum Dis Clin North Am 1998;24:305. [PMID: 9606761]

Lu TS et al: Concurrent acute gouty and gonococcal arthritis. Lancet Infect Dis 2002;2:313. [PMID: 12062998]

Treatment

A. ANTIBIOTICS

1. Selection and use—Whenever possible antibiotics should be chosen based on the antibiotic sensitivities of the specific organisms that have been cultured from the infection site. Consultation with infectious disease experts is prudent for unusual or resistant organisms or if a lengthy course of therapy is anticipated. Because patterns of bacterial resistance to antibiotics vary from region to region, these experts work closely with local clinical laboratories to establish locally specific bacterial sensitivity profiles. Also infectious disease experts are often more closely attuned to the latest clinical research regarding antibiotic treatment of musculoskeletal infections (information that is not usually encountered in the primary orthopedic literature), and the continually changing patterns of bacterial resistance. For example *Staphylococcus epidermidis* is becoming increasingly resistant to methicillin, and certain strains of enterococci and *S aureus* are resistant to vancomycin. Resistance to second- and third-generation cephalosporins is emerging in some gram-negative bacilli, and penicillin resistance is increasing in *Bacteroides* and *Clostridium* species. Even if an organism is sensitive to a given antibiotic, addition of a second antibiotic may be necessary to lessen the risk of treatment failure due to the development of antibiotic resistance.

Antibiotic therapy is usually continued for 6 weeks for patients with septic arthritis or osteomyelitis. In acute pediatric infections caused by sensitive organisms, a shorter course of therapy may be sufficient. In patients with multiple medical problems, retained orthopedic hardware, or persistent open wounds, a longer course of therapy may be required.

Erythrocyte sedimentation rates (ESR) and C-reactive protein (CRP) levels should be serially checked weekly or semiweekly to monitor the success of treatment. A patient with persistently elevated ESR and CRP levels toward the end of planned antibiotic treatment may have an incompletely treated infection. Persistence of the infection may be due to the retention of orthopedic hardware, the incomplete debridement of necrotic tissue, the immunocompromised status of the host, or the development of antibiotic resistance by the causative bacteria. Ideally, surgical reexploration should be performed on these patients and tissue samples should be recultured after the patient is off antibiotics to determine if additional treatment is required.

Occasionally, antibiotics must be given for palliation rather than cure. Chronic suppressive antibiotic therapy may be appropriate in selected patients with severe immunocompromise, those who are not surgical candidates, or those with stable joint prostheses infected by sensitive organisms. Close monitoring of these patients is necessary to detect possible antibiotic resistance.

For example, an 80-year-old female with a history of a revision total hip arthroplasty 10 years previously underwent a girdlestone arthroplasty 5 years ago to treat septic loosening of the prosthesis. All components were removed, the bones debrided, and antibiotic beads were placed in the acetabulum (Figure 8–2). During this time a severe hematologic bleeding disorder was diagnosed that prohibited further surgery. Her lateral hip incision incompletely healed, and she developed a mature deep sinus that tracked down to the cut end of the femur. The antibiotic beads could not be retrieved through this opening. She also developed a new sinus tract in her medial thigh. These wounds were treated with daily absorptive alginate dressings and occasionally she had debridement of the sinus tracts in clinic to prevent them from closing. When the sinus tracts closed the undrained pus rapidly created a pressurized abscess that resulted in a prompt increase in local inflammation, bacteremia, and acute febrile illness. Her infection was suppressed using culture-specific oral antibiotics for staphylococcal and enterococcal bacteria. Over the past 5 years she has lived with her infection and has controlled her pain with oral narcotics. She is able to stand to transfer and walk short distances with a walker.

2. Intravenous route of administration—Use of a peripheral intravenous central catheter (PICC) line is now the standard intravenous (IV) access for extended antibiotic therapy. PICC lines can be inserted by qualified nursing personnel in an outpatient setting, and the

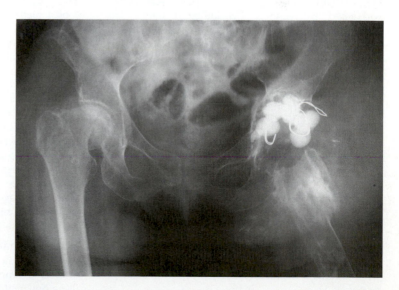

Figure 8–2. AP pelvic radiograph depicting the Girdlestone arthroplasty and retained antibiotic beads in the left hip area, and a painless malunion of a subcapital fracture of the right hip.

placement of the line can be confirmed by a chest radiograph. Specialized personnel in the radiology department can also place PICC lines using ultrasound to identify suitable veins and fluoroscopy to ensure appropriate catheter placement with the tip of the catheter in the superior vena cava. A subclavian central line such as a Hickman catheter is used as a backup if peripheral access cannot be established. These catheters are generally placed in an operating room setting with the patient heavily sedated or under general anesthesia.

Most home health agencies are expert in managing PICC lines and administering antibiotics to patients in a home setting. Portable, computerized IV pumps with replaceable drug cartridges are often used to automate the delivery of antibiotics throughout a 24-hour period.

3. Methicillin-resistant *Staphylococcus aureus*— Methicillin-resistant *Staphylococcus aureus* (MRSA) is the most common resistant bacteria encountered in orthopedic practice. A 6-week course of vancomycin (1 g IV every 12 h) is the current standard treatment for MRSA. However, this drug has relatively poor bone penetration, and it requires close monitoring because, rarely, it can be the cause of nephrotoxicity and ototoxicity. Establishing therapeutic drug levels by adjusting the dose and interval of treatment should be performed based on drug peak and trough levels. Generally, if the peak level is too high, the dose has to be lowered; and if the trough is too high, the interval between doses has to be lengthened. Dosing has to be adjusted in patients with renal insufficiency based on creatinine clearance and one daily dose or one dose every other day is not uncommon in this setting. Toxicity is more likely to occur if the trough level remains above the acceptable range. Many infectious disease experts treat MRSA with a two-drug regimen, often adding rifampin to vancomycin. Newer antibiotics such as linezolid (Zyvox) are now being introduced for MRSA.

B. SURGERY

1. Septic arthritis—Complete surgical evacuation of a purulent effusion offers the best protection against cartilage destruction in patients with acute infectious pyarthrosis. The greatest risk of cartilage damage comes from proteolytic enzymes produced by the recruited polymorphonuclear leukocytes rather than from direct action of the bacteria. Although serial needle aspirations may accomplish this goal in the acute setting, surgical drainage, irrigation, and drain tube placement are more efficient and better tolerated by the patient. Whenever technically possible arthroscopy is preferred, especially when dealing with septic arthritis of the knee joint. Limited open arthrotomy may also be used because the synovium need not be extensively debrided in acute infections.

In chronic septic arthritis a pannus of hypertrophic synovium forms that must be surgically debrided to ensure successful treatment. Debridement debulks the bacterial load and decreases the production of inflammatory agents that destroy cartilage.

2. Osteomyelitis—Successful treatment of bone and soft-tissue infections requires the surgical removal of all nonviable tissue and foreign debris. Necrotic tissue shelters bacteria from access by white blood cells and from therapeutic concentrations of antibiotics. In acute open fractures all devitalized soft tissue and all free bony fragments that are completely denuded of periosteum must be removed from the wound. Although buckshot and isolated bullets do not need to be removed from gun-shot victims, thorough exploration of the bullet wounds is necessary to remove any embedded bullet wadding and clothing fragments. In chronic osteomyelitis the sequestrum must be completely removed although the involucrum should be left in place. Involucrum is viable reactive tissue that has a generous vascular supply and contributes to the mechanical stability of the bone.

Skin, subcutaneous fat, and muscle should be sharply debrided until they bleed freely. The appearance of viable cancellous bone is easily discerned by the presence of bleeding trabecular surfaces. It is more difficult to tell the viability of cortical bone because of its normally sparse vascularity. Biologic dyes such as fluorescein and isosulfan blue and flow Doppler examination have been used intraoperatively to estimate the vascularity of cortical bone. However, visual inspection for punctate bleeding remains the simplest and most popular method of determining the viability of cortical bone. The "paprika sign" should be apparent after water-cooled high-speed burring of all exposed cortical surfaces to ensure that all dead bone tissue has been removed (Figure 8–3).

Occasionally infections are so severe or are located in such unforgiving anatomic locations that amputation is the best method of surgically curing the infection. For example a 60-year-old male with insulin-dependent diabetes and extensive peripheral vascular disease, developed a rapidly worsening heel infection that exposed his calcaneus (Figure 8–4). During physical examination a Q-tip could easily probe exposed cancellous bone of the calcaneus and subtalar joint. A subtotal calcanectomy with free flap coverage after peripheral arterial bypass would have been necessary for any chance of infection control and limb salvage. The patient elected to proceed with a recommended below-knee amputation.

3. Implantable antibiotics—An excellent method to supplement the IV administration of systemic antibiotics is to implant local antibiotics into the wound using polymethylmethacrylate bone cement as a carrier.

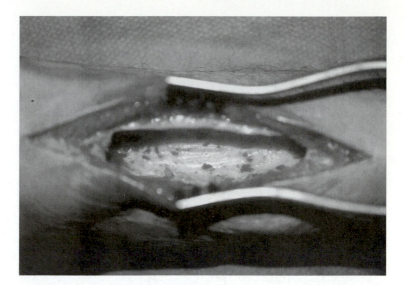

Figure 8–3. Intraoperative photograph of the "paprika sign," representing punctate bleeding from the endosteal surface of a tibia that has just undergone aggressive debridement with a high-speed burr.

Antibiotic "spacers" and "beads" have the added advantage of provisionally filling dead spaces so that bacteria-rich fluids do not accumulate and thwart the host's defenses. Intraoperatively, methacrylate powder is thoroughly mixed with powdered antibiotics and then made into a dough by adding the liquid methacrylate monomer. The antibiotic dough can be fashioned into a string of beads using gauge-5 wire or No. 5 nonabsorbable suture (Figure 8–5). Antibiotic-laden cement spacers can be molded into a disk shape like a hockey puck for the knee joint after removal of a total knee prosthesis. Also cement spacers can be molded into the shape of a femoral head and secured to the femur using a rush rod that has been placed in the femur. Palacos cement has been shown to have superior antibiotic elution characteristics when compared with other bone cements. Vancomycin and tobramycin are commonly used in combination to treat presumed staphylococcal infections. A standard recipe in a patient without renal insufficiency is to mix one full bag of Palacos with 2 g of vancomycin and 3.6 g of tobramycin. Scoring the surface of a spacer and using numerous small beads rather than a few large beads increases the overall surface area of the antibiotic cement implant, enhances the elution of the antibiotics, and results in higher local concentrations of antibiotics. Initially the local serum

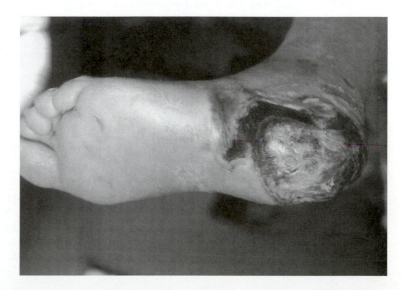

Figure 8–4. Calcaneus ulcer with exposed bone and blackened eschar.

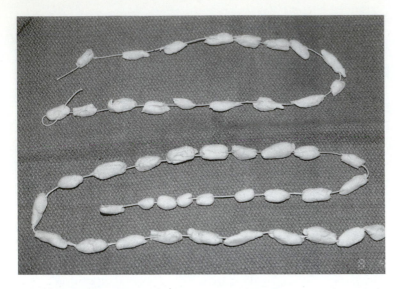

Figure 8–5. Two strings of antibiotic beads have been molded onto a No. 5 braided nonabsorbable suture with the knotted ends incorporated into the outermost beads.

concentrations may be as much as a hundred times the minimal inhibitory concentration for *Staphylococcus.* After 3 weeks the antibiotic concentrations drop below the minimal inhibitory concentration. Although spacers and beads have been left in place indefinitely, it is a good practice to remove them after the infection has been treated to ensure that the cement does not act as a foreign body and precipitate a new infection.

4. Soft-tissue and bone reconstruction—Assuming musculoskeletal infections have been comprehensively treated with antibiotics and debridement, bone reconstruction can proceed in a standard fashion. Total joints can be reimplanted, and structural bone defects can be filled with bone graft. Intercalary long bone defects can be spanned with bone transport techniques, vascularized structural bone autotransplants supported by external fixators, or even structural allografts secured with intramedullary rods.

Expeditious soft-tissue coverage is the first reconstructive priority in the contemporary management of acute open fractures. Rotation, pedicled, or free flaps are used to accomplish wound closure. Early flap reconstruction also ensures a good vascular supply to the injured area that promotes bone healing and resistance to local infection. If definitive bone fixation must be delayed until after complete debridement and soft-tissue coverage has been accomplished, provisional stabilization of the bone can be achieved with orthotics, skeletal traction, or external fixation.

Occasionally an acute infection develops after orthopedic fixation of a fracture. Assuming good soft-tissue coverage of the fracture area, the patient is treated with antibiotics, and the implanted hardware is left in place

until the fracture heals. Once biologic union of the fracture has been achieved, surgical debridement of the wound and removal of the fixation hardware can be performed without having to be concerned about a mechanically unstable bone.

Historically the Papineau technique was used for the reconstruction of bony defects caused by infected nonunions. Debridement of dead bone and "saucerization" of the soft tissues was followed by placing cancellous bone graft into the open wound. Through a process of soft-tissue granulation and replacement of the bone graft by adjacent healthy bone, the defect could close by secondary intention and yield a structurally sound union of the bone. However, the process requires vigilant daily wound care and infection control, takes as long as bone transport for segmental defects and is not always successful. The techniques of bone and soft-tissue reconstruction mentioned earlier have largely replaced this technique in developed countries.

C. ADJUNCTIVE THERAPIES

1. Local wound care—Newer alginate dressing materials are more absorbant and may be left in place for 24 h. Saline wet-to-dry dressings are used for initial mechanical debridement of wounds that contain necrotic material and must be changed every 6 h. Antiseptic solutions such as hydrogen peroxide, povidone-iodine, isopropyl alcohol, and sodium hypochlorite (Dakin's solution, 5% NaClO) are now used only for the first few days until the bacterial load is reduced and necrotic tissue has been debrided. Extended use of these caustic agents inhibits fibrogenesis. Instead, petroleum gel or topical antibiotic cream are placed on the wounds to keep the tissues from desiccating and to promote fibroblast growth.

Treatment of open wounds has been transformed using a new method that employs a sealed sponge dressing to which a negative pressure is applied using a portable pump (Figure 8–6). An open-cell sponge is cut to fit the shape of the wound and is secured by an airtight plastic dressing (see Figure 8–12d and e). The sponge is connected to a vacuum pump by way of a plastic tube. When the pump is activated a partial vacuum is generated within the wound. The porous sponge partially collapses, causing contraction of the walls of the wound. All drainage fluids are sucked out through the sponge and tubing and are collected in a container located in the pump unit. The wound is kept quite clean, and the dressing is changed every 2–3 days. The units are portable and can be serviced by visiting nurses in an outpatient setting.

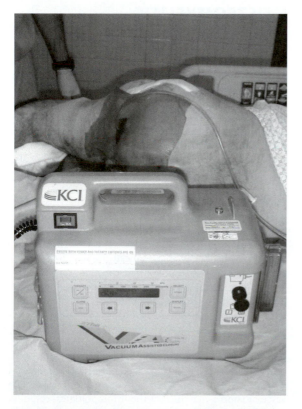

Figure 8–6. Portable wound suction pump (AKA wound *vacuum-assisted closure* device, or VAC). Note the tubing that runs from the pump to a black sponge placed in a patient's ischial decubitus.

2. Hyperbaric oxygen—Hyperbaric oxygen (HBO) therapy is used to treat a variety of orthopedic disorders. Specialized diving chambers have been developed for medical purposes to expose patients to 100% oxygen at 2 or more atmospheres of pressure. During an HBO treatment superphysiologic concentrations of oxygen from the lungs are dissolved into the serum. These high serum oxygen levels have been shown to stimulate neoangiogenesis, to sustain hypoxic tissues, to support the activity of phagocytic white blood cells, and inhibit infections caused by anaerobic bacteria. It does not cause oxygen to be absorbed from the skin or wound surface, and it does not revitalize tissue that has already become necrotic. Therefore, an adequate vascular inflow to the wound is necessary for HBO to work. When appropriately indicated, HBO can be a useful adjunct to good medical and surgical wound management.

Acute problems that can be helped by HBO include severe crush injury, compromised muscle flaps, and necrotizing fasciitis. Each of these conditions is characterized by soft tissues that have become acutely hypoxic and are at risk for infection. "Acute" HBO protocols usually require higher pressures (2.4–3 atm) and more frequent sessions (two to three times a day) for several days. To be effective an acute HBO treatment protocol must be started as soon as possible after the injury, because a 48-h delay in initiating HBO can render it ineffective.

Chronic wounds that can be helped by HBO are primarily related to chronic ischemic ulcers that are not due to peripheral vascular disease, venous stasis disease, or pressure necrosis. Diabetic foot ulcers in particular may benefit from "chronic" HBO protocols: 2 atm for 90 min daily for 20+ days. The older literature includes uncontrolled studies that expound the utility of treating chronic osteomyelitis with HBO. However, newer reconstruction techniques that have been devised, including free flaps for soft-tissue coverage and bone transport for bone defect restoration, have empowered the surgeon to perform more comprehensive debridement and more aggressive wound closure. Better surgical management has been found to result in better cure rates for chronic osteomyelitis.

3. Nutritional support—Patients with severe infections and large wounds have increased nutritional and caloric needs. Nutritional depletion can be measured using the following tests: albumin, prealbumin, total protein, total lymphocyte count, and anergy panel (see Table 8–3). Dietary supplementation to restore normal healing in a compromised host may be accomplished using enteral tube feedings or parenteral infusions.

Azad N et al: Nutrition survey in an elderly population following admission to a tertiary care hospital. CMAJ 1999;161:511. [PMID: 10497606]

Centers for Disease Control and Prevention: Vancomycin resistant Staphylococcus aureus-Pennsylvania, 2002. JAMA 2002;288:2116.

Connolly LP et al: Acute hematogenous osteomyelitis of children: assessment of skeletal scintigraphy-based diagnosis in the era of MRI. J Nucl Med 2002;43:1310. [PMID: 12368368]

Gristina AG et al: The glycocalyx, biofilm, microbes, and resistant infection. Semin Arthroplasty 1994;5:160. [PMID: 10155159]

Hall BB et al: Anaerobic osteomyelitis. J Bone Joint Surg (Am) 1983;65:30.

Hiramatsu K: Vancomycin-resistant Staphylococcus aureus: A new model of antibiotic resistance. Lancet Infect Dis 2001;1:147. [PMID: 11871491]

Jacobson JA: Musculoskeletal sonography and MR imaging. A role for both imaging methods. Radiol Clin North Am 1999;37:713. [PMID: 10442077]

Jenson JE et al: Nutrition in orthopaedic surgery. J Bone Joint Surg (Am) 1982;64:1263.

Jones S et al: Cephalosporins for prophylaxis. J Bone Joint Surg (Am) 1985;67:921.

Kartsonis N et al: Efficacy of caspofungin in the treatment of esophageal candidiasis resistant to fluconazole. J Acquir Immune Defic Syndr 2002;31:183. [PMID: 12394797]

Ledermann HP et al: Pedal abscesses in patients suspected of having pedal osteomyelitis: analysis with MR imaging. Radiology 2002;224:649. [PMID: 12202694]

Mader JT, Wilson KJ: Comparative evaluation of cefamandole and cephalothin in the treatment of experimental Staphylococcus aureus osteomyelitis in rabbits. J Bone Joint Surg (Am) 1983;65:507.

Mazza A: Ceftriaxone as short-term antibiotic prophylaxis in orthopedic surgery: a cost-benefit analysis involving 808 patients. J Chemother 2000;12 Suppl 3:29. [PMID: 11432680]

Neut D et al: Biomaterial-associated infection of gentamicin-loaded PMMA beads in orthopaedic revision surgery. J Antimicrob Chemother 2001;47:885.

Perea S, Patterson TF: Antifungal resistance in pathogenic fungi. Clin Infect Dis 2002;35:1073. [PMID: 12384841]

Petty W et al: The influence of skeletal implants on the incidence of infection: Experiments in a canine model. J Bone Joint Surg Am 1985;67:1236.

Schmidt AH, Swiontkowski MF: Pathophysiology of infections after internal fixation of fractures. J Am Acad Orthop Surg 2000;8:285. [PMID: 11029556]

Shirtliff ME, Mader JT: Acute septic arthritis. Clin Microbiol Rev 2002;15:527. [PMID: 12364368]

Sonne-Holm S et al: Prophylactic antibiotics in amputation of the lower extremity for ischemia. J Bone Joint Surg Am 1985;67:80.

Stewart PS, Costerton JW: Antibiotic resistance of bacteria in biofilms. Lancet 2001;358:135. [PMID: 11463434]

Stott NS: Review article: Paediatric bone and joint infection. J Ortho Surg (Hong Kong) 2001;9:83. [PMID: 12468850]

Stumpe KD et al: FDG positron emission tomography for differentiation of degenerative and infectious endplate abnormalities in the lumbar spine detected on MR imaging. AJR Am J Roentgenol 2002;179:1151. [PMID: 12388490]

Tarkowski A et al: Current Status of pathogenetic mechanisms in staphylococcal arthritis. FEMS Microbiol Lett 2002;217:125. [PMID 12480095]

Tomas MB et al: The diabetic foot. Br J Radiol 2000;73:443. [PMID: 10844873]

Turpin S, Lambert R: Role of scintigraphy in musculoskeletal and spinal infections. Radiol Clin North Am 2001;39:169. [PMID: 11316353]

van de Belt H: Infection of orthopedic implants and the use of antibiotic-loaded bone cements. A review. Acta Orthop Scand 2001;72:557. [PMID: 11817870]

Vandecasteele SJ et al: New insights in the pathogenesis of foreign body infections with coagulase negative staphylococci. Acta Clin Belg 2000;55:148. [PMID: 10981322]

Zhuang H et al: Exclusion of chronic osteomyelitis with F-18 fluorodeoxyglucose positron emission tomographic imaging. Clin Nucl Med 2000;25:281. [PMID: 10750968]

Zhuang H et al: Persistent non-specific FDG uptake on PET imaging following hip arthroplasty. Eur J Nucl Med Mol Imaging 2002;29:1328. [PMID: 12271415]

OSTEOMYELITIS

Classification Systems

Several classification systems have been used to describe osteomyelitis. The traditional system divides bone infections according to the duration of symptoms: acute, subacute, and chronic (Table 8–5). Acute osteomyelitis is identified within 7 to 14 days of onset. Acute infections are most frequently associated with hematogenous seeding of bones in children. However, adults may also develop acute hematogenous infections especially around implanted metal prostheses and fixation hardware. The duration of subacute osteomyelitis is between several weeks and several months. Chronic osteomyelitis is a bone infection that has been present for at least several months. It is associated with an epicenter of bone necrosis called a sequestrum that is generally encased in vascular reactive bone called an involucrum.

Another system developed by Waldvogel categorizes bone infections based on etiology and chronicity: hematogenous, contiguous spread (with or without concomitant vascular disease) and chronic (see Table 8–5). Hematogenous and contiguous spreading infections may be acute although the latter is associated with trauma or preexisting localized soft-tissue infections such as diabetic foot ulcers. Compromise in soft-tissue vascular supply may inhibit the immunological response to an infection. Therefore, Waldvogel created this subcategory to acknowledge the increased difficulty in treating infections in hosts with compromised vascularity.

Cierny and Mader developed a staging system for osteomyelitis that is classified by the anatomic extent of the infection and by the physiologic status of the host

Table 8–5. Classification systems for osteomyelitis.

Traditional system

Type	Time of onset
Acute	≤ 2 weeks
Subacute	Weeks to months
Chronic	≥ 3 months

Waldvogel system

Hematogenous
Arising from contiguous infection
   No vascular disease
Vascular disease present
Chronic

Cierny-Mader system

Anatomic extent of infection
1. Medullary only (acute hematogenous)
2. Superficial cortex (contiguous spread or soft tissue trauma)
3. Localized (cortical and medullary, mechanically stable)
4. Diffuse (cortical and medullary, mechanically unstable)
5. Subtype by host's physiologic status

A	Healthy
Bs	Compromised due to systemic factors
B1	Compromised due to local factors
B1s	Compromised due to both local and systemic factors
C	Treatment worse than the disease

---

rather than by chronicity or etiology (see Table 8–5 and Box 8–1). The four stages are characterized by the pattern of bony involvement of the infection in order of increasing complexity: stage 1—medullary only, stage 2—superficial cortex only, stage 3—localized medullary and cortical, and stage 4—diffuse medullary and cortical (see Box 8–1). The latter two categories are best distinguished by the presence or absence of mechanical compromise of the involved bone. Localized infections have not created an unstable bone. However, diffuse infections have sufficiently weakened the bone that surgical stabilization of the bone is necessary.

Host factors that mitigate healing are subcategorized into three groups: A—healthy host, B—compromised host, C—"incurable" host where the treatments that would be necessary to cure the disease are worse than living with the symptoms of the disease itself. A good example is an ambulatory diabetic smoker with peripheral vascular disease that has a stage 3 infection in a mechanically stable femur. Appropriate local wound care and suppressive antibiotic therapy may indeed be preferable to extensive surgical debridement that would risk destabilizing the bone, worsening a nonhealing soft-tissue wound, and increasing the risk of an above knee amputation.

Systemic factors that compromise the host include diabetes mellitus, immunosuppression (eg, corticosteroid or cyclosporin usage), immune disease (eg, AIDS), malnutrition (often associated with alcohol or IV drug abuse), renal or hepatic failure, chronic hypoxia, and extremes of age. Local factors include peripheral vascular disease, venous stasis disease, chronic lymphedema, extensive soft-tissue scarring, radiation fibrosis, arteritis, diabetic dysvascularity of small vessels, neuropathy, and tobacco use.

Belzunegui J et al: Musculoskeletal infections in intravenous drug addicts: Report of 34 cases with analysis of the microbiological aspects and pathogenic mechanisms. Clin Exp Rheumatol 2000;18:383. [PMID: 10895378]

Casado E et al: Musculoskeletal manifestations in patients positive for human immunodeficiency virus: Correlation with CD4 count. J Rheumatol 2001;28:802. [PMID: 11327254]

Gilad J et al: Polymicrobial polyarticular septic arthritis: A rare clinical entity. Scand J infect Dis 2001;33:381.

ACUTE OSTEOMYELITIS

1. Acute Hematogenous Osteomyelitis

Acute hematogenous osteomyelitis (AHO) is most frequently encountered in the metaphysis of long bones in children. Clinically patients have the signs and symptoms of an acute inflammation. Pain is usually localized although it may radiate to adjacent regions of the body. For example if a child complains of knee pain, the hip joint must be thoroughly evaluated for the possibility of septic arthritis. If a bone in the leg is infected, the child may limp or stop walking altogether. A child will also demonstrate guarding of an infected arm, refusing to use it and holding it to her side. Exam usually reveals local tenderness and occasionally limited motion of an adjacent joint, but swelling and redness are less frequent. Systemic signs of fever and chills may be present and infants may be irritable or lethargic and uninterested in eating.

Serology will characteristically show dramatic elevations in the CRP and the ESR. The white blood cell count (WBC) is usually elevated, and a left shift may be apparent. Peripheral blood cultures will grow the offending organism in up to one half of acutely infected children.

Plain radiographs taken early in the course of disease are usually negative. After a week or two radiographs may reveal a radiolucent lesion and periosteal elevation. Reactive sclerosis will be absent because it is encountered only in chronic bone infections. Technetium bone scan will show increased activity on soft tissue and delayed bone images. CT may show a radiolucent area in cancellous bone and signs of periosteal elevation. MRI will show early inflammation of bone marrow

BOX 8–1. THE CIERNEY AND MADER STAGING SYSTEM.

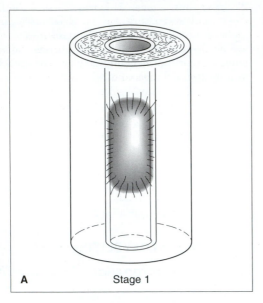

A   Stage 1

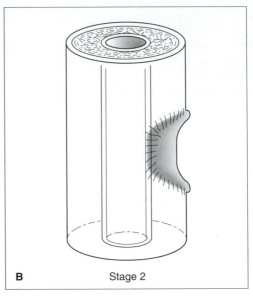

B   Stage 2

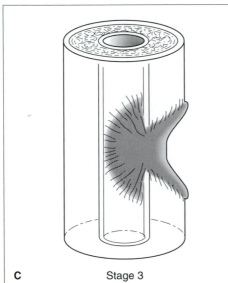

C   Stage 3

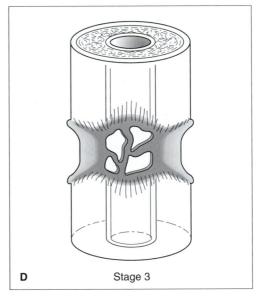

D   Stage 3

The Cierny and Mader staging system for osteomyelitis is classified by the anatomic extent of the infection and by the physiologic status of the host rather than by chronicity or etiology. The four stages are characterized by the pattern of bony involvement of the infection in order of increasing complexity: stage 1—medullary only, stage 2—superficial cortex only, stage 3—localized medullary and cortical, and stage 4—diffuse medullary and cortical.

with inflammation of the periosteum and adjacent soft tissues as the infection progresses. In later stages abscess formation may be seen as a signal void on gadolinium contrast images.

The clinical and radiologic appearance of AHO may be similar to inflammatory neoplasms such as acute lymphocytic leukemia, Ewing's sarcoma, and Langerhans' cell histiocytosis (AKA eosinophilic granuloma). Therefore, a biopsy may be required to distinguish an infection from a tumor.

Standard evaluation of a patient with suspected AHO includes a needle or open biopsy to obtain tissue for culture *and* histology and subsequent initiation of empiric antibiotics. If an abscess is identified, thorough irrigation and local debridement through a small cortical window should be performed. Once the culture results and sensitivities have been obtained, the final antibiotic regimen may be selected. Six weeks of antibiotic therapy are usually indicated. In pediatric patients with sensitive staphylococcal infections, 2 weeks of parenteral antibiotics may be followed by 4 weeks of oral antibiotic therapy. Close clinical follow-up is necessary to ensure that the patient's inflammatory symptoms are resolving. Serial ESR and CRP should return to normal within the treatment period.

If the patient does not improve, temporary discontinuation of antibiotics may be necessary prior to performing a surgical exploration to culture the infected site. Often antibiotics, even those to which the bacteria are resistant, may suppress the bacteria enough that they will not grow in culture. Although a 2-week waiting period off of antibiotics, which is customary for cases of chronic osteomyelitis, may not be tolerated by patients with acute osteomyelitis, even waiting for several days may increase the culture yield. This further highlights the potential problems of beginning an empiric regimen using inappropriate antibiotics and then having difficulty obtaining productive cultures. Either a delay in treatment will occur or the patient will have to be placed on several antibiotics to cover all possible organisms.

In patients with stable prosthetic joints who acquire an acute hematogenous infection due to a sensitive organism, thorough soft-tissue debridement, exchange of the polyethylene liner or temporary substitution of the polyethylene with a molded antibiotic spacer, and 6 weeks of IV antibiotic therapy confer a salvage rate approaching 50%.

Clinical Example

A 13-year-old female complained of acute knee pain beginning 7 days earlier when arising from sleep. Her pain worsened to the point where she had to stay at home from school because she could not walk. On exam her thigh was tender, and her hip and knee motion severely restricted due to pain, but there was no knee effusion. Her temperature was 100.9°F. The serum white blood cell count was 17,000 with a left shift, and the ESR was four times normal. Plain films of the femur were normal. An MRI of the thigh showed significant inflammation of the marrow and adjacent soft tissues on T_2-weighted images (Figure 8–7A). Intraoperatively the midfemur was exposed, a hole was drilled in the femur and a collection of pus was aspirated from the marrow cavity (Figure 8–7B). Irrigation was performed through the drill hole and the wound closed over a drain. *Staphylococcus aureus* was cultured, and the patient was successfully treated with 6 weeks of IV antibiotics.

2. Acute Osteomyelitis Due to Puncture Wound

Acute osteomyelitis must be considered in the evaluation of a patient who has suffered a deep puncture wound. The feet and hands are the most frequent sites of these injuries. The soft tissue wound may appear insignificant. It may be difficult to detect a foreign body made of wood or plastic on plain radiography, and wound exploration for a foreign body in a clinic setting is frequently unrewarding. Please refer to Chapter 9 (Foot and Ankle Surgery) and Chapter 10 (Hand Surgery) for further information.

Clinical Example

An 11-year-old male punctured his foot when he stepped on a sharp object. Initial radiographs of the foot showed no evidence of a foreign body (Figure 8–8A). In retrospect a small puncture wound can be visualized in the middistal diaphysis. He was initially treated with a limited irrigation and debridement in the emergency department and discharged on oral antistaphylococcal antibiotics. Two weeks later the arch of his foot became swollen and drainage emanated from the puncture wound (Figure 8–8B). He was admitted to the hospital and placed empirically on triple IV antibiotics. Superficial swabs of the wound grew *Pseudomonas.*

A technetium bone scan identified a significant uptake of radiotracer in the distal aspect of the first metatarsal compared with the opposite normal foot (Figure 8–8C). New radiographs of the foot depicted a circular region of osteolysis with a slight elevation of the adjacent periosteum (Figure 8–8D). The patient underwent a thorough irrigation and debridement in the operating room. No foreign body was identified. Deep cultures of the wound revealed *Mycobacterium fortuitum,* a rapidly growing *Mycobacterium* other than

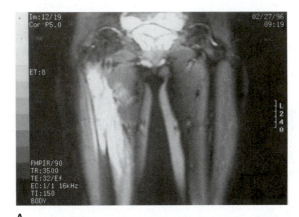

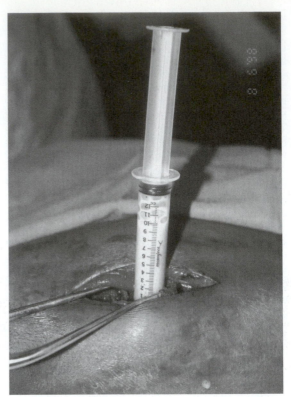

A   **B**

Figure 8–7. **A.** T_2-weighted MRI of the thigh, showing marrow edema in the femur and surrounding muscula-ture. **B.** Aspiration of the medullary cavity of the femur produces 10 mL of pus in the syringe.

tuberculosis (MOTT). He clinically improved within several days of beginning oral clarithromycin and con-tinued this treatment for nine months.

This case illustrates the need to obtain accurate wound cultures in order to choose appropriate antibi-otic therapy. Superficial cultures often reveal skin con-taminants that are not representative of the organisms actually causing the infection. When infections do not respond to routine empiric antibiotic therapy, it is al-ways important to consider surgical exploration to ob-tain deep cultures of the wound for mycobacterium and fungal organisms as well as for aerobic and anaerobic organisms.

Agrawal A et al: Cryptococcal arthritis in an immunocompetent host. J S C Med Assoc 2000;96:297. [PMID: 10933007]

Babhulkar SS, Pande SK: Unusual manifestations of osteoarticular tuberculosis. Clin Ortho 2002;398:114. [PMID: 11964639]

Caspofungin: new preparation. A last resort for invasive aspergillo-sis. Prescrire Int 2002;11:142. [PMID: 12378745]

Centers for Disease Control and Prevention, Reported Tuberculo-sis in the United States, 1995. August, 1996.

Centers for Disease Control and Prevention. Guidelines for pre-venting the transmission of *Mycobacterium tuberculosis* in health care facilities. MMWR Morb Mortal Wkly Rep 1994; 43(RR-13):1.

Chan ED, Iseman MD: Current medical treatment for tuberculo-sis. BMJ 2002;325:1282. [PMID: 1248250]

Dhillon MS et al: Tuberculosis of the sternoclavicular joints. Acta Orthop Scand 2001;72:514. [PMID: 11728080]

Hansen BL, Andersen K: Fungal arthritis. A review. Scan J Rheu-matol 1995;24:248. [PMID: 7481591]

Nolan CM, Goldberg SV: Treatment of isoniazid-resistant tuber-culosis with isoniazid, rifampin, ethambutol and pyrazi-namide for 6 months. Int J Tuberc Lung Dis 2002;6:952. [PMID: 12475140]

Silber JS et al: Insidious destruction of the hip by Mycobacterium tuberculosis and why early diagnosis is critical. J Arthroplasty 2000;15:392. [PMID: 10794239]

SUBACUTE OSTEOMYELITIS

Subacute infections are often associated with pediatric patients. These infections are usually caused by organ-isms of low virulence and are associated with muted

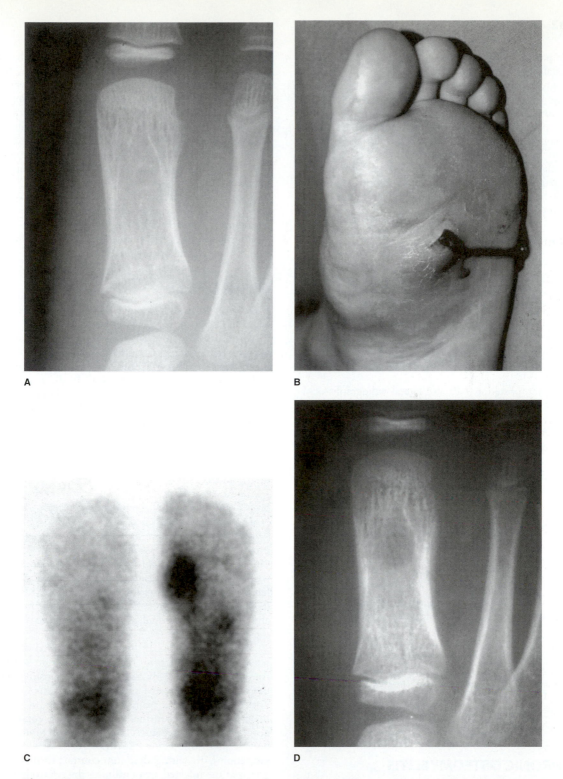

Figure 8–8. **A.** Initial plain radiograph of the first metatarsal. **B.** Preoperative view of the puncture wound. **C.** Bone phase of a technetium bone scan of the feet. **D.** Follow-up, radiograph of the first metatarsal taken 2 weeks after Figure 8–8A.

symptoms. Ultimately the infection appears to reach a stalemate with the host's defenses and does not progress. Subacute osteomyelitis shares some of the radiographic characteristics of both acute and chronic infections. Like acute osteomyelitis, regions of osteolysis and periosteal elevation may be present. Like chronic osteomyelitis, a circumferential zone of reactive sclerotic bone may be visualized. When subacute osteomyelitis affects the diaphysis of a long bone it may be particularly difficult to distinguish from Langerhans cell histiocytosis (AKA eosinophilic granuloma) or Ewing's sarcoma.

Clinical Example

A 14-year-old male presented with a 2-month history of left ankle pain and swelling that occurred when he jumped off a farm trailer. His symptoms persisted although some improvement was reported. He denied any fever, chills, or night sweats and could walk without assistance. On exam he was still tender and focally erythematous over the anterior region of the ankle. WBC was normal and the ESR was only slightly elevated.

Anteroposterior (AP) and lateral radiographs of the tibia show mixed areas of radiodensity and radiolucency in the metaphysis and a slightly raised periosteum (Figures 8–9A and B). Axial T_2-weighted MRI shows marrow edema and periosteal elevation—identified as the outer dark ring just superficial to the cortex. A halo of inflammation surrounds the raised periosteum (Figure 8–9C). Coronal T_2-weighted MRI shows the periosteal elevation along the metadiaphysis and the marrow edema extending as far proximally as the midtibia (Figure 8–9D). During open surgical biopsy, purulent material was encountered within the metaphysis but not along the periosteal surface or in the ankle joint. Thorough irrigation and debridement of the area was performed with primary closure of the incision over a drain. The patient was subsequently cured of his subacute nonresistant *S aureus* infection with 6 weeks of IV nafcillin.

Mader JT et al: Antibiotic therapy for musculoskeletal infections. Instr Course Lect 2002;51:539. [PMID: 12064145]

Stengel D et al: Systematic review and meta-analysis of antibiotic therapy for bone and joint infections. Lancet Infect Dis 2001; 1:175. [PMID: 11871494]

Vinod MB et al: Duration of antibiotics in children with osteomyelitis and septic arthritis. J Paediatr Child Health 2002; 38:363. [PMID: 12173997]

CHRONIC OSTEOMYELITIS

Chronic osteomyelitis is the result of untreated acute or subacute osteomyelitis. It can occur hematogenously, iatrogenically, or as a result of penetrating trauma. Chronic infections are often associated with orthopaedic metal implants used to replace joints, fuse spine segments, or fix fractures. Direct intraoperative inoculation or subsequent hematogenous seeding of metal or dead bone surfaces may provide a haven for the bacteria protecting them from white blood cells and effective concentrations of antibiotics. Therefore, removal of the metal and dead bone are necessary in addition to appropriate antibiotics to eradicate chronic osteomyelitis.

Surgical debridement of necrotic bone for infection control is akin to curettage of a benign bone tumor. A recent study validating the Cierny-Mader classification system substaging A and B was reported. Debridements were wide marginal or intralesional.

Clinical Example

A 62-year-old male sustained a closed femur fracture when he fell from a ladder 40 years ago. His fracture was fixed with an intramedullary rod that was subsequently removed after the fracture healed. Unfortunately the patient's leg became infected postoperatively and a draining sinus tract developed adjacent to the fracture site. Subsequently he had several local debridements when oral antibiotics would not resolve his symptoms. He enjoyed extended asymptomatic intervals of up to 14 years between successive debridements. For the last 4 years he had an intermittently draining sinus tract and occasional bouts of pain relieved with brief courses of oral ciprofloxacin.

At the time of presentation he had had a fever of 38.5°C and increasing leg pain and swelling for 1 week. Once the sinus tract opened up and began to drain pus, he defervesced and his leg symptoms modestly improved although it was still difficult for him to walk. On physical examination the sinus tract was probed with a Q-tip, which easily reached the surface of the femur. Serologic exam yielded these results: CRP = 7.5 (≤ 0.5 is normal), ESR = 38 (0–15 mm Hg is normal), and WBC = 7.9 (normal 5–10 k). A sensitive *S aureus* was cultured.

Radiographs depict an irregularly expanded callus of sclerotic bone at the prior fracture site (Figure 8–10A). An indium-labeled WBC scan was focally positive (Figure 8–10B). CT showed small free fragments of bone not connected to the main shaft (Figure 8–10C). The main fragment was further outlined using computer-generated sagittal reconstructions and was thought to be a sequestrum (Figure 8–10D). A T_1-weighted fat saturation MRI with gadolinium contrast further characterized the infected area outlining the relatively small area of focal inflammation (Figure 8–10E).

Curettage of the femur produced a 3.5-cm sequestrum (Figure 8–10F). A water-cooled high-speed

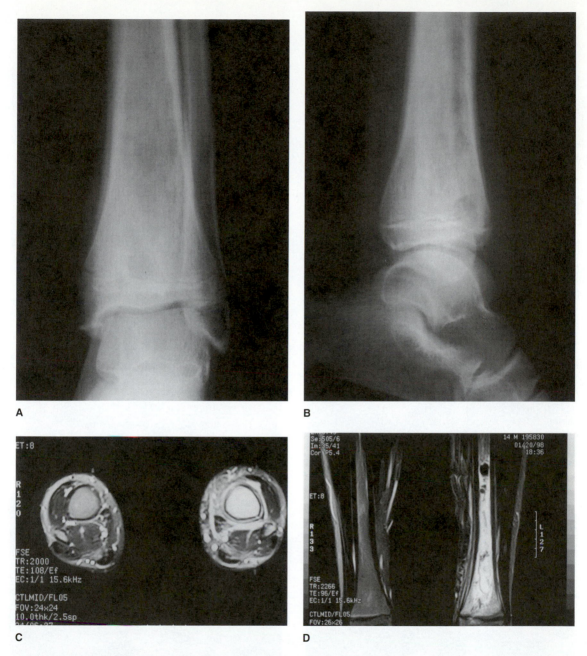

Figure 8–9. **A.** AP radiograph of the distal tibia. **B.** Lateral radiograph of the distal tibia. Notice focal region of osteopenia immediately above the growth plate. **C.** Axial T_2-weighted MRI of both tibias in the region of the distal metaphysis shows marrow edema and periosteal elevation and inflammation on the affected left side. **D.** Coronal T_2-weighted MRI of both tibias shows extensive marrow edema and periosteal inflammation ascending to the midtibia on the affected side.

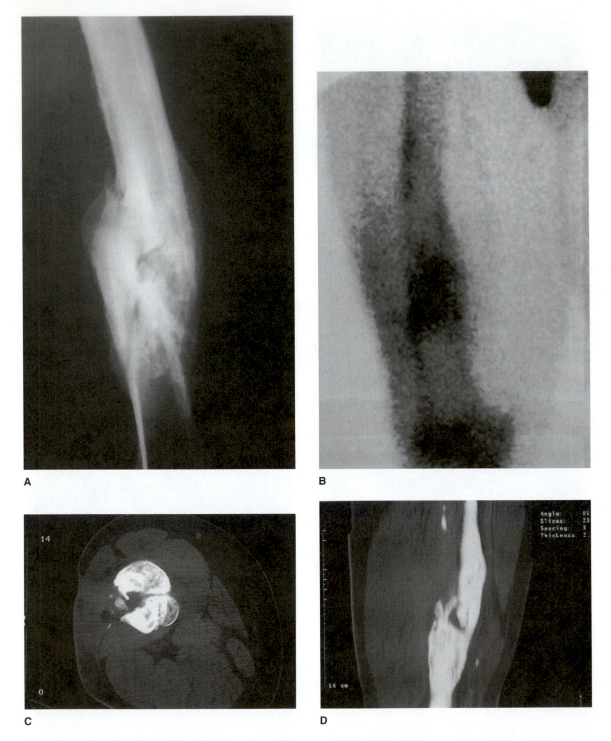

Figure 8–10. **A.** Lateral radiograph of the femur. **B.** Indium-labeled WBC bone scan. **C.** Axial CT scan of the infected area. **D.** Computer-reformatted CT with sagittal image of the femur.

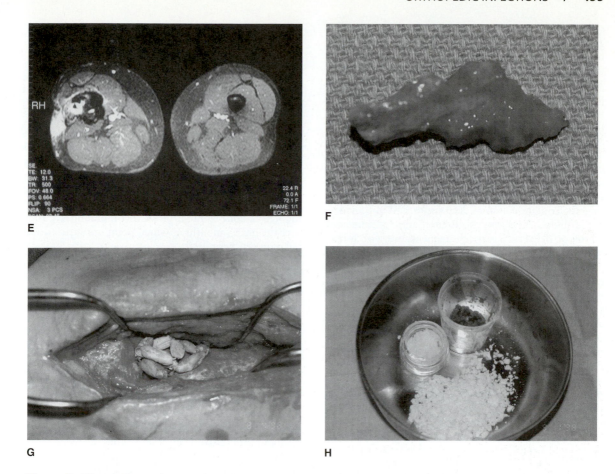

Figure 8–10. **E.** An axial T$_1$-weighted fat-saturated MRI with gadolinium contrast. **F.** Sequestrum. **G.** Beads placed in the operative wound. **H.** Ingredients used to bone graft the bone defect (clockwise from bottom: allograft cancellous bone chips, demineralized bone matrix, autograft iliac crest bone).

burr was used to extensively debride the adjacent cortical bone until it bled freely. A string of antibiotic beads were made on a No. 5 nonabsorbable braided suture using 2 g of vancomycin powder, 3 g of tobramycin powder, and one bag of polymethylmethacrylate bone cement (see Figure 8–5). The beads were counted and snugly placed into the cavity in a way that they could easily be retrieved later (Figure 8–10G). The adjacent soft tissues were curetted to remove necrotic material but the sinus tract was not closed or excised. Operative cultures grew sensitive *S aureus* and a 6-week course of intravenous Nafcillin (2 g q4h) was begun as an outpatient. A visiting nurse administered the antibiotic through a PICC line using a programmable computerized pump.

Three weeks later the beads were removed and a mixture of posterior iliac crest bone graft, demineralized bone matrix, and allograft cancellous bone chips were placed into the cavity (Figure 8–10H). Further cultures of the wound were sterile. At the conclusion of his antibiotic therapy, his ESR and CRP had returned to normal values, his sinus tract had completely healed and he was asymptomatic.

OSTEOMYELITIS DUE TO OPEN FRACTURES

Osteomyelitis due to trauma may present acutely or chronically. In acute cases the signs of infection may be masked by the local open wound and may be delayed by the use of empiric antibiotics and surgical debridement that is not complete. Similar bone changes can be seen on radiographic imaging even in the presence of fractures and fixation hardware. Open wounds where the bone is exposed must undergo comprehensive irrigation and debridement in the operating room. Foreign material including road dirt, clothing, and bullet shell wadding must be completely removed, and all necrotic areas of the soft tissues must be excised. If a fracture is present, all fracture fragments that have been completely stripped of their blood supply must also be removed. Viable bone fragments where the periosteum is still attached, may be left in the wound but must be carefully monitored. Pulsatile lavage using at least 6 L of saline, with or without antibiotics, is a proven adjunct to sharp surgical debridement. In cases of large soft-tissue defects, early flap coverage is ideal to prevent ongoing contamination of deep tissues and to provide a robust blood supply to the injured area for enhanced antibiotic delivery. Serial debridements every 48 h may be necessary in order to establish the viability of injured tissues and to ensure that complete removal of all devitalized tissue has been accomplished. In cases where soft-tissue coverage must be delayed, a wound vacuum-assisted closure device (VAC) is an ideal way to manage the wound. This system is easy to apply and only needs to be changed every 2–3 days. Because the pump is portable and the wound is sealed and dry, patient acceptance is high. For these reasons wound VAC system has largely replaced open continuous irrigation systems that are more labor-intensive to maintain and less well tolerated by the patient.

Fractures can heal even in the presence of a soft-tissue or bone infection. If an acute infection is present in an open wound where a fracture has been fixed with a rod or plate, it must be determined if the soft and bony tissues are viable. If they are viable, the fixation hardware should be left in place until the fracture heals. If necrotic redebridement to remove all areas of necrosis must first be performed even if the fixation hardware has to be replaced. If there is a large defect in the bone after comprehensive debridement, the bone should be held to length with an external fixator until the infection is resolved. Placement of temporary antibiotic beads may help to provide local antibiotic delivery and eliminate the "dead space." Then reconstruction with autograft, vascularized bone graft, or bone transport may be performed.

Chronic osteomyelitis due to open trauma may often be associated with a healed fracture and an open wound where the bone or fixation hardware may be exposed.

The hardware must be removed and the site of infection must be treated like any chronic osteomyelitis with thorough bone debridement, use of local antibiotic beads, and systemic intravenous antibiotics. Once the infection is controlled, bone grafting or other reconstruction of the defect may take place, often in association with a local or free flap to reconstruct the soft tissue defect.

Clinical Example

A 42-year-old female sustained an open fracture of the proximal third of her tibia. She underwent debridement and fracture fixation with a 10-hole plate. The fracture healed after 6 months but remained painful and began to drain purulent material from three sinus tracts (Figure 8–11A). A lateral radiograph shows the tibia before and after plate removal and debridement using a water-cooled high-speed burr (Figures 8–11B and C). The tibia was then packed with a string of antibiotic beads and primarily closed. Half way through the 6-week course of intravenous antibiotic therapy the beads were removed (Figure 8–11D) and the defect bone grafted. Graft incorporation occurred over the next 3 months at which point unrestricted ambulation was permitted.

SQUAMOUS CELL CARCINOMA ARISING FROM A CHRONIC OSTEOMYELITIS

On rare occasion squamous cell carcinoma may arise in the chronically infected granulation tissue that is adjacent to a chronically infected bone. The patient has usually had stable chronic osteomyelitis for many years. The tumor can be difficult to visually distinguish from the granulation tissue from whence it arose. The focus of carcinoma will appear to be an exuberance of proliferative, lobulated, and friable "granulation tissue." A recent and progressive worsening of the soft-tissue defect in an otherwise stable case of chronic osteomyelitis is a clue that carcinoma has developed. Liberal sampling of the wound can easily be done in a clinic setting with a disposable skin punch biopsy trephine used by dermatologists for skin biopsies. Histologic examination of the biopsy specimens enables the pathologist to readily distinguish between squamous cell carcinoma and chronic granulation.

Staging studies, including contrast CT scan of the chest, abdomen, and pelvis; technetium total body bone scan; and PET scan, are used to detect other sites of disease. PET is particularly helpful in detecting regional and systemic lymphatic spread of the tumor. Wide surgical excision of the primary site and any positive lymph nodes are necessary to render the patient surgically free of disease. Adjunctive radiotherapy for local control and chemotherapy for systemic control are used in conjunction with surgical excision in most cases.

Clinical Example

A 49-year-old male presented with a 30-year history of ischial decubitus ulcers and rectal fistulas. He had had spinal meningitis during infancy resulting in severe paraparesis, hypoesthesia, and incontinence of bowel

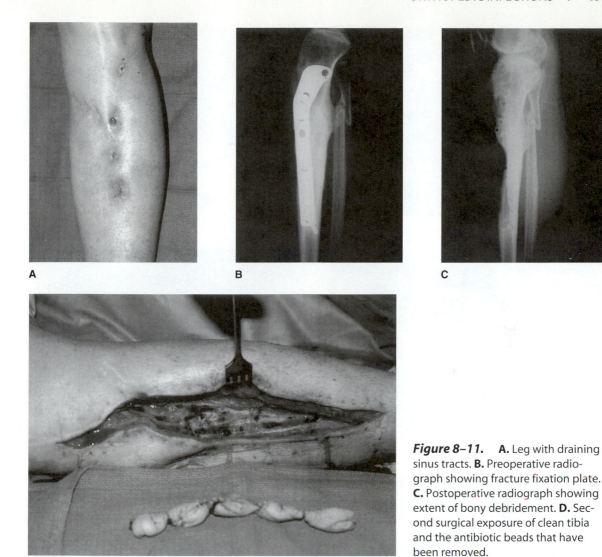

Figure 8–11. **A.** Leg with draining sinus tracts. **B.** Preoperative radiograph showing fracture fixation plate. **C.** Postoperative radiograph showing extent of bony debridement. **D.** Second surgical exposure of clean tibia and the antibiotic beads that have been removed.

and bladder. Despite a long series of local debridement procedures, muscle flaps, and skin grafts; his buttock region remained open to some degree during this entire time. More recently he was concerned about a reactivation of his ischial osteomyelitis. On physical exam a 15-cm region of friable sponge-like neogranulation was identified adjacent to a scarred ulcer overlying the ischium (Figure 8–12A). Plain films suggested chronic reactive changes in the ischium due to infection and prior surgery. Punch biopsies of the concerning area of neogranulation revealed squamous cell carcinoma. CT of the chest abdomen and pelvis were negative except for enlarged inguinal lymph nodes. The patient under-

went a permanent diverting colostomy and inguinal and retroperitoneal lymph node dissection. All lymph nodes were negative. Subsequently the tumor was radically excised, including a partial excision of the ischium (Figures 8–12B and C). A wound VAC was used for local wound care (Figures 8–12D and E). Eight weeks later the wound edges had retracted, and normal healthy granulation tissue covered the bony defect (Figure 8–12F). The area was subsequently covered with skin graft to achieve complete healing.

Fitzgerald RH et al: Local muscle flaps in the treatment of chronic osteomyelitis. J Bone Joint Surg (Am) 1985;67:175.

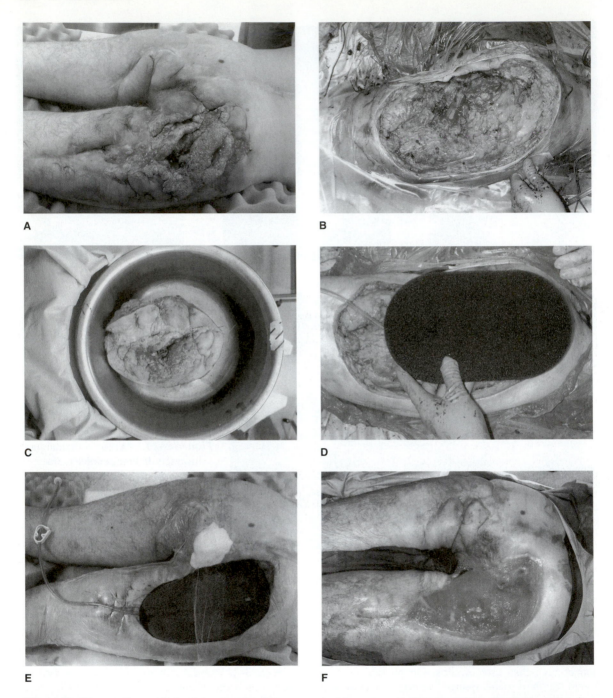

Figure 8–12. **A.** Photograph of chronic ulcerative wound with neogranulation tissue laterally. **B.** Wound and tumor bed after wide excision of the carcinoma. **C.** Tumor/wound specimen, 18 cm in diameter. **D.** Wound VAC sponge being measured over wound. **E.** Wound VAC sponge in place partially contracting wound. **F.** Eight weeks after wound VAC and antibiotic therapy. Bed ready for skin grafting.

Gonzalez MH et al: Free tissue coverage of chronic traumatic wounds of the lower leg. Plast Reconstr Surg 2002;109:592. [PMID: 11818841]

Kuokkanen HO et al: Radical excision and reconstruction of chronic osteomyelitis with microvascular muscle flaps. Orthopedics 2002;25:137. [PMID: 11871378]

Moroni A et al: State of the art review: techniques to avoid pin loosening and infection in external fixation. J Ortho Trauma 2002;16:189. [PMID: 11880783]

Strauss MB, Bryant B: Hyperbaric oxygen. Orthopedics 2002;25: 303. [PMID: 11918035]

Wieland AJ et al: The efficacy of free tissue transfer in the treatment of osteomyelitis. J Bone Joint Surg (Am) 1984;66:181.

■ SEPTIC ARTHRITIS

Diagnosis

There is no formal classification system for septic arthritis. Most joint infections are acute rather than chronic, monoarticular rather than polyarticular, and arise from a hematogenous source of organisms rather than by direct inoculation or extension from an adjacent infection. The most important clinical question that often arises is whether the patient's inflamed joint is due to an infection or due to a noninfectious inflammatory process. Inflammatory arthropathies are numerous and patients often require systemic medical treatment to control the joint symptoms. They are often categorized as seropositive (for rheumatoid factor) or seronegative. Common conditions include crystal arthropathies (gout and pseudogout), autoimmune disorders with joint involvement (RA, systemic lupus erythematosus, and inflammatory bowel disease). Finally arthropathy from osteoarthritis and avascular necrosis may present with inflammatory symptoms and mimic an indolent infection.

Diagnosis of septic arthritis is much more dependent on arthrocentesis for synovial fluid analysis (see Table 8–4) and culture than it is on radiologic imaging. Early plain radiographs are usually normal. Ultrasound is better at diagnosing increased fluid within a joint space but is not specific as to the cause. Many of the radiographic features of bone scan, CT, and MRI are nonspecific and leave the diagnosis of septic arthritis in question.

ACUTE SEPTIC ARTHRITIS

Hematogenous septic arthritis commonly affects patients with compromised immunologic defense mechanisms. The underlying source of infection can frequently be determined, and blood cultures are positive in about half of patients. Patients at risk include those with specific immune deficiencies from HIV or chemotherapy; those with chronic disease, including RA, gout, renal failure, and sickle cell disease; and intravenous drug abusers. Patients with known arthropathy from other causes are also at increased risk for superimposed infections. Patients routinely complain of severe pain with passive motion of the affected joint. Rest pain, guarding, swelling, erythema, and heat become more pronounced as the infection progresses. Fever and chills are not sensitive indicators of septic arthritis.

The most common joint affected by hematogenous septic arthritis is the knee. The hip, ankle, wrist, shoulder, and elbow follow in frequency of involvement. The differential diagnosis includes Charcot joint, gout, pseudogout, RA, and other inflammatory arthropathies. The diagnosis is tentatively made on joint fluid analysis (see Table 8–4).

Although infections often spread from joints to affect adjacent metaphyseal bone, tumors seldom do except at the sacroiliac joint. Surgical decompression and irrigation of all large joints is preferred to serial needle aspirations. In the acute setting arthroscopy is ideal for culturing synovial tissue, thoroughly irrigating the joint space and for placement of an indwelling drainage tube.

Clinical Example

A 53-year-old female with RA and a painful left hip, presented with a 3-week history of rapidly worsening groin pain, slight fever, and lethargy. Degenerative narrowing of the hip joint is seen on a prior AP radiograph (Figure 8–13A). Although the patient's WBC was normal the hematocrit was only 18! Her groin was extremely tender and any motion of the hip joint elicited excruciating pain. The patient was admitted to the hospital directly from the clinic. A bone scan showed intense activity in the region of the hip (Figure 8–13B). A CT of the pelvis outlines a loculated soft-tissue mass anterior to the femoral head displacing the femoral artery and vein medially (Figure 8–13C). Using CT guidance, the region was aspirated, and a pigtail catheter was inserted to drain the abscess cavity. MRI with T_1 fat-saturated sequences and gadolinium contrast further characterized the infection, revealing significant inflammation in the femoral head and an effusion of the hip joint (Figure 8–13D). A plain radiograph at that time showed a dramatic collapse of the femoral head (Figure 8–13E). A Girdlestone arthroplasty was performed, and the remainder of the femoral head was submitted for histologic analysis (Figure 8–13F). An antibiotic spacer was orthotopically placed to stabilize the femur and the wound was closed over drains (Figure 8–13G). A 6-week course of IV antibiotics was given. Afterward, the hip was surgically reexamined and no evidence of persistent infection was seen

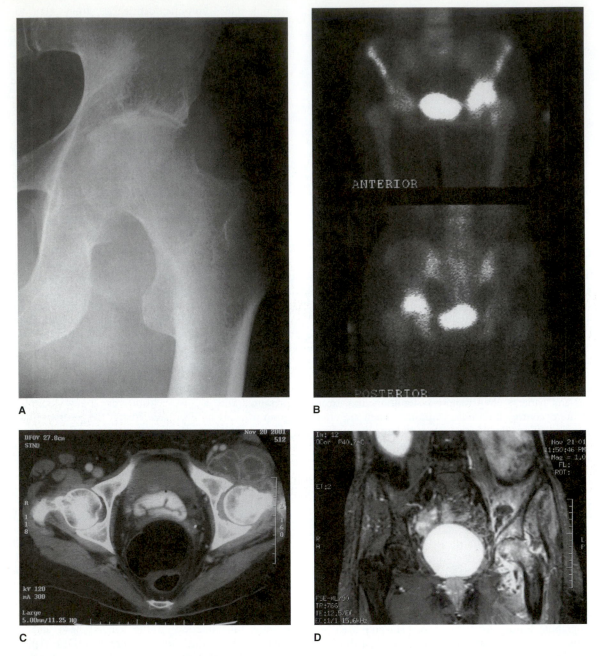

Figure 8–13. **A.** Initial AP radiograph of hip joint with narrowed cartilage due to rheumatoid arthritis. **B.** Technetium bone scan shows intense activity in region of left hip. **C.** CT scan shows loculated soft-tissue mass anterior to the femoral head displacing the femoral artery and vein medially. **D.** T_1-weighted fat-saturated MRI with gadolinium contrast showing intense inflammation around hip joint and in acetabulum and femoral head. A retroperitoneal abscess is depicted in the enlarged iliopsoas muscle by a dark central area of signal void surrounded by a halo of bright inflammation.

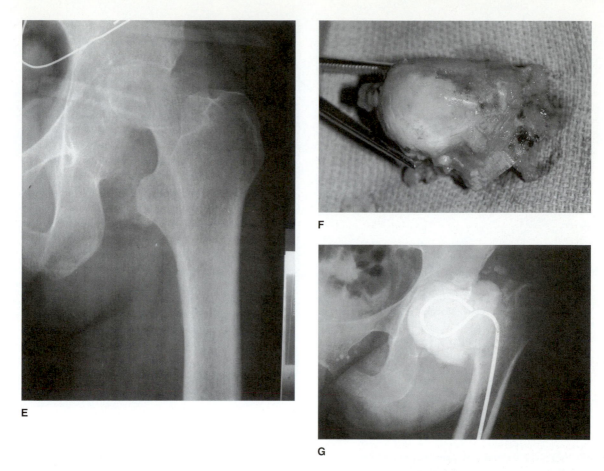

Figure 8–13. **E.** Preoperative plain radiograph showing extensive collapse of the weight bearing portion of the femoral head. **F.** Surgical specimen showing flattened femoral head (*upper portion*). Note the cut surface of the neck (*lower right*). **G.** Radiograph of an antibiotic spacer molded around a rush rod that has been implanted in the femoral canal.

grossly or by frozen section analysis. At that time a total hip prosthesis was successfully implanted.

CHRONIC SEPTIC ARTHRITIS

Unlike acute septic arthritis, which is intensely painful, chronic septic arthritis presents with indolent joint symptoms that are often muted by oral or intra-articular injections of anti-inflammatory medications and that may be attributed to coexistent chronic joint arthritis. Immunocompromised patients are susceptible to less virulent and slower growing organisms such as atypical mycobacteria and fungus. These organisms may solicit a subdued chronic inflammatory response that generates less pain and joint effusion, resulting in a delay in diagnosis.

Clinical Example

A 52-year-old male with AIDS on retroviral therapy presented with a 4-month history of arthritic pain and effusion in his knee and a 1-week history of an enlarging painful mass on the medial aspect of his knee (Figure 8–14A). One year earlier he had been diagnosed with a large popliteal abscess in the same leg caused by *S epidermidis* that was successfully treated with surgical drainage and 6 weeks of intravenous antibiotics. Exam revealed focal swelling, warmth, erythema, and restricted motion due to pain. During arthrotomy the medial swelling was found to communicate directly with the knee joint. Intraoperative findings included a large quantity of pus, extensive erosion of cartilage, and chronic proliferative synovial tissue (Figure 8–14B). After irrigation and de-

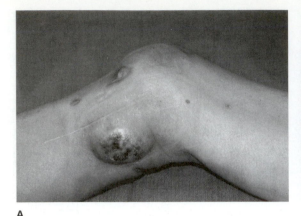

A

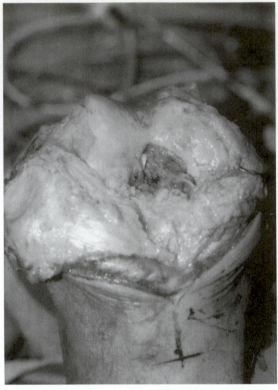

Figure 8–14. **A.** A large focal erythematous soft-tissue swelling and a longitudinal scar from prior surgical drainage of a popliteal abscess are seen along the medial aspect of the knee. **B.** With the patella everted to the left the articular surfaces of the femur are seen at the top and the hypertrophic synovium is seen below. Note the complete loss of cartilage on the medial femoral condyle to the right.

B

bridement, the wound was primarily closed over drainage catheters. Cultures grew *Candida albicans* and the patient was treated with fluconazole (Diflucan).

Even though this patient's symptoms appeared to be acute, he actually had chronic septic arthritis, that likely began 4 months previously when he began having arthritic pain. Because he was immunocompromised, his inflammatory symptoms were muted, causing a delay in clinical presentation. Unusual pathogens are a hallmark of immunocompromised patients. Therefore, it is essential to acquire mycobacterial and fungal cultures in addition to aerobic and anaerobic bacterial cultures. Unless the cause of immunosuppression is known, a comprehensive diagnostic survey must be undertaken to identify the underlying causes, including cancer, severe malnutrition, immune disorders, and chronic viral infection.

Aubry A et al: Sixty cases of Mycobacterium marinum infection: Clinical features, treatment, and antibiotic susceptibility of the causative isolates. Arch Intern Med 2002;162:1746. [PMID: 12153378]

Biviji AA et al: Musculoskeletal manifestations of human immunodeficiency virus infection. J Am Acad Orthop Surg 2002;10: 312. [PMID: 12374482]

Brna JA, Hall RF Jr: Acute monoarticular herpetic arthritis: A case report. J Bone Joint Surg Am 1984;66:623. [PMID: 6707045]

Gordon SC, Lauter CB: Mumps arthritis. A review of the literature. Rev Infect Dis 1984;6:338.

Kujula G, Newman JH: Isolation of echovirus type II from synovial fluid in acute monocytic arthritis. Arthritis Rheum 1985;28:98.

Le Dantec C et al: Occurrence of mycobacteria in water treatment lines and in water distribution systems. Appl Environ Microbiol 2002;68:5318. [PMID: 12406720]

Mylonas AD et al: Natural History of Ross River virus-induced epidemic polyarthritis. Med J Aust 2002;177:356. [PMID: 12358577]

Ray CG et al: Acute polyarthritis associated with active Epstein-Barr virus infection. JAMA 1982;248:2990.

SEPTIC ARTHRITIS DUE TO ADJACENT INFECTION

Contiguous spread of infection to a joint most commonly occurs in pediatric patients with AHO or in adults with chronic wounds such as ischial decubiti and diabetic foot ulcers. Chronic soft-tissue and bone infections may extend into joints in adults as well. Of particular concern is occurrence in patients who are immunocompromised or insensate.

Clinical Example

A 28-year-old-male with paraplegia and a long-standing history of sacral and ischial decubiti presented with a 2-week history of fevers, anemia, and increased spasticity of the lower extremities. Two large fist-sized decubiti, one over the sacrum and one over the right ischium, were observed (Figure 8–15A). The underlying bone was easily palpated at the base of both of these ulcers. Further examination with a probing finger revealed a deep sinus that tracked to the posterior aspect of the femoral head. Plain films revealed a chronically dislocated hip with cephalad migration of the femur and concomitant destruction of the ilium (Figure 8–15B). Axial CT scan showed air within and surrounding the dislocated femoral head (Figure 8–15C). MRI with in-

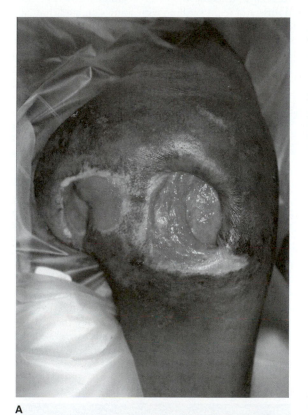

A

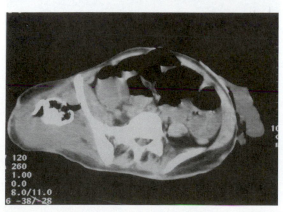

C

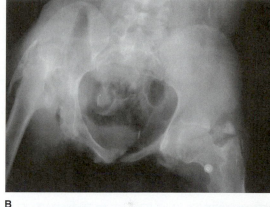

B

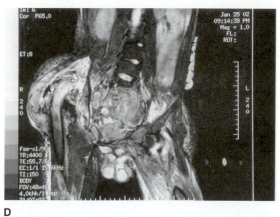

D

Figure 8–15. **A.** Large sacral and right ischial ulcer. **B.** AP radiograph of the pelvis. **C.** CT scan of pelvis. **D.** MRI with inversion recovery sequence of pelvis.

version recovery sequencing depicted extensive inflammation of the femur, the ilium, an the surrounding gluteal musculature (Figure 8–15D). An extensive surgical debridement of the acetabulum, removal of the proximal femur was performed through the lateral ulcer. A wound VAC was placed on both ulcers, and culture specific antibiotics were administered. The patient refused a hip disarticulation with an anterior thigh flap that would close both ischial and sacral decubiti, and he was subsequently treated with chronic oral antibiotic suppression and daily wound packing.

Caksen H et al: Septic arthritis in childhood. Pediatr Int 2000; 42:534. [PMID: 11059545]

Perry CR: Septic arthritis. Am J Orthop 1999;28:168. [PMID: 10195840]

Salter RB et al: The protective effect of continuous passive motion on living articular cartilage in acute septic arthritis. Clin Orthop 1981;159:223.

Shirtliff ME, Mader JT: Acute septic arthritis. Clin Microbiol Rev 2002;15:527. [PMID: 12364368]

Swan A et al: The value of synovial fluid analysis in the diagnosis of joint disease: a literature survey. Ann Rheum Dis 2002;61: 493. [PMID: 12006320]

■ SOFT-TISSUE INFECTIONS

CELLULITIS

Skin infections are common, and it is important to distinguish cellulitis from noninfectious rashes and from deeper infections that have a component of cellulitis, such as osteomyelitis, septic arthritis, myositis, and necrotizing fasciitis. Stasis dermatitis may visually mimic

cellulitis. Patients often present with a rash over areas of increased peripheral edema. Unlike patients with cellulitis, these patients do not have a fever or elevated WBC.

Clinical Example

A 43-year-old male fell 3 weeks ago, injuring his leg. He presented with progressively worsening pain and swelling in his thigh. On examination, cellulitis of the anterior and lateral thigh was manifested by erythema, diffuse and tense swelling with shiny skin, and dramatic pain with knee flexion and tenderness with light palpation (Figure 8–16A). No swelling or erythema of the calf or foot was noted, and distal pulses and sensation were intact. Plain radiographs of the femur were normal. Doppler ultrasound ruled out a deep venous thrombosis but identified diffuse swelling of the muscle compartment. A T_2-weighted MRI depicted characteristic expansion of the subcutaneous tissues with feathery streaks of increased water content circumferentially. It also revealed an underlying fluid collection within the vastus lateralis and intermedius (Figure 8–16B). Surgical inspection of this fluid revealed pus from an underlying myositis. An intramuscular hematoma from nonpenetrating trauma to the thigh had become hematogenously seeded with *S aureus*. The infection caused an expanding abscess with myositis and superficial cellulitis. Culture acquisition, serial irrigation and debridement with open packing, and antibiotic therapy were started. Delayed primary closure and 6 weeks of culture-sensitive IV antibiotics cured the patient's infection. It is important to note in this case that the cellulitis was manifested after the leg began to swell, indicating clinically that the cellulitis was a secondary finding. In this circumstance a search for an underlying cause was necessary to understand the source of infection.

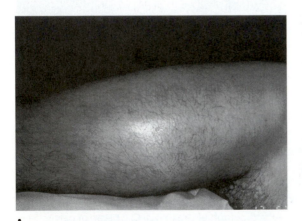

A

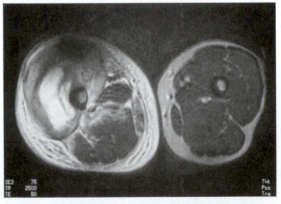

B

Figure 8–16. **A.** Cellulitis and diffuse thigh swelling. **B.** Axial T_2-weighted MRI of the thigh.

PYOMYOSITIS

Pyomyositis is usually due to hematogenous spread of bacteria rather than direct inoculation via penetrating trauma. Usually there is very limited muscle necrosis and a very vascular fibrous reactive capsule contains the abscess. Open exploration with copious irrigation, limited debridement, and primary wound closure over a surgical drain is the surgical treatment of choice. Evaluation for contiguous spread to bone or joint must be performed. Aspiration for culture and insertion of a pigtail catheter for drainage can be done with ultrasound or CT guidance.

Clinical Example

A 6-year-old male presented with a 2-week history of a posterior thigh mass. Focal tenderness and swelling were present, but no erythema was noted (Figure 8–17A). Further inspection revealed numerous insect bites around his ankle and leg that had become open pustules due to vigorous scratching. A T_1-weighted fat-saturated MRI with gadolinium clearly characterized a fluid collection represented by a black signal void (Figure 8–17B). A halo of increased signal uptake along the rim of the fluid collection represents intense localized inflammation. The patient underwent surgical exploration, and pus was easily expressed from the thigh. The wound was debrided, irrigated, and a surgical drainage tube was placed. The wound was primarily closed. Staining revealed gram-positive cocci in clusters, and cultures grew a sensitive *S aureus*. Intravenous antibiotics were initiated, and the patient's symptoms rapidly improved. A week later he was discharged to home with 5 weeks of oral antibiotic that cured his infection.

BURSITIS

Occasionally a bursa will become infected by hematogenous spread or due to open trauma to the overlying skin. The patient complains of pain and stiffness and possibly a fever. A tender, inflamed bursal region is seen clinically with significant erythema and swelling. Because these findings may also occur in acute exacerbations of rheumatism and flair-ups of gout, the patient must be carefully questioned regarding a possible history of these diagnoses. For example, aspiration of a soft, inflamed olecranon tophus may yield fluid that is strikingly similar to pus. Gram stain and polarized microscopy are necessary to identify negatively birefringent crystals.

If infectious bursitis is identified within the first several days, an oral course of antibiotics may successfully treat the infection. If skin erythema spreads and the bursa fills with fluid, the patient must be admitted to the hospital to aspirate and culture the bursal fluid and to begin empiric IV antibiotics. If the infection does not begin to clinically resolve within 48 h, surgical bursectomy and primary closure of the wound over a drain should be performed.

Clinical Example

An 18-year-old female skinned her knee on the gym floor during a game of basketball 1 week prior to presentation. She was noted on exam to have a dramatically painful, swollen, and erythematous prepatellar region with only slight loss of knee motion. A small central eschar, indicative of a floor burn, was observed (Figures 8–18A,B). Gram stain of the aspirate from the prepatellar bursa revealed gram-positive cocci in clus-

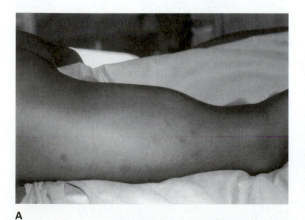

A

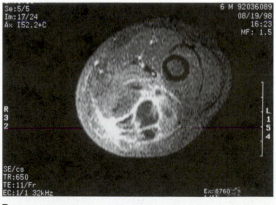

B

Figure 8–17. **A.** Prone patient with focal swelling of the posterior region of the midthigh. Note the insect bites scarring the skin. **B.** T_1-weighted MRI with gadolinium contrast showing dark signal void in center of abscess.

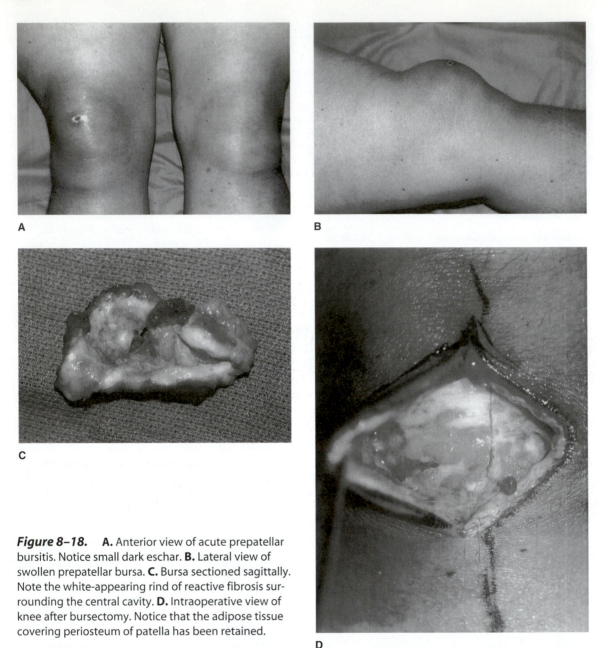

Figure 8–18. **A.** Anterior view of acute prepatellar bursitis. Notice small dark eschar. **B.** Lateral view of swollen prepatellar bursa. **C.** Bursa sectioned sagittally. Note the white-appearing rind of reactive fibrosis surrounding the central cavity. **D.** Intraoperative view of knee after bursectomy. Notice that the adipose tissue covering periosteum of patella has been retained.

ters. Despite 2 days of IV antistaphylococcal antibiotic therapy, the inflammation worsened. A complete bursectomy was performed (Figure 8–18C). A layer of normal appearing fatty tissue was left to cover the surface of the patella (Figure 8–18D), and the wound was closed over a surgical drain. Subsequently the inflammation quickly improved within 3 days, and the pa-

tient was sent home with 3 weeks of culture-specific antibiotics.

NECROTIZING FASCIITIS

Necrotizing fasciitis is a rare but extremely aggressive, life-threatening, soft-tissue infection of the subcuta-

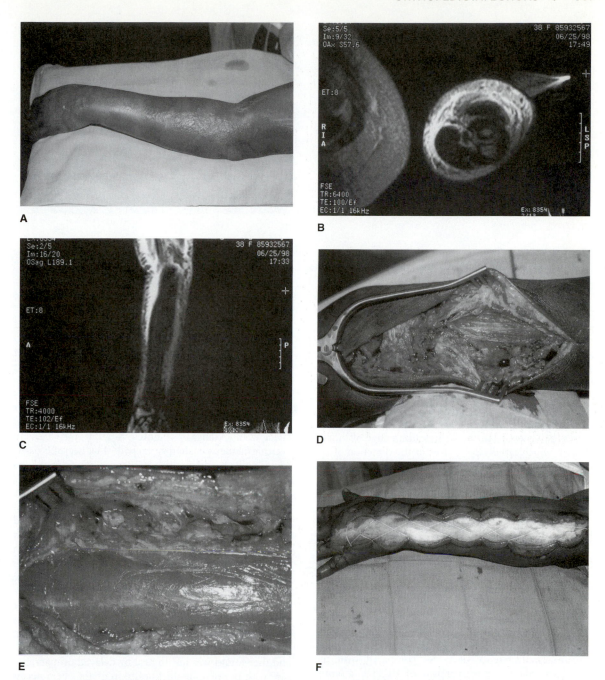

Figure 8–19. **A.** A small draining puncture wound is noted at the middorsum of the hand, and an extensive erythematous rash covers the forearm. **B.** Axial MRI inversion recovery sequence showing circumferential subcutaneous inflammation. **C.** Sagittal MRI inversion recovery sequence showing subcutaneous inflammation but absence of inflammation in muscle tissue. **D.** Dorsal forearm incision revealing extensive subcutaneous necrosis. **E.** Necrosis in subcutaneous tissues but not in muscle tissue. **F.** Open packing of wound with saline-dampened gauze sponges secured with staples and sterile rubber bands in a shoelace fashion.

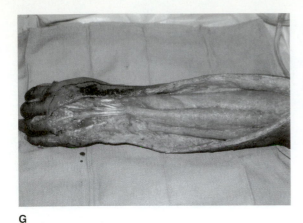

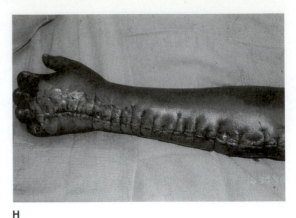

G

H

Figure 8–19. **G.** Appearance of viable wound after 1 week of serial debridements, antibiotics, and hyperbaric oxygen treatments. **H.** Delayed primary closure with interrupted retention sutures.

neous and fascial tissues often encountered in diabetic patients. The muscle tissues are generally spared. Clinical examination of the skin reveals streaking erythema and sometimes small blisters, arising in the region of an incidental puncture wound. Local induration is always found and occasionally subcutaneous crepitance due to gas in the soft tissues is encountered. Air in the soft tissues can usually be seen on plain radiographs in gas-producing clostridial infections (see Figure 8–1). Serial exams are necessary to track the leading edge of the infection, which rapidly progresses in the direction of venous drainage. Emergent surgical debridement of devitalized tissues (sometimes necessitating amputation) along with antibiotics and intensive care treatment for hypotension are required to prevent death.

Clinical Example

A 38-year-old female with a history of insulin-dependent diabetes mellitus sustained a penetrating trauma to the dorsum of her wrist while using scissors. Two days later she presented to the emergency room with a very painful arm and an infected stab wound that was draining serous fluid, an erythematous rash that extended from the wound to her elbow, and an increase of her forearm circumference of 6 cm compared with the other arm. She had a temperature of 101.5°F, a serum WBC of 22,000 with a left shift, and normal plain radiographs of the forearm.

The patient was admitted to the hospital and started empirically on a ticarcillin with clavulanate potassium

(Timentin) and gentamicin. However, after 24 h the arm pain progressively worsened, and the rash advanced above the elbow (Figure 8–19A). MRI showed significant soft-tissue edema in the subcutaneous tissues but not in the muscle compartments (Figures 8–19B and C). Concerned about an uncontrolled necrotizing fasciitis, surgical exploration was emergently performed. Although most of the skin and all of the muscle tissues were viable, necrosis of the subcutaneous tissues and fascia was extensive (Figures 8–19D and E). All necrotic tissue was sharply excised. The necrotic tissue could easily be distinguished because it was friable to palpation. Normal-appearing tissue was firmer, and a finger could not easily dissect the plane between the subcutaneous tissue and the fascia. The wound was copiously irrigated with a pulsatile lavage device and packed open with moist gauze dressings secured with sterile rubber bands and staples in a shoelace fashion (Figure 8–19F). Gram-positive cocci in chains was identified intraoperatively, and the antibiotics were switched to oxacillin and clindamycin. Hyperbaric oxygen treatments using an acute protocol of 2.4 atm for 90 min tid was begun, and daily surgical debridements were performed for 3 days (Figure 8–19G). Some skin died and was debrided. The patient's infection cleared, and the wound was left to heal by delayed primary closure with use of split-thickness skin grafts where necessary (Figure 8–19H).

Foot & Ankle Surgery

Jeffrey A. Mann, MD, Loretta B. Chou, MD, & Steven D. K. Ross, MD

This chapter will discuss the diagnosis and treatment of common acquired and congenital deformities of the foot, arthritis and other pain syndromes affecting the foot, neurologic disorders, and diabetic and rheumatoid manifestations of the foot. Biomechanic principles of the foot and ankle are described, and common sports injuries of the foot and ankle are also discussed. Traumatic injuries to the foot and ankle are discussed in Chapter 3, Musculoskeletal Trauma Surgery.

BIOMECHANIC PRINCIPLES OF THE FOOT & ANKLE

The following is a limited discussion of the biomechanic principles governing the foot and ankle during the gait cycle. The physician must have a clear understanding of these principles to accurately evaluate problems affecting the foot and ankle. Once normal biomechanic function is understood, anatomic and functional abnormalities are more easily detected.

Gait

Gait is the orderly progression of the body through space while expending as little energy as possible. As the body moves through a gait cycle, forces are generated actively, by action of the body's muscles, and passively, by the effects of gravity on the body. To accommodate these forces, the foot is flexible at the time of heel strike, when it must absorb the impact of the body against the ground, and rigid at the time of toe-off, when it must assist in moving the body forward. The magnitude of the forces on the foot increases significantly as the speed of gait increases. For example, when an individual is walking, the initial force with which the foot meets the ground is approximately 80% of body weight, whereas when an individual is jogging, it is approximately 160%. The peak force against the foot during walking is approximately 110% of body weight, whereas for jogging it is approximately 240%. This marked increase probably contributes to some of the injuries seen in runners.

The Walking Cycle

The walking cycle is discussed more extensively in Chapter 1, but pertinent aspects relating to the foot will be discussed here (Figure 9–1).

Observation of the patient while walking may give the clinician insight into the cause of a gait anomaly (Figure 9–2). For example, equinus deformity resulting from spasticity or contracture may cause the toe to make initial contact with the ground rather than the heel. At 7% of the gait cycle, the foot is usually flat on the ground, but spasticity or tightness of the Achilles tendon will cause this to be delayed. At 12% of the cycle, the opposite foot toes off and the swing phase begins. Heel rise of the standing foot begins at 34% of the cycle, as the swinging leg passes the standing limb. Heel rise may be premature in spasticity or prolonged in weakness of the gastrocsoleus muscle. Heel strike of the opposite foot occurs at 50% of the cycle, ending the period of single-limb support; this may occur sooner if there is weakness of the contralateral calf muscle. Toe-off of the opposite foot occurs at 62% of the cycle, at the beginning of the swing phase. These markers of the gait cycle should be kept in mind when observing gait, so pathologic conditions may be identified.

Motions of the Foot & Ankle

The names for various motions about the foot and ankle may be confusing and may be used incorrectly. The motions that occur at the ankle joint are dorsiflexion and plantar flexion. The motions of the heel medially and laterally, which occur in the subtalar joint, are inversion (varus) and eversion (valgus), respectively. The motion occurring at the transverse tarsal joint (talonavicular and calcaneocuboid) is adduction, which is movement toward the midline, and abduction, which is movement away from the midline.

Supination and pronation are terms for two different combinations of movements, but unfortunately these terms are sometimes used in the literature interchangeably. Pronation refers to dorsiflexion of the ankle joint, eversion of the subtalar joint, and abduction of the transverse tarsal joint. Supination is the opposite, namely, plantar flexion of the ankle joint, inversion of the subtalar joint, and adduction of the transverse tarsal joint.

The nomenclature may also be confusing when such terms as forefoot varus and forefoot valgus are used (Figure 9–3). Forefoot varus or valgus is an anatomic deformity that is observed when the hindfoot is placed in neutral position. Neutral position is achieved when the calcaneus is aligned with the long axis of the tibia and

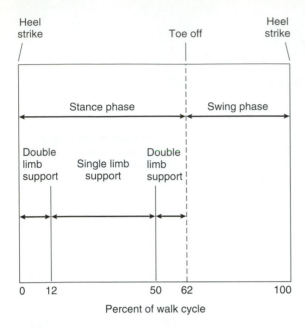

Figure 9–1. Phases of the walking cycle. Stance phase constitutes approximately 62% and swing phase 38% of the cycle. (Reproduced, with permission, from Mann RA, Coughlin MJ: *The Video Textbook of Foot and Ankle Surgery*. St. Louis: Medical Video Productions, 1991.)

the head of the talus is covered with the navicular bone. Forefoot varus deformity is present when the lateral aspect of the forefoot is in greater plantar flexion than the medial aspect. With a flexible deformity, the foot will lie flat on the floor during stance, but with a fixed deformity, excessive weight is borne on the lateral side of the

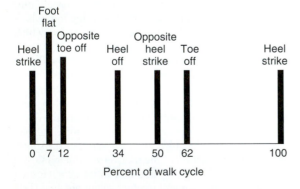

Figure 9–2. Events of the walking cycle. (Reproduced, with permission, from Mann RA, Coughlin MJ: *The Video Textbook of Foot and Ankle Surgery*. St. Louis: Medical Video Productions, 1991.)

foot. As a result, as the weight passes onto the forefoot region, the calcaneus goes into valgus position, and this may result in lateral impingement against the fibula if severe. In forefoot valgus deformity, the medial side of the foot has greater plantar flexion than the lateral side, and this results in excessive weight bearing by the first metatarsal head. To accommodate for this deformity, the calcaneus assumes a varus position, and this may result in a feeling of instability at the ankle joint.

Mechanisms of the Foot During Weight Bearing

As mentioned previously, the normal foot is flexible at the time of heel strike to absorb the impact of striking the ground. As a result, the subtalar joint literally collapses into a position of valgus, causing internal rotation of the tibia and resulting distally in unlocking of the transverse tarsal (talonavicular and calcaneocuboid) joint. Thus, the forefoot is more flexible. The only muscle group that is functioning about the foot and ankle during heel strike is the anterior compartment muscle group, which helps to control the initial rapid plantar flexion following heel strike by an eccentric or lengthening contraction. The flexibility of the foot is greatest at about 7% of the cycle, and a series of changes is then initiated. With the foot fixed to the ground, the body passes over the foot, which lifts the heel up and forces the metatarsophalangeal joints into extension. As this occurs, the foot is converted into a rigid lever that supports the body at the time of toe-off. The mechanisms that bring about conversion of the foot from a flexible to a rigid structure are (1) the tightening of the plantar aponeurosis, (2) the progressive external rotation of the lower extremity, which begins at the pelvis and is passed distally across the ankle joint into the subtalar joint, and (3) the stabilization of the transverse tarsal joint, which results from the progressive inversion of the subtalar joint.

Joints About the Foot & Ankle

A. ANKLE JOINT

The ankle joint consists of the articulation of the talus with the tibia and fibula, with a range of motion of 15 degrees of dorsiflexion and 55 degrees of plantar flexion. The anterior compartment muscles of the leg, the tibialis anterior, and the toe extensors, control plantar flexion of the ankle joint at the time of initial ground contact and provide dorsiflexion of the ankle joint during swing phase. If this muscle group does not function, a footslap is observed at the time of heel strike, and a dropfoot occurs during swing phase. The greatest force across the ankle joint during walking has been calculated to be about 4½ times body weight; this force is present at 40% of the walking cycle.

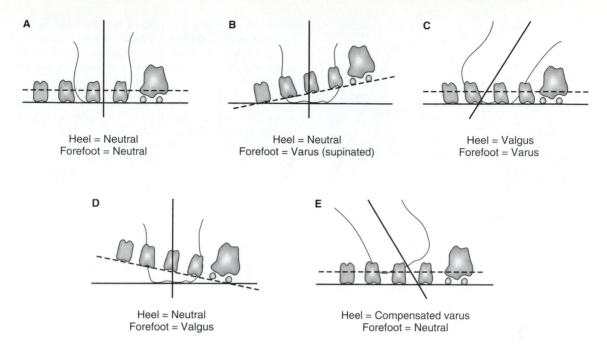

Figure 9–3. Biomechanics of foot posture. **A:** Normal alignment: forefoot perpendicular to heel. **B:** Forefoot varus (uncompensated): lateral aspect of forefoot plantar flexed in relation to medial aspect. **C:** Forefoot varus (compensated): with the forefoot flat on the floor, the heel assumes a valgus position. **D:** Forefoot valgus (uncompensated): medial aspect of forefoot plantar flexed in relation to lateral aspect. **E:** Forefoot valgus (compensated): with the forefoot flat on the floor, the heel assumes a varus position. (Reproduced, with permission, from Mann RA, Coughlin MJ: *The Video Textbook of Foot and Ankle Surgery.* St. Louis: Medical Video Productions, 1991.)

B. Subtalar Joint

The subtalar joint is the articulation between the talus and the calcaneus. The primary joint surface is the posterior facet, with much smaller middle and anterior facets. The motion of this joint is inversion of approximately 30 degrees and eversion of approximately 10 degrees. The tibialis posterior causes inversion and the peroneus brevis eversion at the subtalar joint. At the time of initial ground contact, eversion is a passive mechanism and occurs because of the shape of the articulations and their ligamentous support. Inversion occurs both actively and passively at the time of toe-off. Active control is achieved by the gastrocsoleus and posterior tibial muscles, and passive inversion occurs by the action of the plantar aponeurosis, the external rotation of the lower extremity, and the oblique metatarsal break.

C. Talonavicular Joint and Calcaneocuboid Joint

These two joints functionally act as a unit known as the transverse tarsal joint. Motion at the transverse tarsal joint is approximately 10 degrees of abduction and approximately 15 degrees of adduction. The head of the talus is firmly seated into the navicular at the time of toe-off, adding stability to the foot. The stability of the transverse tarsal joint is controlled by the position of the subtalar joint. When the subtalar joint is in an inverted position, the axes of these two joints are nonparallel, giving rise to increased stability of the hindfoot. When the calcaneus is in an everted position at the time of heel strike, these joints are parallel to one another, thereby giving rise to increased flexibility of these joints (Figure 9–4). The clinical implication is that when carrying out a subtalar arthrodesis, placement of the subtalar joint into a varus position locks the transverse tarsal joint, causing increased stiffness of the forefoot and, frequently, discomfort. When the hindfoot is everted into a position of 5–7 degrees of valgus, the flexibility of the transverse tarsal joint is maintained. This allows the forefoot to be more supple and makes ambulation easier.

D. Metatarsophalangeal Joints

The motion at these joints is between 50 and 70 degrees of dorsiflexion and 15–25 degrees of plantar flexion. The role of the metatarsophalangeal joints during

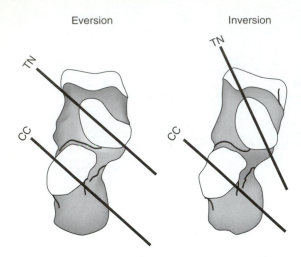

Eversion   Inversion

Figure 9–4. The function of the transverse tarsal joint as described by Elftman demonstrates that when the calcaneus is in eversion, the resultant axes of the talonavicular and calcaneocuboid joints are parallel or congruent. When the subtalar joint is in an inverted position, the axes are incongruent, giving increased stability to the midfoot. (Reproduced, with permission, from Mann RA, Coughlin MJ: *The Video Textbook of Foot and Ankle Surgery*. St. Louis: Medical Video Productions, 1991.)

gait is discussed in the section on Deformities of the First Toe.

E. THE PLANTAR APONEUROSIS

Although the plantar aponeurosis is not an articulation per se, it probably plays the predominant role in the overall stability of the foot. The plantar aponeurosis arises from the tubercle of the calcaneus and passes distally to insert into the base of each proximal phalanx (Figure 9–5). As the metatarsophalangeal joints pass into dorsiflexion in the last half of the stance phase, the rigidity of the plantar aponeurosis forces the metatarsal heads into a plantarward direction, which raises the longitudinal arch. This is known as a windlass mechanism. The now-rigid foot provides support to the body for the push-off phase of gait. Secondarily, this mechanism also helps bring about inversion of the subtalar joint.

F. GAIT ABNORMALITIES

The following is a brief description of the more common gait abnormalities.

1. Dropfoot gait—In dropfoot gait, there is lack of ankle dorsiflexion, resulting in plantar flexion at the ankle joint. When walking, these patients adopt a step-page-type gait. This gait pattern is manifested by increased flexion of the hip and knee to enable the swinging leg to clear the ground. If this compensatory mechanism does not occur, the patient may catch the toes on the ground.

2. Equinus gait—An equinus gait pattern is one in which the ankle joint is fixed in plantar flexion throughout the entire gait cycle. This may result from a stroke or head injury, trauma to the lower extremity, or a congenital deformity, and often is associated with tightness of the posterior capsule. This gait pattern is characterized by forefoot floor contact (no heel contact). The anterior loading of the foot results in a back knee thrust, which may, over a long period of time, result in a hyperextension deformity of the knee. A weak quadriceps muscle may accentuate this problem.

3. Cavus deformity—A cavus deformity is an excessive elevation of the longitudinal arch. A moderate decrease in the range of motion of the foot usually accompanies this deformity. In addition, the hindfoot is often in a varus posture and the forefoot in valgus posture. This is most frequently observed in Charcot-Marie-Tooth disease but may also be seen in poliomyelitis and occasionally as a late result of calf compartment syndrome. The deformity significantly diminishes the overall surface available for weight bearing in these patients. Clawing of the toes may further reduce contact with the ground. Thus, the gait pattern in these patients is altered, with increased pressure on the heel at initial ground contact, followed by increased pressure along the lateral side of the foot and underneath the first metatarsal head as the gait cycle progresses.

4. Pes planus deformity—The patient with a pes planus deformity demonstrates just the opposite of cavus deformity; the foot is too flexible. At the time of initial ground contact, there is excessive valgus of the hindfoot and in severe cases breaking down of the longitudinal arch with an associated abduction of the forefoot. This results in an increased weight-bearing surface and often easy fatigability because of the lack of adequate support of the longitudinal arch.

Cavanaugh PR: The biomechanics of lower extremity action in distance running. Foot Ankle 1987;7:197.

Mann RA: Biomechanics of the foot and ankle. In Mann RA, Coughlin MJ (editors): *Surgery of the Foot and Ankle*. St. Louis: Mosby-Year Book, 1993.

Mann RA et al: Running symposium. Foot Ankle 1981;1:190.

Saunders JBDM et al: The major determinants in normal and pathologic gait. J Bone Joint Surg Am 1953;35:543.

Stiehl JB: *Inman's Joints of the Ankle*. Philadelphia: Williams and Wilkins, 1991.

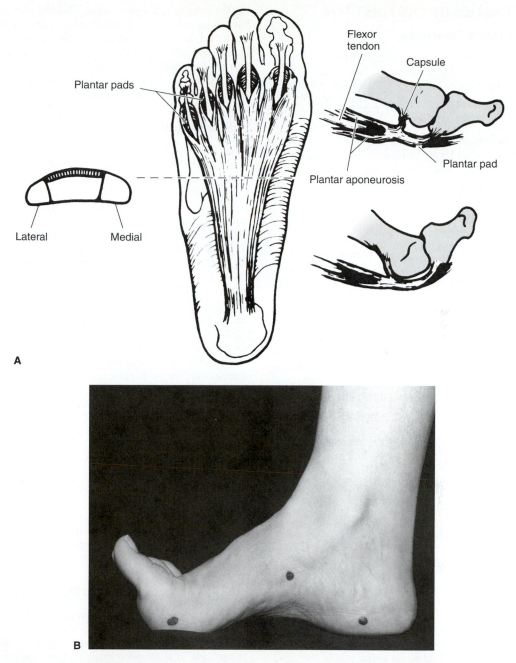

Figure 9–5. Windlass mechanism. **A:** The plantar aponeurosis, which arises from the tubercle of the calcaneus, divides and inserts into the base of each of the proximal phalanges. **B:** Dorsiflexion of the metatarsophalangeal joints wraps the plantar aponeurosis around the metatarsal head, depressing the metatarsal heads and elevating the longitudinal arch. (Reproduced, with permission, from Mann RA, Coughlin MJ: *The Video Textbook of Foot and Ankle Surgery.* St. Louis: Medical Video Productions, 1991.)

DEFORMITIES OF THE FIRST TOE

Biomechanic Principles

The first metatarsophalangeal joint functions mainly as a weight-bearing structure and stabilizer of the medial aspect of the longitudinal arch. The static stability of the first metatarsophalangeal joint is provided by the collateral ligaments and the strong plantar plate, which consists of the plantar aponeurosis and the joint capsule. Added dynamic stability is provided by the abductor hallucis and adductor hallucis muscles, which insert along the medial and lateral sides of the metatarsal head, respectively. No muscle inserts into the metatarsal head per se, and therefore it is suspended in a sling of muscles and tendons. This allows the metatarsal head to be pushed in a medial or lateral direction, depending on the deviation of the proximal phalanx.

As previously discussed, the plantar aponeurosis forces the metatarsal heads into plantar flexion during the last third of the stance phase of the walking cycle. As a result, pressure that is present under the metatarsal heads is transferred to the toes, especially the hallux (see Figure 9–5). If this windlass mechanism for the hallux is lost as occurs in a bunion deformity, then pressure is no longer transferred to the toes but remains beneath the metatarsal heads. Metatarsalgia results from this transfer of load, especially beneath the lesser metatarsal heads. The second metatarsal frequently bears the load because the weight-bearing ability of the first metatarsal is disrupted.

Any type of surgical procedure that disrupts this mechanism may result in the development of transfer lesions as well. This problem can be seen after the Keller arthroplasty, in which the base of the proximal phalanx is removed, or after prosthetic replacement of the first metatarsal joint. Metatarsal osteotomy with excessive shortening (> 5–7 mm) or dorsiflexion of the first metatarsal may also cause this problem.

Normal Anatomy

The first metatarsophalangeal joint consists of the articulating surfaces of the metatarsal head and the base of the proximal phalanx. On the plantar aspect of the foot beneath the metatarsal head are the two sesamoid bones, which are embedded in the dual tendons of the flexor hallucis brevis and lie on either side of the crista. Medially and laterally, the collateral ligaments stabilize the metatarsophalangeal joint, and toward the plantar surface, they blend with the adductor and abductor hallucis tendons along the lateral and medial sides of the joint. Further toward the plantar surface, the sesamoids are stabilized by the firm attachment of the encapsulating plantar aponeurosis, which inserts into the base of the proximal phalanx. Plantar to the sesamoids passes the flexor hallucis longus tendon. Dorsally, the extensor hallucis longus tendon is stabilized by a medial and lateral hood mechanism similar to that present in the hand, and the extensor digitorum brevis muscle inserts into the proximal phalanx along the lateral aspect of the joint. Normal motion of the metatarsophalangeal joint consists of dorsiflexion and plantar flexion.

Hallux Valgus

The most common deformity of the metatarsophalangeal joint is hallux valgus or "bunion" deformity, which results from the lateral deviation of the proximal phalanx and the resultant medially directed pressure exerted against the metatarsal head. The medial eminence becomes prominent as the proximal phalanx drifts into a valgus position. Attenuation of the medial joint capsule and contracture of the lateral joint capsule occur. As the metatarsal head is pushed medially, the sesamoids, which are firmly anchored by the adductor hallucis tendon and transverse metatarsal ligament, slowly erode the crista. Eventually the sesamoids subluxate from underneath the first metatarsal, with the fibular sesamoid lying in the first web space. The extensor hallucis longus and flexor hallucis longus, which insert into the base of the distal phalanx, also deviate in a lateralward direction and contribute to the progressive hallux valgus deformity. As the deformity becomes more severe, both the extrinsic and intrinsic muscles lie lateral to the longitudinal axis of the first metatarsophalangeal joint, thereby further enhancing the deformity. As the deformity becomes more severe, pronation of the great toe occurs. Attenuation of the weakest portion of the capsule (the dorsomedial aspect) allows the abductor hallucis tendon to slide beneath the metatarsal head and rotate the proximal phalanx into a position of pronation. More rapid progression of the deformity may occur in a small percentage of patients whose first metatarsocuneiform joint demonstrates a significant degree of instability.

Etiology of Hallux Valgus Deformity

Hallux valgus deformity occurs in women approximately 10 times more frequently than in men. The incidence is also significantly higher in persons who wear shoes than in those who do not. The conclusion can therefore be made that a major contributing cause of hallux valgus deformity is wearing tight, pointed-toed shoes that women often wear. Other factors that may contribute to hallux valgus are congenital deformity or predisposition, severe flatfoot deformity, chronic tightness of the Achilles tendon, spasticity, hypermobility of the first metatarsocuneiform joint, and systemic disease such as rheumatoid arthritis.

Clinical Findings

A. HISTORY

The clinical evaluation of hallux valgus deformity begins with a careful history to obtain the chief complaint. The chief complaint may be primarily medial eminence pain, plantar first metatarsal or lesser metatarsal head pain, impingement upon the second toe, resultant deformities of the lesser toes, or the inability to wear certain shoes. The examiner should ask about factors that seem to aggravate the discomfort, the patient's occupation and level of athletic endeavors, and what type of shoe is most commonly worn.

B. PHYSICAL EXAMINATION

The physical examination starts with the patient in a standing position to observe the degree of deformity of the great toe and lesser toes. The overall posture of the foot is noted. The patient's gait is observed, looking for evidence of abnormal ground contact or early heel rise, which would indicate possible tightness of the Achilles tendon. In the seated position, the range of motion of the ankle, subtalar, transverse tarsal, and metatarsophalangeal joints is noted. The neurovascular status of the foot is carefully assessed, noting venous stasis changes. Doppler studies are obtained if there is any question regarding the circulatory status of the foot. The plantar aspect of the foot is examined for abnormal callus formation, particularly beneath the metatarsal head and along the medial aspect of the great toe.

The motion of the first metatarsophalangeal joint is carefully observed in its deformed position and after the toe is carefully brought back toward normal alignment. Restriction of motion gives the clinician insight into the degree of surgical correction that can be obtained at the joint without impairing motion of the joint. The first metatarsocuneiform joint is examined for hypermobility by moving it in a dorsomedial and plantolateral direction.

C. IMAGING STUDIES

The radiographic evaluation consists of weight-bearing anteroposterior, lateral, and oblique radiographs. From these radiographs, the following measurements are made:

(1) The hallux valgus angle is the angle created by the intersection of the lines that longitudinally bisect the proximal phalanx and first metatarsal. A normal angle is less than 15 degrees (Figure 9–6A).

(2) The intermetatarsal angle is defined as the angle created by the intersection of the lines bisecting the first and second metatarsal shafts. This angle should be less than 9 degrees.

(3) The distal metatarsal articular angle measures the relationship of the distal articulating surface of the first metatarsal to the long axis of the metatarsal. Normally there is less than 10 degrees of lateral deviation (Figure 9–6B).

(4) A determination is made as to whether or not the first metatarsophalangeal joint is congruent or incongruent. A congruent joint is one in which no lateral subluxation of the proximal phalanx occurs on the metatarsal head; an incongruent joint is one in which lateral subluxation of the proximal phalanx on the metatarsal head does occur (Figure 9–7).

(5) The shape of the metatarsocuneiform joint is observed, looking for evidence of excessive medial deviation of this articulation. This observation alerts the examiner to the fact that hypermobility may be present.

(6) The presence of arthrosis of the metatarsophalangeal joint is evaluated, as characterized by narrowing or osteophyte formation about the joint.

(7) The size of the medial eminence is measured by a line drawn down the medial aspect of the first metatarsal shaft.

(8) The presence of a hallux valgus interphalangeus is characterized by lateral deviation of the proximal or distal phalanx, or both, in relation to a line drawn across the base of the proximal phalanx. Normal is considered up to approximately 10 degrees of lateral deviation.

Treatment

A. NONOPERATIVE TREATMENT

The patient should be encouraged to wear shoes of adequate size and shape. This simple form of management may relieve most symptoms.

A variety of pads are available to address symptoms that occur due to the bunion deformity. Pads may be placed in the first web space or over the median eminence to help take pressure off of a painful median eminence. Pads are also available that can be placed underneath the metatarsal heads to take pressure off painful calluses or sesamoids.

If after adequate conservative management the patient continues to have discomfort, surgical intervention may be considered. Surgery is not performed for cosmetic reasons or to allow patients to wear fashionable shoes, but rather to correct a symptomatic structural deformity.

Juvenile hallux valgus deformity presents a significant problem in management, but as a general rule, conservative management should be continued until

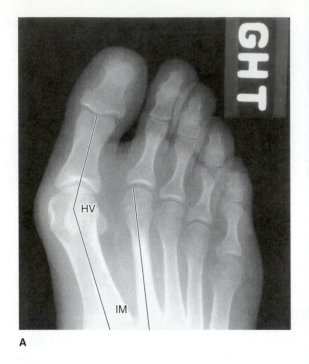

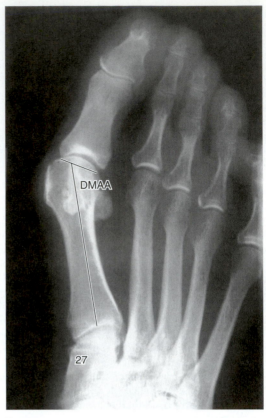

Figure 9–6. Radiologic evaluation. **A:** Hallux valgus (HV) and intermetatarsal (IM) angles. **B:** Distal metatarsal articular angle (DMAA = 27). (Reproduced, with permission, from Mann RA, Coughlin MJ: *The Video Textbook of Foot and Ankle Surgery.* St. Louis: Medical Video Productions, 1991.)

growth has been completed, after which surgery may be considered. Extra care must be taken into consideration in the juvenile population where cosmetic appearance may play a greater role in the patient's or parents' desire for surgery.

Hallux valgus surgery is generally contraindicated in high-performance athletes or dancers until they are no longer able to perform at the level necessary to continue in their vocation or avocation. Premature surgery in these individuals may diminish their special abilities.

B. SURGICAL TREATMENT:

1. Algorithm for surgical treatment—If surgery is being considered, the patient's chief complaint, the physical findings, and the radiographic measurements must be correlated to enable the surgeon to select the best procedure. No single procedure will succeed for all hallux valgus deformities, and careful preoperative planning is essential.

The following factors need to be considered in the decision-making process:

(1) patient's chief complaint;

(2) physical findings;

(3) degree of hallux valgus and intermetatarsal angle;

(4) distal metatarsal articular angle;

(5) congruency or incongruency of the metatarsophalangeal joint;

(6) presence of arthrosis of the joint;

(7) degree of pronation of the hallux;

(8) age of the patient;

(9) circulatory status; and

(10) patient expectations for outcome of operation.

The algorithm (Figure 9–8) divides hallux valgus deformities into three main groups: those with a congruent joint, those with an incongruent joint, and those

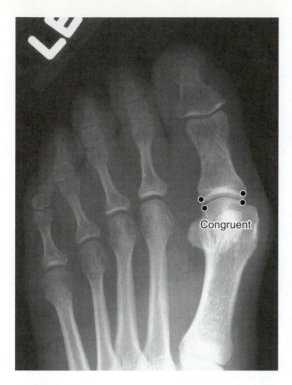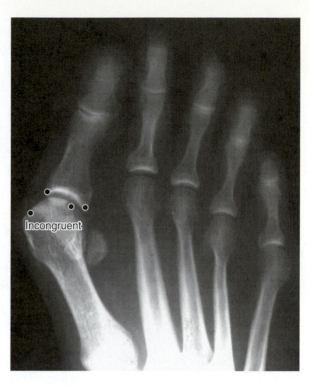

Figure 9–7. **Left:** Congruent joint. **Right:** Incongruent joint. (Reproduced, with permission, from Mann RA, Coughlin MJ: *The Video Textbook of Foot and Ankle Surgery*. St. Louis: Medical Video Productions, 1991.)

associated with degenerative joint disease. The algorithm lists the operative procedure that may best correct the deformity within each classification. Although no one scheme is all-inclusive, this algorithm is helpful in organizing the treatment plan.

In using this algorithm, the first question to ask is if the deformity is congruent or incongruent. A congruent metatarsophalangeal joint implies that the goal is mainly treatment of an enlarged medial eminence, and little or no correction of the stable metatarsophalangeal is required. For the congruent joint, a chevron procedure or Akin procedure with removal of the medial eminence usually results in satisfactory correction.

If the deformity is incongruent to the degree that the proximal phalanx is subluxed laterally on the metatarsal head, a procedure that moves the proximal phalanx back onto the metatarsal head is required. The procedure of choice depends upon the severity of the deformity (see Figure 9–8).

If the first metatarsocuneiform joint is hypermobile, the distal soft-tissue procedure with a metatarsocuneiform arthrodesis should be considered. Generally, in the patient with advanced hallux valgus deformity and degenerative joint disease, arthrodesis of the joint is indicated. If routine hallux valgus repair is attempted in

the patient with advanced arthrosis, stiffness of the metatarsophalangeal joint frequently results. Use of a prosthetic replacement, as a general rule, will not produce a satisfactory long-term result, particularly in active individuals.

2. Surgical procedures—

a. Distal soft-tissue procedure—The distal soft-tissue procedure was previously referred to as the McBride procedure, which was first modified by DuVries and subsequently modified further and given its current designation. The procedure is indicated for mild hallux valgus deformity, usually with an intermetatarsal angle of less than 12–13 degrees and a hallux valgus deformity of less than 30 degrees. Within this range of deformity, a satisfactory outcome can usually be anticipated from this procedure.

The procedure requires releasing the soft-tissue contracture on the lateral side of the metatarsophalangeal joint, including the lateral joint capsule, the adductor hallucis tendon, and the transverse metatarsal ligament (Figure 9–9). On the medial side of the metatarsophalangeal joint, the medial eminence is removed 2–3 mm medial to the sagittal sulcus and in line with the medial aspect of the metatarsal shaft. The capsule on the me-

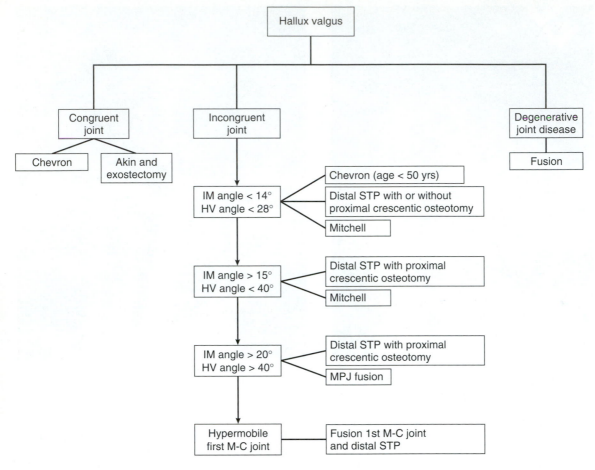

Figure 9–8. Algorithm for hallux valgus deformities. STP = soft-tissue procedure, M-C = metatarsocuneiform, and MPJ = metatarsal phalangeal joint. (Redrawn, with permission, from Mann RA, Coughlin MJ: *The Video Textbook of Foot and Ankle Surgery.* St. Louis: Medical Video Productions, 1991.)

dial side of the joint is plicated to hold the toe in correct alignment. Postoperatively, the patient is maintained in a firm compression dressing, which is changed on a weekly basis for 8 weeks. During this period, the patient is permitted to ambulate in a postoperative shoe.

The most common complication consists of recurrence of the deformity, usually because the deformity was too severe to be corrected by the procedure. In these cases, a metatarsal osteotomy added to the distal soft-tissue procedure would complete the correction.

Hallux varus deformity is a medial deviation of the proximal phalanx on the metatarsal head, a complication that may occur in approximately 5–7% of cases. This deformity is usually a result of excessive excision of the medial eminence or fibular sesamoidectomy, which causes joint instability. Occasionally, the medial joint

capsule is overplicated or the lateral joint capsule fails to attain adequate strength. Mild hallux varus deformity, up to 7–10 degrees, usually is of no clinical significance unless the joint is also hyperextended.

b. Distal soft-tissue procedure with proximal metatarsal osteotomy—The addition of the proximal metatarsal osteotomy to the distal soft-tissue procedure significantly expands the capability of this procedure to correct hallux valgus deformity. If the intermetatarsal angle exceeds 13 degrees, the degree of deformity between the first and second metatarsal will prevent adequate correction of alignment of the metatarsophalangeal joint with the distal soft-tissue procedure alone. Realignment of the fixed bony deformity present between the first and second metatarsals permits the combined procedure to be used for deformities with up to

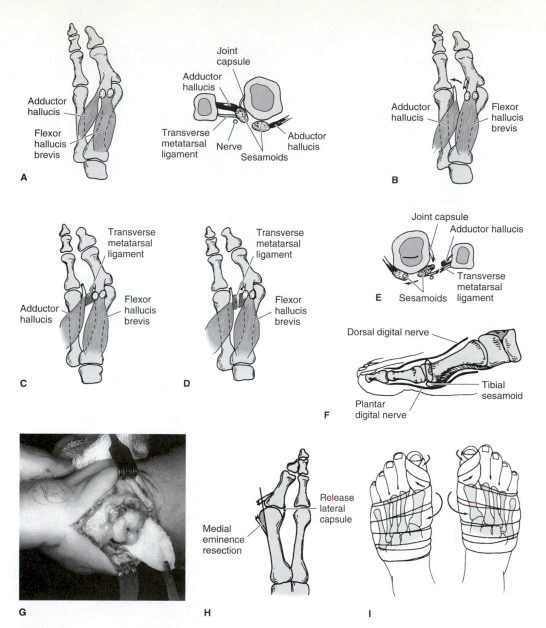

Figure 9–9. Distal soft-tissue procedure. **A:** The adductor tendon inserts into the lateral aspect of the fibular sesamoid and into the base of the proximal phalanx. **B:** The adductor tendon has been removed from its insertion into the lateral side of the fibular sesamoid and base of the proximal phalanx. **C:** The transverse metatarsal ligament is passed from the second metatarsal into the fibular sesamoid. **D:** The transverse metatarsal ligament has been transected. **E:** The three contracted structures on the lateral side of the metatarsophalangeal joint have been released. **F:** The medial capsular incision begins 2–3 mm proximal to the base of the proximal phalanx, and a flap of tissue measuring 3–8 mm is removed. **G:** The medial eminence is exposed by creating a flap of capsule that is based proximally and plantarward. **H:** The medial eminence is removed in line with the medial aspect of the first metatarsal. **I:** The postoperative dressings are critical. Note that the metatarsal heads are firmly bound with the gauze, and that the great toe is rotated so as to keep the sesamoids realigned beneath the metatarsal head. This necessitates dressing the right great toe in a counterclockwise direction and the left great toe in a clockwise direction when one is standing at the foot of the bed. (Reproduced, with permission, from Mann RA, Coughlin MJ: *The Video Textbook of Foot and Ankle Surgery*. St. Louis: Medical Video Productions, 1991.)

50 degrees of hallux valgus and a 25-degree inter-metatarsal angle.

In carrying out this operative procedure, the distal soft-tissue procedure is performed as described earlier. The metatarsal osteotomy is carried out through a third incision, which is centered over the dorsal aspect of the base of the metatarsal shaft. The most commonly used osteotomy is a crescentic-shaped osteotomy whose concavity is directed proximally (Figure 9–10). This enables the surgeon to rotate the metatarsal head laterally as the metatarsocuneiform joint is pushed in a medial-ward direction. This usually results in approximately 2–3 mm of lateral displacement of the osteotomy site. Stabilization is carried out with a screw, which passes from distal to proximal. Other types of osteotomies have been used to realign the first metatarsal, including oblique, chevron-shaped and closing wedge osteotomies.

Postoperatively, the treatment is the same as for the distal soft-tissue procedure, with 8 weeks of dressing changes and immobilization in a postoperative shoe. As a general rule, cast immobilization is not necessary.

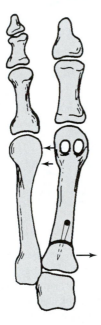

Figure 9–10. The osteotomy site is reduced by pushing the proximal fragment medially with a small freer while pushing the metatarsal head laterally. This locks the lateral side of the osteotomy site so the internal fixation can be inserted. (Reproduced, with permission, from Mann RA, Coughlin MJ: *The Video Textbook of Foot and Ankle Surgery.* St. Louis: Medical Video Productions, 1991.)

The postoperative results following the distal soft-tissue procedure with proximal osteotomy result in greater than 90% patient satisfaction. The addition of the osteotomy does create an increased risk of complications. Dorsiflexion of the osteotomy site may occur, but this is usually not of clinical significance. Nonunion of the osteotomy may develop in 1% of cases. Excessive lateral displacement of the metatarsal head can result in hallux varus deformity, which is more resistant to treatment than when osteotomy is not included.

c. Chevron procedure—The chevron procedure is usually indicated for hallux valgus deformity of less than 30 degrees, with an intermetatarsal angle of less than 12 degrees. The distal metatarsal articular angle should not be more than 12 degrees, or complete correction will not be obtained. The operative procedure is based upon lateral translation of the metatarsal head, along with plication of the medial joint capsule. The joint is approached surgically through a medial incision, the capsule opened, and the medial eminence removed. A chevron-shaped cut with the apex based distally is carried out and translated laterally approximately 3–4 mm. The medial bony prominence created by the shift of the metatarsal head is excised and the medial joint capsule plicated. The osteotomy site is fixed with a pin or a screw (Figure 9–11).

Postoperatively, the foot is firmly bandaged for 6–8 weeks, and the patient is permitted to ambulate in a postoperative shoe. If a pin has been used for fixation, it is removed after 4 weeks.

Uniformly good results have been reported following a chevron procedure. If it is used to correct a deformity that is too severe, the outcome may be unsuccessful. The most serious complication, occurring in 1–2% of cases, is avascular necrosis of the metatarsal head, which is probably the result of extensive stripping of the soft tissue surrounding the head. As with any type of osteotomy, the distal fragment is capable of migrating either too far laterally or medially, giving rise either to hallux varus deformity or recurrent hallux valgus deformity. Occasionally, arthrofibrosis of the joint is noted, resulting in significant joint stiffness.

d. Akin procedure—The Akin procedure consists of a medial closing wedge osteotomy at the base of the proximal phalanx. This procedure is used along with simple excision of the median eminence or with a chevron procedure to correct a hallux valgus deformity with a congruent joint. The Akin procedure is indicated for a hallux valgus deformity of less than 25 degrees, with an intermetatarsal angle of 12 degrees or less.

The operative procedure consists of a medial approach to the base of the proximal phalanx and the me-

Figure 9–11. Chevron procedure. **A:** The apex of the chevron osteotomy starts in the center of the metatarsal head and is brought proximally. The plantar aspect of the line of the osteotomy should be proximal to the joint capsule, thereby avoiding the sesamoid bones. **B:** The osteotomy site is displaced laterally 20–30% of the width of the shaft. (Reproduced, with permission, from Mann RA, Coughlin MJ: *The Video Textbook of Foot and Ankle Surgery.* St. Louis: Medical Video Productions, 1991.)

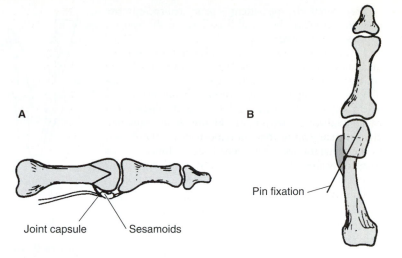

Joint capsule   Sesamoids

Pin fixation

dian eminence. After removing the median eminence in line with the metatarsal, a wedge of bone is removed from the medial aspect of the proximal phalanx. The osteotomy is closed down and stabilized internally with sutures or wires, or externally with a K-wire. Dressings are applied for 6–8 weeks postoperatively.

e. **Keller procedure**—The Keller procedure is reserved for the older, less active patient, in a patient prone to skin problems, or in the case of an arthritic joint. This procedure is contraindicated in an active person.

The procedure consists of removal of the base of the proximal phalanx, which decompresses the metatarsophalangeal joint, and excision of the medial eminence. An attempt is made to reapproximate the intrinsic muscles that have been detached by placing them into the remaining stump of bone (Figure 9–12). As a rule, a longitudinal pin is used to stabilize the operative site for approximately 4 weeks.

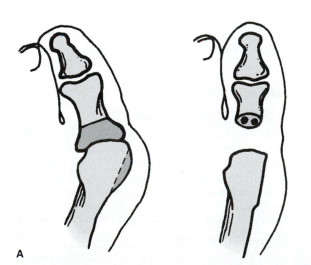

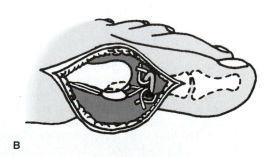

A   B

Figure 9–12. Keller procedure. **A:** The medial eminence is removed in line with the medial aspect of the metatarsal shaft. The proximal third of the proximal phalanx is removed. **B:** An attempt is made to reapproximate the plantar and medial capsular structures to the remaining base of the proximal phalanx. (Reproduced, with permission, from Mann RA, Coughlin MJ: *The Video Textbook of Foot and Ankle Surgery.* St. Louis: Medical Video Productions, 1991.)

Postoperatively, the patient is permitted to ambulate in a postoperative shoe, and dressings are changed for approximately 6 weeks.

Results in the older patient with low functional demand are satisfactory. If the procedure is used in a younger patient, a certain degree of instability and loss of weight bearing by the first metatarsophalangeal joint occurs, because the base of the proximal phalanx has been removed. There is significant loss of foot function, and a transfer lesion may develop beneath the second metatarsal head because the great toe no longer carries adequate weight. Often, the metatarsophalangeal joint becomes cocked upward and into varus.

f. Arthrodesis of the first metatarsophalangeal joint—Arthrodesis of the first metatarsophalangeal joint is indicated in the patient with hallux valgus who also has advanced degenerative arthrosis of the joint, or as a salvage procedure following a previously failed surgical attempt to realign the metatarsophalangeal joint. The procedure is also indicated in the patient with advanced hallux valgus deformity that cannot be corrected by the previously described procedures. Hallux valgus deformity in which the proximal phalanx is subluxed more than 50% of the metatarsal head, or one with a significant degree of stiffness about the metatarsophalangeal joint should be considered for fusion.

The arthrodesis is carried out by creating two flat surfaces or a ball-and-socket type of configuration. The arthrodesis site is stabilized with an interfragmentary screw and plate, or Steinmann pins if the bone stock is poor. The position of the arthrodesis is critical. The joint should be placed in 15–20 degrees of valgus and 10–15 degrees of dorsiflexion in relation to the ground or the plantar aspect of the foot. In relation to the first metatarsal shaft, which is inclined plantarward approximately 15 degrees, it should be in approximately 30 degrees of dorsiflexion (Figure 9–13). Any pronation that is present must also be corrected at the same time.

The patient must wear a postoperative shoe until arthrodesis occurs in 10–12 weeks. The unreliable patient should be treated in a short leg walking cast until fusion has occurred.

The main complication associated with arthrodesis of the first metatarsophalangeal joint is malposition. If the toe is not placed into adequate dorsiflexion or valgus, excessive stress occurs against the interphalangeal joint, which may result in a painful arthritic condition of the joint. The fusion rate is approximately 95%. Occasionally, the degree of valgus and dorsiflexion is correct but the toe is left in a pronated position, which will result in pressure along the medial side of the interphalangeal joint and possible discomfort.

The patient's gait following arthrodesis of the first metatarsophalangeal joint in proper alignment is most

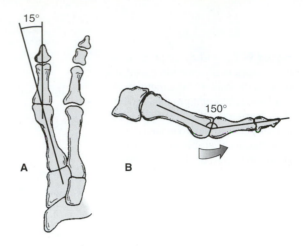

Figure 9–13. Arthrodesis of the first metatarsophalangeal joint. **A:** The joint is placed into about 15 degrees of valgus. **B:** The joint is placed into approximately 10–15 degrees of dorsiflexion in relation to the floor, which is approximately 25–30 degrees of dorsiflexion in relation to the first metatarsal shaft. (Reproduced, with permission, from Mann RA, Coughlin MJ: *The Video Textbook of Foot and Ankle Surgery.* St. Louis: Medical Video Productions, 1991.)

satisfactory. These patients are able to roll over the fusion site and have little or no difficulty carrying out everyday activities. Squatting is the only activity that is difficult because the toe must be in full dorsiflexion when this activity is carried out. Patients are able to return to most types of athletic activities, although at a somewhat slower pace.

Hallux Rigidus

A. General Considerations

Hallux rigidus or first metatarsophalangeal joint arthritis is a relatively common problem, often affecting people at a much younger age than arthritis of other joints. Hallux rigidus is seen in patients from their 30s onward. The reason why arthritis of this joint is seen in younger patients is unclear but may be associated with an unrecognized chondral injury to the metatarsal head.

B. Clinical Findings

Patients present with complaints of joint stiffness and pain with dorsiflexion of the joint. The symptoms are worse with increased physical activities. Patients also complain of a painful dorsal prominence over the metatarsal neck that makes shoe wear uncomfortable. Radiographs show varying degrees of joint space narrowing and, invariably, a large osteophyte on the dorsal aspect of the metatarsal neck.

C. Conservative Treatment

Conservative treatment consists of NSAIDs and wearing a stiff-soled shoe with a deep toe box. In older, sedentary, patients, these measures are usually adequate. In more active individuals, however, surgical treatment is usually indicated.

D. Surgical Treatment

Several surgical treatment methods are available for treating hallux rigidus. Resection of the dorsal bone spur, known as cheilectomy, is efficacious and the least intrusive surgical option. Approximately 25% of the dorsal aspect of the metatarsal head is removed along with the bone spur, and a thorough synovectomy of the joint is performed. Postoperatively, patients regain up to 50% of their dorsiflexion and are generally quite satisfied with their decreased levels of pain and improved physical abilities. This procedure is less likely to have a favorable outcome on joints with advanced arthritis.

A resection arthroplasty (Keller procedure) can be used on older, less active patients, but has a high rate of complications, as previously discussed. Prosthetic replacement of the arthritic first metatarsophalangeal joint can be used in older, lower demand patients but has been shown to have high rates of failure in younger, more active individuals.

First metatarsophalangeal joint arthrodesis provides predictable pain relief and longevity for advanced arthritis. The drawback is that of lost motion at the joint. However, patients can remain quite active with a first metatarsophalangeal joint fusion as described previously.

Sesamoid Disorders

A. General Considerations

The two sesamoid bones on the plantar aspect of the first metatarsophalangeal joint can become painful for a variety of reasons. Fractures, osteonecrosis, arthritis, and subluxation can affect these small bones. Often they can become painful for no clear reason, a condition referred to as sesamoiditis.

B. Clinical Findings

The patient with a painful sesamoid complains of discomfort on the plantar aspect of the foot, directly under the affected bone. The pain is worse with weight-bearing activities. The history may be significant for a trauma to the toe causing a fracture, but most commonly, the pain has an insidious onset.

C. Physical Examination

The painful sesamoid is determined by direct palpation. Postural abnormalities of the foot that may be contributing to the condition are evaluated. For example, hallux valgus deformity may cause a subluxation of the sesamoid from its normal articulation with the plantar aspect of the metatarsal head, causing pain.

D. Radiographic Findings

Radiographs of the foot are taken, including a skyline or sesamoid view, which is a tangential view of the sesamoid metatarsal head articulation. Abnormalities may be seen, such as subluxation of the sesamoids in the case of hallux valgus, fragmentation as seen in osteonecrosis, or joint space narrowing seen in the case of arthritis. Displaced fractures are easy to determine, but nondisplaced fractures may be difficult to distinguish from a bipartite sesamoid that is a normal finding. A bone scan may be helpful in the case of normal radiographs to diagnose osteonecrosis or sesamoiditis.

E. Treatment

If an acute injury has occurred and radiographs are consistent with a fracture of the sesamoid, then a short leg walking cast is placed. If symptoms came on gradually, a stiff-soled shoe is used, with a soft pad placed just proximal to the sesamoids to take the pressure off the involved area. Usually the majority of symptoms will resolve in a matter of weeks, although some degree of discomfort may persist for several months. If 6–12 months of conservative treatment has not relieved the symptoms, the affected sesamoid can be removed, which will relieve the pain.

Alvarez R et al: The simple bunion: Anatomy at the first metatarsophalangeal joint of the great toe. Foot Ankle 1984;4:229.

Coughlin MJ, Abdo RV: Arthrodesis of the first metatarsophalangeal joint with Vitallium plate fixation. Foot Ankle Int 1994;15:18.

Coughlin MJ: Hallux valgus. J Bone Joint Surg 1996;78:932.

Coughlin MJ: Juvenile hallux valgus etiology and treatment. Foot Ankle Int 1995;16:682.

Dreeben S, Mann RA: Advanced hallux valgus deformity: Long-term results utilizing the distal soft-tissue procedure and proximal metatarsal osteotomy. Foot Ankle Int 1996;17:142.

Easley ME et al: Prospective, randomized comparison of proximal crescentic and proximal chevron osteotomies for correction of hallux valgus deformity. Foot Ankle Int 1996;17:307.

Mann RA, Donatto KC: The chevron osteotomy: A clinical and radiographic analysis. Foot Ankle Int 1997;18:255.

Mann RA, Coughlin MJ: Adult hallux valgus. In Mann RA, Coughlin MJ (editors): *Surgery of the Foot and Ankle.* St. Louis: Mosby-Year Book, 1993.

Mann RA et al: Hallux valgus repair utilizing a distal soft-tissue procedure and proximal metatarsal osteotomy: Long-term follow-up. J Bone Joint Surg Am 1992;74:124.

Plattner PF, Van Manen JW: Results of Akin type proximal phalangeal osteotomy for correction of hallux valgus deformity.
Orthopaedics 1990;13:989.

Richardson EG: Keller resection arthroplasty. Orthopedics 1990;
13:1049.

Tourne Y et al: Hallux valgus in the elderly: Metatarsophalangeal
arthrodesis of the first ray. Foot Ankle Int 1997;18:195.

DEFORMITIES OF THE LESSER TOES

The most common problems involving the four lesser
toes include mallet toe, hammer toe, clawtoe, and hard
and soft corns. More proximally, at the metatarsophalangeal joint, subluxation or dislocation of the joint
may occur. All of these conditions alter the shape of the
foot and at times make wearing shoes difficult. Furthermore, in the patient with an insensitive foot, ulcerations may form over the bony prominences of these deformities.

The most common cause of clawtoe, hammer toe,
and mallet toe deformities are the long-term use of
tightly fitting footwear. These deformities may also
result from chronic neurologic problems, including
Charcot-Marie-Tooth disease, rheumatoid or psoriatic
arthritis, degenerative disk disease, compartment syndrome, and diabetic neuropathy. Additional predisposing factors are a wide foot or an abnormally long second ray and occasionally postural abnormalities of the
foot. Any problem that disturbs the balance between
the intrinsic muscles of the foot and the extrinsic flexors
and extensors can also cause these deformities.

Anatomy & Pathophysiologic Findings

The metatarsophalangeal joint is stabilized on the plantar aspect by a consolidation of the plantar capsule and
plantar aponeurosis (plantar plate) and medially and
laterally by the collateral ligaments. Plantar flexion of
the metatarsophalangeal joint is affected by the intrinsic
muscles, the interossei, and lumbricals, whose lines of
action pass plantarward to the axis of the metatarsophalangeal joint. The flexor digitorum brevis and flexor
digitorum longus muscles produce plantar flexion of
the proximal interphalangeal and distal interphalangeal
joints, respectively. On the dorsal aspect of the joint,
the extensor digitorum longus and brevis tendons and
the extensor hood or sling constitute the extensor
mechanism. This mechanism causes dorsiflexion of the
metatarsophalangeal joint and can cause extension of
the distal interphalangeal and proximal interphalangeal
joints if the proximal phalanx is in a neutral or plantar-
flexed position. When the metatarsophalangeal joint is
hyperextended, the ability of the extensor hood to
extend the distal interphalangeal and proximal interphalangeal joints is significantly diminished. Chronic
hyperextension of the metatarsophalangeal joint even-

tually leads to fixed flexion deformities at the interphalangeal joints. As a general rule, a fixed deformity is significantly more bothersome to the patient than a flexible deformity.

1. Mallet Toe Deformity

A mallet toe is a flexion deformity of the distal interphalangeal joint. It may be a fixed or flexible deformity.
In general, the deformity involves the second toe, usually because of its excessive length in relation to the adjacent toes.

Clinical Findings

A. SYMPTOMS AND SIGNS

A mallet toe tends to cause pain over the dorsal aspect
of the distal interphalangeal joint, or occasionally at the
tip of the toe from striking the ground. This may result
in a callus or, in cases associated with neuropathy, an
ulceration. Occasionally, the nail itself is deformed if
the pressure has been chronic.

The initial physical examination is carried out with
the patient standing to evaluate the severity of the deformity and ascertain whether deformities are present
in other toes. The interphalangeal joint is then carefully
palpated to determine whether the deformity is fixed or
flexible. If the distal interphalangeal joint is flexible,
plantar flexion of the ankle will permit the joint to be
straightened out completely. As the ankle joint is
brought into dorsiflexion, however, the deformity recurs. In the case of a fixed deformity, ankle motion will
not affect the deformity.

B. IMAGING STUDIES

Radiographic evaluation will confirm the clinical findings of the flexion deformity of the distal interphalangeal joint.

Treatment

A. CONSERVATIVE MANAGEMENT

The patient should be encouraged to obtain a shoe with
a wide enough toe box to accommodate the deformed
toe. An extra-depth shoe may be necessary if the deformity is too severe. If the main complaint is pain under
the tip of the toe, a small pad can be placed underneath
the toe to keep it from striking the ground, or lamb's
wool can be wrapped around the toe.

B. SURGICAL TREATMENT

Surgical treatment of a flexible mallet toe deformity requires release of the flexor digitorum longus tendon.
This is carried out under local anesthesia by incising the

tendon on the plantar aspect of the toe at the level of the middle phalanx. This usually results in resolution of the problem.

A fixed mallet toe deformity requires a condylectomy, which is carried out through an elliptical incision made over the dorsal aspect of the distal interphalangeal joint. Along with the ellipse of skin, the extensor tendon is excised, the collateral ligaments released, and the distal portion of the middle phalanx removed. The distal phalanx is reduced and held in place either with a 0.045-in. Kirschner wire for 4 weeks or with Telfa bolsters (Figure 9–14).

Good results may be expected following this procedure. The most common complication occurs because a contracture of the flexor digitorum longus tendon was not appreciated prior to surgery, or because insufficient bone was removed from the middle phalanx to adequately decompress the deformity.

2. Hammer Toe Deformity

A hammer toe deformity is a plantar flexion deformity of the proximal interphalangeal joint, which may either be fixed or flexible. It is frequently associated with varying degrees of hyperextension of the metatarsophalangeal joint. A flexion deformity of the distal interphalangeal joint usually accompanies a hammer toe, but an extension deformity is occasionally observed.

Clinical Findings

A. SYMPTOMS AND SIGNS

Clinical evaluation is similar to that of a mallet toe deformity, with care taken to distinguish between a fixed or flexible deformity. Also, the metatarsophalangeal joints of each toe are evaluated for hyperextension deformities. Callus formation or even an ulcer may be present over the extensor surface of the proximal interphalangeal joint. Metatarsophalangeal joint correction

may be necessary to alleviate the hammer toe. Similarly, a significant hallux valgus deformity that is impinging on the second toe may require treatment to make room for correction of the hammer toe.

B. IMAGING STUDIES

Radiographs help in the evaluation of proximal interphalangeal flexion deformity, hyperextension deformity at the metatarsophalangeal joint, and hallux valgus deformity. It is critical that all joints be assessed when hammer toe correction is being considered.

Treatment

A. CONSERVATIVE MANAGEMENT

The conservative management of hammer toe deformities is foremost that of proper shoe wear, as previously emphasized. In addition, toe sleeves are available that pad the painful callus.

Conservative management becomes more difficult if a significant fixed deformity is present, particularly if it is associated with extension of the metatarsophalangeal joint or a significant hallux valgus deformity.

B. SURGICAL TREATMENT

Surgical decision making regarding the hammer toe hinges on whether (1) the deformity is fixed or flexible, (2) any deformity of the metatarsophalangeal joint needs to be corrected concomitantly, and (3) a space must be created for the toe by correcting the hallux valgus deformity.

1. Flexible hammer toe deformity—A flexible hammer toe deformity is corrected with the Girdlestone flexor tendon transfer. In this procedure, the long flexor tendon is harvested from the plantar aspect of the foot, brought up on either side of the extensor hood mechanism, and sutured into the extensor hood with the toe held in approximately 5 degrees of plantar flexion and the ankle in plantar flexion (Figure 9–15). This causes

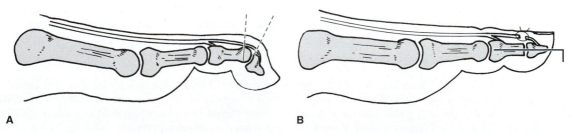

A   **B**

Figure 9–14.   Mallet toe repair. **A:** Resection of condyles of the middle phalanx. **B:** Intramedullary Kirschner wire fixation. (Reproduced, with permission, from Mann RA, Coughlin MJ: *The Video Textbook of Foot and Ankle Surgery.* St. Louis: Medical Video Productions, 1991.)

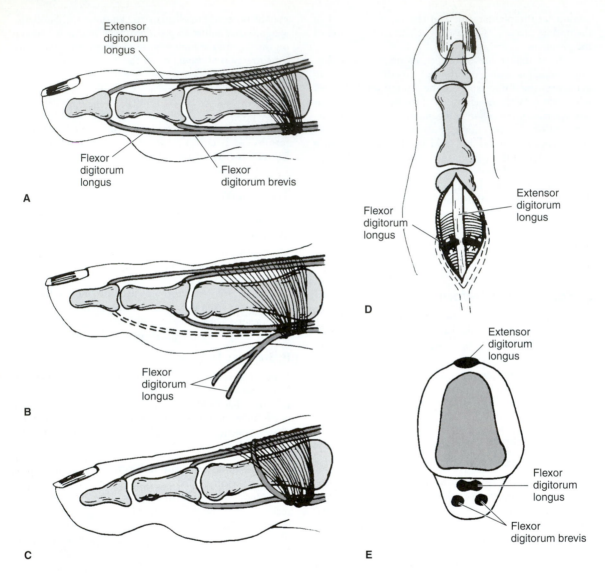

Figure 9–15. Flexor tendon transfer for flexible hammer toe deformity. **A:** Lateral view of lesser toe. **B:** The long flexor is detached from its insertion and is delivered through the proximal plantar wound. It is split longitudinally along the median raphe. **C:** Each limb is transferred dorsally on either side of the proximal phalanx and is secured on the dorsal aspect. **D:** Dorsal view after tendon transfer. **E:** Cross section showing flexor digitorum longus tendon in sheath. (Reproduced, with permission, from Mann RA, Coughlin MJ: *The Video Textbook of Foot and Ankle Surgery.* St. Louis: Medical Video Productions, 1991.)

the long flexor tendon to act as an extensor of the interphalangeal joints and a flexor of the metatarsophalangeal joint, thereby correcting the deformity. A soft dressing is applied and a postoperative shoe is worn for 4 weeks, after which ambulation is allowed.

2. Fixed hammer toe deformity—The DuVries proximal phalangeal condylectomy is used for the fixed

deformity. This procedure is identical to that described for treatment of the mallet toe deformity, but involves the proximal interphalangeal joint instead of the distal interphalangeal joint (Figure 9–16).

3. Complications—The main complication observed with either procedure is inadequate correction of the deformity, usually because of failure to appreciate a

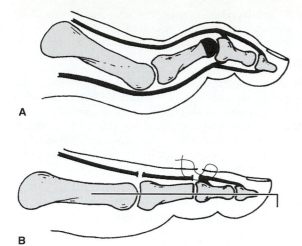

Figure 9–16. Fixed hammer toe repair. **A:** Resection of the head of the proximal phalanx. **B:** Intramedullary Kirschner wire fixation. (Reproduced, with permission, from Mann RA, Coughlin MJ: *The Video Textbook of Foot and Ankle Surgery.* St. Louis: Medical Video Productions, 1991.)

contracture of the flexor digitorum longus tendon at the time of surgery.

3. Clawtoe Deformity

Clawtoe deformity involves both the metatarsophalangeal and interphalangeal joints and may be flexible or fixed. Clawtoe deformity can be disabling, particularly in the patient with a neuromuscular disorder. This deformity is characterized by marked dorsiflexion of the metatarsophalangeal joint, which results in pain secondary to chafing over the interphalangeal joints against the shoe and pain beneath the metatarsal heads because the metatarsal heads are forced into plantar flexion. In contrast to hammer toe or mallet toe deformities, which usually involve a single toe, clawtoe deformity usually involves all of the lesser toes. An associated deformity of the great toe may occur as well.

Clinical Findings

A. Symptoms and Signs

The clinical evaluation is similar to that described for the previous lesser toe deformities. The metatarsal heads are palpated, as the fat pad may be displaced distally and the skin beneath the metatarsal heads may be atrophic. Callosities may be present on the extensor surface of the proximal interphalangeal joints and on the plantar aspect of the metatarsophalangeal joints.

B. Imaging Studies

Radiographs demonstrate the deformity, which is present at the metatarsophalangeal and interphalangeal joints. The posture of the entire foot needs to be evaluated, looking for the presence of a cavus-type foot deformity, characterized by increased dorsiflexion pitch of the calcaneus and increased plantar flexion of the first metatarsal.

Treatment

A. Conservative Management

An extra-depth shoe reduces the pressure on the lesser toes, and arch supports placed under the metatarsal head area may relieve the pain. Flexible mild deformities can be treated with shoe inserts placed immediately proximal to the metatarsophalangeal joints. These can have the effect of balancing the extensors and flexors of the toes.

B. Surgical Treatment

The type of operative intervention depends upon the nature of the deformity. Flexible deformities can be treated with the Girdlestone flexor tendon transfer. In addition, however, the extensor tendons usually must be lengthened to permit correction of the metatarsophalangeal joints to neutral plantar flexion.

A concomitant fixed contracture of the proximal interphalangeal joint requires a DuVries proximal phalangeal condylectomy as well as the Girdlestone tendon transfer procedure. Furthermore, release of the dorsal capsule, collateral ligaments, and extensor tendon is performed at the metatarsophalangeal joint. Postoperative management for the patient with clawtoe deformity is the same as discussed earlier for hammer toe deformity.

Following this surgical procedure no active motion of the toes occurs. The toes are usually well aligned in a plantigrade position. The marked deformity of the proximal interphalangeal joints has been relieved so that they no longer strike the top of the shoe. The main problems that can occur after surgery are (1) failure to adequately correct a fixed hammer toe deformity by use of the tendon transfer and (2) failure to adequately release the fixed deformity at the metatarsophalangeal joint, resulting in recurrence of the deformity.

4. Hard Corn & Soft Corn (Clavus Durum & Clavus Mollum)

A corn is a keratotic lesion that forms over a bony prominence on the lesser toes because of excessive pressure on the skin. A hard corn occurs most commonly over the dorsal and lateral aspect of the fifth toe, usually over the lateral condyle of the proximal phalanx. A soft corn represents a keratotic lesion in a web space and is so named because maceration results from moisture between the toes. The soft corn may occur anywhere along the toe where a bony excrescence is present and frequently occurs in the fourth web space between the base of the proximal phalanx of the fourth toe and the medial condyle of the head of the proximal phalanx of the fifth toe. At times, an ulceration may occur because of the extent of the maceration.

Treatment

A. CONSERVATIVE MANAGEMENT

The main objective of conservative management is reducing pressure on the bony prominences. Footwear with a large toe box can relieve this pressure. Debridement or shaving of the lesion reduces pain. The procedure can frequently be carried out by younger patients without assistance, but this becomes increasingly difficult in older individuals because of decreasing flexibility and poor eyesight. Skin compromise, especially in the diabetic patient, must be avoided. At times, soft pads or lamb's wool can be placed around the toe to minimize pressure on the involved area, but the patient must wear a shoe with an adequate toe box to accommodate such modalities.

B. SURGICAL TREATMENT

1. Surgical treatment of the hard corn—The hard corn, over the fifth toe, is managed surgically by removing the distal portion of the proximal phalanx and occasionally the dorsolateral aspect of the proximal portion of the middle phalanx. The longitudinal incision is made over the dorsal aspect so that the scar will not chafe against the shoe. The extensor tendon is split, the collateral ligaments cut, and the condyle exposed. With a bone cutter, the distal portion of the proximal phalanx is generously removed and the edges smoothed with a rongeur. Following closure, a compression dressing is applied for several days. The toe is taped to the adjacent fourth toe for 8 weeks.

Removal of excessive bone is the major complication, which causes the small toe to become too floppy, creating a nuisance for the patient.

2. Surgical treatment for the soft corn—Soft corns are treated surgically by making an incision over the lesion and using a small rongeur to remove the underlying bony excrescence. This is a simple procedure and almost invariably results in satisfactory resolution of the problem.

3. Syndactyly—Because the soft corn is caused by pressure on the skin, removal of the skin between the toes can resolve the problem. Syndactyly is a procedure by which the skin is removed between the fourth and fifth toes and the two toes are sutured together to eliminate the problem of a soft corn in the web space. Although the soft corn can usually be managed with a condylectomy, as described earlier, occasionally a great deal of maceration or ulceration precludes treating it only with a condylectomy. In these cases, syndactyly is indicated. Occasionally, a floppy fifth toe from previous surgery can be stabilized by syndactyly.

5. Subluxation & Dislocation of the Metatarsophalangeal Joint

Dorsal subluxation or dislocation of the metatarsophalangeal joint occurs because of weakening of the supporting plantar capsule and collateral ligament structures, which maintain the stability of the metatarsophalangeal joint. Secondary changes such as hammer toe may occur in the toe itself. Pain usually occurs either beneath the metatarsophalangeal joint or over the dorsal aspect of the toe as it strikes the top of the shoe.

Etiologic Findings

The most common cause of a subluxed or dislocated joint is probably a progressive hallux valgus deformity pressing against the second toe. Over time, subluxation and eventual dislocation of the second metatarsophalangeal joint can occur.

A nonspecific synovitis, isolated to the metatarsophalangeal joint and usually involving the second metatarsophalangeal joint, is the next most common cause. The clinical picture is one of generalized swelling about the metatarsophalangeal joint that subsides over a period of 3–6 months, followed by progressive subluxation and eventual dislocation of the joint. Occasionally, subluxation or dislocation of the metatarsophalangeal joint may result from trauma.

Arthritic conditions such as rheumatoid or psoriatic arthritis can cause subluxation or dislocation at multiple joints. Advanced neuromuscular disorders may cause severe subluxation of the metatarsophalangeal joint, but dislocation is unusual.

A variant of this condition results from attenuation of collateral ligaments on one side of the metatarsophalangeal joint. The cause may be idiopathic but occasionally may follow a steroid injection into the area. The metatarsophalangeal joint, instead of subluxing in a dorsalward direction, deviates medially or occasionally laterally, crossing over the adjacent toe. This again is most common in the second metatarsophalangeal joint.

When the toe deviates in a medialward direction and crosses over the great toe, the patient may have difficulty wearing shoes.

Clinical Findings

A. SYMPTOMS AND SIGNS

Patients complain of pain on the dorsal and plantar aspects of the affected joint. They may note swelling as well, and will complain of an associated hammer toe or lateral deviation of the toe if present. The degree of deformity is evaluated with the patient in a standing and sitting position. The affected metatarsophalangeal joint is palpated for active synovitis, flexibility of the joint, and degree of subluxation.

The dorsal-plantar stability of the joint is evaluated by holding the proximal phalanx between the examiner's fingers and moving it dorsally and plantarward, similar to a Lachman's test of the knee. If a significant hallux valgus deformity is associated with crossover of the second toe on the first toe, then the hallux valgus requires evaluation.

B. IMAGING STUDIES

The radiographs of the foot reveal the extent of the subluxation or dislocation. The severity of the hallux valgus is evaluated, and changes about the articular surface of the joint are observed. In rheumatoid arthritis, multiple joint involvement is noted.

Treatment

A. CONSERVATIVE MANAGEMENT

Conservative management consists of using a shoe with a wide enough toe box to accommodate the deformity and prescribing a well-molded, soft orthotic device to relieve pressure on the metatarsal head. Unfortunately, this may raise the forefoot, causing impingement on the toe box area of the shoe and some discomfort. A series of cortisone injections into the affected joint may be performed. No more than three injections are given, and at least 1 month is allowed between injections. If the patient cannot be adequately accommodated with these modalities, surgical intervention may be indicated. A significant hallux valgus deformity indicates the need for correction to make a space for second toe correction. Failure to treat both problems will result in recurrence.

B. SURGICAL TREATMENT

The subluxed metatarsophalangeal joint with a flexible hammer toe is treated by releasing the dorsal contracture of the extensor tendons and joint capsule, followed by a Girdlestone flexor tendon transfer, as previously described. This will usually bring the toe into better alignment, although the patient will lose some selective voluntary control of the toe, but this is usually not of any significance. If a fixed hammer toe is present, a proximal phalanx condylectomy is added to the procedure.

The more severe, complete dorsal dislocation of the metatarsophalangeal joint is a difficult surgical problem. In the past this has been treated by an aggressive release of the dorsal joint capsule and collateral ligaments, and synovectomy of the metatarsophalangeal joint. The distal one third of the metatarsal head is removed to decompress the joint. Accompanying hammer toe procedures are performed to correct the invariably present fixed hammer toe.

A longitudinal Kirschner wire stabilizes the correction for 2 weeks. After pin removal, motion is started at the metatarsophalangeal joint. This procedure results in significant joint stiffness and possible resubluxation of the joint.

Recently, an osteotomy of the metatarsal neck has been used to treat dislocated or advanced subluxation of the metatarsophalangeal joint. An oblique osteotomy is performed, starting at the metatarsal neck and aimed proximally at a shallow angle to the metatarsal shaft, creating a long osteotomy site. Once the osteotomy is complete, the metatarsal head is slid proximally to the appropriate level that will allow the joint to assume a reduced position. The amount of shortening is usually between 4.0 mm and 6.0 mm. The osteotomy is fixed with a single 2.5-mm or smaller diameter cortical screw. Accompanying hammer toe procedures are then performed if necessary. Good short-term results have been noted with this procedure without the complication of joint stiffness as occurs with previously described procedures.

Repair of the medially or laterally dislocated metatarsophalangeal joint can be a technically difficult problem. Satisfactory correction can be achieved with one of two techniques. A soft-tissue release of the joint capsule can be performed on the side to which the toe deviates, allowing realignment of the toe. Alternatively, a closing-wedge osteotomy at the base of the proximal phalanx can also achieve good realignment of the toe. Severe deformities can be corrected with an oblique metatarsal neck osteotomy, previously described for treatment of dorsally subluxated metatarsophalangeal joints. The technique is identical, although some soft-tissue balancing may need to be added to the procedure.

Coughlin MJ: Operative repair of the mallet toe deformity. Foot Ankle Int 1995;16:109.

Coughlin MJ, Mann RA: Lesser toe deformities. In Mann RA, Coughlin MJ (editors): *Surgery of the Foot and Ankle.* St. Louis: Mosby-Year Book, 1993.

Fourtin PT, Myerson MS: Second metatarsophalangeal joint instability. Foot Ankle Int 1995;16:306.

Lehman DE, Smith RW: Treatment of symptomatic hammer toe with a proximal interphalangeal joint arthrodesis. Foot Ankle Int 1995;16:535.

Mizel MS, Michaelson JD: Nonsurgical treatment of monarticular nontraumatic synovitis of the second metatarsophalangeal joint. Foot Ankle Int 1997;18:424.

Mizel MS, Yodlowski ML: Disorders of the lesser metatarsophalangeal joints. J Am Acad Orthop Surg 1995; 3:166.

Myerson MS, Shereff MJ: The pathologic anatomy of claw and hammer toes. J Bone Joint Surg Am 1989;71:45.

REGIONAL ANESTHESIA FOR FOOT & ANKLE DISORDERS

Regional anesthesia of the foot and ankle is a valuable tool in the surgeon's armamentarium. Most procedures below the ankle can be performed without general anesthesia, making them amenable to an outpatient surgery setting and eliminating the hazards of central nervous system depression. Pain develops gradually as the anesthesia wears off, and the analgesic requirements of the patient are thereby reduced significantly.

Digital Block

A. INDICATIONS

Digital block is suitable for procedures used in the toes, such as treatment of nail disorders, correction of hammer toe or mallet toe, tendon releases, and some metatarsophalangeal joint procedures.

B. TECHNIQUE

Short- and longer-term anesthesia is provided by digital block using a 1:1 mixture of 1% lidocaine hydrochloride and 0.25% bupivacaine. A short, 25-gauge needle is used to inject approximately 1.5 mL on either side of the toe within the subcutaneous layer between the skin and deeper fascia. The needle is then passed toward the plantar aspect of the toe to anesthetize the digital nerves. Both sides of the toe should be anesthetized. Anesthesia should be administered before the operative site is prepared to allow the 15 min necessary for the block to take effect before starting a procedure.

Ankle Block

A. INDICATIONS

Ankle block anesthesia is commonly used for operations on the forefoot and midfoot, such as bunion procedures, neuroma excision, metatarsal osteotomies, and tarsometatarsal fusions. If more than one lesser toe procedure is being performed, an ankle block is preferred to multiple digital blocks. Ankle block anesthesia is not recommended for hindfoot procedures, such as hindfoot fusions or ankle arthroscopy.

B. TECHNIQUE

The successful ankle block must anesthetize the posterior tibial nerve, superficial branch of the deep peroneal nerve, sural nerve, saphenous nerve, and superficial peroneal nerve. The posterior tibial nerve requires a larger, 3-cm, 22- or 25-gauge needle and approximately 7–10 mL of a 1:1 mixture of 1% lidocaine hydrochloride and 0.25% bupivacaine. The landmark for the posterior tibial nerve behind the malleolus is approximately two finger-breadths proximal to the tip of the malleolus and along the medial border of the Achilles tendon (Figure 9–17). The needle is inserted perpendicular to the shaft of the tibia until the posterior cortex of the tibia is palpated with the tip of the needle. The needle is then withdrawn approximately 2 mm. Approximately 7–10 mL of anesthetic agent is injected into this area after aspiration is done to confirm that the needle is not in a vessel.

To anesthetize the deep peroneal nerve, the site of the injection is located by palpating the extensor hallucis and extensor digitorum longus tendons at the level of the navicular. The deep peroneal nerve lies just lateral to the dorsalis pedis artery. The 25-gauge needle is inserted and advanced to bone and then withdrawn 1–2 mm, aspiration is attempted, and approximately 5 mL of anesthetic is injected (Figure 9–18).

The saphenous nerve is identified one to two finger-breadths proximal to the tip of the medial malleolus and just posterior to the saphenous vein. A 25-gauge needle is inserted and 3 mL of anesthetic injected (Figure 9–19).

The sural nerve is blocked approximately 1–1.5 cm distal to the tip of the lateral malleolus and can often be palpated in the subcutaneous fat. A 25-gauge needle is inserted and approximately 3–5 mL of anesthetic injected.

The superficial peroneal nerve branches are blocked starting two finger-breadths proximal and anterior to the tip of the lateral malleolus, and the injection is carried out below the subcutaneous veins but above the long extensor tendons in a ring-type block. Approximately 5 mL of anesthetic agent is used. The anesthesia for ankle block takes effect within 15–20 min.

Coughlin MJ: Peripheral anesthesia. In Mann RA, Coughlin MJ (editors): *Surgery of the Foot and Ankle,* Mosby-Year Book, 1993.

Lee TH et al: Regional anesthesia in foot and ankle surgery. Orthopedics 1996;19:577.

Rongstad K et al: Popliteal sciatic nerve block for postoperative analgesia. Foot Ankle Int 1996;17:378.

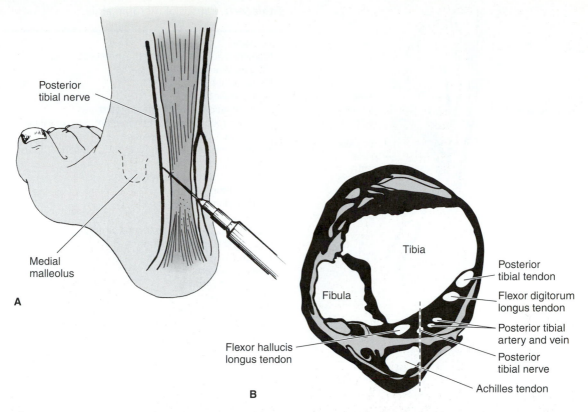

Figure 9–17. **A:** Anesthetic technique. Posterior approach to posterior tibial nerve along medial border of Achilles tendon. **B:** A cross section of the tibia at the level of the ankle shows the posterior tibial nerve to be in a line directly deep to the medial border of the Achilles tendon and 2–3 mm superficial to the posterior cortex of the tibia. (Reproduced, with permission, from Mann RA, Coughlin MJ: *The Video Textbook of Foot and Ankle Surgery.* St. Louis: Medical Video Productions, 1991.)

Sarrafian SK: Regional anesthesia of the midfoot. In Jahss MH (editor): *Disorders of the Foot,* 2nd ed. Philadelphia: WB Saunders, 1990.

METATARSALGIA

Metatarsalgia is a general term for pain arising from the metatarsal head region. The center of pressure during normal gait is initially applied to the heel and progresses along the plantar aspect of the foot. For more than 50% of the stance time, the pressure is concentrated beneath the metatarsal head area. This extended period of pressure can cause bothersome pain. A precise diagnosis is necessary in metatarsalgia to direct treatment toward the specific cause.

Etiologic Findings

Metatarsalgia encompasses a broad spectrum of conditions with various causes arising out of the anatomic structures in the area. It may be associated with abnormalities of the metatarsal head subluxation or dislocation of the metatarsophalangeal joints, systemic diseases, dermatologic lesions, soft-tissue disorders, or iatrogenic causes. Table 9–1 lists the various causes of metatarsalgia and the differential diagnoses that should be considered in evaluating these patients.

Clinical Findings

A. SYMPTOMS AND SIGNS

The clinical evaluation begins with a careful history directed toward delineating the precise location of the pain. The physical examination of the foot and lower extremity begins with the patient standing. Any deformities of the toes are noted, such as clawing of the toes, a long second ray, or swelling around any of the joints. The patient should be evaluated for a postural problem of the foot, such as a flat foot or cavus foot. The plantar

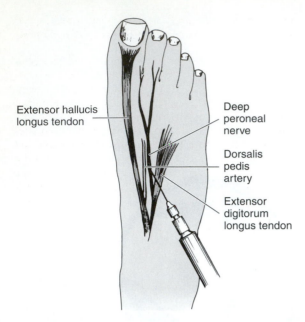

Figure 9–18. Anesthetic technique. Dorsal approach to deep peroneal nerve. (Reproduced, with permission, from Mann RA, Coughlin MJ: *The Video Textbook of Foot and Ankle Surgery.* St. Louis: Medical Video Productions, 1991.)

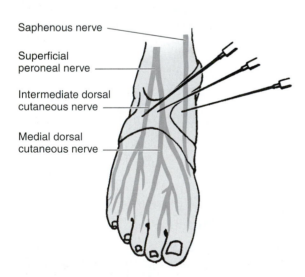

Figure 9–19. Anesthetic technique. Superficial nerve branches over anterior ankle. (Reproduced, with permission, from Mann RA, Coughlin MJ: *The Video Textbook of Foot and Ankle Surgery.* St. Louis: Medical Video Productions, 1991.)

Table 9–1. Causes of metatarsalgia.

Bone causes
   Prominent fibular condyle of the metatarsal head
   Long metatarsal
   Morton's foot
   Hypermobile first ray
   Posttraumatic malalignment of metatarsals
   Abnormal foot posture such as forefoot varus or valgus,
      cavus foot, or equinus deformity
   Systemic disease, rheumatoid arthritis, psoriatic arthritis
Dermatologic lesions
   Wart, seed corn, hyperkeratosis of the skin
Soft tissue disorders
   Atrophy of the plantar fat pad
   Sequelae of a crush injury
   Plantar scars secondary to trauma or surgery
Metatarsophalangeal joint disorders
   Subluxed or dislocated joint
   Freiberg's infraction
   Nonspecific synovitis
Iatrogenic causes
   Residuals of metatarsal surgery
   Transfer lesion due to previous surgery
   Hallux valgus surgery, eg, shortening or dorsiflexion of the
      metatarsal

aspect of the foot is carefully evaluated for evidence of callus formation. The metatarsal heads are palpated individually to assess for generalized plantar fat pad atrophy, a prominent fibular condyle, synovitis, or possibly a transfer lesion beneath a metatarsal head resulting from previous forefoot surgery.

B. Imaging Studies

The radiographic evaluation includes weight-bearing anteroposterior, lateral, and oblique views of the foot. Occasionally, a "skyline view" of the metatarsal heads (obtained with the metatarsophalangeal joints in dorsiflexion) is helpful to evaluate their overall alignment, particularly in cases resulting from previous surgery, by demonstrating the height of the metatarsal heads.

Treatment

A. Conservative Management

Conservative management is directed at relieving the pressure beneath the area of maximum pain. Initially, the patient must obtain a shoe of appropriate style and adequate size to allow an orthotic device to be inserted. A lace-type shoe with a soft sole material and an adequate toe box is appropriate. High-heeled shoes, loafers, or tight shoes are inappropriate, as they have decreased volume for the foot and may cause increased pressure against the involved area. As a general rule, the softer the orthotic device the more comfortable the patient. A hard acrylic orthotic device is not particularly comfortable for the patient and should usually be avoided.

B. Surgical Treatment

The surgical management of metatarsalgia depends on the cause and will be covered under different sections of this chapter. In general, pain from a bony prominence can be relieved by a partial ostectomy or osteotomy, dermatologic lesions such as warts can often be burned off with liquid nitrogen or excised, or pain caused by a subluxated metatarsophalangeal joint can be corrected with tendon transfer. The outcome depends on the severity of the problem and the type of surgical intervention required to correct it.

KERATOTIC DISORDERS OF THE PLANTAR SKIN

Friction and pressure over bony prominences, particularly on the plantar skin, can often result in callus formation. Modest callus formation is normal, but more extensive callus formation, particularly on the plantar aspect of the foot, may become symptomatic and occasionally quite disabling.

Etiologic Findings

Many of the intractable plantar keratoses arise from the bony abnormalities presented in Table 9–1.

Clinical Findings

A. Symptoms and Signs

A careful history of the problem is extremely important, especially if the patient has had multiple surgical procedures. The patient's activities, type of shoes that exacerbate or relieve the pain, how often the lesion needs to be trimmed, and the type of orthotic devices that have been used are all important factors. The physical examination, however, is the most important single factor in the diagnosis of intractable plantar keratoses. First, the overall posture of the foot needs to be evaluated to determine whether the condition is the result of a postural abnormality. Specifically, a rigid plantar-flexed first metatarsal could cause a diffuse callus beneath the first metatarsal head, or a hypermobile first ray that fails to support the medial forefoot may result in generalized callus formation beneath the lesser metatarsal heads. Varus posture of the forefoot (the lateral aspect of the

foot in greater plantar flexion than the medial aspect) may result in callus formation beneath the fifth metatarsal head.

The nature of the callus itself is important because it helps to determine the cause of the problem. A well-localized lesion beneath the metatarsal head is often caused by a prominent fibular condyle on the second or third metatarsal. A diffuse callus is usually associated with a long metatarsal. The callus may have arisen after trauma or surgery in which an adjacent metatarsal has been dorsiflexed, thereby increasing the weight-bearing load of the metatarsal. A callus on the bottom of the foot must be differentiated from a plantar's wart, which can occasionally mimic a plantar callosity. Shaving the lesion will reveal bleeding from end arteries in a plantar's wart, while a keratotic lesion consists only of hyperkeratotic tissue.

B. Imaging Studies

Routine weight-bearing radiographs are performed and are correlated with the clinical findings in evaluation of these patients.

Treatment

A. Conservative Management

A wide, soft lace-up shoe is recommended, often with the addition of a soft metatarsal support. The orthotic device usually consists of a soft pad, as demonstrated in Figure 9–20. It is usually not necessary for an orthotic device to be fabricated early in the treatment of metatarsalgia, as the less expensive, commercially available pads are sufficient in most cases.

B. Surgical Treatment

The surgical management of metatarsalgia depends upon the cause of the condition. The following causes of intractable plantar keratoses may respond to surgical intervention.

Localized intractable plantar keratosis beneath a metatarsal head is usually caused by a prominent fibular condyle. It occurs most frequently underneath the second metatarsal but may also be found underneath the third and fourth metatarsals. Surgical treatment involves plantar condylectomy in which 30% of the plantar region of the metatarsal head is removed, thereby removing the sharp bony prominence (Figure 9–21). This procedure results in predictable pain relief of the affected toe, although 5–10% of patients will develop a transfer lesion beneath the adjacent metatarsal head.

A diffuse callus beneath the second metatarsal that is the result of a dorsiflexed or hypermobile first metatarsal can be treated with dorsiflexion osteotomy done at the base of the second metatarsal. If the lesion

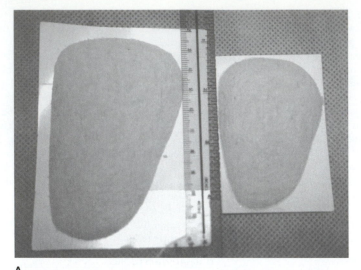

A

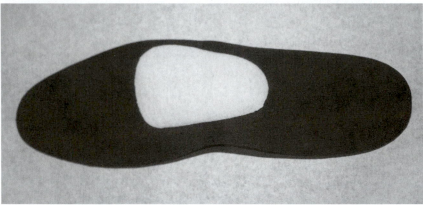

B

Figure 9–20. **A:** A metatarsal pad may help to redistribute weight bearing and re-lieve symptoms. **B:** A soft insole may be added to help absorb pressure and allow transfer of the metatarsal pad from one shoe to another. (Reproduced, with permis-sion, from Mann RA, Coughlin MJ: *The Video Textbook of Foot and Ankle Surgery.* St. Louis: Medical Video Productions, 1991.)

is the result of an excessively long metatarsal, it may be shortened to the level of a line drawn between the adjacent metatarsal heads, thereby reestablishing a smooth metatarsal pattern. If the callus is a result of a dislocated metatarsophalangeal joint, the joint must be surgically reduced, using one of the techniques previously described, to alleviate the chronic downward pressure against the metatarsal head. All of these surgical procedures to eliminate a callus are fairly successful, although the possibility of a transfer lesion developing is approximately 5–10%.

Occasionally, a well-localized callus is present beneath the tibial sesamoid. This can be treated surgically by shaving the plantar third of the sesamoid. This alleviates the callus in almost all cases, with the only significant complication being caused by inadvertent disruption of the plantar medial cutaneous nerve during the surgical approach to the sesamoid.

Bunionettes are caused by prominence of the fifth metatarsal head and may lead to metatarsalgia. A diffuse callus beneath the fifth metatarsal head can be treated with a midshaft metatarsal osteotomy to bring it

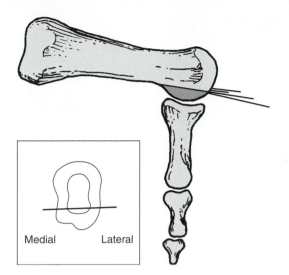

Figure 9–21. A plantar condylectomy is performed with resection of one fourth to one third of the plantar surface of the metatarsal head. (Reproduced, with permission, from Mann RA, Coughlin MJ: *The Video Textbook of Foot and Ankle Surgery.* St. Louis: Medical Video Productions, 1991.)

out of its plantar-flexed position. This will usually alleviate the condition. It is unusual for a transfer lesion to occur beneath the fourth metatarsal head.

At times, the fifth metatarsal head is too prominent on the lateral aspect of the foot rather than the plantar aspect. In these cases, a chevron osteotomy of the fifth metatarsal head, displacing it in a medialward direction, will alleviate the condition (Figure 9–22), sometimes with slight loss of motion of the metatarsophalangeal joint.

A subhallux sesamoid can cause a small callus beneath the interphalangeal joint of the great toe and be quite bothersome to the patient. Surgical excision of the sesamoid is indicated, with good results and little or no disability.

Coughlin MJ: Etiology and treatment of the bunionette deformity. Instr Course Lect 1990;39:37.

Dreeben SM et al: Metatarsal osteotomy for primary metatarsalgia: Radiographic and Pedobarographic study. Foot Ankle 1989; 9:214.

Idusuyi OB et al: Oblique metatarsal osteotomy for intractable plantar keratosis: Ten-year follow-up. Foot Ankle Int 1998;6: 351.

Mann RA, Chou LB: Surgical management for intractable metatarsalgia. Foot Ankle Int 1995;16:322.

Mann RA, Coughlin MJ: Keratotic disorders of the plantar skin. In Mann RA, Coughlin MJ (editors): *Surgery of the Foot and Ankle.* St. Louis: Mosby-Year Book, 1993.

Mann RA, Wapner K: Tibial sesamoid shaving for treatment of intractable plantar keratosis under the tibial sesamoid. Foot Ankle 1992;13:196.

DIABETIC FOOT

Approximately 14 million people in the United States are diabetic, and foot problems are the most common cause for hospitalization of this population. More than half of all nontraumatic amputations of limbs are done in diabetics. One report showed a 68% incidence of foot disorders in a large diabetic clinic. Treatment of the diabetic who presents with foot problems requires a team approach, involving the primary care physician, vascular surgeon, orthopedic surgeon, infectious disease specialist, orthotist, diabetic nurse specialist, and, whenever possible, the patient's family members.

Pathophysiologic Findings

The most frequent problem faced by the diabetic is breakdown of the skin of the foot (Figure 9–23). The cause of foot ulcers is multifactorial but stems from diminished sensation resulting from neuropathic disease. Unappreciated local stresses are placed on the skin externally by poorly fitting shoes and internally by skeletal abnormalities. Other neurologic problems exacerbate the condition. Autonomic neuropathy causes dry skin and cracks in the dermis, which may become portals of entry for infection. Reactive hyperemia, which normally helps to clear infections, is blunted by autonomic neuropathy. Motor neuropathy affects the intrinsic muscles of the foot and may lead to clawtoe deformities. The metatarsal heads and proximal interphalangeal joints become prominent and predispose to ulcerations (Figure 9–24). Diabetic patients are more likely to develop atherosclerotic disease, which decreases global blood flow to the extremity and can prevent healing of an ulcer. Other factors that affect skin healing in diabetics include nutritional deficiencies, diminished microcirculation, and lowered resistance to infection.

History

When a diabetic patient presents with a possible foot infection, the presence of symptoms, such as swelling and erythema, and the character of any present drainage is assessed. The length of time that these symptoms have been present is also determined. A past history of foot infections is sought, previous or current antibiotic usage is detailed, and any recent trauma to the foot is noted. A history is taken about the severity of the patient's diabetes, including how long ago the diabetes was diagnosed, whether the patient is taking insulin, what other organ systems are involved, and the degree of neuropathy that is present in the patient's feet.

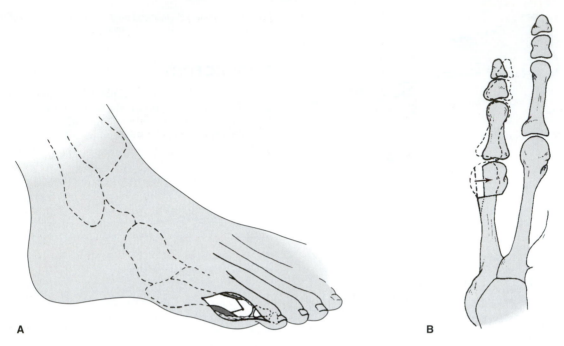

A

B

Figure 9–22. **A:** Lateral view of chevron fifth metatarsal osteotomy. **B:** Diagram following completion of this procedure. (Reproduced, with permission, from Mann RA, Coughlin MJ: *The Video Textbook of Foot and Ankle Surgery.* St. Louis: Medical Video Productions, 1991.)

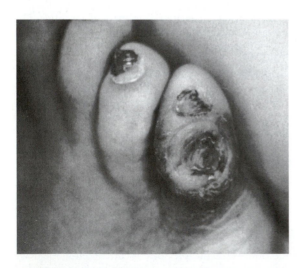

Figure 9–23. Ulceration over the dorsolateral aspect of the fifth toe as the result of pressure from a shoe. (Reproduced, with permission, from Mann RA, Coughlin MJ: *The Video Textbook of Foot and Ankle Surgery.* St. Louis: Medical Video Productions, 1991.)

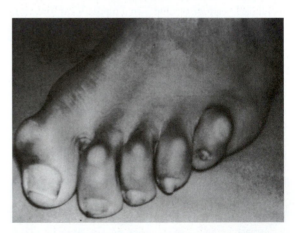

Figure 9–24. Clawtoe deformity involves hammer toe deformity associated with dorsiflexion of metatarsophalangeal joint. (Reproduced, with permission, from Mann RA, Coughlin MJ: *Surgery of the Foot and Ankle,* 6th ed. St. Louis: Mosby-Year Book, 1993.)

Clinical Findings

A. GENERAL EXAMINATION

Examination of the diabetic patient should begin with inspection of the shoe for internal and external wear patterns. The leg and foot are inspected for overall appearance of skin, hair growth, perfusion, pulses, and color to assess the extent of neuropathic problems.

B. SKIN BREAKDOWN

Any bony prominences are recognized as areas of potential skin breakdown. The most common prominences are located under the metatarsal heads, on the dorsum of proximal interphalangeal joints, under the medial sesamoid, at the base of the fifth metatarsal, under the medial arch in a Charcot foot, and over the medial eminence of the hallux (Figure 9–25). Neurologic examination should test light touch, pin-prick sensation, vibratory sensation, and proprioception. Ulcers should be carefully documented and evaluated for evidence of infection in the adjacent soft tissues. Open wounds should be probed to evaluate the extent of involvement of deeper structures, such as tendons, joints, and bony surfaces.

C. VASCULAR FINDINGS

Vascular evaluation is essential in the diabetic patient and should include more than just palpation of pulses. The overall potential for healing of foot lesions in a diabetic is related to the ischemic index. This index is obtained by dividing the blood pressure measurement in the brachial artery by that in the dorsalis pedis and posterior tibial arteries, as measured by Doppler ultrasound with a calf cuff. If the index is 0.45 or greater, there is a 90% chance that a foot ulcer will heal. Lower indices are an indication for a vascular surgery consultation. It must be kept in mind, however, that falsely elevated values of blood pressure in the foot may result from calcification of major blood vessels. Thus, apparent vascular insufficiency in the light of an adequate ischemic index also warrants a vascular surgery consultation.

D. IMAGING STUDIES

Radiographic studies should include weight-bearing x-ray films of both feet and ankles if indicated. Plain radiographs can help identify bony prominences that predispose the patient to ulcer formation, and osteomyelitis or changes consistent with a neuropathic foot may be identified. Early Charcot (neuropathic) joint changes may be difficult to differentiate from osteomyelitis. The four D's of neuropathic joints are helpful in delineating more advanced cases: debris, destruction, dislocation, and densification.

The presence of infection may be delineated on serial radiographs as bony changes and osteolysis progressing over a several-week period. A technetium bone scan is sensitive in detecting early osteomyelitis but is quite nonspecific. Magnetic resonance imaging (MRI) can demonstrate bone and soft-tissue changes, such as edema or the extent of an abscess cavity, but cannot definitively distinguish Charcot changes from osteomyelitis.

Classification & Treatment of Diabetic Foot Ulcers

The Rancho Los Amigos Hospital classification of diabetic foot ulcers (Figure 9–26) is based on the depth of tissue affected and extent of the foot involved. Treatment choice depends on the grade of ulcer (Figure 9–27). Table 9–2 shows treatment based on classification of foot ulcers.

As a general rule in treating infections of the foot, a balance must be struck between salvage of tissue and foot function. A healed amputation at a more proximal level is more advantageous to the patient than leaving a marginally viable area of the foot that requires constant wound care.

Large wounds should not be left to heal by secondary intention. Split-thickness skin grafts, especially on the sole of the foot or over an amputation site are prone to breakdown.

A. SURGICAL TREATMENT FOR RELIEVING BONY PROMINENCES

As previously stated, a major goal of surgical procedures in the ulcerated or "at risk" foot is to relieve bony prominences that cause pressure on the skin. These prominences are located at several common sites.

The hallux may have a prominence beneath the metatarsal head, on the plantar-medial aspect of the interphalangeal joint, or over the median eminence secondary to a bunion deformity (Figure 9–28). A prominence caused by the medial sesamoid can be relieved by complete removal of the sesamoid. If this does not adequately relieve the prominence, a dorsiflexion osteotomy or resection of the metatarsal head can be performed. Ulcers found over the plantarmedial aspect of the interphalangeal joint can often be relieved by simple excision of the prominent medial condyles or by resection of the entire joint. A prominence over the median eminence can be addressed with a routine bunion procedure.

The diabetic patient is subject to clawtoe deformities resulting from motor neuropathy, causing prominences under the metatarsal heads and over the dorsum of the proximal interphalangeal joints. Depending on the severity, treatment varies from reduction of the metatarsophalangeal joints and proximal interphalangeal arthroplasties to resection of the metatarsal heads and interphalangeal fusions.

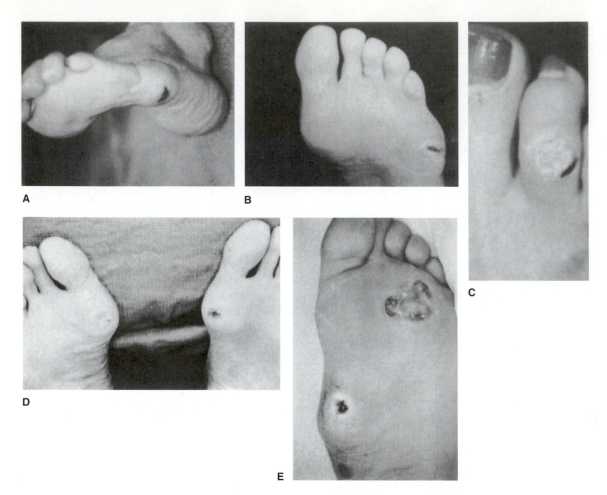

Figure 9–25. Examples of pressure ulceration at various locations on bony prominences. **A:** Fifth metatarsal base. **B:** Fifth metatarsal head. **C:** Dorsum of the proximal interphalangeal joint of a hammer toe. **D:** Medial sesamoid, first metatarsal head. **E:** Exostosis of a midfoot (type 1) Charcot joint, as well as intermediate metatarsal heads. (Reproduced, with permission, from Brodsky JW: The Diabetic Foot. In Mann RA, Coughlin MJ: *Surgery of the Foot and Ankle,* 6th ed. St. Louis: Mosby-Year Book, 1993.)

A collapsed longitudinal arch from Charcot changes causes the classic rocker-bottom foot with prominences along the plantar and medial aspects of the midfoot. This can be addressed with a simple exostectomy for a mild deformity, or an appropriate osteotomy or arthrodesis for a more complex deformity.

B. TREATMENT OF OSTEOMYELITIS

Osteomyelitis is a common complication present in a grade 2 or 3 diabetic foot ulcer. The infection is seldom eradicated without surgical debridement of the bone. Frequently, more radical treatment than simple exostectomy is required. For example, infection of a proximal phalanx is usually treated by resection of the phalanx. Osteomyelitis of the metatarsal may require ray amputation if more than just the head is involved. If multiple metatarsals are infected, a transmetatarsal amputation is often the best treatment.

Osteomyelitis of the midfoot is a complication of a collapsed Charcot foot. The treatment options for such an infection include wide local debridement with exostectomy or a Syme's amputation. Similarly, osteomyelitis of the calcaneus is usually treated with a below-knee amputation, though a partial calcanectomy and less commonly a Syme's amputation can be attempted.

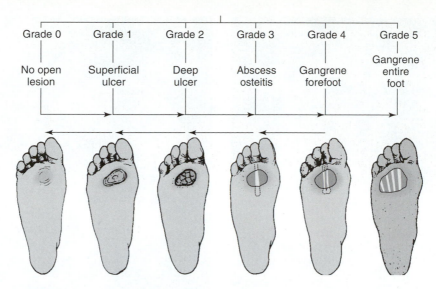

Figure 9–26. The original Rancho Los Amigos classification by Wagner and Meggitt presented the first widely referenced classification of diabetic foot lesions. Two concepts included in this classification are now in need of revision, in light of further experience. The first is the concept that all lesions of the diabetic foot from grade 1 ulcers to grade 5 gangrene occur along a natural continuum. Although this may often be true for the grade 1 ulcer, which progresses to the grade 3 lesion of osteomyelitis, this is not the case with grades 4 and 5. Grades 4 and 5 are vascular lesions or descriptions of the vascular status of the foot and are not necessarily related to the progression of the lesser grades. The ischemic lesions of grades 4 and 5 may exist separately from the lesser grades or coincide with any of them, including a forefoot that is otherwise grade 1 (ie, a superficial lesion). Vascular pathologic changes can and should be graded also, but there is not necessarily a relationship between the depth of ulcerative lesions (ie, grades 0, 1, 2, and 3) and the dysvascularity of the foot (ie, grades 4 and 5). Moreover, the grade 5 foot is truly no longer a foot problem but belongs in the domain of salvage of the proximal portion of the leg. The second concept that needs to be refined is that there are not necessarily pathways backward and forward from each grade of lesion (eg, grade 4 feet [partial gangrene] cannot be reversed to grade 3). (Reproduced, with permission, from Brodsky JW: The Diabetic Foot. In Mann RA, Coughlin MJ [editors]: *Surgery of the Foot and Ankle*, 6th ed. St. Louis: Mosby-Year Book, 1993.)

C. TREATMENT OF CHARCOT FOOT

A Charcot joint is also referred to as a neuropathic, neurotrophic, or neuroarthropathic joint. Diabetes is by far the leading cause of Charcot joints. A Charcot foot has several distinct characteristics. Marked destruction of joint surfaces is evident with collapse of joint spaces, often accompanied by dislocations of one or more joints (Figure 9–29). Calcification or bony debris is present in the periarticular soft tissues. Pain is minimal or considerably less than would be expected given the degree of destruction. The cause of Charcot joints remains controversial. The traditional theory is that repetitive trauma to an insensitive foot causes the joint destruction. Recent findings attribute the massive bony resorption sometimes found in Charcot joints to increased vascularity secondary to abnormal sympathetic reflexes. Both of these factors probably play a role in Charcot arthropathy.

A patient with a Charcot foot will present with a fracture, subluxation, or dislocation of one or more of their joints. They may have a red, hot, swollen foot,

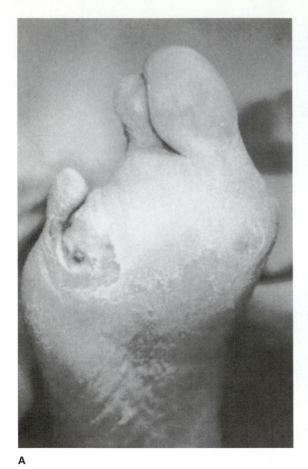 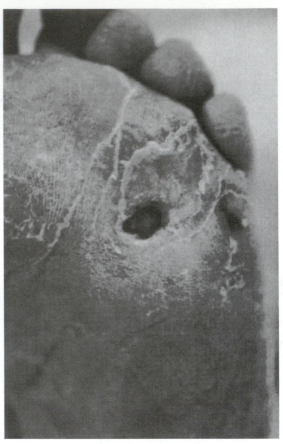

A   **B**

Figure 9–27. Comparison of grade 1 (**A**) and grade 2 (**B**) ulcers (new depth and ischemia classification). Note the exposed deep tissues of the grade 2 ulcer. (Reproduced, with permission, from Brodsky JW: The Diabetic Foot. In Mann RA, Coughlin MJ [editors]: *Surgery of the Foot and Ankle,* 6th ed. St. Louis: Mosby-Year Book, 1993.)

which may cause difficulty in distinguishing Charcot foot from cellulitis, osteomyelitis, or an abscess. This clinical picture is referred to as **acute Charcot joint.** Roentgenographic studies may be normal or may show early destructive changes. Infection can usually be ruled out by clinical examination and laboratory testing. Computed tomographic (CT) scan and MRI are usually not helpful in distinguishing a Charcot foot from osteomyelitis, unless an abscess cavity is present.

A chronic or subacute Charcot foot is identified primarily by its irregular shape. Physical examination shows little acute inflammation or erythema but rather evidence of chronic swelling of the affected area. Radiographs show marked joint destruction, subluxation, or dislocation, and periarticular soft-tissue calcification and new bone formation. Multiple bony protuberances, with or without overlying ulcerations, are usually pres-

ent. The classic rocker-bottom foot results from collapse of the longitudinal arch and subluxation at the midtarsal joints. The joints most commonly involved with Charcot changes are the tarsometatarsal joints, followed by the talonavicular and calcaneocuboid joints (Figure 9–30). The phalanges and subtalar joint are rarely involved.

1. Principles of treatment—There are several important principles to follow in the treatment of Charcot joints. The primary goal is to limit joint destruction and preserve normal bony anatomy to prevent soft-tissue ulceration.

2. Treatment of acute phase—For a patient who presents in the acute phase of Charcot joint, the initial treatment should be immobilization and elevation of the foot. This can best be achieved with a non-

Table 9–2. Classification and treatment of diabetic foot ulcers.

Grade	Classification	Treatment
0	Foot is "at risk" for developing ulcer. Skin remains intact, but underlying bone deformity places foot at risk for skin breakdown.	Proper footwear plus other preventive measures such as patient education, and surgical correction as described in text.
1	Lesion affects skin only	Outpatient dressing changes or total contact cast. Antibiotics usually not necessary.
2	Deep lesions that involve underlying tendons, bones, or ligaments (Figure 9–26).	Surgical debridement and hospitalization for aggressive wound care and intravenous antibiotics. Goal is conversion to grade 1 ulcer.
3	Abscess or esteomyelitis present as complication of ulcer.	Emergency surgery for drainage of acute infection. Wound often left open, with dressing changes performed until definitive closure or amputation is done at a later date.
4	Gangrene is present in the toes or forefoot.	Appropriate amputation.
5	Entire foot is gangrenous.	Appropriate amputation.

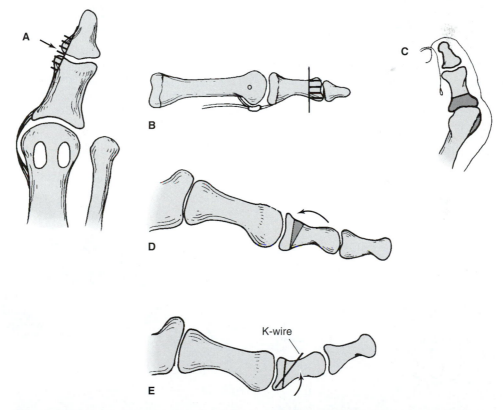

Figure 9–28. Four procedures for recalcitrant ulceration over the condyles of the interphalangeal joint of the hallux. **A:** Reduction of the condyles of the joint. **B:** Resection of the interphalangeal joint. **C:** Modified Keller procedure (resection of the base of the proximal phalanx). **D:** Dorsiflexion osteotomy of the base of the proximal phalanx. **E:** Kirschner wire fixation of dorsiflexion osteotomy. (Reproduced, with permission, from Brodsky JW: The Diabetic Foot. In Mann RA, Coughlin MJ [editors]: *Surgery of the Foot and Ankle,* 6th ed. St. Louis: Mosby-Year Book, 1993.)

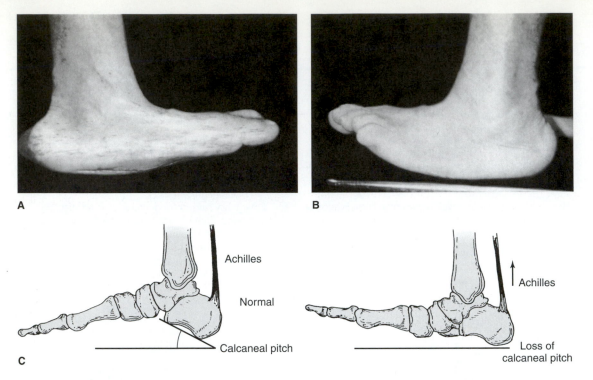

Figure 9–29. **A** and **B:** The classic rocker-bottom Charcot foot, with collapse and then reversal of the longitudinal arch. **C:** Loss of the normal calcaneal pitch, or angle relative to the floor in patients with Charcot collapse of the arch. This leads to a mechanical disadvantage for the Achilles tendon. (Reproduced, with permission, from Brodsky JW: The Diabetic Foot. In Mann RA, Coughlin MJ [editors]: *Surgery of the Foot and Ankle,* 6th ed. St. Louis: Mosby-Year Book, 1993.)

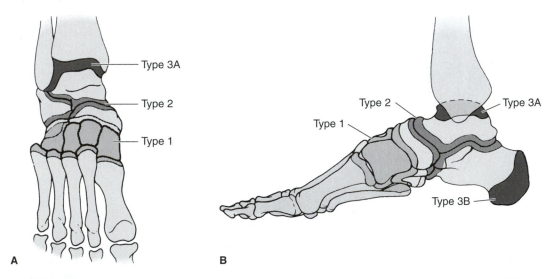

Figure 9–30. Anteroposterior (**A**) and lateral (**B**) views of the foot, demonstrating the anatomic classification of Charcot joints of the tarsus. Type 1: midfoot, involving the tarsometatarsal and naviculocuneiform joints. Type 2: hindfoot, involving the subtalar, talonavicular, or calcaneocuboid joints. Type 3A: ankle, involving the tibiotalar joint. Type 3B: Os calcis, involving a pathologic fracture of the calcaneus. (Reproduced, with permission, from Brodsky JW: The Diabetic Foot. In Mann RA, Coughlin MJ [editors]: *Surgery of the Foot and Ankle,* 6th ed. St. Louis: Mosby-Year Book, 1993.)

weight–bearing total contact cast. The skin must be checked at weekly intervals initially to look for breakdown. Surgery is never attempted on the acute Charcot foot, unless necessitated by infection. Once the acute phase subsides, the immobilization can be accomplished by means of an ankle-foot orthosis or other appropriate removable support. Custom-made shoes can then be fitted to adjust to the bony prominences.

3. Treatment of subacute phase—Surgery can be performed once the foot has stabilized, and there is no ongoing bony destruction. Operations address the bony prominences that have been created by Charcot destruction and collapse. Often, simple removal of a prominence is all that is required, and, sometimes, fusion of one or several joints is necessary. One of the most common foot deformities is a collapsed arch and rocker-bottom deformity from subluxation of multiple joints in the midfoot. Usually, an exostectomy of the prominent bones on the plantar aspect of the midfoot is sufficient. Alternatively, an osteotomy and arthrodesis of the midfoot can be performed to realign the foot and reconstitute the arch in cases where a simple exostectomy is inadequate (Figure 9–31). This procedure has a high complication rate and an extended time to achieve union. Not infrequently, amputation may result. In the case of Charcot involvement of the ankle joint, retrograde intramedullary nailing has been shown to be successful in achieving union but also has significant complication rates.

Apelqvist J et al: Long term costs for foot ulcers in diabetic patients in a multi-disciplinary setting. Foot Ankle Int 1995;16:388.

Brodsky JW: The diabetic foot. In Mann RA, Coughlin MJ (editors): *Surgery of the Foot and Ankle.* St. Louis: Mosby-Year Book, 1993.

Early JS, Hansen ST: Surgical reconstruction of the diabetic foot: A salvage approach for a mid foot collapse. Foot Ankle Int 1996;17:325.

Johnson JE et al: Prospective study of bone, indium-111-labeled white blood cell, and gallium-67 scanning for the evaluation of osteomyelitis in the diabetic foot. Foot Ankle Int 1996; 17:10.

Myerson MS et al: Management of mid foot diabetic neural arthropathy. Foot Ankle Int 1994;15:233.

Perry JE et al: The use of running shoes to reduce plantar pressures in patients who have diabetes. J Bone Joint Surg 1995;778:1819.

Pinzur MS, Kelikian A: Charcot ankle fusion with a retrograde locked intramedullary nail. Foot Ankle Int 1997;18:699.

Schon LC, Marks RM: The management of neural arthropathic fracture-dislocations in the diabetic patient. Orthop Clin North Am 1995;25:375.

Wagner FW Jr: A classification and treatment program for diabetic, neuropathic, and dysvascular foot problems. Instr Course Lect 1979;28:143.

Weinstein D et al: Evaluation of magnetic resonance imaging in the diagnosis of osteomyelitis and diabetic foot infections. Foot Ankle 1993;14:18.

DISORDERS OF THE TOENAILS

Occasional toenail problems occur in the younger age group. Trauma such as stubbing the toe or, more frequently, improper nail care can initiate ingrown toenails. This is usually the result of tearing off a toenail, which leaves the nail too short and predisposes it to become ingrown.

Toenail problems in the older age-group are more varied, including an incurvating nail or a thickened hypertrophied nail associated with a chronic fungal infection, an ingrown nail resulting from improper nail cutting, and on rare occasions a subungual exostosis.

Etiologic Findings

The anatomy of the toenail is demonstrated in Figure 9–32. The nail unit consists of four components: the proximal nail fold, the nail matrix, the nail bed, and the hyponychium. The area in which most of the problems occur is the lateral or medial nail groove, where an ingrown nail occurs at the level of the nail bed or hyponychium.

Clinical Findings

A. SYMPTOMS AND SIGNS

The history of most nail problems is not complex and usually quickly defines the nature of the problem.

1. Infection of the toenails—Infection of the toenails usually begins slowly, with erythema and swelling along the lateral side of the nail, followed by increasing pain and drainage, and finally the development of granulation tissue, usually in response to the foreign body reaction of the nail itself.

2. Mycotic nail—In the case of the mycotic (fungal) nail, there is usually a long, slow history of development of deformation of the nail, often with medial or lateral deviation of the nail, marked hypertrophy, and increased pain when wearing shoes. At times, an incurvated nail condition develops in which one or both edges of the nail slowly curve inward, resulting in pinching of the nail plate. This may cause a localized infection, or it may be that just the sheer pressure of the nail against the skin is the cause of the pain.

3. Subungual exostosis—The patient who develops subungual exostosis usually notes pain evolving beneath the toenail over a long period. Erosion of the nail from below occurs because of the pressure of the exostosis against the nail itself. Often, the patient does not seek help until there is actual breakdown of the tissue, giving rise to a rather ugly-appearing lesion that seems much more ominous than the condition itself.

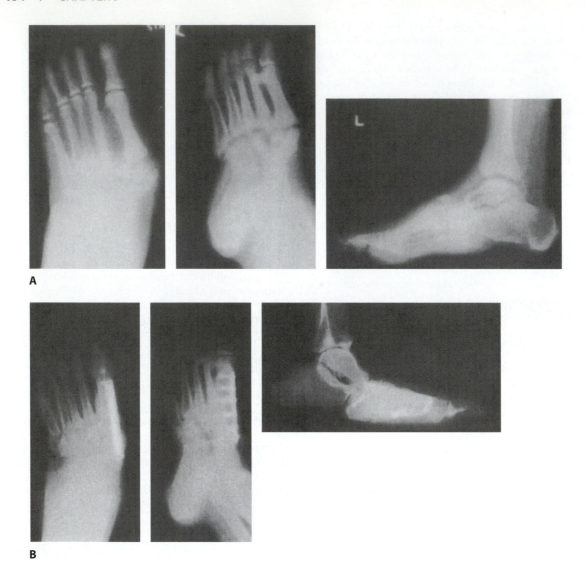

Figure 9–31. **A:** Patient with advanced midfoot Charcot deformity and soft-tissue breakdown over an extruded medial cuneiform. **B:** Limited arthrodesis with internal fixation and iliac grafting to relieve pressure on soft tissue and reestablish weight bearing of the first ray. (Reproduced, with permission, from Brodsky JW: The Diabetic Foot. In Mann RA, Coughlin MJ [editors]: *Surgery of the Foot and Ankle,* 6th ed. St. Louis: Mosby-Year Book, 1993.)

B. IMAGING STUDIES

The only time a radiograph is necessary when evaluating a toenail problem is for subungual exostosis, which is clearly seen with a lateral view.

Treatment

A. CONSERVATIVE MANAGEMENT

1. Chronic ingrown toenail—For the chronic ingrown toenail, the margin of the nail is often cut on an oblique angle to relieve the pressure of the nail against the skin. This procedure, along with local care and occasionally systemic antibiotics, usually permits the condition to resolve. It is important, however, to explain to the patient the necessity of permitting the nail to grow out over the ungual labia, to depress it and prevent the ingrown nail from recurring.

2. Chronic onychophosis of the nail—Chronic onychophosis of the nail must be kept debrided. If an

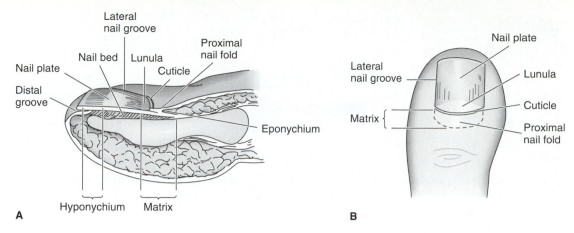

Figure 9–32. **A:** Cross section of the toe demonstrates the components of the toenail and supporting structures. **B:** The proximal nail is covered by the proximal nail fold and cuticle. The lunula is the main germinal area. (Reproduced, with permission, from Mann RA, Coughlin MJ: *The Video Textbook of Foot and Ankle Surgery*. St. Louis: Medical Video Productions, 1991.)

ingrown nail occurs, the margins must be trimmed to relieve the pressure against the skin.

3. Subungual exostosis—Subungual exostosis is not treated conservatively unless there is a surrounding infection.

B. Surgical Treatment

1. Ingrown toenail—The surgical management of the ingrown toenail consists of the Winograd procedure. In this procedure, the medial or lateral margin of the offending nail is removed to prevent the margin of the nail from growing into the labia. The nail matrix is removed as thoroughly as possible to prevent the possible growth of a nail horn, which occurs in about 5% of cases.

2. Chronic ingrown toenail or onychophosis—Surgical avulsion of the toenail for a chronic ingrown nail problem, or onychophosis, usually is not satisfactory; as the nail regrows, it once again becomes ingrown. Medical therapy will not prevent recurrence of an ingrown toenail.

3. Chronic infection—If there is severe distortion of the nail caused by chronic infection, the nail and the nail bed can be removed in their entirety. This usually results in a horny base where the nail existed, and this is often a satisfactory outcome. A nail horn may grow, which patients do not appreciate, and may require removal.

The terminal Syme's amputation can be carried out to eliminate the nail and matrix completely (Figure 9–33). Although results are usually satisfactory, some patients do not like the appearance of the toe or absence of the toenail because of its somewhat bulbous appearance. The terminal Syme's procedure is carried out under digital block. An elliptical incision is made over the distal end of the toe, removing the nail and its matrix in their entirety. The distal portion of the distal phalanx is removed and the edges smoothed. The tip of the toe is defatted and loosely sutured. In this manner, the nail is completely removed and soft tissue covers the area of the former nail bed. The only significant complication associated with this procedure is the regrowth of some nail matrix beneath the healed flap, which will result in an abscesslike lesion that must be drained and the nail matrix excised. This may be a resistant problem, requiring more than one debridement over a period of years.

4. Subungual exostosis—Surgical management of subungual exostosis requires lifting up the nail, identification of the exostosis, and complete removal of the exostosis and its stalk. The dissection must be carefully carried out and the entire exostosis removed to prevent recurrence. The nail bed is placed back onto its bed.

Coughlin MJ: Toenail abnormalities. In Mann RA, Coughlin MJ (editors): *Surgery of the Foot and Ankle*. St. Louis: Mosby-Year Book, 1993.

Gupta AK, Scher RK, De Doncker P: Current management of onychomycosis: An overview. Dermatol Clin 1997;15:121.

Mann RA, Coughlin MJ: Toenail abnormalities. In Mann RA, Coughlin MJ (editors): *The Video Textbook of Foot and Ankle Surgery*. St. Louis: Video Medical Productions, 1990.

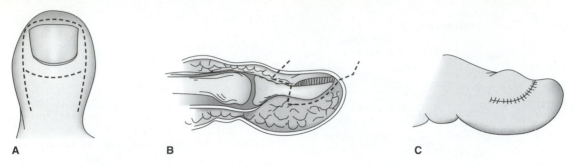

A   **B**   **C**

Figure 9–33. Syme's amputation of toenail. **A:** Elliptical or rectangular incision is centered over the nail bed and matrix. **B:** The distal half of the distal phalanx is resected. **C:** Excess skin is resected, and skin edges are approximated. (Reproduced, with permission, from Mann RA, Coughlin MJ: *The Video Textbook of Foot and Ankle Surgery*. St. Louis: Medical Video Productions, 1991.)

NEUROLOGIC DISORDERS OF THE FOOT

1. Interdigital Neuroma

An interdigital neuroma is a painful affliction involving the plantar aspect of the forefoot. It usually involves the second or third interspace and is characterized by a well-localized area of pain on the plantar aspect of the foot that radiates into the web space. The symptoms are usually aggravated by ambulation and relieved by rest. As a rule, wearing a tight-fitting shoe aggravates the pain, and walking barefoot often relieves it.

Etiologic Findings

The precise cause of interdigital neuroma has not been determined. It occurs in women about 10 times more frequently than men, and, as a result, high-fashion shoe wear has been implicated. Several studies demonstrate that the changes in the nerve appear to occur just distal to the transverse metatarsal ligament. This finding has given rise to the hypothesis that the neuroma results from the constant traction of the nerve against the ligament as the toes are brought into a dorsiflexed position, a theory that would explain the higher incidence in women wearing high-heeled shoes. Although this condition is called **interdigital neuroma,** it is not a neuroma per se. The pathologic changes involve actual degeneration of the nerve tissue associated with deposition of fibrin in the surrounding tissue (Figure 9–34).

Clinical Findings

A. SYMPTOMS AND SIGNS

Overall alignment of the toes is observed with the patient in a standing position. Occasionally, an associated cyst in the web space will cause deviation of the toes that is evident only in a standing position. Mechanical pressure from the cyst causes neuritic symptoms.

The patient is then seated and the foot carefully examined. The patient with a neuroma demonstrates well-localized tenderness between the two metatarsal heads. The third interspace is more frequently involved than the second, and it is extremely rare to have involvement of the first or fourth web space. Pain over the metatarsophalangeal joint itself is caused by disease involving the metatarsophalangeal joint and is not associated with a neuroma. Therefore, it is important to distinguish pain in the interspace from pain affecting the metatarsophalangeal joint.

In approximately 75% of neuroma patients, the clinical symptoms are reproduced by firmly palpating the web space, resulting in dysesthesia in the involved

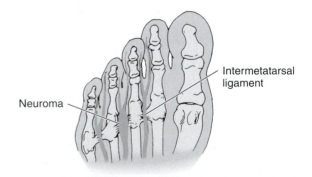

Intermetatarsal ligament

Neuroma

Figure 9–34. An interdigital neuroma impingement occurs beneath the intermetatarsal ligament. (Reproduced, with permission, from Mann RA, Coughlin MJ: *The Video Textbook of Foot and Ankle Surgery*. St. Louis: Medical Video Productions, 1991.)

web space. Often in the third interspace, a palpable click can be noted as the metatarsal heads are squeezed together while pressure is being applied to the plantar aspect of the foot. This helps to confirm the clinical diagnosis. Sensory deficit is rarely associated with interdigital neuroma.

B. IMAGING STUDIES

Radiographs are not helpful in the diagnosis of an interdigital neuroma but may reveal pathology at the metatarsophalangeal joint as the cause of the patients symptoms.

Treatment

A. CONSERVATIVE MANAGEMENT

Conservative management begins with wearing a wider, soft-soled shoe to accommodate the foot without mediolateral compression and lowering the heel. A soft metatarsal support is placed in the shoe proximal to the area of the neuroma, thereby spreading the metatarsal heads and lifting them off the bottom of the shoe. Approximately one third of patients will respond to this treatment. Steroid injection into the web space can be helpful in resolving the neuroma but is not without hazard. Atrophy of the surrounding fat tissue and occasionally rupture of a collateral ligament may occur, resulting in deviation of the toe.

B. SURGICAL TREATMENT

Surgical excision of the nerve is indicated if conservative treatment fails. A 2.5-cm dorsal approach incision is made in the midline of the involved web space and carried down to the transverse metatarsal ligament, which is cut. The nerve is noted to lie just beneath the transverse metatarsal ligament. A nerve that is quite thickened is reassuring evidence that the correct diagnosis has been made; however, a nerve of normal thickness should still be removed if the clinical diagnosis of neuroma has been made from other evidence. The nerve is freed up distally and proximally, transected proximal to the metatarsal head, and then dissected out distally, where it is cut just past its bifurcation. Care is taken not to disrupt the surrounding fatty tissue or intrinsic muscles. A compression dressing is used for 3 weeks after routine wound closure, and ambulation is permitted in a postoperative shoe. Decreased sensation in the toes on either side of the web space is noted postoperatively in 60% of patients.

Approximately 80% of patients are totally satisfied with the results of the procedure, whereas 20% obtain little or no relief. The precise cause of this failure rate is a bit of an enigma. Obviously in some patients, the diagnosis was incorrectly made and the metatarsophalangeal joint was actually involved.

C. RECURRENT NEUROMA

A recurrent neuroma is indeed a true neuroma that has resulted following the transection of the common digital nerve on the plantar aspect of the foot. True neuritic symptoms occur in some cases in which transection was not proximal enough or the nerve ending was adherent and trapped beneath the metatarsal head. Careful percussion of the plantar aspect to elicit the Tinel's sign can frequently localize the cut end of the nerve (bulb neuroma). If the severed nerve can be clinically well localized, re-exploration for the neuroma is carried out usually through a dorsal approach. The neuroma is identified and transected to a more proximal level, and symptoms are relieved in 60–70% of patients.

2. Tarsal Tunnel Syndrome

Tarsal tunnel syndrome is a compressive neuropathy of the posterior tibial nerve as it passes behind the medial malleolus. The tarsal tunnel is formed by the fibroosseous tunnel resulting from the flexor retinaculum as it wraps around the posterior aspect of the medial malleolus (Figure 9–35). Tarsal tunnel syndrome causes poorly localized dysesthesias on the plantar aspect of the foot. The symptom complex is often aggravated by activity and relieved by rest. Some patients complain mainly of nocturnal dysesthesias.

Etiologic Findings

Tarsal tunnel syndrome may arise from a space-occupying lesion within the tarsal tunnel (eg, a ganglion, synovial cyst, or lipoma) or distally against one of the two terminal branches: the medial or lateral plantar

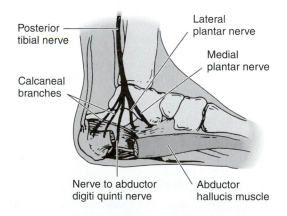

Figure 9–35. Posterior tibial nerve and major branches. (Reproduced, with permission, from Mann RA, Coughlin MJ: *The Video Textbook of Foot and Ankle Surgery.* St. Louis: Medical Video Productions, 1991.

nerve. It occasionally follows severe trauma to the lower extremity probably because of edema or scarring. Other causes are severe venous varicosities, tenosynovitis, or a tumor within the nerve. In more than half of the cases, however, the precise cause cannot be determined.

Clinical Findings

A. Symptoms and Signs

The diagnosis is entertained after obtaining a history of paresthesias or burning in the tibial nerve distribution. Careful evaluation of the patient in the standing and sitting positions is necessary to check posture and increased fullness, thickening, or swelling in the involved tarsal tunnel area. Careful percussion may elicit a Tinel's sign over the posterior tibial nerve in the tarsal tunnel or distally along the divisions of the posterior tibial nerve (the medial calcaneal nerve, and medial and lateral plantar nerves).

Muscle weakness is usually not observed, but loss of sensation and two-point discrimination may be occasionally detected.

Electrodiagnostic studies should be carried out to help confirm the diagnosis of tarsal tunnel syndrome. Nerve conduction velocities along the medial plantar nerve to the abductor hallucis muscle (latency < 6.2 ms) and of the lateral plantar nerve to the abductor digiti quinti (latency usually < 7 ms) should be within 1 ms of each other, otherwise indicating nerve compression in the tarsal tunnel. Motor-evoked potentials that demonstrate a decreased amplitude and increased duration are also felt to be indicative of tarsal tunnel syndrome. The most accurate study for tarsal tunnel syndrome appears to be sensory nerve conduction velocity, although this is also the least reproducible study.

The definitive diagnosis of tarsal tunnel syndrome should be based upon (1) the clinical history of ill-defined burning, tingling pain in the plantar aspect of the foot, (2) positive physical findings of Tinel's sign along the course of the nerve, and (3) electrodiagnostic studies. If all three factors are not positive, the diagnosis of tarsal tunnel syndrome should be suspect. MRI may be quite useful in demonstrating the presence of a space-occupying lesion.

Treatment

A. Conservative Management

The tarsal tunnel syndrome should be managed with anti-inflammatory medications and an occasional steroid injection into the tarsal tunnel area. Aspiration and injection of a cyst or ganglion may be attempted but is rarely successful. Immobilization in a polypropylene ankle-foot orthosis may also be useful.

B. Surgical Treatment

Surgical intervention can be considered if conservative management fails. Approximately 75% of patients operated on for tarsal tunnel syndrome are satisfied with the result. The other 25% may continue to have varying degrees of discomfort. The surgical release uses an incision behind the medial malleolus that is carried distally to about the level of the talonavicular joint. The investing retinaculum is exposed and released. The posterior tibial nerve is identified proximal to the tarsal tunnel area and carefully traced distally behind the medial malleolus. The division into its three terminal branches is identified. Because the medial calcaneal branch passes from the posterior aspect of the lateral plantar nerve, the dissection should be carried out along its dorsal aspect. There may be one or more medial calcaneal branches. The medial plantar nerve should be traced distally until it passes through the fibro-osseous tunnel in the abductor hallucis muscle. The lateral plantar nerve should be traced behind the abductor hallucis muscle until it passes toward the lateral aspect of the foot. A preoperative Tinel's sign distal to the tarsal tunnel area requires that the area be carefully explored to determine whether there is a ganglion or cyst within the tendon sheath as a cause of the tarsal tunnel syndrome.

Postoperatively, a compression dressing is applied and weight bearing is prohibited for 3 weeks, before progressive ambulation is permitted.

The results following tarsal tunnel release depend on the pathologic symptom that is found at the time of surgery. Removal of a space-occupying lesion usually relieves all of the symptoms. Involvement of a single nerve branch, such as the medial or lateral plantar nerve, also portends good results after surgery. If more diffuse pain is felt throughout the foot before surgery, and no definite constriction on the nerve is found at exploration, only one half to two thirds of patients can be expected to experience pain relief.

3. Traumatic Neuromas About the Foot

A traumatic neuroma about the foot presents a difficult problem in management because footwear can cause constant irritation of the neuroma. The most frequent cause of traumatic neuroma in the foot is previous surgery. Despite caution in making incisions about the foot, many lesser and occasionally major nerve trunks can be injured. The dorsal aspect of the foot is most frequently involved (Figure 9–36).

Clinical Findings

The clinical evaluation begins with a careful history of the problem and an evaluation of the area involved to

The results following resection of a traumatic neuroma are quite variable. Initial relief from removing the traumatic neuroma is routine, but unless the nerve is buried where it will not be exposed to pressure, the symptoms may recur in time. It is therefore preferable to bury the end of the nerve into bone, if possible. Resection of most neuromas will accentuate a sensory deficit, but this is usually not a significant clinical problem.

4. Entrapment of the Superficial Branch of the Deep Peroneal Nerve

Osteophyte formation at the talonavicular or metatarsocuneiform joint may entrap the superficial branch of the deep peroneal nerve as it passes beneath the extensor retinaculum. Patient complaints are of dysesthesias on the foot or difficulty in wearing shoes, depending upon the location of the entrapment.

The superficial branch of the deep peroneal nerve passes onto the dorsum of the foot between the extensor hallucis longus and extensor digitorum longus tendons. It continues beneath the extensor retinaculum, coursing along the dorsal surface of the talus and navicular, and more distally across the metatarsocuneiform joints. Osteophyte formation at any point along the course of the nerve may cause sufficient pressure against the nerve to cause an entrapment problem.

Clinical Findings

A. Symptoms and Signs

The clinical evaluation begins with a careful history regarding the patient's complaint of dysesthesias over the dorsum of the foot. The physical examination demonstrates tingling along the course of the superficial branch of the deep peroneal nerve, which radiates into the first web space. Often the precise location of the nerve entrapment can be identified by careful palpation and by rolling the nerve across the involved bony prominence.

B. Imaging Studies

Radiographs usually reveal the offending osteophytes, often along the area of the talonavicular or metatarsocuneiform joints. Placing a radiographic marker at the area of maximum tenderness can help to identify the bony prominence.

Treatment

A. Conservative Management

Conservative management consists of attempting to keep the pressure off the involved area, either by padding the tongue of the shoe or by trying to create a pad that will not put pressure directly upon the nerve.

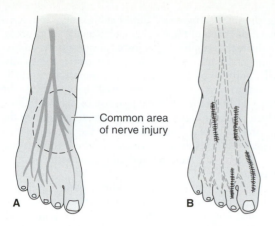

Figure 9–36. **A:** Common area of traumatic nerve entrapment. **B:** Frequent incisions that may lead to entrapment of dorsal sensory nerves. (Reproduced, with permission, from Mann RA, Coughlin MJ: *The Video Textbook of Foot and Ankle Surgery*. St. Louis: Medical Video Productions, 1991.)

determine the precise location of the neuroma, which is essential for proper treatment. Rarely is any type of electrodiagnostic study indicated, and radiographs are not usually necessary.

Treatment

A. Conservative Management

Attempts to relieve pressure on the neuroma with a large shoe or a carefully designed pad may be of benefit. Occasionally a cortisone injection into the area may help, particularly when a small nerve is involved. Surgical intervention is indicated if conservative measures fail.

B. Surgical Treatment

Careful planning must be undertaken prior to the excision of a traumatic neuroma. The exact location of the neuroma and the area of sensitivity proximal to it must be determined. The incision must be made as precisely as possible to identify the neuroma and trace the nerve proximally into an area that would not be affected by pressure from shoes and boots. The neuroma is excised, leaving enough nerve to bring the cut end into an area of minimal pressure. The cut end is buried into an excavation in bone, if possible, or beneath a muscle such as the extensor digitorum brevis muscle. When carrying out a resection of the sural nerve, it is important, particularly in an individual who wears heavy work boots, that the end of the nerve is brought proximally enough so that the top of the boot will not press upon the nerve, resulting in continued symptoms.

If these measures fail, decompression of the nerve will usually bring about satisfactory resolution of the condition.

B. SURGICAL TREATMENT

Depending upon the area of entrapment (talonavicular or metatarsocuneiform), a slightly curved incision is made and carried down through the retinaculum to expose the nerve. Great caution must be taken during the approach so that the nerve is not inadvertently damaged. The nerve is carefully lifted off of its bed, exposing the osteophytes, which are removed with a rongeur. The bone surfaces are coated with bone wax prior to laying the nerve back on its bed. After wound closure in layers, the foot is immobilized for approximately 3 weeks in a postoperative shoe.

The results following release of the superficial portion of the deep peroneal nerve are usually satisfactory. Because the nerve itself usually is not damaged by the entrapment, a favorable outcome is expected.

Bailie DS, Kelikian AS: Tarsal tunnel syndrome: Diagnosis, surgical technique, and functional outcome. Foot Ankle Int 1998; 2:65.

Baxter DE: Functional nerve disorders. In Mann RA, Coughlin MJ (editors): *Surgery of the Foot and Ankle.* St. Louis: Mosby-Year Book, 1993, pp. 559-573.

Beskin JL: Nerve entrapment syndromes of the foot and ankle. J Am Acad Orthop Surg 1997;5:261.

Cimino WR: Tarsal tunnel syndrome: Review of the literature. Foot Ankle 1990;11:47.

Mann RA: Static nerve disorders. In Mann RA, Coughlin MJ (editors): *Surgery of the Foot and Ankle.* St. Louis: Mosby-Year Book, 1993.

Mann RA, Reynolds JD: Interdigital neuroma: A critical clinical analysis. Foot Ankle 1983;3:238.

Okafor B, et al: Treatment of Morton's neuroma by neurolysis. Foot Ankle Int 1997;5:284.

Pfeiffer WH, Cracchiolo A III: Clinical results after tarsal tunnel decompression. J Bone Joint Surg 1994;76A:1222.

RHEUMATOID FOOT

The foot is involved in 90% of patients with long-standing rheumatoid arthritis, and the involvement is almost always bilateral. The forefoot is most commonly involved, but deterioration of the subtalar joint has been noted in about 35% of patients and of the ankle joint in about 30%.

Etiologic Findings

The changes in the forefoot are caused by the chronic synovitis, which destroys the supporting structures about the metatarsophalangeal joints. The joint capsules are distended and the ligaments destroyed. When these structures no longer function to provide stability

for the joint, progressive dorsal subluxation and eventual dislocation of the metatarsophalangeal joints occur. As the metatarsophalangeal joints progress from subluxation to dislocation, the plantar fat pad is drawn distally, and the base of the proximal phalanx eventually comes to rest on the metatarsal head. Thus, the metatarsals are forced into a position of plantar flexion, which results in significant callus formation beneath the metatarsal heads. The changes at the metatarsophalangeal joints result in imbalance of the intrinsic muscles, and severe hammer toe and clawtoe deformities may result.

Significant midfoot and hindfoot pathology is also found in patients with rheumatoid arthritis. A severely flattened longitudinal arch can result from long-standing subtalar joint involvement with subluxation of the joint. Pain with less severe deformity is present in isolated talonavicular involvement of the midfoot.

Clinical Findings

A. SYMPTOMS AND SIGNS

The clinical evaluation of the rheumatoid patient begins with a careful history of the disease and the medications the patient is taking and an attempt to ascertain whether the disease process is currently in an active or a quiescent stage. It is important to obtain some indication of the patient's wound-healing capacity in the foot or elsewhere in the body.

The vascular status of the foot and quality of the skin is noted. The feet are assessed with the patient standing, which will often demonstrate marked deformities of multiple joints or localized involvement of only one or two joints. Flattening of the longitudinal arch and any hindfoot valgus are evaluated. The patient is then seated and a careful evaluation of all the joints about the foot and ankle is carried out to determine precisely the degree to which they are affected. Careful palpation of the metatarsophalangeal joints will often demonstrate the degree of the synovial activity as well as the degree of stability of the joints. The plantar aspect of the foot is inspected for the callus formation and past or present ulcerations. Flattening of the longitudinal arch and any hindfoot valgus are evaluated.

B. IMAGING STUDIES

Radiographs help to assess the number of joints involved and the degree of involvement. Bilateral involvement is frequently asymmetric.

Treatment

A. CONSERVATIVE MANAGEMENT

Conservative management includes medical management, carried out by the patient's rheumatologist. The patient should wear an extra-depth shoe with a Plasti-zote liner to reduce pressure on the metatarsal heads and the toes, which may be severely contracted dorsally. Frequently, the patient is quite comfortable in this shoe and does not require further treatment. With significant hindfoot involvement, an ankle-foot orthosis may be required to help relieve pain.

B. Surgical Treatment

The main goal of surgical management of the forefoot is to create a stable foot that will alleviate the pain beneath the metatarsal head region (Figure 9–37). Arthrodesis of the first metatarsophalangeal joint is the procedure used, with the joint placed in approximately 15 degrees of dorsiflexion in relation to the floor and approximately 15 degrees of valgus position. The lesser metatarsophalangeal joints are corrected by release of

the extensor tendons and resection arthroplasty. The metatarsal heads are excised to decompress the metatarsophalangeal joints, and the fat pad is brought back down onto the plantar aspect of the foot. The hammer toes are corrected by closed osteoclasis, which results in satisfactory realignment. The toes and metatarsophalangeal joint area are stabilized with longitudinal Kirschner wires postoperatively for approximately 4 weeks.

The results of this rheumatoid forefoot repair are most gratifying in that about 90% of patients will be satisfied with the results. There are few complications, though the blood supply to the toes is always of concern because the procedure is extensive. Occasionally, wound healing is delayed, particularly if the patient is taking high dosages of corticosteroids. A callus may re-form beneath a metatarsal head because of new bone formation about the end of the resected metatarsal.

If only a single joint is involved with the rheumatoid process, a less extensive procedure is carried out. Treatment may be isolated to a fusion of the first metatarsophalangeal joint or an arthroplasty of a lesser metatarsophalangeal joint with closed osteoclasis of the lesser toe. For isolated talonavicular rheumatoid arthritis with no significant deformity of the arch, an isolated talonavicular fusion is adequate. If much deformity is present because of subtalar joint subluxation, a triple arthrodesis is required. Ankle joint involvement is treated with ankle joint fusion. The details of the surgical procedures are described elsewhere in this chapter.

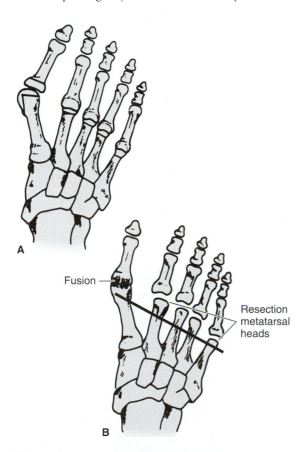

Cracchiolo A III: Surgery for rheumatoid disease. Part I. Foot abnormalities in rheumatoid arthritis. Instr Course Lect 1984; 33:386.

Haynu T et al: Arthroplasty for rheumatoid forefoot deformities by a shortening oblique osteotomy. Clin Orthop 1997;338:131.

Harper MC, Tisdel CO: Talonavicular arthrodesis for the painful adult acquired flat foot. Foot Ankle Int 1996;17:658.

Mann RA, Schakel ME: Surgical correction of rheumatoid forefoot deformities. Foot Ankle Int 1995;16:1.

McGarvey SR, Johnson KA: Keller arthroplasty in combination with resection arthroplasty of the lesser metatarsophalangeal joints in rheumatoid arthritis. Foot Ankle 1988;9:75.

Thompson FM, Mann RA: Arthritides. In Mann RA, Coughlin MJ (editors): *Surgery of the Foot and Ankle.* Mosby-Year Book, 1993.

Vainio KI: The rheumatoid foot: A clinical study with pathological and roentgenological comments. Clin Orthop 1991;265:4.

Figure 9–37. **A:** Resection of metatarsal heads. **B:** Symmetric resection of metatarsal heads minimizes recurrence of intractable plantar keratoses. (Reproduced, with permission, from Mann RA, Coughlin MJ: *The Video Textbook of Foot and Ankle Surgery.* St. Louis: Medical Video Productions, 1991.)

HEEL PAIN

Heel pain usually occurs on the plantar aspect of the heel but may also occur on the posterior aspect. When evaluating the patient for heel pain, the clinician must attempt to define as precisely as possible the location and, hence, the cause of the pain.

The causes of heel pain are presented in Table 9–3. The causes are quite variable and need to be carefully defined, so that the proper treatment can be chosen.

Clinical Findings

A. Symptoms and Signs

The clinical evaluation begins with a careful history of the onset and location of the pain. The patient's activities and types of footwear that aggravate and relieve the pain are discussed. Specific inquiry regarding radiation of pain proximally in the lower extremity may suggest lumbar disk disease as the cause. Patients active in sports should be questioned regarding significant changes in their level of activity because heel pain often is the result of increased stress on the foot.

The cause of the patient's heel pain can usually be determined by palpating the area of maximum tenderness. Plantar fasciitis, the most common cause of heel pain, usually has an area of maximum pain along the plantar medial aspect of the heel, which corresponds to the origin of the plantar fascia at the medial calcaneal tuberosity. Sometimes the pain extends distally along the plantar fascia toward the metatarsal heads. The pain is usually worsened with dorsiflexion of the toes. Achilles tendinitis typically occurs at one of two discreet sites; at the calcaneal insertion, or centered 3.0–4.0 cm proximal to the insertion. Insertional Achilles tendinitis is characterized by pain over bony prominences or spurs located at the posterior superior aspect of the calcaneus. Noninsertional Achilles tendinitis is usually associated with a thickened tendon and often quite severe pain to palpation of the thickened area.

Table 9–3. Causes of heel pain.

Causes of plantar heel pain
  Plantar fascitis
  Atrophy of heel pad
  Posttraumatic, eg, calcaneal fracture
  Enlarged calcaneal spur
  Neurologic conditions such as tarsal tunnel syndrome or
    entrapment of nerve to abductor digiti quinti
  Degenerative disk disease with radiation toward heel
  Systemic disease, eg, Reiter's syndrome, psoriatic arthritis
  Acute tear of plantar fascia
  Calcaneal apophysitis
Causes of posterior heel pain
  Retrocalcaneal bursitis
  Achilles tendinitis
  Haglund's deformity
  Degeneration of Achilles tendon insertion

Tarsal tunnel syndrome with involvement of the medial calcaneal branches should be investigated by careful percussion of the posterior tibial nerve. Evidence of degenerative disk disease requires careful testing of motor function and sensation more proximally in the calf.

B. Imaging Studies

Radiographs may demonstrate a large plantar calcaneal spur or a calcification at the insertion of the Achilles tendon. Alternatively, the posterosuperior aspect of the calcaneus may be too prominent and protrude into the Achilles tendon, a condition known as Haglund's disease or Haglund's deformity. A bone scan will sometimes reveal increased activity about the calcaneus, as may be seen in systemic diseases such as Reiter's syndrome. MRI scan may help to delineate the degree of the Achilles tendon degeneration present in cases of Achilles of tendinitis and can help to identify discontinuity of the tendon if this is in question.

Treatment

A. Conservative Management

The conservative management of heel pain depends upon the specific cause. Because many causes are related to abnormal stress on the foot, the basic principles involve reducing the stress on the involved area. Activity modification, footwear with a softer, more resilient heel, use of a soft orthotic device under the longitudinal arch to relieve some of the pressure on the region of pain, use of soft padding beneath the heel in the form of a heel cup, and, at times, cast immobilization are all modalities that may help. Nonsteroidal anti-inflammatory medications are often useful as is physical therapy to teach stretching exercises of the Achilles tendon and plantar fascia. Ultrasound therapy for plantar fasciitis and Achilles tendinitis can also be occasionally useful. The use of a night splint to help keep the Achilles tendon and plantar fascia stretched often relieves the acute pain patients experience when they first get up in the morning.

In general, the treatment of heel pain is often prolonged, requiring a great deal of patience on the part of the physician and patient. It is important to explain to the patient the nature of the problem and the fact that it is often a chronic condition that requires many months to resolve.

B. Surgical Treatment

A patient in whom symptoms cannot be controlled after 9–12 months of conservative management for plantar fasciitis may be a candidate for release of the plantar fascia and excision of a plantar heel spur if present. The success rate is approximately 75%. Caution must be exercised with the approach to the medial side of the heel to avoid damage to the medial calcaneal branch. Disruption of this nerve will cause an area of heel numbness, and possibly a troublesome neuroma along the medial side of the heel. An endoscopic approach for plantar fascia release has been described in patients who do not have a plantar heel spur that requires removal.

Surgical treatment of Achilles tendinitis is offered if 6–9 months of conservative measures do not help to eliminate symptoms. Insertional Achilles tendinitis is treated with debridement of degenerative tendon and excision of bone spurs. If a Haglund's deformity is present, it is also resected. Non-insertional Achilles tendinitis is treated with debridement of degenerative tendon. In either case, if the majority of the tendon is nonviable, it must be resected and the Achilles tendon reconstructed using the flexor digitorum longus or flexor hallucis longus tendon.

Baxter DE, Pfeffer GB: Treatment of chronic heel pain by surgical release of the first branch of the lateral plantar nerve. Clin Orthop 1992;279:229.

Bordelon RL: Heel pain. In Mann RA, Coughlin MJ (editors): *Surgery of the Foot and Ankle.* St. Louis: Mosby-Year Book, 1993.

Daly PJ et al: Plantar fasciotomy for intractable plantar fasciitis: Clinical results and biomechanical evaluation. Foot Ankle 1992;13:188.

Gill LH: Plantar fasciitis: Diagnosis and conservative management. J Am Acad Orthop Surg 1997;5:109.

Murphy GA et al: Biomechanical consequences of sequential plantar fascia release. Foot Ankle Int 1998;19:149.

Reeve F et al: Endoscopic plantar fascia release: A cross-sectional anatomic study. Foot Ankle Int 1997;18:398.

Sammarco GJ, Helfrey RB: Surgical treatment of recalcitrant plantar fasciitis. Foot Ankle Int 1996;17:520.

ARTHRODESIS ABOUT THE FOOT & ANKLE

General Considerations

A. GOALS OF ARTHRODESIS

Arthrodesis is surgical fixation of a joint to obtain fusion of the joint surfaces. Arthrodesis about the foot and ankle can be effective in achieving the following goals:

(1) elimination of joint pain;

(2) creation of a plantigrade foot;

(3) stabilization of the foot or ankle when adequate muscle function is lacking, as in residual poliomyelitis or loss of the longitudinal arch secondary to rupture of the posterior tibial tendon; and

(4) restoration of function by salvaging a situation in which no reasonable reconstructive procedure is available, as in fusion of the first metatarsophalangeal joint after failed hallux valgus repair.

B. PRINCIPLES OF ARTHRODESIS

An arthrodesis about the foot and ankle requires adherence to these general principles:
list-numbered-first:

(1) To be effective, the arthrodesis must produce a plantigrade foot. If the hindfoot or forefoot is malaligned, a less than satisfactory clinical result will be seen.

(2) Broad, cancellous bony surfaces must be placed into apposition.

(3) The arthrodesis site should be stabilized with rigid internal fixation, preferably with interfragmentary compression.

(4) When correcting malalignment of the foot, it is imperative that the hindfoot be placed into 5–7 degrees of valgus and the forefoot in neutral position with regard to abduction, adduction, pronation, and supination.

(5) The surgical approaches should be carried out in such a way as to minimize the risk of damage to the nerves.

C. EFFECTS OF ARTHRODESIS ON JOINT MOTION

Following ankle arthrodesis, residual dorsiflexion and plantar flexion movement occurs within the subtalar and transverse tarsal joints, and additional, compensatory motion may develop over time. Arthritic changes in these joints may become symptomatic following ankle arthrodesis, and in time, extension of the fusion may be required.

The subtalar joint and transverse tarsal joints must be viewed as a joint complex similar to the universal joint of a car. Movement in these joints is interrelated. After subtalar arthrodesis, inversion and eversion is lost, but transverse tarsal joint motion is minimally affected. Arthrodesis of either the talonavicular or calcaneocuboid joint, however, will eliminate most of the subtalar joint motion because rotation must occur around the talonavicular and the calcaneocuboid joint for subtalar motion to occur.

A triple arthrodesis eliminates the subtalar and transverse tarsal joint motion, causing increased stress upon the ankle joint and the midtarsal joints distal to the fusion site. A small percentage of patients will develop degenerative changes in the ankle joint following triple arthrodesis. It is imperative, therefore, to carefully evaluate the ankle joint prior to carrying out a triple arthrodesis.

Arthrodesis of the tarsometatarsal joints will not significantly affect motion of the foot and ankle, but a certain degree of stiffness is noted through the midtarsal area following this fusion. Fusion of the first metatarsophalangeal joint places added stress on the interphalangeal joint of the great toe, particularly with poor alignment. Although up to 40% of patients may develop degenerative changes in this joint, they are rarely of clinical significance.

D. DISADVANTAGES OF ARTHRODESIS

Although arthrodesis is an effective reconstructive tool, the resulting loss of motion places increased stress on the surrounding joints, making them more prone to developing arthritis or worsening preexisting degenerative changes. Thus, correction of a problem without arthrodesis is preferable whenever possible, such as with an osteotomy, tendon transfer, or both.

Ankle Fusion

A. INDICATIONS

The main indications for ankle arthrodesis are the following:

(1) arthrosis of the ankle joint usually secondary to a previous ankle fracture, although primary arthrosis does occur;

(2) changes secondary to rheumatoid arthritis; and

(3) malalignment of the ankle joint as the result of an epiphyseal injury or previous fracture.

B. TECHNIQUE

The surgical approach preferred by the authors is a transfibular approach (Figure 9–38). The incision begins along the fibula, approximately 10 cm proximal to the tip of the fibula, and is carried distally along the shaft of the fibula and then curves toward the base of the fourth metatarsal. In this way, the incision avoids the sural nerve posteriorly and the superficial peroneal nerve dorsally. The flaps that are created are full thickness, to lessen the possibility of wound-healing problems. The dissection is carried across the anterior aspect of the ankle joint, to the medial malleolus and along the lateral aspect of the neck of the talus. Posteriorly, the fibula and the posterior aspect of the ankle joint are exposed, while distally the subtalar joint and sinus tarsi area are exposed. The fibula is removed approximately 2 cm proximal to the joint, after which a cut is made in the distal tibia, starting approximately 2 mm proximal to the joint surface (Figure 9–39). This cut should be made as perpendicular as possible to the long axis of the tibia and should extend to the medial malleolus but not through it. The foot is placed into a plantigrade position and a cut made in the dome of the talus parallel to the cut in the tibia, thereby creating two flat surfaces

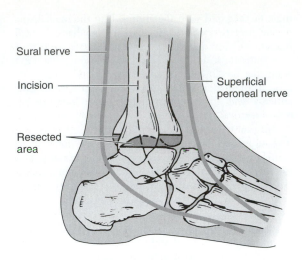

Figure 9–38. Technique for ankle arthrodesis. Skin incision is placed between superficial peroneal nerve and sural nerve. (Reproduced, with permission, from Mann RA, Coughlin MJ: *The Video Textbook of Foot and Ankle Surgery.* St. Louis: Medical Video Productions, 1991.)

and correcting any malalignment. At this point, the ankle should be aligned in neutral position, insofar as dorsiflexion and plantar flexion are concerned, and at about 5 degrees of valgus. The degree of rotation should be equal to that of the opposite extremity, which is usually 5–10 degrees of external rotation. If the two joint surfaces do not easily oppose each other, it is because the medial malleolus is too long, and the

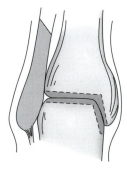

Figure 9–39. The fibula is excised approximately 2–2.5 cm proximal to the ankle joint, and the distal portion of the tibia cut, producing a flat cut perpendicular to the long axis of the tibia. (Reproduced, with permission, from Mann RA, Coughlin MJ: *The Video Textbook of Foot and Ankle Surgery.* St. Louis: Medical Video Productions, 1991.)

malleolus should be exposed through a dorsomedial incision and the distal centimeter removed.

The two flat surfaces should now be in total apposition, with little or no pressure being exerted. Temporary fixation is obtained by inserting two 0.062 K-wires. Interfragmentary compression is gained with two 6.5-mm cancellous screws, one of which starts in the sinus tarsi area and the other in the lateral process. These screws should be parallel to each other and should penetrate the medial cortex of the tibia side, to gain adequate interfragmentary compression (Figure 9–40). Following insertion of the screws, there should be rigid fixation of the arthrodesis site. Because the joint surfaces are fully opposed, there is no room for bone grafting. The wound is closed over a suction device.

In the immediate postoperative period, a firm compression dressing incorporating plaster splints is applied. After swelling is decreased, a short leg cast is applied and weight bearing is not allowed for 6 weeks. Weight bearing is then allowed with the short leg cast in place for another 6 weeks. Arthrodesis generally occurs following 12 weeks of immobilization.

C. Complications

Nonunion of the ankle joint, although uncommon, does occur. Using the surgical technique described earlier, a fusion rate of 90% can be anticipated. If nonunion occurs, bone grafting and further internal fixation may be required.

Malalignment of the ankle joint with the foot in too much internal rotation is poorly tolerated and often requires revision surgery. Excessive plantar flexion causes a back knee thrust and eventually some knee discomfort; excessive dorsiflexion causes increased stress on the

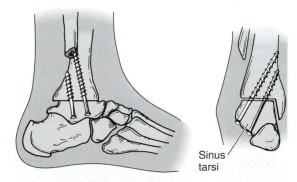

Figure 9–40. Diagram demonstrating placement of the 6.5-mm screws across the arthrodesis site. (Reproduced, with permission, from Mann RA, Coughlin MJ: *The Video Textbook of Foot and Ankle Surgery.* St. Louis: Medical Video Productions, 1991.)

heel (that can usually be treated with adequate padding); varus deformity may cause subtalar joint instability; excessive valgus causes stress on the medial aspect of the knee joint.

It is extremely important not to place any pin or screw across the subtalar joint for fear of damaging the posterior facet, which may lead to arthrosis.

D. Special Considerations

Avascular necrosis of the talus requires excision and bone grafting because avascular bone will not heal. Bone grafting may also be necessary when attempting to carry out a fusion after a severely comminuted pilon fracture because the bone is often relatively avascular.

Total Ankle Arthroplasty

Total ankle arthroplasty is an alternative to ankle arthrodesis for painful arthrosis of the ankle joint. Advantages include a maintenance of some ankle joint motion and thus less stress on adjacent joints. Unfortunately the results using a variety of implants have not held up over time, especially when compared with ankle joint fusions. However, two newer prostheses have shown promising early and medium-term results, and long-term results are being awaited before widespread use of either prosthesis is advocated.

Subtalar Arthrodesis

A. Indications

The main indications for subtalar arthrodesis are the following:

(1) arthrosis of the subtalar joint, usually following a calcaneal fracture, but occasionally for primary arthrosis of the joint;

(2) varus or valgus deformity secondary to rheumatoid arthritis;

(3) varus deformity secondary to residual clubfoot or possibly following compartment syndrome;

(4) unstable subtalar joint secondary to poliomyelitis, a neuromuscular disorder, or tendon dysfunction such as posterior tibial tendon dysfunction; and

(5) symptomatic talocalcaneal coalition without secondary changes in the talonavicular or calcaneocuboid joints.

B. Technique

The incision for subtalar arthrodesis begins at the tip of the fibula and is carried distally toward the base of the fourth metatarsal. As the incision is deepened, the sural nerve or one of its branches should be carefully noted and retracted. Small "twigs" of nerve may be present that unfortunately may be cut and give rise to a painful neuroma. The sinus tarsi area is exposed by reflecting the extensor digitorum brevis muscle distally. The use of a laminal spreader in the subtalar joint will enhance the exposure.

The articular cartilage is removed from the joint surfaces, which include the middle and posterior facets. The bony joint surfaces are then deeply feathered or scaled using a small osteotome. These cuts through the subchondral bone will greatly enhance the possibility of fusion. The area around the floor of the sinus tarsi and anterior process region can be carefully shaved to obtain local bone graft for the fusion.

The alignment of the subtalar joint is critical. It must be aligned into approximately 5–7 degrees of valgus position, producing a supple transverse tarsal joint. If it is placed in varus position, the foot is stiff and the patient will walk on the side of the foot.

Rigid fixation of the subtalar joint is achieved by using a 7-mm cannulated interfragmentary screw starting at the posterior tip of the calcaneus and passing into the body or neck of the talus. The guide pin is first placed up into the posterior facet, the subtalar joint is then manipulated into proper alignment, and the guide pin is passed into the talus. The alignment of the screw is verified on radiograph, and the screw inserted.

Following adequate internal fixation, the local bone graft is packed into the sinus tarsi area. Additional bone may be obtained from the area of the medial malleolus, or occasionally the iliac crest, although the latter site significantly adds to the morbidity of the procedure.

Postoperatively, a firm compression dressing incorporating plaster splints is applied. A short leg cast is applied, and weight bearing is not allowed for 6 weeks. The cast is changed and weight bearing is allowed for another 6 weeks. Twelve weeks of immobilization generally achieves an arthrodesis.

C. COMPLICATIONS

Nonunion of the subtalar joint is uncommon, although it can occur. Careful surgical technique and heavy scaling of the joint surfaces can help to prevent this complication. If nonunion occurs, bone grafting and added fixation are required to attempt to achieve a solid union.

Misalignment of the subtalar joint may also be a complication. An excessive valgus deformity following subtalar fusion may result in impingement laterally against the fibula or peroneal tendons. It will also cause excessive stress along the medial aspect of the midfoot, and occasionally the knee joint. A varus deformity of the subtalar joint imparts rigidity to the transverse tarsal joint, resulting in stiffness of the forefoot. This also increases pressure along the lateral aspect of the foot, particularly in the area of the base of the fifth metatarsal.

D. SPECIAL CONSIDERATIONS

The patient with rheumatoid arthritis or posttraumatic complications may have lateral subluxation of the calcaneus in relation to the talus, which usually requires CT scanning for identification. The calcaneus must be displaced medially at operation to align it with the lateral aspect of the talus and place it under the tibia in a proper weight-bearing position. If the calcaneus is fused with significant lateral deviation, the abnormal alignment places added stress on the ankle and midfoot region.

Special attention to the peroneal tendons is necessary when a subtalar arthrodesis is done to correct an old calcaneal fracture. Protrusion of the lateral wall of the body of the calcaneus from the healed fracture results in impingement on the peroneal tendons beneath the fibula. This protrusion must be carefully excised when the subtalar fusion is carried out, so that the lateral aspect of the talus and calcaneus are in line. Further, the peroneal tendon sheath should be dissected subperiosteally off the calcaneus to provide tendon sheath to protect the peroneal tendons from the raw, bony surface of the calcaneus.

Occasionally a bone block distraction arthrodesis of the subtalar joint is performed in cases of severe deformity after a calcaneus fracture. If the talus has assumed a horizontal position because of flattening of Böhler's angle, this can cause limited ankle joint dorsiflexion. Placing a tricortical block of iliac crest into the posterior facet of the subtalar joint will help to improve the overall alignment of the hind foot and regain ankle joint dorsiflexion.

Talonavicular Arthrodesis

A. INDICATIONS

Talonavicular arthrodesis is indicated in the following conditions:

(1) posttraumatic injury, rheumatoid arthritis, or primary arthrosis;

(2) unstable talonavicular joint secondary to rupture of the posterior tibial tendon, rheumatoid arthritis, or ligamentous injury about the talonavicular joint; and

(3) in conjunction with double or triple arthrodesis of the hindfoot.

B. TECHNIQUE

The talonavicular joint is approached through a medial or dorsomedial incision that starts in the region of the naviculocuneiform joint and extends to the neck of the talus. The soft tissues are stripped from around the joint and the articular cartilage removed with a curet or curved osteotome. Distraction of the joint by placing a towel clip into the navicular often facilitates exposure and debridement of the joint. Correct alignment of the talonavicular joint is extremely critical because this fusion essentially eliminates motion in the subtalar joint. The fusion position of the subtalar joint is 3–5 degrees of valgus with the forefoot in a plantigrade position (Figure 9–41). After the foot has been properly aligned to correspond to the opposite foot, fixation of the joint is carried out. Proper alignment of this joint is particularly critical when treating the laterally subluxed talonavicular joint in the patient with a ruptured posterior tibial tendon. The internal fixation is carried out by using interfragmentary compression with a single large

screw (6.5 mm), or 2 smaller screws (4.0 mm), or by using multiple staples.

Postoperatively the patient is immobilized in a non-weight–bearing cast for 6 weeks followed by a weight-bearing cast for an additional 6 weeks.

The talonavicular joint has a relatively high incidence of nonunion, which is probably the result of the difficulty in exposing the joint. If the joint is also approached medially to gain additional exposure, the surfaces can be well scaled, and the fusion rate should approach 90%.

C. COMPLICATIONS

Complications of nonunion and misalignment are similar to those discussed for subtalar joint fusion.

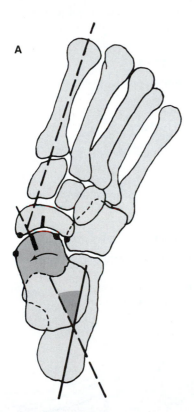

Flatfoot deformity

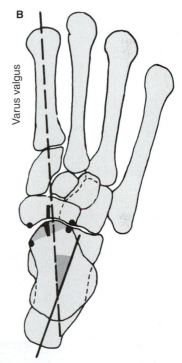

Varus valgus

Long axis of talus
through first metatarsal

Figure 9–41. Talonavicular fusion. **A:** Changes that occur in the talonavicular joint with a flatfoot deformity. Note that the head of the talus deviates medially as the forefoot deviates laterally into abduction. **B:** The forefoot has been brought into adduction so that the navicular is once again centered over the head of the talus. (Reproduced, with permission, from Mann RA, Coughlin MJ: *The Video Textbook of Foot and Ankle Surgery.* St. Louis: Medical Video Productions, 1991.)

D. SPECIAL CONSIDERATIONS

An isolated talonavicular joint fusion will usually produce a satisfactory result, particularly in relatively sedentary patients older than 50 years. In younger, more active individuals with no other affliction (eg, rheumatoid arthritis), consideration should be given to including the calcaneocuboid joint at the same time to obtain a more stable transverse tarsal joint and enhance the fusion of the talonavicular joint through added stability.

Double Arthrodesis (Calcaneocuboid & Talonavicular Joints)

A. INDICATIONS

In recent years, double arthrodesis has evolved as a procedure that provides the same degree of stability to the foot as a triple arthrodesis (Figure 9–42). By locking the transverse tarsal joint (calcaneocuboid and talonavicular), further subtalar motion is prevented because these three joints function together. This procedure is also indicated in the younger, active patient in whom an isolated talonavicular fusion is contemplated because it gives added stability to the foot.

Indications for double arthrodesis are as follows:

(1) arthrosis of the talonavicular and calcaneocuboid joints (eg, following trauma);

(2) unstable talonavicular and calcaneocuboid joint following rupture of the posterior tibial tendon or neuromuscular disease when a flexible subtalar joint is present; and

(3) arthrosis of the talonavicular joint or calcaneocuboid joint in an active individual, usually younger than 50 years of age, to give the midfoot a greater degree of stability.

B. TECHNIQUE

The talonavicular joint is approached through a medial or dorsomedial incision, as previously described, and the calcaneocuboid joint is approached through the same incision along the lateral side of the foot as was described for subtalar fusion. Once these joints are exposed, the joint surfaces are denuded of articular cartilage and the subchondral bone heavily feathered.

The alignment when carrying out a double arthrodesis is extremely critical because once this fusion has been achieved, the subtalar joint or the transverse tarsal joint no longer move. Therefore, the foot must be placed into a plantigrade position prior to the fixation of the arthrodesis site. The desired position is 5 degrees of valgus of the calcaneus, neutral abduction and adduction of the transverse tarsal joint, and correction of any forefoot varus that is present. This alignment creates a plantigrade foot. The fixation of the talonavicular joint is done first with the insertion of a screw (6.5 mm) or screws (4 mm) or possibly the use of multiple staples. The calcaneocuboid joint is then fixed the same way. Postoperative care is the same as for other foot fusions.

C. COMPLICATIONS

Complications of nonunion and malalignment are similar to those discussed for subtalar joint fusion.

Triple Arthrodesis

The triple arthrodesis is a fusion of the talonavicular, calcaneocuboid, and subtalar joints (Figure 9–43). In the past, it was the procedure of choice for all hindfoot problems, before isolated fusions became more accepted. Now, this procedure is still commonly used when limited fusions are inadequate.

A. INDICATIONS

Indications for triple arthrodesis are as follows:

(1) arthrosis secondary to trauma involving the subtalar, talonavicular, or calcaneocuboid joints;

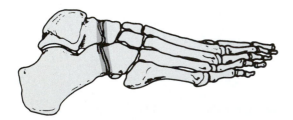

Figure 9–42. Double arthrodesis consisting of a talonavicular and calcaneocuboid fusion. (Reproduced, with permission, from Mann RA, Coughlin MJ: *The Video Textbook of Foot and Ankle Surgery.* St. Louis: Medical Video Productions, 1991.)

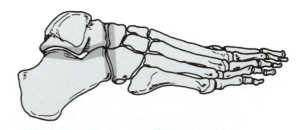

Figure 9–43. Diagram of a triple arthrodesis. (Reproduced, with permission, from Mann RA, Coughlin MJ: *The Video Textbook of Foot and Ankle Surgery.* St. Louis: Medical Video Productions, 1991.)

(2) arthrosis or instability of the talonavicular or calcaneocuboid joints in association with a fixed deformity of the subtalar joint;

(3) instability of the foot secondary to posterior tibial tendon dysfunction with a fixed subtalar joint that cannot be realigned by a double arthrodesis;

(4) unstable hindfoot secondary to poliomyelitis, nerve injury, or rheumatoid arthritis;

(5) symptomatic, unresectable calcaneonavicular bar; and

(6) malalignment of the hindfoot secondary to trauma such as a crush injury or compartment syndrome.

B. TECHNIQUE

The triple arthrodesis is carried out as previously described for subtalar fusion and talonavicular fusion. The foot is fixed after manipulation back into a plantigrade position (3–5 degrees of valgus of the subtalar joint), neutral position as far as abduction and adduction of the transverse tarsal joint, and correction of forefoot varus. Postoperative care is the same as for subtalar fusion.

C. COMPLICATIONS

The main complication is failure of fusion of one of the joints, but this is uncommon, as the successful fusion rate exceeds 90%. The talonavicular joint is most likely to have nonunion. Malalignment of the foot or forefoot may require revision and technically is a difficult procedure. The sural nerve may become entrapped or disrupted through the lateral approach.

Tarsometatarsal Arthrodesis

Arthrodesis in the tarsometatarsal area may involve a single tarsometatarsal joint, usually the first joint, or multiple joints. The fusion mass not infrequently will extend proximally to include the intertarsal bones and sometimes even the naviculocuneiform joints. A careful determination of the involved joints is important when considering a tarsometatarsal fusion for a patient with posttraumatic disorders. At times, in addition to the plain radiograph, a CT scan and bone scan may be necessary to help in precisely defining the involved area.

A. INDICATIONS

The indications for a tarsometatarsal fusion are as follows:

(1) hypermobility of the first metatarsocuneiform joint associated with a hallux valgus deformity in a small percentage of patients with a bunion deformity;

(2) arthrosis involving one or more of the tarsometatarsal joints either resulting from trauma or as a primary disease process; and

(3) arthrosis associated with a deformity resulting from an old Lisfranc fracture-dislocation.

B. TECHNIQUE

The surgical approach to the first metatarsocuneiform joint is through a dorsomedial longitudinal incision to expose the joint. If multiple joints are involved, the second incision is centered over the second metatarsal, through which the lateral side of the first and all of the second and third metatarsocuneiform joints can be adequately viewed (Figure 9–44). The incision must be sufficiently long to permit adequate exposure of the joints and must be extended proximally if the naviculocuneiform joints are going to be fused as well. Cautious dissection is necessary, as there are numerous superficial nerves as well as the neurovascular bundle (dorsalis pedis and superficial branch of the deep peroneal nerve) passing over the area of the second metatarsocuneiform joint in this approach. If the fourth and fifth metatarsocuboid joints are to be fused, then a third longitudinal incision is made over this area to enable adequate exposure. The articular cartilage is carefully removed from the tar-

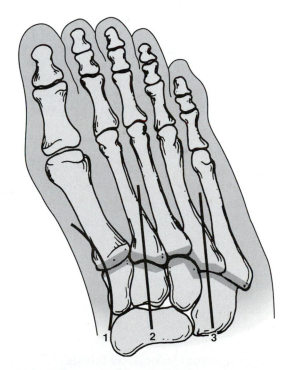

Figure 9–44. Longitudinal incisions used for a tarsometatarsal arthrodesis. (Reproduced, with permission, from Mann RA, Coughlin MJ: *The Video Textbook of Foot and Ankle Surgery.* St. Louis: Medical Video Productions, 1991.)

sometatarsal and intertarsal joints, depending on the extent of the fusion mass. The bones are heavily feathered to create a good environment for healing. If a deformity is present (usually an abduction deformity of the foot or possibly dorsiflexion), it should be corrected. The first metatarsocuneiform joint is aligned and fixed using 4-mm cancellous screws or a dorsomedial plate. Interfragmentary longitudinal compression of the other joints is obtained to prevent possible nonunion. The screw pattern found to be most useful for the first metatarsocuneiform joint is one brought from the dorsal aspect of the cuneiform directed distally, and a second screw from the dorsal aspect of the metatarsal base directed proximally, crossing the metatarsocuneiform joint. Care must be taken to also correct any dorsiflexion or abduction deformity that is present.

Postoperatively, the joint is placed in a short leg, non-weight–bearing cast for 6 weeks, and then in a weight-bearing cast for another 6 weeks.

C. COMPLICATIONS

The possibility of nonunion exists, but with interfragmentary compression this risk is minimized. If nonunion occurs, bone grafting may be required as well as improved internal fixation. When multiple tarsometatarsal joints are fused, there is a moderate amount of swelling and tension placed against the incisions. It is critical postoperatively to use a compression dressing to minimize the risk of swelling and prevent possible wound sloughing. If sloughing occurs, it must be treated appropriately, and, occasionally, skin grafting is required.

A tarsometatarsal fusion involving multiple joints may cause a plantar callus because one of the metatarsals has been placed in a position of too much plantar flexion. Osteotomy at the base of the metatarsal may be necessary to realign the metatarsal.

Staples should be avoided as a means of internal fixation of the tarsometatarsal joints because they have a tendency to cause dorsiflexion of the metatarsals, and plantar callosities may result.

First Metatarsophalangeal Joint Arthrodesis

See the discussion of hallux valgus at the beginning of the chapter.

Interphalangeal Joint Arthrodesis (Hallux Arthrodesis)

A. INDICATIONS

Interphalangeal joint arthrodesis is usually indicated for the following problems:

(1) arthrosis, usually secondary to trauma or occasionally following a first metatarsophalangeal joint arthrodesis; and

(2) stabilization of the interphalangeal joint when carrying out a transfer of the extensor hallucis longus into the neck of the first metatarsal (first toe Jones procedure).

B. TECHNIQUE

The interphalangeal joint is approached through a dorsal transverse incision centered over the joint. Usually, an ellipse of skin is removed, exposing the ends of the involved joints. Using a small power saw, the end of the distal portion of the proximal phalanx and the proximal portion of the distal phalanx are removed, placing the distal phalanx into approximately 5–7 degrees of plantar flexion and 3–4 degrees of valgus position. Internal fixation is achieved by using a longitudinal screw (4 mm) or crossed K-wires, or both.

A postoperative shoe is used, with weight bearing allowed as tolerated until fusion occurs, usually in 8 weeks.

C. COMPLICATIONS

Nonunion of interphalangeal joint fusion is uncommon. If it does occur, it often is asymptomatic and does not require treatment. If it is symptomatic, usually the fusion will need to be revised because the area is too small for adequate bone grafting.

Buck P et al: The optimum position of arthrodesis of the ankle. J Bone Joint Surg Am 1987;69:1052.

Carr JB et al: Subtalar distraction bone block fusion for late complications of os calcis fractures. Foot Ankle Int 1988;9:81.

Clain MR, Baxter DE: Simultaneous calcaneal cuboid and talonavicular fusion: Long term follow up study. J Bone Joint Surg Am 1994;76:133.

Harper MC, Tisdel CL: Talonavicular arthrodesis for the painful adult acquired flat foot. Foot Ankle Int 1996;17:658.

Kitaoka HB, Patzer GL: Clinical results of the Mayo total ankle arthroplasty. J Bone Joint Surg 1996;78:1658.

Komenda GA et al: Results of arthrodesis of the tarsometatarsal joints after traumatic injury. J Bone Joint Surg 1996;78:1665.

Mann RA: Arthrodesis of the foot and ankle. In Mann RA, Coughlin MJ (editors): *Surgery of the Foot and Ankle.* St. Louis: Mosby-Year Book, 1993.

Mann RA et al: Isolated subtalar arthrodesis. Foot Ankle Int 1998; 19:511.

Mann RA et al: Mid-tarsal and tarsometatarsal arthrodesis for primary degenerative osteoarthrosis or osteoarthrosis after trauma. J Bone Joint Surg 1996;78:1376.

Mann Ra, Rongstad KM: Arthrodesis of the ankle: A critical analysis. Foot Ankle Int 1998;19:3.

Ouzounian TJ: Triple arthrodesis. Foot Ankle Clin 1996;1:133.

Schon LC, Bell W: Fusions of the transverse tarsal and mid-tarsal joints. Foot Ankle Clin 1996;1:99.

CONGENITAL FLATFOOT

Congenital flatfoot is the term used to describe a flat-foot present since birth. The condition may not be apparent during the early years of life but is usually identified toward the end of the first or during the second decade. The typical asymptomatic flexible flatfoot is probably a normal variant of the longitudinal arch. This deformity must be differentiated from the symptomatic flexible or semiflexible flatfoot, which usually will become symptomatic in the early teen years. These individuals have a fairly flexible foot until adolescence, when the foot often becomes somewhat more rigid and often symptomatic.

The patient with a tarsal coalition will frequently present with a peroneal spastic flatfoot, usually around the age of 10–12 years. A tarsal coalition is the union of two or more tarsal bones, usually occurring between the calcaneus and the navicular or between the talus and the calcaneus. Coalitions may not become symptomatic until adulthood, brought on by a sudden twisting injury of the foot, although this mechanism rarely causes peroneal spasm.

Flatfoot associated with an accessory navicular bone usually becomes symptomatic in the early to mid-teenage years and may be unilateral or bilateral. Residual congenital deformity from conditions such as clubfoot or congenital vertical talus are present from birth and are discussed in Chapter 11, Pediatric Orthopedic Surgery.

The patient with generalized dysplasia such as Marfan's syndrome or Ehlers-Danlos syndrome may present with flatfoot. A generalized ligamentous laxity will be present from the time of birth, and the diagnosis is usually already known.

Clinical Findings

A. Symptoms and Signs

The clinical evaluation begins with the patient in a standing position. In all cases of congenital flatfoot the longitudinal arch flattens when the patient is standing. In the case of tarsal coalition with peroneal spastic flatfoot, the calcaneus is in a severe fixed valgus position. A tarsal coalition or an accessory navicular may be unilateral, as well as the residuals of a congenital deformity such as clubfoot or congenital vertical talus. The symptomatic and asymptomatic flexible flatfoot and the generalized dysplasia are present bilaterally.

The physical examination of these patients is extremely important. The asymptomatic flexible flatfoot will usually demonstrate a satisfactory range of motion and no contracture of the Achilles tendon. The symptomatic flexible flatfoot, however, will almost invariably demonstrate an equinus contracture. To adequately test for tightness of the Achilles tendon, the head of the talus is covered with the navicular, after which the foot is brought up into dorsiflexion with the knee extended. If the foot is brought into dorsiflexion, permitting lateral subluxation of the talonavicular joint, the examiner often is fooled into thinking that dorsiflexion is adequate when indeed it is not.

The patient with tarsal coalition usually demonstrates restricted hindfoot motion secondary to peroneal spasm due to the cartilaginous or bony bar. The peroneal tendons can actually be felt to be bow-strung behind the fibula, not permitting any passive or active inversion of the subtalar joint to occur. On occasion, clonus can be elicited. As a rule, stressing of these joints causes the patient increased discomfort. In flatfoot associated with an accessory navicular, pain is present over the prominence. Frequently, stressing of the posterior tibial tendon aggravates the condition. The patient with residual congenital deformity often demonstrates a certain degree of stiffness of the foot and, not infrequently, varying degrees of deformity of the remainder of the foot. The patient with generalized dysplasia demonstrates marked hypermobility of all the joints, with no contractures whatsoever.

B. Imaging Studies

The radiographic evaluation is useful in differentiating the various types of flatfoot. In almost all cases, the lateral view shows a lack of normal dorsiflexion pitch of the calcaneus, which is approximately 20 degrees or more. In symptomatic flexible flatfoot, the calcaneus may even be in a mild degree of equinus position. On the lateral radiograph, a line drawn through the long axis of the talus and first metatarsal will demonstrate an angle of more than 30 degrees in severe flatfoot, 15–30 degrees in moderate flatfoot, and 0–15 degrees in mild flatfoot (Figure 9–45).

The calcaneonavicular coalition is best observed on an oblique radiograph and is identified as a bridge from the anterior process of the calcaneus to the inferior lateral aspect of the navicular (Figure 9–46). The subtalar or talocalcaneal bar is best demonstrated on a CT scan taken in the coronal plane (Figure 9–47). Flatfoot associated with an accessory navicular demonstrates the accessory bone along the medial side of the navicular, but occasionally a medial oblique view is necessary to outline the size of the fragment (Figure 9–48). In a patient with a residual congenital deformity, such as a clubfoot or congenital vertical talus, the changes about the foot will often be sufficient to make the diagnosis fairly obvious. The patient with generalized dysplasia often demonstrates complete collapse of the longitudinal arch.

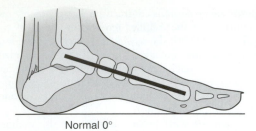

Normal 0°

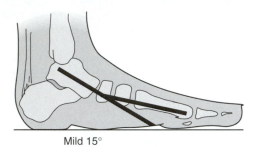

Mild 15°

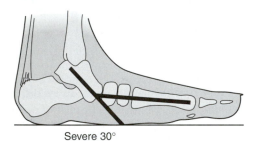

Severe 30°

Figure 9–45. Measurement of flatfoot deformity by using the lateral talometatarsal angle: 0 degrees, normal; 1–15 degrees, mild; 16–30 degrees, moderate; greater than 30 degrees, severe. (Reproduced, with permission, from Bordelon RL: Foot Ankle 1980;1:143.)

Treatment

A. CONSERVATIVE MANAGEMENT

Conservative management is undertaken for congenital flatfoot deformities. A longitudinal arch support may benefit the patient but is usually not necessary for the asymptomatic flexible flatfoot. For symptomatic flexible flatfoot, a semirigid longitudinal arch support and Achilles stretching exercises may be of some benefit.

The tarsal coalition can be treated conservatively with a short leg walking cast, followed by a polypropylene ankle-foot orthosis or a University of California Biomechanics Laboratory (UCBL) insert. If adequate pain relief is achieved, further treatment is not neces-

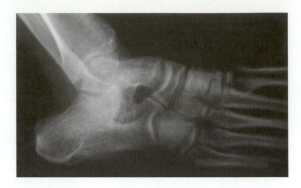

Figure 9–46. Oblique view of the foot at 45-degree angle demonstrating calcaneonavicular coalition. (Reproduced, with permission, from Mann RA, Coughlin MJ: *Surgery of the Foot and Ankle,* 6th ed. St. Louis: Mosby-Year Book, 1993.)

sary. Flatfoot with an accessory navicular may respond to modification of the shoe to relieve some of the pressure from the involved area. Occasionally, the use of a longitudinal arch support will relieve the pressure.

Residual flatfoot resulting from congenital problems can be treated with an ankle-foot orthosis or UCBL insert if symptomatic. The patient with generalized dysplasia usually does not require any treatment at all.

B. SURGICAL MANAGEMENT

Surgical procedures are never appropriate for asymptomatic flatfoot. Symptomatic flexible or semiflexible flat-

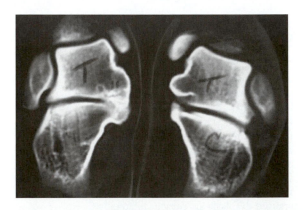

Figure 9–47. CT scan demonstrating osseous coalition on one side (left) and fibrous coalition on the other (right). (Reproduced, with permission, from Mann RA, Coughlin MJ [editors]: *Surgery of the Foot and Ankle,* 6th ed. St. Louis: Mosby-Year Book, 1993.)

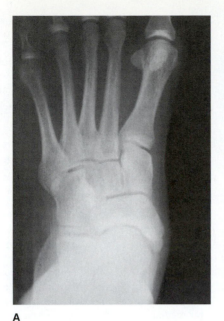 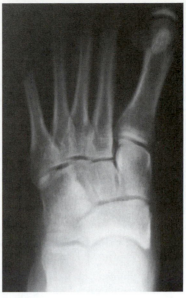

A   B

Figure 9–48. Large accessory navicular. **A:** Preoperatively, a cartilaginous plate is loose and painful. **B:** One year postoperatively. (Reproduced, with permission, from Mann RA, Coughlin MJ [editors]: *Surgery of the Foot and Ankle,* 6th ed. St. Louis: Mosby-Year Book, 1993.)

foot occasionally is treated surgically, particularly if equinus contracture is observed after age 5 or 6 years. A significant equinus contracture may benefit from lengthening of the Achilles tendon. A lateral column lengthening procedure, such as an Evans calcaneal osteotomy, is indicated in cases of symptomatic flexible flatfoot that have failed conservative management. This procedure helps to correct heel valgus and forefoot abduction and should be done as late into growth as possible to avoid disturbing open growth centers. Rarely should a triple arthrodesis be carried out because this leaves a young patient with a very stiff foot.

A tarsal coalition that does not respond to conservative management may require resection. The surgical approach to the calcaneonavicular bar is identical to that of the subtalar joint. The bar is carefully outlined and then resected in its entirety. Talocalcaneal coalitions are resectable throughout the adolescent years, if less than 20% of the posterior facet of the subtalar joint is involved or if the coalition is confined only to the middle facet. More extensive involvement of the subtalar joint in an adolescent or any bar in an adult patient is an indication for subtalar arthrodesis. The approach is through a medial incision centered over the middle facet, and caution is taken to carefully reflect the tendons and posterior tibial nerve. The extent of the coalition is identified, and it is resected to expose the area of normal-appearing articular cartilage. Bone wax is applied to the edges or a free fat graft is inserted to prevent re-formation of the bar. Flatfoot associated with an accessory navicular may require excision of the accessory navicular and plication of the posterior tibial tendon (Kidner procedure). This fairly successful operation is usually carried out during the late adolescent years.

Residual congenital deformity or generalized dysplasias usually will not require surgical management. In severe cases, a triple arthrodesis is indicated after the foot has matured.

Bordelon RL: Flatfoot in children and young adults. In Mann RA, Coughlin MJ, eds: *Surgery of the Foot and Ankle.* Mosby-Year Book: St. Louis; 1993.

Evans D: Calcaneo-valgus deformity. J Bone Joint Surg 1979;57: 270.

Gonzalez P, Kumar SJ: Calcaneonavicular coalition treated by resection and interposition of the extensor digitorum brevis muscle. J Bone Joint Surg 1990;72:71.

McCormack TJ et al: Talocalcaneal coalition resection: A ten year follow up. J Pediatr Orthop 1997;17:13.

ACQUIRED FLATFOOT DEFORMITY

Acquired flatfoot deformity is a condition affecting a foot that at one time had a normal functioning longitudinal arch. Over time, the arch has progressively flattened, leading to a varying amount of symptoms. This deformity is different from congenital flatfoot deformity, which has been present since birth. Acquired flatfoot deformity in the adult is multifactorial and may be attributed to the following:

(1) posterior tibial tendon dysfunction;

(2) arthrosis of the tarsometatarsal joints, which may be primary or secondary to a previous Lisfranc fracture or dislocation;

(3) Charcot changes in the midfoot resulting from a peripheral neuropathy; or

(4) talonavicular collapse resulting from trauma or rheumatoid arthritis.

The preceding clinical problems are manifested by deformities affecting different areas of the midfoot. These deformities may include dorsal subluxation of the talonavicular joint and tarsometatarsal joints, abduction of the forefoot, valgus deformity of the rearfoot, or all three. The extent of the deformity varies widely and is usually progressive. Acquired flatfoot deformity may or may not affect a patient bilaterally.

Clinical Findings

A. SYMPTOMS AND SIGNS

A careful history is important to help distinguish between differing causes of acquired flatfoot deformity. Usually, no specific traumatic event is recalled by the patient who presents with dysfunction of the posterior tibial tendon. In about half of patients with tarsometatarsal joint arthrosis, a Lisfranc fracture-dislocation has occurred, whereas the other half has primary arthrosis. The patient with Charcot foot usually gives a relevant history of the cause of their peripheral neuropathy, such as diabetes. The patient with collapse of the talonavicular joint usually either has sustained prior trauma or has rheumatoid arthritis, which results in disruption of the spring ligament complex. The physical examination begins by observing the foot with the patient standing, observing for unilateral or bilateral flattening of the longitudinal arch. Also evaluate for varying degrees of abduction of the forefoot and hindfoot valgus. When the patient is asked to stand on tiptoe, the involved calcaneus remains in valgus position rather than inverting, as normally occurs. When the patient is viewed from the posterior aspect, more toes are visible laterally on the involved foot than the uninvolved foot.

The patient with posterior tibial tendon dysfunction demonstrates little or no active inversion strength. Usually, the posterior tibial tendon is thick and swollen and there is increased warmth and pain to palpation over the tendon sheath.

Arthrosis of the tarsometatarsal joints creates a deformity of abduction of the forefoot with varying degrees of dorsiflexion, giving rise to a rather prominent medial cuneiform. Not infrequently, palpable osteophytes are present on the dorsal and plantar aspect of the tarsometatarsal joints.

A Charcot foot presents with varying degrees of swelling and deformity. In the early stages, the foot demonstrates generalized swelling and increased warmth, with loss of sensation in a stocking-glove distribution. Deformity may vary from a mild flat foot to a severe rocker-bottom deformity. It is important to palpate for bony prominences on the medial and plantar aspects of the foot that make it at risk for ulcerations.

In the patient with rheumatoid arthritis, most of the changes occur within the talonavicular joint. In this case, the head of the talus is often palpable on the plantar medial aspect of the foot. When the subtalar joint is more involved, a fixed valgus deformity is usually present as well.

The posttraumatic deformity may vary, depending on precisely which joints are involved. If trauma has led to a collapse of the navicular, the longitudinal arch is flattened with little forefoot abduction, and the head of the talus is often palpable on the plantar medial aspect of the foot. Usually there is little or no motion in the hindfoot and midfoot joints.

B. IMAGING STUDIES

Radiographs usually differentiate the cause of the problem. In the patient with posterior tibial tendon dysfunction, there may be sagging of the talonavicular joint or abduction of the navicular on the head of the talus. The patient with tarsometatarsal joint arthrosis demonstrates typical degenerative changes at the affected joints, along with varying degrees of lateral and dorsal subluxation of the joints. Patients with Charcot foot also demonstrate one of several characteristic changes seen in the neuropathic foot. Often the bone destruction and joint dislocation are dramatic (Figure 9–49). The patient with rheumatoid arthritis demonstrates the typical destructive changes observed with this disease process, with loss of the bony architecture.

Treatment

A. CONSERVATIVE MANAGEMENT

Conservative management is aimed at providing support to the longitudinal arch and ankle with a polypropylene ankle-foot orthosis. The orthosis must be shaped to accommodate any prominences that

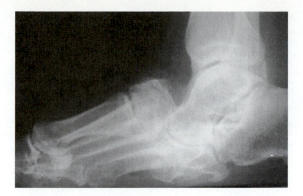

Figure 9–49. Charcot midfoot changes resulting in joint dislocations and a rocker-bottom deformity of the foot.

might be present. Unfortunately, these prominences present the potential for skin breakdown, particularly in the neuropathic foot. A rocker-bottom-type shoe with an adequate toe box is sometimes indicated to give the patient a smoother gait pattern.

B. SURGICAL TREATMENT

The surgical management of these various conditions is specific for each problem. Posterior tibial tendon dysfunction with a satisfactory range of motion of the joints of the hindfoot and midfoot can be treated with reconstruction of the posterior tibial tendon, using a flexor digitorum longus tendon. A calcaneal osteotomy can be added if a significant valgus deformity of the heel is present. Alternatively, a lateral column lengthening, consisting of a calcaneal-cuboid distraction arthrodesis, can be used to correct a flexible flat foot with significant abduction of the forefoot. Tendon transfer is contraindicated for a fixed deformity, but a subtalar or triple arthrodesis would be indicated.

The patient with Charcot foot is treated in a short leg cast until the acute process subsides, after which a polypropylene ankle-foot orthosis is used. Occasionally, a bony prominence that continues to cause skin breakdown may be excised to permit the patient to use an ankle-foot orthosis. In extreme rocker-bottom deformities, midfoot correction with an osteotomy may be required. The rheumatoid patient usually requires stabilization of the involved area with triple arthrodesis or subtalar fusion, depending upon where the main problem has occurred.

The posttraumatic foot with involvement of the navicular or talonavicular joint requires triple arthrodesis, which may need to be extended distally to include the cuneiform area as well.

The patient with arthrosis of the tarsometatarsal joints will respond well to surgical management by realigning the foot and carrying out arthrodesis of the involved joints.

Chen CH et al: Isolated talonavicular arthrodesis for talonavicular arthritis. Foot Ankle Int 2001;22:633.

Funk DA et al: Acquired adult flatfoot secondary to posterior tibial tendon pathology. J Bone Joint Surg Am 1986;68:95.

Guyton GP et al: Flexor digitorum longus transfer and medial displacement calcaneal osteotomy for posterior tibial tendon dysfunction: A middle-term clinical follow-up. Foot Ankle Int 2001;22:627.

Mann RA: Flatfoot in adults. In Coughlin MJ, Mann RA (editors): *Surgery of the Foot and Ankle.* St. Louis: Mosby, Inc., 1999.

Mann RA, Thompson FM: Rupture of the posterior tibial tendon causing flatfoot: Surgical treatment. J Bone Joint Surg Am 1985;67:556.

Schon LC et al: Charcot neuroarthropathy of the foot and ankle. Clin Orthop 1998;349:116.

Simon SR et al: Arthrodesis as an early alternative to nonoperative management of Charcot arthropathy of the diabetic foot. J Bone Joint Surg Am 2000;82:939.

Thomas RL et al: Preliminary results comparing two methods of lateral column lengthening. Foot Ankle Int 2001;22:107.

CAVUS FOOT

Cavus foot deformity is characterized by an abnormal elevation of the longitudinal arch, with resulting decrease in the plantar weight-bearing area and stress concentrated on the metatarsal heads. The condition may be aggravated by clawing of the toes, further reducing the forefoot weight-bearing area. Generalized stiffness of the joints is common, causing the patient to avoid prolonged use of the foot.

Etiologic Findings

The various causes of cavus foot deformity include the following:

(1) anterior horn cell disease such as poliomyelitis, diastematomyelia, and spinal cord tumor;

(2) nerve disorders such as Charcot-Marie-Tooth disease and spinal dysraphism;

(3) muscular diseases such as muscular dystrophy;

(4) long tract and central diseases such as Friedreich's ataxia and cerebral palsy;

(5) idiopathic conditions such as residual clubfoot, arthrogryposis, and cavus foot of undetermined cause; and

(6) posttraumatic disorders following injuries such as compartment syndrome or crush injury.

Anatomy

Cavus foot deformity is extremely variable in its presentation, from mild to extremely severe degree of cavus. The types of deformities can be classified based upon the localizing of the area of deformity:

1. Posterior cavus deformity—This deformity mainly involves the calcaneus, which has a dorsiflexion pitch angle of greater than 40 degrees measured on a weight-bearing lateral radiograph. Normally, the dorsiflexion pitch to the calcaneus is approximately 20 degrees.

2. Anterior cavus deformity—In anterior cavus deformity, there is a forefoot equinus deformity with the hindfoot in a neutral position. The anterior cavus may be localized, mainly involving the first and second metatarsal, or it may be more global, with the entire forefoot in a position of plantar flexion.

3. Combined cavus deformity—In a combined cavus deformity, which is the most severe, there are both anterior and posterior components.

Clinical Findings

A. Symptoms and Signs

A careful history regarding the onset of the condition and progression is important. A detailed family history should also be obtained because idiopathic cavus deformity does tend to run in families. Progression of deformity should be ascertained, particularly in the adolescent, because this may indicate a spinal cord abnormality or neoplasm. Activity level and ambulation should also be carefully evaluated as markers of progression of neural or muscular disease.

The degree of deformity of the foot must be examined with the patient in a standing position. This will also reveal any evidence of atrophy of the calf muscles, as would be seen in Charcot-Marie-Tooth disease, clubfoot, or arthrogryposis. The range of motion of the joints of the foot and ankle should be carefully measured and the muscle strength recorded. The degree of deformity and flexibility of the rearfoot, forefoot, metatarsophalangeal joints, and lesser toes must be ascertained. The presence of a tight plantar fascia should also be noted.

B. Imaging Studies

Weight-bearing radiographs of the foot and ankle should be obtained to help classify the type of cavus deformity and formulate a treatment plan.

Treatment

A. Conservative Management

Conservative care is tailored to the severity of the cavus deformity. Mild deformities may only require a softer-soled shoe. Significant clawing of the lesser toes may require an extra-depth shoe. A custom-made Plastizote liner with a built-in arch support helps to decrease the stress on the metatarsal heads. A significant motor deficit may require an ankle-foot orthosis to stabilize the ankle. Most cases of cavus foot can be managed with conservative modalities.

B. Surgical Treatment

Surgical treatment for the cavus foot is aimed at correcting the site of the deformity. The most frequent pattern consists of plantar flexion of the first metatarsal, contracture of the plantar fascia, and varus deformity of the calcaneus. These problems respond to release of the plantar fascia, dorsiflexion osteotomy of the first and perhaps second metatarsal, and lateral closing wedge osteotomy (Dwyer procedure) of the calcaneus to correct the varus deformity. Fusion of the joints is avoided to maintain as much flexibility of the foot as possible (Figure 9–50).

A more severe deformity involving dorsiflexion of the calcaneus can be treated with sliding osteotomy of the calcaneus (Samilson procedure), correcting any varus deformity with a lateral closing wedge osteotomy and releasing the plantar fascia (Figure 9–51). Forefoot deformity is treated with osteotomy of the first and sometimes second metatarsal. In some patients, transfer of the peroneus longus tendon into the brevis and lengthening of the posterior tibial tendon will provide dynamic muscle balance for the foot.

Severe deformities not amenable to procedures that will retain joint motion require triple arthrodesis. A Siffert beak-type triple arthrodesis corrects the deformity because the navicular is mortised under the head of the talus to help reduce the elevation of the longitudinal arch (Figure 9–52). A first metatarsal osteotomy may need to be added to the procedure as well.

The lesser toes may have either fixed or flexible clawtoe deformities. Flexible deformity often responds to release of the extensor tendons and a Girdlestone flexor tendon transfer. If a fixed deformity is present, a DuVries phalangeal condylectomy corrects the hammer toe, followed by extensor tendon release and the Girdlestone procedure.

Hyperextension of the first metatarsophalangeal joint is corrected by interphalangeal arthrodesis of the hallux and transfer of the extensor hallucis longus tendon into the neck of the first metatarsal (Jones procedure) (Figure 9–53).

Breusch SJ et al: Function after correction of a clawed great toe buy a modified Robert Jones transfer. J Bone Joint Surg (Br) 2000:82-B:250.

Mann RA: Pes cavus. In Coughlin MJ, Mann RA (editors): *Surgery of the Foot and Ankle.* St. Louis: Mosby, Inc., 1999.

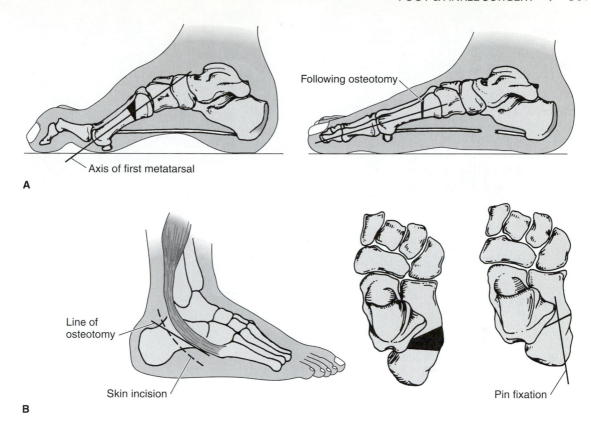

A

B

Figure 9–50. Technique for correction of cavus foot. **A:** For first metatarsal osteotomy, a dorsally based wedge of bone has been removed approximately 1 cm distal to the metatarsocuneiform joint. The plantar fascia is released. Dorsiflexion of the osteotomy site helps correct the cavus deformity by flattening the arch. **B:** Heel varus is corrected by a closing wedge calcaneus osteotomy. (Reproduced, with permission, from Mann RA, Coughlin MJ: *The Video Textbook of Foot and Ankle Surgery.* St. Louis: Medical Video Productions, 1991.)

Siffert RS, del Torto U: "Beak" triple arthrodesis for severe cavus deformity. Clin Orthop 1983;181:64.

Sammarco GJ, Taylor R: Cavovarus foot Treated with combined calcaneus and metatarsal osteotomies. Foot Ankle Int 2001;22:19.

ORTHOTIC DEVICES FOR THE FOOT & ANKLE

Orthotic devices are used to redistribute stresses on the foot as it makes contact with the ground and to accommodate for abnormal function of defective muscles or ligaments. This is achieved by controlling the posture of the foot and padding certain areas to relieve pressure and provide increased comfort for the foot. Orthoses are also used to limit motion in arthritic joints, making them less painful. The orthotic device may be attached to the sole of the shoe, may be in-serted inside the shoe as an insole, may cup the foot (UCBL insert), or may extend across the ankle to hold the entire foot and ankle in place (ankle-foot orthosis).

Orthotic Shoe Sole Devices

A variety of heel and sole corrections are available to accommodate foot postural abnormalities. A medial or lateral heel or sole wedge (or a combination of both) can help control excessive pronation or supination from weak tendons, ligamentous instability, or fixed deformities. A wide heel is used to increase the stability of the subtalar joint. A rocker sole helps to stabilize the forefoot in the case of a fracture or arthritis and is also helpful to a patient with an ankle fusion to allow a more normal gait pattern.

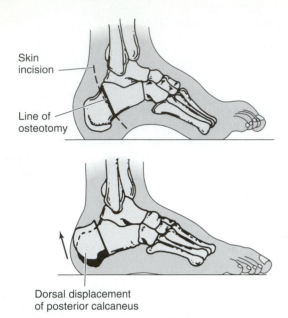

Skin incision

Line of osteotomy

Dorsal displacement of posterior calcaneus

Figure 9–51. Techniques of calcaneal osteotomy. In the treatment of pes cavus, the osteotomy permits the calcaneus to be moved into a more dorsal position and, if necessary, to be closed laterally to correct heel varus. (Reproduced, with permission, from Mann RA, Coughlin MJ: *The Video Textbook of Foot and Ankle Surgery.* St. Louis: Medical Video Productions, 1991.)

Orthotic Insole Devices

Insole orthotic devices can be used for flexible deformities to alter the posture of the foot, and for fixed deformities to redistribute stress. The simplest device is a soft liner for a shoe or boot made out of a high-density foam material. Other simple orthoses include a soft felt pad to relieve pressure on the metatarsal heads or a combination of materials to produce a more rigid support to help control a forefoot deformity such as forefoot varus or valgus deformity. Orthotic devices take up space in the shoe, and the patient may need a larger or deeper shoe.

UCBL Insert (University of California Biomechanics Laboratory Insert)

The principle of the UCBL insert is to correct a foot deformity such as flatfoot by stabilizing the calcaneus in neutral position and molding the orthosis to block abduction of the forefoot. Posting along the medial aspect may compensate for forefoot varus. In theory, this orthotic device is excellent for controlling the rearfoot and forefoot, but two caveats apply to the use of this

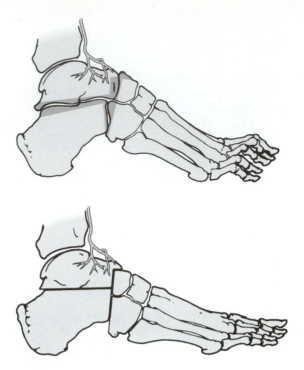

Figure 9–52. A diagram of a beak-type triple arthrodesis. This mortises the navicular underneath a portion of the head of the talus to allow rotation of the distal portion of the foot, permitting flattening of the longitudinal arch and correction of the cavus deformity. (Reproduced, with permission, from Mann RA, Coughlin MJ: *The Video Textbook of Foot and Ankle Surgery.* St. Louis: Medical Video Production, 1991.)

device. The first is that the foot must be flexible, as correction of a rigid deformity is impossible. The second is that a bony prominence can chafe against the polypropylene material, resulting in pain or skin breakdown over the prominence.

Ankle-Foot Orthosis

An ankle-foot orthosis (AFO) is a molded polypropylene device that passes along the posterior aspect of the calf and then onto the plantar aspect of the foot to the metatarsal heads. Alterations are made in a variety of ways to accommodate the patient's problem (Figure 9–54). Ankle problems such as arthrosis or dorsiflexion weakness require adequate rigidity to eliminate ankle joint motion. An orthosis for a subtalar joint problem should have enough flexibility to provide ankle joint motion but must be rigid enough to immobilize the subtalar joint. When the problem involves the transverse tarsal joint, the AFO can be fabricated to permit

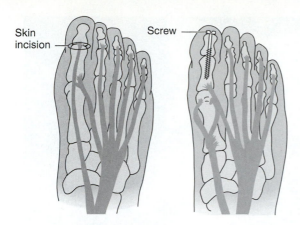

Figure 9–53. Diagram of the first toe Jones procedure. This procedure moves the pull of the extensor hallucis longus tendon from the great toe into the neck of the metatarsal. An interphalangeal arthrodesis of the hallux is carried out. (Reproduced, with permission, from Mann RA, Coughlin MJ [editors]: *Surgery of the Foot and Ankle.* St. Louis: Mosby-Year Book, 1993.)

some ankle joint motion but maintain immobilization of the transverse tarsal joint area, usually by blocking abduction of the forefoot. When managing tarsometatarsal arthritis, the footpiece is carried to the tips of the toes. Again, a significant fixed bony deformity results in pressure points, making fitting of the device difficult. If the patient has loss of sensation, careful construction and padding are essential to minimize the risk of ulcers forming over a bony prominence. In cases of marked instability or discomfort, an anterior shell can be added to the ankle-foot orthosis, and the brace is extended proximally to create a patellar tendon bearing surface.

Double Upright Orthosis

The double upright orthosis with a hinged ankle may be used when individuals require stability but are engaged in physically demanding activities. The double upright orthosis is somewhat more cumbersome than the ankle-foot orthosis but provides rigid immobilization. The hinge mechanism of the ankle joint may be changed, depending upon the nature of the patient's problem. The ankle joint can be "free," which allows dorsiflexion and plantar flexion to occur, or it can be "fixed" to prevent plantar flexion past 90 degrees. This brace can be modified with a spring load to provide dorsiflexion for the patient with dropfoot resulting from paralysis, but should not be used for the patient with spasticity, because it may accentuate the spasticity.

Prescriptions for Orthotic Devices

The following are typical prescriptions for orthotic devices.

A. Metatarsalgia or Atrophy of Plantar Fat Pad

1. Treatment—A full-length, well-molded orthosis for metatarsal arch support is used to relieve pressure under the metatarsal heads. Use soft insole material.

2. Explanation—In the treatment of metatarsalgia or atrophy of the plantar fat pad, a full-length orthosis is needed that is molded to the plantar aspect of the foot and built up just proximal to the metatarsal heads to relieve pressure on them. The material should be soft to provide extra cushioning for the foot.

B. Ruptured Posterior Tibial Tendon with Moderately Severe Flexible Flatfoot Deformity

1. Treatment—Ankle-foot orthosis, with Trimline cut to permit 30% ankle joint motion, is molded to reestablish the longitudinal arch and built up on the lateral aspect of the footpiece to block abduction of the forefoot.

2. Explanation—With a moderately advanced flexible flatfoot deformity, an in-shoe orthotic device alone will not provide sufficient support; the ankle-foot orthosis is needed to provide adequate stability. Some ankle joint motion is included, which makes ambulation more comfortable for the patient. The longitudinal arch is molded to support the foot in a plantigrade position, and the lateral aspect of the ankle-foot orthosis is built up to prevent the forefoot from moving into an abducted position. By blocking abduction, the amount of pressure needed beneath the longitudinal arch to prevent it from collapsing is decreased.

C. Posterior Tibial Tendon Insufficiency with Mild Flatfoot Deformity and 5 Degrees of Forefoot Varus Deformity

1. Treatment—Use a well-molded longitudinal arch support, with a 5-degree varus post and a 3-degree medial heel lift.

2. Explanation—Insufficiency of the posterior tibial tendon that has not produced a significant foot deformity can be treated with a well-molded longitudinal arch support. The 5-degree varus forefoot post compensates for the fixed forefoot varus, and the 3-degree heel lift likewise helps tilt the hindfoot from valgus deformity closer to neutral position.

D. Dropfoot Secondary to Peroneal Nerve Injury

1. Treatment—An ankle-foot orthosis with a full footpiece is molded to the longitudinal arch.

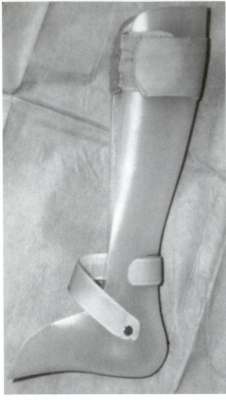
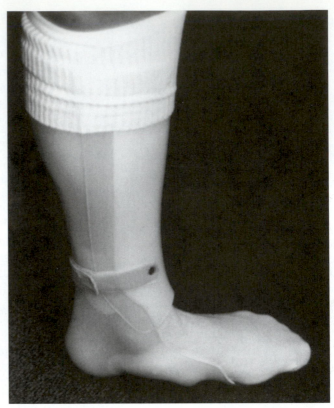

A

B

Figure 9–54. Types of ankle-foot orthoses. **A:** A standard ankle-foot orthosis with a trim line cut to maximum stability of the ankle joint. If the trim line is cut more posteriorly, there would be some give at the ankle joint. **B:** An anterior shell has been added to the ankle-foot orthosis to increase the stability of the foot and ankle within the brace. (Reproduced, with permission, from Mann RA, Coughlin MJ [editors]: *Surgery of the Foot and Ankle,* 6th. ed. St. Louis: Mosby-Year Book, 1993.)

2. Explanation—A dropfoot secondary to a peroneal nerve injury responds well to an ankle-foot orthosis with a full footpiece. The footpiece supports the toes so they do not drop and makes it easier for the patient to put on shoes.

E. DIABETIC NEUROPATHY WITH CLAWFOOT DEFORMITY

1. Treatment—An extra-depth shoe with a molded Plastizote liner is backed with a pelite material.

2. Explanation—The patient with clawfoot deformity requires a shoe that has extra height in the toe box. The extra-depth shoe provides enough room for the toes, so they will not chafe against the top of the shoe. The molded Plastizote liner is an excellent means of provid-

ing full contact to the plantar aspect of the foot. Plastizote has a tendency to "bottom out," and by backing the material with a pelite liner or some comparable material, the life expectancy of the Plastizote is extended significantly.

Bordelon RL: Orthotics, shoes, and braces. Orthop Clin North Am 1989;20:751.

Pfeffer G et al: Comparison of custom and prefabricated orthoses in the initial treatment of proximal plantar fasciitis. Foot Ankle Int 1999;20:214.

Raikin SM et al: Biomechanical evaluation of the ability of casts and braces to immobilize the ankle and hindfoot. Foot Ankle Int 2001;22:214.

Van Schie C et al: Design criteria for rigid rocker shoes. Foot Ankle Int 2000;21:833.

LIGAMENTOUS INJURIES ABOUT THE ANKLE JOINT

Ankle ligament injuries represent the most common musculoskeletal injury; therefore, accurate assessment and treatment of these injuries are important. The lateral collateral ligament complex is most commonly injured, but damage to other important structures around the ankle joint should not be overlooked. For example, syndesmosis ligament and subtalar joint injuries are often mistaken for lateral collateral sprains. These ligaments may be injured in conjunction with lateral collateral sprains or as isolated injuries. Medial ankle injuries, such as deltoid and spring ligament complex sprains, may occur in conjunction with lateral ligament sprains, and should not be overlooked when focusing on the lateral ligament injury.

Functional Anatomy

The lateral collateral ligament structure of the ankle consists of three distinct ligamentous bands, namely, the anterior and posterior talofibular ligaments (ATFL and PTFL) and the calcaneal fibular ligament (CFL).

When the ankle joint is in plantar flexion, the ATFL is in line with the fibula and is therefore placed under stress with an inversion injury and often damaged. Conversely, when the ankle joint is in dorsiflexion, the CFL is in line with the long axis of the fibula and is therefore subject to injury. If the applied stress is severe, both the ATFL and the CFL may be torn, no matter the position of the ankle joint. The syndesmosis ligament complex tethers the tibia and fibula together and is injured by an external rotational force to the foot. The deltoid ligament is the sole medial stabilizer of the ankle joint. An isolated deltoid ligament injury can occur with an eversion or external rotation force on the foot. The deltoid ligament can also sustain injury in conjunction with a syndesmosis ligament injury, with lateral ankle sprains, or with a concomitant fibula fracture.

Clinical Findings

A. Classification

Lateral collateral ankle ligament injuries are divided into three degrees of severity. A grade I sprain is confined to the ATFL and demonstrates no instability. A grade II sprain involves injury to both the ATFL and CFL, with mild laxity of one or both ligaments. A grade III sprain involves injury and significant laxity of both the ATFL and CFL.

B. Symptoms and Signs

A past history of injuries of the ankle and problems with chronic ankle ligament instability should be ascertained.

A careful physical examination is important to evaluate the degree of involvement of each ligament and to rule out injury to any adjacent bony or soft-tissue structures. The ATFL, CFL, and syndesmosis ligaments are palpated for tenderness. To rule out other sources of pathology, pain should be sought in the area of the anterior process of the calcaneus, the lateral process of the talus, the base of the fifth metatarsal, along the subtalar joint, and along the course of the peroneal tendons. All of these structures are subject to injury from an inversion stress on the foot.

A patient with a significant medial joint pain with or without lateral ligament pain should be evaluated for an injury to the posterior tibial tendon or osteochondral fracture of the medial talar dome.

Assessment of ankle ligament stability requires clinical and radiographic stress examinations. To perform an anterior drawer maneuver, which tests stability of the ATFL, the ankle is placed in 30 degrees of equinus, and the ankle is pulled in an anterior and slightly internally rotated direction (Figure 9–55). A feeling of subluxation will be present if a significant ligament injury has occurred. A talar tilt maneuver is performed by placing an inversion stress on the heel. With the foot in plantar flexion, this tests the stability of the ATFL. With the foot in neutral or dorsiflexion, a talar tilt maneuver tests the stability of the CFL. If clinical instability is suggested by either maneuver, radiographic confirmation can be performed, with comparison to the unaffected ankle.

Injury to the syndesmosis ligament complex is suspected if the region between the distal anterior tibia and fibula is tender to palpation. If extensive swelling is present more than two centimeters proximal to the ankle joint, syndesmosis rupture is a strong possibility. Pain elicited by squeezing the tibia and fibula together in the mid calf is diagnostic of a syndesmosis ligament tear. A syndesmosis ligament injury is also suspected if external rotation of the foot is painful.

C. Imaging Studies

Standard anteroposterior, lateral, and oblique radiographs of the ankle should be obtained to rule out a fracture of the fibula, talus, or calcaneus. If ligament laxity is suggested on clinical examination, stress radiographs should be obtained. An anteroposterior view is taken while a talar tilt maneuver is performed, and a lateral view is taken while an anterior drawer maneuver is performed. More than 10 degrees of tilt and more than 5–7 mm of anterior drawer are considered abnormal.

If a syndesmosis ligament injury is suspected, careful attention must be paid to the joint spaces to rule out widening of the ankle mortise. If instability is sus-

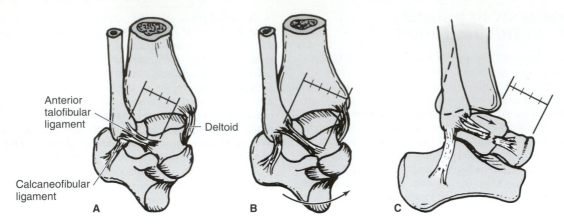

Figure 9–55. Mechanics of carrying out a stress test of the lateral ankle ligaments. **A:** Normal anatomic alignment, which demonstrates the checkrein effect of the anterior talofibular ligament on the talus. **B:** The stress test for the calcaneofibular ligament is carried out by firmly inverting the calcaneus. **C:** The anterior talofibular ligament is tested by placing the ankle joint in neutral position and applying an anterior pull with slight medial rotation. (Reproduced, with permission, from Mann RA, Coughlin MJ [editors]: *Surgery of the Foot and Ankle,* 6th. ed. St. Louis: Mosby-Year Book, 1993.)

pected, a stress radiograph is performed by externally rotating the foot with the tibia held still.

MRI or CT scan may be helpful in some instances if there is a high index of suspicion for an accompanying injury. Osteochondral injuries to the talus should be ruled out with an MRI scan. If a talus or calcaneus fracture is suspected, either MRI or CT scan may be of benefit.

Treatment

A. Conservative Management

Acute grade I ligament tears are treated with a lateral stabilizing ankle brace, ice, and avoidance of painful activities. Immediate full weight-bearing is allowed, as are non-weight–bearing physical activities, such as bicycling and swimming. The brace can be discontinued in 1 month.

Grade II ligament tears are treated with protected weight bearing and a lateral stabilizing ankle brace. The patient can begin non-weight–bearing exercise (stationary bicycle) after 7 days, along with peroneal strengthening exercises. Weight-bearing exercise (jogging) may resume after 2–3 weeks.

In a grade III ligament tear, the ankle is immobilized with a removable walking cast for 3–4 weeks. This is followed by a period of physical therapy consisting of range-of-motion exercises, peroneal strengthening, and proprioception training using a biomechanical ankle platform system (BAPS) board.

Treatment of isolated deltoid ligament sprains depends on the severity of the injury and is similar to lateral ligament injuries. Mild injuries can be treated with immediate mobilization and rapid return to activity, whereas more severe injuries should be casted for 3–4 weeks.

Syndesmosis ligament tears, if mild, can be treated with weight bearing in a cast or brace, and close follow-up to assess for widening of the ankle joint mortise. If the interosseous membrane is damaged, as evidenced by massive swelling of the leg proximal to the ankle joint, treatment depends on the radiographic appearance of the ankle. If the mortise has not widened, the patient is kept non-weight–bearing in a cast for 6 weeks, with close radiographic follow-up. If initial or follow radiographs show a widened mortise, the patient requires surgical repair of the syndesmosis ligaments with temporary screw placement until the ligaments have healed.

B. Surgical Treatment

The surgical treatment of an acute ligamentous injury is indicated only for the occasional elite athlete. Most ligamentous injuries, even grade III sprains, will heal sufficiently with no significant disability if properly attended. On the other hand, even less severe ankle sprains may cause chronic pain or functional instability if left untreated.

The indication for a lateral ligament reconstruction is functional ligament instability, which is primarily a clinical diagnosis. A patient with ligament instability complains of recurrent sprains that occur with sports activities or even with activities of daily living, despite 4–6 months of physical therapy and use of a lateral stabilizing brace. A patient with functional ligament instability also complains of difficulty walking on uneven ground.

Although many lateral ankle reconstruction procedures have been described for chronic lateral ankle ligament instability, a Broström repair is the procedure of choice. This is an anatomic repair that is highly effective and has lower morbidity than other procedures that harvest the peroneus brevis tendon. The Broström procedure is a soft-tissue ligamentous repair in which the ATFL and CFL are plicated and reattached to their anatomic positions (Figure 9–56). The repair is reinforced by bringing up a portion of the inferior extensor retinaculum.

Chronic lateral ankle pain following an ankle sprain may be caused by a previously undiagnosed condition rather than chronic ankle instability. The differential diagnosis for chronic ankle pain is similar to that following an acute injury, and would also include subtalar joint instability, and dislocating or torn peroneal ten-

dons. Impingement of scar tissue in the lateral gutter between the talus and fibula may also cause chronic lateral ankle pain. In addition to a careful physical examination, an MRI or CT scan may be helpful for distinguishing between these possible causes of pain.

Surgical treatment may help to relieve symptoms of chronic pain, once an accurate diagnosis has been made. Chondral or osteochondral fractures of the talus can be treated with arthroscopic or open debridement or pinning. Subtalar joint instability is addressed with a Broström procedure. A fracture of the anterior or lateral process of the talus is either removed if it is small, or fixed if it is a large fragment. Tears or dislocations of the peroneal tendons are repaired or stabilized. Scar tissue in the lateral gutter can be treated with arthroscopic debridement.

DiGiovanni BF et al: Associated injuries found in chronic lateral ankle instability. Foot Ankle Int 2000;21:809.

Krips R et al: Long-term outcome of anatomical reconstruction versus tenodesis for the treatment of chronic anterolateral in-

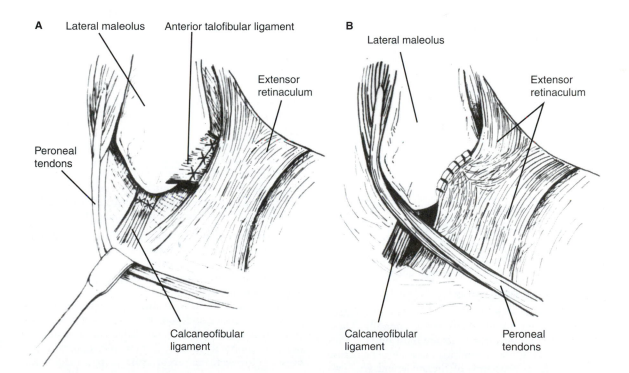

Figure 9–56. Modified Broström anatomic reconstruction. **A:** Imbrication of anterior talofibular and calcaneofibular ligaments. **B:** Imbrication of inferior extensor retinaculum to reinforce the repair. (Reproduced, with permission, from Coughlin MJ, Mann RA [editors]: Surgery of the Foot and Ankle, 7th ed. St. Louis: Mosby, 1999. Modified from Renstrom, Trevino S: In Operative techniques in sports medicine, vol 2, no 1, Philadelphia: WB Saunders, 1994.)

stability of the ankle joint: A multicenter study. Foot Ankle Int 2001;22:415.

Liu SH, Baker CL: Comparison of lateral ankle ligamentous reconstruction procedures. Am J Sports Med 1994;22:313.

Lofvenberg R et al: The outcome of non-operated patients with chronic lateral instability of the ankle: A 20 year follow up study. Foot Ankle Int 1994;15:165.

Messer TM et al: Outcome of the modified Broström procedure for chronic lateral ankle instability using suture anchors. Foot Ankle Int 2000;21:996.

Miller CD et al: Deltoid and syndesmosis ligament injury of the ankle without fracture. Am J Sports Med 1995; 23:746.

Pijnenburg ACM et al: Treatment of ruptures of the lateral ankle ligaments: A meta-analysis. J Bone Joint Surg Am 2000;82: 761.

ARTHROSCOPIC EXAMINATION OF THE FOOT & ANKLE

Arthroscopy is an important tool for use in diagnosis and treatment of foot and ankle disorders. With developments in instrumentation, more ankle joint conditions can be treated arthroscopically. Arthroscopy of the subtalar joint has also become an accepted method for diagnosing and treating some subtalar joint abnormalities.

Advantages of Arthroscopy over Open Arthrotomy

Arthroscopy of the ankle joint offers distinct advantages over open exploration. The entire joint can be better visualized through the arthroscope, including the lateral and medial gutters and the posterior aspect of the joint. Dynamic studies can be performed to stress ligaments or identify areas of soft-tissue or bony impingement. Furthermore, the low morbidity of arthroscopy allows rapid rehabilitation.

Indications

Indications for ankle joint arthroscopy are listed in Table 9–4. In addition, arthroscopic examination can be used as a diagnostic tool in some instances when the precise cause of ankle pain remains in question.

A. THERAPEUTIC INDICATIONS

1. Loose bodies—Intra-articular loose bodies are usually easy to identify and remove arthroscopically. These bony or cartilaginous fragments are most often the result of trauma or osteochondritis dissecans. They cause pain or locking symptoms of the ankle and are diagnosed on plain radiographs, CT, or MRI scan.

2. Ankle joint infection—Arthroscopic irrigation, drainage, and synovectomy have proved to be an excellent method of treating ankle joint infections.

Table 9–4. Proven indications for ankle arthroscopy.

Loose body removal
Irrigation and debridement for infection
Shaving of small osteophytes
Debridement of localized general synovitis
Debridement of osteochondral fractures
Debridement of osteochondritis dissecans lesions
Debridement of soft-tissue impingement

3. Synovitis—Synovitis may be present as a result of inflammatory arthritis (rheumatoid arthritis) or neoplastic diseases (pigmented villonodular synovitis), following trauma, or for unknown reasons (idiopathic). Whether the synovitis is localized or diffuse, arthroscopic debridement of inflamed synovium will often relieve symptoms. Synovectomy is more easily and thoroughly performed arthroscopically.

4. Osteophyte formation—Repetitive trauma or early osteoarthritis can lead to osteophytic formation on the anterior lip of the tibia and the neck of the talus. These lesions can cause pain and limited ankle joint dorsiflexion and can be removed arthroscopically with a high-speed burr.

5. Other lesions within the joint—Chondral or osteochondral lesions, whether caused by trauma or osteochondritis dissecans, can be treated arthroscopically. This may involve debridement of loose cartilage flaps, drilling of subchondral bone, or pinning of large osteochondral fragments.

Patients who present with ankle pain over the anterolateral joint line and a history of a severe ankle sprain or recurrent sprains may have impingement of scar tissue in the lateral gutter between the talus and fibula. This entity responds well to arthroscopic debridement of scar tissue from the lateral gutter.

6. Controversial indications—Arthroscopic debridement of the arthritic ankle joint has not proved to be beneficial for generalized arthritis but may help for localized degenerative changes accompanied by early osteophyte formation.

Arthroscopically assisted fixation of ankle fractures has been described and potentially allows for more accurate realignment of the joint surfaces and identification of chondral lesions that would otherwise be missed. However, the use of arthroscopy in the treatment of most routine ankle fractures is probably not indicated.

Techniques of arthroscopically assisted ankle arthrodesis have been described, and several studies have been published. This technique causes less morbidity and allows a shorter time to fusion with good fusion rates. However, this is a technically demanding procedure and cannot be used to correct any joint deformity.

B. DIAGNOSTIC INDICATIONS

Ankle arthroscopy can be a valuable diagnostic tool when the cause of symptoms remains unclear (Table 9–5). Chronic ankle pain or swelling that remains refractory to conservative measures and has not been diagnosed by conventional imaging studies may warrant arthroscopic exploration to help make a diagnosis. Chondromalacia or inflamed synovium may be causing such symptoms, and neither may be demonstrated on imaging studies, including MRI. Patients with episodes of locking, stiffness, or instability for which a cause cannot be found may be aided by diagnostic ankle arthroscopy. Loose bodies, cartilage flaps, or arthrofibrosis may be contributing to such symptoms, all of which can be addressed arthroscopically (see Table 9–5).

Technique

The patient is placed supine on the operating table with the foot positioned to allow access from all directions. This can be achieved with the foot placed off the edge of the bed or with the thigh held flexed in a well-padded thigh holder (Figure 9–57). General or spinal anesthesia is necessary for full relaxation of the extremity.

The use of distraction greatly enhances arthroscopic procedures, providing better views of the structures of the joint and allowing tools to be introduced into the joint. Noninvasive distractors with padded straps over the foot and heel are the most commonly used types of distractor. (see Figure 9–57). Invasive distractors require placement of pins or screws through the tibia proximally and the calcaneus or talus distally. Stronger distraction forces can be obtained in this manner, but the morbidity is higher.

Most ankle arthroscopies are performed using two anterior portals: anterolateral and anteromedial (Figure

Table 9–5. Refractory conditions diagnosed by arthroscopy.

Chondromalacia
Synovitis
Locking of the joint
Chronic stiffness
Instability
Loose bodies
Cartilage flaps
Arthrofibrosis

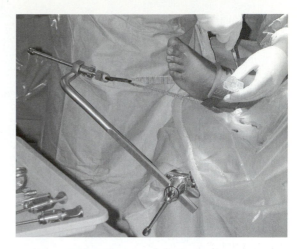

Figure 9–57. Soft strap type of distractor used during ankle arthroscopy.

9–58). A posterolateral portal is usually established as well for outflow or to access the posterior aspect of the joint. Thorough knowledge of the anatomy of the tendons, nerves, and vessels is essential to prevent damage to any of these structures with portal placement. The anterolateral portal is placed just lateral to the tendon of the peroneus tertius muscle, taking care to avoid branches of the superficial peroneal nerve. The anteromedial portal is placed just medial to the anterior tibial tendon, taking care to avoid the saphenous nerve and vein, which usually can be palpated. The posterolateral portal is placed just lateral to the Achilles tendon. The sural nerve and small saphenous vein lie in close proximity to this portal.

Initially, the entire joint is explored in a systematic manner, to ensure that abnormalities are not overlooked. The entire cartilaginous surface of the talus and tibia are examined. The medial and lateral gutters are explored, paying special attention to tibiotalar and talofibular articulations. The synovium is inspected for inflammation. Ligamentous structures are identified, specifically the deltoid and talofibular ligaments, which are observed closely for signs of laxity while varus and valgus forces are applied. Loose bodies are carefully searched for throughout the examination.

After a thorough diagnostic examination has been performed, therapeutic maneuvers are undertaken. This may consist of synovial biopsy or resection, resection or drilling of abnormal cartilaginous surfaces, resection of scar tissue, or other procedures.

Postoperatively, a compression dressing is applied with a posterior splint for 5 to 7 days to allow the portals to heal. Weight bearing is then progressed as tolerated, and activities are advanced to normal.

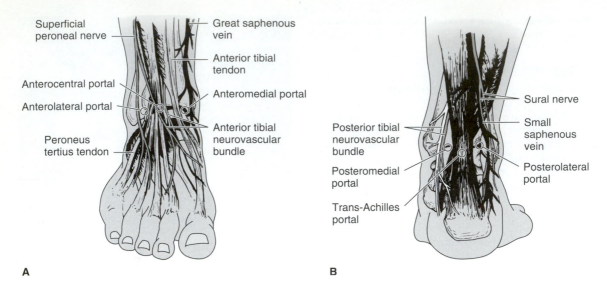

Figure 9–58. **A:** The anterior portals used for ankle arthroscopy are illustrated. The anterocentral portal is not used. **B:** The posterolateral portal is the only posterior portal utilized for ankle arthroscopy. (Reproduced, with permission, from Ferkel, RD: Arthroscopy of the Ankle and Foot, in Mann RA, Coughlin MJ [editors]: *Surgery of the Foot and Ankle,* 6th ed. St. Louis: Mosby-Year Book, 1993.)

Complications

Although several complications have been reported, the most common is nerve damage associated with portal placement. Either hypesthesias or neuroma formation may be seen. Damage to arteries and tendons is less common. Postoperative joint infection, draining sinuses, and soft-tissue or bone infections at the sites of pin distractors are uncommon complications of ankle arthroscopy.

Subtalar Joint Arthroscopy

The subtalar joint is technically challenging for arthroscopy, given its complex shape and the difficulty distracting the joint. Subtalar joint arthroscopy is indicated for several conditions involving the subtalar joint. Talocalcaneal interosseous ligament tears, chondral lesions, synovitis, and focal degenerative changes may respond to arthroscopic debridement of the subtalar joint.

For subtalar joint arthroscopy, the patient can either be placed prone with a bump under the ipsilateral hip or placed in the lateral decubitus position. Two portals are used over the anterolateral subtalar joint, approximately 1.5 cm apart. The anterior and lateral portions of the posterior facet and the interosseous ligament can be visualized from these portals. A third portal is placed posterolaterally, for outflow and for visualization of the posterior aspect of the joint. For additional details about the technique of subtalar joint arthroscopy, the reader is referred to the references.

Bonnin M, Bouysset M: Arthroscopy of the ankle: Analysis of results and indications on a series of 75 cases. Foot Ankle Int 1999;20:744.

Chaytor ER, Conti SF: Arthroscopy of the foot and ankle: Current concepts review. Foot Ankle Int 1998;19:184.

Ferkel RD: Arthroscopy of the ankle and foot. In Coughlin MJ, Mann RA (editors): *Surgery of the Foot and Ankle.* St. Louis: Mosby, Inc., 1999.

Frey C et al: Arthroscopic evaluation of the subtalar joint: Does sinus tarsi syndrome exist? Foot Ankle Int 1999;20:185.

Kim SH, Ha KI: Arthroscopic treatment for impingement of the anterolateral soft tissues of the ankle. J Bone Joint Surg Br 2000;82-B;1019.

O'Brien TS et al: Open versus arthroscopic ankle arthrodesis: A comparative study. Foot Ankle Int 1999;20:368.

Schimmer RC et al: The role of ankle arthroscopy in the treatment strategies of osteochondritis dissecans lesions of the talus. Foot Ankle Int 2001;22:895.

Thordarson DB et al: The role of ankle arthroscopy on the surgical management of ankle fractures. Foot Ankle Int 2001;22:123.

van Dijk CN et al: A prospective study of prognostic factors concerning the outcome of arthroscopic surgery for anterior ankle impingement. Am J Sports Med 1997; 25:737.

■ TENDON INJURIES

Tendon injuries about the foot and ankle are common causes of disability. This is due to the fact that large forces are acting on these tendons in a repetitive fashion during walking and running activities. The tendons cross the ankle joint at an acute angle, which further predisposes them to injury. Injury to tendons may be caused by acute trauma, such as in Achilles tendon ruptures, or may be due to chronic strain, such as posterior tibial tendon dysfunction.

ACHILLES TENDON INJURIES

Achilles tendon abnormalities are extremely common, especially among active men and women age 30–50 years. The primary disorders are Achilles tendinitis, either insertional or noninsertional, and Achilles tendon ruptures. Achilles tendinitis was previously discussed in the section on heel pain.

1. Achilles Tendon Rupture

Pathogenesis

The mechanism of injury is usually mechanical overload from an eccentric contraction of the gastrocsoleus muscle complex. This occurs as a sudden, forceful dorsiflexion of the foot as the gastrocsoleus is contracted. The tear usually occurs 3–6 cm proximal to the insertion of the Achilles tendon, at the site of its poorest blood supply (Figure 9–59). At times, a history of inter-

mittent pain in the tendon is elicited, suggestive of a prior tendinitis. The typical patient is 30–50 years old and a recreational ("weekend warrior") athlete. These factors suggest that insufficient conditioning of the musculotendon unit plays a role in the injury. The most common sports activities leading to Achilles tendon ruptures are basketball, racket sports, soccer, and softball.

Clinical Findings

A. SYMPTOMS AND SIGNS

The diagnosis of Achilles tendon rupture is usually made from the history. The patient describes sudden pain in the heel after attempting a pushing-off movement. It is often accompanied by an audible pop, and immediate weakness is noted in the affected leg. On physical examination, a palpable defect is often present in the tendon. Ankle plantar-flexion is markedly weak compared with the unaffected side, but is possible, as other tendons that cross the ankle joint can plantar-flex the foot. A positive Thompson's test is diagnostic of complete Achilles tendon rupture. This is performed with the patient prone and the affected knee bent 90 degrees. Squeezing the calf causes plantar flexion of the foot if the Achilles tendon is intact or partially torn but not if there is complete rupture of the tendon.

B. IMAGING STUDIES

Plain radiographs are not helpful in diagnosing Achilles tendon tear, unless there is an avulsion off the calcaneus with a fragment of bone, an uncommon condition. MRI is extremely sensitive in diagnosing this disorder

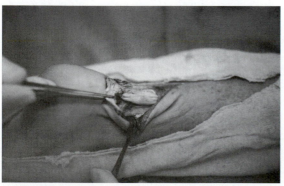
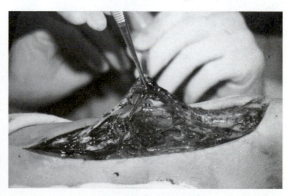

A   B

Figure 9–59. Examples of acute Achilles tendon ruptures. **A:** Complete rupture with minimal fraying of the tendon. **B:** Achilles tendon rupture with marked fraying of the tendon. (Reproduced, with permission, from Plattner P, Mann RA: Disorders of Tendons, in Mann RA, Coughlin MJ [editors]: *Surgery of the Foot and Ankle,* 6th ed. St. Louis: Mosby-YearBook, 1993.)

and in determining if some tendon remains in continuity (Figure 9–60). However, MRI is rarely needed since physical exam is usually diagnostic of Achilles tendon rupture.

Treatment

Methods for treating Achilles tendon rupture include primary repair using open or percutaneous techniques, or cast immobilization. Surgical repair is recommended for active individuals, in the case of a rerupture, or if the injury is greater than 2 weeks old. The primary risk of surgical repair is wound healing in a small percentage of patients.

Cast treatment for Achilles tendon ruptures is recommended for more sedentary individuals, patients who are at increased risk of developing wound problems, or high-risk surgical patients. The primary risk of cast immobilization is a higher chance of rerupture. For the vast majority of patients, either treatment method will result in a good outcome.

A. Nonsurgical Treatment

Once an acute rupture is diagnosed, the patient should be placed in a gravity equinus cast. A below-knee cast is adequate in a reliable patient. If there is a question as to whether the tendon edges are properly apposed in the cast, an MRI scan be done, although this is not routine. After 4 weeks, the cast is changed, with correction of approximately half of the previous equinus. Over the next 4 weeks, the patient is brought down to neutral with serial casts. Once at neutral, the patient is given a removable walking cast for 4 weeks. Supervised strengthening activities are then begun.

B. Surgical Treatment

The surgical approach is on the medial side of the Achilles tendon sheath. The frayed edges of the tendon are debrided. The foot is positioned in equinus position equal to the resting equinus of the opposite ankle. Two heavy nonabsorbable sutures are woven through 3–4 cm of each tendon edge using a Bunnell or Kessler stitch (Figure 9–61). The repair can be reinforced with lighter, absorbable sutures at the site of the tear. If the plantaris tendon is intact, it can be harvested and used to reinforce the repair.

Postoperatively, a hard cast is used for 3 weeks, followed by a removable cast with adjustable ankle motion. Over the next 2–3 weeks, the joint should be gradually brought out of equinus. Weight bearing is then allowed, and range-of-motion exercises are begun.

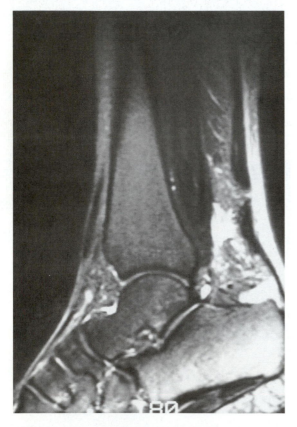

Figure 9–60. MRI of Achilles tendon rupture.

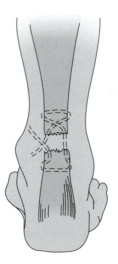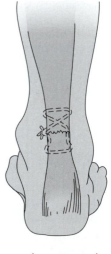

Figure 9–61. Suture techniques used to reapproximate the ruptured Achilles tendon. (Reproduced, with permission, from Mann RA, Coughlin MJ [editors]: *Surgery of the Foot and Ankle,* 6th ed. St. Louis: Mosby-Year Book, 1993.)

The cast is discontinued at 6 to 8 weeks, and supervised strengthening exercises are performed.

A percutaneous method of Achilles tendon repair is described in the references.

C. Treatment of Chronic Ruptures or Reruptures

Chronic Achilles tendon ruptures, more than 6 weeks old, or reruptures of previously treated injuries are challenging reconstruction problems because of retraction and degeneration of the tendon ends. A number of different procedures have been described to address this problem, including a variety of synthetic and interpositional grafts (Figure 9–62).

Small defects can be bridged by turning down a strip of gastrocnemius fascia, which is sutured into the distal tendon stump. Larger defects can be treated by using a V-Y lengthening of the gastrocnemius aponeurosis. If the deficit is too large for V-Y lengthening, transfer of the flexor hallucis longus tendon can be performed. The tendon of the flexor hallucis longus is transected distally in the foot, and the distal segment is tenodesed to the flexor digitorum longus to maintain flexion of the great toe. The proximal tendon is secured through a drill hole in the calcaneus. A central slip of the Achilles tendon is advanced to bridge the gap, and then the repair is reinforced by securing it to the flexor hallucis (Figure 9–63).

The postoperative course for these procedures includes 6 weeks non-weight–bearing and a total of 3 months in a cast.

POSTERIOR TIBIAL TENDON INJURIES

This topic is covered in the section on acquired flatfoot deformities.

PERONEAL TENDON INJURIES

Peroneal tendon injuries fall into the categories of peroneal tendonitis, peroneal tendon tears, and peroneal tendon subluxation or dislocation.

1. Peroneal Tendonitis

Pathogenesis

Inflammation of the peroneal tendons may be caused by acute trauma, inflammatory arthropathy conditions, or repetitive motion. Traumatic events that may induce tendonitis include a direct blow to the posterolateral ankle, a fracture of the calcaneus or fibula, or an inversion sprain of the ankle. Most cases are at least partially due to repetitive motion injury from recurrent rubbing of the peroneal tendons on the distal end of the fibula. Some studies have shown an association between tendonitis and hypertrophy of the peroneal tubercle. Tendonitis of the peroneus longus is often associated with

inflammation of the os peroneum, a small sesamoid bone located in the tendon where it curves around the lateral border of the cuboid.

Clinical Findings

A. Symptoms and Signs

Pain and swelling are located along the course of the peroneal tendons. The symptoms are made worse with activity, and improve with rest and NSAIDs. The onset may be insidious, or it may be associated with an acute injury. Physical examination usually demonstrates pain with resisted eversion of the foot.

B. Imaging Studies

An MRI scan may help to distinguish between tendonitis and a tendon tear, although small tears may not be identified on an MRI.

Treatment

A. Nonsurgical

If symptoms are mild, the recommended treatment includes NSAIDs, activity modification and an ankle brace. Four to six weeks of cast immobilization is used for more advanced symptoms or for patients who do not respond to initial treatment. Occasionally, a single corticosteroid injection is given into the tendon sheath.

B. Surgical

Operative intervention is recommended for patients who fail conservative treatment. The tendon sheath is explored, inflamed synovium is removed, and the tendons are carefully explored to look for tears or stenotic lesions. Postoperatively, early range of motion is encouraged for simple synovectomy.

2. Peroneal Tendon Tears

Pathogenesis

The majority of peroneal tendon tears are attritional in nature, due to mechanical irritation within the fibular groove. The peroneus longus tendon, which lies posterior, places pressure on the brevis tendon. Also, a sharp lateral edge of the fibula may predispose to a longitudinal split of the tendons. Laxity of the tendon sheath and subluxation of the tendons out of the fibular groove may contribute to tears as well. Acute tears of the peroneal tendons occur rarely, and there is almost certainly some degree of pre-existing degenerative changes within the tendon.

Clinical Findings

Clinical presentation is similar to that of peroneal tendonitis, with pain and swelling along the tendon

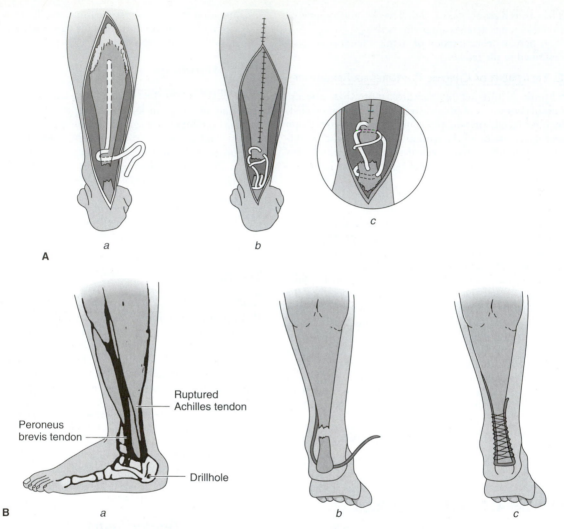

Figure 9–62. Various methods of reconstruction for untreated Achilles tendon ruptures. **A:** Repair using fascial strip from proximal gastrocsoleus complex. *a:* Distally based fascial strip is passed transversely through proximal tendon fragment. *b:* The strip is woven across the gap. *c:* Enlarged diagram of *b*. **B:** Repair using peroneus brevis tendon. The peroneus brevis is isolated and detached from its insertion into the fifth metatarsal. *a:* A transverse drill hole is placed in the calcaneus. *b:* The peroneus brevis is transferred through the drill hole. *c:* The tendon is sutured to itself and to the Achilles tendon proximally and distally. (**A:** Reproduced, with permission, from Bosworth DM: J Bone Joint Surg Am 1956;38:111. **B:** Reproduced, with permission, from Plattner, P, Mann, RA: Disorders of Tendons, in Mann RA, Coughlin MJ [editors]: *Surgery of the Foot and Ankle,* 6th ed. St. Louis: Mosby-Year Book, 1993.)

sheath, and pain with resisted eversion of the foot. An MRI scan may be helpful to demonstrate a tear.

Treatment

A. Nonsurgical

Treatment is identical to that of peroneal tendonitis.

B. Surgical

In the case of an MRI-documented peroneal tendon tear, surgical repair is indicated except in sedentary individuals. At surgery, both tendons are carefully examined, the fibula is explored for a sharp edge, and the sheath is evaluated for laxity. The tendon is repaired with nylon or prolene suture. Areas with significant de-

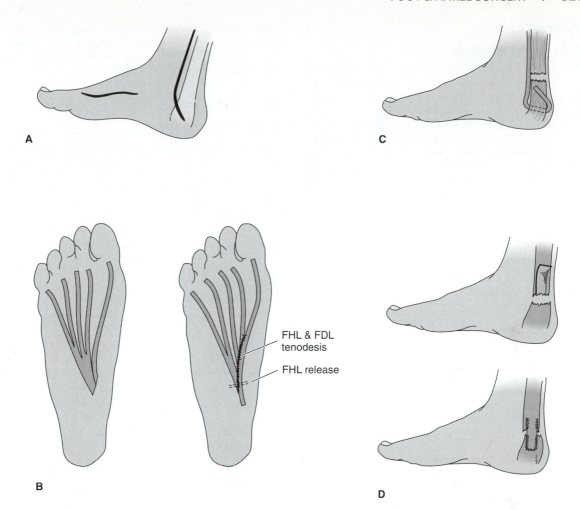

A

B

C

D

FHL & FDL
tenodesis

FHL release

Figure 9–63.   Delayed repair of ruptured Achilles tendon using flexor digitorum longus transfer. **A:** Operative technique demonstrating incisions. **B:** Tenodesis of the flexor digitorum longus stump to the flexor hallucis longus. **C:** Flexor digitorum longus pulled through drill hole in calcaneus. **D:** Augmentation of spanned gap by turndown of fascial strip from gastrocsoleus complex. (Reproduced, with permission, from Plattner, P and Mann RA: Disorders of Tendons, in Mann RA, Coughlin, MF [editors]: *Surgery of the Foot and Ankle,* 6th ed. St. Louis: Mosby-Year Book, 1993.)

generation are removed. Postoperatively, the ankle is immobilized for 3–4 weeks, then gentle range of motion is started. Weight bearing is allowed after 6 weeks.

3. Peroneal Tendon Subluxation and Dislocation

Pathogenesis

Peroneal tendon dislocation is caused by a sudden forceful dorsiflexion motion of the ankle combined with a si-multaneous strong contraction of the peroneal musculature. This mechanism injures the superior peroneal retinaculum, which holds the peroneal tendons in place along the posterior edge of the distal fibula. The retinaculum is rarely ruptured; rather it is stripped off the fibular insertion or avulsed with a small piece of fibular cortex. This allows for the creation of a false pouch and laxity of the retinaculum, allowing the peroneal tendons to dislocate anteriorly. If this condition goes unrecognized, either the tendons remain dislocated, or they relocate with the propensity for recurrent subluxation or dislocation.

Clinical Findings

A. SYMPTOMS AND SIGNS

The patient usually recalls an acute episode of trauma and frequently the sensation of the tendon dislocating. Pain and swelling is localized to the peroneal tendon sheath around the tip of the fibula. With recurrent subluxation, a feeling of dislocation may also be felt, but most commonly the patient feels as though they are recurrently spraining their ankle. In either setting, resisted eversion of the ankle elicits pain, and possibly causes the tendons to subluxate. Unfortunately, many acute peroneal tendon dislocations go unrecognized as lateral ankle sprains.

B. IMAGING STUDIES

Radiographs may show a small piece of bone lateral to the distal fibula, indicative of avulsion of the retinaculum. MRI scan usually details the injury well if careful attention is paid to this area.

Treatment

A. NONSURGICAL

Treatment of acute peroneal tendon dislocations consists of casting in plantarflexion and inversion for 3 weeks, followed by a walking cast for 3 weeks. Cast treatment has at least a 50% failure rate. Once a tendon is chronically dislocated or recurrently subluxates, no treatment will keep it in position.

B. SURGICAL

Surgical repair is recommended for an athletic individual following an acute dislocation of their peroneal tendons. It is also recommended for patients with recurrent dislocation if their physical activities are significantly restricted. The procedure consists of repairing the superior peroneal retinaculum to the fibula, either through drill holes or with suture anchors. In the case of attenuated retinaculum due to chronic dislocations, the repair can be reinforced with a strip of Achilles or by rerouting the calcaneofibular ligament over the tendons. At the time of surgical repair, the tendons are inspected for tears. Postoperatively, the patient is immobilized in a cast for 6 weeks.

ANTERIOR TIBIAL TENDON RUPTURE

Pathogenesis

Rupture of the anterior tibial tendon occurs infrequently, and most often in an older patient. The mechanism is either chronic rubbing against the inferior edge of the extensor retinaculum, or rubbing against an exostosis at the first metatarsocuneiform joint. The rupture usually occurs at the distal 2–3 cm of tendon. Trau-matic ruptures can occur due to sudden forced plantarflexion against a contracted anterior tibial muscle. The anterior tibial tendon can also be lacerated by the edge of the tibia when it is fractured.

Clinical Findings

A. SYMPTOMS AND SIGNS

Patients with a degenerative rupture present with complaints of pain and swelling over the anterior ankle. They sense the foot slapping down, or catching their foot on the ground when they walk. Frequently, patients present after the symptoms have been present for several months. In the case of acute trauma, pain and swelling are usually more severe. Physical exam is notable for weakness of ankle dorsiflexion, often with a palpable mass over the anterior ankle joint.

B. IMAGING STUDIES

If the diagnosis is in doubt, MRI scan can accurately determine if the tendon is ruptured.

Treatment

A. NONSURGICAL

In the case of a less active patient, nonsurgical treatment appears to give equal functional results to surgical repair. Cast immobilization is followed by long-term use of an ankle-foot orthosis.

B. SURGICAL

Acute tendon rupture or laceration of the tendon in an active individual should be surgically repaired. Chronic ruptures that are symptomatic usually require reconstruction using an extensor tendon graft or tendon transfer because the distal stump is usually too degenerated to perform a primary repair.

Brandes CB, Smith RW: Characterization of patients with primary peroneus longus tendinopathy: A review of twenty-two cases. Foot Ankle Int 2000;21:462.

Jaakkola JI et al: Early ankle motion after triple bundle technique repair vs casting for acute Achilles tendon rupture. Foot Ankle Int 2001;22:979.

Lim J et al: Percutaneous vs open repair of the ruptured Achilles tendon—A prospective randomized controlled study. Foot Ankle Int 2001;22:559.

Ma GW, Griffith TG: Percutaneous repair of acute closed ruptured Achilles tendon. A new technique. Clin Orthop 1988;128:247.

Coughlin MJ: Disorders of tendons. In Coughlin MJ, Mann RA (editors): *Surgery of the Foot and Ankle.* St. Louis: Mosby, Inc., 19993.

Porter DA et al: Primary repair without augmentation for early neglected Achilles tendon ruptures in the recreational athlete. Foot Ankle Int 1997;18:557.

OSTEOCHONDRAL LESIONS OF THE TALUS

Osteochondral lesions of the talus (OLT) are defects of cartilage and subchondral bone in the dome of the talus. More sophisticated imaging techniques have made diagnosis of this entity more precise, and advancement in arthroscopic methods have expanded treatment options for this difficult problem.

Pathogenesis

OLTs, also known as osteochondritis dissecans lesions, may occur as a result of trauma or may be long-standing conditions that are ischemic in origin. The majority of lesions are located either posteromedially or anterolaterally on the talar dome. Posteromedial lesions are more common, and are usually deeper lesions involving subchondral bone. Their origin is thought to involve ischemia, often with an episode of trauma exacerbating the underlying condition. The anterolateral lesions are a result of a single traumatic episode or repetitive trauma from lateral ankle sprains. These lesions tend to be shallower and often purely cartilaginous.

Clinical Findings

A. Symptoms and Signs

Patients usually present with several months of ankle pain following a routine ankle sprain. Sometimes they recount a history of recurrent sprains to the ankle. The pain is usually located over the anterior aspect of the ankle on the side of the lesion, but it may be diffuse. Occasionally there is a sensation of locking in the ankle. A high index of suspicion is necessary, as OLTs can be misdiagnosed as a chronic ankle sprain. See the section on ligamentous injuries about the ankle joint for a complete discussion on the differential diagnosis of chronic ankle pain.

B. Imaging Studies

Radiographs are often normal in OLTs. MRI scan is the imaging procedure of choice for determining the size, location, and extent of bony or cartilaginous involvement (Figure 9–64).

Treatment

A. Nonsurgical

A trial of cast immobilization is warranted if the MRI scan shows no evidence of a displaced lesion.

B. Surgical

The surgical treatment method depends on the type of lesion. Acutely or recently displaced lesions can be reduced and pinned with an absorbable pin by either

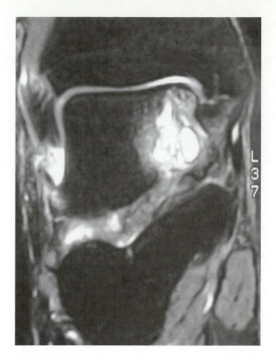

Figure 9–64. MRI scan of extensive osteochondral lesion of the talus.

open or arthroscopic methods. Purely cartilaginous lesions can be curetted to a stable rim and drilled to stimulate vascular ingrowth and fibrocartilage formation. Lesions with bony involvement should be aggressively curetted, bone-grafted, and drilled, either open or arthroscopically. A medial malleolar osteotomy is often required to access a posteromedial OLT. If a bony lesion has intact overlying cartilage, drilling and bone grafting can be performed through the talus, thereby sparing the overlying cartilage. Postoperatively, patients are kept non-weight–bearing for 4 weeks, but early range of motion is encouraged.

New techniques have been developed for lesions that have failed traditional treatment methods. Osteochondral autograft or allograft bone plugs can be used to replace bone and cartilage defects. Autograft plugs are generally harvested from the ipsilateral knee. Autologous chondrocyte implantation has also been used to a limited extent for OLTs. Short-term follow-up data is encouraging, but no long-term data are available for either of these newer techniques.

Ferkel RD: Osteochondral lesions of the talus. In Ferkel RD (editor): Arthroscopic surgery: The foot and ankle. Philadelphia: Lippincott-Raven, 1996.

Giannini S et al: Autologous chondrocyte transplantation in osteochondral lesions of the ankle joint. Foot Ankle Int 2001;22: 513.

Hangody L et al: Mosaicplasty for the treatment of osteochondritis dissecans of the talus: Two to seven year results in 36 patients. Foot Ankle Int 2001;22:552.

Hepple S et al: Osteochondral lesions of the talus: A revised classification. Foot Ankle Int 1999;20:789.

Tol JL et al: Treatment strategies in osteochondral defects of the talar dome: A systematic review. Foot Ankle Int 2000;21: 119.

Hand Surgery

Michael S. Bednar, MD, & Terry R. Light, MD

Function of the Hand

The hand is a vital part of the human body, allowing humans to directly interact with their environment. The functional capabilities of the hand are many because the hand is ultimately an end organ of the human mind. The hand's enormous capacity for adaptability has allowed primitive humans to make stone tools and modern humans to pilot complex aircraft.

The human hand is capable of **prehension,** which involves approaching an object, grasping it, modulating and maintaining grasp, and ultimately releasing the object. When a **power grasp** is used, the object is pushed by the flexed fingers against the palm, while the thumb metacarpal and proximal phalanx stabilize the object. When an object is held with a **precision pinch pattern,** the object is secured between the pulp of the thumb distal phalanx and the index finger or index and middle fingers.

The hand can touch objects or other human beings while sensing temperature, vibration, and texture. This quality of **tactilegnosis** is sophisticated enough to allow blind individuals to read the pattern of small elevations that distinguish one Braille letter from another. The hand is also an instrument of communication, whether by making a gesture, playing a musical instrument, drawing, writing, or typing.

General Considerations in Treatment of Hand Disorders

Treatment of hand disorders requires an understanding of normal anatomy and its common variations. Treatment usually attempts to restore the normal anatomy, but when that is not possible, the goal should be restoration of maximal function. The appearance of the hand is of concern to most individuals because the hand is usually uncovered and exposed to the scrutiny of others. Imperfections are often a source of embarrassment. Effective treatment requires a mature balancing of the need for normal function and normal appearance of the hand. Complex reconstruction that restores prehension but results in a hideous appearance of the hand will be ineffective if the patient is so reluctant to expose the hand that he or she avoids using it. Conversely, a functionless stiff finger leading to awkward motion of an otherwise supple hand may cause the patient more embarrassment than amputation.

DIAGNOSIS OF DISORDERS OF THE HAND

History

When a patient seeks evaluation of a hand disorder, the physician should ask many general questions as well as questions specific to hand function and injury. The chief complaint as perceived by the patient should be summarized in one or two sentences. The patient's hand dominance, age, gender, and occupation should be noted, as well as any hobbies that require hand dexterity or strength. The time of onset of symptoms should be recorded. If injury is the cause of discomfort, the date and mechanism of injury should be noted and whether the injury occurred at the work place. The patient should be questioned about prior treatment and their perception of its effectiveness.

Complaints should then be further detailed, such as the nature of pain (sharp, aching, dull, or burning), whether night symptoms are present, and whether the pain is worse upon awakening in the morning or after a full day of work. The patient should be asked whether symptoms include numbness or tingling. Specific motor difficulties, such as trouble in writing or removing jar tops, should be noted. If the patient complains mainly of unilateral symptoms, the examiner should ask if similar symptoms are occurring on the opposite side. Finally, because the hand is an exposed area of the body, the impact of altered appearance should be discussed.

The medical history should include any prior hand injuries and any systemic diseases such as rheumatoid arthritis or other inflammatory arthropathies, diabetes, other endocrine disorders, renal disease, or vascular disease. Women of childbearing age should be questioned about recent pregnancies.

A careful history will suggest the correct diagnosis in approximately 90% of patients with hand problems.

Examination of the Hand

A. GENERAL EXAMINATION

Examination of the hand should begin with observation. Vascular status can be assessed by noting the color of the fingers. Some hint of nerve function can be obtained by observing pseudomotor function as revealed by sweatiness or dryness of the fingers. The extent of injury is suggested by the degree of swelling and ecchymosis. The posture of the digits and the wrist may signal the possibility of tendon or bone disruption. Normally, a cascade of increased digital flexion is noted when ulnar digits are observed next to radial digits (Figure 10–1).

A diagram of the hand is often helpful in documenting the abnormality. Laceration sites, previous scars, amputated fingers, and subjective areas of decreased sensation can be noted on the diagram.

Next, the hand, wrist, and forearm are gently palpated. The temperature and moisture of the fingers should be noted. When the skin is blanched in the paronychial region, circulation should return within 3 s. Areas of tenderness on palpation are carefully noted.

B. RANGE OF MOTION

The passive and active range of motion of the shoulder, elbow, forearm, wrist, and hand are evaluated. The normal range of motion of the wrist and fingers is indicated in Table 10–1. In documenting range of motion, active extension should be to the left and active flexion to the right. When the range of passive extension and flexion is different from that of active motion, the passive range of motion values are noted in parentheses next to the corresponding active range of motion values.

C. MUSCLE FUNCTION

The integrity of individual muscles should be documented. The flexor digitorum profundus to each finger is tested by stabilizing the middle phalanx and asking the patient to flex the distal interphalangeal joint (Figure 10–2). The flexor digitorum superficialis of each finger is tested by keeping all fingers except the one to be tested in full extension. The patient is then asked to flex the finger at the proximal interphalangeal joint (Figure 10–3). The function of the flexor pollicis longus is tested simply by asking the patient to flex the interphalangeal joint of the thumb.

The function of the extrinsic extensors is tested by asking the patient to extend the metacarpophalangeal joints of the fingers. If the examiner simply asks the patient to open the hand, the proximal and distal inter-

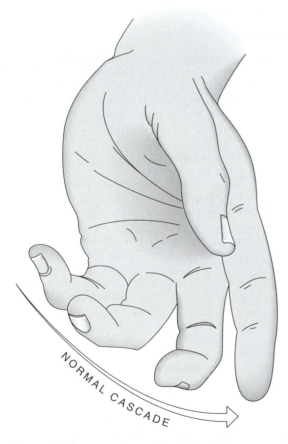

NORMAL CASCADE

Figure 10–1. Normal cascade of digital flexion posture. When the wrist is in slight extension and the fingers are at rest, there is progressively less flexion from the little finger to the index finger. (Reproduced, with permission, from Carter PR: *Common Hand Injuries and Infections.* Philadelphia: WB Saunders, 1983.)

Table 10–1. Normal range of motion in joints of arm and hand.

Elbow: Extension and flexion 0°/135°
Forearm: Supination and pronation 90°/90°
Wrist: Flexion and extension 80°/70°
       Radial deviation and ulnar deviation 20°/30°
Finger
  MP: Extension and flexion 0°/90°
  PIP: Extension and flexion 0°/110°
  DIP: Extension and flexion 0°/65°
Thumb
  CMC: Extension and flexion 50°/50°
      Abduction and adduction 70°/0°
    MP: Extension and flexion—variable, up to 0°/90°
    IP: Extension and flexion—variable, up to 0°/90°

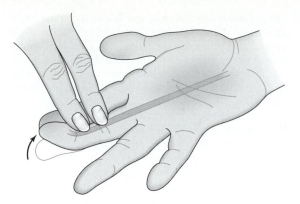

Figure 10–2. Testing of flexor digitorum profundus integrity. If the distal interphalangeal joint can be actively flexed while the proximal interphalangeal joint is stabilized, then the profundus tendon has not been severed. (Reproduced, with permission, from American Society for Surgery of the Hand: *The Hand: Examination and Diagnosis,* 2nd ed. New York: Churchill Livingstone, 1983.)

phalangeal joints may be extended by contraction of the interosseous muscles, and this may mislead the examiner to conclude that digital extension is normal. Interosseous muscle function is screened by asking the patient to abduct the fingers. The examiner then palpates the contraction of the hypothenar and the first dorsal interosseous muscles.

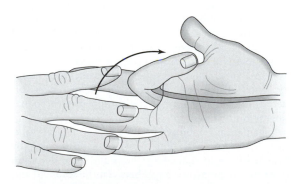

Figure 10–3. Testing of flexor digitorum superficialis integrity. If the proximal interphalangeal joint can be actively flexed while the adjacent fingers are held completely extended, the sublimis tendon has not been severed. (Reproduced, with permission, from American Society for Surgery of the Hand: *The Hand: Examination and Diagnosis,* 2nd ed. New York: Churchill Livingstone, 1983.)

D. SENSORY FUNCTION

Examination of sensory function requires evaluation of the integrity of the median, ulnar, and radial nerves as well as the component proper digital nerves to each side of the finger. Each of the major nerves has an autogenous sensory zone, an area of the hand that is supplied predominantly by that nerve (Figure 10–4). The autogenous zone of the median nerve is the pulp of the index finger, whereas the ulnar nerve provides sensory fibers from the pulp of the little finger. The skin on the dorsum of the first web space is innervated by the superficial branch of the radial nerve.

1. Two-point discrimination—The integrity of each digital nerve may be evaluated using either a blunt-tipped caliper or an unfolded paper clip to test two-point discrimination. The two points of the testing instrument are held apart at a measured distance. The examiner alternates between touching the skin with one or two points. The points may be either touched (static two-point discrimination) or longitudinally moved (moving two-point discrimination) against the skin on either the radial or ulnar side of the finger. The points

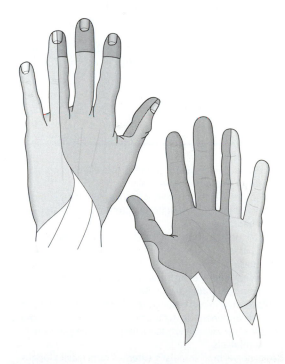

Figure 10–4. Sensory distribution in the hand. Light shading = ulnar nerve; medium shading = radial nerve; darkest shading = median nerve. (Reproduced, with permission, from Way LW, ed: *Current Surgical Diagnosis & Treatment,* 10th ed. Stamford: Appleton & Lange, 1994.)

should be pressed against the finger until the skin just begins to blanch. The two-point discrimination value is the smallest distance between the two points that the patient can correctly detect in two out of three trials. Because of the increased sensory cues provided by movement, moving two-point discrimination will usually have a value less than or equal to static two-point discrimination. Static two-point discrimination is normal if the distance is less than 7 mm, impaired if 7–14, and absent if 15 mm or more.

E. Motor Function

Examination of motor function may be organized by considering groups of muscles within specific nerve domains (Table 10–2). Proximally, the median nerve innervates the pronator teres, flexor carpi radialis, palmaris longus, and flexor digitorum superficialis. The anterior interosseous nerve branch of the median nerve innervates the flexor digitorum profundus of the index and middle fingers, flexor pollicis longus, and pronator quadratus muscles. The motor branch of the median to the thenar musculature innervates the opponens pollicis, abductor pollicis brevis, and superficial portion of the flexor pollicis brevis. The index- and long-finger lumbricals are innervated by branches running with the sensory nerve branches of the median nerve to the index and middle fingers.

The ulnar nerve innervates the flexor carpi ulnaris and flexor digitorum profundus of the ring and little fingers proximally. Within the hand, the ulnar nerve innervates the hypothenar musculature, flexor digiti quinti, and abductor digiti quinti. The deep motor branch of the ulnar nerve innervates the dorsal and palmar interosseous muscles, lumbricals to the ring and little fingers, deep portion of the flexor pollicis brevis, and adductor pollicis muscles.

The radial nerve innervates the triceps, brachioradialis, extensor carpi radialis longus and brevis, supinator, and anconeus muscles. The posterior interosseous division of the radial nerve then distally innervates the extensor digitorum communis, extensor indicis proprius, extensor digiti minimi, extensor carpi ulnaris, abductor pollicis longus, and extensor pollicis longus and brevis.

Muscle strength should be graded according to the British muscle grading system based on a scale of 0 to 5, with 5/5 being normal strength, 4/5 less than normal strength but with ability to resist a fair amount of resistance, 3/5 resistance against gravity, 2/5 resistance with gravity eliminated, and 1/5 only a trace or flicker of contraction without significant motion.

Diagnostic Studies

A number of different studies may be helpful in establishing the proper diagnosis in a patient with hand or wrist pain. The choice of technique should be based on a careful history and physical examination.

A. Imaging Studies

In most instances, radiographic evaluation includes anteroposterior and lateral films. The importance of obtaining a true lateral radiograph cannot be overemphasized because many disorders, particularly interphalangeal joint subluxation and carpal instability, are not evident on oblique views. Oblique views may be useful in defining phalangeal fracture patterns. Tangential views are useful in assessing a carpometacarpal boss.

Stress views allow assessment of ligamentous stability. This is particularly useful in the evaluation of collateral ligament stability of the thumb metacarpophalangeal joint.

Ligamentous stability of the wrist may also be evaluated by radial and ulnar deviation views and by clenched-fist grip views. Grip views and ulnar deviation views may demonstrate a gap between the scaphoid and the lunate that is not apparent on simple anteroposterior and lateral studies.

B. Electrodiagnostic Studies

Electrodiagnostic studies include both nerve conduction studies and electromyography. Nerve conduction studies measure both motor (proximal to distal) and sensory (distal to proximal) conduction. Electromyography allows evaluation of muscle function.

Table 10–2. Innervation of the hand and forearm.

Median nerve
    Proximal median nerve: pronator teres, flexor carpi radialis, flexor digitorum superficialis
    Anterior interosseous nerve: flexor pollicis longus, index and middle flexor digitorum profundus, pronator quadratus
    Distal median nerve: index and middle lumbrical, opponens pollicis, abductor pollicis brevis, flexor pollicis brevis
Ulnar nerve
    Proximal ulnar nerve: flexor carpi ulnaris, ring and small flexor digitorum profundus
    Distal ulnar nerve: flexor digiti minimi, abductor digiti minimi, opponens digiti minimi, volar and dorsal interossei, flexor pollicis brevis, adductor pollicis, ring and small lumbricals
Radial nerve: brachioradialis, extensor carpi radialis longus, supinator, anconeus
Posterior interosseous nerve: extensor carpi radialis brevis, extensor digitorum communis, extensor indicis proprius, extensor digiti minimi, extensor carpi ulnaris, abductor pollicis longus, extensor pollicis longus, extensor pollicis brevis

C. Computed Tomography Scan

A computed tomography (CT) scan allows excellent visualization of the distal radioulnar joint. The relationship of the distal ulna to the sigmoid notch should be viewed in pronation, neutral, and supination. CT scanning may be helpful in ascertaining displacement and healing of scaphoid fractures.

D. Magnetic Resonance Imaging

Magnetic resonance imaging (MRI) provides direct visualization of soft-tissue structures. The integrity of the transverse carpal ligament may be evaluated. This is particularly helpful in patients with persistent symptoms following carpal tunnel release. Evaluation of tumors and avascular necrosis is also facilitated by MRI.

New generation MRI scanners are better in evaluating triangular fibrocartilage complex and intracarpal ligament tears.

E. Bone Scan

The technetium-99 MDP bone scan is a useful physiologic test in the evaluation of unexplained hand or wrist pain. This test can rule out bone involvement and can be used to localize inflammatory processes for further study with anatomic imaging techniques (Figure 10–5).

F. Wrist Arthrographic Studies

Arthrographic studies of the wrist allow evaluation of the integrity of three different soft-tissue stabilizing structures: the scapholunate ligament, lunotriquetral ligament, and triangular fibrocartilage complex. A single radiocarpal injection tests the competence of each of the three structures to prevent dye from escaping from the radiocarpal space (Figure 10–6). If dye is noted in the distal radioulnar joint, the triangular fibrocartilage complex is perforated. If dye is noted at the midcarpal level, disruption of the scapholunate or lunotriquetral ligament is present. Because tears of the triangular fibrocartilage complex or ligaments may create a one-way valve phenomenon, separate midcarpal and distal radioulnar joint injections may reveal disruptions not apparent from the radiocarpal injection.

G. Wrist Arthroscopy

Arthroscopic examination of the wrist allows for direct visualization of articular surfaces, wrist ligaments, and the triangular fibrocartilage complex. The effect of stress maneuvers on intercarpal kinematics may be directly observed by these studies. Wrist arthroscopy is particularly helpful in the debridement or repair of the triangular fibrocartilage complex tears. Partial tears of either the scapholunate or lunotriquetral ligaments may be debrided. Intra-articular fracture of the distal radius may be anatomically aligned and pinned under direct observation.

Jansen JC, Adams BD: Long-term outcome of nonsurgically treated patients with wrist pain and a normal arthrogram. J Hand Surg [Am]. 2002;27(1):26. [PMID: 11810610]

Osterwalder JJ et al: Diagnostic validity of ultrasound in patients with persistent wrist pain and suspected occult ganglion. J Hand Surg Am 1997;22:1034.

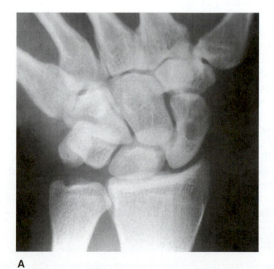
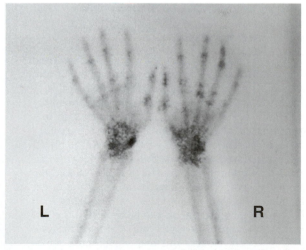

A **B**

Figure 10–5. Radiograph (**A**) and bone scan (**B**) demonstrating increased activity in the region of the scaphoid in a woman with a symptomatic cyst.

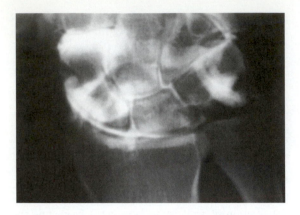

Figure 10–6. Arthrogram injection of dye into the radiocarpal joint flows into the midcarpal joint, demonstrating a perforation of the scapholunate or lunotriquetral ligament.

Potter HG, Weiland AJ: Magnetic resonance imaging of triangular fibrocartilage complex lesions. J Hand Surg [Am]. 2002;27 (2):363. [PMID: 11901408]

SPECIAL TREATMENT PROCEDURES FOR HAND DISORDERS

1. Replantation

Replantation is the reattachment of a body part that has been totally severed from the body, without any residual soft-tissue continuity. Revascularization is the reconstruction of damaged blood vessels to prevent an attached but ischemic body part from becoming necrotic.

Initial Care of Patient

Appropriate treatment of the patient and the ischemic or detached body part requires coordinated initial care and prompt referral to a surgeon at a center capable of mobilizing resources for early surgical care. The initial treating physician should place the amputated part in a sponge soaked with either normal saline or Ringer's lactate solution. The wrapped part should then be placed into a plastic bag, which is sealed and immersed in an ice-water solution. Under no circumstances should the amputated part be placed directly into ice water or exposed to dry ice.

A compressive dressing should be applied to the amputation stump. No attempt should be made to ligate bleeding vessels, because this may compromise subsequent neurovascular repair. If the amputated part is not cooled, ischemia is poorly tolerated and successful revascularization is unlikely after 6 h. Cooled parts may be replanted up to 12 h after injury.

Indications & Contraindications

Replantation is indicated for severed thumbs or multiple digits, transmetacarpal hand amputations, wrist- or distal forearm-level amputations, and amputations of almost any body part in a child. In more proximal levels of amputation, only sharp or moderately avulsed parts can be considered for replantation. The more proximal the amputation, the greater the amount of ischemic muscle mass and the more urgent the need for revascularization.

Contraindications to replantation include severely crushed or mangled parts; multilevel amputation; amputations in patients with arteriosclerotic vessels; amputations in patients with other serious injuries or diseases; and amputations with prolonged warm ischemic times, particularly at proximal levels.

In adults, replantation of an individual finger proximal to the insertion of the flexor digitorum superficialis is usually contraindicated because of the likelihood of poor function. Stiffness of these replanted fingers is caused by simultaneous zone 2 flexor tendon disruption, phalangeal fracture, and extensor tendon disruption. Replantation at this level may be considered in children or for aesthetic reasons.

Surgical Procedure

The preferred method of anesthesia is a scalene or axillary block because these techniques provide a sympathetic block resulting in vasodilation. The surgical sequence of replantation begins with a wide surgical exposure that allows identification and isolation of arteries, veins, and nerves. The soft tissue is then meticulously debrided. The bone is shortened and solid internal fixation is achieved, so that early postoperative motion may be instituted.

The extensor tendons are repaired first and then the flexor tendons. Anastomosis of one or preferably two arteries is then performed, followed by repair of the nerves and anastomosis of the veins. Two veins should be repaired for each artery repaired. Skin should be closed loosely, with care taken to approximate soft tissue over repaired vessels and nerves.

In replantations proximal to the distal forearm, fasciotomies of all compartments should be performed. The patient should be returned to the operating room in 48–72 h, so that the wound may be reevaluated and additional necrotic tissue debrided.

Postoperative Care

Postoperatively, the hand is protected in an elevated, loose, bulky dressing. Anticoagulation with one of a variety of medications should be given in the perioperative period to diminish the likelihood of anastomosis thrombosis. Low-molecular-weight dextran for 5–7 days and aspirin are among the recommended regimen. Some patients, particularly children, may require sedation to decrease the chance of arterial spasm in the early postoperative period. Vasospastic agents such as nicotine, caffeine, theophylline, and theobromine should be restricted for the first few weeks after replantation or revascularization. The patient should be placed on a broad-spectrum antibiotic for 5–7 days. Clinical monitoring of the replanted or revascularized parts may be supplemented with a pulse oximeter, laser Doppler, or temperature probe.

In those replanted or revascularized parts that show impending failure by change in color, capillary refill, or tissue turgor, the dressing should be loosened. Hand position should be changed to relieve pressure on the part. Patients may be given a heparin bolus of 3000–5000 units. The patient must be well hydrated and the room warm. If no improvement is seen after 4–6 h, the patient may be returned to the operating room for exploration of the anastomoses. Vascular revision is most successful when carried out within 48 h of injury.

Technical problems involving vascular anastomoses are most often caused by thrombosis, an ill-placed suture occluding the lumen, poor proximal flow secondary to spasm, or undetected intimal vessel damage. If vascular damage is found, a larger segment of the vessel should be resected and a vein graft interposed. If failure appears secondary to poor venous outflow, the intermittent application of leeches (*Hirudo* spp) for 1–5 days may be helpful in allowing reestablishment of adequate venous drainage.

Prognosis

Approximately 85% of replanted parts remain viable. Sensory recovery with two-point discrimination of 10 mm or less occurs in approximately 50% of adults. Patients often complain of cold intolerance during the first 2 or 3 years after replantation. Range of motion in replanted digits is largely dependent on the level of injury and usually averages 50% of the normal side.

In most children, normal sensation will be regained after digital replantation, and the epiphyseal plates will remain open and achieve approximately 80% of normal longitudinal growth. Although the functional results are more promising in children, the viability rate is lower because of the greater technical demands of the small vessel anastomoses and the greater sympathetic tone.

Because nerves transected in the proximal arm must regenerate over the considerable length of the limb, only limited motor return is seen in the forearm and hand in proximal limb replantations in adults. One potential benefit of a proximal upper limb replantation may be converting a traumatic above-elbow amputation to an assistive limb with elbow control. Replantation may provide dramatic restoration of hand function when the level of initial amputation is either in the distal forearm or at the wrist level (Figure 10–7).

2. Amputation

The purpose of amputation is to preserve maximal function consistent with bone loss and to achieve an aesthetically acceptable appearance. Priority should be given to preserving functional length, minimizing scar and joint contractures, and preventing the development of symptomatic neuromas.

Phalangeal Amputation

Digital amputation may be carried out through a phalanx or an interphalangeal joint. If the amputation is through the proximal or distal interphalangeal joint, the distal articular surface is contoured to remove the palmar condylar prominences. If the normal insertion of a tendon has been amputated, the tendon should be pulled distally, severed proximally, and allowed to retract. The flexor and extensor tendons should never be sewn over the amputation bone end to provide soft-tissue coverage. Nerves should be identified, drawn distally, and transected proximally to prevent the development of a neuroma adherent to the skin scar. If possible, the thick well-padded skin of the palmar surface of the finger should be used to cover the amputation stump. A nontender, shortened, well-padded digit is preferable to a poorly covered, slightly longer, tender digit.

Ray Resection

Amputations through the proximal portion of the proximal phalanx or at the metacarpophalangeal joint of the index or little finger may leave an unsightly bony prominence on the border of the palm, and amputations at a similar level in the middle or ring finger may create an awkward interdigital gap that allows small objects to fall through the palm. Ray resection may be employed to close traumatic wounds, remove dysfunctional or dysesthetic digits, or treat malignant tumors. The aesthetic and functional advantages of ray resection must be balanced against the loss of palmar breadth and, hence, diminution of grip strength.

Index-ray resection creates a normal-appearing web between the middle finger and the thumb. Similarly, resection of the little-finger metacarpal will leave a smooth ulnar contour. Little-finger ray resection is contraindicated in patients who prefer maximal grip strength over cosmesis. Resection of the middle- or

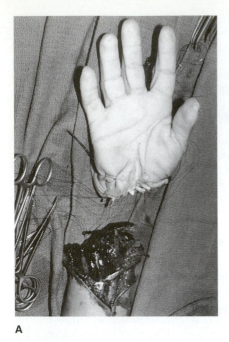
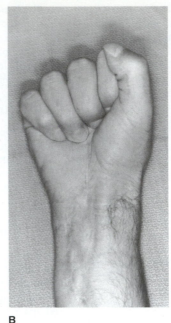
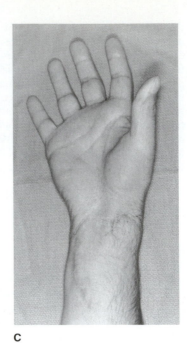

A   B   C

Figure 10–7. Replantation of hand. Intraoperative view (**A**). Following operation, flexion (**B**) and extension (**C**) are restored.

ring-finger ray should be accompanied by either soft-tissue coaptation or metacarpal transposition. Resection of the middle ray through the proximal metacarpal metaphysis allows transposition of the corresponding distal portion of the index ray to the middle-ray position (Figure 10–8). Ring-finger ray resection may be closed by either osteotomizing the little-finger metacarpal and moving it to the ring-finger base or by pulling the little finger radialward across the hamate by tight repair of the deep transverse intermetacarpal ligament between the middle and little fingers.

Steichen JB, Idler RS: Results of central ray resection without bony transposition. J Hand Surg Am 1986;11:466.

■ DISORDERS OF THE MUSCULATURE OF THE HAND

Anatomy

Control of digital posture requires a complex balance of extrinsic and intrinsic muscle forces. Extrinsic muscles have their origin outside of the hand and their insertion on the hand or carpus, whereas intrinsic muscles have both origin and insertion within the hand. Extrinsic

muscles are either flexors or extensors, and intrinsic muscles contribute to both digital flexion and extension.

A. EXTRINSIC EXTENSOR MUSCLES

The extrinsic extensors run through six different fibro-osseous retinacular compartments at the wrist level (Figure 10–9A). The first (most radial) compartment contains the abductor pollicis longus and the extensor pollicis brevis. The abductor pollicis longus inserts at the base of the thumb metacarpal and radially abducts the thumb, whereas the extensor pollicis brevis inserts on the dorsum of the proximal aspect of the proximal phalanx of the thumb and actively extends the metacarpophalangeal joint of the thumb.

The second extensor compartment contains the extensor carpi radialis longus and the extensor carpi radialis brevis. The extensor carpi radialis longus, inserting on the index metacarpal, dorsiflexes and radially deviates the wrist, and the extensor carpi radialis brevis, inserting into the base of the middle metacarpal, provides balanced wrist dorsiflexion.

The third compartment contains the extensor pollicis longus, which runs longitudinally down the forearm through the third compartment and turns abruptly radialward about Lister's tubercle, a dorsal prominence on the distal radius. Because its insertion is on the distal phalanx, the extensor pollicis longus provides forceful

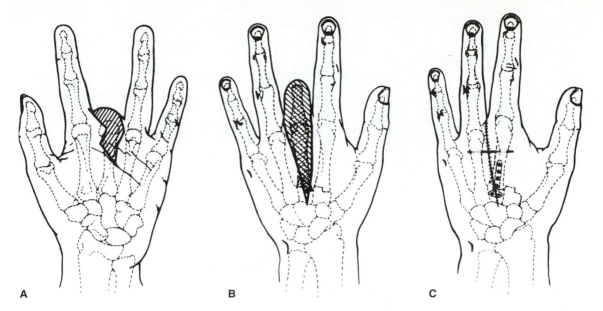

Figure 10–8. Middle-ray resection and index-ray transposition. **A:** Converging chevron incisions reduce palmar skin and soft-tissue redundancy. **B:** Corresponding step-cut osteotomies are fashioned in both the index and middle metacarpal proximal metaphyses. **C:** The transposed index finger is fixed to the middle finger with a plate and is further stabilized with Kirschner wire into the ring-finger metacarpal. (Reproduced, with permission, from Chapman MW, ed: *Operative Orthopaedics,* vol 2. Baltimore: Lippincott, 1988.)

extension of the thumb interphalangeal joint. The oblique course of the extensor pollicis longus tendon provides a significant adduction component to the pull of the extensor pollicis longus.

The fourth extensor compartment contains the extensor indicis proprius and the extensor digitorum communis, whereas the fifth compartment contains the extensor digiti quinti. These three muscles each have a role in digital extension at the metacarpophalangeal, proximal interphalangeal, and distal interphalangeal joints of the fingers. The principal bony insertion of the extrinsic digital extensors is on the dorsal proximal aspect of the middle phalanx. Metacarpophalangeal joint extension is provided by extrinsic extensor force transmitted through the sagittal bands. Distal interphalangeal joint extension is achieved through the conjoined lateral bands that are composed of tendinous slips from the extrinsic and intrinsic tendons.

The extensor indicis proprius inserts on the index finger ulnarly to the extensor digitorum communis. The extensor digitorum communis inserts on the index, middle, ring, and, in some cases, little fingers. The extensor digiti quinti tendon inserts on the little finger ulnarward to the extensor digitorum communis insertion.

The extensor carpi ulnaris tendon runs through the sixth compartment and inserts at the base of the little-finger metacarpal. It provides wrist extension and ulnar deviation.

The individual extensor digitorum communis tendons of the middle, ring, and little fingers are tethered together by juncturae tendinum over the dorsum of the hand proximal to the metacarpophalangeal joint (Figure 10–9B). The extensor indicis proprius tendon may be recognized at the wrist level as possessing the most distal muscle belly of any of the digital extensor tendons.

The digital extensor tendons are stabilized over the midline of the metacarpophalangeal joint by their attachment to sagittal band fibers (Figure 10–10). The sagittal band fibers insert onto the volar proximal phalanx and onto the lateral borders of the volar plate. The sagittal band fibers form a sling that allows proximal extrinsic extensor tension to be transmitted to the proximal phalanx, permitting metacarpophalangeal joint extension without a tendinous insertion onto the proximal phalanx. With rupture or attenuation of the sagittal band fibers, the extrinsic extensor tendon sublux ulnarly relative to the metacarpal head. By holding the extrinsic extensor tendon balanced over the prominence of the metacarpal head, the sagittal bands normally keep the extrinsic extensor as far as possible away from the center of rotation of the metacarpophalangeal

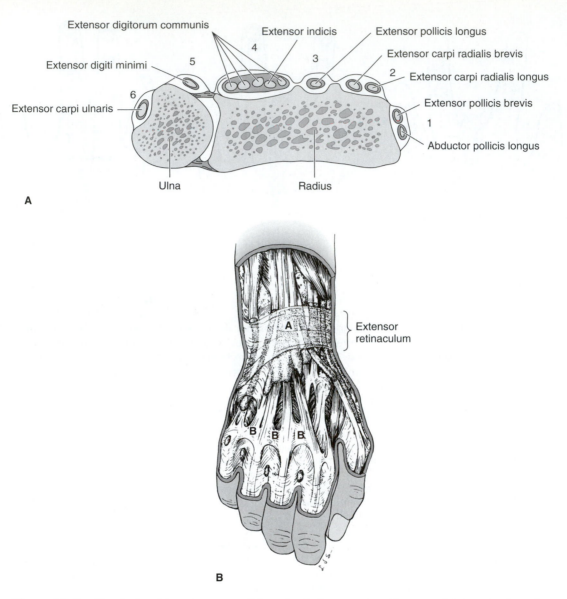

Figure 10–9. The six dorsal compartments of the wrist. **A:** Cross-section of pronated right wrist viewed from distal to proximal. (Reproduced, with permission, from Reckling FW et al: *Orthopaedic Anatomy and Surgical Approaches.* St Louis: Mosby-Year Book, 1990.) **B:** Dorsal view. A = extensor retinaculum over the compartments; B = juncturae tendinum (conexus intertendineus). (Reproduced, with permission, from Way LW, ed: *Current Surgical Diagnosis & Treatment,* 10th ed. Stamford: Appleton & Lange, 1994.)

joint, thereby giving it the greatest mechanical efficiency.

B. Extrinsic Flexor Muscles

The extrinsic digital flexors are the flexor digitorum profundus and the flexor digitorum superficialis. The

flexor digitorum profundus inserts on the proximal volar aspect of the distal phalanx, flexing the distal interphalangeal joint as well as the proximal interphalangeal and metacarpophalangeal joints. The flexor digitorum superficialis acts as a flexor of the proximal interphalangeal and metacarpophalangeal joints. It lies

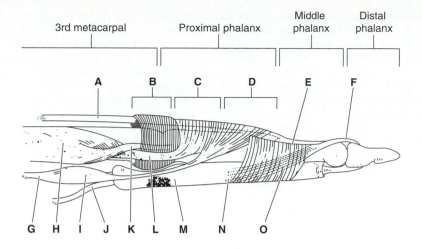

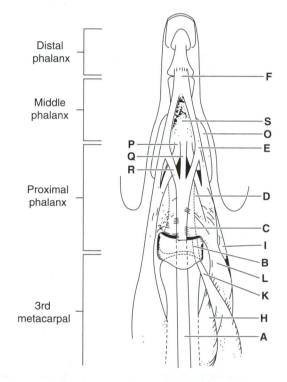

A. Common extensor tendon
B. Sagittal bands
C. Transverse fibers of the interossei
D. Oblique fibers of the interossei
E. Lateral conjoined tendon
F. Terminal tendon
G. Flexor digitorum profundus tendon
H. Interosseous muscle (second dorsal) deep head
I. Lumbrical muscle
J. Tendon of flexor digitorum superficialis
K. Medial tendon, superficial head of second dorsal interosseous
L. Lateral tendon of deep head of second dorsal interosseous
M. Fibrous flexor pulley
N. Oblique retinacular ligament
O. Transverse retinacular ligament
P. Medial interosseous band
Q. Central slip of the common extensor
R. Lateral slip of the common extensor
S. Triangular ligament

Figure 10–10. Extensor hood mechanism. The dorsal hood apparatus provides points of insertion of both extrinsic extensors and intrinsic muscles of the hand. (Modified and reproduced, with permission, from Way LW, ed: *Current Surgical Diagnosis & Treatment,* 10th ed. Stamford: Appleton & Lange, 1994.)

palmar to the flexor digitorum profundus tendon in the palm, splits at the level of the metacarpophalangeal joint, and passes dorsal to the flexor digitorum profundus tendon before reattaching or inserting into the middle phalanx. Although the extrinsic flexors provide metacarpophalangeal joint flexion, this is achieved only after most of their excursion has been expended flexing the interphalangeal joints.

C. INTRINSIC MUSCLES

The intrinsic muscles that control finger posture are the dorsal and palmar interossei, lumbricals, and hypothenar muscles. These muscles are responsible for primary flexion, abduction, and adduction of the metacarpophalangeal joints and primary extension of the proximal interphalangeal and distal interphalangeal joints.

The index metacarpal is abducted by the first dorsal interosseous muscle and adducted by the first palmar interosseous muscle. The middle finger is radially abducted by the second dorsal interosseous muscle and ulnarly abducted by the third dorsal interosseous muscle. The ring finger is adducted by the second volar interosseous muscle and abducted by the fourth dorsal interosseous muscle. The little finger is adducted by the third volar interosseous muscle and abducted by the abductor digiti quinti muscle.

The first, second, and fourth dorsal interossei have both superficial and deep muscle bellies, with the superficial belly giving rise to a tendon of insertion on the proximal phalanx tubercle. The deep muscle belly inserts into the hood of the dorsal aponeurosis and thus contributes to metacarpophalangeal joint flexion and proximal and distal interphalangeal joint extension. The third dorsal interosseous usually has a single muscle belly, which inserts into the dorsal hood apparatus. The insertion of the volar interosseous muscles is also into the hood apparatus (see Figure 10–10).

All interosseous muscles pass palmar to the axis of motion of the metacarpophalangeal joint and dorsal to the transverse intermetacarpal ligament. Their tendinous insertions are into the lateral band fibers, which pass dorsal to the axis of motion of the proximal and distal interphalangeal joints. When the metacarpophalangeal joint is flexed, the interossei are less effective in extending the interphalangeal joints than when the metacarpophalangeal joint is in extension or slight flexion.

The four lumbrical muscles insert into the radial lateral band of the dorsal hood aponeurosis of each finger. The lumbricals originate from the flexor digitorum profundus tendons of the corresponding finger. Their course is more volar than that of the dorsal or palmar interosseous muscles because they lie palmar to the transverse intermetacarpal ligament. The lumbrical muscles modulate flexor and extensor digital tone and

may have a role in digital proprioception. Contraction of the profundus muscle belly draws the profundus tendon proximally and thus pulls the lumbrical origin proximally, simultaneously increasing tension on the dorsal hood fibers that extend the proximal and distal interphalangeal joints. Contraction of the lumbrical muscle draws the proximal profundus distally and reduces tension on the flexor digitorum profundus at the distal interphalangeal joint, so that distal interphalangeal joint extension is facilitated.

The abductor digiti quinti, like the first, second, and fourth interossei, has two tendons of insertion. One of these tendons inserts directly onto the bone of the abductor tubercle along the ulnar aspect of the little-finger proximal phalanx, and the other insertion is into the dorsal hood apparatus. The flexor digiti quinti inserts onto the ulnar tubercle at the base of the proximal phalanx but does not insert into the dorsal hood apparatus. The primary function of the flexor digiti quinti is flexion of the metacarpophalangeal joint.

D. DORSAL HOOD APPARATUS

The dorsal hood apparatus, frequently referred to as the extensor mechanism, is the confluence of intrinsic and extrinsic tendon insertions on the dorsal aspect of the finger (see Figure 10–10). Through dorsal hood attachments, the extrinsic extensor muscles extend the metacarpophalangeal joint, the intrinsic muscles flex the metacarpophalangeal joint, and both the intrinsic and extrinsic muscles extend the proximal and distal interphalangeal joints.

Extension of the metacarpophalangeal joint is achieved through the action of the extrinsic extensor tendons pulling through the sagittal band sling mechanism, which lifts up the proximal phalanx. Flexion of the metacarpophalangeal joint is achieved both by the tendinous insertion of the intrinsics on the proximal phalanx and by a similar sling effect with oblique fibers of the intrinsic mechanism blending into the hood and converging at the level of the central slip to create a sling, which flexes the metacarpophalangeal joint. Additionally, the flexor digitorum profundus and superficialis secondarily flex the metacarpophalangeal joint.

Extension of the proximal interphalangeal joint is achieved through the action of the central slip, which is the bony insertion of the extrinsic digital extensors on the middle phalanx. In addition, the intrinsic muscles contribute to proximal interphalangeal joint extension through medial slips from the lateral band, which run centrally to insert on the proximal dorsal aspect of the middle phalanx as part of the central slip.

Distal interphalangeal joint extension is achieved through both intrinsic and extrinsic forces pulling through the radial and ulnar conjoined lateral bands, which merge to form the terminal tendon insertion.

The intrinsic contribution to the conjoined lateral band is through its insertion into the lateral band. The extrinsic contribution to distal interphalangeal joint extension occurs through lateral slip fibers that diverge from the central slip over the dorsum of the proximal phalanx and join the lateral band to form the conjoined lateral band. The conjoined lateral bands from the radial and ulnar side converge distally as the terminal tendon inserting on the distal phalanx.

DISRUPTION OF EXTENSOR MUSCLE INSERTIONS

1. Sagittal Band Disruption

Anatomy & Clinical Findings

The sagittal band fibers transmitting extrinsic extensor power may be disrupted by laceration or, more often, may become attenuated because of underlying synovitis of the metacarpophalangeal joint, as occurs in rheumatoid arthritis. When the sagittal band fibers along either the radial or ulnar aspect of the dorsal hood become attenuated, the extensor tendon may sublux into the valley between the adjacent metacarpal heads. Because the subluxed extrinsic extensors are mechanically less effective at extending the metacarpophalangeal joint, full active extension of this joint may be lost. This phenomenon occurs commonly in rheumatoid arthritis. It also may result from tearing of the sagittal band fibers with torquing activity such as occurs in the middle finger with pitching a baseball.

Treatment

An acute tear of the radial sagittal band may be treated by splinting. If this is ineffective, surgical repair may be indicated. Chronic injuries are treated by releasing the ulnar sagittal band and recentralizing the extensor tendon by placing a strip of the tendon around the radial collateral ligament.

2. Boutonnière Deformity

Anatomy & Clinical Findings

When the central slip is disrupted because of laceration, closed rupture, or elongation secondary to synovitis of the proximal interphalangeal joint, the direct bony insertion of the extrinsic extensors on the middle phalanx is lost. When the insertion of the medial slips from the lateral band is also lost, active proximal interphalangeal joint extension will be lacking. The finger will rapidly be drawn into a position of proximal interphalangeal joint flexion as the unopposed motion of the flexor dig-

itorum sublimis and profundus draws the finger into flexion (Figure 10–11). The lateral bands migrate apart as the finger is flexed and are drawn into a progressively more palmar position, eventually coming to lie palmar to the axis of flexion of the joint. In the subluxed position, the lateral bands become a deforming force contributing to the tendency of the finger to flex at the proximal interphalangeal joint.

With central slip disruption, the force normally transmitted through the central slip to the middle phalanx from both extrinsic extensor and intrinsic muscles bypasses the proximal interphalangeal joint and is refocused on the distal interphalangeal joint, amplifying the force of extension of this joint and hyperextending it. Because the distal interphalangeal joint is relatively resistant to active flexion, contraction of the flexor digitorum profundus muscle primarily flexes the proximal interphalangeal joint and is relatively ineffective in flexing the distal interphalangeal joint, unless the proximal interphalangeal joint is supported in maximal extension. The digit rapidly assumes the boutonnière deformity posture of proximal interphalangeal joint flexion and distal interphalangeal joint hyperextension.

Treatment

Because the proximal interphalangeal joint is at the center of the complex balance of the intrinsic and extrinsic forces, restoration of proper balance and tension on the central slip may be technically difficult. When the central slip is acutely lacerated, it should be directly repaired and the joint pinned in full extension for 3–6 weeks to protect the integrity of the repair. Closed ruptures of the central slip, if diagnosed acutely, should be treated with 6 weeks of splinting of the proximal interphalangeal joint in full extension. When diagnosis is delayed even a few weeks, a fixed flexion contracture of the proximal interphalangeal joint is usual.

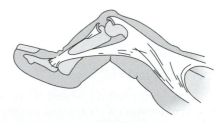

Figure 10–11.   Boutonnière deformity caused by loss of active proximal interphalangeal extension secondary to loss of the central slip insertion on the proximal dorsal middle phalanx. (Reproduced, with permission, from Way LW, ed: *Current Surgical Diagnosis & Treatment,* 10th ed. Stamford: Appleton & Lange, 1994.)

Surgical treatment of closed rupture of the central slip in a finger that has developed a fixed flexion contracture is frequently disappointing because the surgical procedure must both release the contracture on the palmar aspect of the joint and augment proximal interphalangeal joint extension on the dorsal aspect. A better strategy employs prolonged splinting to diminish the extent of the fixed proximal interphalangeal joint flexion contracture. Among the variety of splints available for this, the Capener splint and the Joint Jack splint are particularly useful. Serial casting of the finger with a circumferential digital cast that is changed every few days may also be helpful in bringing the proximal interphalangeal joint into extension. During the period of splinting, the patient should be instructed to carry out active flexion of the distal interphalangeal joint, with the middle phalanx supported in extension. Care should be taken that splints and casts are fashioned to allow and encourage distal interphalangeal joint flexion. Once full proximal interphalangeal joint extension is achieved, splinting should be continued on a full-time basis for an additional 6–12 weeks. In many instances, this will achieve sufficient tightening of the central slip to permit satisfactory active proximal interphalangeal joint extension.

If active extension cannot be restored with prolonged splinting, several operative interventions may be considered. The first, a Fowler type of tenotomy, obliquely divides the dorsal hood apparatus over the middle phalanx, proximal to the terminal tendon insertion. This diminishes distal interphalangeal joint hyperextension and may improve active proximal interphalangeal joint extension by refocusing intrinsic and extrinsic forces at the more proximal joint.

Alternatively, other surgical techniques attempt to more directly augment proximal interphalangeal joint extension, either by shortening the central slip or by mobilizing portions of one or both lateral bands. Though such techniques may increase active extension of the joint, they often do so at the loss of full proximal interphalangeal joint flexion.

3. Mallet Finger

Anatomy & Clinical Findings

Mallet finger deformity reflects the loss of normal extensor force transmission via the terminal tendon insertion onto the distal phalanx. The unopposed flexor digitorum profundus pulls the distal joint into flexion (Figure 10–12). The usual mechanism of injury involves sudden passive flexion of the actively extended distal interphalangeal joint. Disruption of the terminal tendon may be entirely confined to the tendon or may

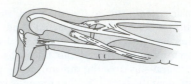

Figure 10–12. Mallet finger deformity is secondary to loss of terminal tendon insertion on the distal phalanx. (Reproduced, with permission, from Way LW, ed: *Current Surgical Diagnosis & Treatment,* 10th ed. Stamford: Appleton & Lange, 1994.)

involve an avulsed fracture fragment from the dorsal lip of the distal phalanx proximal articular surface.

Because the avulsed fragment includes the terminal tendon insertion, the clinical appearance of soft tissue and bony mallet fingers will be similar. The distal joint will rest in flexion, a posture that cannot be actively changed. Full passive extension of the distal interphalangeal joint will be possible.

Treatment

A radiograph should be obtained to determine whether a fracture is present and, more importantly, whether subluxation of the joint has occurred. If the joint is without subluxation, splinting is recommended even if a small fracture site gap remains in the articular surface. The distal interphalangeal joint should be splinted in extension continuously for 8 weeks, and the finger may then be tested. If residual drooping of the distal joint is noted, an additional 2–4 weeks of splinting is required.

INTRINSIC PLUS & INTRINSIC MINUS POSITIONS

Together, the interossei and lumbricals flex the metacarpophalangeal joints and extend the proximal and distal interphalangeal joints. Hence, the posture of the hand in which the metacarpophalangeal joints are flexed and the proximal and distal interphalangeal joints are extended is known as the **intrinsic plus position** (Figure 10–13). This is an ideal position for splinting the hand because the collateral ligaments of the metacarpophalangeal and interphalangeal joint are fully stretched. It has been termed the **position of safety,** or **position of advantage,** for immobilization of the hand.

The normal excursion of the intrinsic muscles is sufficient to allow simultaneous passive positioning of the metacarpophalangeal joints in extension while the prox-

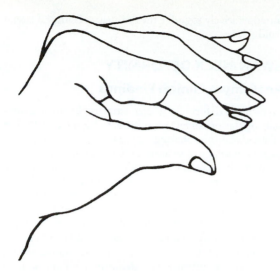

Figure 10–13. Intrinsic plus position.

imal and distal interphalangeal joints are flexed. This posture, known as the **intrinsic minus position,** requires full relaxation of the intrinsic muscles (see Figure 10–13, Figure 10–14). When the intrinsic muscles are paralyzed, the hand tends to assume this same posture (clawhand). Although the extrinsic extensors have fibers that ultimately provide proximal and distal interphalangeal joint extension, their excursion is expended in unopposed metacarpophalangeal joint hyperextension. Thus, the hand devoid of intrinsic power is unable to achieve active extension of the proximal and distal interphalangeal joints, unless the metacarpophalangeal joint is flexed by other means.

Treatment

Surgical correction of the intrinsic minus hand must either prevent hyperextension of the metacarpophalangeal joint passively or restore active control of metacarpophalangeal joint flexion. This may be achieved either by tenodesis or capsulodesis across the metacarpophalangeal joint or by an active tendon transfer. Once control of the joint has been restored, extrinsic extensors usually can effectively open the hand at the proximal and distal interphalangeal joints. If active proximal interphalangeal joint extension is not possible through the extrinsic extensors when the metacarpophalangeal joint is flexed, then tendon transfer for metacarpophalangeal joint flexion should be inserted into the digital lateral bands. This augments proximal interphalangeal joint extension and provides metacarpophalangeal joint flexion.

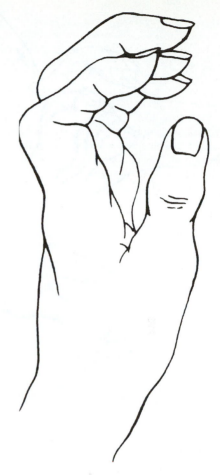

Figure 10–14. Intrinsic minus position secondary to low median and ulnar nerve palsies.

INTRINSIC MUSCLE TIGHTNESS
Anatomy & Clinical Findings

When the lumbricals and interossei become contracted and overly tight, the limitation of their excursion will not permit full simultaneous metacarpophalangeal joint extension and interphalangeal joint flexion. The **intrinsic tightness test** was originally described by Finochietto and later by Bunnell (Figure 10–15). It is accomplished by first determining that the metacarpophalangeal and interphalangeal joints each have a full range of passive joint motion in a reduced position. The metacarpophalangeal joint is then passively held in an extended position while the examiner attempts to passively flex the proximal and distal interphalangeal joints. If full passive flexion of the proximal and distal interphalangeal joints

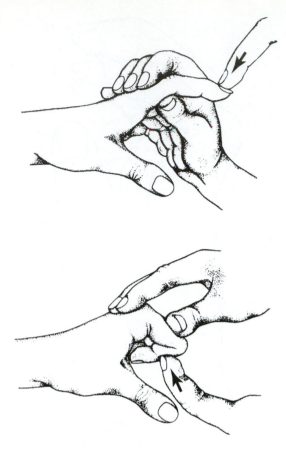

Figure 10–15. Intrinsic tightness test is performed by flexing the proximal interphalangeal joint with the metaphalangeal joint extended and flexed. Tightness to proximal interphalangeal flexion occurs with the metaphalangeal joint extended. (Reproduced, with permission, from Green DP, ed: *Operative Hand Surgery,* 2nd ed. New York: Churchill Livingstone, 1988.)

is not possible in this position, the intrinsic muscles are deemed tight.

Causes of intrinsic muscle tightness include conditions as diverse as rheumatoid arthritis, head injury, and crush injury of the hand.

Treatment

Surgical treatment of intrinsic tightness may be carried out as an isolated procedure or in combination with metacarpophalangeal joint reconstruction. The intrinsic force is diminished either by intrinsic muscle tenotomy or by resection of a triangular segment of one or both lateral bands. The intrinsic tightness test may be used

intraoperatively to judge the adequacy of surgical lateral band release.

SWAN-NECK DEFORMITY

Anatomy & Clinical Findings

Swan-neck deformity is characterized by hyperextension of the proximal interphalangeal joint and flexion of the distal interphalangeal joint (Figure 10–16). The pathophysiology of swan-neck deformity involves either primary or secondary stretching or disruption of the volar plate's restraint on proximal interphalangeal joint extension. Synovitis of the proximal interphalangeal joint secondary to rheumatoid arthritis may distend the joint. This renders the volar plate relatively incompetent to prevent proximal interphalangeal joint hyperextension. Overly forceful intrinsic muscle contraction (as occurs with an intrinsic plus deformity) will transmit an abnormally high force through the central slip, hyperextending the proximal interphalangeal joint. Once this has occurred, the dorsal hood apparatus is relatively ineffective in extending the distal interphalangeal joint, resulting in the posture of distal interphalangeal joint flexion.

In some fingers, a fixed extension contracture or ankylosis of the proximal interphalangeal joint may occur as a consequence of swan-neck deformity. In other fingers, the proximal interphalangeal joint will remain supple but will rest in a hyperextended posture.

Treatment

Surgical treatment of swan-neck deformity secondary to intrinsic tightness requires diminishing intrinsic muscle

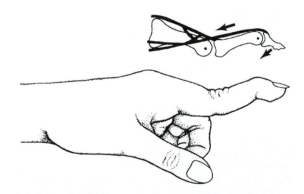

Figure 10–16. Swan-neck deformity. (Reproduced, with permission, from American Society for Surgery of the Hand: *The Hand: Examination and Diagnosis,* 2nd ed. New York: Churchill Livingstone, 1983.)

force, usually through resection of a triangle of the proximal lateral band and dorsal hood. A new "check-rein" to proximal interphalangeal joint extension is created, either through tenodesis of one slip of the flexor digitorum superficialis or tenodesis in which one of the lateral bands is rerouted volar to the center of rotation of the proximal interphalangeal joint, recreating the sagittal oblique retinacular ligament.

Riordan, DC, Harris C Jr: Intrinsic contracture in the hand and its surgical treatment. J Bone Joint Surg Am 1954; 36:10.

Smith RJ: Intrinsic contracture. In Green DP, ed: *Operative Hand Surgery*. New York: Churchill Livingstone, 1988.

■ DISORDERS OF THE TENDONS OF THE HAND

FLEXOR TENDON INJURY

Anatomy

The extrinsic flexors of the finger consist of the flexor digitorum profundus and the flexor digitorum superficialis. The flexor digitorum profundus originates from the proximal ulna and the interosseous membrane. In the forearm, it divides into two muscle groups, the most radial component supplying the index finger and the ulnar component supplying the middle, ring, and little fingers. The flexor digitorum profundus and the flexor pollicis longus muscles form the deep compartment of the volar forearm. As the flexor digitorum profundus and flexor pollicis longus tendons travel through the carpal tunnel, they occupy the floor of the carpal tunnel.

The tenosynovial sheath of the flexor pollicis longus is continuous with the radial bursa, and the tenosynovial sheath to the little finger is continuous with the ulnar digital bursa. In some patients, these two bursae communicate, allowing a so-called **horseshoe abscess** to spread between the thumb and little finger if infection occurs in the flexor tendon sheath of either one of these digits.

The lumbricals originate from the radial side of the index, middle, ring, and little fingers in the palm. The profundus tendon passes through the bifurcation of the flexor digitorum superficialis before inserting into the proximal palmar base of the distal phalanx. The innervation of the flexor digitorum profundus of the index and middle fingers is through the anterior interosseous branch of the median nerve, whereas the profundus of the ring and little fingers is innervated by

the ulnar nerve. The profundus provides digital flexion at both the proximal and distal interphalangeal joints.

The flexor digitorum superficialis has two heads: the radial head originates from the proximal shaft of the radius and the humeral ulnar head from the medial humeral epicondyle and coronoid process of the ulna. Each digit has a corresponding independent superficialis muscle. As the superficialis tendons pass through the carpal tunnel, the tendons of the middle and ring fingers are more superficial and central than those of the index and little fingers. In the proximal aspect of the finger, the flexor digitorum superficialis tendon bifurcates around the flexor digitorum profundus at the beginning of the A_2 pulley. The flexor digitorum superficialis tendon slips then reunite distally at Camper's chiasm, with about half of the fibers staying on the ipsilateral side and half crossing to the contralateral side of the finger. The tendon then inserts via radial and ulnar slips into the proximal metaphysis of the middle phalanx. The entire flexor digitorum superficialis muscle receives innervation from the median nerve. The primary function of the superficialis is digital flexion at the proximal interphalangeal joint.

The flexor pollicis longus originates from two heads: The radial head takes origin from the proximal radius and interosseous membrane, and an accessory head originates from the coronoid process of the ulna and from the medial epicondyle of the humerus. In the palm, the flexor pollicis longus tendon transverses between the abductor pollicis and the flexor pollicis brevis. The flexor pollicis longus inserts into the proximal base of the distal phalanx and is innervated by the anterior interosseous branch of the median nerve. The flexor pollicis longus flexes both the interphalangeal and metacarpophalangeal joints of the thumb.

As the flexor tendons pass distal to the metacarpal neck, they enter the fibro-osseous tunnel, or digital flexor sheath. The fibro-osseous tunnel extends distally to the proximal aspect of the distal phalanx. The tendinous sheath consists of annular pulleys, which provide mechanical stability, and cruciate pulleys, which provide flexibility (Figure 10–17). The first, third, and fifth annular pulleys (A_1, A_3, and A_5) are located over the metacarpophalangeal, proximal interphalangeal, and distal interphalangeal joints, respectively, and the second and fourth pulleys (A_2 and A_4) are situated over the middle portion of the proximal and middle phalanges. The A_2 and A_4 pulleys are the most important in maintaining the mechanical advantage of the flexor tendons.

The tenosynovium which lines the fibro-osseous tunnel supplies both nutrition and lubrication to the poorly vascularized flexor tendons. Proximal to the sheath, the tendons are well vascularized by the peritenon. Within

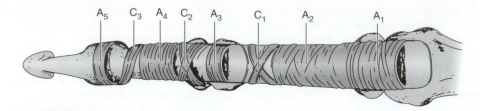

Figure 10–17. Annular (A) and cruciate (C) pulley locations.

the sheath, vascularity is supplied via the vincular system: the vinculum longus and brevis.

Following injury, the flexor tendon heals through both extrinsic and intrinsic mechanisms. Extrinsic healing occurs via cells brought to the site of repair by ingrowth of capillaries and fibroblasts; formation of adhesions follows at the repair site. Intrinsic healing occurs from tendon cells themselves. The goal of flexor tendon repair and postoperative care is to encourage both intrinsic and extrinsic healing without the formation of thick adhesions, which would limit tendon excursion and ultimately result in restricted motion of the finger.

Clinical Findings

The time since injury as well as the mechanism of injury (sharp open injury versus closed avulsion injury) should be noted in the history.

A. NORMAL CASCADE OF FINGERS

The resting posture of the fingers should be observed. Disruption of the normal cascade of increasing flexion in the relaxed fingers as one moves from the index finger to the little finger should arouse suspicion of tendon disruption (Figure 10–18).

B. NORMAL TENODESIS PHENOMENON

Tendon integrity may also be evaluated by taking advantage of the normal tenodesis positioning of the digits, which occurs as the wrist is passively brought through a range of motion and the motion of the fingers is observed. As the wrist is dorsiflexed, the digital extensors relax and the finger flexors become taught, passively flexing the fingers in the normal cascade pattern. When the muscles of the proximal forearm are squeezed, the fingers normally flex involuntarily.

C. TESTING OF INDIVIDUAL TENDONS

Isolated testing of the superficialis and profundus tendons is employed to determine the integrity of each tendon (see Figures 10–2 and 10–3). Note that the flexor digitorum superficialis of the little finger is not

independent of the ring finger in many individuals, either because of cross-connections between the two tendons or because of congenital absence of the tendon. The strength of flexion should be noted as each of the tendons is tested. If the patient is able to flex the finger but experiences pain with flexion and is unable to generate full power against resistance, a partial flexor tendon injury should be suspected.

Treatment

Functional outcomes are equivalent if the repair is done the day of injury (primary repair) or within the first 7–10 days after the injury (delayed primary repair).

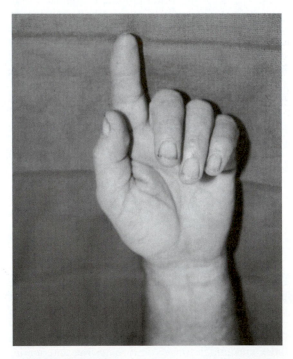

Figure 10–18. If the index finger remains extended when the hand is at rest, its flexor tendons have been severed.

Because repair requires proper visualization of both ends of the tendon, the wound may need to be electively extended. The tendon ends must be gently retrieved, because trauma to the flexor tendon sheath will create adverse scarring. Tendons should not be grasped along their tenosynovial surfaces. The A_2 and A_4 pulleys should be preserved. A maximum of 1 cm may be debrided from the tendons before compromising digital extension. A core suture of either 3-0 or 4-0 braided synthetic material is secured to coapt tendon ends (Figure 10–19). The flexor tendon repair is strengthened by employing four to six strands of suture across the repair site rather than two. A running 6-0 nylon epitendinous suture completes the tendon repair. The role of flexor tendon sheath repair remains controversial.

Because the results and complications of flexor tendon repair vary by level of injury, five zones of injury have been defined (Figure 10–20). Zone I extends from the insertion of the profundus on the distal phalanx to the insertion of the flexor digitorum superficialis on the middle phalanx. The tendon may be directly repaired if the distal stump is large enough, or it may be reinserted to bone. Care must be taken not to advance the tendon more than 1 cm.

Zone II, which extends from the proximal portion of the A_1 pulley to the insertion of the superficialis tendon, contains both the profundus and superficialis tendons in a relatively avascular region. Care must be taken to preserve the vincular blood supply. When both the superficialis and profundus tendons are divided, it is preferable to repair both tendons because greater digital independence of motion may be achieved with a somewhat lower risk of tendon rupture during the rehabilitation period. Repair of the superficialis tendon as well as the profundus tendon also diminishes the likelihood of proximal interphalangeal joint hyperextension deformity.

Zone III injuries are between the proximal edge of the A_1 pulley and the distal edge of the transverse carpal ligament.

In zone IV, the area beneath the transverse carpal ligament, a step-cut release and repair of the transverse

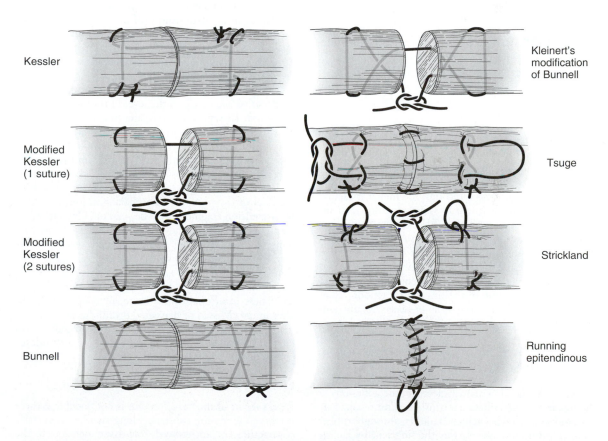

Figure 10–19. Kessler sutures and other types of sutures for flexor tendon repair. (Reproduced, with permission, from Green DP, ed: *Operative Hand Surgery,* 2nd ed. New York: Churchill Livingstone, 1988.)

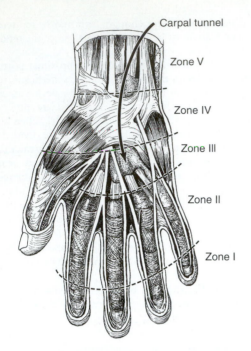

Figure 10–20. Flexor tendon injury zones. (Modified and reproduced, with permission, from Way LW, ed: *Current Surgical Diagnosis & Treatment,* 10th ed. Stamford: Appleton & Lange, 1994.)

carpal ligament should be performed to prevent flexor tendon bowstringing.

Zone I and II injuries of the thumb are handled similarly to those of analogous finger zones. In zone III of the thumb, it is difficult to access the flexor pollicis longus tendon as it passes through the thenar musculature. Options for treatment of injuries at this level include either primary tendon grafting or step-cut lengthening of the tendon in the forearm, so that the repair is distal to the obscuring thenar muscles.

Improved results of flexor tendon surgery in recent years reflect the evolution of postoperative therapy programs. Immobilization of the finger after tendon repair is appropriate only in very young or otherwise uncooperative patients. The wrist should be immobilized at approximately 30 degrees of flexion, the metacarpophalangeal joints at approximately 45 degrees of flexion, and the interphalangeal joints at 0–15 degrees of flexion. A program of passive range-of-motion exercises should be initiated. This will decrease the adhesions at the repair site and enhance intrinsic tendon repair. Passive motion may be achieved either through rubber band splinting to passively flex the finger or by having the patient passively move the finger. At 4–6 weeks following repair, active flexion and extension exercises are

allowed as splinting is discontinued. At 6–8 weeks, passive extension exercises and isolated blocking is encouraged. After 8 weeks, the patient may begin flexion against resistance.

When a four- or six-strand repair is performed, active assisted motion is begun within the first 2 weeks. In this program, the wrist is extended and the fingers are passively flexed. The patient is then asked to actively flex the fingers to hold this position.

With four- and six-strand techniques for flexor tendon repair, active motion can begin earlier than with a two-strand repair. In properly motivated and cooperative patients, an active hold program is begun within the first week. The therapist passively brings the hand into flexion and the patient is asked to maintain the position. Results for this surgical and postoperative program appear superior.

Flexor Tendon Avulsion Injuries

The flexor tendon may be avulsed from its bony insertion, usually by forced extension of the finger while the finger is simultaneously actively flexed. Seventy-five percent of flexor digitorum profundus avulsion injuries involve the ring finger. Such injuries commonly occur in football or rugby, when the athlete grabs an opponent's jersey and a finger is involuntarily extended as the opponent attempts to elude tackle.

Flexor digitorum profundus avulsion injuries may be classified according to the level of profundus tendon retraction. In type 1 injuries, the tendon has retracted proximally from the sheath into the palm. Repair of these injuries should be performed within 10 days to avoid myostatic contracture, which will limit the ability to bring the tendon to its normal insertion without undue tension. In type 2 injuries, the tendon retracts to the level of the proximal interphalangeal joint. A small bony avulsion fragment may be seen on a lateral radiograph of the finger in these injuries. The tendon may be reinserted into the distal phalanx up to 6 weeks after injury. Type 3 injuries involve a distal phalangeal avulsion fragment that is so large that it blocks retraction of the flexor digitorum profundus proximal to the A_4 pulley. These injuries also may be repaired up to 6 weeks after injury. Missed or neglected profundus avulsion injuries, if symptomatic, may be treated by staged tendon reconstruction, distal interphalangeal joint arthrodesis, or tenodesis.

Flexor Tendon Reconstruction

Direct repair of the flexor tendon is not possible if there is loss of the tendon substance, long-standing myostatic contracture, or unresolved soft-tissue defects. If the flexor digitorum superficialis tendon is present with a full active range of proximal interphalangeal joint motion, arthrodesis or tenodesis of the distal interphalangeal joint, creating a "superficialis finger," may be elected. If the patient requires active motion at the distal interphalangeal joint, then tendon grafting will be required. Tendon grafting is usually indicated when both flexor digitorum superficialis and flexor digitorum profundus tendons cannot be repaired.

Primary tendon grafting may be performed when there is satisfactory skin coverage, full passive range of metacarpophalangeal and interphalangeal joint motion, an intact annular pulley system, minimal scarring in the sheath, adequate digital circulation, and at least one intact digital nerve. Possible donor tendon sources include the palmaris longus, plantaris, or toe extensor tendons. The palmaris longus and plantaris tendons are absent in a significant minority of individuals.

A. Surgical Procedure

The donor tendon graft is secured into the distal phalanx. Proximal attachment of the donor tendon to the profundus motor is performed either with a tendon weave or an end-to-end repair. Establishing appropriate tension on the tendon graft is critical. If insufficient tension is placed, a lumbrical plus deformity will occur, reflecting proximal displacement of the lumbrical origin. With this deformity, as the patient pulls the proximal profundus tendon proximally, the lumbrical is placed under tension, and this tension is transmitted to the dorsal hood apparatus, so that the finger will paradoxically extend both the proximal and distal interphalangeal joints. If the tendon graft tension is too tight, then full extension will be impossible. The results of primary tendon grafting are inferior to primary repair in identical circumstances.

Primary tendon repair is contraindicated if the fibro-osseous sheath is extensively scarred or if critical pulleys are absent. Restoration of flexion in such situations will require a staged tendon reconstruction. In stage 1, the tendon remnants are excised from the sheath and joint contractures are released. The A_2 and A_4 pulleys are reconstructed using either a flexor tendon remnant or a strip of the wrist extensor retinaculum. A silicone rod similar in size to the anticipated tendon graft is secured to the distal phalanx and passed within the sheath. Early passive range-of-motion stimulates the development of a pseudosheath surrounding the silicone tendon rod.

The second stage of the procedure occurs at least 3 months after the initial procedure. Full digital passive range of motion and soft-tissue equilibrium must be achieved before the second stage is undertaken. The silicone tendon rod is replaced with a tendon graft. The donor tendon is secured to the distal phalanx and to the donor motor in a manner similar to primary tendon grafting.

B. Complications

1. Adhesions—The most common complication following flexor tendon surgery is formation of adhesions, which may occur in spite of an appropriate therapy program. Tenolysis should be considered when active flexion is restricted despite a normal passive range of motion, in a wound that has reached soft-tissue equilibrium (usually at least 3 months since repair), in a motivated patient.

Ideally, tenolysis should be performed under local anesthesia with intravenous sedation. Elevation of skin flaps allows wide exposure of the sheath. Care is taken to preserve the annular pulleys while adhesions are released between the tendon and the sheath and between the tendon and the phalanges. Evaluation of the adequacy of lysis may be obtained by asking the patient under local anesthesia to actively flex the finger. If regional or general anesthesia is employed, the tendon must be identified at a more proximal level and traction applied to the tendon at this level to confirm the improvement in joint motion.

Active range-of-motion exercise is begun within the first 24 h after surgery. Electrical stimulation of the proximal muscle belly may facilitate early motion.

2. Tendon repair rupture—The second major postoperative complication of flexor tendon repair is rupture of the repair. When the rupture is immediately diagnosed, repair should be attempted a second time, as success rates approach those of uncomplicated primary repair. If rupture is not promptly diagnosed, the ruptured tendon ends must be resected, and either free tendon grafting or staged tendon reconstruction will be necessary to restore active flexion.

3. Failure of staged reconstruction—If staged reconstruction has failed, arthrodesis or amputation of the digit may be considered, particularly when neurovascular compromise occurs.

Coyle MP Jr et al: Staged flexor tendon reconstruction fingertip to palm. J Hand Surg [Am] 2002;27(4):581. [PMID: 12132079]

Doyle JR: Anatomy of the finger flexor tendon sheath and pulley system. J Hand Surg Am 1988;13:473.

Hunter JM, Salisbury RE: Flexor tendon reconstruction in severely damaged hands: A two-stage procedure using a silicone-dacron reinforced gliding prosthesis prior to tendon grafting. J Bone Joint Surg Am 1967;53:829.

Lister GD et al: Primary flexor tendon repair followed by immediate controlled mobilization. J Hand Surg (Am) 1977; 2:441.

Smith RJ, Hastings H II: Principles of tendon transfer to the hand. Instr Course Lect 1980;29:129.

Strickland JW: Development of flexor tendon surgery: Twenty-five years of progress. J Hand Surg [Am] 2000;25(2):214. Review. No abstract available. [PMID: 10722813]

Thurman RT et al: Two-, four-, and six-strand zone II flexor tendon repairs: An in situ biomechanical comparison using cadaver model. J Hand Surg Am 1998;23:261.

Whitaker JH et al: The role of flexor tenolysis in the palm and digits. J Hand Surg (Am) 1977;2:462.

TENOSYNOVITIS

Tenosynovitis may develop about any of the extrinsic flexor or extensor tendons, either throughout their course or, more commonly, at points of constraint by bony fibrous pulleys or retinacular sheaths.

1. deQuervain's Tenosynovitis

Clinical Findings

The abductor pollicis longus and extensor pollicis brevis tendons may become inflamed beneath the retinacular pulley at the radial styloid region. Symptoms are provoked by lifting activity in which the thumb is adducted and flexed while the hand is ulnarly deviated. Activities such as inflating a blood pressure cuff, picking up a new baby out of a crib, or lifting a heavy frying pan off the stove may provoke pain along the radial aspect of the wrist.

The Finkelstein test may be helpful in diagnosing this disorder (Figure 10–21).

Treatment

Initial treatment includes immobilization with a forearm-based thumb spica splint, which prevents both

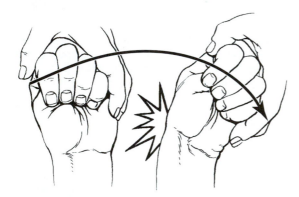

Figure 10–21. Finkelstein maneuver. The patient's thumb is enclosed in the palm. The wrist is then abruptly deviated ulnarward by the examiner. In a positive test, pain is produced on the radial border of the wrist. (Reproduced, with permission, from Lister G: *The Hand: Diagnosis and Indications,* 3rd ed. New York: Churchill Livingstone, 1993.)

wrist deviation and thumb carpometacarpal and metacarpophalangeal joint motion while allowing interphalangeal joint motion. Steroid injection into the first extensor compartment may diminish swelling and pain.

If deQuervain's tenosynovitis is unresponsive to conservative care, surgical release of the overlying retinaculum may be elected. Because most patients with symptomatic disease have more than one abductor pollicis longus slip, it is essential that the extensor pollicis brevis tendon be identified and decompressed. In some cases, the first extensor compartment is divided by a septum, creating two separate tendon sheaths. In such cases, each of the component sheaths must be opened to allow unconstrained tendon gliding.

Injury to the sensory branch of the radial nerve as it runs over the first compartment is a troublesome complication that may overshadow any benefit from tendon decompression. Extreme caution must be exercised in carrying out the skin incision and subcutaneous dissection in this region.

2. Flexor Tenosynovitis (Trigger Finger & Trigger Thumb)

Clinical Findings

Flexor tenosynovitis or tenovaginitis is characterized by pain and tenderness in the palm at the proximal edge of the A_1 pulley (Figure 10–22). Patients frequently note catching or triggering of the affected finger or thumb after forceful flexion. In some instances, the opposite hand must be used to passively bring the finger or thumb into extension. In more severe cases, the finger may become locked in a flexed position. Triggering is often more pronounced in the morning than later in the day. Stenosing tenosynovitis is particularly common in diabetic patients. When multiple digits are involved, the possibility of diabetes should be considered in previously undiagnosed patients.

Treatment

Most triggering digits may be successfully treated by long-acting steroid injection into the flexor sheath. To inject a trigger finger, the needle is inserted at the proximal palmar crease for the index finger and the distal palmar crease for the middle, ring, and small fingers. The needle enters the flexor tendon and pressure is applied to the plunger. The needle is slowly backed out until the needle is between the tendon and the tendon sheath, discerned by loss of plunger resistance. One milliliter of a combination of a short-acting anesthetic and steroid are given. The injection may be repeated if symptoms recur after an initially positive response to injection.

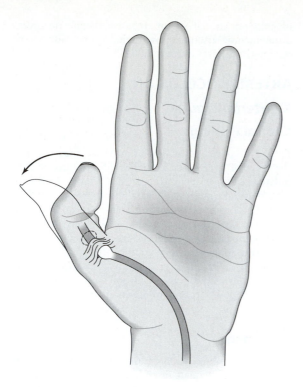

Figure 10–22. Trigger thumb. (Reproduced, with permission, from American Society for Surgery of the Hand: *The Hand: Examination and Diagnosis,* 2nd ed. New York: Churchill Livingstone, 1983.)

Surgical release of the A$_1$ pulley is recommended in digits refractory to steroid injection. Release is accomplished by directly exposing the pulley and longitudinally incising its transversely oriented fibers. The fibers of the A$_2$ pulley must be spared to preserve effective digital flexion. Percutaneous release of the A$_1$ pulley may be done on the middle and ring fingers, especially if they actively lock. In patients with rheumatoid arthritis, the entire annular pulley system should be preserved to prevent further ulnar drift of the fingers. Triggering in these patients is treated by tenosynovectomy and excision of one slip of the flexor digitorum superficialis.

3. Flexor Carpi Radialis Tenosynovitis

Clinical Findings

Flexor carpi radialis tenosynovitis is characterized by pain with wrist motion, particularly active wrist flexion or passive wrist dorsiflexion. Marked tenderness is experienced on palpation of the skin overlying the tendon, particularly over the trapezium.

Treatment

Conservative care includes splinting the wrist in flexion and administration of oral anti-inflammatory medication. If these measures are ineffective, a long-acting steroid may be injected about the tendon at the trapezial level.

Surgical decompression of the flexor carpi radialis is considered if conservative measures are ineffective. Decompression unroofs the tendon sheath in the distal forearm and across the wrist. The fibro-osseous sheath is further decompressed by resection of the palmar ulnar ridge of the trapezium overlying the tendon.

Benson LS, Ptaszek AJ: Injection versus surgery in the treatment of trigger finger. J Hand Surg Am 1997;22:138.

Wilhelmi BJ et al: Trigger finger release with hand surface landmark ratios: An anatomic and clinical study. Plast Reconstr Surg 2001;108(4):908. [PMID: 11547146]

Zingas C et al: Injection accuracy and clinical relief of deQuervain's tendinitis. J Hand Surg Am 1998;22:89.

■ VASCULAR DISORDERS OF THE HAND

Anatomy

The blood supply to the hand comes predominantly through the ulnar and radial arteries. The ulnar artery is larger than the radial artery and provides the primary arterial contribution to the hand. In most hands, the ulnar artery supplies the superficial palmar arch, which provides the principal blood supply to the common and proper digital arteries. The radial artery enters the hand by passing deep to the tendons of the first dorsal compartment over the anatomic snuffbox, dives palmarward between the bases of the first and second metacarpals, and forms the deep palmar arch. The median artery, a remnant of the embryologic vascular supply to the developing upper limb, contributes to the superficial palmar arch in 10% of patients.

The superficial palmar arch is distal to the deep palmar arch. The arterial arch is complete, with total communication between the radial and ulnar arteries, in 34% of hands and incomplete in 20%. The remainder have limited communication between the ulnar and radial arteries in varied configurations. The deep palmar arch runs alongside the motor branch of the ulnar nerve as it travels transversely just palmar to the proximal metacarpal shafts. The princeps pollicis artery is derived from the deep palmar arch in 98% of patients. The deep palmar arch also supplies the deep metacarpal arterial branches, which provide secondary blood flow to the digital arteries.

Clinical Findings

Patients with vascular insufficiency frequently complain of cold intolerance. When color changes occur, paleness or whiteness of the fingers is more suggestive of loss of inflow, whereas redness or bluish discoloration suggests inadequate venous return. Ulcerations of the tips of the fingers may denote ischemia.

The duration of vascular symptoms should be noted. If the abnormality is congenital in origin, changes in symptoms over time should be documented. The occupational history should record whether the patient uses vibrating tools or is subjected to repetitive blunt hand trauma during work. Occupations requiring outdoor work in all seasons (construction) or in a cold environment indoors (butchers) are noted. A history of trauma may suggest arterial or periarterial damage. Any sports activities that involve repeated trauma to the hand should be recorded; golfers, baseball catchers, and handball players are particularly at risk of closed vascular injury. Exposure to vasoconstrictive drugs, and particularly tobacco, should be noted. Other evidence of vascular disease should be sought, as well as diseases with vascular effects such as scleroderma or diabetes. Pulses are palpated, noting thrills or bruits.

A. ALLEN'S TEST

Allen's test allows assessment of the extent of connection between the radial and ulnar arteries through the palmar arches. The examiner compresses both the radial and ulnar arteries at the wrist and then asks the patient to repetitively flex and extend the fingers. After the hand blanches, pressure is released from the radial artery while compression is maintained on the ulnar artery. The examiner observes how long it takes for each of the fingers to regain its pink color. The initial step is repeated with both vessels compressed, and the ulnar artery occlusion is then released while pressure is maintained on the radial artery. Again, examination of the reperfusion of the fingers reveals which digits are primarily supplied through the ulnar artery. In this fashion, the extent of interconnections between the radial and ulnar arteries may be assessed.

B. DIAGNOSTIC STUDIES

Noninvasive vascular diagnostic studies include Doppler scans, which detect the presence of flow; plethysmography, which determines the pulse volume difference between brachial and digital arteries; and cold stress testing, a technique that evaluates the effect of cold on arterial spasm. Invasive diagnostic procedures include arteriography, digital subtraction arteriography, and early-phase radionuclide scans.

ARTERIAL OCCLUSION

1. Arterial Trauma

Clinical Findings

Partial or complete division of an artery may occur as the result of lacerations, acute injection trauma, or cannulation injuries. Hemorrhage from arterial disruption should initially be treated with direct pressure. Total arterial division must be repaired if distal vascularity is inadequate. Partial arterial injuries may bleed profusely because the lacerated vessel ends are tethered to one another and are unable to retract, constrict, and occlude further flow. Partial arterial injury may require resection with or without reconstruction to prevent the formation of aneurysms or arteriovenous fistulas. Injection injury may produce either spasm or occlusion.

Treatment

The primary objective in treating arterial injuries is the restoration of adequate distal blood flow. Attempts may be made to remove distal clots with Fogarty catheters. If this is unsuccessful, clot-dissolving agents such as urokinase, direct or systemic vasodilators, and stellate ganglion blocks may be employed to diminish vascular spasm. Care must be taken when using multiple agents to ensure that they do not interfere with one another. For instance, use of urokinase after an axillary block may produce axillary artery hemorrhage, thereby compounding the problem.

2. Thrombosis

Clinical Findings

The ulnar artery is the most common site of upper extremity arterial thrombosis. This entity, also known as **ulnar hammer syndrome,** is most often the result of repetitive trauma to the hypothenar area of the hand. Patients may complain of a tender pulsatile mass on the ulnar side of the palm. In some instances, presenting symptoms will reflect a low ulnar nerve palsy secondary to compression of the ulnar nerve by the aneurysm at the level of Guyon's canal. Distal vascular insufficiency may be evident in the ring and little fingers.

Treatment

If evaluation demonstrates that all the fingers are well perfused by the radial artery alone, excision of the segment of the ulnar artery containing the aneurysm or thrombosed segment and ligation of the vessel ends will be curative. Division of the vessel may confer a modest sympathectomy effect to the residual ulnar vessel because sympathetic fibers running with the ulnar artery are divided at the time of vessel division. If, however, digital perfusion is inadequate after a vessel segment has been resected and the tourniquet deflated, then vein grafting will be required to reconstruct the ulnar artery.

3. Aneurysm

A distinction should be made between true and false aneurysms. In a true aneurysm, all layers of the arterial wall are involved. These aneurysms are usually caused by blunt trauma but may also be secondary to degeneration or infection. False aneurysms are characterized by partial wall involvement, with periarterial tissues forming a false wall lined by endothelium. False aneurysms are most common following penetrating trauma such as stab wounds.

Both true and false aneurysms should be treated with resection. As mentioned in the immediately preceding section, the necessity of vascular reconstruction is dictated by the adequacy of distal perfusion after tourniquet release.

VASOSPASTIC CONDITIONS

Clinical Findings

Raynaud's phenomenon, Raynaud's disease, and Raynaud's syndrome are often confused. **Raynaud's phenomenon** is a condition in which pallor of the digits occurs with or without cyanosis on exposure to cold. **Raynaud's disease** (primary Raynaud's) is present when Raynaud's phenomenon occurs without another associated or causative disease. Raynaud's disease most commonly occurs in young women and is often bilateral, without demonstrable peripheral arterial occlusion. In severe cases, patients may develop gangrene or atrophic changes limited to the distal digital skin. **Raynaud's syndrome** (secondary Raynaud's) occurs when Raynaud's phenomenon is associated with another disease such as connective tissue disorders (systemic lupus erythematosus), neurologic disorders, arterial occlusive disorders, and blood dyscrasias.

Treatment

All patients with Raynaud's phenomenon experience cyclic episodes of digital pallor alternating with episodes of cyanosis and hyperemia. Treatment includes protection of the hands from cold by the use of gloves or mittens. Patients should be strongly encouraged to cease all cigarette or cigar smoking. Drug treatment attempts to diminish occlusive phenomena.

Alpha-receptor blocking agents, nitroglycerin ointment, nifedipine, and other calcium channel blockers have been demonstrated as effective in decreasing spasm. Digital artery sympathectomy, the surgical stripping of the periarterial tissue of the common digital artery over a short segment at the distal palmar level, may improve circulation to ischemic digits.

Coleman SS, Anson BJ: Arterial patterns in the hand based upon a study of 650 specimens. Surg Gynecol Obstet 1961;113:409.

Ruch DS et al: Arterial reconstruction for radial artery occlusion. J Hand Surg [Am]. 200025(2):282. [PMID: 10722820]

Ruch DS et al: Periarterial sympathectomy in scleroderma patients: Intermediate-term follow-up. J Hand Surg [Am]. 2002;27 (2):258. [PMID: 11901385]

Wilgis EFS: The evaluation and treatment of chronic digital ischemia. Ann Surg 1981;193:6.

■ DISORDERS OF THE NERVES OF THE HAND

PERIPHERAL NERVE INJURY

Anatomy

Peripheral nerves consist of a mixture of myelinated and unmyelinated axons. Motor, sensory, and sympathetic fibers often travel together in a single nerve. Axons are grouped in bundles termed **fascicles,** which are surrounded by perineurium. The fine connective tissue between axons within a fascicle is called **endoneurium.** Fascicles are held together as a nerve by the epineurium. Nerves are considered monofascicular, oligofascicular, or polyfascicular, depending on the number of fascicles. The relationship between fascicles changes along the longitudinal course of the nerve. The degree of fascicular change decreases distally. The mesoneurium, which is the connective tissue surrounding the epineurium, facilitates longitudinal gliding of the nerve.

After a nerve is injured, a number of changes occur. The somatosensory cortex reorganizes so that the area represented by the injured nerve diminishes. The cell body of the lacerated axon increases in size. The production of materials for repair of the cytoskeleton is increased, and the production of neurotransmitters decreases. At the proximal segment of the injured axon, further proximal degeneration occurs based on the severity of the injury. In the axon distal to the laceration, Schwann cells phagocytose the axon, allowing the surrounding myelin tube to collapse.

Within 24 h of injury, axonal sprouting occurs from the proximal stump. Multiple axons in a fascicle form a regenerating unit. The number of axons in the unit decreases with time. Longitudinal growth of the regenerating nerve is dependent on the ability of the axons to adhere to trophic factors in the basal lamina of the Schwann cell. Changes also occur at the distal end of the nerve. At the motor end-plate, the muscle fibers atrophy. The sensitivity and number of acetylcholine receptors increases as their location expands from pits to the entire length of the muscle fiber. If the muscle fiber is reinnervated, both old and new motor end-plates become active. The recovery of strength is greatest after primary nerve repair, less vigorous after repair with nerve grafting, and weakest after direct implantation of the nerve end into muscle. Muscle reinnervation occurs only if the axon reaches the muscle within a year. In contrast, sensory receptors may be effectively reinnervated years after injury.

Nerve injures are classified into three types. (1) **Neurapraxia** is a conduction block that occurs without axonal disruption. Recovery is usually complete within days to a few months. (2) **Axonotmesis** describes an injury in which axonal disruption occurs, with the endoneurial tube remaining in continuity. The intact endoneurial tube provides the regenerating sprouting axons with a well-defined path to the end organs. Because axonal growth occurs at approximately 1 mm/d, recovery will be good but slow. (3) **Neurotmesis** refers to transection of the nerve. Unless the nerve is repaired, the regenerating axons will not find a suitable path and recovery will not occur. The frustrated sprouting axons will form a neuroma at the distal end of the proximal segment of the lacerated nerve.

Diagnostic Studies

Preoperative and postoperative assessment of motor and sensory function include quantitative measurement of pinch and grip strength, static and moving two-point discrimination, and vibration and pressure measurements. Two-point discrimination will reflect innervation density, whereas vibration and pressure measurements will gauge innervation threshold.

Treatment

Nerve repair should be carried out with magnification and microsurgical technique. A tension-free repair provides the ideal environment for nerve regeneration. Tension at the repair site may be diminished by advancement of the nerve (ie, anterior transposition of the ulnar nerve for proximal forearm ulnar nerve laceration) or by limitation of joint motion. If a tension-free repair is impossible, nerve grafting is necessary to bridge the defect in the nerve. Frequently used donor nerves include the sural nerve, the anterior branch of the me-

dial antebrachial cutaneous nerve, and the lateral antebrachial cutaneous nerve.

Primary repair is preferred to nerve grafting because the latter procedure requires two sites of nerve coaptation. Epineurial repair is usually performed under magnification, using 8-0 or 9-0 suture (Figure 10–23A). When a particular fascicular group (eg, motor branch of the median nerve) is recognized as mediating a specific function, it may be repaired separately (Figure 10–23B). Postoperative therapy may include motor and sensory reeducation to maximize the clinical result.

Primary nerve repair is indicated after a sharp nerve division occurs. After avulsion injuries, repair even by nerve grafting cannot be performed until the proximal and distal extent of injury is known. When closed nerve injury occurs, sensory and motor function is closely monitored. If no recovery is seen within 3 months, electrodiagnostic studies are carried out. If no electrical evidence of recovery is documented, the nerve is explored, and neurolysis, secondary nerve repair, or nerve grafting is accomplished.

COMPRESSIVE NEUROPATHIES

Compressive neuropathies are a group of nerve injuries that have common pathophysiology factors and occur at predictable sites of normal anatomic constraint. Nerve dysfunction is the result of neural ischemia in the compressed segment. Symptoms may resolve after release of the anatomic structures producing pressure on the nerve, particularly when compression has been neither severe nor long-standing.

1. Median Neuropathy

Carpal Tunnel Syndrome

A. ANATOMY

Compression of the median nerve within the carpal tunnel is the most common upper extremity compressive neuropathy. The carpal tunnel is that space along the palmar aspect of the wrist anatomically bounded by the scaphoid tubercle and the trapezium radially, the hook of the hamate and the pisiform ulnarly, and the transverse carpal ligament on the palmar side (Figure 10–24).

B. CLINICAL FINDINGS

Carpal tunnel syndrome is often idiopathic. It has been associated with pregnancy, amyloidosis, flexor tenosynovitis, overuse phenomenon, acute or chronic inflammatory conditions, traumatic disorders of the wrist, endocrine disorders (diabetes mellitus and hypothyroidism), and tumors within the carpal tunnel.

Differential diagnosis includes compression of the median nerve or cervical roots in other anatomic loca-

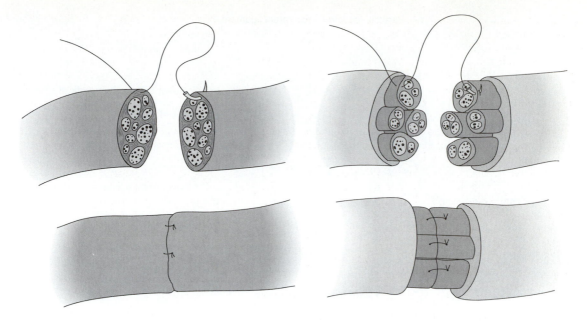

A. Epineurial repair   **B.** Group fascicular repair

Figure 10–23. **A:** Schematic diagram of epineurial repair technique. **B:** Group fascicular repair technique. (Reproduced, with permission, from Mackinnon SE, Dellon AL: *Surgery of the Peripheral Nerve*. Thieme, 1988.)

tions. Diabetic neuropathy may produce symptoms similar to those of carpal tunnel syndrome, and patients with diabetic neuropathy may develop concomitant carpal tunnel syndrome.

1. Symptoms and signs—Most patients complain of numbness in the thumb and index and middle fingers, though many will note that the entire hand feels numb. Pain rarely prevents the affected individual from falling asleep but characteristically awakens the patient from sleep after a number of hours. After a brief period of moving the fingers, most patients are able to return to sleep. Many patients complain of finger stiffness upon arising in the morning.

Discomfort or numbness, or both, may be incited by activities in which the wrist is held in a flexed position for a sustained period of time (eg, holding a steering wheel, telephone receiver, book, or newspaper). Discomfort and pain may radiate from the hand up the arm to the shoulder or neck. The patient may complain of clumsiness when trying to perform tasks such as unscrewing a jar top and may experience difficulty in securely holding onto a glass or cup.

Atrophy of muscles innervated by the median nerve is visible in severe long-standing cases but is uncommon in most cases of recent onset. Weakness of the abductor pollicis brevis muscle may be detected by careful manual muscle testing.

2. Provocative tests—Two provocative tests, Phalen's maneuver and Tinel's sign, are helpful in establishing the diagnosis of carpal tunnel syndrome.

a. Tinel's sign—Tinel's sign is elicited by percussing the skin over the median nerve just proximal to the carpal tunnel; when it is positive, the patient will complain of an electric sensation radiating into the thumb, index, middle, or ring fingers.

b. Phalen's maneuver—Phalen's wrist flexion sign, or Phalen's maneuver, will usually be positive in patients with carpal tunnel syndrome and is thought by many to be even more diagnostic than Tinel's sign. When this maneuver is performed, the elbow should be maintained in extension while the wrist is passively flexed (Figure 10–25). The time is then measured from initiation of wrist flexion to onset of symptoms; onset within 60 s is considered supportive of the diagnosis of carpal tunnel syndrome. Both the time to onset and the location of paresthesias should be recorded.

3. Two-point discrimination test—Two-point discrimination is often diminished in patients with carpal tunnel syndrome. Sensation in the radial aspect of the palm should be normal, however, because the palmar cutaneous branch of the median nerve does not pass through the carpal tunnel.

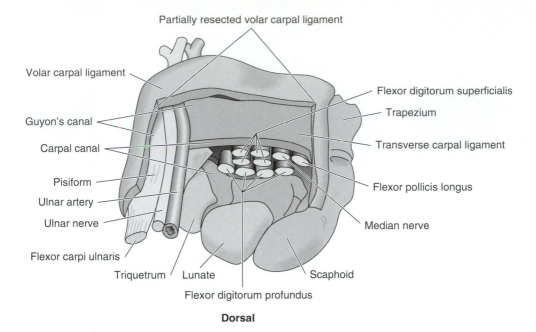

Partially resected volar carpal ligament

Volar carpal ligament

Guyon's canal

Carpal canal

Pisiform

Ulnar artery

Ulnar nerve

Flexor carpi ulnaris

Triquetrum   Lunate

Flexor digitorum profundus

Flexor digitorum superficialis

Trapezium

Transverse carpal ligament

Flexor pollicis longus

Median nerve

Scaphoid

Dorsal

Figure 10–24. Guyon's canal and carpal tunnel and contents. (Cross-section of supinated right wrist, viewed from proximal to distal.) Note the relationship between the transverse carpal ligament and the volar carpal ligament (partially resected). (Reproduced, with permission, from Reckling FW, Reckling JB, Mohn MP: *Orthopaedic Anatomy and Surgical Approaches.* St Louis: Mosby-Year Book, 1990.)

4. Imaging studies—The diagnostic evaluation may include a radiograph of the wrist, including a carpal tunnel view. Electrodiagnostic studies (nerve conduction velocities and electromyography) help localize nerve compression to the wrist and evaluate residual neural and motor integrity. Electromyogram/nerve conduction velocity (EMG/NCV are indicated for patients who have failed conservative care and are considered candidates for surgery. A motor distal latency greater than 3.5–4.0 ms is the best indicator of carpal tunnel syndrome.

C. TREATMENT

1. Conservative measures—Because the pressure within the carpal tunnel increases if the wrist is held in sustained flexion (usual sleep posture) or sustained extension, the initial treatment of carpal tunnel syndrome should include a splint that maintains the wrist in a neutral position at night. Clinical improvement with this simple measure adds further support to the diagnosis of carpal tunnel syndrome. Activities that provoke symptoms may be modified with simple measures such as adjustment of keyboard height and rotation of repetitive job activities.

Injection of steroids into the carpal tunnel will often decrease the inflammatory response around the flexor tendons and diminish symptoms. To inject the carpal tunnel, a 25-gauge, 1½-in. needle is placed at the palmar wrist crease just ulnar to the palmaris longus tendon. If the palmaris longus is absent, a line along the radial border of the ring finger is drawn to the wrist crease. Before placing the needle, patients are told they may experience an electric shock sensation in the fingers. If this sensation occurs, the needle may be in the median nerve, and the injection should not be given. The needle is withdrawn and placed a few millimeters ulnar. When inserting the needle, first the skin is punctured, then a "pop" is felt as the needle passes through the transverse carpal ligament. A mixture of a short-acting anesthetic and steroid is injected. Transient relief of symptoms after injection suggests a greater likelihood of a favorable result after surgical decompression.

2. Surgical treatment—Patients unresponsive to conservative measures may benefit from surgical division of the transverse carpal ligament. This division may be accomplished with either direct open exposure or through an endoscopic approach. The open incision is made in the palm over the transverse carpal ligament, staying

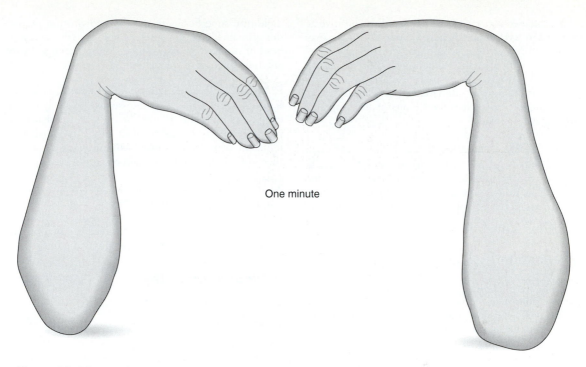

One minute

Figure 10–25. Phalen's maneuver. (Reproduced, with permission, from American Society for Surgery of the Hand, 2nd ed. *The Hand: Examination and Diagnosis.* New York: Churchill Livingstone, 1983.)

ulnar to the axis of the palmaris longus, along the longitudinal axis of the radial border of the ring finger. This incision avoids injury to the palmar cutaneous branch of the median nerve. After longitudinally incising the palmar fascia, the transverse carpal ligament is identified and is longitudinally sectioned under direct observation. Endoscopic division of the transverse carpal ligament avoids a potentially tender palmar incision with either a single wrist portal proximal to the palm or with a combined proximal portal and short midpalmar portal along the axis of the open incision. Although some studies have noted an earlier return to work activities after endoscopic release, the incidence of iatrogenic nerve and tendon injuries may be higher with endoscopic release than with open release. Both types of procedures are accepted ways of treating carpal tunnel syndrome. The decision of which technique to use is based on the surgeon's experience. Endoscopic carpal tunnel release should not be used for recurrent carpal tunnel syndrome.

After surgery, the hand is bandaged for a week. Patients are encouraged to actively move their fingers from the first postoperative day. Wrist motion is begun within the first week. Incisional tenderness most commonly prevents patients from fully using their hands and returning to work with no restrictions for the first

4–8 weeks. If patients have difficulty with hand function 3–4 weeks after surgery, a therapy program is prescribed consisting of desensitization, range of motion, and strengthening.

Pronator Syndrome

A. ANATOMY

The median nerve may be compressed in the proximal forearm by one or more of the following structures: ligament of Struthers, lacertus fibrosus, pronator teres muscle, or proximal fibrous arch on the undersurface of the flexor digitorum superficialis muscle.

B. CLINICAL FINDINGS

Patients with pronator syndrome complain of pain that is usually more severe in the volar forearm than in the wrist or hand. Pain usually increases with activity. Complaints of numbness in the thumb, index, middle, and ring fingers may initially suggest the possibility of carpal tunnel syndrome. Night symptoms are, however, unusual in cases of isolated pronator syndrome.

Examination may reveal sensory and motor deficits similar to those seen in carpal tunnel syndrome, but significant differences may be detected on careful evaluation. Dysesthesia may include the distribution of the palmar cutaneous nerve. Tinel's sign will be positive at the forearm level rather than at the wrist. Phalen's maneuver will not provoke symptoms. Patients may experience pain with resistance to contraction of the pronator teres or flexor digitorum superficialis muscles tested by resistance to forearm pronation or to isolated flexion of the proximal interphalangeal joints of the long and ring fingers.

C. TREATMENT

Evaluation of symptomatic patients should include electrodiagnostic studies if a 6-week course of immobilization fails to effect improvement. Surgical treatment requires generous decompression of all potentially constricting sites.

Anterior Interosseous Syndrome

A. ANATOMY

The anterior interosseous nerve branch divides from the median nerve 4–6 cm below the elbow. This branch of the nerve innervates the flexor pollicis longus, flexor digitorum profundus of the index and middle fingers, and pronator quadratus muscles. The anterior interosseous nerve may be compressed by the deep head of the pronator teres, origin of the flexor digitorum superficialis, palmaris profundus, or flexor carpi radialis. In addition, accessory muscles connecting the flexor digitorum superficialis to the flexor digitorum profundus proximally and Gantzer's muscle (the accessory head of the flexor pollicis longus) may impinge on the anterior interosseous nerve.

B. CLINICAL FINDINGS

Patients with anterior interosseous nerve syndrome complain of inability to flex the thumb interphalangeal joint as well as the index-finger distal interphalangeal joint. In contrast to those with pronator syndrome, these patients will not complain of numbness or pain.

C. TREATMENT

Surgical decompression of the anterior interosseous nerve may be indicated when the syndrome does not spontaneously improve. This requires exploration and division of all potentially compressing structures.

2. Ulnar Neuropathy

Cubital Tunnel Syndrome

A. ANATOMY

The region in which the ulnar nerve is most commonly compressed is at the cubital tunnel along the medial elbow. Compression may occur between the ulnar and humeral origins of the flexor carpi ulnaris or at the proximal border of the cubital tunnel, as the nerve is tethered anteriorly with elbow flexion (Figure 10–26).

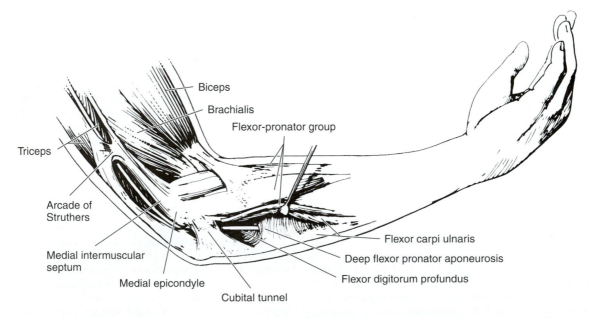

Figure 10–26. Points of constriction of the ulnar nerve at the elbow. (From Amadio PC: Anatomic basis for a technique of ulnar nerve transposition. Surg Radiol Anat 1986;8:155; used, with permission, from Mayo Foundation.)

B. Clinical Findings

Patients with cubital tunnel syndrome most often complain of paresthesia and numbness involving the ring and little fingers. Because symptoms may be aggravated or provoked by full flexion of the elbow, patients may complain of increased symptoms when talking on the telephone. Many patients complain of being awakened at night by the symptoms, most often when sleeping with the elbows flexed. Patients who have weakness of muscles innervated by the ulnar nerve may note clumsiness and lack of dexterity.

1. Provocative tests—

a. Tinel's sign—On physical examination, a positive Tinel's sign is noted with percussion over the ulnar nerve at the elbow. The nerve may be noted to sublux over the medial epicondyle as the arm is brought into flexion.

b. Motor strength—Motor strength should be assessed in intrinsic muscles innervated by the ulnar nerve (first dorsal interosseous muscle) and in extrinsic muscles innervated by the ulnar nerve (flexor digitorum profundus of the little finger).

c. Froment's sign—With weakness of the adductor pollicis muscle innervated by the ulnar nerve, a positive Froment's sign may be observed. As the patient tries to hold a piece of paper placed between the thumb and the index finger, the interphalangeal joint flexes in an attempt to substitute flexor pollicis longus activity for lost adductor pollicis strength.

d. Elbow flexion test—The ulnar nerve may be irritated by fully flexing the elbow with the wrist in the neutral position. The elbow flexion test, a provocative maneuver, is considered positive if paresthesia is elicited in the ring and little fingers within 60 s. The location of the paresthesia and the time between initiation of elbow flexion and the onset of symptoms should be recorded.

C. Treatment

1. Conservative treatment—Conservative treatment may include the use of an elbow pad to protect the nerve from trauma or a splint holding the elbow at approximately 45 degrees of flexion. The splint may be worn continuously or at night only, depending on the frequency and intensity of symptoms.

2. Surgical treatment—Electrodiagnostic studies should be obtained if conservative treatment does not alleviate the symptoms, particularly if residual motor weakness is evident. The reliability of nerve conduction studies at the elbow depends on the ability of the electromyographer to accurately measure the length of the ulnar nerve.

Numerous procedures have been described to relieve ulnar nerve compression at the elbow. These include simple decompression of the ulnar nerve within the cubital tunnel or decompression with anterior transposition of the nerve subcutaneously, intramuscularly, or submuscularly into the flexor pronator mass. When the nerve is transposed, great care must be taken to excise the medial intermuscular septum and to release the aponeurosis between the humeral and ulnar origins of the flexor carpi ulnaris, so as not to provide a new area of impingement.

An alternative surgical strategy involves decompression of the nerve and medial epicondylectomy, which attempts to remove the prominence against which the ulnar nerve is tethered with elbow flexion. After surgery, the arm is placed into a long arm splint with the elbow flexed to 90 degrees. The splint is removed after 1–2 weeks to begin active range-of-motion exercises. Strengthening begins at 4–6 weeks and the patient returns to work with no restrictions of the arm at 8–12 weeks.

Ulnar Tunnel Syndrome

A. Anatomy

The ulnar nerve passes from the forearm into the hand through Guyon's canal (see Figure 10–24). The anatomic confines of Guyon's canal are the pisiform and pisohamate ligament ulnarly, the hook of the hamate and insertion of the transverse carpal ligament radially, and the volar carpal ligament forming the roof of the tunnel.

B. Clinical Findings

Examination should document ulnar nerve sensory and motor integrity. In contrast to the findings in cubital tunnel syndrome, Tinel's sign will be positive at the wrist rather than at the elbow. The region of compression should be delineated by electrodiagnostic studies.

C. Treatment

When splinting is ineffective, surgical decompression should be considered. When symptoms exist in tandem with carpal tunnel syndrome, release of the transverse carpal ligament favorably alters the shape and size of Guyon's Canal. Postoperative care is the same as for carpal tunnel release.

3. Radial Neuropathy

Radial Tunnel Syndrome

A. Anatomy

The radial nerve may become symptomatic if compressed in the region of the radial tunnel. Points of impingement along the radial tunnel, located at the level of the proximal radius, include fibers spanning the radiocapitellar joint, the radial recurrent vessels, the extensor carpi radialis brevis, the tendinous origin of the supinator (arcade of Frohse), and the point at which the nerve emerges from beneath the distal edge of the supinator.

B. CLINICAL FINDINGS

Because radial tunnel syndrome often occurs in combination with lateral epicondylitis, the two diagnoses are frequently confused. Patients with radial tunnel syndrome experience pain over the midportion of the mobile wad (brachioradialis, extensor carpi radialis longus, and extensor carpi radialis brevis muscles), whereas the pain experienced by patients with lateral epicondylitis is located at or just distal to the lateral epicondyle. Patients with radial tunnel syndrome experience pain when simultaneously extending the wrist and fingers while the long finger is passively flexed by the examiner (positive long-finger extension test). Patients with radial tunnel syndrome often also experience pain with resisted forearm supination.

C. TREATMENT

Conservative treatment of radial tunnel syndrome includes measures to avoid forceful extension of the wrist and fingers. The wrist is splinted in dorsiflexion while the forearm is immobilized in supination. Persistent symptoms in spite of splinting may be treated by surgical exploration and decompression of the radial nerve. Concomitant lateral epicondylitis refractory to conservative measures should be treated surgically at the same time that the radial nerve is decompressed.

Posterior Interosseous Nerve Syndrome

A. ANATOMY

The radial nerve branches into the posterior interosseous nerve and the superficial sensory branch of the radial nerve after passing anteriorly to the radiocapitellar joint. The posterior interosseous nerve then passes beneath the origin of the extensor carpi radialis brevis, radial recurrent artery, and arcade of Frohse. The posterior interosseous nerve is most commonly entrapped at the proximal edge of the supinator, though entrapment may occur at either the middle or the distal edge of the supinator muscle.

B. CLINICAL FINDINGS

In contrast to radial tunnel syndrome, patients with posterior interosseous nerve syndrome have significant extrinsic extensor weakness. Pain may be less than in radial tunnel syndrome.

Paralysis may be either partial or complete. Because the brachioradialis, extensor carpi radialis longus, supinator, and often extensor carpi radialis brevis are innervated by the radial nerve prior to the division into the posterior interosseous nerve, these muscles will be spared. Digital extension at the metacarpophalangeal joint will be the principal deficit from loss of extensor digitorum communis, extensor indicis proprius, and extensor digit quinti function.

The differential diagnosis in a patient with spontaneous loss of digital extension should also include multiple tendon ruptures, particularly in patients with rheumatoid arthritis. The **tenodesis effect,** in which the fingers extend as the wrist is passively flexed, is preserved in posterior interosseous nerve syndrome but absent if the extensor tendons have ruptured.

C. TREATMENT

Treatment of posterior interosseous nerve syndrome requires thorough decompression of the nerve. If nerve recovery does not occur, tendon transfers will restore digital extension.

4. Thoracic Outlet Syndrome

Anatomy

The brachial plexus exits the base of the neck and upper thorax through the thoracic outlet. Anatomic boundaries of the outlet are the scalenus anterior muscle anteriorly, the scalenus medius muscle posteriorly, and the first rib inferiorly. Thoracic outlet syndrome, usually resulting from irritation of the C8- and T1-innervated nerves, may be caused by a cervical rib, a fiber spanning from a rudimentary cervical rib, tendinous bands from the scalenus anterior to the medius muscles, or hypertrophic clavicle fracture callus. Poor posture with slumping shoulders or prolonged military brace position have each been implicated as a contributing factor.

Clinical Findings

The symptoms of thoracic outlet syndrome are often vague. They may include pain in the C8-T1 dermatome, with a variable degree of intrinsic muscle weakness. Patients may experience vascular symptoms if the axillary artery is simultaneously being compressed in the thoracic outlet region.

A. PROVOCATIVE TESTS

1. Elevated stress test—Physical examination of the patient with suspected thoracic outlet syndrome should include an elevated stress test, in which the patient's shoulders are kept extended and the arm is externally rotated 90 degrees at the shoulder. The patient is then asked to open and close the hands with the arms elevated for 3 min. Reproduction of symptoms is suggestive of thoracic outlet syndrome.

2. Other tests—Adson's sign and Wright's test may be helpful in determining if vascular compression is present. In a positive Adson's test, the radial pulse is obliterated when the arm is dependent and the head is turned to the affected side. In Wright's test, the pulse is obliterated when the shoulder is abducted, externally rotated, and the head is turned away from the involved shoulder. In addition, this maneuver should reproduce the patient's symptoms. Physical examination should document C8-T1 sensation and intrinsic muscle strength.

B. DIAGNOSTIC STUDIES

Workup of the symptomatic patient should include radiographs of the cervical spine to rule out a cervical rib, electrodiagnostic studies to assess the function of the lower roots, and Doppler studies of the arm in varied positions to assess compression of the axillary artery.

Treatment

Initial treatment includes postural exercises. Patients who are unresponsive to conservative treatment or have demonstrable weakness may benefit from surgical resection of a cervical rib, resection of the first rib, or scalenotomy.

5. Cervical Root Compression

Clinical Findings

Cervical spine root compression may produce peripheral symptoms and findings affecting the hand, causing initial complaints of hand pain or weakness. It is worthwhile to routinely inquire about pain or decreased motion of the cervical spine. If the patient has been involved in an accident involving sudden neck flexion and extension, this too should be noted. Cervical root compression may occur from a herniated cervical disk, cervical spondylosis, intervertebral foraminal osteophytes, or, rarely, a cervical cord tumor.

Patients with cervical root compression more often complain of pain in a radicular rather than a peripheral nerve distribution. In spite of symptoms involving the hand, most patients, when carefully questioned, will be able to distinguish pain that begins in the neck and radiates to the hand from pain that begins in the hand and radiates proximally to the neck. Pain may be exacerbated with neck motion (flexion and extension, lateral bending, or rotation), coughing, or sneezing.

A. SPURLING'S TEST

Physical examination of the patient with cervical radiculopathy will frequently demonstrate a decreased range of neck motion or pain with neck motion. Symptoms may be reproduced with axial compression on the patient's head (positive Spurling's test). Detailed sensory and motor examination may reveal deficits in the domain of one or more roots.

B. DOUBLE CRUSH SYNDROME

Occasional simultaneous presentation of cervical radiculopathy with peripheral entrapment neuropathy has been termed the double-crush syndrome. Whether compression at one level renders a nerve more vulnerable to compressive forces at a second level or whether such cases simply represent two common entities in the same extremity remains the subject of debate.

Treatment

If a nerve is compressed at more than one location, the more symptomatic area is usually treated first. If both areas are equally symptomatic, the simpler of the two operations is chosen.

Gelberman RH et al: Carpal tunnel syndrome: Results of a prospective trial of steroid injection and splinting. J Bone Joint Surg Am 1980;62:1181.

Leffert RD: Anterior submuscular transposition of the ulnar nerves by the Learmouth technique. J Hand Surg (Am) 1982; 7:147.

Lister GD et al: The radial tunnel syndrome. J Hand Surg (Am) 1979;4:52.

Morgenlander JC et al: Surgical treatment or carpal tunnel syndrome in patients with peripheral neuropathy. Neurology 1997;49:1159.

Trumble TE et al: Single-portal endoscopic carpal tunnel release compared with open release: A prospective, randomized trial. J Bone Joint Surg Am. 2002;84-A(7):1107. [PMID: 12107308]

Upton ARM, McComas A: The double crush nerve entrapment syndromes. Lancet 1973;2:359.

■ DISORDERS OF THE FASCIA OF THE HAND

DUPUYTREN'S DISEASE

Dupuytren's disease is a nodular thickening on the palmar surface of the hand (Figure 10–27). It is a progressive condition, affecting the preexisting palmar fascia, resulting from incompletely understood pathologic changes mediated by the myofibroblast. Dupuytren's disease occurs most commonly in patients age 40–60 years. It is observed more often in males, in whom it

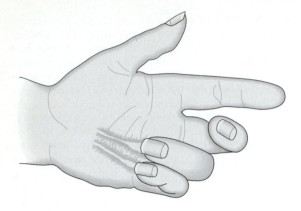

Figure 10–27. Dupuytren's contracture. (Reproduced, with permission, from American Society for Surgery of the Hand: *The Hand: Examination and Diagnosis,* 2nd ed. New York: Churchill Livingstone, 1983.)

appears earlier and is often more aggressive. Flexion contractures most frequently occur at the metacarpophalangeal joints but may also tether the proximal interphalangeal joint and, less commonly, the distal interphalangeal joint. The little and ring fingers and the thumb index web are the most commonly involved areas. Ectopic deposits may occur in the dorsum of the proximal interphalangeal joint (knuckle pads), the dorsum of the penis (Peyronie's disease), and the plantar fascia of the foot (Lederhose's disease).

Epidemiologic Factors

A number of predisposing factors have been identified. The disease most commonly appears in patients of Northern European ancestry and is occasionally encountered in Asians; it is rarer in other racial groups. Dupuytren's disease has been associated with epilepsy medications taken for seizure disorders, with alcoholism, and with diabetes. The relationship of work and trauma to the development of the disease remains controversial. The most aggressive disease occurs in patients who have a family history of disease and in those who have onset of disease before 40 years of age. More severely involved patients may have extensive bilateral involvement and ectopic deposits on the dorsum of the hands and the feet. These patients often undergo surgery at an early age, but extension and recurrence of the disease is common.

Anatomy

Dupuytren's contracture distorts the anatomy of the palmar fascia. Flexion contractures of the metacarpophalangeal joint are caused by pathologic contracture of pretendinous bands at a superficial level. Contracture

of the natatory ligaments produces web space contractures and scissoring of the fingers. The transverse fibers of the palmar aponeurosis are not involved with disease, except at the base of the thumb. In the fingers, the superficial volar fascia, lateral digital sheath, spiral band, and Grayson's ligaments may contract alone or in combination to produce contracture of the proximal interphalangeal joint. When a spiral band contracts, the digital nerve is often displaced palmarly to the band from proximal lateral to distal central in the region of the proximal phalanx.

Treatment

Nonsurgical treatment has not been effective in reversing or halting Dupuytren's disease. The primary indication for surgery is a fixed contracture of more than 30 degrees at the metacarpophalangeal or any flexion contracture at the proximal interphalangeal joint.

Surgical exposure may be achieved through either transverse or longitudinal skin incisions. A transverse incision across the distal palmar skin crease is useful when extensive palmar involvement is anticipated. Transverse incisions may either be sutured if there is little tension or left open to heal by secondary intention. When longitudinal incisions are used to expose the finger, Brunner zigzag incisions are useful. An alternative is a longitudinal incision that is modified for closure by a series of Z-plasty flap transpositions.

The goal of surgical release is to achieve a regional fasciectomy or subtotal palmar fasciectomy that will allow maximal untethered joint motion. A local fasciotomy may occasionally be elected in older, more debilitated patients with severe joint contractures.

Severe or recurrent proximal interphalangeal joint disease may occasionally be best treated with a salvage procedure, usually proximal interphalangeal joint arthrodesis. Amputation may be considered when profound stiffness or neurovascular compromise is present.

Complications

The most common postoperative complication is hematoma, which may expand and compromise skin flaps and act as a nidus for infection. To diminish the possibility of postoperative hematoma, the tourniquet should be released and meticulous hemostasis obtained prior to wound closure. Tight skin closure should be avoided. If flap necrosis occurs, the affected regions should be treated by open dressing changes. If skin loss is extensive, skin graft application may be necessary to gain early wound closure.

Joint stiffness may occur, particularly after extensive surgical release of the proximal interphalangeal joint. Extensive therapy is often necessary, consisting of both active and passive exercises and splinting.

Mild sympathetic dystrophy is not uncommon. For patients who have a more severe form, hospitalization with elevation, sympathetic blocking agents, oral steroids, and intensive therapy may be necessary.

Prognosis

Correction is usually maintained at the metacarpophalangeal joints. Recurrence is more common at the proximal interphalangeal joint, particularly when the extent of initial proximal interphalangeal joint contracture was substantial. Long-term postoperative night splinting may diminish the extent of residual digital flexion contracture.

Al-Qattan MM: The injection of nodules of Dupuytren's disease with triamcinolone acetonide. J Hand Surg [Am]. 2001;26 (3):560. No abstract available. [PMID: 11418926]

Jensen CM et al: Amputations in the treatment of Dupuytren's disease. J Hand Surg Br 1993;18:781.

McCash CR: The open technique in Dupuytren's contracture. Br J Plast Surg 1964;17:271.

McFarlane RM: On the origin and spread of Dupuytren's disease. J Hand Surg [Am]. 2002;27(3):385. Review. [PMID: 12015711]

■ COMPARTMENT SYNDROMES

Compartment syndromes are a group of conditions that result from increased pressure within a limited anatomic space, acutely compromising the circulation and ultimately threatening the function of the tissue within that space.

Recurrent or chronic compartment syndrome results from increased pressure within the compartment with a specific activity, most commonly in athletes during exercise. Symptoms of muscle weakness may be severe enough to stop the exercise program in spite of the patient being asymptomatic between recurrences.

Volkmann's ischemic contracture is the final sequela of acute compartment syndrome in which dead muscle has been replaced with fibrous tissue. Because nerve injury is not always associated with this condition, sensation and intrinsic muscle function may be normal distal to the involved compartment.

Often, there is no associated nerve injury, and thus no sensory deficit or loss of motor function is evident in the domain distal to the involved compartment.

Etiologic Factors

The most common causes of compartment syndrome are fractures, soft-tissue crush injuries, arterial injuries either caused by localized hemorrhage or postischemic swelling, drug overdose with prolonged limb compression, and burn injuries. In most cases, fractures are closed or, if open, are grade 1 injuries, with only limited disruption of compartmental soft-tissue envelopes.

The pathophysiology of compartment syndrome is a consequence of closure of small vessels. Increased compartment pressure increases the pressure on the walls of arterioles within the compartment. Increased local pressure also occludes small veins, resulting in venous hypertension within the compartment. The arteriovenous gradient in the region of the pressurized tissue becomes insufficient for tissue perfusion. Because the elevated pressure within the compartment is insufficient to occlude major arteries as they pass through the compartment, distal pulses usually remain strong in spite of evolving tissue ischemia in the affected soft-tissue compartment.

Clinical Findings

The diagnosis of compartment syndrome is made predominantly on clinical findings. The clinician must have a high index of suspicion whenever a closed compartment has the potential for bleeding or swelling. Compartment syndromes are characterized by pain out of proportion to the initial injury. Pain is often persistent, progressive, and unrelieved by immobilization. Pain may be accentuated by passive stretching of involved muscles. Diminished sensation may be noted in the distribution of the nerve whose compartment is being compressed. This phenomenon is believed to be secondary to nerve ischemia. A third sign is weakness and paralysis of muscles within the compartment. A fourth sign is tenseness of the compartment on palpation. Of the preceding signs and symptoms, pain with passive muscle stretching is the most sensitive in detecting compartment syndrome.

If the diagnosis of compartment syndrome is in question, the clinician is obligated to ascertain the pressure within the potential affected compartments. Various methods are available, including a portable hand-held pressure monitor or a simple modification of a mercury manometer connected to tubing and a three-way stopcock. Although the exact pressure threshold for requiring fasciotomy varies among authors, fasciotomy should be strongly considered whenever the compartment pressure is greater than 30 mm Hg in the forearm. Pressure measurements of the compartments of the hand are difficult to interpret. The decision to perform a fasciotomy of the hand or finger is based solely on clinical judgment.

Treatment

Once the diagnosis of compartment syndrome has been established, fasciotomy of the involved compartment should be performed as soon as possible because elevation of compartment pressure to more than 30 mm Hg for over 8 h causes irreversible tissue death. Prophylactic fasciotomy should also be considered in patients in whom ischemia has been present for more than 4 h. All patients undergoing forearm or arm replantation should undergo fasciotomy at the time of the initial surgical procedure.

The compartment most often requiring release in the upper extremity is the volar compartment of the forearm (Figure 10–28A). The skin incision should extend from the elbow to the carpal tunnel. The preferred skin incision extends from the medial side of the biceps and swings ulnarly toward the medial epicondyle. Care must be taken to incise the lacertus fibrosus at the elbow level. The incision may be extended in a radial direction to allow decompression of the mobile wad. In the distal half of the forearm, the incision runs along the ulnar border. The flap is designed to allow coverage of the median nerve at the conclusion of the procedure when wounds will be left open. The incision is then carried obliquely across the wrist and provides exposure of the carpal tunnel in the proximal palm.

An epimysiotomy of the individual superficial and deep compartment muscle bellies should be performed as needed. Care should be taken to ensure that the deep compartment musculature (the flexor pollicis longus and flexor digitorum profundus muscles) has been completely decompressed. The skin incision should be partially closed over the median nerve in the hand and distal forearm. The proximal wound over muscle should be left open. The patient should be returned to the operating room within 48 h for reevaluation. At the second surgery, dressings are changed and secondary debridement is accomplished if nonviable muscle remains. In some instances, it is possible to close the wound secondarily; in most cases, split-thickness skin grafting of the residual skin defect is a safer alternative.

Decompression of the dorsal forearm when necessary may be accomplished with a dorsal longitudinal incision (Figure 10–28B).

In the hand, the connections between compartments are limited; therefore, each compartment should be released individually. This may be accomplished by two longitudinal dorsal incisions over the index and ring metacarpals. Through these incisions, each of the interosseous compartments can be entered on both the radial and ulnar sides of each metacarpal. Separate volar incisions are needed when decompression of the thenar

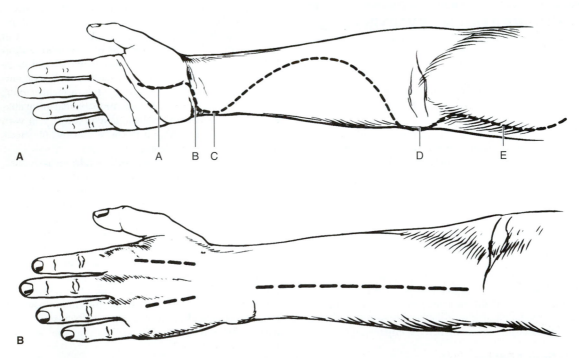

Figure 10–28. **A:** Various skin incisions used for performing a volar arm fasciotomy. **B:** To decompress the dorsal and mobile wad compartments, straight incisions are preferred because fewer veins will be damaged. (Reproduced, with permission, from Green DP, ed: *Operative Hand Surgery,* 2nd ed. New York: Churchill Livingstone, 1988.)

and hypothenar compartments is necessary on the palm of the hand.

In the finger, fasciotomy may be required for treatment of either severe trauma or snakebite injuries. Because compartment pressures in the finger are difficult to measure, the indications for finger fasciotomy are based on the degree of swelling. Midaxial incisions along the ulnar side of the index, middle, and ring fingers and the radial side of the little finger and thumb allow satisfactory digital decompression. Care is taken to retract the neurovascular bundle palmarward, and the fascia between the neurovascular bundle and the flexor tendon sheath are then incised. Wounds are left open postoperatively, and wound closure is achieved either secondarily or with a split-thickness skin graft.

Eaton RG, Green WT: Volkmann's ischemia: A volar compartment syndrome of the forearm. Clin Orthop 1975;113:58.

Gelberman RH et al: Compartment syndromes of the forearm: Diagnosis and treatment. Clin Orthop 1981;161:252.

Matsen F et al: Diagnosis and management of compartmental syndromes. J Bone Joint Surg Am 1980;62:286.

Mubarak S, Carroll N: Volkmann's contracture in children: Aetiology and prevention. J Bone Joint Surg Br 1979;61:285.

■ FRACTURES & DISLOCATIONS OF THE HAND

FRACTURES & DISLOCATIONS OF THE METACARPALS & PHALANGES

Fractures of the metacarpals and phalanges account for approximately 10% of all fractures. More than half of all hand fractures are work-related. Fractures of the border digits, thumb, and little finger are most common, and the most commonly fractured bone is the distal phalanx (45–50% of all hand fractures).

Clinical Findings

Description of a phalangeal or metacarpal fracture should include notation of the bone involved, the location within the bone (base, shaft, or neck), and whether the fracture is open or closed. Further determination should be made as to whether the fracture is displaced or nondisplaced, if it has an intra-articular component, and whether rotational or angular deformity is present.

Because metacarpal or phalangeal rotational malalignment is difficult to evaluate from a radiograph, physical examination is essential. The patient is asked to actively flex the fingers individually and together. Nail rotation, finger direction, and overlapping of the fingers is assessed. Associated vascular, nerve, and tendon injuries, as well as the adequacy of soft-tissue coverage, also should be evaluated.

Treatment

Treatment of metacarpal and phalangeal fractures requires accurate fracture diagnosis, reduction, sufficient immobilization to maintain the fracture reduction, and early motion of the uninvolved fingers to prevent stiffness. Immobilization should usually place the hand in an intrinsic plus, or safe, position to avoid secondary joint contracture (see Figure 10–13). Immobilization for phalangeal fractures should rarely exceed 3 weeks and for metacarpal fractures 4 weeks. Because radiologic union will usually lag behind clinical union in the hand, initiation of digital motion should not be delayed until clear radiologic union is seen, because residual stiffness is likely.

The fixation required to maintain fracture reduction is directly dependent upon the fracture characteristics. Stable fractures may be treated by either buddy taping the affected finger to an adjacent finger and allowing early motion or with a brief period of splint immobilization. Repeat radiographs are done at 7–10 days to document maintenance of fracture reduction. Initially displaced unstable fractures that require closed reduction to achieve proper alignment will require external immobilization with a cast or splint.

When external immobilization is impossible or unlikely to maintain fracture reduction, internal fixation is required. Internal fixation techniques useful in the management of hand fractures include Kirschner wire fixation, interosseous wiring, tension band wiring, interfragmentary screw fixation, or fixation with plates and screws. Kirschner wire fixation is versatile but lacks the rigidity of other techniques. Additional stability may be achieved by combining Kirschner wire fixation with tension band wires. Interfragmentary screws provide ideal fixation for long oblique fractures, in which the obliquity of the fracture is more than two times the diameter of the fractured bone. Plates and screws in the hand are particularly helpful in open metacarpal fractures with bone loss. When segmental bone loss occurs, initial treatment includes debridement of an associated open wound and maintenance of skeletal length with either internal or external fixation. After the soft-tissue coverage has been ensured, bony graft reconstruction may be coupled with definitive internal fixation.

1. Physeal Fractures

Approximately one third of all fractures of the immature skeleton involve the epiphysis. Salter-Harris physeal fractures are divided into five types. Type 1 fractures, which shear through the growth plate without extension into the epiphysis or metaphysis, may be effectively treated with simple immobilization. Type 2 fractures, in which a metaphyseal fracture fragment is attached to the epiphysis, can usually be reduced in a closed fashion and immobilized with a splint. One of the more common type 2 fractures is the so-called extraoctave fracture at the base of the proximal phalanx of the little finger, which is caused by ulnar deviation of the finger. Reduction may be accomplished by metacarpophalangeal joint flexion and little finger radial deviation. Type 3 and 4 fractures are intra-articular injuries. When displaced, these fractures require open reduction to achieve restoration of the articular surface and physis. Type 5 fractures are uncommon in the phalanges, occurring most often in the finger metacarpals as a result of axial compression. Type 5 crush injuries to the growth plate may provoke either partial or complete fusion of the physis and thereby lead to an angular deformity or a shortened finger.

2. Distal Phalanx Fractures

Distal phalangeal fractures occur most often in the middle finger and the thumb. These fractures usually result from a crushing injury, such as occurs with a misdirected hammer striking a thumb holding a nail or a protruding middle finger distal phalanx caught in a closing door.

Precise reduction of distal phalangeal fracture fragments is not required in closed injuries, unless the articular surface is involved. Treatment consists of splinting the bone and distal interphalangeal joint for protection and pain relief. While the distal interphalangeal joint is splinted, motion should be encouraged at the metacarpophalangeal and proximal interphalangeal joints. Splint protection may be discontinued at 3 weeks.

Nail matrix injuries are often associated with open distal phalanx fractures. Proper treatment of these fractures requires removal of the nail, irrigation of the fracture and nail bed, and nail bed repair with fine absorbable sutures. Fracture reduction is usually accomplished by nail matrix repair and replacement of the nail. In rare cases, pin fixation of markedly displaced distal phalanx fractures may be required. After nail bed repair, either the original nail, a nail prosthesis, a piece of aluminum suture package, or a piece of gauze should be interposed between the nail roof and the nail bed to prevent synechia formation.

Displaced open distal phalangeal epiphyseal injuries are most often caused by flexion of the distal phalanx with the apex at the dorsal physis. Often, the nail is avulsed dorsal to the eponychia. Treatment requires nail removal, irrigation, reduction of the fracture, and nail bed repair. Failure to appreciate the open nature of a displaced type 1 fracture of the distal phalanx may result in chronic osteomyelitis of the distal phalanx.

3. Proximal & Middle Phalanx Fractures

Angulation of fractures of the proximal and middle phalanges reflects the tendon forces inserting on the bone. The middle phalanx has an extensor force transmitted to it by the central slip attaching dorsally and proximally. The terminal extensor tendon inserts dorsally and distally into the terminal phalanx, providing a secondary dorsiflexion force. The flexor digitorum superficialis inserts volarly over the middle three fifths of the middle phalanx. Therefore, middle phalanx fractures that occur proximal to the flexor digitorum superficialis insertion angulate with the fracture apex dorsally; fractures that occur distal to this insertion will angulate with the apex palmarly. All proximal phalangeal fractures angulate with the apex palmarly because of the force of lateral bands that pass palmarward to the axis of the metacarpophalangeal joint and dorsalward to the axis of the proximal interphalangeal joint.

Adhesions involving the flexor or extensor tendons are a major complication of proximal and middle phalangeal fractures. Fracture displacement increases the likelihood of tendon adherence and limitation of joint motion. Malunion or malrotation of the fractures may require secondary correction.

Early appropriate treatment of these fractures attempts to prevent complications. In a stable nondisplaced or impacted fracture, only temporary splint protection is required, followed by dynamic splinting such as buddy taping. Careful radiographic follow-up is needed to document maintenance of the reduction. Patients who require closed reduction and immobilization should have the forearm, wrist, and injured digits as well as an adjacent digit immobilized in a plaster cast or gutter splint.

4. Metacarpal Fractures

Metacarpal Head Fractures

Intra-articular fractures of the metacarpal head require open reduction and internal fixation if more than 20–30% of the joint surface is involved. Realigned articular fracture fragments may be held in place with either a Kirschner wire or small screw. Fractures with marked comminution of the metacarpal head distal to the ligament origin may not be amenable to precise internal fixation and may be treated with early immobilization with distraction traction.

Metacarpal Neck Fractures

Metacarpal neck fractures are most frequent in the little finger, though they may occur in any metacarpal. Metacarpal neck fractures result from a direct blow, either delivered to the hand or by the hand to a solid object (animate or inanimate). Comminution of the volar cortex results in collapse deformity with apex dorsal angulation (Figure 10–29). Greater residual fracture angulation may be accepted in the ring and little fingers because the greater mobility in the ulnar carpometacarpal joints allows greater compensatory motion. The flexion and extension arc is 15 degrees in the ring finger carpometacarpal joint and 30 degrees in the little finger.

Fracture site angulation of more than 10 degrees should not be accepted in the index and middle fingers. Fractures of the ring and little fingers with initial angulation of less than 15 degrees should be immobilized in a gutter splint for 10–14 days. When angulation is 15–40 degrees, reduction should be accomplished before an ulnar gutter splint immobilization is employed for 3 weeks. With angulation of more than 40 degrees, extensor lag may be noted at the proximal interphalangeal joint, and the patient may complain of a "marble" in the palm when making a fist. If reduction cannot be maintained, fixation may be employed.

Metacarpal Shaft Fractures

Metacarpal shaft fractures result from a direct blow or crushing injury. Dorsal angulation of the fracture fragments is secondary to the interosseous muscle forces. The closer the fracture is to the carpometacarpal joints, the greater the lever arm and, hence, the less angulation can be tolerated. Less shortening occurs in isolated fractures of the middle and ring finger metacarpals than in

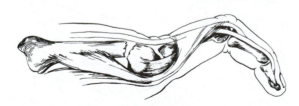

Figure 10–29. Boxer's fracture. If the angulation in a metacarpal neck fracture is severe, clawing may result when the patient attempts to extend the finger. This is a good clinical test to supplement the evaluation of the severity of the angulation as seen radiographically. (Reproduced, with permission, from Rockwood CA Jr et al, ed: *Fractures in Adults,* 3rd ed. Baltimore: Lippincott, 1991.)

the index or little fingers because the deep intermetacarpal ligaments tether the metacarpal distally. Isolated metacarpal fractures may be treated with cast or splint immobilization for 4–6 weeks. Displaced metacarpal shaft fractures may be fixed percutaneously with a longitudinal pin or by percutaneously pinning the fractured metacarpal to an adjacent metacarpal. Skeletal fixation is essential if metacarpal rotational deformity cannot entirely be corrected with closed treatment because modest metacarpal malrotation will result in substantial digital overlap. Dorsal angulation of more than 10 degrees in index and middle metacarpals and more than 20 degrees in ring and little metacarpals, shortening of more than 3 mm, or multiple displaced metacarpal fractures should be treated with operative intervention. Long spiral fractures may be effectively fixed with multiple screws, and transverse fractures are usually most securely fixed with dorsally applied plates. When two or more metacarpals are simultaneously fractured, the splinting effect of the intact adjacent metacarpals is lost. Secure fixation with screws or plates should be employed in at least one of the injured metacarpals.

5. Joint Injuries

Distal Interphalangeal Joint

The most common intra-articular fracture of the distal interphalangeal joint is a bony mallet finger, in which a portion of the articular surface is avulsed by the extensor tendon. Most bony mallet injuries can be treated with splinting in extension for 6 weeks. Indications for fixation of these fractures are controversial. Internal fixation should be considered in fractures that include articular surface loss greater than 30% and subluxation of the joint.

Dislocation of the distal interphalangeal joint is uncommon without an associated fracture. Closed reduction with temporary splint protection allows early mobilization to begin within 7–10 days.

Condylar Fractures

Condylar fractures may occur in either the proximal or middle phalanges. These fractures are most often athletic injuries. Anteroposterior, lateral, and oblique radiographs are necessary to identify the fracture fragments. If the injury is inadequately appreciated, angulation of the finger and joint incongruity may lead to degenerative arthritis. Displaced fracture should be openly reduced and internally fixed if the condylar fracture is displaced by more than 2 mm. If both condyles are fractured, they must be precisely secured together and then secured to the phalangeal shaft. The collateral ligament insertion to the condyle must be preserved as it is the only blood supply to the fragment. Permanent loss of motion may be anticipated in complex condylar fractures.

Proximal Interphalangeal Joint Dislocation & Fracture-Dislocation

Dorsal dislocations of the proximal interphalangeal joint are more common than palmar or lateral dislocations. Dorsal dislocations may be separated into three types (Figure 10–30). In type 1 dislocations, a hyperextension injury avulses the volar plate from the base of the middle phalanx, whereas the collateral ligaments partially split from the middle phalanx and the joint surface is intact. Type 2 dislocations are dorsal dislocations similar to type 1 injuries, except that a larger portion of the collateral ligament is torn. In type 3 injuries, a dorsal dislocation occurs with proximal retraction of the middle phalanx. A portion of the middle phalangeal palmar base may be sheared away. Stable fracture-dislocations are associated with fractures in which less than 40% of the middle phalanx base has been fractured. Unstable fracture-dislocations have more than 40% bone fracture involvement and are associated with complete loss of collateral ligament stability.

Treatment of proximal interphalangeal joint dislocations depends on the dislocation type. Stable type 1 and 2 injuries should be treated by closed reduction and immobilization in a dorsal splint in 30 degrees of flexion for 1–2 weeks. While in the splint, patients are encouraged to actively flex the proximal interphalangeal joint. After reduction and splinting, a radiograph should document the reduction. After 2–3 weeks, the splint is re-

moved. The finger may be buddy taped to an adjacent finger during sports for the next month.

Unstable fracture-dislocations should be treated with closed reduction. Considerable flexion (> 75 degrees) may be necessary to achieve reduction. Again, radiographs must document congruent joint reduction. When a reduction is possible, the splint is straightened by 10 degrees each week until approximately 6 weeks after reduction, when splinting may be discontinued. If closed reduction cannot be achieved, open reduction is required. When a single, large, palmarly displaced articular fragment is present, internal fixation may be attempted. If the fracture is comminuted, however, either volar plate arthroplasty or an axial traction technique that allows early controlled passive joint motion is necessary.

Lateral proximal interphalangeal dislocation is six times more common on the radial than on the ulnar side. These dislocations are associated with avulsion of the volar plate, extensor mechanism, or a portion of the phalangeal base. After the joint is reduced, the residual joint stability should be assessed by observing the active range of motion. Stable fracture-dislocations are immobilized at 5–10 degrees of flexion for 3 weeks, and then active range-of-motion activities are allowed.

Palmar proximal interphalangeal dislocations are unusual. The condyle of the proximal phalanx may buttonhole between the central slip and the lateral bands. Closed reduction may be attempted by applying traction to the fingers after flexing both the metacarpophalangeal and proximal interphalangeal joints. If closed reduction is successful, the digit should be splinted for 3–6 weeks to allow healing of the extensor rent. If closed reduction is unsuccessful, open reduction

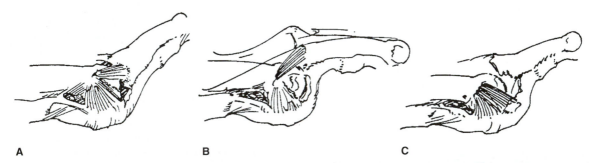

A   **B**   **C**

Figure 10–30. Various dorsal dislocations of the proximal interphalangeal joint. **A:** Type 1 (hyperextension). The volar plate is avulsed, and an incomplete longitudinal split occurs in the collateral ligaments. The articular surfaces maintain congruous contact. **B:** Type 2 (dorsal dislocation). There is complete rupture of the volar plate and a complete split in the collateral ligaments, with the middle phalanx resting on the dorsum of the proximal phalanx. The proximal and middle phalanges lie in almost parallel alignment. **C:** Type 3 (fracture-dislocation). The insertion of the volar plate, including a portion of the volar base of the middle phalanx, is disrupted. The major portion of the collateral ligaments remains with the volar plate and flexor sheath. A major articular defect may be present.

will be necessary to free the condyle from the rent in the extensor mechanism.

Metacarpophalangeal Joint

Dorsal metacarpophalangeal dislocations most commonly involve either the index or little finger. The volar plate is ruptured proximally from the metacarpal by hyperextension injury. If the joint is subluxed and the volar plate has not yet become interposed, closed reduction may be achieved by flexion of the joint. Traction across the subluxated metacarpophalangeal joint can turn a reducible joint into an irreducible, dislocated joint. Once the joint has dislocated, the volar plate has become interposed between the dislocated articular surfaces. The injury is termed **complex** or **irreducible,** and open reduction is required to extract the volar plate from between the articular surfaces (Figure 10–31). Open reduction may be accomplished through either a palmar or dorsal approach. If the palmar approach is used, care should be taken to avoid injury to the radial digital nerve of the index finger or the ulnar digital nerve of the small finger. The A$_1$ pulley is incised to release the tension of the flexor tendons on the volar plate. If the dorsal approach is used, the volar plate is longitudinally incised.

Postoperatively, the metacarpophalangeal joint is immobilized in approximately 30 degrees of flexion for 3–5 days. Splinting with active motion is then continued for 3 weeks.

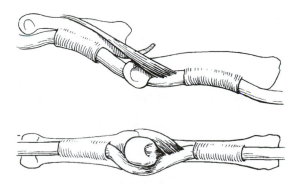

Figure 10–31. Complex dislocation of the metacarpophalangeal joint. In the upper, lateral diagram, the palmar plate is locked between the head of the metacarpal and the base of the proximal phalanx. In the lower diagram, an anterior view, the head of the metacarpal can be seen trapped between the flexor digitorum profundus on one aspect and the lumbrical on the other. (Reproduced, with permission, from Lister G: *The Hand: Diagnosis and Indications,* 3rd ed. New York: Churchill Livingstone, 1993.)

Although lateral dislocations of the metacarpophalangeal joint are rare, isolated radial collateral ligament ruptures may occur. These injuries should also be immobilized in approximately 30 degrees of flexion for 3 weeks. The fingers should be protected from ulnar stress for an additional 3 weeks. Unstable index and middle finger radial collateral ligament tears should be surgically repaired.

Finger Carpometacarpal Joints

Sprains and fracture-dislocations may involve any of the carpometacarpal joints. Sprains of the index- and middle-finger carpometacarpal joints may occur with palmar flexion and torsion. If tenderness is localized to the carpometacarpal joint and careful radiographs fail to demonstrate fracture, a sprain may be diagnosed.

Treatment of acute sprain injuries consists of 3–6 weeks of immobilization. If localized pain persists, steroid injection may be considered. Chronic pain at the index middle trapezoid capitate joint may be treated with either carpal boss excision or arthrodesis of the carpometacarpal joint. Carpometacarpal fracture-dislocations of the ring and little fingers are usually secondary to direct or longitudinal blows. Dorsal dislocations are more common than volar dislocations. Oblique views with partial pronation and supination may be required to clearly visualize the carpometacarpal joint. Closed reduction may be achieved with longitudinal distraction. The reduction may be maintained by percutaneous Kirschner wire fixation. When fracture-dislocation of the little-finger metacarpal articular surface shears off a fragment of the hamate, displacement of the metacarpal shaft is likely. Because of forces of the extensor carpi ulnaris and the hypothenar muscles, the metacarpal shaft tends to displace proximally and angulate palmarly. Longitudinal traction and percutaneous Kirschner wire fixation of the ring- and little-finger metacarpals will stabilize these fractures. Open reduction is necessary for an irreducible dislocation or for chronic fracture-dislocations. If the patient develops degenerative arthritis of the hamate metacarpal joint, arthrodesis of the ring or small finger carpometacarpal joint (or both) is well tolerated.

Thumb Metacarpophalangeal Joint

The most common injury to the metacarpophalangeal joint is sprain of the ulnar collateral ligament of the thumb (gamekeeper's thumb, skier's thumb). This injury occurs when the thumb is forced into radial deviation, stressing the ulnar collateral ligament. When the ulnar collateral ligament tears from its phalangeal insertion, the adductor aponeurosis may become interposed between the retracted ligament, preventing healing of the ligament to the proximal phalanx with closed treatment (Stener's lesion). Evaluation of the integrity of the ligament may be made by radially stressing the flexed metacarpophalangeal joint under local anesthesia. Radial deviation that is more than 30 degrees from that of the opposite thumb is diagnostic of a totally disrupted, incompetent ligament.

Closed treatment of a partial ligament tear may be accomplished with a thumb spica splint for 3–4 weeks. Complete disruption of the ligament requires surgical exploration and reattachment to the bone. Avulsion of the ulnar collateral ligament may also occur with a bony fragment. If the fragment is greater than 15% of the articular surface or if the avulsed fragment is displaced more than 5 mm, open repair of the ligament is recommended.

Chronic symptomatic ulnar collateral ligament injuries may be repaired if the residual ligament is of sufficient quality. Supplementation of the repair with either tendon transfer or tendon grafting may be useful. In patients who have developed traumatic arthritis or if ligament reconstruction is not deemed feasible, arthrodesis of the metacarpophalangeal joint is preferred.

Thumb Carpometacarpal Joint

Four patterns of thumb metacarpal fracture are most commonly encountered.

A. BENNETT'S FRACTURE

Bennett's fracture is an intra-articular fracture in which the small volar radial fragment of the metacarpal articular surface remains attached to the anterior oblique ligament, while the remainder of the metacarpal articular surface and shaft is displaced proximally, radially, and into adduction in response to the force of the adductor pollicis and abductor pollicis longus muscles (Figure 10–32). Acute Bennett's fractures may often be reduced by traction and pressure on the proximal metacarpal, with slight pronation. The reduction may then be stabilized by percutaneous pin fixation through the metacarpal shaft into either the fragment or the trapezium. If satisfactory reduction cannot be achieved by closed means, open reduction and internal fixation are required.

B. ROLANDO'S FRACTURE

Rolando's fracture is a comminuted T or Y intra-articular fracture. When large fragments are present, open reduction and internal fixation is possible. When the joint is highly comminuted, cast immobilization, traction, or limited open reduction and internal fixation with cast immobilization may be employed.

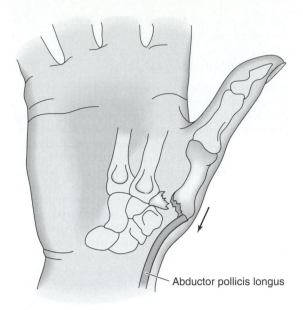

Abductor pollicis longus

Figure 10–32. Bennett's fracture. The first metacarpal shaft is displaced by the pull of the muscle. (Reproduced, with permission, from American Society for Surgery of the Hand: *The Hand: Examination and Diagnosis,* 2nd ed. New York: Churchill Livingstone, 1983.)

C. EXTRA-ARTICULAR FRACTURE

Extra-articular fractures are much less likely to develop traumatic arthritis. Because of the mobility of the carpometacarpal joint of the thumb, significant angulation (> 30 degrees) can be accepted without functional loss.

D. EPIPHYSEAL FRACTURE

Epiphyseal fractures of the thumb metacarpal are treated like other Salter-Harris fractures.

Belsky MR et al: Closed reduction and internal fixation of proximal phalangeal fractures. J Hand Surg Am 1984;9:725.

Eaton R, Malerich M: Volar plate arthroplasty of the proximal interphalangeal joint: A review of ten years' experience. J Hand Surg (Am) 1980;5:260.

Kiefhaber TR, Stern PJ: Fractures dislocations of the proximal interphalangeal joint. J Hand Surg Am 1998;23:368.

Page SM, Stern PJ: Complications and range of motion following plate fixation of metacarpal and phalangeal fractures. J Hand Surg Am 1998;23:827.

WRIST INJURIES

Scaphoid Injuries

The scaphoid is the most commonly fractured bone in the carpus. Anatomically, the scaphoid may be divided into proximal, middle, and distal thirds. The middle third is termed the **waist.** The scaphoid tubercle forms a distal volar prominence. Because the scaphoid articulates with four carpal bones and the radius, most of its surface is composed of articular cartilage. Therefore, the vascular supply to the scaphoid comes through a narrow nonarticular region in the waist. Most of the blood supply to the scaphoid enters distally. In approximately one third of fractures at the waist level, there is diminished flow to the proximal pole. This may result in avascular necrosis of the proximal pole of the scaphoid. Almost 100% of proximal pole fractures will develop aseptic necrosis.

Middle third fractures account for approximately 70% of scaphoid fractures, proximal pole fractures for 20%, and distal pole fractures for the rest.

Cast immobilization is recommended in the treatment of all nondisplaced scaphoid fractures, which are fractures with less than 2 mm of displacement and no fracture site angulation. On average, middle third fractures will heal in 6–12 weeks, distal third fractures in 4–8 weeks, and proximal third fractures in 12–20 weeks. When initial radiographs demonstrate fracture displacement, open reduction and internal fixation is required to prevent malunion. Internal fixation is accomplished with either smooth Kirschner wires or a buried compression screw. Because of the significant time to union in proximal pole fractures, some surgeons recommend primary fixation of these fractures even when nondisplaced. Recent studies have supported percutaneous fixation of nondisplaced waist fractures to decrease the period of cast immobilization.

Delayed union may be treated with either prolonged casting or open reduction, curettage, and bone grafting. Nondisplaced ununited fractures may be treated by excavation of the scaphoid and placement of a volar corticocancellous bone graft (**Matti-Russe procedure**). If fracture site angulation or collapse is present, a cortical cancellous volar graft is employed to correct the deformity. The graft must be stabilized with either a buried compression screw or Kirschner wires. If the proximal pole is avascular and no significant radiocarpal arthritis is present, revascularization of the scaphoid with a vascularized bone graft from the dorsal radius should be performed.

Although excision of the ununited scaphoid and replacement with a silicone implant was favored by many authors in the past, silicone particulate-induced synovitis has developed in many cases. Silicone carpal implant is no longer a recommended treatment. Once degenerative arthritis is evident at the radiocarpal joint, salvage procedures include proximal row carpectomy, scaphoid excision and midcarpal arthrodesis, or total wrist arthrodesis.

Lunate & Perilunate Dislocations

Lunate and perilunate dislocations are the result of a powerful force causing disruption of the ligamentous support about the lunate. The mechanism of these injuries is usually dorsiflexion, ulnar deviation, and intercarpal supination. Mayfield has defined four stages of disruption. Stage 1 injuries demonstrate disruptions of the scapholunate ligament. Stage 2 injuries also include tears of the ligaments dorsal to the lunate. In stage 3 injuries, the arc of disruption extends across the lunotriquetral ligament. Stage 4 injuries have total disruption of the entire lunate ligamentous support. The sequence of injuries is paralleled by a progression of clinical entities from scapholunate dissociation to perilunate dislocation to lunate dislocation.

When the entire carpus except the lunate dislocates and the lunate remains normally seated in the lunate fossa of the radius, the abnormality is termed **perilunate dislocation** (Figure 10–33). When the relationship between the carpus and the radius is preserved but the lunate is dislocated palmarward into the carpal tunnel, the condition is termed **lunate dislocation.** Both lunate and perilunate dislocations imply disruption of ligamentous connections between the scaphoid and the lunate, between the capitate and the lunate, and between the lunate and the triquetrum. Although the lunate is bound to the scaphoid by the scapholunate ligament and to the triquetrum through the lunotriquetral ligament, the interval between the lunate and the capitate known as the space of Poirier lacks direct ligamentous connection.

A variant of perilunate dislocation is **transscaphoid perilunate dislocation.** With this injury, the arc of disruption passes through the scaphoid rather than the scapholunate ligament. The disruption then passes between the proximal scaphoid and the capitate, between the capitate and the lunate, and between the lunate and the triquetrum.

Intercarpal ligamentous disruptions will heal if the normally connected bones are maintained in an anatomic relationship. Intercarpal dislocations should be reduced initially in a closed fashion. Reduction is usually achieved by longitudinal traction and direct pressure on the dislocated carpal bone or bones. Occasionally, anatomic alignment of the carpus can be achieved and maintained with closed reduction and cast application. In most instances, however, open reduction, pin fixation, and direct ligamentous repair is necessary to secure anatomic reduction. Surgical treatment of perilunate and lunate dislocations often requires both palmar and dorsal approaches. Through the dorsal approach, intercarpal alignment is visualized, adjusted, and stabilized. The palmar approach is employed to release the median nerve at the carpal tunnel and to repair the rent in the space of Poirier.

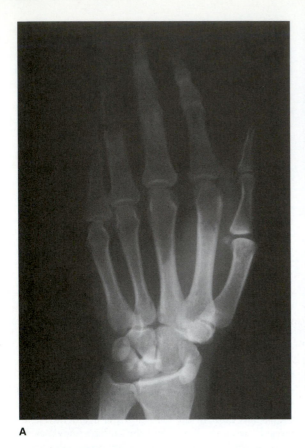

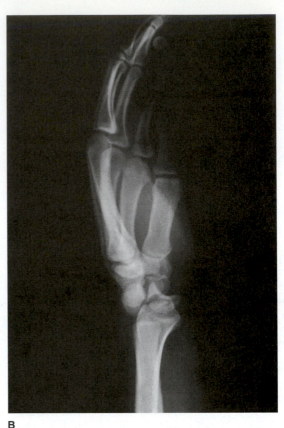

A

B

Figure 10–33. Perilunate dislocation: Anteroposterior view (**A**); lateral view (**B**).

Kienbock's Disease

Kienbock's disease results from ischemic necrosis of the lunate. The cause of the condition is the subject of extensive debate. It is more common in patients with a negative ulnar variance, in which the ulna is shorter than the radius. It is unclear whether the relatively shorter ulna alters and increases the force transmitted to the lunate through the lunate fossa of the radius or whether the altered stress causes the lunate to be shaped in a more triangular and less cuboid or trapezoidal configuration.

Kienbock's disease may be classified based upon the extent of collapse (Figure 10–34). Stage I disease demonstrates a linear compression fracture but an otherwise normal-appearing architecture and density. MRI studies will show poor vascularity of the lunate in stage I (Figure 10–35). In stage II disease, on plain films, the density is abnormal. By stage III, lunate collapse is present. Stage III disease is subdivided into stage IIIA, in which the lunate is collapsed but carpal height remains normal, and stage IIIB, in which the lunate is collapsed

and carpal height is also abnormal. At stage IV, extensive osteoarthritic changes are present.

The current recommendations for the treatment of Kienbock's disease include radial shortening osteotomy for ulnar-negative or neutral variance when no carpal collapse is present. If the patient initially demonstrates a positive ulnar variance, recommendations consist of either a capitate shortening osteotomy or an intercarpal arthrodesis of the scaphoid, trapezium, and trapezoid. A new technique is to restore the anatomic height of the lunate with a vascularized bone graft and additional cancellous bone. In stage IIIB and IV wrists, consideration is given to either proximal row carpectomy or wrist arthrodesis. Silicone replacement of the lunate is no longer routinely advised for Kienbock's disease.

Carpal Instability

To properly determine the orientation of the carpus, true anteroposterior and lateral radiographs are required. The anteroposterior view should be obtained

Stage I

Stage II

Stage III

Stage IV

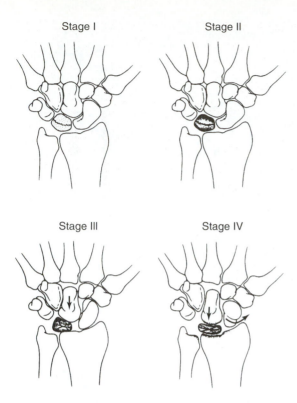

Figure 10–34. Staging of Kienbock's disease (after Lichtman). Stage I: Routine radiographs (posteroanterior, lateral) are normal, but tomography may show a linear fracture, usually transverse through the body of the lunate. MRI will confirm avascular changes. Stage II: Bone density increase (sclerosis) and a fracture line are usually evident on the posteroanterior radiograph. Posteroanterior and lateral tomograms demonstrate sclerosis, cystic changes, and often a clear fracture. There is no collapse deformity. Stage III: Advanced bone density changes are present, with fragmentation, cystic resorption, and collapse. The diagnosis is evident from posteroanterior radiograph. Tomograms (posteroanterior and lateral) show the degree of lunate infractation and amount of fracture displacement. Proximal migration of the capitate is present, and there is mild to moderate rotary alignment of the scaphoid. Stage IV: Perilunate arthritic changes are present, with complete collapse and fragmentation of the lunate. Carpal instability is evident, with scaphoid malalignment and capitate displacement into the lunate space. (Reproduced, with permission, from Rockwood CA Jr et al, eds: *Fractures in Adults,* 3rd ed. Baltimore: Lippincott, 1991.)

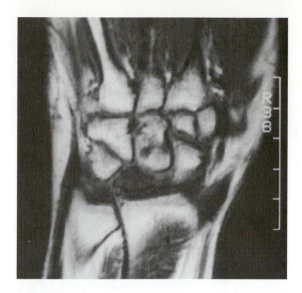

Figure 10–35. MRI showing Kienbock's disease.

with the forearm positioned in neutral rotation to allow a precise standardized evaluation of the relationship between the distal radius and the distal ulna. When the ulna is shorter than the radius, the term **negative ulnar variance** is used, and when the ulna extends further distally than the radius, the term **positive ulnar variance** is used.

The anteroposterior radiograph should demonstrate the close relationship of the scaphoid and the lunate. Normally, the ossified portions of these two bones are separated by their abutting respective articular cartilage shells, creating a radiographic "gap" of 3 mm or less. A gap of more than 3 mm is considered abnormal and is indicative of separation of these two bones secondary to ligamentous disruption. When the scapholunate gap is abnormally wide on a standard radiograph, the abnormality is referred to as **static scapholunate dissociation** (Figure 10–36). When the standard anteroposterior radiograph is normal but an anteroposterior radiograph taken with the fingers squeezing tightly to form a fist reveals an abnormal gap, the condition is referred to as **dynamic scapholunate dissociation.**

The lateral radiograph should be obtained with the wrist in a neutral position, neither flexed nor extended. The lateral radiograph is often overlooked because of the projected superimposition of shadows. This normal overlapping allows measurement of a number of angles between bones. Normally, the middle metacarpal, capitate, lunate, and radius are collinear. The long axis of the radius is readily defined. Establishing the relationship of the scaphoid to the radius requires defining a line drawn along the most palmar portions of the distal

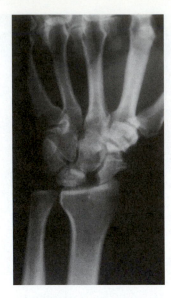

Figure 10–36. Anteroposterior view of static scapholunate dissociation.

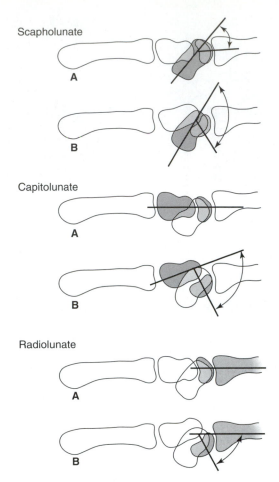

Figure 10–37. Carpal angle measurements are of considerable aid in identifying carpal instability patterns. **A** = normal angle; **B** = abnormal angle seen in dorsiflexion instability. The capitolunate angle should theoretically be 0 degrees with the wrist in neutral position, but the range of normal probably extends to as much as 15 degrees. The scapholunate angle may be the most helpful; an angle of greater than 80 degrees is definite evidence of dorsiflexion instability. The radiolunate angle is abnormal if it exceeds 15 degrees. (Reproduced, with permission, from Green DP, ed: *Operative Hand Surgery*, 2nd ed. New York: Churchill Livingstone, 1988.)

and proximal poles of the scaphoid. The axes of the radius and the scaphoid intersect, forming the **radioscaphoid angle** (Figure 10–37). This angle is usually between 40 and 60 degrees. When the angle is greater than 60 degrees, the scaphoid is abnormally flexed.

The orientation of the lunate viewed on the lateral radiograph is derived by first establishing a line between the most distal palmar and dorsal lips of the lunate. A second line is then drawn perpendicular to the first line, establishing the axis of the lunate. The angle between the radial and lunate axes (**radiolunate angle**) is normally less than 15 degrees.

The orientation of the lunate seen on the lateral radiograph normally reflects a ligamentous balancing of the influences of the adjacent scaphoid and triquetrum. The scaphoid tends to tether the lunate into flexion through the scapholunate ligament, whereas the triquetrum tends to tether the lunate into extension (dorsiflexion) through the lunotriquetral ligament. When the scapholunate ligament is disrupted, the scaphoid tends to flex excessively, and the lunate, under the unopposed influence of the triquetrum, dorsiflexes (**dorsal intercalated segment instability [DISI]**) (Figure 10–38). When the lunotriquetral ligament is disrupted, the lunate, under the unopposed influence of the scaphoid, is flexed (**volar intercalated segment instability [VISI]**). The optimal treatment for DISI is currently an area of intense interest. Acute ligamentous disruption is usually treated with direct ligamentous

reapproximation and repair. When ligamentous repair is not possible but degenerative changes have not occurred, ligamentous reconstruction, dorsal capsular ligamentodesis, or intercarpal fusions may be considered.

Degenerative arthritis occurs in wrists subjected over time to loads applied to noncongruently articulating

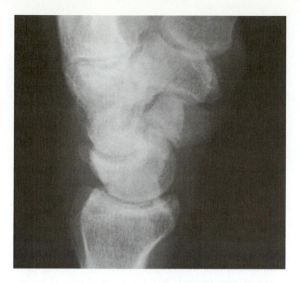

Figure 10–38. Lateral radiograph of dorsal intercalated segment instability.

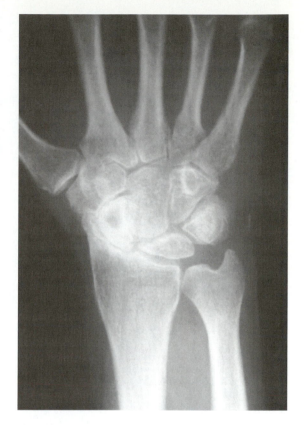

Figure 10–39. Scapholunate advanced collapse pattern.

carpal bones. The **scapholunate advanced collapse pattern** (SLAC wrist) describes the evolution of degenerative arthritis resulting from disruption of the scapholunate ligament (Figure 10–39). The earliest evidence of degenerative change is seen at the radioscaphoid joint, and with time, degenerative change progresses to include the capitate lunate articulation. When radioscaphoid change is present but the articular surface of the capitate retains its normal articular cartilage, proximal row carpectomy (removal of the scaphoid, lunate, and triquetrum) will allow preservation of wrist motion as the capitate head shifts proximally to articulate within the lunate fossa of the distal radius. When degenerative change is present at the capitate lunate portion of the midcarpal joints in addition to radioscaphoid change, the scaphoid may be excised and intercarpal fusion of the capitate, lunate, triquetrum, and hamate accomplished. This selective intercarpal fusion procedure provides motion through the residual radiolunate articulation. Complete wrist fusion provides reliable pain relief while permanently sacrificing wrist motion.

Distal Radioulnar Joint

The distal radioulnar joint (DRUJ) is composed of two joints. The proximal and distal articulations of the ulna and radius allow forearm rotation. The ulna also articulates with the ulnar carpus through the triangular fibrocartilage complex (TFCC). Approximately 20% of the load from the hand to the forearm passes through the ulnocarpal joint. Problems at the DRUJ are related to one or both of these joints.

When the ulnar variance is positive, the patient may develop an ulnocarpal impaction syndrome. This often presents with pain on the ulnar side of the wrist, particularly with ulnar deviation. Radiographs may be positive for degenerative changes of the distal ulna and ulnar lunate. Treatment consists of shortening the ulna. This may be done by removing 2–3 mm of the ulnar head (wafer procedure) either by open method, by arthroscope, or by an ulnar-shortening osteotomy, performed in the diaphyseal ulna, and fixed with a plate and screws. After the wafer procedure, patients often complain of ulnar pain for a prolonged (3–6 month) period. Approximately 50% of patients who have an ulnar shortening osteotomy will require plate removal.

Another source of ulnar-sided wrist pain is a tear of the TFCC. Tears are divided into degenerative and traumatic types. Degenerative tears are usually related to ulnocarpal impaction. Traumatic tears usually occur after a twisting injury of the wrist. Central tears and tears near the radial attachment are usually treated with an arthroscopic debridement. Tears in the well-vascularized periphery of the TFCC are treated with arthroscopic or open repair. After repair, patients are maintained in a long arm cast for 6 weeks to allow cartilage healing.

Arthritis between the radius and ulna can be caused by traumatic, degenerative, or inflammatory arthritis. Treatment consists of hemiresection or complete excision of the ulnar head (Darrach's procedure). An alternative treatment is fusion of the DRUJ with creation of a pseudarthrosis of the distal ulna (Suave-Kapandji procedure). This is particularly useful in the presence of ulnar translocation of the carpus.

One of the most difficult problems to treat is instability of the DRUJ. Instability is usually the result of trauma, but it may occur after an excessive distal ulna resection. In treating DRUJ instability, it must first be determined that no malunions are present in the radius and ulna. A number of operations have been designed to stabilize the distal ulna, all with varying degrees of success.

Adams BD, Berger RA: An anatomic reconstruction of the distal radioulnar ligaments for posttraumatic distal radioulnar joint instability. J Hand Surg [Am]. 2002;27(2):243. [PMID: 11901383]

Berger RA: The anatomy of the ligaments of the wrist and distal radioulnar joints. Clin Orthop. 2001;(383):32. Review. [PMID: 11210966]

Blatt G: Capsulodesis in reconstructive hand surgery: Dorsal capsulodesis for the unstable scaphoid and volar capsulodesis following excision of the distal ulna. Hand Clin 1987; 3:81.

Cohen MS, Kozin SH: Degenerative arthritis of the wrist: Proximal row carpectomy versus scaphoid excision and four-corner arthrodesis. J Hand Surg [Am]. 2001;26(1):94. [PMID: 11172374]

Gelberman RH et al: Ulnar variance with Kienbock's disease. J Bone Joint Surg Am 1975;57:674.

Linscheid RL et al: Traumatic instability of the wrist. J Bone Joint Surg Am 1972;54:1612.

Mayfield JK et al: Carpal dislocations: Pathomechanics and progressive perilunar instability. J Hand Surg (Am) 1980;5:226.

Palmer A, Werner FW: The triangular fibrocartilage complex of the wrist: Anatomy and function. J Hand Surg (Am) 1981;6:153.

Rettig ME et al: Open reduction and internal fixation of acute displaced scaphoid waist fractures. J Hand Surg [Am]. 2001;26 (2):271. [PMID: 11279573]

Shin AY et al: Treatment of isolated injuries of the lunotriquetral ligament. A comparison of arthrodesis, ligament reconstruction and ligament repair. J Bone Joint Surg Br. 2001;83 (7):1023. [PMID: 11603516]

Steinmann SP et al: Use of the 1,2 intercompartmental supraretinacular artery as a vascularized pedicle bone graft for difficult scaphoid nonunion. J Hand Surg [Am]. 2002;27(3):391. [PMID: 12015712]

Walsh JJ et al: Current status of scapholunate interosseous ligament injuries. J Am Acad Orthop Surg. 2002;10(1):32. Review. [PMID: 11809049]

Watson HK, Ballet FL: The SLAC wrist: Scapholunate advanced collapse pattern of degenerative arthritis. J Hand Surg Am 1984;9:358.

Wyrick JD et al: Motion-preserving procedures in the treatment of scapholunate advanced collapse wrist: Proximal row carpectomy versus four-corner arthrodesis. J Hand Surg Am 1995; 20:965.

■ FINGERTIP INJURIES

SOFT-TISSUE INJURIES

Because of the importance of the fingertip in providing a contact surface for sensate prehension, injuries to the fingertip may result in significant disability. The pulp of the fingertip is covered by tough, highly innervated skin, anchored to the phalanx by fibrous septa. The dorsum of the fingertip is composed of the nail and nail bed.

Treatment

The goals in treatment of fingertip injuries are to provide adequate sensation, minimal tenderness, satisfactory appearance, and full joint motion. Preservation of length should be integrated with the previously mentioned goals.

The choice of treatment is dependent on the size and location of the defect. The mechanism of injury (sharp, crushing, or avulsion), whether bone is exposed, and the angle of loss are all important considerations in planning treatment.

A. OPEN WOUND CARE

The simplest treatment is open wound care. This is indicated in most injuries in children and in defects of 1 cm^2 or less in adults. The wound is thoroughly cleansed. Bone is shortened so that it is covered by soft tissue and the length of the bone is the same as the length of the nail bed. Dressings are changed until the wound is healed. The disadvantages of the open method are the possibility of stump tenderness and prolonged healing time. Advantages include the ability to initiate and preserve full digital motion.

B. COMPOSITE GRAFTING

Replacement of the amputated part as a composite graft (skin and subcutaneous tissue) is indicated in children and selected adults with sharp distal amputations. When successful, this treatment gives the best appearance. The disadvantages, however, are unpredictability of the viability of the part, with recovery delayed by failure and secondary procedures.

C. MICROVASCULAR REPLANTATION

Microvascular replantation is possible in selected sharp amputations distal to the distal interphalangeal joint. Disadvantages include the expense of complex surgery and the time lost from work.

D. PRIMARY SHORTENING AND CLOSURE

Primary shortening and closure is indicated when more than 50% of the distal phalanx has been lost or the nail matrix has been irreparably damaged. This one-stage procedure allows for immediate mobilization. In performing the procedure, the end of the distal phalanx bone should be trimmed to provide a tension-free closure. The nail bed should be trimmed as far proximal as the bone. If the nail bed is pulled over the end of the shortened bone, a hook-shaped nail will result. Neurectomy of digital nerves under traction allows the nerve ends to retract from scar tissue into proximal soft tissue.

E. SKIN GRAFTING

Skin grafting may also be employed to obtain closure if no bone is exposed. Split-thickness grafts may be placed on a less well vascularized bed. Split-thickness grafts contract more than full-thickness grafts. As the graft shrinks, the area of sensory loss also shrinks. The appearance and durability of scar tissue may be less than ideal, however.

Full-thickness skin grafts provide more durable coverage and better appearance. Care should be taken to match the pigmentation of the skin at the donor and recipient sites. The ulnar border of the hand provides an ideal donor source. Full-thickness grafts require a better vascularized bed to ensure survival.

F. SKIN FLAPS

Local advancement skin flaps are useful in the treatment of fingertip injuries.

1. V-Y advancement skin flaps—V-Y advancement skin flaps may advance palmar tissue or unite two lateral skin flaps. These skin flaps are helpful in the management of transverse or dorsal oblique amputations in which soft-tissue tip coverage is needed and further skeletal shortening deemed undesirable. Complete separation of the vertical septa between the skin and the bone is required to mobilize skin flaps for advancement. The septa between the flap and the proximal skin must then be divided. Traction on the flap will help differentiate the septa from vessels and nerves.

2. Moberg palmar advancement flap—Defects of up to 1.5 cm on the thumb may be covered by a palmar advancement flap known as the Moberg flap. Bilateral midlateral incisions dorsal to the neurovascular bundles of the thumb allow mobilization of the flap from the flexor tendon sheath. The flap may be maximally advanced by flexion of the thumb interphalangeal joint. When additional coverage is required, the skin of the flap may be transversely divided at the metacarpophalangeal crease, the distal portion of the flap may be advanced further, and a skin graft may be placed between the distal flap and the proximal flap. Disadvantages of this flap include the possibility of interphalangeal joint flexion contracture and the potential for dorsal tip necrosis if dorsal vascular branches to the digit are injured.

3. Regional skin flaps—Regional skin flaps are considered when fingertip skin has been lost but nail and bone have been preserved.

  a. Cross-finger flap—The cross-finger flap is the most commonly used. Skin is elevated from the dorsum of the adjacent finger, with care being taken not to incise the extensor paratenon. The skin is then rotated palmarward and sewn to the palmar defect of the involved finger. The donor region on the donor finger is skin grafted. The transposed flap is divided from the donor finger after 2 weeks. Joint stiffness is a potential complication in both the donor and recipient digits. The creation of a defect on a normal digit is another disadvantage.

  b. Thenar flap—The thenar flap may be used in children and young adults in whom the potential for joint stiffness is less. More subcutaneous fat is transferred with a thenar flap than with a cross-finger flap. Thenar skin flaps usually result in good matching of color and texture with the pulp.

■ NAIL BED INJURIES

Clinical Findings

Nail bed injuries, often neglected, should be carefully attended to because the nail enhances sensibility, provides protection and fine manipulation of the finger, and gives the finger a normal appearance. The nail bed may be injured by subungual hematoma, nail matrix laceration, avulsion of the nail matrix from the nail fold, or complete loss of the nail matrix.

Treatment

When a subungual hematoma involves more than 50% of the subungual area, the nail should be removed and the nail bed laceration repaired with fine absorbable suture. Either the nail is replaced or a dressing is placed under the nail fold to prevent synechia formation with resultant splitting of the nail. Nail bed defects are treated with split-thickness nail bed grafts taken from either an adjacent uninjured fingernail or a toenail.

When nail bed injuries occur with an open distal phalangeal fracture, consideration should be given to pin fixation of the fracture because this will stabilize the nail repair.

Caution is required in the treatment of nail bed injuries in children, who often suffer injury from having a fingertip slammed in a door. The nail often lies dorsal to the nail fold, and a small subungual hematoma is noted. If a radiograph is obtained, usually a physeal fracture of the distal phalanx is observed. Because the nail bed laceration communicates with the physeal fracture, this injury represents an open fracture and must be treated appropriately. The nail should be removed and the fracture site irrigated. Often, an interposed portion of the nail bed must be extracted from between the fragments of the physeal fracture. If the fracture is unstable, pin fixation will facilitate nail bed repair. Failure to appreciate the open nature of this pediatric injury may result in osteomyelitis of the distal phalanx.

Atasoy E et al: Reconstruction of the amputated fingertip with a triangular volar flap: A new surgical procedure. J Bone Joint Surg Am 1970;52:921.

Kappel DA, Burech JG: The cross-finger flap: An established reconstructive procedure. Hand Clin 1985;1:677.

Macht SD, Watson HK: The Moberg advancement flap for digital reconstruction. J Hand Surg (Am) 1980;5:372.

■ THERMAL INJURY

ACUTE BURN INJURY

Degree of Injury

A. First-Degree Burns

Burns are characterized by the depth of skin injury. First-degree burns involve only the epidermis. Patients usually present with swollen red areas, and care is symptomatic.

B. Second-Degree Burns

Second-degree burns involve both the epidermis and the superficial portion of the dermis. These burns may be identified by skin blistering and blanching of the skin when pressure is applied. Second-degree burns are subdivided into superficial and deep burns. Superficial second-degree burns are treated with topical antibiotics such as silver sulfadiazine. The extremity is elevated and the hand splinted in the intrinsic plus position. With the wrist in 30 degrees of extension, the metacarpophalangeal joint is flexed and the interphalangeal joints are extended. The thumb should be maintained in an abducted position to prevent contracture of the first web space. The patient should begin a vigorous therapy program emphasizing active range of motion as soon as it is tolerated. Compression garments may be required for swelling after reepithelialization.

In deep second-degree burns, excision of the remaining portion of the skin and application of a skin graft does not produce long-term results superior to those achieved with spontaneous healing. Therefore, the treatment of deep second-degree burns should be similar to that of superficial second-degree burns.

C. Third-Degree Burns

Third-degree burns involve the entire epidermis, dermis, and a portion of the subcutaneous region. These burns result in waxy dry regions often having a nontender central area, caused by burning of the neural tissue. Third-degree burns should be treated with excision within the first 3–7 days and a split-thickness skin graft of the involved areas.

D. Fourth-Degree Burns

In addition to involvement of the skin, fourth-degree burns involve deep tissues, including muscle, tendon, and bone. Often, the only effective treatment for these burns is amputation of the involved part, with appropriate soft tissue coverage of the residual stump.

Complications

A. Neurovascular Complications

The neurovascular status of the burned hand should be carefully monitored. Massive swelling will necessitate release of compartments of the hand and forearm. Digital releases are best performed by longitudinal releases along the ulnar border of the index, middle, and ring fingers and along the radial border of the thumb and little finger. Longitudinal incisions on the dorsal hand allow decompression of interosseous muscle compartments. Incisions are made along the medial and lateral aspects of the arm and forearm.

B. Late Complications

1. Joint contractures—Joint contractures are the most common complications of upper extremity burns. At the elbow, these are most often flexion contractures. Treatment consists of soft-tissue release and either skin grafting of open regions or rotation of local skin flaps. Elbow motion may also be limited by the development of heterotopic ossifications. Excision of the ossification may be successful if delayed until the area of ossification has matured 1½–2 years after the burn injury. Because the area of most intense heterotopic ossification is posteromedially, care must be taken to protect the ulnar nerve during elbow release surgery.

2. Wrist and hand contractures—Wrist contracture may tether the hand into either a flexed or extended position, depending on the region of the burn. In the fingers, burns usually involve the thin skin on the dorsum of the finger, often disrupting the central slip insertion onto the middle phalanx. The loss of active proximal interphalangeal joint extension combined with dorsal hand burns may result in development of a "claw" deformity, with flexion contractures of the proximal interphalangeal joints and hyperextension contracture at the metacarpophalangeal joint.

Treatment of metacarpophalangeal joint extension contracture usually requires release of the dorsal scar, addition of a dorsal skin graft, and dorsal capsular release. The most predictable treatment of severe proximal interphalangeal joint contracture in the burn patient is arthrodesis of the proximal interphalangeal joint. Proximal interphalangeal flexion contractures may also occur secondary to scarred volar skin. In such cases, soft tissue release may be accomplished with either Z-plasty flap transposition or by palmar scar excision and full-thickness skin graft application.

Adduction contracture, the most common thumb deformity in the burned hand, may be difficult to fully resolve. The extent of release required depends upon the degree of contracture. A modest adduction contracture may be effectively treated with Z-plasty of the thenar skin to regain adequate abduction in the first web space. With more severe contracture, release of the adductor pollicis from its origin or at its insertion and release of the first dorsal interosseous muscle origin from the thumb metacarpal may be required. If web space skin coverage is inadequate after muscle release, full-thickness skin grafting or local or distant skin flaps may be needed.

Ideally, first web space contracture should be avoided. This is done by carefully maintaining the first web space during the initial phases of burn treatment. When the extent of web space burn is severe and the normal first web cannot be maintained with dressings, an external fixator should be placed, spanning the thumb and index-finger metacarpals.

ELECTRICAL BURNS

The extent of injury in electrical burns is proportional to the amount of current that passes through the involved portion of the body. Ohm's law states that the amount of current is equal to the voltage divided by the resistance. Therefore, for a given voltage, those structures that have a lower resistance will conduct a greater amount of current. The relative resistance of structures in the arm from least resistance to greatest resistance is as follows: nerve, vessel, muscle, skin, tendon, fat, and bone. Alternating current is more injurious than direct current. Because of its frequency, alternating current produces muscle tetany in the finger flexors, which may prevent the patient from releasing the grasped current source. The duration of contact plays a direct role in the severity of injury because a longer contact period will result in more electrical energy passing through the body.

Clinical Findings

The greatest current density occurs at the entrance and exit wounds, usually apparent as charred areas that are blackened and surrounded by a gray-white zone, an area of tissue necrosis in which the tissue is still intact but will die. These areas are surrounded by a red zone, in which there is a variable extent of vessel thrombosis, coagulation, and necrosis.

High-voltage, or **arc, burns** are noted more for their degree of thermal than electric injury. Arc burns may extend across flexor surfaces from the hand to the wrist or from the forearm to the arm. Arc burns are usually associated with a high temperature of 3000–5000 °C.

It is often difficult to precisely assess the extent of tissue necrosis in burn wounds at the time of initial presentation. All burn patients should be examined for fractures, particularly cervical spine fractures, as electrical burn patients may have been thrown a distance by the current. The possibility of either compartment syndrome or concomitant peripheral nerve injury must also be considered. Patients should be admitted to an intensive care unit and monitored for cardiac arrhythmia, renal failure, sepsis, secondary hemorrhage, and neurologic complications to the brain, spinal cord, or peripheral nerves.

Treatment

Treatment for upper extremity burns consists of initially debriding clearly nonviable tissue. Fasciotomy and nerve decompression should be done as indicated by examination. A second debridement is then performed in 48–72 h, for tissue in the gray-white zones. Debridement should be continued every 48–72 h until a stable wound has been achieved. The extent of necrosis often appears to increase with each successive debridement. This phenomenon reflects both an underestimation of the extent of initial injury and progressive vascular thrombosis. After all necrotic tissue has been debrided, reconstruction is accomplished with either local or distant skin flaps or amputation.

CHEMICAL BURNS

The severity of chemical burns is directly proportional to the concentration and penetrability of the offending agent, the duration of skin exposure, and the mechanism of contact. Destruction will continue until either the chemical combines with the tissue or the agent is neutralized by an applied secondary agent or washed from the skin surface. The mainstay of treatment of chemical burns of the skin is water irrigation.

Two notable exceptions are hydrofluoric acid and white phosphorous chemical burns. In hydrofluoric acid burns, the agent cannot be removed with water. Calcium gluconate 10%, either applied to the skin as a gel or injected subcutaneously, is required to neutralize the acid. Patients with hydrofluoride burns experience severe pain seemingly out of proportion to the injury. White phosphorus burns, also refractory to water irrigation, are treated with 1% copper sulfate solution.

Iatrogenic chemical burns may occur with extravasation of chemotherapeutic agents administered intravenously. Chemotherapeutic agents are classified as **vesicants,** which include doxorubicin and vincristine and have a high probability of causing skin necrosis, and **nonvesicants,** which include cyclophosphamide. Management of both types of injury requires early surgical debridement of the region of extravasation. Secondary wound coverage may be obtained with either split-thickness skin grafting or skin flap coverage.

COLD INJURY (FROSTBITE)

Clinical Findings

Frostbite occurs as the result of cellular injury when the cell membrane is punctured by ice crystals formed in the extracellular space. With the formation of ice crystals, osmotic gradients develop, leading to cell dehydration and electrolyte disturbances. A vascular component to the damage also is present, and patients may develop severe vasoconstriction as a result of increased sympathetic tone. Vessel endothelial injury may cause thrombosis. With capillary endothelial damage, leakage occurs into the extracellular space, resulting in hemoconcentration and sludging within the capillary system.

Frostbite injuries may be classified as either superficial or deep. Superficial frostbite involves only the skin and usually heals spontaneously, whereas deep frostbite damages both the skin and subcutaneous structures (Figure 10–40). As with burn injuries, the depth of the area of necrosis is difficult to determine initially.

Treatment

The initial treatment of frostbite consists of rewarming the part and providing pain relief. The core body tem-

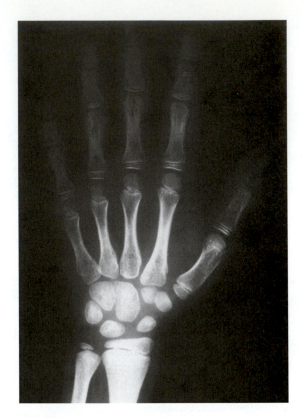

Figure 10–40. Radiograph of deformities of the fingers of the left hand in a 12-year-old girl caused by frostbite incurred at the age of 2 years. Note destruction of epiphyses of middle and distal phalanges of all fingers and deformity of epiphysis of proximal phalanx of little finger. Osseous changes in right hand were similar.

perature should be restored and the frozen extremity rapidly rewarmed in a water bath at 38–42 °C. Because rapid rewarming induces considerable pain, it should be delayed until adequate analgesia can be administered. After rewarming, treatment should include elevation of the hand, local wound care, and dressing changes. Frequent whirlpool debridement and active range-of-motion exercises should be instituted. The role of anticoagulants and sympathectomy in increasing blood flow is controversial.

Long-Term Sequelae

Long-term sequelae depend on the extent of initial injury. Adult patients may develop osteoarthritis of the interphalangeal joints. Skeletally immature patients may develop epiphyseal destruction, with digital shortening, nail dysplasia, and joint destruction. Severe injuries may produce intrinsic muscle atrophy or vasospastic syndrome secondary to increased sympathetic tone. Vasospasm may lead to severe pain, coldness, or edema of the finger; trophic changes leading to decreased nail or hair growth; or Raynaud's phenomenon. In severe injuries, mummification of nonviable portions of the fingers may become apparent. Amputation or surgical debridement of these mummified parts should usually be delayed 60–90 days, unless local infection develops. This delay allows maximal reepithelialization beneath the nonviable tissue.

Dibbell DG et al: Hydrofluoric acid burns of the hand. J Bone Joint Surg Am 1970;52:931.

Woo SH, Seul JH: Optimizing the correction of severe postburn hand deformities by using aggressive contracture releases and fasciocutaneous free-tissue transfers. Plast Reconstr Surg 2001;107(1):1. [PMID: 11176593]

■ HIGH-PRESSURE INJECTION INJURY

Injection machinery used in industry may create pressures of 3000–10,000 psi. The amount of pressure reflects both the design of the nozzle aperture and the distance between the nozzle and the finger. Virtually all patients who sustain injuries with pressures of over 7000 psi require amputation.

Clinical Findings

Injection injuries usually puncture the palmar digital pulp, track to the flexor tendon sheath, and fill the tendon sheath with the injected material. These injuries have a particularly poor prognosis. Injections into the palm have a somewhat better prognosis because the site of the material is unconfined by fascial planes. Prognostic factors include the time interval from injury to treatment, as well as the amount and type of material injected. Whereas paint injection may cause more necrosis of the finger, grease injection will more often lead to fibrosis of the finger. The amputation rate for paint injection injuries is approximately 60% and 20% for grease injection injuries.

The examiner must be wary of the relatively innocuous-appearing entrance wound at the time of initial presentation. Initial pain may be modest but increases with time as more distal swelling and early necrosis occur.

Treatment

The effectiveness of corticosteroids administered every 6 h remains controversial in the treatment of injection injuries. Patients should be brought to the operating room soon after the injury occurs. Thorough debridement of all injected material is attempted. This is easier when the injected material is pigmented. Nonpigmented materials such as kerosene or turpentine are considerably more difficult to thoroughly remove. The hand should be splinted in the safe position. Sympathetic blocks may be helpful in managing pain. Repeat debridement should be done if there is any question of the adequacy of the initial procedure.

Although injection injuries may appear relatively simple, these are severe injuries that will compromise function and result in amputation. The seriousness of these injuries should be recognized at the time of presentation.

Gelberman RH et al: High-pressure injection injuries of the hand. J Bone Joint Surg Am 1975;57:935.

Failla JM, Linden MD: The acute pathologic changes of paint-injection injury and correlation to surgical treatment: A report of two cases. J Hand Surg Am 1997;22:156.

■ INFECTIONS OF THE HAND

Felon

A felon is an abscess of the pulp space of the distal phalanx. Vertical septa between the skin and the bone create small closed compartments within the pulp space. Infection in this region produces localized erythema, swelling, and throbbing pain.

Treatment of these infections requires incision and drainage, with release of the vertical septa to completely decompress the pulp space (Figure 10–41). A drain is placed in the wound, the hand is elevated, and intravenous antibiotics are administered.

Paronychia

Paronychia is the most common digital infection. The paronychia is the gutter along both the radial and ulnar borders of the fingernail. The eponychium is the roof of the nail over the nail lunula. Paronychial infections may be classified as acute or chronic.

A. ACUTE INFECTION

Acute infections are most often caused by *Staphylococcus aureus*. They begin as a localized cellulitis, with erythema around the nail. Untreated, this cellulitis may progress to an abscess at the nail margin.

Treatment of early infection includes warm soaks and oral antibiotics. Once an abscess has formed, inci-

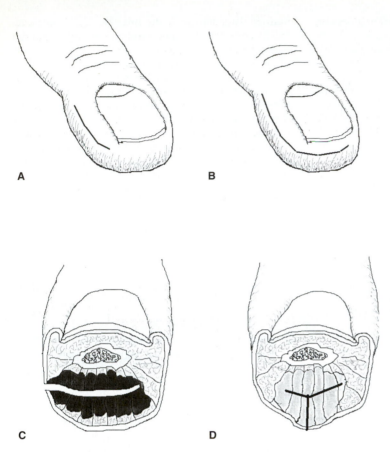

Figure 10–41. Incisions for drainage of felons. **A:** Unilateral longitudinal approach that should be used for most felons. It is generally made on the ulnar side of the finger, unless it is the little finger, to preserve sensation. **B:** The hockey stick, or dJ, incision should be reserved for extensive or severe abscess or felon. **C:** The incision must decompress the longitudinal septa, but should not go through-and-through. **D:** The felon that points volarly may be decompressed through a longitudinal, midline incision, which is preferable due to less risk to sensory nerves. A transverse incision may also be made but there is risk of damage to the digital nerves. (Courtesy of HB Skinner, ©copyright 2002.)

sion and drainage is required. To adequately debride the region, either an incision is made in the abscess and the abscess packed, or a portion of the lateral nail is removed and the abscess decompressed.

B. CHRONIC INFECTION

Chronic paronychial infections are most often caused by *Candida* spp. These occur commonly in patients who work with their hands in water, such as bartenders or dishwashers. Patients may have repeated episodes of acute infection in addition to chronic infection.

Treatment of chronic infection may be accomplished by eponychial marsupialization, excision of a segment of the eponychia without incision of the nail roof. Simultaneous nail removal may increase the effectiveness of marsupialization.

Web Space Abscess

Web space abscesses most often occur after palmar puncture wounds. The infection spreads from the palm along the path of least resistance to the dorsal web

space. Treatment requires dorsal and palmar incision, drain placement, open wound care, and appropriate antibiotic coverage.

Flexor Suppurative Tenosynovitis

Kanavel described four cardinal signs of acute suppurative tenosynovitis: (1) pain on passive digital extension, (2) flexed position of the digit, (3) symmetric swelling of the digit, which may include the palm, and (4) tenderness with palpation along the flexor tendon sheath. Acute suppurative tenosynovitis of the flexor pollicis longus sheath may extend into the thenar space. Likewise, infections in the flexor sheath of the little finger may extend into the ulnar bursa. In some patients, coalescence between the radial and ulnar bursas may allow infection to track in a horseshoe pattern, extending from the thumb to the little finger.

Treatment of acute suppurative tenosynovitis requires incision, irrigation, and drainage. Although an extensive midlateral incision may be used, limited incisions are preferred. Short incisions over the proximal (metacarpophalangeal joint region) and distal (distal interphalangeal region) margins of the flexor tendon sheath allow thorough sheath irrigation (Figure 10–42). The sheath is opened distally and a small tube (16-gauge catheter or No. 8 pediatric feeding tube) is inserted. A drain is placed in the flexor sheath through the proximal wound. Irrigation of the finger is performed with 5 mL of saline injected every 2 h. Intravenous antibiotics are administered, and the hand is elevated.

Two days after surgery the dressing is changed. Swelling should be significantly decreased. The catheter is removed, and the patient is encouraged to begin active range-of-motion exercises.

Bite Injuries

Although bite wounds may initially appear harmless, a bite may inoculate deep tissues with virulent organisms.

A. CAT AND DOG BITES

Because the small puncture wounds of cat bites are more often disregarded than the large tearing wounds of dog bites, late sequelae are most common after cat bites. Cat and dog bites frequently harbor *Pasteurella multocida,* an organism best treated with ampicillin, penicillin, or a first-generation cephalosporin. Acute animal bites may be treated with incision and drainage and an initial course of intravenous antibiotics in the emergency room followed by oral antibiotics.

B. HUMAN BITES

Most human bite wounds result from a fist striking a tooth, which readily penetrates the skin, subcutaneous tissue, extensor tendon, and capsule of the metacarpophalangeal joint (Figure 10–43). Human bites often contain *Eikenella corrodens,* an organism best treated with penicillin or ampicillin. Human bite wounds should be excised and drained, and intravenous antibiotic therapy instituted. Arthrotomy of the metacarpophalangeal joint and irrigation is necessary if this injury is suspected.

C. SPIDER BITES

Although most spider bites are innocuous, the bite of a brown recluse spider requires early wide excision to control the locally injected toxin.

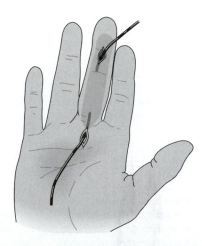

Figure 10–42. Drainage and closed irrigation for flexor sheath infection. The antibiotic solution drips in through the distal catheter and drains out through the proximal one. (Reproduced, with permission, from Way LW, ed: *Current Surgical Diagnosis and Treatment,* 10th ed. Stamford: Appleton & Lange, 1994.)

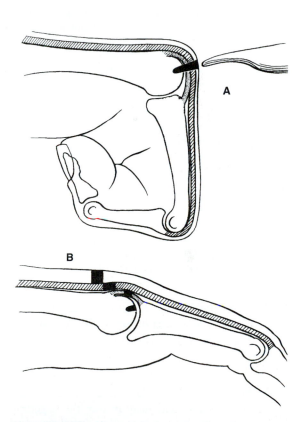

Figure 10–43. Human bite wound of metacarpophalangeal joint. **A:** The tooth pierces the clenched fist of the attacker, penetrating skin, tendon, joint capsule, and metacarpal head. **B:** When the finger is extended by swelling and at surgery, the four puncture wounds do not correspond. (Reproduced, with permission, from Lister G: *The Hand: Diagnosis and Indications,* 3rd ed. New York: Churchill Livingstone, 1993.)

Infection Caused by Unusual Organisms

A. Atypical Mycobacterial Infection

Mycobacterium marinum infection may present as a chronically inflamed finger that has been punctured by the spine or a fin of a saltwater fish. Successful culture of the organism is difficult but is most likely at a temperature of 30–32 °C. Antitubercular drug therapy is effective in treating and eradicating these infections.

B. Gram-Negative Infection

Because of the risk of a gram-negative infection following mutilating farm injuries or injuries with possible fecal contamination, these patients should be treated with broad-spectrum antibiotics.

C. Anaerobic Infection

When *Clostridium perfringens* infection occurs after hand injury, immediate wide fasciotomy and intravenous penicillin should be instituted. Hyperbaric oxygen therapy may be helpful. If infection cannot be adequately controlled, amputation may be necessary to avoid death.

The possibility of *Clostridium tetani* contamination must be remembered with any puncture wound. Initial evaluation of all patients with penetrating wounds must include questioning about tetanus inoculation. If inoculation is not up to date, antitoxin should be administered.

D. Gonorrhea

A patient who presents with an isolated septic joint or tenosynovitis without a history of puncture wound may have a hematogenous gonorrheal infection. Treatment consists of culturing the involved organism on the appropriate media and treatment with penicillin or tetracycline.

E. Necrotizing Fasciitis

The causative agent in necrotizing fasciitis is most commonly hemolytic *Staphylococcus.* Treatment consists of wide surgical debridement to the fascia and appropriate antibiotics.

F. Herpetic Whitlow

Herpes simplex infections may involve the fingertips. They are most common in medical or dental personnel who care for the oral tracheal area and are also seen in small children. It may be difficult to distinguish these lesions from acute bacterial infections of the fingers. Close examination reveals the presence of groups (crops) of vesicles, with surrounding erythema. Aspiration of a vesicle will reveal clear fluid. Serial viral titers will confirm the diagnosis. In contrast to bacterial infections, however, herpetic whitlow should not be incised, but should simply be treated with splinting and elevation.

Abrams RA, Botte MJ: Hand infections: Treatment recommendations for specific types. J Am Acad Orthop Surg 1996;4:219.

Arons MS et al: *Pasteurella multocida:* The major cause of hand infections following domestic animal bites. J Hand Surg (Am) 1982;7:47.

Bednar MS, Lane LB: Eponychial marsupialization and nail removal for surgical treatment of chronic paronychia. J Hand Surg Am 1991;16:314.

Chuinard RG, D'Ambrosia RD: Human bite infections of the hand. J Bone Joint Surg Am 1977;59:416.

Neviaser RJ: Closed tendon sheath irrigation for pyogenic flexor tenosynovitis. J Hand Surg (Am) 1978;3:462.

■ ARTHRITIS OF THE HAND

OSTEOARTHRITIS

Osteoarthritis is a slowly progressive polyarticular disorder of unknown cause, predominantly affecting the hands and large weight-bearing joints. Clinically, osteoarthritis is characterized by pain, deformity, and limitation of motion. Focal erosions, articular cartilage space loss, subchondral sclerosis, cyst formation, and peripheral joint osteophytes are evident on radiographic examination.

Epidemiologic Factors

The disease occurs commonly in older individuals, with approximately 80–90% of adults over age 75 years showing radiographic evidence of osteoarthritis. The most powerful determinants of developing osteoarthritis of the hand are female gender, increasing age, and positive family history.

The most frequently involved hand joints are the distal interphalangeal joints, carpometacarpal joint of the thumb (Figure 10–44), and proximal interphalangeal joints. The bony enlargement commonly seen in the osteoarthritic distal interphalangeal joint is often referred to as **Heberden's nodes,** whereas osteoarthritic enlargement at the proximal interphalangeal joint is known as **Bouchard's nodes.**

Secondary osteoarthritis may develop in the hand as the result of trauma, avascular necrosis, prior inflammatory arthritis, or metabolic disorders.

Clinical Findings

Patients often complain of activity-induced or work-related pain. Most patients experience periods of exacerbation and remission. Functional limitations result from pain, weakness, loss of motion, and deformity.

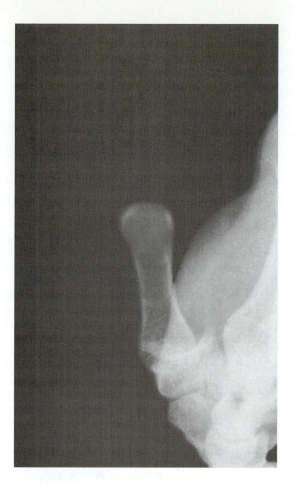

Figure 10–44. Osteoarthritis of the carpometacarpal joint of the thumb.

Tenderness and enlargement of the distal and proximal interphalangeal joints are noted on examination. Axial compression of the thumb trapeziometacarpal with a circumduction motion (**grind test**) will reproduce pain. As the disease progresses, radial subluxation of the thumb metacarpal on the trapezium may develop, leading to adduction deformity of the metacarpal.

Treatment

Nonoperative treatment includes oral nonsteroidal anti-inflammatory medication, long-acting intra-articular steroid injection, and splint immobilization.

The primary indication for surgery is pain unresponsive to oral medication and splinting. Distal interphalangeal joint arthrodesis relieves pain, corrects deformity, and resolves joint instability. Because the severely arthritic distal interphalangeal joint is often stiff, the additional loss of motion occasioned by

arthrodesis is usually well tolerated. The distal interphalangeal joint is fused in 10–15 degrees of flexion, a position in which the fingernail is parallel with the axis of the middle phalanx.

At the proximal interphalangeal joint, pain is the primary indication for surgery. Implant arthroplasty may be helpful in relieving pain and retaining motion in the ring and little fingers. The motion attained from implant arthroplasty is less in the proximal interphalangeal joints than in the metacarpophalangeal joints. Implant arthroplasty is usually avoided in the index- or middle-finger proximal interphalangeal joint because of residual instability to lateral or key pinch.

Arthrodesis effectively relieves pain at the proximal interphalangeal joint and provides pinch stability. The ideal position of arthrodesis varies from the radial to the ulnar digits. The index-finger proximal interphalangeal joint is usually fused at 40 degrees of flexion, the middle finger at 45 degrees, the ring finger at 50 degrees, and the little finger at 55 degrees.

At the trapeziometacarpal joint, conservative treatment includes a hand-based thumb spica splint with the interphalangeal joint left free, cortisone injections, warm soaks, and nonsteroidal anti-inflammatory drugs. Many patients with advanced degenerative changes on radiograph will obtain good pain relief with conservative therapy.

The primary indication for surgery is persistent pain. Trapezium resection arthroplasty relieves pain at the trapeziometacarpal joint and allows retention of full metacarpal motion. Either the distal half of the trapezium or the entire trapezium may be resected, depending on whether the patient has isolated trapeziometacarpal arthritis or pantrapezial arthritis. A tendon interposition is done using either the flexor carpi radialis or portion of the abductor pollicis longus. The tendon is placed through a drill hole in the articular surface of the thumb metacarpal to suspend the thumb. The remaining tendon is rolled into an "anchovy" and placed in the space of the excised trapezium. These two interventions prevent impingement of the metacarpal on the scaphoid. After surgery, the thumb is immobilized in a cast for 4 weeks followed by a thumb spica splint for 2–4 weeks.

Arthrodesis of the thumb carpometacarpal joint is an alternative to trapeziectomy and suspension sling arthroplasty. With the joint fused, patients are unable to lay their hand flat on a table. However, pain relief is excellent, and it may be the procedure of choice for a young laborer.

RHEUMATOID ARTHRITIS

Rheumatoid arthritis is a chronic inflammatory disease of unknown cause. The combined effect of tenosynovitis and synovitis on joints and periarticular tissues results in progressive joint destruction and deformity. Rheumatoid arthritis affects 0.3–1.5% of the population, and women are two to three times more commonly affected than men.

Clinical Findings

Evaluation of the hand affected by rheumatoid arthritis is often complex. The goal is to differentiate which of the patient's many problems—pain, weakness, or mechanical dysfunction—is most significant. Specifically, an evaluation is made of tendon rupture, adherence, or triggering and nerve compression symptoms. The most common nerve compression syndromes are compression of the median nerve at the wrist and compression of the radial nerve at the elbow. The appearance of rheumatoid nodules and ulnar drift deformity at the metacarpophalangeal joint may be disturbing to the patient. Rheumatoid nodules occur in 20–25% of patients with rheumatoid arthritis. Treatment of these conditions is not a priority unless erosion, pain, or infection is present.

Treatment

The shoulder, elbow, forearm, wrist, and hand should be individually examined. The goal of surgical reconstruction is restoration of a functional upper extremity, not just a functional hand. Indications for surgical intervention include relieving pain, slowing the progression of disease, improving function, and improving appearance.

Surgical treatment may be classified as either preventive or corrective. Preventive options include tenosynovectomy and synovectomy. Corrective procedures include tendon transfers, nerve decompression, soft-tissue reconstruction, and arthrodesis.

Synovectomy is most often considered in patients who have mild disease and are under good medical control but have persistent synovitis in one or two joints. Contraindications to synovectomy include rapidly progressive disease, multiple joint involvement, and underlying joint destruction.

A. ELBOW RECONSTRUCTION

Synovitis of the elbow joint may cause pain, joint destruction, and radial nerve compression. Nodules or bursas are common over the olecranon. Surgical treatment of the rheumatoid elbow includes radial head excision and synovectomy. As the disease progresses, consideration may be given to total elbow arthroplasty.

B. WRIST RECONSTRUCTION

Rheumatoid arthritis frequently involves the wrist and occurs in a predictable pattern. On the radial side of the wrist, the radioscaphocapitate and the radiolunatotriquetral ligaments are attenuated, permitting rotatory displacement of the scaphoid. Scapholunate dissociation is followed by radiocarpal collapse.

On the ulnar side of the wrist, the ulnar carpal ligaments become attenuated, allowing the carpus to drift radially. Attenuation of the distal radioulnar joint allows the head of the ulna to displace dorsally, producing **caput-ulnae syndrome.** The extensor carpi ulnaris tendon displaces volarly. These changes lead to supination of the carpus on the radius, ulnar translocation of the carpus, and a concomitant radialward displacement of the metacarpals (Figure 10–45). The carpus may also dislocate volarly beneath the radius.

Surgical treatment consists of extensor tenosynovectomy, with transposition of the dorsal retinaculum over the wrist joint to reinforce the capsule, and wrist synovectomy. The extensor carpi ulnaris tendon can be relocated from a volar to a dorsal position.

If pain is present over the distal ulna or if rupture of the little- or ring-finger extensor tendon results from a sharp prominence of the distal ulna, then resection of the distal ulna is performed. Fusion of the rheumatoid wrist provides stability and may increase function. Either a total wrist arthrodesis or a radiolunate arthrodesis may be elected, depending on the extent of midcarpal joint involvement.

C. HAND RECONSTRUCTION

Triggering of the digits is a common problem caused by flexor tenosynovitis. The A_1 pulley should not be incised in the treatment of rheumatoid trigger digits. Loss of the true A_1 pulley will increase the tendency of the fingers to drift ulnarward. Instead, tenosynovectomy and excision of the ulnar slip of the sublimis tendon should be considered.

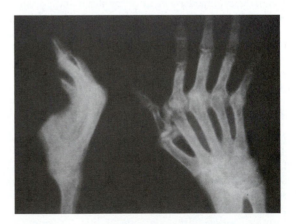

Figure 10–45. Radialward displacement of the metacarpals in rheumatoid arthritis.

If flexor tendon rupture occurs, treatment may include tendon transfer, bridge grafting, or joint fusion. The flexor tendon that most commonly ruptures is the flexor pollicis longus as it rubs over an osteophyte on the volar aspect of the scaphotrapezial joint (**Mannerfelt's lesion**). Extensor tendon ruptures are caused by attrition of the common extensor tendon of the ring and little fingers over the distal ulna (**Vaughn-Johnson syndrome**).

Treatment of the arthritic hand depends on the joints involved. The distal interphalangeal joint is usually best treated by arthrodesis. At the proximal interphalangeal joint, synovectomy may be performed if synovitis is isolated to the proximal interphalangeal joint without multiple joint involvement. Alternatives for the more involved joint are arthroplasty or arthrodesis.

At the metacarpophalangeal joint, inflammation of the synovium may cause the extensor mechanism to sublux ulnarly because of attenuation of the radial sagittal band. The mechanism may be relocated to improve function of the joint. For isolated joints without significant destruction, synovectomy may be performed. As destruction of the joint progresses, resection arthroplasty is required (Figure 10–46). This is the most common indication for silicone arthroplasty in the hand. Subluxation and ulnar drift alone are not absolute indications for arthroplasty if satisfactory function of the hand remains. Arthroplasty will not increase the range of motion of the metaphalangeal joints, but it will change its arc. Because most patients have severe flexion and ulnar deviation of the joints, arthroplasty is designed to give them a more functional range of motion, especially for grasping large objects. Because the implants will break with extensive use, silicone arthroplasty is indicated in the low-demand hand and is therefore better suited to rheumatoid than osteoarthritic patients.

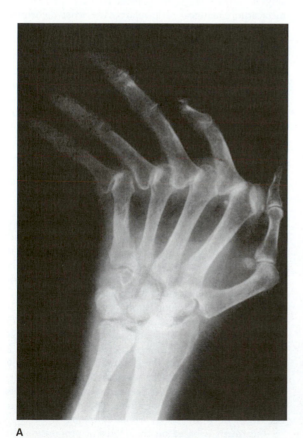

A

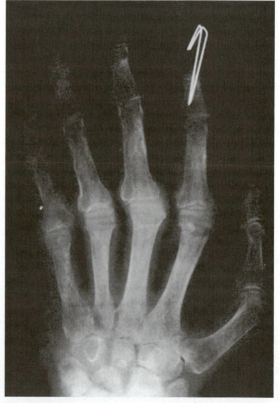

B

Figure 10–46. **A:** Preoperative view of metacarpophalangeal joint in rheumatoid arthritis. **B:** Following resection arthroplasty.

1. Boutonnière deformity—In addition to arthritis, various finger deformities occur related to soft-tissue damage. At the proximal interphalangeal joints, the most common is boutonnière deformity. Because of proximal interphalangeal joint synovitis, the central slip is either elongated or ruptured, which allows the proximal interphalangeal joint to flex and the lateral bands to volarly sublux. As the lateral bands migrate below the proximal interphalangeal joint axis, they become active proximal interphalangeal flexors rather than extensors. In addition to increasing the proximal interphalangeal joint deformity, the relative shortening of the extensor mechanism leads to distal interphalangeal joint hyperextension. Treatment of mild boutonnière deformities, which are passively correctable, consists of synovectomy and splinting. Lateral band reconstruction may be considered to relocate the bands dorsal to the axis of rotation. Alternatively, tenotomy of the terminal slip may be done to allow relaxation of the extensor mechanism and prevent hyperextension of the distal interphalangeal joint. Once moderate deformity of the proximal interphalangeal joint occurs (30- to 40-degree flexion deformity, with a flexible joint and preservation of the joint space), consideration may be given to reconstruction of the central slip as well as lateral band reconstruction and terminal tendon tenotomy. In the final stage of boutonnière deformity, the joint deformity becomes fixed, and the best form of treatment is arthroplasty or fusion.

2. Swan-neck deformity—Swan-neck deformities consist of hyperextension at the proximal interphalangeal joint and flexion at the distal interphalangeal joint. The mechanism of swan-neck deformity is terminal tendon rupture or attenuation, with secondary hyperextension of the proximal interphalangeal joint resulting from overpulling of the central slip or proximal interphalangeal joint hyperextension caused by laxity of the volar plate, rupture of the flexor digitorum superficialis, or intrinsic tightness. The most common of these mechanisms is intrinsic tightness secondary to metacarpophalangeal joint synovitis.

Swan-neck deformities are divided into four stages. In stage 1, the joints are supple in all positions. Treatment consists of splinting, distal interphalangeal joint fusion, or soft-tissue reconstruction to limit proximal interphalangeal joint hyperextension. In stage 2, proximal interphalangeal flexion is limited because of intrinsic tightness. Intrinsic release with or without reconstruction of the metacarpophalangeal joint may be of benefit. In stage 3, proximal interphalangeal joint motion is limited in all positions, yet the joint is still preserved. Mobilization of the lateral bands may help to relieve this deformity. Finally, in stage 4, the proximal interphalangeal joint is arthritic. Either proximal inter-

phalangeal arthrodesis or arthroplasty should be considered for stage 4 joint destruction.

3. Synovitic metacarpophalangeal joint deformity—The metacarpophalangeal joints always sublux volarly and ulnarly. This deformity results from synovial invasion of the collateral ligaments with secondary laxity, volar and ulnar forces that are normally present on the joint, augmentation of these forces by radial deviation of the wrist, attenuation of the radial sagittal band (allowing ulnar subluxation of the extensor tendon), and contracture of the intrinsic muscles. Treatment of the synovitic metacarpophalangeal joint consists of medical management and splinting. When the joint space is not narrowed, surgical synovectomy may provide some relief. Once moderate joint destruction or volar subluxation and ulnar deviation occurs, the decision about surgery is based on the function of the hand. When the patient is still able to use the hand for activities of daily living, splinting and other assistive aids are provided. Once loss of function occurs, metacarpophalangeal arthroplasty is considered. In performing metacarpophalangeal arthroplasty, the wrist deformity should first be corrected and all soft-tissue releases required to relieve the subluxing forces should be performed. Reconstruction of the stabilizing radial collateral ligament of the index finger should be done, and the extensor tendon should be relocated. Postoperatively, extensive splinting and therapy will be required to hold the hand in proper position. Therapy consists of an outrigger splint holding the wrist in dorsiflexion and the metaphalangeal joints in full extension and neutral radial-ulnar alignment. The splint is worn full time for 6 weeks and part time for 3 months. The patient wears a resting pen splint at night for 1 year.

D. THUMB RECONSTRUCTION

Three patterns of rheumatoid thumb deformities have been defined. In type 1 deformity, the metacarpophalangeal joint is flexed while the interphalangeal joint is hyperextended and the thumb metacarpal is secondarily abducted. In type 2 and 3 deformities, carpometacarpal subluxation leads to metacarpal adduction. In type 2 deformities, interphalangeal joint hyperextension develops with metacarpophalangeal flexion, and in type 3 deformities, the metacarpophalangeal joint is hyperextended and the interphalangeal joint is flexed. Type 2 deformities are unusual. Type 1 deformities are usually initiated by synovitis of the metacarpophalangeal joint, leading to attenuation of the extensor pollicis brevis tendon, intrinsic muscle tightness, and ulnar and volar displacement of the extensor pollicis longus.

Treatment is based on the degree of progression. In type 1 deformities, if the metacarpophalangeal and interphalangeal joints are passively correctable, synovectomy and extensor reconstruction may be performed. If the metacarpophalangeal joint flexion deformity is fixed, arthrodesis or arthroplasty of the joint is considered. When fixed metacarpophalangeal flexion and interphalangeal extension deformities are present simultaneously, the interphalangeal joint is fused and the metacarpophalangeal joint is replaced with an arthroplasty or also undergoes arthrodesis.

Type 3 deformities are analogous to swan-neck deformities of the fingers. The carpometacarpal joint disease allows dorsal and radial subluxation of the joint, with secondary adduction contraction of the metacarpal and hyperextension of the metacarpophalangeal joint. Treatment with minimal metacarpophalangeal deformity (stage 1) or passively correctable metacarpophalangeal deformity (stage 2) consists of splinting and carpometacarpal arthroplasty or fusion. Once the metacarpophalangeal deformity becomes fixed (stage 3), first web release and carpometacarpal arthroplasty are required.

E. SURGICAL PRIORITIES

When multilevel deformity is present, consideration should be given to combined procedures. If wrist and metacarpophalangeal deformities are both present, the wrist should be fused prior to or simultaneously with metacarpophalangeal joint reconstruction. When both metacarpophalangeal and proximal interphalangeal joint deformities are present, motion-preserving procedures such as arthroplasty should be carried out at the metacarpophalangeal joint. Treatment of concomitant proximal interphalangeal joint involvement depends on the stage of deformity. Mild to moderate proximal interphalangeal joint deformities can either be ignored or treated by closed manipulation and pin fixation. With severe deformity, arthrodesis of the proximal interphalangeal joint should be performed.

In all cases, attempts should be made to perform multiple operations in a single setting. These patients often require numerous procedures for multiple joints of the upper and lower extremities, and surgical and rehabilitation time must be used judiciously.

Other Inflammatory Arthritides

Other inflammatory conditions related to rheumatoid arthritis may affect the hand, producing joint destruction and deformity.

A. JUVENILE RHEUMATOID ARTHRITIS

In juvenile rheumatoid arthritis, early epiphyseal closure occurs as a result of synovitis and increased periarticular blood flow. Narrowing of phalangeal and metacarpal medullary canals makes implant arthroplasty difficult. The metacarpophalangeal joints may deviate radially rather than ulnarly.

B. ARTHRITIS MUTILANS

In arthritis mutilans, marked bone loss occurs, but the soft-tissue envelope is preserved. Early joint fusion is required to avoid progressive bone loss.

C. SYSTEMIC LUPUS ERYTHEMATOSUS

Systemic lupus erythematosus affects periarticular soft tissue, resulting in joint laxity with secondary dysfunction. Synovitis is minimal in lupus, and therefore the articular cartilage is preserved. Soft-tissue reconstruction is ineffective, and joint fusions are preferable to restore stability and function. The exception to this is the metacarpophalangeal joints, where implant arthroplasty may be used, even though normal articular cartilage will be sacrificed.

D. PSORIATIC ARTHRITIS

Psoriatic arthritis presents deformities similar to that of rheumatoid arthritis. The hand has a marked tendency to become stiff. In psoriatic arthritis, the metacarpophalangeal joints become stiff in extension, as opposed to their behavior in rheumatoid arthritis, where they become stiff in flexion.

Burton RI, Pellegrini VD Jr: Surgical management of basal joint arthritis of the thumb. Part II. Ligament reconstruction with tendon interposition arthroplasty. J Hand Surg Am 1986; 11:324.

Dolphin JD: Extensor tenotomy for chronic boutonnière deformity of the finger: Report of two cases. J Bone Joint Surg Am 1965;47:161.

Littler JR, Eaton RG: Redistribution of forces in correction of boutonnière deformity. J Bone Joint Surg Am 1967;49:1267.

Millender LH, Nalebuff EA: Reconstructive surgery in the rheumatoid hand. Orthop Clin North Am 1975;6:709.

Steichen J et al: Results of surgical treatment of chronic boutonnière deformity: An analysis of prognostic factors. In Strickland JW, Steichen JB (editors): *Difficult Problems in Hand Surgery.* Mosby, 1982.

■ HAND TUMORS

Nearly all mass lesions in the hand or wrist are benign conditions. Foreign body granulomas, epidermoid inclusion cysts, and neuromas are usually related to prior trauma.

Ganglions and fibroxanthomas arise adjacent to joints or tendon sheaths.

Ganglion

Ganglions are the most common soft-tissue tumors of the hand and wrist. They are cystic structures filled with a mucinous fluid but without a synovial or epithelial lining. In most cases, a stalk can be identified communicating between the cyst and an adjacent joint or tendon sheath. The three most common locations for ganglions are the wrist, digital flexor sheath, and distal interphalangeal joint (Figure 10–47).

A. DORSAL WRIST GANGLION

Dorsal wrist ganglions arise from the dorsal capsule of the scapholunate joint. Small firm dorsal ganglions may be barely palpable but highly symptomatic, whereas large ganglions are often soft and only mildly symptomatic. Aspiration and steroid injection may provide transient symptomatic relief, but recurrence is frequent. Symptomatic lesions can be surgically excised, with expectation of cure if care is taken to excise the stalk of the lesion with a capsular window from the lesion's origin. Because these lesions arise from the dorsal portion of the scapholunate ligament, care must be taken to preserve the ligament or a scapholunate dissociation may occur.

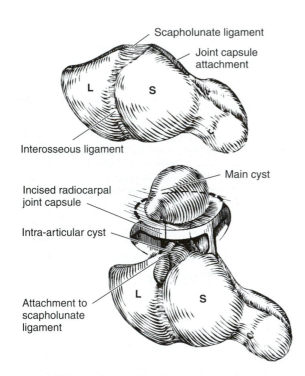

Figure 10–47. The ganglion and scapholunate attachments are isolated from the remaining uninvolved joint capsule (not shown). (Reproduced, with permission, from Green DP, ed: *Operative Hand Surgery,* 2nd ed. New York: Churchill Livingstone, 1988.)

B. PALMAR WRIST GANGLION

Palmar wrist ganglions present as swellings on the palmar radial aspect of the wrist. These lesions arise from either the palmar radioscaphoid or palmar scaphotrapezial joint. Surgical resection of the palmar radial ganglion requires mobilization and protection of the adjacent radial artery.

C. FLEXOR SHEATH GANGLION

Flexor sheath ganglions present as firm mass lesions over the palmar aspect of the flexor sheath. The mass is usually between 3 and 8 mm in diameter and is often so firm that it is presumed to be a bone exostosis. Treatment of symptomatic lesions is accomplished with aspiration or excision.

D. MUCOUS CYST

Mucous cysts are ganglions arising from the distal interphalangeal joint. The neck of the ganglion arises either radially or ulnarly to the extensor terminal tendon. Treatment is excision with debridement of the joint osteophyte. If the skin is thinned, a local rotation flap is required for soft-tissue coverage after excision.

Fibroxanthoma

Fibroxanthomas are also known as **giant cell tumors of tendon sheath** or **tendon sheath xanthomas.** These slowly enlarging, firm lesions are usually painless. They are usually fixed to deep tissues, more often on the palmar aspect of the hand or finger. Surgical resection requires delineation of adjacent nerves that may be displaced, compressed, or encircled by a fibroxanthoma.

Epidermoid Inclusion Cyst

Epidermoid inclusion cysts are usually the result of previous trauma such as a puncture wound, stab wound, or laceration. Epidermal cells become embedded in the subcutaneous tissue, evolving into a gradually enlarging pearllike mass. Eventually, the mass becomes noticeable, particularly when it is located over the palmar aspect of the pulp. Surgical treatment is excision of the mass without rupture.

Foreign Bodies

Foreign bodies may act as a nidus, inciting the development of a surrounding granuloma. This may be associated with a local inflammatory reaction or frank infection. Treatment consists of excision.

Neuromas

Neuromas are a normal response to nerve transection. Neuromas are inevitable in all amputations of the hand. If the neuroma enlargement of the distal end of the proximal segment of the transected nerve is in an area of palmar pulp contact, the lesion may be highly symptomatic. Treatment alternatives include neuroma revision or rerouting of the neuroma to a location away from contact stress.

■ CONGENITAL DIFFERENCES

Congenital hand differences occur in approximately 1 in 1500 live births. The term **differences** is favored by many recent authors because it is less offensive to patients and their parents than the more widely used terms abnormality, anomaly, or malformation.

Many congenital hand differences are part of a well-delineated association or syndrome. The abnormality may suggest that other regions of the body or organ systems be evaluated. When a baby is seen with bilateral total absence of the radius and normal or very mildly hypoplastic thumbs, the possibility of **thrombocytopenia with aplastic radii syndrome** should be considered and a platelet count obtained. Radial absence may also be associated with the VATER syndrome: vertebral, anal, tracheal, esophageal, and renal defects.

A number of frequently encountered conditions such as cleft hand are inherited as autosomal-dominant traits. The expertise of an experienced geneticist is invaluable in providing counsel to families considering additional children and to patients wishing to know the likelihood that their offspring would be affected by the disorder.

The two most commonly encountered conditions are syndactyly and polydactyly. In Caucasian populations, syndactyly is more common, and in Africa-American populations, polydactyly is the most commonly encountered congenital hand anomaly.

Syndactyly

Syndactyly, the webbing together of digits, is simple if soft tissue alone is involved and complex if bone or nails are joined (Figure 10–48). Surgical release of syndactyly requires the use of local flaps to create a floor for the interdigital web space and a partial surface for the adjacent sides of the separated digits. Residual defects along the sides of the separated fingers are covered with full-thickness skin grafts. Surgery is indicated when the webbing occurs a few millimeters distal to the

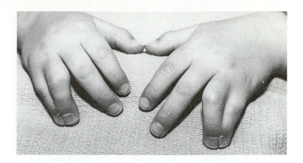

Figure 10–48. Bilateral complex syndactyly of the ring and little fingers.

usual point of separation of the fingers and the webbing prohibits full use of the fingers. Surgery is usually performed at the age of 6–12 months.

Polydactyly

Radial polydactyly is usually manifest as thumb duplication. When two thumbs are present in the same hand, they are rarely both normal in size, alignment, and mobility (Figure 10–49). The more ulnarward of

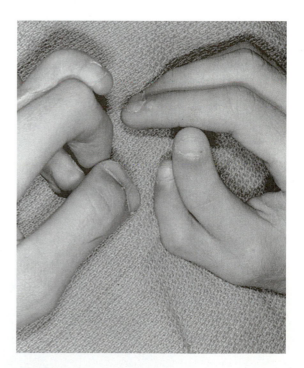

Figure 10–49. Thumb polydactyly.

the two thumbs is usually better developed than the more radialward thumb. The level of bifurcation varies from a wide distal phalanx with two nails, to two digits each possessing a metacarpal and a proximal and distal phalanx. In the most common form of thumb duplication, a single broad metacarpal supports two proximal phalanges, each of which support a distal phalanx. Reconstruction requires merging of elements of both component digits. Usually the ulnar thumb is maintained. If the duplication occurs at the metacarpophalangeal joint, the radial collateral ligament is preserved with the metacarpal and attached to the proximal phalanx of the ulnar thumb. Surgery is usually performed at the age of 6 to 12 months.

Partial or Absent Structures

Absence or partial deficiency of the radius results in inadequate support of the hand and carpus. The unsupported hand angulates radially. Stretching of contracted radial soft-tissue structures is accomplished through repeat manipulation, casting, or splinting. The hand is surgically reoriented onto the end of the ulna by a centralization procedure.

Absence of the thumb or severe hypoplasia of the thumb may be treated by pollicization of the index finger. This procedure shifts the index finger to the thumb position and repositions the index-finger extrinsic extensor tendons as well as the dorsal and palmar interosseous tendons to provide balanced control of the shifted digit.

Light TR, Manske PR: Congenital hand malformations and deformities of the hand. Instr Course Lect 1989;38:31.

American Society for Surgery of the Hand: *The Hand: Examination and Diagnosis.* New York: Churchill Livingstone, 1983.

Pediatric Orthopedic Surgery

11

George T. Rab, MD

The scope of pediatric orthopedics ranges from congenital anomalies to injuries in the older adolescent. The pathophysiologic manifestations of many of these disorders differ from analogous adult problems because of the added dimension of growth. The physician's relationship with the pediatric patient generally occurs in the context of a protective family environment, in contrast to the more independent relationship the physician may form with an adult. The natural tendency for children to be active and the remarkable regenerative processes of the immature skeleton frequently make formal rehabilitation unnecessary following surgery or recuperation after serious injury.

Guidelines for Pediatric Orthopedics

The following rules may be helpful when applying general orthopedic principles to the child:

(1) A growing bone normally tends to remodel itself toward the adult configuration. This process occurs faster in younger children and in deformities near the ends of bone. Remodeling is faster when deformity is in the plane of motion of the nearest joint.

(2) Skeletal deformities worsen as abnormal growth continues (eg, following permanent damage to the growth plate), especially near rapidly growing areas such as the knee. This characteristic is exaggerated in younger children.

(3) Children tolerate long-term immobilization better than adults and tend to recover soft-tissue mobility spontaneously following most injuries.

(4) Fracture healing is usually more rapid and predictable in the actively growing skeleton than in the adult skeleton.

(5) Joint surfaces in children are generally more tolerant of irregularity than those of the adult. Although degenerative arthritic changes may follow childhood injury, there is often an asymptomatic interval of many decades before the process becomes clinically evident.

(6) Many "deformities," such as metatarsus adductus, internal tibial torsion, and genu valgum (knock-knee), are actually physiologic variations that spontaneously correct with growth. Thus, the clinician must distinguish between conditions that need no treatment and those requiring early intervention.

GROWTH DISORDERS

General skeletal growth is discussed in detail in Chapter 1.

1. Limb-Length Inequality

Limb-length inequality may reflect either a congenital deficiency or any of a wide variety of acquired conditions (Table 11–1). Upper extremities of unequal length are usually only of cosmetic interest and can easily be compensated for by modifying clothing. In the lower extremities, however, length discrepancies may be severe enough—greater than 1 in. (2.5 cm)—to limit function and require treatment. Lesser discrepancies can be managed with a shoe lift.

Treatment

A. CALCULATION OF LIMB LENGTH AT MATURITY

Clinical management of limb-length inequality in pediatric patients should include calculation of projected lengths at maturity. Several mathematical methods, based on skeletal age, gender, and normal growth rates, are available. The following general rule can be used to estimate the extent of future growth: The average growth rate of the distal femur and proximal tibia is 10–12 mm/year and 5–6 mm/year, respectively, with growth continuing until age 14 in females and age 16 in males.

B. SURGICAL TREATMENT

1. Epiphysiodesis—The simplest surgical procedure to treat pediatric bone-length discrepancies is epiphysiodesis (premature surgical closure of the growth plate). In the longer limb, this is performed by curetting or drilling the physis, or inserting small bone grafts across the medial and lateral edges of the plate. Epiphysiodesis is usually performed at the distal femoral physis, proximal tibial physis, or both, because they are rapidly growing and easily accessible surgically. The remaining open physes in the limb allow for continued growth but

Table 11–1. Causes of limb-length inequality.

Infectious causes
    Osteomyelitis
    Septic arthritis
Neoplastic causes
    Arteriovenous malformations
    Hemangioma
Neuromuscular causes
    Cerebral palsy
    Isolated limb paralysis
    Poliomyelitis
Traumatic causes
    Malunion of long bones
    Physeal injury
Other causes
    Avascular necrosis of femoral head (and physis)
    Congenital amputations
    Legg-Calvé-Perthes disease

at a slower rate. The exact timing of epiphysiodesis is crucial to attaining equal limb lengths at skeletal maturity. Timing is calculated by the same method used to predict ultimate adult leg length. The effectiveness of epiphysiodesis requires that bone still be growing and that accurate data be collected on this growth for several years (ie, scanograms for leg-length measurement, skeletal age).

2. Femoral shortening—If a child has reached the age when bone growth will be insufficient to make epiphysiodesis practical, the long leg may be shortened at skeletal maturity by femoral shortening. This may be performed as an open procedure by removing a segment of femur and fixing the bone with a plate and screws. It may also be done as a closed procedure, using an intramedullary femoral rod introduced through a buttock incision for fixation. A cylindric segment of femur is cut out of the bone using intramedullary saws, and the bone is pushed aside to allow the femur to shorten over the rod. The excised bone segment eventually resorbs.

3. Other techniques—Leg-length inequalities projected to be 6 cm or more generally do not respond well to the previously described treatments, which in these cases may lead to unacceptably short stature or limb segments. Although some discrepancies are so severe that amputation of the foot and prosthetic fitting are required, newer techniques of bone lengthening have proved highly successful in treating these children (see Chapter 1).

Anderson M et al: Growth and predictions of growth in the lower extremities. J Bone Joint Surg Am 1963;45:1.

Moseley CF: Assessment and prediction in leg-length discrepancy. Instr Course Lect 1989;38:325.

Little DG et al: A simple calculation for the timing of epiphysiodesis. J Pediatr Orthop 1996;16:173.

Paley D: Current techniques of limb lengthening. J Pediatr Orthop 1988;8:73.

2. Dwarfism & Other Disorders of Growth

Orthopedic disorders often accompany dwarfism (achondroplasia, multiple epiphyseal dysplasia) or other syndromes (Down syndrome, Marfan's syndrome). The classification of skeletal syndromes and dysplasias is undergoing rapid change as knowledge is gained using molecular biologic and genetic techniques. A detailed review of these conditions is outside the scope of this work; Table 11–2 lists some of these conditions and the major orthopedic problems associated with them.

Smith DW: Recognizable Patterns of Human Malformation. 5th ed. Philadelphia: WB Saunders, 1997.

Sponseller PD et al: The thoracolumbar spine in Marfan syndrome. J Bone Joint Surg 1995; 77A:867.

INFECTIOUS PROCESSES

1. Hematogenous Osteomyelitis

Osteomyelitis, an infection of bone tissue, usually occurs in the marrow cavity but sometimes affects the cortex as well. In children, it is most commonly the result of hematogenous spread, frequently following an upper respiratory infection or partially treated distant infection. Direct inoculation of bacteria into an open fracture or penetrating wound can also lead to infection and may resemble other serious bacterial infections in children (Table 11–3).

Clinical Findings

Acute bacterial hematogenous osteomyelitis in the metaphysis occurs following sludging of bacteria-laden blood in the venous sinusoids. As the infection progresses, edema fluid and infected purulent tissue invade the porous cortex and elevate the periosteum, which is highly resistant to infection because of its extreme vascularity. The pressure of the pus beneath the richly innervated periosteum causes localized pain. Eventually, if the infection is untreated, the periosteum itself ruptures, and infected tissue spills into the surrounding soft tissue or ruptures the skin (Figure 11–1).

    The accumulated purulence in the metaphysis and under the periosteum creates an efficient avascular culture medium in the cortex between them. This dead cortex is called sequestrum, and, if it is large, surgical removal may be required to control the infection.

Table 11–2. Orthopedic involvement in selected syndromes and dwarfing conditions.

Achondroplasia
   Short limbs; genu varum; exaggerated lumbar lordosis; spinal stenosis; ligamentous laxity
Apert's syndrome
   Foot deformities; hand and foot polydactyly
Arthrogyposis
   Severe joint stiffness, contractures, and dislocations; resistant clubfoot
Cleidocranial dysplasia
   Absent clavicles; coxa vara
Diastrophic dysplasia
   Severe clubfoot; joint dislocations; joint stiffness; cervical kyphosis; scoliosis
Down syndrome
   Cervical (C1–C2) instability; hip dislocation; ankle valgus; ligamentous laxity
Enchondromatosis
   Asymmetric multiple enchondromas in long bones; limb-length inequality; angulation of long bones
Fibrous dysplasia
   Multiple fibrous lesions in bone; limb bowing or shortening; occasional endocrine disorders
Larsen's syndrome
   Hip, knee, and radial head dislocations; severe cervical kyphosis and instability; scoliosis
Marfan's syndrome
   Scoliosis
Metaphyseal chondrodysplasia
   Moderate dwarfing; genu varum; ligamentous laxity; cervical instability
Multiple epiphyseal dysplasia
   Mild dwarfism; joint surface deformities with premature osteoarthritis; angular limb deformities
Multiple hereditary exostoses
   Mild dwarfing; osteochondroma (external enlargements) at all long bone ends
Osteogenesis imperfecta
   Bone fragility and multiple fractures; bowing of bones; scoliosis; mild to moderate dwarfing
Spondyloepiphyseal dysplasia
   Severe dwarfing; coxa vara; genu valgum; scoliosis; odontoid hypoplasia, instability, and deformity

Table 11–3. Common pathogens in pediatric bone and joint infections.

Osteomyelitis
   Group A *Streptococcus*
   Salmonella (with sickle cell)
   Staphylococcus aureus
Septic joint
   Escherichia coli (neonatal)
   Group A *Streptococcus*
   Haemophilus influenzae (age 6–24 months) in non-HIB immunized patients
   Neisseria gonorrhoeae (adolescent)
   Pneumococcus
   Proteus (neonatal)
   Staphylococcus aureus
   Streptococcus fecalis (neonatal)
Soft-tissue infection
   Escherichia coli (neonatal)
   Group A *Streptococcus*
   Proteus
   Pseudomonas
   Staphylococcus aureus
   Streptococcus fecalis (neonatal)

The elevated periosteum responds to infection by producing a shell of periosteal new bone called involucrum, which provides some stability to the infected bone and rarely becomes infected itself.

Pain and tenderness at the infection site are universal signs, limping is common, and frequently the child is irritable. Fever and leukocytosis are common but not universal, and the erythrocyte sedimentation rate (ESR) is almost always elevated, usually to 50 mm/h or more.

Clinical examination is usually sufficient to make the diagnosis; occasionally bone scans may be required to help localize lesions. Although the diagnosis is usually clear, osteomyelitis should be suspected if a child has bone pain in the absence of other systemic signs but has recently received antibiotic treatment for other conditions.

Treatment

A. Early Treatment

Treatment depends on the duration of symptoms and findings on radiograph. If the infection is detected

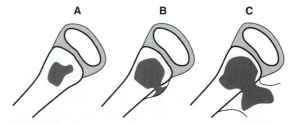

Figure 11–1. Hematogenous osteomyelitis in children. Cellulitic phase (**A**) can exude through the cortex, raising periosteum (**B**). Late rupture into soft tissues (**C**) is rare, unless infection is untreated.

early, no visible radiograph changes usually are apparent except for soft-tissue swelling. In that case, intravenous and, later, oral antibiotics may resolve the infection. Aspiration of the metaphysis should be done for culture before beginning antibiotic therapy. Up to 30–40% of cultures may be negative despite other clear evidence of bacterial infection; in that case, empiric treatment (usually with antistaphylococcal antibiotics) is appropriate.

B. Treatment for Advanced Infection

In advanced cases, lytic defects or osteoporosis may be present, and periosteal reaction may be visible on radiograph; such cases require open drainage and debridement of the infected metaphysis. Treatment must be continued until there is no evidence of residual infection because bacteria can survive in bone tissue that is not well perfused with antibiotic. In such cases, a 3-month prolonged regimen of oral antibiotics will minimize the possibility of chronic osteomyelitis.

Scott RJ et al: Acute osteomyelitis in children: A review of 116 cases. J Pediatric Orthop 1990;5:649.

Hamdy RC et al: Subacute hematogenous osteomyelitis: Are biopsy and surgery always necessary? J Pediatr Orthop 1996;16:220.

2. Septic Joint

Septic arthritis in children, like osteomyelitis, usually is hematogenous in origin. The bacterial complications are similar to those seen in bone infections (see Table 11–3). Septic joints frequently follow upper respiratory infections; they may be delayed in onset by a week or more and may present in an attenuated form when a previous infection has been partially treated.

Clinical Findings

The classic septic joint in a child presents a dramatic picture: The joint is splinted by muscle spasm, and motion of even a few degrees causes extreme pain. There may be effusion, but findings may be less striking if antibiotics have been used in the recent past. During this acute inflammatory phase, children are more comfortable if the involved joint is immobilized.

Although white blood cell counts and the ESR are usually elevated, the definitive diagnosis of septic joint requires aspiration and synovial fluid analysis. Sterile aspiration does not harm the joint and should be done immediately when the diagnosis is suspected. Aspiration of deep joints such as the hip may require radiographic control.

Synovial white blood cell counts range from 50,000/μL (in nonpyogenic infections such as *Neisseria gonorrhoeae*) to over 250,000/μL (*Staphylococcus aureus*). This white cell response, with the concomitant high level of lysosomal enzyme release, is most destructive of articular cartilage in septic joints. Although synovial fluid cultures give definitive guidance for therapy, antibiotic treatment can initially be based on results of Gram staining. In addition, immunochemical tests may offer rapid identification of certain pathogens.

Treatment

Treatment always includes drainage of the joint. In easily accessible joints such as the finger or knee, certain low-grade infections may respond well to repeated aspirations. In most cases, however, surgical drainage by arthrotomy or arthroscopy is preferable.

Antibiotics easily cross the synovial membrane and are continued until the joint inflammation is resolved, usually for at least 3 weeks. Intravenous administration is used initially but may often be followed by oral medication once the temperature, sedimentation rate, and leukocyte count return to normal.

Shaw B, Kasser J: Acute septic arthritis in infancy and childhood. Clin Orthop 1990;256:212.

Green NE, Edwards K: Bone and joint infections in children. Orthop Clin North Am 1987;18:555.

Wall EJ: Childhood osteomyelitis and septic arthritis. Curr Opin Pediatr 1998;10:73

Kim HKW et al: A shortened course of parenteral antibiotic therapy in the management of acute septic arthritis of the hip. J Pediatr Orthop 2000;20:44.

3. Septic Hip

Septic hip is one of the true surgical emergencies in pediatric orthopedics. It must be differentiated from transient synovitis of the hip, which is a benign condition (see the section on Transient Synovitis of the Hip).

Septic hip requires rapid diagnosis by aspiration and immediate surgical drainage. A delay of even 4–6 h can result in avascular necrosis of the femoral head. Splinting the joint with a spica cast may be required to prevent late subluxation of the hip.

Because of the unique structure and blood supply of this joint (Figure 11–2), purulence within the joint capsule can cause thrombosis of epiphyseal vessels and necrosis of the proximal femoral epiphysis. Neglected septic hips may subluxate or dislocate because of effusion and laxity caused by hyperemia. For these reasons, septic hip (or osteomyelitis of the proximal femur) always requires surgical drainage. An anterior approach is preferred to reduce the risk of vascular injury.

Septic hip in a growing child is also a special orthopedic case because the femoral neck (which is intraarticular) is actually the anatomic metaphysis of the proximal femur. It is thus susceptible to hematogenous

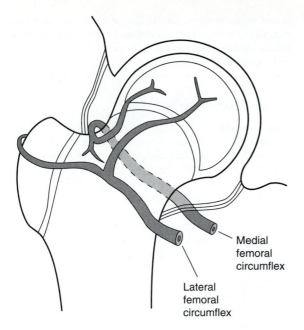

Figure 11–2. The blood supply of the proximal femur is unusual because the capsule interferes with the direct routing of blood vessels. The epiphyseal vessels emerge distal to the capsule and course up the surface of the femoral neck, rendering them susceptible to injury, thrombosis, or blockage by increased intra-articular pressure.

Medial femoral circumflex

Lateral femoral circumflex

osteomyelitis, which may rupture into the hip joint and cause sepsis.

A common clinical problem is the differentiation between septic and hip and transient synovitis of the hip. Juvenile arthritis may occasionally be included in the differential. Table 11–4 highlights differences in the conditions.

Choi IH, et al: Sequelae and reconstruction after septic arthritis of the hip in infants. J Bone Joint Surg 1990;72A:1150.

4. Puncture Wounds of the Foot

Sneakers and tennis shoes offer little protection from nail punctures of the plantar surface of the foot. The penetrating nail may carry *Pseudomonas* bacteria (which have been shown to contaminate the soles of tennis shoes) into the plantar fascia.

The symptoms of *Pseudomonas* infection include redness, swelling, and pain that persist longer than 1 week. Surgical incision and drainage of the abscess are usually curative. Interestingly, prophylactic use of antibiotics does not seem to lessen the chance of developing late abscess.

5. Skeletal Tuberculosis

As in the adult, *Mycobacteria* organisms may invade the pediatric skeleton by hematogenous spread to bone or synovium while the initial pulmonary infection goes undetected. The most common sites of invasion are the hip and spine. Tuberculosis should be considered, and skin tests performed, in children suffering from chronic atypical musculoskeletal infections, particularly if the child is immunosuppressed.

Clinical Findings

Hip involvement is characterized by a chronic limp associated with a flexion contracture. In addition, muscle atrophy of the thigh may be striking. Radiographic examination discloses osteoporosis, joint narrowing, and irregular erosions.

Spine involvement may include paraspinal abscess (best visualized by CT scan or MRI), vertebral destruction, or kyphosis, which may be severe and lead to paralysis.

Table 11–4. Clinical differential diagnosis of inflammatory hip conditions.

	Septic Hip	Transient Synovitis of Hip	Juvenile Arthritis of Hip
Pain	Severe	Moderate-severe	Moderate
Gait	Cannot walk	Limp or cannot walk	Limp
Fever	Common	No	No or low-grade
Radiograph	Negative	Negative	Joint narrowing
WBC	Elevated	Normal	Normal-elevated
Aspirate	Turbid; 5000–250,000 WBC; bacteria present	Normal	25,000–50,000 WBC with monocytes
Treatment	Urgent surgical drainage; antibiotics	Symptomatic	Salicylates, rest, physical therapy

WBC = white blood cells.

Treatment

Treatment of skeletal tuberculosis consists of combination chemotherapy, with surgical debridement in resistant cases. Occasionally, surgical fusion of joints or spine may be required.

Watts HG, Lifeso RM: Tuberculosis of bones and joints (current concepts review). J Bone Joint Surg 1996;78A:288.

6. Discitis In Children

Discitis is a low-grade inflammatory process involving the intervertebral disc, usually in the lumbar spine. It affects children at any age, although it is most frequent in ages 2–6. The disorder is caused by hematogenous bacterial seeding, with the most common cultures growing *Staphylococcus aureus* from disc aspirate. The classic presentation in a toddler is refusal to walk; pain is not a prominent symptom in this age group. Older children (up to early teen-years) may have either back or abdominal pain.

Clinical Findings

Small children may have limitation of passive hyperextension of the spine (in the prone position) with no other findings. Older children have splinting of the paraspinous muscles and pain with percussion. The ESR may be normal or elevated; those patients with an elevated ESR are more likely to have bacterial growth if cultures are done. Aspirate cultures may be negative in up to 40% of patients. Radiographs at first are normal but eventually demonstrate disc space narrowing with sclerosis of adjoining end-plates, best visualized on spot lateral views. Bone scan is positive in those children with negative radiographs.

Treatment

Management depends on the severity of clinical findings because a large number of discitis patients have self-limited disease and spontaneously improve. Children with sepsis or elevated ESR may benefit from disc aspiration and culture. Less ill children are usually treated with empiric antistaphylococcal oral antibiotics for 6 weeks. Pantaloon spica cast may occasionally be required for symptom relief. Long-term outcome is universally favorable, although occasional spontaneous fusion of the disc space occurs.

METABOLIC DISORDERS

1. Rickets & Ricketslike Conditions

Nutritional rickets is a dietary deficiency of vitamin D that interferes with skeletal ossification. In the United States, vitamin supplementation of food and milk has virtually eliminated the dietary form of rickets. Numerous ricketslike metabolic conditions persist with orthopedic consequences, however.

Renal Osteodystrophy

Renal osteodystrophy, a disorder of calcium, phosphorus, and vitamin D and of parathyroid function in children with chronic renal disease, has potentially serious skeletal manifestations. In transplantation patients, the condition can be aggravated by chronic illness and antimetabolite or steroid usage.

Osteoporosis, leading to compression fractures of the spine, is a common complication. Delayed healing of fractures is also common. Inadequate metaphyseal ossification during skeletal growth results in wide irregular cartilaginous growth plates, which tend to slip slowly, sometimes producing grotesque hip, knee, and ankle deformities. Such deformities are usually best treated only after transplantation or other improvement in renal status. Occasionally, severe functional disabilities may require osteotomy to correct deformity before renal transplantation. Healing may be delayed, however, and the condition may recur.

Hypophosphatemic Rickets

Hypophosphatemic rickets (vitamin D-resistant rickets) is an dominant X-linked condition in which vitamin production and metabolism are normal but renal tubular loss of phosphate interferes with skeletal ossification. The major manifestations are a mild-to-moderate decrease in stature and bowing of the lower extremities.

The medical history usually discloses a parent or sibling with short stature and bowlegs. In addition, serum phosphorus is reduced, and serum calcium is normal. Radiographic examination discloses characteristic widening of growth plates, funnel-like beaking of the metaphyses, and curvature of the femoral and tibial shafts, which are normally straight.

Medical treatment with megadoses of vitamin D and phosphorus supplementation may not be curative. Functionally disabling deformities can be corrected by multiple-level osteotomies, which usually require bilateral surgery. Because postosteotomy healing is delayed and recurrence of deformity is common until maturity, surgery should be postponed until adolescence, if possible.

Mankin HJ: Rickets, osteomalacia, and renal osteodystrophy: An update. Orthop Clin North Am 1990;21:81.

HIP DISORDERS

1. Transient Synovitis of the Hip

Transient synovitis of the hip is a benign nontraumatic, self-limited disorder that mimics septic hip in clinical presentation. The physician confronting this condition must exclude septic hip, which is a surgical emergency.

Although the cause of transient synovitis is unclear, evidence suggests it is associated with immune responses to viral or bacterial antigens, mediated through the synovial membrane. Synovial fluid rapidly accumulates under pressure in the hip joint, and there may be severe pain from capsular distension. The fluid is resorbed within 3–7 days, with no long-term sequelae.

Clinical Findings

As with septic hip, upper respiratory tract infections often precede transient synovitis by a few days to 2 weeks. The hip contains excess synovial fluid and is held in flexion, abduction, and external rotation because this is the joint's position of maximum capacity. The joint may be sore and resistant to movement, but subluxation does not occur. Usually, the patient will allow careful passive movement.

Radiographs reveal only capsular swelling, and effusion may be detected on ultrasound. Leukocytosis is absent, and the ESR is not elevated.

Although experienced physicians frequently suspect transient synovitis based only on clinical examination, aspiration of the hip following confirmation of needle position by radiograph is the safest approach. Synovial fluid will not show elevation of the white blood cell count, and bacterial cultures will be negative.

Treatment

Treatment of transient synovitis includes simple analgesics and splintage, usually by bed rest, until symptoms resolve.

The early stages of Legg-Calvé-Perthes disease (see section on Legg-Calvé-Perthes Disease) may include a synovial stage that, until the development of characteristic radiograph findings, is indistinguishable from transient synovitis. Typically, the pain is less severe than in transient synovitis, the children are a bit older (> age 4–5 years), and there is no history of recent illness.

There is no evidence that transient synovitis leads to Legg-Calvé-Perthes disease itself.

Kocher MS et al: Differentiating between septic arthritis and transient synovitis of the hip in children: An evidence-based clinical prediction algorithm. J Bone Joint Surg 1999;81A:1662.

Haueisen DC et al: The characterization of transient synovitis of the hip in children. J Pediatr Orthop 1986;6:11.

2. Developmental Dysplasia of the Hip

Developmental dysplasia of the hip is one of the most serious problems in pediatric orthopedics. The neonatal hip is a relatively unstable joint because the muscle is undeveloped, the soft cartilaginous surfaces are easily deformed, and the ligaments are lax. Exaggerated positioning in acute flexion and adduction in utero may occur, especially in breech presentation. This may cause excess stretching of the posterior hip capsule, which renders the joint unstable after delivery. Laxity may reflect family history or the presence of maternal relaxin in the fetal circulatory system.

This relative instability may lead to asymptomatic subluxation (partial displacement) or dislocation (complete displacement) of the hip joint. Displacement of the femoral head in the infant is proximal (posterior and superior) because of the pull of the gluteal and hip flexor muscles. In the subluxated hip, asymmetric pressure causes progressive flattening of the posterior and superior acetabular rim and medial femoral head (dysplasia is the term to describe these structural deviations from normal).

In the completely dislocated hip, dysplasia also occurs because normal joint development requires concentric motion with normally mated joint surfaces. The shallow deformed dysplastic joint surfaces predispose to further mechanical instability and the inexorable progression of undetected, and therefore untreated, developmental dysplasia of the hip.

Developmental dysplasia of the hip (DDH) occurs in approximately 1 in 1000 live births in whites, is less common in blacks, and may be more common in certain ethnic groups such as North American Indians. In all groups, this disorder is more likely if certain risk factors are present, such as positive family history, ligamentous laxity, breech presentation (and, by association, cesarean section), female gender, large fetal size, and first-born status. Dislocations may be bilateral but are more often unilateral and on the left side.

Clinical Findings

Reversal of dysplasia and subsequent normal hip development depend on early detection of DDH. Early detection is made more challenging by lack of a definitive test or finding on examination. Moreover, because this disorder is painless, there are no symptoms in the infant. Detection of bilateral dislocations may be particularly difficult.

Radiographs are usually not useful in newborn infants, because the femoral head is composed of radiolucent cartilage. Ultrasound examination is helpful, but before 8–10 weeks of age, false-positive results are common. The test is expensive, and interpretation requires comprehensive training. Thus, the best test for this disorder is careful physical examination at birth, repeated at each well-baby check until the child is walking normally. A high index of suspicion is mandatory, especially if risk factors are present.

A. TESTS FOR DYSPLASIA

Several examination maneuvers require a quiet relaxed infant and commonly produce false-negative findings. Although it is imperative to detect subluxated or dislocated hips, it is also helpful to identify the very lax (unstable) but still located hip. This type of joint may either dislocate later or exhibit subtle dysplasia during growth that can cause premature osteoarthritis.

1. Asymmetric skin folds—A dislocated hip displaces proximally, causing the leg to be marginally shorter. This occasionally leads to the accordion phenomenon, with wrinkling of thigh skin folds. The most significant fold is between the genitals and gluteus maximus region. This test is not very reliable, frequently producing false-positive and false-negative results (Figure 11–3A).

2. Galeazzi's test—With the child lying on a flat surface, flex the hips and knees so the heels rest flat on the table, just distal to the buttock (Figure 11–3B). A dislocated hip is signaled by relative shortening of the thigh compared with the normal leg, as shown by the difference in knee height level. This test is almost always useless in children under 1 year of age and is negative if dislocation is bilateral.

3. Passive hip abduction—The flexed hips are gently abducted as far as possible (Figure 11–3C). If one or both hips are dislocated, the femoral head (the pivot point during abduction) is posterior, causing relative tightness of the adductor muscles. Asymmetric abduction or limited abduction (usually less than 70 degrees from the midline) is a positive finding. When the hip is lax (dislocatable but not dislocated), the abduction test will be normal despite the presence of subluxation or dislocation.

4. Barlow's test—This is a provocative test that picks up an unstable but located hip; it is unsuitable for a dislocated hip. The flexed calf and knee are gently grasped in the hand, with the thumb at the lesser trochanter and fingers at the greater trochanter (knee flexion relaxes the hamstrings). The hip is adducted slightly and gently pushed posteriorly with the palm (Figure 11–3D, F). Detection of "pistoning," or the sensation of the femoral head subluxating over the posterior rim of the acetabulum, is a positive finding.

5. Ortolani's test—This test detects hips that are already dislocated. The flexed limb is grasped as in Barlow's test, above. The hip is abducted while the femur is gently lifted with the fingers at the greater trochanter

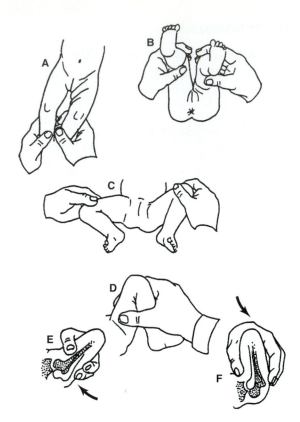

Figure 11–3. Clinical examination of developmental dislocation of the hip. In all pictures, the child's left hip is the abnormal side. **A:** Asymmetric skin folds. **B:** Galeazzi's test. **C:** Limitation of abduction. **D, E, F:** Ortolani's and Barlow's tests (see text).

(Figure 11–3D, E). In a positive test, there will be a sensation of the hip reducing back into the acetabulum. Reduction is felt but not heard: The old concept of a "hip click" is incorrect. Ortolani's test may be negative at age 2–3 months, even when the hip is dislocated, because of the development of soft-tissue contracture.

B. IMAGING STUDIES

In the infant, diagnosis is made by physical examination alone, and radiographs are generally unnecessary. Dysplasia, instability, and dislocation may appear on ultrasound studies, which can allow visualization of hip contour and stability before ossification is present. Sonography is a dynamic examination that requires an experienced interpreter, and there can be false positives prior to 6–10 weeks of age. Radiographs may be used at any age, but the absence of ossified structures renders them inaccurate in the newborn. After 4–6 months, when the ossific nucleus appears in the femoral head, radiographs are more helpful. Because much of the skeleton is cartilaginous at this age, certain lines and angles may be drawn on x-ray films to allow estimates of geometric parameters (Figure 11–4). These may suggest evidence of acetabular dysplasia (a more vertical slope of the acetabular roof, measured as the acetabular index), femoral dysplasia (small or absent ossification center in the femoral head), or lateral superior displacement of the femoral head.

Increased femoral anteversion (external rotation of the femoral head and neck) is often present in DDH but not visible. Increased anteversion may be seen as an

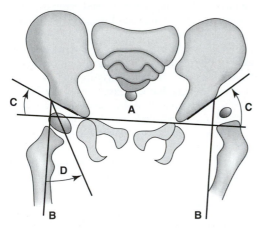

Figure 11–4. Lines drawn for measurement in developmental dysplasia of the hip. In the figure, the patient's left hip (on the right of the figure) is the subluxated one. **A:** Hilgenreiner's line is a horizontal line of the pelvis, drawn between the triradiate cartilages. The proximal femoral ossification center should be below this line. **B:** Perkins's line is a vertical line (perpendicular to Hilgenreiner's line) drawn down from the lateral edge of the acetabulum. The femoral head ossification center, as well as the medial beak of the proximal metaphysis, should fall medial to this line. **C:** The acetabular index is the angle between Hilgenreiner's line and a line joining the acetabular center (triradiate) with the acetabular edge as it intersects Perkins's line. It measures acetabular depth and should be below 30 degrees by 1 year of age and below 25 degrees by 2 years of age. **D:** The center-edge angle is the angle between Perkins's line and a line joining the lateral edge of the acetabulum with the center of the femoral head. It is a measure of lateral subluxation that becomes smaller as the hip subluxates laterally. Normal is 20 degrees or greater.

increase in relative femoral neck valgus in the older child.

C. Detection of Dysplasia in Older Child

As the infant grows older, many diagnostic maneuvers that are positive in a young infant become negative because soft-tissue changes accommodate the displaced structures. Thus, Ortolani's and Barlow's signs can be negative, even in the face of grossly abnormal hip development, making detection particularly difficult (especially between 4 and 15 months). The first signs of developmental dysplasia may then not be recognized until the child begins to walk and demonstrates a waddling gait with excessive lumbar lordosis. Radiographs at this age are diagnostic.

Treatment

Treatment of DDH should be initiated as soon as the diagnosis is suspected. Early treatment is generally successful, whereas a delay in treatment may result in permanent dysplastic changes. Exact treatment depends on patient age at presentation and degree of involvement. Regardless of age, treatment may fail, and the physician may need to institute a more complex treatment plan. The current recommendations are as follows:

A. Age 0–6 Months

A dislocated hip at this age may spontaneously reduce over 2–3 weeks if the hip is held in a position of flexion. This is best accomplished with the Pavlik harness (Figure 11–5), a device that holds the hips flexed at 100 degrees and prevents adduction but does not limit further flexion. Movement in the harness is beneficial for the joint and helps to achieve gradual reduction and stabilization of the hip. The Pavlik harness presents a low risk of avascular necrosis (see section of Avascular Necrosis of the Hip). This treatment should not be continued beyond 3–4 weeks if there is no improvement. The failure rate of the Pavlik harness is approximately 10%.

In this age group, the rare patient with a located hip but also dysplasia or ligamentous instability may also be treated in a Pavlik harness or another abduction device.

B. Age 6–15 Months (Before Walking)

Gentle reduction of the dislocation under a general anesthetic and maintenance of a located position for 2–3 months in a spica cast usually stabilize the joint. Even after the hip is stable, any residual dysplasia must be treated by bracing or surgery. In the past, prereduction skin traction was thought to reduce the risk of avascular necrosis. It is now believed that adequate hip flexion and limited abduction in the spica cast is the

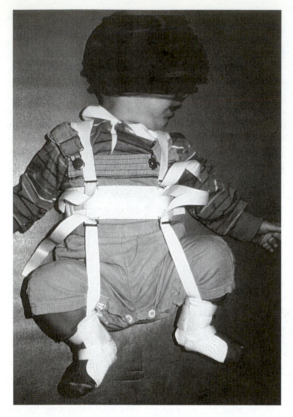

Figure 11–5. The Pavlik harness, a device used for treatment of hip dislocation, subluxation, and dysplasia.

most important safety factor, and many surgeons no longer use traction.

C. AGE 15 MONTHS TO 2 YEARS

In toddlers or young children in whom closed reduction has failed, open reduction of the hip is required. Femoral-shortening osteotomy may be required at the time of open reduction to reduce soft-tissue tension and minimize the risk of avascular necrosis. Severe flattening of the acetabulum with distortion of the normal spherical femoral head shape is found on opening the hip. The limbus (acetabular rim) may be flattened and inverted, and the ligamentum teres is always hypertrophic. Fibrofatty tissue occupying the center of the acetabulum must be removed. After reduction, the position is maintained by capsular repair (capsulorrhaphy) and a cast, until stability is achieved. Prolonged bracing or surgery is often required to resolve the residual dysplasia that accompanies untreated dysplasia in this group of children.

D. AGE ABOVE 2 YEARS

Significant residual dysplasia is present in children with DDH who are untreated at this age. Dysplasia may also persist despite successful reduction performed by any method at an earlier age. The dysplasia may be accompanied by a limp, and radiographs show a high acetabular index (more vertical acetabular roof), increased valgus of the femoral neck, and subluxation of the femoral head.

Surgical correction of dysplasia creates a stable mechanical environment that permits remodeling to a more normal joint during growth. The procedure involves bony procedures, either on the acetabular or femoral sides of the joint, or on both sides. Acetabular procedures such as the Salter or Pemberton osteotomies reduce the acetabular index and increase the mechanical stability of the joint.

Femoral osteotomy corrects the anteversion and femoral neck valgus that characterize femoral dysplasia. The exact selection of osteotomy site may be based on maximum radiographic dysplasia or on the individual surgeon's preference. All of the osteotomies require that the femoral head be spherical and the hip joint concentrically reduced before an attempt can be made to correct the dysplasia. In general, the osteotomy should address the site of dysplasia, that is, acetabular dysplasia is not ideally treated with femoral osteotomy. Nevertheless, femoral osteotomy, if performed before age 4 years, will stimulate a dysplastic shallow acetabulum to remodel into a more normal shape. This occurs because the femoral osteotomy renders the hip joint more stable, thus allowing the normal mechanisms of growth to take over. Similarly, patients will exhibit a progressive decrease in femoral dysplasia following successful acetabular osteotomy.

1. Salter osteotomy—Salter osteotomy is a surgical procedure to redirect the acetabulum in DDH (Figure 11–6). Animal models demonstrate that residual hip dysplasia is accompanied by acetabular malrotation and deficiency in the anterolateral acetabular rim. Salter osteotomy corrects this deficiency by rotating the acetabular region anteriorly and laterally.

The procedure is indicated in children 18 months to 10 years of age in whom concentric reduction of the hip has been achieved. It is used to correct moderate acetabular dysplasia and can improve the acetabular index by 15 degrees. It may also be used to stabilize the hip at the time of open reduction. The pelvis above the hip joint is exposed subperiosteally. A transverse cut is made, using a wire saw, from the sciatic notch to the anteroinferior iliac spine, and the entire distal fragment (including the acetabulum) is spun on the pivot points of the notch and the pubic symphysis. This redirects the entire dysplastic acetabulum to a more horizontal

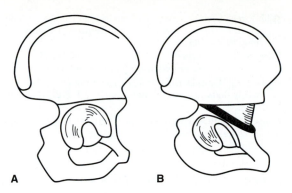

Figure 11–6. Salter innominate osteotomy, used for managing acetabular dysplasia. After a transverse cut is made above the acetabulum (**A**), the acetabular fragment is rotated forward and outward (**B**) to improve acetabular coverage.

stable position. A bone graft and pins hold the osteotomy open until it heals. A spica cast is used for 6 weeks to protect the graft during healing.

Salter osteotomy requires a second operation to remove the fixation pins. Because the geometric reorientation afforded is limited, there may be residual dysplasia. In addition, failure to achieve a concentric reduction before pelvic osteotomy usually renders the procedure ineffective.

2. Pemberton osteotomy—Indications for Pemberton osteotomy (Figure 11–7) are similar to those of the Salter osteotomy, and frequently one or the other is selected according to the surgeon's experience or preference. The Pemberton procedure is particularly suited

for correction of the long "stretched out" dysplastic acetabulum because it reduces the capacity of an overly spacious acetabulum. This is done by cutting above the acetabular roof, down to the flexible triradiate cartilage (the growth plate of the center of the acetabulum). The roof fragment is then pried down to a more horizontal position and held in place by wedging a bone graft into the resulting defect. The fold thus produced in the center of the acetabulum may cause temporary stiffness. In younger children, this quickly remodels, but it is the major reason many surgeons do not perform this procedure on children older than 7–8 years.

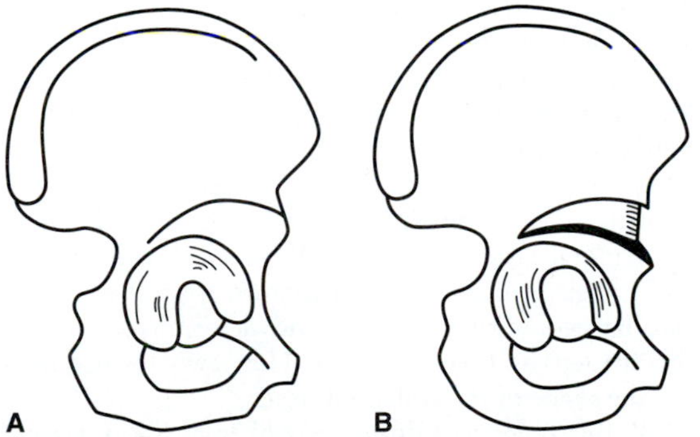

Like the Salter procedure, Pemberton osteotomy requires concentric reduction before it is performed. For the Pemberton osteotomy, the pelvis is exposed above the joint. Under radiographic guidance, a curved osteotome is used to cut the pelvic bone from the acetabular roof down to the triradiate cartilage (the central growth plate of the acetabulum). The flexible cartilage allows the fragment to be hinged down over the femoral head, producing a more horizontal acetabular roof. A bone graft from the upper ilium wedges into the osteotomy site to maintain correction, and a spica cast is used until healing, which takes about 6 weeks.

Rarely, early extrusion or graft collapse occurs, and transient stiffness may be seen in older children. Because there is no internal fixation, a second procedure is unnecessary.

3. Femoral osteotomy—Femoral osteotomy (Figure 11–8) may be used to correct severe increased femoral anteversion or coxa valga (a high neck-shaft angle), conditions that are sometimes seen in residual DDH.

Figure 11–7. Pemberton pericapsular iliac osteotomy. An osteotomy cut is made above the acetabulum down to the flexible triradiate cartilage (**A**). The fragment is pried down to improve acetabular coverage and held with a bone graft (**B**).

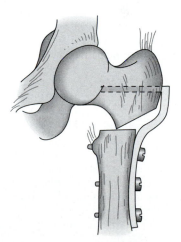

Figure 11–8. Femoral osteotomy is performed at the intertrochanteric level and fixed with a plate and screws.

The procedure is particularly indicated when radiographs taken with the hip in abduction and external rotation show improvement in the overall congruency of the hip. Redirection of an anteverted proximal femur in valgus angulation will stimulate spontaneous improvement in dysplastic acetabula in children younger than 4 years.

Femoral osteotomy is performed using a lateral approach, with the cut made across the intertrochanteric region of the femur. This site is chosen both because it is distal to the blood supply of the femoral head and because the cancellous bone heals easily. A metal blade-plate is placed in the proximal (femoral neck) fragment, usually after positioning with a provisional guide wire. The femoral neck fragment is rotated into a more horizontal position (varus) and is then internally rotated to correct excessive anteversion. The exact degree of correction is determined by preoperative radiograph positioning to achieve maximum congruence and correction of radiographic dysplasia. The plate portion is then clamped to the shaft of the bone and fixed with screws. A spica cast is usually used to supplement fixation.

After healing (6 weeks), the patient may resume walking. A Trendelenburg limp is common for 1–2 years after femoral osteotomy because of the geometric distortion of the relationship between the joint and insertion of the abductor muscles. This resolves as the femur remodels with growth and does not present a long-term problem.

Avascular Necrosis of the Hip

If a reduction maneuver for DDH has been forceful or if there is tension in the soft tissues around the hip, the resulting compression of the joint may cause transient blockage of the blood supply to the femoral head. The subsequent death of the ossific nucleus and proximal growth plate of the femur (avascular necrosis) is a complication of treatment rather than of the disorder itself. A well-recognized cause of avascular necrosis is exaggerated forced abduction in the spica cast used after closed or open reduction. Avascular necrosis may be mild (involving a small fraction of the ossific nucleus), in which case it may go undetected and be of little significance. At the other extreme, avascular necrosis may lead to complete femoral head death and loss of future growth at the proximal physis. As it revascularizes, a dead femoral head may deform significantly, subluxate further, and require abduction bracing or osteotomy. Thus, it can cause leg-length inequality or early osteoarthritis of the hip. The best treatment for avascular necrosis is prevention.

Bennett JT, MacEwen GD: Congenital dislocation of the hip: Recent advances and current problems. Clin Orthop 1989; 247:15.

Bialik V et al: Clinical assessment of hip instability in the newborn by an orthopedic surgeon and a pediatrician. J Pediatr Orthop 1986;6:703.

Kalamchi A, MacFarlane R III: The Pavlik harness: Results in patients over three months of age. J Pediatr Orthop 1982;2:3.

Segal LS et al: Avascular necrosis after treatment of DDH: The protective influence of the ossific nucleus. J Pediatr Orthop 1999;19:177.

Zionts LE, MacEwen GD: Treatment of congenital hip dislocation in children between the ages of one and three years. J Bone Joint Surg Am 1986;68:829.

3. Legg-Calvé-Perthes Disease

Legg-Calvé-Perthes disease (LCP, Perthes disease) is a serious but self-limited pediatric hip disorder. Although its cause is unknown, the disease is thought to be related to avascular necrosis of the hip. It affects children age 4–10 years and is somewhat more common in boys. Children with the disease are often small for their age and have retarded bone age. The disease is generally unilateral. If it is bilateral, other conditions such as Gaucher's disease or multiple epiphyseal dysplasia must be considered. Recent investigations have suggested that some cases of LCP might be related to a variety of transient or permanent hypercoagulation states. This research has not yet been confirmed in multiple centers. Surprisingly, trauma is not considered a causative factor in LCP.

Although early radiographs may be negative, they eventually show fragmentation, irregularity, and collapse of part or all of the femoral head ossification center (Figure 11–9). The few pathologic specimens that have been examined suggest that multiple rather than single episodes of avascular necrosis occur over a period of months. Early bone scans may show a filling defect corresponding to areas of necrosis, and magnetic resonance imaging (MRI) is typical of avascular necrosis. The disease has a characteristic course (see Figure 11–9). Initially, the avascular episodes are silent and the child is asymptomatic. As the bone of the proximal femoral epiphysis dies, it is revascularized. Osteoclasts remove dead bone while osteoblasts simultaneously lay down new bone on the dead trabeculas (a process known as "creeping substitution"). During this phase, the femoral head is mechanically weak. Fragmentation and collapse of the bony structure may then occur, causing geometric flattening and deformity of the ossific nucleus and femoral head. The newly formed bone has the shape of the collapsed head.

At this point, continued growth may allow gradual remodeling and improvement of the femoral head shape until maturity. The symptomatic collapse phase rarely exceeds 1–1½ years, but full revascularization and remodeling may continue silently for several years thereafter.

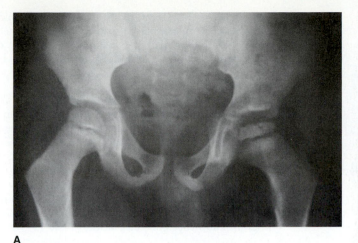

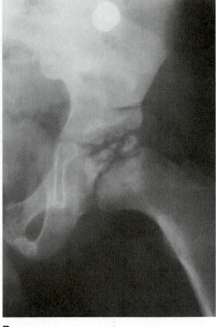

Figure 11–9. Legg-Calvé-Perthes disease. **A:** Central necrotic fragment with collapse. **B:** Same patient after healing and partial remodeling.

Clinical Findings and Classification

A. SYMPTOMS AND SIGNS

The clinical presentation of LCP in a child age 4–10 years is usually a painless limp. If pain is present, it may be mild and referred to the thigh or knee. Physical examination discloses atrophy of the thigh on the affected side and, usually, limited hip motion. The typical patient has a flexion contracture of 0–30 degrees, loss of abduction compared with the opposite side (in severe cases, no abduction beyond 0 degrees), and loss of internal rotation of the hip.

B. IMAGING STUDIES

Radiographs may be negative at first, probably because the initial softening of the femoral head is sufficient to cause symptoms but insufficient to change the radiographic appearance of the femoral head. The eventual characteristic collapse of portions of the femoral head is diagnostic of the disease, however.

The exact extent of necrosis, which is usually estimated in fourths of the head using the Catterall classification (Figure 11–10), is helpful in determining whom to treat. It may require additional radiographs.

An alternative radiograph classification uses the lateral one third of the femoral epiphysis (the "lateral pillar"). Collapse of this structure suggests a poor prognosis for late deformity, whereas maintenance of pillar height correlates with good long-term results. Partial collapse suggests an intermediate prognosis. The difficulty with all classification systems is their reproducibility and the need to delay until the collapse phase before the exact extent of involvement is clear.

There is little value in bone scans or MRI in the clinical management of LCP.

Treatment Options

A. NO TREATMENT

Children with bone age less than 5 years and children who exhibit relatively minor involvement (less than half of the femoral head) rarely need treatment. In these children, so much of the femoral head is cartilage, and therefore unaffected by necrosis, that mechanical collapse does not markedly decrease sphericity. Also, younger children have tremendous remodeling potential, and minor collapse can be outgrown before

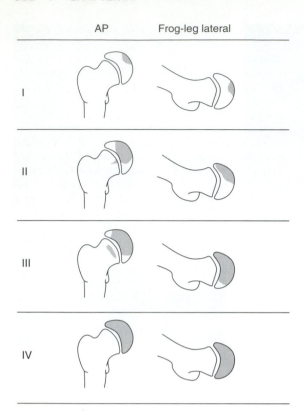

AP   Frog-leg lateral

I

II

III

IV

Figure 11–10. The Catterall classification is used to determine probable course and prognosis of Legg-Calvé-Perthes disease. It is based on progressive involvement of approximate fourths of the femoral head.

maturity. Older children who exhibit some radiograph changes but have excellent range of motion may require only observation and serial reexamination.

B. NONOPERATIVE AND OPERATIVE TREATMENT

The issues surrounding selection of patients with LCP who need treatment are as highly controversial as the treatment itself. Most experts agree that children who maintain excellent motion (particularly abduction greater than 30 degrees in the absence of flexion contracture) may not require intervention. In children older than 4–5 years with significant collapse or progressive loss of abduction, treatment is frequently recommended.

There is no evidence that use of crutches or relief of weight bearing has any effect on femoral head collapse in this disease. For those children requiring it, however, treatment should minimize the effects of collapse and reduction of the subluxation that often occurs when the femoral head deforms. This is best achieved by abduc-

tion of the hip until subluxation resolves. The "molding" action of the acetabular shape is thought to help improve the contour of the collapsing femoral head. Abduction can be accomplished nonoperatively by holding the legs in abduction (Petrie) casts or using an ambulatory brace (Figure 11–11).

Operative procedures are advocated by some and include varus femoral osteotomy and Salter osteotomy, which have been adapted from hip dysplasia treatment to control the subluxation seen in some cases of LCP. Healing usually occurs within 18 months.

Despite many studies, there is still no consensus for the best method of treatment; some patients do well without treatment, while others have a poor result after aggressive treatment. Prognosis can often be predicted from the knowledge of certain factors (Table 11–5).

Catterall A: The natural history of Perthes disease. J Bone Joint Surg Br 1971;53:37.

Cooperman DR et al: Factors relating to hip joint arthritis following three childhood diseases—juvenile rheumatoid arthritis, Perthes disease, and postreduction avascular necrosis in congenital hip dislocation. J Pediatric Orthop 1986;6:706.

Glueck CJ et al: Protein C and S deficiency, thrombophilia, and hypofibrinolysis: Pathophysiologic causes of Legg-Perthes disease. Pediatr Res 1994;35:383.

Herring JA: The treatment of Legg-Calvé-Perthes disease. A critical review of the literature. J Bone Joint Surg Am 1994;76:448.

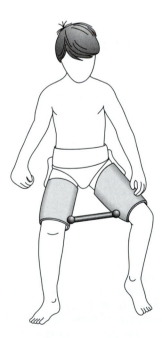

Figure 11–11. Abduction bracing is one method used for ambulatory treatment of Legg-Calvé-Perthes disease.

Table 11–5. Factors in long-term prognosis for patients with Legg-Calvé-Perthes disease.

Relative Prognosis	Good	Poor
Age at diagnosis	< 5 years	> 8–9 years
Hip Motion[a]	Maintained (abduction > 30°)	Stiff (abduction < 15°)
Extent of involvement	< 50% of femoral head	> 50% or total femoral head
Radiograph features	Little or no subluxation	Subluxation, lateral calcification

[a]During first year of treatment.

McAndrew MP, Weinstein SL: A long-term follow-up of Legg-Calvé-Perthes disease. J Bone Joint Surg Am 1984;66:860.

4. Slipped Capital Femoral Epiphysis

Slipped capital femoral epiphysis is an adolescent hip disorder characterized by displacement of the femoral head on the femoral neck. Displacement changes the geometry of the upper end of the femur and hinders hip function (Figure 11–12). This disorder is one of the main causes of premature osteoarthritis in young adults.

Slipped capital femoral epiphysis usually affects both male and female adolescents age 11–13 years. In 25–30% of patients, the condition is bilateral, although both legs are not always affected simultaneously. The typical patient is overweight-often markedly so—and is in either late prepuberty or early puberty. Rarely, the patient is tall, asthenic, and rapidly growing.

This disorder occurs at a time when the cartilage physis of the proximal femur is thickening rapidly under the influence of growth hormone. The vigorous secretion of sex hormone has not yet begun, however, so the mechanical effect of sex hormones on closure and stabilization of the growth plate is absent. This combination of thick growth plate cartilage (weaker than bone and subject to shear), lack of sexual maturity (which would stabilize the physis), mechanical stress (caused by obesity), and the peculiar anatomic mechanics of the hip joint renders the growth plate susceptible to slippage.

The direction of the slip is always posterior and often medial, and the mechanical bases of chronic and acute disorders are the same. In chronic slipped capital femoral epiphysis, the most common form (90% of patients), the femoral head slips insidiously at the growth plate over the course of several months. In the acute form, the femoral head is suddenly displaced, a condition that can be superimposed on chronic changes. Displacement may occur during normal activity or following minor trauma.

Because slipped capital femoral epiphysis is a progressive disorder and the prognosis depends on the severity of the slippage, early detection and prompt treatment are imperative.

Clinical Findings

A. SYMPTOMS AND SIGNS

The onset of chronic slipped capital femoral epiphysis is usually insidious, with a history of a painful limp for 1 to several months prior. The pain is characteristically aching and located in the thigh or knee rather than the hip. This referred pain to the knee is responsible for many misdiagnoses. Patients may be seen for knee pain and dismissed as normal after a negative knee examination and radiographs. A high index of suspicion is required to detect slipped capital femoral epiphysis in the obese limping adolescent complaining of knee pain. The change in hip range of motion is usually diagnostic. Loss of abduction and internal rotation of the hip are evident, although these may be difficult to identify in the grossly overweight child. There is almost always a characteristic obligatory external rotation of the hip

AP

Frog-leg lateral

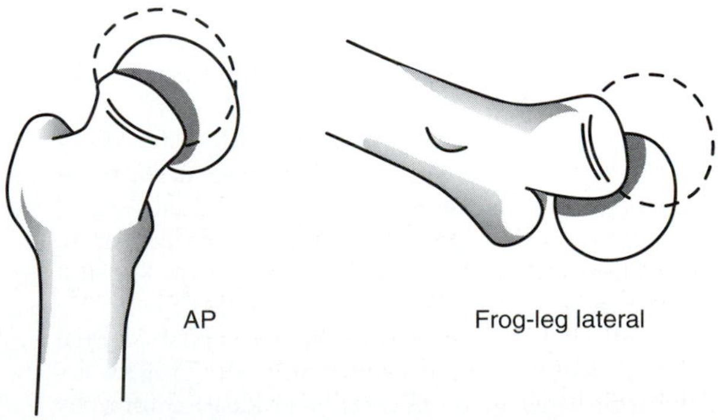

Figure 11–12. Anteroposterior (AP) and frog-leg views of a slipped epiphysis. The dotted lines show the normal position of the femoral head.

when it is flexed because of the distorted hip anatomy caused by the disorder. The femoral head is posterior to its normal position, so the flexed hip must externally rotate to keep the head within the acetabulum.

Acute slipped capital femoral epiphysis is accompanied by severe pain and limping, which may render the patient immobile. The onset is sudden, following little or no trauma, and examination discloses a painful, guarded, restricted range of hip motion. An acute slip is analogous to an epiphyseal fracture. In its "unstable" form, the patient will be unable to bear weight, and there is a high rate of avascular necrosis. In its "stable" form, the sudden increase in displacement is painful, but limited weight-bearing is possible and the risk of avascular necrosis appears to be lower.

B. IMAGING STUDIES

Slipped capital femoral epiphysis can be difficult to detect on standard anteroposterior radiograph (Figure 11–13). A frog-leg lateral view is the best for detecting mild forms because slippage is always posterior. A radiograph also shows changes suggesting acute or chronic forms, information that may be critical to management of the disorder.

Establishing the severity of slippage is important in determining treatment and prognosis. Severity is estimated by the percentage of femoral neck left exposed: slippage of less than 25% of neck width is mild; 25–50% is moderate; and more than 50% is severe.

Treatment

Slipped capital femoral epiphysis is usually a progressive disease that requires prompt surgical treatment. Because the changes in the chronic form occur so slowly, it is impossible to manipulate the femoral head into a better position. Treatment consists of fixing the slip in its current position and preventing progression. This is done by inserting one or more screws or pins across the growth plate, regardless of the severity of the slip (pinning in situ).

Following surgery, aching rapidly resolves, and during the remaining 2–3 years of skeletal growth, the extent of remodeling of the distorted proximal femur may be considerable, leading to an improved range of motion.

Acute slips, if unstable, may be gently reduced before fixation, but the risk of further damage to the tenuous blood supply of the proximal femur and subsequent avascular necrosis is always significant. For this reason, many surgeons accept the position of an acute slip and pin it in situ.

In some cases, high-grade slipped capital femoral epiphysis will not remodel sufficiently with growth, despite treatment. In these cases, a residual, chronically

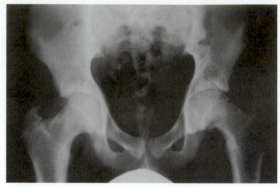

A

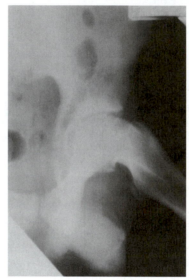

B

Figure 11–13. Radiograph diagnosis of left slipped capital femoral epiphysis. **A:** Anteroposterior film shows subtle medial displacement of left epiphysis, best appreciated by drawing a line (Klein's line) along the lateral side of the normal and abnormal femoral neck. The slipped epiphysis does not protrude lateral to this line. **B:** Frog-leg lateral radiograph clearly demonstrates posterior displacement.

painful limp is present, requiring correction by proximal femoral osteotomy. The osteotomy site may be at the level of the slip; this is mechanically effective but relatively risky for the blood supply. Alternatively, osteotomy can be performed at the trochanteric level; this is a safer procedure for correction of the functional deformity but does not resolve the exact anatomic deformity.

Complications

A. CHONDROLYSIS

In addition to the problems of impingement of the anterior metaphyseal prominence, which can impede motion, some patients with slipped capital femoral epiphysis develop chondrolysis, a poorly understood degeneration of the hip articular cartilage. It may be painful and may progress to severe joint narrowing and degenerative changes within 6 months.

During chondrolysis, cartilage is replaced by fibrous tissue, the joint capsule thickens and contracts, and joint motion is lost. Typically, the joint stiffens in flexion, abduction, and external rotation. Radiographs disclose joint narrowing, irregularity, and subchondral sclerosis, as well as regional osteoporosis from disuse.

Chondrolysis can result from iatrogenic malposition (permanent penetration) of pins or screws used for fixation of slipped capital femoral epiphysis. Although brief penetrations during surgery are probably common and cause no complications, unrecognized permanent pin penetration is disastrous. Chondrolysis also appears without obvious penetration and occasionally is detected in patients before treatment begins.

Chondrolysis is treated by nonsteroidal anti-inflammatory medications, aggressive physical therapy and range-of-motion exercises, and observation. About half of patients eventually recover satisfactory painless motion. The other half may require hip fusion for symptomatic relief.

B. AVASCULAR NECROSIS

Patients with an acutely slipped capital femoral epiphysis can develop avascular necrosis of the femoral head (see section on Developmental Dysplasia of the Hip). Because such patients are teenagers, the prognosis is poor, although some patients with partial head involvement regain a painless hip after a 1–2 years of symptoms. Some patients with painless but abnormal range of motion may be treatable by intertrochanteric osteotomy to reorient the arc of motion. Long-term pain following avascular necrosis is treated by hip fusion.

C. PROGNOSIS

A slipped epiphysis is a major cause of early osteoarthritis. In general, the higher the degree of slip, the earlier the degenerative changes begin. In fact, a statistical increase in degenerative arthritis is evident even in the radiographically normal hip of patients with a contralateral slipped epiphysis. This suggests that subclinical bilateral involvement is more common than recognized.

Carney BT et al: Long-term follow-up of slipped capital femoral epiphysis. J Bone Joint Surg 1991;73A:667.

Canale ST: Problems and complications of slipped capital femoral epiphysis. Instr Course Lect 1989;38:281.

Koval KJ et al: Treatment of slipped capital femoral epiphysis with a cannulated screw technique. J Bone Joint Surg 1989;71A:1370.

Morrissey RT: Principles of in situ fixation in chronic slipped capital femoral epiphysis. Instr Course Lect 1989;38:257.

Siegel DB et al: Slipped capital femoral epiphysis. A quantitative analysis of motion, gait, and femoral remodeling after in situ fixation. J Bone Joint Surg 1991; 73A:659.

FOOT DISORDERS

1. Metatarsus Adductus

Metatarsus adductus (metatarsus varus) is the most common foot deformity in the newborn infant, occurring in 5 in 1000 live births, frequently bilaterally. Although it is usually isolated, several apparently unrelated deformities (such as DDH) are statistically more likely to occur in the presence of this disorder. The cause is unknown but might be related to "uterine packing."

Clinical Findings

The hallmark of the deformity is medial deviation of the forefoot, with the apex of the deformity at the midtarsal region. The hindfoot is normal. Frequently, a deep skin crease is evident at the medial border of the foot, suggesting that the deformity has been present for some time. The adducted forefoot usually can be passively corrected to a neutral position but occasionally is fairly rigid. When the examining physician places a hand on the forefoot so as to hide it, the ankle has full movement.

Treatment

Metatarsus adductus tends to be self-correcting. Even severe cases generally resolve by 12–18 months of age without treatment. Nevertheless, many orthopedists use passive stretching to reassure parents that the child is being treated. Indeed, there is some evidence that passive correction and serial plaster casting can speed resolution of the disorder. Recurrence after brief casting is frequent in young children, and, in any case, it is necessary to wait for spontaneous resolution. Therefore, treatment for metatarsus adductus is usually not recommended.

Farsetti P et al: The long-term functional and radiographic outcomes of untreated and non-operatively treated metatarsus adductus. J Bone Joint Surg 1994;76A:257.

2. Congenital Clubfoot

Congenital clubfoot (equinovarus foot; talipes equinovarus) is a severe fixed deformity of the foot (Figure

11–14). It is characterized by fixed ankle plantar flexion (equinus), inversion and axial internal rotation of the subtalar (talocalcaneal) joint (varus), and medial subluxation of the talonavicular and calcaneocuboid joints (adductus). Severe cavus may be present, with a medial and plantar midfoot crease. Whether unilateral or bilateral, the deformity is more common in males, although when it occurs in females, it tends to be more severe.

The incidence in the newborn population is 1 in 1000, with increased risk for families in which even distant members have the deformity. There is considerable evidence that clubfoot is an inherited trait, but the disorder appears to reflect polygenetic expression, and exact inheritance patterns are unclear. Although most are isolated deformities and are considered idiopathic, clubfoot may frequently be present in association with a wide variety of syndromes that affect the musculoskeletal system.

Clinical Findings

A. SYMPTOMS AND SIGNS

Clinical diagnosis of clubfoot is uncomplicated. Because it is a rigid deformity, clubfoot cannot be passively corrected, as can metatarsus adductus. Frequently, the foot is so severely internally rotated and inverted that the sole faces superiorly. Occasionally, the plantar flexion of the ankle is not obvious, because the

posterior tip of the calcaneus is small, high, and difficult to palpate. Clubfoot is always associated with a permanent decrease in calf circumference related to fibrosis of the calf musculature. This may not be obvious at birth but becomes more apparent after the child begins to walk.

Special attention should be paid to the presence of spine deformity, caudal dimpling, or midline spinal hairy patches, all of which may imply a neurogenic component. Thus, the examining physician should carefully search for features of other deformities or syndromes.

B. IMAGING STUDIES

Increasingly, clubfoot is suspected from prenatal ultrasound examination. Radiographs are rarely of value in the initial clubfoot evaluation because the bones of the foot are minimally ossified at birth. Radiographs become more important if the physician is considering surgical intervention or if the child has reached walking age, and radiographs can quantify the completeness of correction achieved by casting or surgery.

The typical radiographic findings of incompletely treated clubfoot include the following features:

(1) presence of hindfoot plantar flexion,

(2) lack of the normal angular relationship between the talus and calcaneus ("parallelism" of talus and calcaneus), and

(3) residual medial subluxation or displacement of the navicular on the talus and the cuboid on the calcaneus (Figure 11–15).

Treatment

A. CONSERVATIVE TREATMENT

Clubfoot always requires treatment, which should begin at birth. The initial approach is passive manipulation and positioning to the corrected position. In the

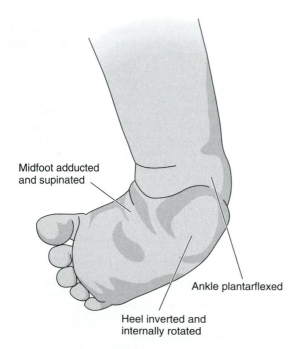

Midfoot adducted and supinated

Ankle plantarflexed

Heel inverted and internally rotated

Figure 11–14. Clinical appearance of congenital right clubfoot.

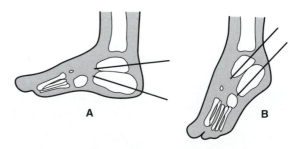

A   B

Figure 11–15. Diagrammatic appearance of radiograph in clubfoot. **A:** Normal foot. **B:** Clubfoot.

United States, the majority of orthopedists use serial manipulation and casting, usually at 1-week intervals in the first month of life, and at 1- to 2-week intervals thereafter. In other parts of the world, strapping (with adhesive tape) or splinting with a variety of braces are popular methods (in addition to serial casting) for maintaining the manipulated correction. There is no evidence for the superiority of either method.

Although nonoperative treatment may be conceptually similar to training a bonsai tree, in that the joints are carefully held in a corrected position during growth, the analogy is limited. In clubfoot, the ligaments and joint capsules are severely contracted and thickened and, unlike supple tree limbs, may not "stretch" despite carefully executed manipulation and casting. In addition, the manipulation that encourages tension in these shortened ligaments may produce damaging compressive forces on delicate cartilaginous anlages of future tarsal bones. For these reasons, many surgeons limit nonoperative treatment to 12 weeks and then reassess the degree of correction attained. If clinical and radiologic evidence indicates significant correction, casting continues. Otherwise, surgery is required. Failure of nonoperative treatment is common, particularly in girls (where the deformity is often more severe) and in bilateral cases.

B. SURGICAL TREATMENT

Surgical correction of all clubfoot deformities is generally performed in one stage. At times, the casting has corrected most of the midfoot deformity, and simple posterior release (ankle capsulotomy and Achillis tendon lengthening) are all that is required. Frequently, the surgeon must consider correction of the entire group of deformities through a comprehensive, extensive surgical approach.

One common approach uses the "Cincinnati" incision, which extends from the navicular bone medially, around the superior portion of the heel, to the cuboid bone laterally (Figure 11–16). During surgery, the medial posterior tibial neurovascular bundle must be identified and protected. The tendons of the posterior tibialis, flexor digitorum longus, flexor hallucis longus, and Achilles tendon are Z-lengthened. The capsules of the talonavicular joint, subtalar (talocalcaneal) joint, and posterior ankle joint are released to allow repositioning of the bones of the hindfoot and midfoot.

The navicular is usually subluxated medially on the head of the talus and must be repositioned onto its normal location. The calcaneus is both inverted and internally rotated on the talus. This is corrected by manually derotating the subtalar joint and tilting the calcaneus back into a neutral position. These corrections are usually held in place after reduction by inserting small Kirschner wires, which are removed after 4–6 weeks.

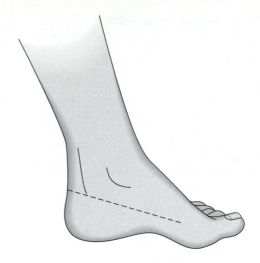

Figure 11–16. Cincinnati incision used for surgical correction of clubfoot.

The ankle is repositioned by dorsiflexion to neutral prior to repair of the lengthened Achilles tendon. Postoperative casting allows the gaping capsule to re-form with the bones of the clubfoot in their appropriate, corrected position.

C. COMPLICATIONS

Early complications of clubfoot surgery are rare, but the rate of recurrence within 3 years is 5–10%. If surgical release is too aggressive, overcorrection with late heel valgus and an overlengthened heel cord can occur.

Clubfoot surgery is conceptually straightforward, but in actuality it is among the most difficult procedures in children's orthopedics because of the judgment required to assess the extent of intraoperative release.

Occasionally, some form of bracing is used postoperatively after the cast is removed. Mild recurrence of deformity is fairly common, and even when deformity is permanently corrected, the foot will always remain smaller and stiffer than normal and calf circumference will be reduced. Families must be informed of this possibility early in treatment so that they have realistic expectations about the outcome.

Irani RN, Sherman MS: The pathological anatomy of club foot. J Bone Joint Surg Am1963;45:45.

Ponseti IV. Congenital Clubfoot. Fundamentals of Treatment. Oxford University Press, Oxford, New York, 1996.

Turco VJ: Resistant congenital club foot: One-stage posteromedial release with internal fixation: A follow-up report of a fifteen-year experience. J Bone Joint Surg Am 1979;61:805.

Yamamoto H et al: Non-surgical treatment of congenital clubfoot with manipulation, cast, and Denis Browne splint. J Pediatr Orthop 1998:18:538.

3. Calcaneovalgus Foot

Calcaneovalgus foot is generally considered to be a "uterine packing" problem in which the foot is markedly dorsiflexed at birth so the dorsum of the foot sits against the anterior surface of the tibia (Figure 11–17). The hindfoot is usually in moderate eversion (valgus) as well. Although some flexibility is present with the deformity, there is resistance to full motion: Most cases will not allow ankle plantar flexion beyond a right angle.

Despite its dramatic appearance, calcaneovalgus foot corrects spontaneously within 2–3 months. Although some orthopedists brace or apply serial casts and many recommend stretching exercises, all true calcaneovalgus feet will resolve without treatment.

Congenital Vertical Talus

Calcaneovalgus foot must be differentiated from a much rarer condition known as congenital vertical talus (congenital rocker-bottom foot, congenital complex pes valgus). In this deformity, although the foot appears to lie against the anterior tibia, the hindfoot is actually plantar-flexed because of contracture of the posterior calf muscles. To accommodate plantarflexion of the hindfoot and dorsiflexion of the forefoot, the midfoot joints (talonavicular and calcaneocuboid joints) must subluxate or dislocate dorsally.

Congenital vertical talus often accompanies genetic disorders, syndromes such as arthrogryposis, or neuromuscular disorders such as spina bifida. It is occasionally found in otherwise normal infants, however. Treatment is usually surgical, although serial casting may be used initially.

4. Cavus Foot

Cavus foot is a foot with an abnormally high arch. Although it is difficult to ascribe a particular threshold of arching beyond which treatment is necessary, most deformities are dramatic enough to make diagnosis straightforward (Figure 11–18).

Frequently, cavus foot accompanies hindfoot varus deformity (cavovarus foot), and there may be clawing of the toes and demonstrable weakness of ankle or foot muscles. In addition, calluses beneath the metatarsal heads and heel skin are common.

Clinical Findings

One of the most common symptoms of cavus foot is anterior ankle pain, sometimes associated with toe

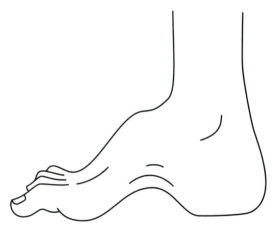

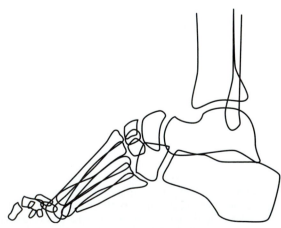

Figure 11–18. Cavus foot: clinical appearance and radiographic appearance.

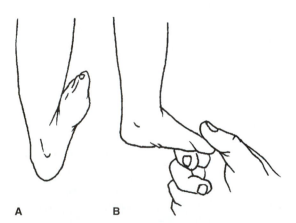

A   **B**

Figure 11–17. Calcaneovalgus foot as it appears in relaxed position (**A**) and maximally plantar-flexed (**B**).

walking. This paradoxic situation occurs because of the pathologic anatomy of the cavus foot. The forefoot is severely plantar-flexed on the hindfoot, requiring marked ankle dorsiflexion to compensate. When the cavus becomes too severe, ankle dorsiflexion is blocked, leading to anterior ankle impingement and pain. The inability to dorsiflex further compromises forefoot clearance, and, eventually, only the metatarsals can contact the floor. This can be misinterpreted as ankle plantarflexion contracture, leading to unnecessary (and possibly harmful) heel cord release.

The cause of cavus foot is usually muscle imbalance in a growing foot. Thus, cavus is rarely found in early childhood but is fairly frequent after age 8–10 years. Although intrinsic muscle weakness is a major cause of cavus foot, weakness of the peroneal or anterior tibialis muscles has also been implicated. Cavus foot is rarely found in the absence of an underlying neuromuscular condition.

Cavus foot is a "marker" for neuromuscular disease. Diagnosis requires a thorough search for the underlying cause and may require neurologic consultation, spinal MRI, and electromyographic (EMG) studies. Table 11–6 lists common neuromuscular causes of cavus foot.

Treatment

Conservative treatment of cavus foot includes accommodation by shoe modifications or inserts. These modalities will not actually correct the condition; severe deformity requires surgical correction by triple arthrodesis (hindfoot fusion in a corrected position). Tendon transfers may be necessary to restore muscle balance.

Levitt RL et al: The role of foot surgery in progressive neuromuscular disorders in children. J Bone Joint Surg Am 1973;55: 1396.

McCluskey WP et al: The cavovarus foot deformity. Etiology and management. Clin Orthop 1989; 247:27.

Table 11–6. Common neuromuscular causes of cavus foot.

Cerebral palsy
Charcot-Marie-Tooth disease
Compartment syndrome
Diastematomyelia
Friedrich's ataxia
Muscular dystrophy
Spinal cord tumor
Spinal dysraphism (spina bifida)

5. Pes Planus (Flatfoot)

Flatfoot refers to loss of the normal longitudinal arch of the medial foot. Many cases of flatfoot are inherited, and a careful family history may uncover other persons with the condition. The foot is usually flexible, so the arch appears when the foot is not bearing weight. Hindfoot valgus (heel eversion) is often present. In severe cases, flatfoot may be painful, but this aspect of the deformity is often overemphasized.

Clinical Findings

Physical determination of the flexibility of the flatfoot requires careful examination. Subtalar motion is usually normal. In feet that exhibit a flat arch and valgus heel while standing, examination from the posterior aspect frequently discloses a normal arch and varus heel by muscle action when the patient stands on tiptoe. If these signs of a flexible flatfoot are not present, alternative diagnoses such as tarsal coalition (see section on Tarsal Coalition) should be considered. The physician should also look for painful plantar calluses.

Standing radiographs disclose loss of the normal medial longitudinal arch and may show mild lateral subluxation of the talonavicular joint as well. In severe chronic cases, degenerative, talonavicular spurring may be present.

Treatment

Symptomatic treatment (shoe modifications, arch supports, and plantar inserts) is appropriate because no long-term treatment can alter the anatomic features of the disorder. Posterior tibial advancement, subtalar joint elevation or fusion, and elongation osteotomy of the lateral calcaneal neck may not provide reproducible, predictable resolution of the problem.

Sullivan JA: Pediatric flatfoot: Evaluation and management. J Am Acad Orthop Surg 1999;7:44.

6. Tarsal Coalition

Tarsal coalition is a congenital connection between two or more tarsal bones. Coalitions may be fibrous, cartilaginous, or bony. Usually, coalitions occur between two bones and are cartilaginous in early life but eventually ossify (or nearly ossify) as the foot matures. Frequently bilateral, coalitions often follow an autosomal-dominant inheritance pattern.

The most common sites for tarsal coalition are between the calcaneus and the navicular laterally (Figure 11–19) and between the talus and the calcaneus medially.

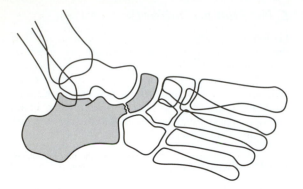

Figure 11–19. Calcaneonavicular tarsal coalition is best seen on oblique radiograph projection.

Clinical Findings

Symptoms of tarsal coalition may include foot pain and stiffness as the lesion begins to ossify during early adolescence. The resulting stiffness and abnormal intertarsal movement patterns in the hindfoot lead to progressive loss of subtalar motion and fixed valgus (eversion) of the heel. Tarsal coalition is often called "peroneal spastic flatfoot" because the peroneals appear to be protectively overactive. As the lesion matures, pain may diminish but stiffness increases, and the abnormal valgus posture persists.

This diagnosis should be suspected in adolescents with foot pain, valgus heel, and decreased subtalar motion. Lateral anteroposterior and oblique radiographs of the foot will confirm the diagnosis of calcaneonavicular coalition, but special subtalar radiographs (Harris views), CT scan, or MRI may be necessary to delineate medial talocalcaneal lesions.

Treatment

Not all coalitions require treatment. The decision to initiate treatment depends on the severity of pain, stiffness, and fixed valgus. Conservative treatment consists of casting to reduce pain and peroneal spasm. If this fails, the coalition can be surgically resected and the resultant space filled with autologous fat or muscle to prevent recurrence. In late or neglected cases with pain or deformity, hindfoot fusion by triple arthrodesis is effective treatment for both symptoms.

Kulic SA, Clanton TO: Tarsal Coalition. Foot Ankle Int 1995; 17:286.

Mosier KM, Asher M: Tarsal coalitions and peroneal spastic flat foot: A review. J Bone Joint Surg Am 1984;66:976.

Wechsler RJ et al: Tarsal coalition: Depiction and characterization with CT and MR imaging. Radiology 1994;193:447.

7. Toe Deformities

Toe deformities occur as isolated conditions, in association with similar hand deformities, and as part of other syndromes. The more commonly found deformities are presented here, with mention of associated hand problems.

Simple Syndactyly

Simple syndactyly, a connection of two or more toes, is the most common toe deformity. The webbing is complete, or a proximal fraction of the web is absent. This disorder demonstrates a strongly familial inheritance pattern and causes no symptoms. It is rarely treated in the foot. In the hand, however, surgical separation is required to restore normal finger function.

Acrosyndactyly

Acrosyndactyly is joining of the tip of two or more toes distally with an open web. It is most commonly seen in conjunction with oligohydramnios, congenital soft-tissue constriction bands, and congenital amputations (Streeter's dysplasia).

In the hand, acrosyndactyly interferes with independent finger function and should be treated surgically (usually at about 6–12 months of age). In the foot, it is usually asymptomatic and may be left untreated.

Polydactyly

Polydactyly is the presence of more than five digits on either the hands or the feet. It is frequently hereditary and often bilateral. Duplication of the thumbs may mirror duplication of the great toes, and both generally require surgical treatment. Both preaxial (duplication of medial toes and radial digits) and postaxial polydactyly (duplication of the lateral toes or ulnar digits) often accompany genetic syndromes and should prompt the physician to look for other symptoms.

8. Constriction Bands (Amniotic Bands)

During gestation, protein-laden amniotic material can condense around limb segments. These amniotic bands may indent delicate embryonic tissues, causing constriction rings or even necrosis and resorption of the distal segment (congenital amputation). Constriction bands may be isolated or associated with Streeter's dysplasia. The syndactyly of Streeter's dysplasia differs from simple syndactyly in that the distal, rather than proximal, web is obliterated (acrosyndactyly). It is thought to be an acquired, rather than hereditary, condition, caused by shearing of the delicate tips of the embryonic digits, followed by conjoined healing of distal digits.

Constriction bands may be very deep and circumferential and occasionally must be released surgically by Z-plasty immediately after birth to avoid postnatal necrosis. Usually, only half of the circumference of a band is released at one time, to protect any remaining blood supply in the other half. Recently, reports of successful one-stage resection and Z-plasty of constriction bands suggest that the remaining blood supply is probably subfascial and interosseous.

9. Adolescent Bunions (Hallux Valgus)

Although bunion (prominence of the medial metatarsophalangeal joint of the great toe) is rare in children, this troublesome deformity often requires treatment. It is frequently hereditary, usually seen in early adolescence, and almost always found in conjunction with a wide forefoot caused by varus (medial deviation) of the first metatarsal shaft (metatarsus primus varus). The wide forefoot allows severe lateral deviation of the great toe (hallux valgus), causing the prominent base of the great toe to rub against the inside of the shoe to create a painful bunion (Figure 11–20).

Although conservative measures may relieve discomfort, many adolescent bunions are progressive and require surgical management. Surgery must address each aspect of the deformity. The surgeon must trim the bunion, correct the varus angulation of the first metatarsal by osteotomy, and centralize and balance the hallux valgus by lengthening the adductor hallucis muscle. There is a fairly high incidence of recurrence of the deformity following surgery.

Thompson GH: Bunions and deformities of the toes in children and adolescents. AAOS Instr Course Lect 1996;45:355.

TORSIONAL & ANGULAR DEFORMITIES OF THE KNEE & LEG

Torsional (rotational) and angular deformities are a major source of referrals to the pediatric orthopedic surgeon (Figure 11–21). Most of these patients are young (< 5 years) and have internal rotational deformities resulting in a "pigeon-toed" gait.

The internal rotation, which can occur at the level of the thigh, leg (shin), or foot, is a cosmetic problem. There is little evidence that any of the torsional "deformities" are harmful to the child or cause significant disability in the adult. Angular deformities (usually varus or valgus at the knee) are also usually benign, although careful evaluation and workup, including radiograph or other imaging modalities, occasionally disclose conditions requiring treatment. Nevertheless, most torsional

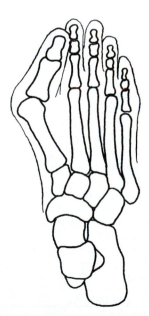

Figure 11–20. Adolescent bunion (hallux valgus) is generally accompanied by a wide forefoot with splaying of the first metatarsal (metatarsus primus varus).

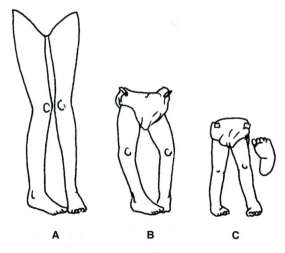

Figure 11–21. The major causes of clinical in-toeing include increased femoral anteversion (**A**), internal tibial torsion (**B**), and metatarsus adductus (**C**).

and angular deformities are physiologic variations of normal anatomy, and correct spontaneously over time.

Increased Femoral Anteversion

The normal femoral neck does not lie exactly in the frontal (coronal) plane but rather projects anteriorly from the plane at an angle called the angle of anteversion (Figure 11–22). Infants have anteversion of as much as 40 degrees, but this angle gradually reduces with growth, so that normal adult femurs exhibit anteversion of 15 degrees. In some children, this gradual regression is slow or incomplete, causing the child to have "excessive" anteversion compared with an average child of the same age. This excessive anteversion produces a relative increase in internal femoral rotation. The clinical manifestation of this increased internal rotation and decreased external rotation of the hip is in-toeing during walking.

Observation of the walking child discloses internal rotation of the entire femur by the medial position of the patella. Although parents may consider this pigeon-toed gait unsightly, increased femoral anteversion is a normal variant that has no effect on function.

Increased femoral anteversion gradually decreases, with improvement in in-toeing, until age 9 years. Subsequently, persistent in-toeing in the adult becomes more likely. Increased femoral anteversion requires no treatment.

Internal Tibial Torsion

Some infants are born with a relatively dramatic internal twisting (torsion) of the tibia that makes the foot and ankle appear markedly rotated inward, relative to

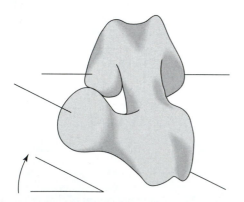

Figure 11–22. The angle of anteversion describes the inclination of the femoral neck forward of (anterior to) the frontal plane.

the axis of the knee. This internal tibial torsion is usually bilateral, frequently familial, and inevitably a normal variant in the wide torsional range seen in infants.

Internal tibial torsion can be clinically measured by comparing the bimalleolar axis (imaginary line connecting the medial and lateral malleoli of the ankle) with the frontal plane of the knee as determined by the position of the patella.

Torsion of 30–40 degrees is not uncommon in the newborn. When the child starts to walk, torsion can cause significant in-toeing, which, in turn, causes excessive tripping.

With growth, internal tibial torsion spontaneously resolves, and normal foot position and walking eventually occur. Some children improve by 24 months of age but may require up to 4 years for full resolution of the torsion. Internal tibial torsion requires no treatment. There is no scientific evidence that braces or shoe modifications alter the natural correction of the deformity.

Metatarsus Adductus

Metatarsus adductus may cause apparent in-toeing in the young child, leading to its inclusion as a torsional deformity. It is described in the previous section on the foot (Table 11–7).

Staheli LT et al: Lower extremity rotational problems in children. Normal values to guide management. J Bone Joint Surg 1985;67A:39.

Bowlegs, Knock-Knee, & Genu Varum

Many infants have bilateral symmetric bowing of the legs, which may persist in the first 1–2 years of walking before developing into an exaggerated knock-kneed condition. The knock-knee is most dramatic at age 3–6 years, when it is known as physiologic genu valgum. At this time, the anatomic angle may be as high as 15 degrees of valgus. The genu valgum then gradually remodels spontaneously to the adult average value of 5–7 degrees of valgus.

Bowing of the legs in infants and excessive valgus of the knees in 6-year-olds are normal phenomena that require no treatment, although parents may have to be reassured that the condition is benign. The rare case of bowing that persists beyond 3 years of age may require further evaluation or treatment. Following are disorders that cause bowing.

A. INTERNAL TIBIAL TORSION

Internal tibial torsion may masquerade as bowing when the child walks with the feet forward and the knees rotated externally rather than internally. As the laterally facing knees flex, they give the appearance of bowlegs. Careful physical examination discloses internal tibial

Table 11–7. In-toeing summary.

	Metatarsus Adductus	**Internal Tibial Torsion**	**Internal Femoral Torsion (Increased Femoral Anteversion)**
Age at resolution	12 months	3–4 years	9–10 years
Leg position	Femur and tibia normal	Patella forward; Foot/ankle internally rotated	Patella internally rotated
Hip examination	Normal	Normal	Internal rotation exceeds external rotation

torsion, which spontaneously resolves by age 4 years. As the torsion corrects, the apparent bowlegs disappear.

B. BLOUNT'S DISEASE

Also known as tibia vara, Blount's disease is a poorly understood loss of medial tibial physeal growth that causes progressive bowing of the leg (Figure 11–23). It may occur as early as 3 years of age and can be bilateral or unilateral. If unilateral, the condition may be suspected earlier because it is obvious by comparison with the other leg. Excessive loading of the knee by early walking in heavy children with physiologic bowing of the legs may contribute to the development of Blount's disease, but this has not been proved. It occurs in all racial groups but is particularly common in blacks and Hispanic children.

Diagnosis of Blount's disease is based on radiographic evidence of decreased medial tibial physeal growth. Later, the medial articular surface is distorted and the medial physis fuses. This allows progressive angular deformity to develop as the lateral growth plate continues elongating while the medial side is tethered.

Mild cases of Blount's disease may spontaneously improve. Although some orthopedists recommend bracing to assist the process, there is no consensus that this is necessary or effective.

Severe or progressive cases of Blount's disease require surgical correction by tibial osteotomy to regain the normal physiologic valgus angle of the knee. Surgery reduces the physiologic load on the medial tibial plateau and may allow normal growth. Often, slight overcorrection of the bowing ensures load reduction, and the resulting valgus slowly resolves as the child grows.

Recently, surgical treatment early in life has become popular, and many orthopedists recommend osteotomy after age 3–4 years if radiographic changes are present. In early cases, surgical correction may cause reversal of the radiographic findings. Once physeal bridging occurs, however, there is no alternative to repeated surgical correction of angular deformity and leg-length inequality until growth ceases at maturity. Controlled studies of the issues involved in treatment of Blount's disease by bracing and surgery are not available.

C. RICKETS

Metabolic disorders of calcium intake can decrease the rate of calcification and ossification of physeal cartilage, causing the development of "softer" bones that are prone to bowing. Vitamin and calcium dietary supplements have virtually eliminated nutritional rickets in the United States. Hypophosphatemic rickets (an X-linked–dominant inherited condition) may present with bilateral symmetric bowing of the legs, however. Children with hypophosphatemic rickets are short and have decreased serum phosphorus levels (with normal

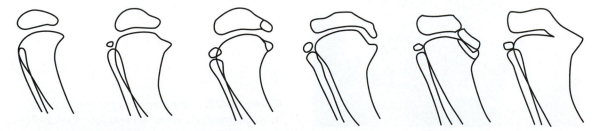

Figure 11–23. The Langenskiöld diagrammatic classification of radiographic changes in Blount's disease (infantile tibia vara). The higher grades are associated with permanent closure of the medial tibial physis, which leads to progressive varus and internal rotation deformity with growth.

serum calcium levels) because of chronic renal tubular wasting of phosphate. Radiographs reveal wide irregular flared physes and generalized bowing of the long bones of the leg (Figure 11–24).

Treatment with phosphate and massive doses of vitamin D supplements improves the radiographic appearance of the physes. There is disagreement over whether treatment has a meaningful effect on the bowing of long bones, however. Occasionally, surgical correction may be required if bowing is severe.

The variety and severity of bowing preclude definite rules and guidelines for surgical treatment of hypophosphatemic rickets. Because bone healing is slower than normal and recurrence of deformity is common with growth, corrective surgery before maturity should only be performed when angular deformity interferes markedly with walking or other functions. It may be necessary to repeat procedures at skeletal maturity, after which correction is lasting.

Fraser RK et al: Medial physeal stapling for primary and secondary genu valgum in late childhood and adolescence. J Bone Joint Surg 1995;77B:733.

Heath CH, Staheli LT: Normal limits of knee angle in white children—genu varum and genu valgum. J Pediatric Orthop 1993;13:259.

Langenskild A, Riska EB: Tibia vara (osteochondrosis deformans tibiae): A survey of seventy-one cases. J Bone Joint Surg Am 1964;46:1405.

Tibial Bowing & Pseudarthrosis

The tibia has a propensity to exhibit congenital angular deformities (bowing of the tibial shaft), which, although rare, are significant. The direction of the bowing is important in both diagnosis and prognosis and is usually detectable at birth. Bowing direction is described by the apex of the bow, not the direction of displacement of the distal part (Figure 11–25).

A. CONGENITAL POSTEROMEDIAL BOWING OF TIBIA

Congenital posteromedial bowing of the tibia is a unilateral birth deformity of the distal fourth of the tibia. The apex of the bow is posteromedial, and often a skin dimple is present over the area. Because of the angle of bowing (often approximately 50 degrees) and the proximity to the ankle joint, the clinical appearance often mimics calcaneovalgus foot. The spatial position of the

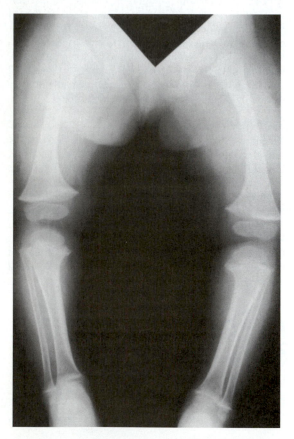

Figure 11–24. Hypophosphatemic rickets. Radiographs demonstrate bowing of long bones and flared, irregular physes (see text).

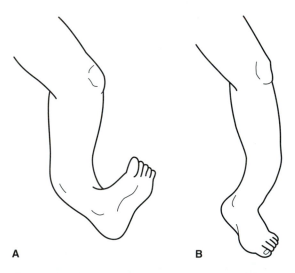

A   **B**

Figure 11–25. The major types of tibial bowing. **A:** Posteromedial bowing. The angulation will spontaneously correct, but with limb-length inequality. **B:** Anterolateral bowing. This disorder will eventually progress to spontaneous tibial fracture with resistant pseudarthrosis (see text).

ankle joint, however, and not the foot itself, is responsible for the deformity. Radiographs of posteromedial bowing disclose the curvature of the distal tibia, often with sclerosis in the underlying section of bone.

Despite its dramatic appearance, posteromedial tibial bowing corrects spontaneously in all cases. Some authors recommend casting to bring the dorsiflexed foot down to plantigrade position, but because the actual deformity is not related to the foot, this advice is not logical: Patients who are never casted resolve as quickly as those who are.

The tibial curvature remodels enough by 3 years of age that the limb appears cosmetically straight, although some bowing may be evident on radiograph for 5–8 years. All patients with posteromedial bowing will be left with a leg-length discrepancy. At maturity, the involved limb will be relatively as much shorter than the longer limb as it was at birth. Therefore, although the angular deformity needs no treatment, long-term follow-up and treatment of limb inequality will be necessary in all cases.

Pseudarthrosis of Tibia

B. Congenital Anterolateral Bowing of Tibia and Congenital

Congenital anterolateral bowing of the tibia and congenital pseudoarthrosis of the tibia represent the other extreme of tibial bowing. For reasons not understood, anterolateral bowing in the distal third of the tibia and fibula is associated with inevitable progressive sclerosis and atrophy of the tibial shaft underlying the deformity. The ultimate fate of this atrophic abnormal bone is spontaneous fracture, which does not heal as readily as most fractures in children do (ie, pseudoarthrosis). Some children with this condition are born with a tibial fracture, whereas others simply have anterolateral bowing and sclerosis at birth, with fractures occurring at up to 8–10 years. In about 30% of cases, coexisting neurofibromatosis is present.

All children with variations of this disorder will require treatment. Because the prognosis is worse for those whose fracture occurs at a younger age, treatment methods will vary. If anterolateral bowing is present but fracture has not occurred, protective bracing might be indicated. The first tibial fracture may heal in children 8 years or older following prolonged casting or casting and surgical bone grafting (with or without internal fixation).

Bone grafting in children whose fracture occurs before age 3 years almost always fails, although repeated attempts to graft have had some success.

The dismal results with conventional treatment of congenital pseudoarthrosis of the tibia in younger patients have prompted some surgeons to try innovative treatments. Electrical stimulation, free microvascular transfer of the fibula, and Ilizarov transport of normal bone to the defect have all been reported to improve the success of treatment. So much surgery may be required to achieve a functional result, however, that many patients eventually undergo amputation to achieve rapid return to the normal functional activities of childhood.

Morrissey RT: Congenital pseudarthrosis of the tibia: Factors that affect results. Clin Orthop 1982;166:21.

Paley D et al: Treatment of congenital pseudarthrosis of the tibia by the Ilizarov technique. Clin Orthop 1992; 280:81.

Pappas AM: Congenital posteromedial bowing of the tibia and fibula. J Pediatr Orthop 1984;4:525.

Tudisco C et al. Functional results at the end of skeletal growth in 30 patients affected by congenital pseudarthrosis of the tibia. J Pediatric Orthop-b; 2000,9:94.

KNEE DISORDERS

1. Discoid Meniscus

The normal menisci of the knee are semilunar in shape and wedge-shaped in cross-section. They deepen the flat tibial articular surface to allow "cupping" of the rounded femoral condyles. The medial meniscus is longer and narrower than the lateral meniscus.

Rarely, the lateral meniscus remains congenitally round (or discoid) instead of acquiring its normal semilunar shape (Figure 11–26). This reduces its cupping function and may cause some instability of either the lateral compartment of the knee or hypermobility of the lateral meniscus itself.

Clinical Findings

The classic physical finding of discoid meniscus is loud clicking over the lateral meniscus during flexion and extension of the knee. This clicking is usually painless but may be accompanied by aching or effusion. Discoid meniscus may be suspected on radiograph by widening of the lateral knee compartment, a subtle increase in subchondral sclerosis laterally, and convexity of the lateral tibial articular surface. Confirmation is attained on

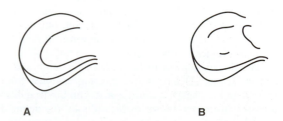

Figure 11–26. **A:** Normal lateral meniscus. **B:** Discoid lateral meniscus, which may cause clicking, effusion, or pain.

arthrography or MRI. The abnormal mechanical function of discoid lateral meniscus make it susceptible to tears, particularly in children over 10 years of age.

Treatment

In the past, symptomatic discoid menisci were treated by total lateral meniscectomy, but the resultant late degenerative knee changes dictated a far more conservative course. Current practice is to avoid treatment unless symptoms are significant and disabling. If treatment is required, the safest approach appears to be arthroscopic removal of the central portion of the discoid shape, thus "sculpting" the lateral meniscus into a roughly semilunar form.

Washington ER III et al: Discoid lateral meniscus in children. Long-term follow-up after excision. J Bone Joint Surg 1995; 77A:1357.

2. Chondromalacia

Patellar chondromalacia and patellar subluxation are common in active adolescents, particularly in females who have small patellas and a slight exaggeration of knee valgus and quadriceps ("Q") angle. Meniscal and ligament injuries are managed as in the adult, although these injuries are not as common in children.

A somewhat more conservative approach to suspect internal knee derangements is warranted in most children. The diagnostic accuracy of both physical exam and complex imaging studies (such as MRI) is surprisingly low in children. False-positive MRIs are particularly typical in children.

These disorders are described in Chapter 3, Musculoskeletal Trauma Surgery, and Chapter 4, Sports Medicine.

3. Osteochondritis Dissecans

In osteochondritis dissecans, a poorly understood disorder of the distal femoral condyle ossification center, a portion of the joint surface softens, shears, or separates through the articular cartilage and underlying bone (Figure 11–27). This disorder is common, but not exclusive, in children age 8–14 years; however, it is an infrequent problem in the adult.

The disease appears to be caused by a combination of two factors: (1) mechanical shearing or injury from activity and (2) femoral condyle susceptibility (fragility) resulting from immature ossification of the femoral condyle (which can be quite irregular in children). The importance of each factor depends on age. Athletic trauma seems more important in older children and

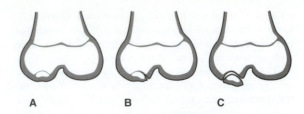

Figure 11–27. Various forms of the osteochondritis dissecans lesion found in children. **A:** Defect in ossification center without cartilage defect. **B:** Lesion with a hinged flap. **C:** Complete separation of bone and cartilage, which can lead to loose body in the knee joint.

adults, while in younger children, ossification defects render the femoral condyle more susceptible to minor repetitive injury.

Clinical Findings

A. SYMPTOMS AND SIGNS

Symptoms and physical findings can be highly variable. Younger children may have an asymptomatic radiographic abnormality of condylar fragmentation or may simply have a vague aching after strenuous activity. Older children and adults may have pain, effusion, and locking or catching if the affected fragment actually separates and becomes a loose body in the knee joint.

B. IMAGING STUDIES

Plain radiographs show an irregular fragment of the surface that is usually sclerotic but may be osteopenic. It is often necessary to obtain tangential views of the condyle such as notch views. Occasionally, the defect is visible only on lateral projection. Always obtain contralateral comparison views. Ossification "defects" that mimic osteochondritis dissecans may be normal ossification fronts, seen to be bilateral and symmetric.

In children older than 11–12 years, MRI or arthrography is used to determine whether the underlying bone alone is involved or whether there is an actual separation of overlying cartilage. Although these studies are helpful in refining treatment strategy in this age group, they are seldom useful in younger children.

Treatment

Young children with asymptomatic osteochondritis dissecans need not be treated, because most of these lesions heal spontaneously. In preadolescents with symptoms or with large lesions seen on radiographs, simple immobilization with either a knee immobilizer or cylinder cast for 6 weeks frequently heals the defect and eliminates symptoms.

Sometimes immobilization is not effective, though. If the lesion is large and accompanied by cartilage separation or displacement, or if the skeleton has reached maturity, treatment may be the same as in the adult. This includes arthroscopic debridement and stabilization of the loose fragment using pins for internal fixation.

Hefti F et al: Osteochondritis dissecans: A multicenter study of the European Pediatric Orthopedic Society. J Pediatric Orthop-b 1999;8:231.

4. Ligament & Epiphyseal Injury

Children who have not reached skeletal maturity have far fewer major ligament injuries of the knee than do older children and adults. Smaller children tend to participate in lower impact activities and sports, and their lack of muscle bulk (which increases during adolescence) limits body acceleration and the force of collision. In addition, ligaments are relatively strong in the immature skeleton compared with bone or cartilaginous physes. Therefore, physeal fractures and bony avulsions of ligament attachments are more likely than traumatic ruptures of the ligaments themselves.

Residual instability may occur in the child's knee after varus or valgus injury. In the adult, such instability would be considered clinical evidence of ligament injury. In children, however, the physis rather than the ligament may be the site of failure. Instability can be caused by a physeal fracture that hinges open rather than the joint opening (Figure 11–28). It is important in such cases to obtain a stress radiograph to ascertain the site of injury because the treatment may vary significantly depending upon the structures involved.

Major intra-articular disruptions of the knee joint (meniscal tear or cruciate ligament injury) are rare in children. Detection may be delayed because symptoms may be less severe than in the adult and their presence not given as much weight in the differential diagnosis. Meniscus injury, particularly when peripheral, may lend itself to arthroscopic repair because of the excellent blood supply in children. Anterior cruciate rupture can be difficult to manage surgically in children because the anatomic sites of the tibial or femoral physes limit the options for reattachment. With the exception of cruciate injuries, most childhood knee ligament injuries are treatable by 2–4 weeks of splinting, and return to function, as tolerated by pain. Physical therapy is rarely necessary in children aged less than 15 years.

Many childhood intra-articular lesions go undetected or undiagnosed. A review of the major signs, symptoms, diagnostic procedures, and treatment options can be found in Chapter 4, Sports Medicine.

Finally, it should be remembered that not all effusions in the knee are traumatic, particularly in younger children. Because children at play are always suffering minor injuries, a history of injury may be inaccurate. The physician must remember to consider septic arthritis and pauciarticular juvenile rheumatoid arthritis in the differential diagnosis of effusion.

OSGOOD-SCHLATTER DISEASE

The proximal tibial physis contains a transverse component that contributes to longitudinal growth and an anterior tongue that contains the attachment of the patellar tendon. In preadolescent and adolescent children (usually males), the distal tip of this tongue may undergo fragmentation from chronic tensile stress, and enlarges from the resultant hyperemic response; this is known as Osgood-Schlatter disease. As the tibial tubercle becomes increasingly prominent, a painful bursa can form over it.

Clinical Findings

Symptoms vary from mild aching at the tubercle to severe pain with patellar function and exaggerated bursal tenderness. Radiographs of the lateral proximal tibia show the characteristic fragmentation (Figure 11–29).

Treatment

Treatment is symptomatic, including analgesics, knee pads to avert direct pressure, quadriceps stretching, avoidance of sports activities, and brief casting or

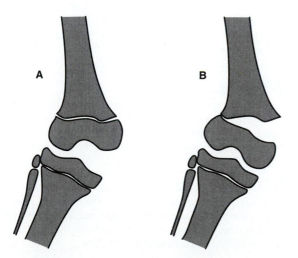

Figure 11–28. Stress radiograph of the unstable knee in an immature patient may reveal ligament rupture (**A**) or separation of the femoral physis (**B**).

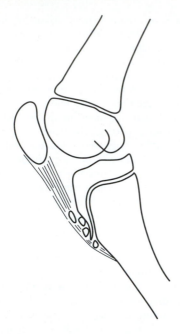

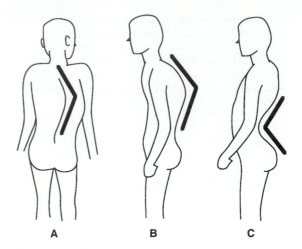

Figure 11–30. Definitions of spinal deformities. **A:** Scoliosis. **B:** Kyphosis. **C:** Lordosis. Frequently, a combination of deformities occur in individual patients (ie, kyphoscoliosis).

Figure 11–29. Osgood-Schlatter disease. The radiographs would show characteristic fragmentation of the tibial tubercle apophysis, similar to diagram.

splinting for painful cases. The disorder resolves spontaneously when the physis closes at skeletal maturity. There is no evidence that physical activity within the limits of pain is harmful to the child with Osgood-Schlatter disease.

Davids JR: Pediatric knee. Clinical assessment and common disorders. Pediatr Clin North Am 1996;43:1067.

Krause BL et al: Natural history of Osgood-Schlatter disease. J Pediatric Orthop 1990;10:65.

SPINAL CURVATURE

Spinal curvature may occur in any age group and present with variable findings. Curvatures may be idiopathic, congenital, or accompany a wide variety of neuromuscular disorders, tumors, and infections. Curvatures may be small and nonprogressive or may worsen and require aggressive treatment. Sometimes, spinal curvature is the first clue to important underlying disease.

Types of Curvatures (Figure 11–30)

A. SCOLIOSIS

Scoliosis is a lateral spinal curvature in the frontal plane, best appreciated by physical examination from the patient's back and by anteroposterior radiographs. Curvatures may be single or multiple and are described by the direction of their convexity. In a flexible spine, the presence of a single (more rigid) curvature can lead to physiologic compensatory curvatures in the opposite direction, above and below the primary curvature. True scoliosis always includes a rotational component that may not be fully appreciated on radiograph and generally includes a lordotic component as well (see section on Lordosis). Surprisingly, lateral curvature is often undetected externally. The rotation of vertebrae that accompanies scoliosis is the physical feature that allows clinical detection.

B. KYPHOSIS

Kyphosis is a forward (flexed) curvature of the spine in the sagittal plane, best appreciated from the side and by lateral radiographs. If kyphosis is acutely angular, a posterior prominence called a gibbus may be evident in the sagittal plane.

C. LORDOSIS

Lordosis is a hyperextension deformity of the spine, most common in the lumbar spine but also often accompanying scoliosis. Lumbar lordosis may be secondary to flexion contracture of the hip.

Detection of Curvature

Although spinal curvatures may be detected first during routine radiograph, most lesions are best diagnosed by physical examination. Spinal examination should proceed according to the following specific protocol:

(1) Place the patient in the standing position (Figure 11–31).

(2) Check the level of the pelvis and look for obvious asymmetry of the rib, scapula, neck, and shoulder height (leg-length inequality can cause apparent scoliosis, which disappears when the short leg is elevated on blocks).

(3) Level the pelvis by seating the child on a firm surface if the pelvis cannot be leveled while standing. This is the case in children with hip contracture from neuromuscular disease.

(4) Have the child bend forward, carefully noting any asymmetric prominence of the lumbar paraspinous muscle, rib cage, or scapula, which suggests the rotational portion of scoliosis. The magnitude of asymmetry corresponds to the severity of the curvature, with convexity of the curvature directed toward the most prominent side.

(5) From the side, check for prominence of the spine that might indicate kyphosis, both in the upright and forward-bending position.

(6) Use radiographs to assess type, severity, and location of the curvature and to look for underlying lesions. Because primary scoliosis and kyphosis curvatures are always stiffer than uninvolved spine segments, bending radiographs may reveal which curvatures are "structural" and which are more flexible compensations (secondary curvature). The Cobb method is usually used to measure curvatures (Figure 11–32). The degree of tilt between the most affected vertebral end plates describes curvature magnitude.

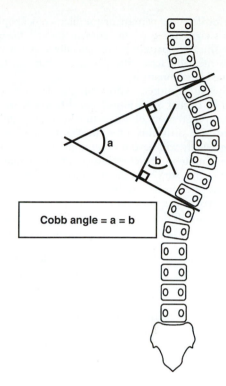

Figure 11–32. The Cobb method of measurement is commonly used to assess spinal curvature. It measures the angle between the far (top and bottom) end plates of the most inclined vertebrae. To allow the measurement lines to fit on the radiograph, lines at 90-degree angles to the end-plates are often drawn, and their relative angles measured. Geometrically, these angles are the same.

Scoliosis

A. IDIOPATHIC SCOLIOSIS

Idiopathic scoliosis has no apparent underlying cause. It is most common in early adolescent girls, although it can be found in either gender at any age. Typically, adolescent idiopathic scoliosis is a convex curvature to the right in the thoracic portion of the spine (right thoracic curvature pattern). Patients with atypical curvature patterns and idiopathic curvature in younger children may require more extensive testing (eg, EMG, MRI) before the cause can be definitively designated idiopathic.

Many idiopathic curvatures progress in magnitude with growth and continue to do so until skeletal maturity. Therefore, the clinician must determine if the curvature is progressing and if the spine is still growing. Radiographs document progression, and observations

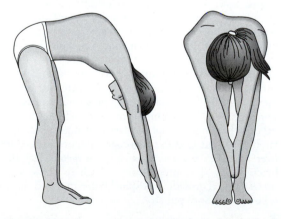

Figure 11–31. Examination of the spine for deformity is best carried out by observing for asymmetry and deformity as the patient bends forward (see text).

of the ossification pattern of the iliac crest apophysis (Risser's sign) are used to estimate skeletal maturity. This ossification pattern begins laterally at puberty and spreads medially across the ilium, capping and fusing with the bone at maturity.

Growing children with progressive curvatures should be treated. A variety of spinal braces is available to treat progression of idiopathic scoliosis. Children who mature with curvatures smaller than 35–40 degrees generally will have no symptoms and no progression in adulthood. If a curvature progresses despite adequate bracing, surgery is the treatment of choice. Some curvatures are too rigid to brace effectively and can only be observed if they are relatively small. If curve magnitude exceeds 40 degrees, bracing will generally be ineffective and surgical correction is the treatment of choice.

Surgery for scoliosis corrects the deformity using metal rods that can be configured to push, pull, distract, or compress portions of the spine with curvature. The involved spinal segments are then fused together using iliac or allograft bone. Typically, a posterior fusion of the laminas and facets is sufficient for most cases of idiopathic scoliosis. Severe cases may also require anterior fusion through the thorax or retroperitoneal space.

B. Congenital Scoliosis

Congenital scoliosis is caused by malformations of vertebral shape. It does not refer to the age of the patient: newborns can have idiopathic scoliosis, despite being born with spinal curvatures. Congenital vertebral malformations generally occur in early embryonic life (before 7 weeks) and are thought to represent errors in formation or segmentation of the spinal segments that originate from primitive mesenchymal condensations of embryonic cells (Figure 11–33).

Curvatures can originate when vertebral parts fail to form (eg, hemivertebrae, wedge vertebrae, butterfly ver-

tebrae) or when embryonic somites fail to segment properly into individual vertebrae (eg, block vertebrae, unilateral unsegmented bar). Because of the embryonic timing of this process, children with congenital scoliosis frequently have abnormalities of other organ systems that form during the same embryonic period (eg, cardiac and renal systems).

Diagnosis of congenital scoliosis must be followed by a careful cardiac examination and by ultrasound or intravenous pyelography evaluation of the kidneys. Although neural tube damage is relatively rare, careful imaging of the spinal canal (MRI, EMG) may be required, especially if surgery is contemplated.

Congenital scoliosis may encompass one or many deformed vertebrae, and different types of vertebral abnormalities are often seen in the same patient. Sometimes, two deforming vertebrae "cancel each other out" and no curvature is visible. For this reason, prediction of progression of the scoliosis depends on serial radiographs. If progression occurs, bracing is usually the first treatment, although surgery is indicated if progression is not halted by external means. Curvatures caused by unilateral unsegmented bars have such a strong tendency to progress that they should be treated by surgery as soon as they are detected.

C. Neuromuscular Scoliosis

Neuromuscular scoliosis includes a diverse group of curvature patterns that occur in association with various neuromuscular diseases. The cause varies with the disease. For example, scoliosis in children with cerebral palsy is usually caused by a combination of spasticity (overactivity of muscle) and weakness. Scoliosis in children with muscular dystrophy is the result of severe progressive muscle weakness that eliminates the paraspinous stability of the spinal column. Scoliosis in infants with spina bifida (myelomeningocele) is frequently congenital (see previous discussion) or associated with the development of a syrinx (central cystic fluid collection) in the spinal cord, a process similar to hydrocephalus.

Patients with neuromuscular scoliosis often develop curvatures at an early age, when surgical treatment is either impossible or would result in severe stunting of spinal growth. It is common to treat such children by daytime bracing, despite the fact that bracing alone is rarely sufficient to eliminate progression or the need for later surgery. In such cases, some surgeons feel that bracing may slow progression enough to allow additional skeletal growth, and spinal correction and fusion is postponed until puberty.

D. Other Scolioses

Childhood scoliosis can be associated with benign tumors of the spine, usually osteoid osteoma and os-

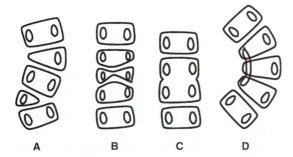

Figure 11–33. Vertebral anomalies of congenital scoliosis. **A:** Hemivertebra. **B:** Butterfly vertebra. **C:** Block vertebra. **D:** Unilateral unsegmented bar.

teoblastoma. Treatment of the tumor is usually curative, although long-standing lesions may require fusion as well.

Neurofibromatosis is associated with both scoliosis and kyphosis and characteristically leads to short high-grade curvatures requiring surgical treatment.

Gupta P et al: Incidence of neural axis abnormalities in infantile and juvenile patients with spinal deformity. Spine 1998;23: 206.

Kyphosis

Kyphosis may be congenital, traumatic, or acquired. Some patients with kyphosis need no treatment, whereas others require immediate surgical attention.

A. POSTURAL KYPHOSIS (POSTURAL ROUNDBACK)

Postural kyphosis is a variation of normal posture and is a cosmetic problem. There is no associated underlying disease, and the spine is flexible and capable of hyperextension. Although it may be worrisome to parents, there is little scientific evidence that it requires, or responds to, treatment.

B. SCHEUERMANN'S KYPHOSIS

Scheuermann's kyphosis is a disorder of growth of the vertebral end plates that affects adolescents, particularly boys, and produces a progressive rigid forward curvature of the thoracic spine. Less commonly, it involves the lumbar spine, causing decreased lumbar lordosis (relative kyphosis). It is often moderately painful. Radiographs show wedging of vertebral bodies, irregularity of the end plates, and kyphosis (Figure 11–34).

Lumbar Scheuermann's kyphosis responds to symptomatic treatment with nonnarcotic pain medications or a supportive lumbar corset. Thoracic involvement with pain or kyphosis of 15–20 degrees greater than normal can be managed with a Milwaukee brace. Brace treatment is usually effective in controlling pain and producing structural correction of the kyphosis. It can sometimes be used at night only so it will not have to be worn during school hours.

Scheuermann's disease is the exception to the general rule that spinal bracing must be done during the growth phase to improve deformity. Patients as old as 18 years will show improvement with the Milwaukee brace. Severe cases (40 degrees excessive kyphosis) may require surgical correction by spinal instrumentation and fusion.

C. CONGENITAL KYPHOSIS

Congenital kyphosis is an important group of diseases, which, like congenital scoliosis, may be caused by failure of formation of vertebrae (hemivertebrae) or failure

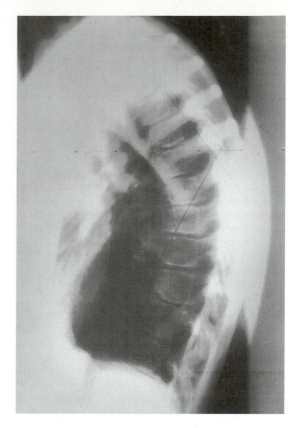

Figure 11–34. Scheuermann's kyphosis is characterized by vertebral wedging, end-plate changes, and kyphosis.

of embryonic segmentation (anterior unsegmented bar). In most cases, the lesion tends to cause uneven growth, so that kyphosis gradually increases as the spine elongates. This can produce bowstringing of the spinal cord over the kyphotic prominence and eventually cause paraplegia. For this reason, any progressive congenital kyphosis must be fused to prevent neurologic complications, regardless of the child's age.

D. TRAUMATIC KYPHOSIS

Traumatic kyphosis is a traumatic compression of vertebrae that may lead to either cosmetic or symptomatic kyphosis. This may be prevented by early surgical stabilization of high-grade unstable traumatic spinal injuries.

E. INFECTIOUS KYPHOSIS

Infectious kyphosis refers to septic destruction of vertebral bodies, which can lead to severe kyphosis. In particular, tuberculous vertebral osteomyelitis can produce soft-tissue abscess, high-grade kyphosis, a sharp gibbus, and paraplegia. Bacterial infection can mimic this, although dramatic deformities are far more unusual.

Treatment includes chemotherapy, surgical debridement and drainage, decompression of the spinal cord, and spinal fusion to prevent further deformity.

Treatment

A. BRACING

Bracing can be used to slow progression of spinal curvatures, prevent progression, or improve underlying structural deformities. Many different types of braces have been devised, each with its own advocates and specific applications (Figure 11–35). When the goal is to provide postural support, slow progression, or postpone (but not prevent) surgery, a polypropylene body jacket, or "clam-shell" brace, may suffice for waking or sitting hours.

Long-term braces designed to arrest progression must be custom molded for the patient, with pads placed to exert appropriate pressure to reduce deformity. Depending on the anatomic level of the curvature, they may be positioned under the arm or may extend to the neck (Milwaukee brace). This type of brace is usually worn 24 h a day.

All braces must be modified or replaced to accommodate growth. In general, bracing is only effective with flexible curvatures in growing children.

B. SURGICAL TREATMENT

Surgical intervention is indicated for curvatures that progress despite adequate conservative treatment (usually bracing). It is also required when spinal compression is imminent (tuberculous kyphosis, congenital kyphosis) or when a curvature is so severe that bracing is impossible and future progression likely.

1. Surgical stages—Surgery involves two separate stages: correction and stabilization. After posterior exposure of the spine, correction is achieved with a variety of mechanical internal fixation devices. Usually, these are rods with hooks, screws, wires, or other mechanisms to distract, compress, or bend spinal segments. Correction is rarely complete because mechanical and safety considerations limit the force that can be applied. Once correction is obtained, the cortex of spine is removed and bone graft is placed over the raw bone. Subsequently, solid fusion occurs within 6 months, permanently stabilizing the spine (Figure 11–36).

2. Treatment of severe curvatures—For small curvatures, posterior instrumentation and fusion are sufficient. Some large idiopathic curves and neuromuscular curves require anterior release and bone grafting to render enough acute flexibility for curvature correction, and enough late stability for dependable fusion. Occasionally, fusion may fail, causing a pseudarthrosis that may be painful or may allow progression of a previously corrected curvature. In this case, fusion must be repeated.

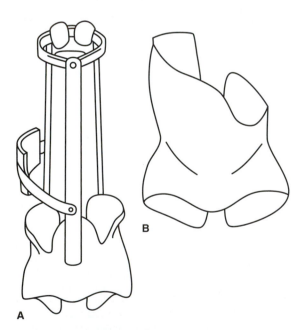

A   **B**

Figure 11–35. Two popular brace styles used for the treatment of spinal deformity are the Milwaukee brace (**A**) and the low-profile (Boston-type) brace (**B**).

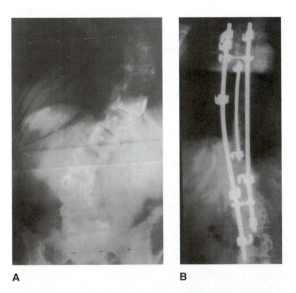

A   **B**

Figure 11–36. Treatment of a scoliotic curve by instrumentation and fusion. Preoperative view (**A**) and postoperative view (**B**).

Lonstein JE: Adolescent idiopathic scoliosis: Screening and diagnosis. Instr Course Lect 1989;38:105.

Tolo VT: Surgical treatment of adolescent idiopathic scoliosis. Instr Course Lect 1989;38:143.

Weinstein SL, Ponseti IV: Curve progression in idiopathic scoliosis. J Bone Joint Surg Am 1983;65:455.

NEUROMUSCULAR DISORDERS

Because muscle weakness or imbalance will change the underlying structure of a growing skeleton, neuromuscular diseases of children often require orthopedic evaluation. Treatment may be required to reverse skeletal deformity and contracture or to effect functional improvement.

Many childhood neuromuscular diseases require coordinating the services of the pediatrician, neurologist, physiatrist, therapist, educator, social worker, nurse, and parent.

1. Cerebral Palsy

Cerebral palsy is a static encephalopathy in a growing child. Although it is often birth-related, the term also includes childhood head injury, stroke, metabolic brain conditions, and degenerative neurologic conditions.

The challenges to physicians evaluating cerebral palsy are making an accurate diagnosis and detecting correctable conditions. It is essential that functional evaluation of the child's condition take into account the need for education, communication, socialization, and mobility.

Types of Cerebral Palsy

The common, though not universal, hallmark of most cases of cerebral palsy is spasticity. Diagnosis of spasticity can be direct (increased tone, increased deep tendon reflexes, clasp-knife rigidity, and clonus) or inferred (shortening of muscles, contractures of joints, joint dislocations, and scoliosis). There are several categories of cerebral palsy.

A. Hemiplegia

Hemiplegia is spasticity involving only one side of the body. It may be mild or severe and typically is more pronounced in the distal skeleton (hand and foot-ankle). Hemiplegia is usually caused by congenital loss of portions of the parietal, contralateral cerebral cortex. This loss may reflect vascular insufficiency, trauma, or porencephalic cysts.

Many patients with hemiplegia have normal development and intelligence. Children with hemiplegia frequently walk at a normal age, although sometimes with marked posturing of the involved side. Right hemiplegia (left cerebral cortex) may involve Broca's area and thus cause speech deficits. Because sensory and motor cortex areas are contiguous, hemiplegia is strongly associated with abnormalities of sensation and proprioception in the affected limbs. This may prove more disabling than the spasticity because a child may not appreciate an insensate limb as part of overall "body image."

B. Diplegia

Diplegia, or diplegic cerebral palsy, is an encephalopathy usually associated with prematurity. It is characterized by relatively symmetric involvement of the lower extremities and lesser involvement of the upper extremities. Prematurity is often accompanied by intracerebral hemorrhage and periventricular leukomalacia, which lead to edema and necrosis in the region of the trigone. This involvement of the pyramidal tract and associated basal ganglia is the main cause of diplegia.

Most diplegic children exhibit primary spasticity with a variety of less obvious neurologic symptoms, including ataxia, rigidity, and athetosis (dystonia). Many have normal intelligence (if the cortex is spared) but may suffer developmental delays caused by damage to associative fibers in the brain. Although they may initially be hypotonic ("floppy"), most diplegic patients develop high tone and spasticity by 12–18 months of age.

Diplegia is usually more severe in the lower extremities and is relatively symmetric. Many children with diplegia eventually walk, exhibiting a crouching gait characterized by flexed, internally rotated hips, flexed knees, and plantar-flexed ankles.

C. Quadriplegia

Quadriplegia (total body involvement) often occurs in children who suffer birth asphyxia, metabolic encephalopathy, or encephalitis. Severe spasticity, seizures, mental retardation, joint contractures, and scoliosis are typical but not always individually present in this type of cerebral palsy. Children with quadriplegia are particularly susceptible to spontaneous hip dislocations (because of hip muscle imbalance) and high-grade scoliosis. Both of these conditions interfere with sitting and may require surgery. Most quadriplegic patients require wheelchair assistance and do not walk.

D. Mixed Neurologic Involvement

Mixed neurologic involvement of extrapyramidal portions of the brain can cause athetosis, dystonia, ballismus, and ataxia. Many children with cerebral palsy exhibit subtle signs of some of these disorders, in addition to spasticity. In some children, one of these signs may predominate, but spasticity is absent. In general, prognosis varies with the anatomy of involvement.

Treatment

It is important before treating cerebral palsy that specific goals be set for the patient. Although the most important goals are not orthopedic, the surgeon may help the patient to achieve them. Increased mobility, for instance, may facilitate achieving a variety of nonorthopedic goals. Especially important are the patient's ability to communicate, move independently, and socialize. Orthopedic treatment may improve sitting position in the wheelchair or improve walking by releasing muscles or joints.

Many children benefit from physical or occupational therapy during the first few years of life. Although the exact role of such therapy in cerebral palsy remains undefined, therapists often help parents and children deal more effectively with the complex problems presented by the disease. Therapists also help parents and children set realistic goals for the future.

Bracing or surgery may be required to control effects of spasticity on individual joints and to decrease spasticity, correct dislocation or contracture, or control scoliosis. Surgery is ineffective in the case of extrapyramidal neurologic symptoms. A variety of nonorthopedic treatments are also used for cerebral palsy. Selective dorsal rhizotomy, a neurosurgical procedure to cut a portion of the posterior roots of the lumbar spinal cord, may reduce spasticity in selected patients by interrupting the reflex arc. Botulinum toxin injection (or phenol injection) into the motor end-plate region of a muscle will temporarily interrupt the nerve supply, relaxing a spastic muscle for several months and allowing therapy or other evaluation. Oral baclofen can reduce overall spasticity. Intrathecal baclofen, delivered by a subcutaneous pump, may offer relaxation of troublesome lower extremity muscle tension in both dystonic and spastic patients.

Hip subluxation is common in quadriplegia, and pelvic radiographs in young quadriplegic patients are needed to detect early, reversible involvement. Subluxation may be treated in children younger than 3–4 years by adductor muscle release, which improves abduction. Rarely, the anterior obturator nerve (which innervates the adductor longus muscle) is resected in order to weaken the adductors. In older children, bony reconstruction by varus-derotation osteotomy and acetabular reorientation or supplementation may be necessary to correct the bone malformation that results from the force of spastic muscles on the growing skeleton. Children who develop hip subluxation often develop scoliosis as well (see section on Scoliosis).

A. ADDUCTOR RELEASE

Adductor release may be done as an open procedure (usually by myotomy or transverse sectioning of the adductor longus and a portion of the adductor brevis) or by percutaneous adductor tenotomy (section of the tendon origin of the adductor longus at the pelvis). The exact technique and amount of release is dictated by the severity of contracture and other factors. When done for hip subluxation, adductor release is most effective before age 3–4 years. It should be sufficient to allow hip abduction of 70–80 degrees on the operating table. When frank subluxation is present, some surgeons perform an anterior obturator neurectomy in addition to the adductor myotomy. This open procedure removes a segment of the obturator nerve that supplies the released adductor longus muscle, so the muscle remains loose after spontaneously reattaching after surgery.

Obturator neurectomy must be carefully used because it can cause excessive weakening of the adductors and, subsequently, late hip abduction contracture. After each of these procedures, the patient is casted in abduction for 3–4 weeks to allow muscle healing in the new elongated position.

Dynamic spasticity or joint contracture (the result of chronic spasticity) can interfere with walking in children with hemiplegia or diplegia. This may be treated by bracing involved joints in a functional position or by surgical lengthening of the muscle-tendon unit. Such "muscle releases" can be done by complete tenotomy, tendon Z-lengthening (common at the Achilles tendon), or lengthening of the aponeurosis of a muscle, which is often done for the iliopsoas or hamstrings (Figure 11–37).

It is convenient to combine multiple procedures for children with cerebral palsy. For example, a typical hemiplegic with a tip-toe (equinus) gait may benefit from lengthening the Achillis tendon to make the foot plantargrade. A typical diplegic patient with a crouching gait may benefit from hip flexor, hamstring, and Achillis tendon lengthenings performed bilaterally during a single operation. The exact timing and extent of surgery are controversial among experts in cerebral palsy. Three-dimensional computerized gait analysis, performed in motion laboratories, can guide the surgeon.

B. MUSCLE RELEASE FOR DYNAMIC DEFORMITY

Muscle releases for dynamic deformity may be done in several ways, depending on the specific muscle, the presence of contracture, and the surgeon's preference. The goal is to weaken selectively spastic muscles to reduce their abnormal influence while not lengthening them so much that the opposite deformity occurs. The more common procedures are described here.

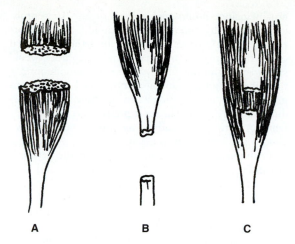

Figure 11–37. Schematic representation of surgical options for muscle release or lengthening in cerebral palsy. **A:** Myotomy; **B:** tenotomy; **C:** aponeurotomy.

1. Achilles tendon lengthening—Achilles tendon lengthening is usually done by Z-lengthening of the distal tendon. Cuts for Z-lengthening can be either open or percutaneous. The ankle is carefully dorsiflexed just beyond neutral to allow the tendon fibers to slide into an elongated position. The surgeon must avoid over-lengthening (a matter of judgment), because an excessively weakened gastrocnemius-soleus group hinders walking and can actually encourage a deeper crouching gait.

2. Gastrocnemius lengthening—Gastrocnemius lengthening is required in patients whose gastrocnemius is considerably more spastic than the soleus. In such cases, ankle dorsiflexion is limited and ankle clonus occurs when the knee is extended, but free dorsiflexion occurs when the knee is flexed. In such patients, the gastrocnemius alone may be released by approaching the musculotendinous junction in the calf and sectioning the aponeurosis or by release of the insertion of the gastrocnemius where it attaches to the soleus and Achilles tendon. This effectively recesses the muscle, selectively weakening it while retaining soleus strength for push-off during walking.

3. Hamstring lengthening—Hamstring lengthening is indicated when the hamstrings are tight (limited straight-leg raising) and knee flexion is persistent during the stance phase of gait (crouching gait). Usually, the distal medial and lateral hamstrings are released, but procedures vary widely among surgeons. On the medial side, the gracilis and semitendinosus tendons are long and are usually Z-lengthened or tenotomized (trans-versely released). The semimembranosus is lengthened by transverse incision of its aponeurosis, which allows the interior muscle fibers to stretch and lengthen. Laterally, both heads of the biceps femoris can be managed by aponeurotic lengthening as well. The procedure must be done carefully to avoid cutting or stretching the sciatic or peroneal nerves. The leg is splinted or casted in extension for 3–4 weeks to allow soft-tissue healing.

4. Iliopsoas lengthening—The hip flexors (psoas and iliacus) may be released at the insertion of the conjoined tendon into the lesser trochanter, usually done in sitters also undergoing adductor release for spastic hip subluxation. If the child is walking and less weakening of hip flexion is desired, the psoas tendon alone can be sectioned at the level of the pelvic brim, retaining the iliacus portion of the muscle for strength.

DeLuca PA: The musculoskeletal management of children with cerebral palsy. Pediatr Clin North Am 1996;43:1135.

2. Myelomeningocele (Spina Bifida)

Myelomeningocele is a complex birth defect affecting the spinal cord and central nervous system. Although the cause is not fully understood, there is a significant hereditary component. Lack of maternal folic acid has been identified as one causative factor.

Embryologic Defect

The basic embryologic defect is a failure of complete tubulation and dorsal closure of the embryonic neural tube and placode, including incomplete closure of the skin over the spinal cord, resulting from lack of induction. In its mildest form, this spinal dysraphism consists of a simple spina bifida occulta or isolated meningocele (protrusion of spinal membranes, but not nerve, outside of the spinal canal, without neurologic deficit). The more severe varieties include herniation of membranes and nervous tissue through large dorsal bony and skin defects at birth and hydrocephalus with cerebral malformations (Figure 11–38).

Myelomeningocele can occur at any spinal level but usually is seen between levels T12 and S2. Because neural tissue fails to form properly, the child is paraplegic and insensate below the level of the dysraphism. The clinical determination of neurologic level is most easily accomplished by describing the last muscles contracting under active voluntary motor control (Table 11–8). This may be difficult because of anatomic variability, the age of the child, and other central nervous system involvement.

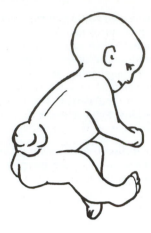

Figure 11–38. Spina bifida (myelomeningocele). The sac includes dysplastic spinal cord and membrane elements, and must be surgically closed in the first days of life. Hydrocephalus and congenital scoliosis are commonly associated.

Treatment of Orthopedic Problems

Orthopedic problems associated with myelomeningocele include clubfoot or congenital vertical talus, torsional deformities of the legs, contractures, hip dislocations, and scoliosis. The lack of sensation may allow extensive pressure sores to develop, or painless fractures may go undetected by patients. The health defects of children with spina bifida, in addition to their paralysis,

Table 11–8. Muscle function at neurologic levels in myelomeningocoele (spina bifida).

Neurologic Level	Functions	Muscles Active
T12	Hip flexion (weak)	Iliopsoas (weak)
L1	Hip flexion	Iliopsoas
L2	Hip adduction (weak)	Adductor longus, brevis (weak)
L3	Hip adduction	Adductors
	Knee extension (weak)	Quadriceps (weak)
L4	Knee extension	Quadriceps
	Ankle dorsiflexion	Anterior tibialis (variable)
L5	Knee flexion	Medial hamstring
	Hip abduction	Tensor fascia lata
S1	Knee flexion	All hamstrings
	Ankle plantar flexion	Gastrocnemius-soleus
S2	Toe flexion	Flexor digitorum longus

usually include nonmusculoskeletal organ system problems such as hydrocephalus or Arnold-Chiari malformation (brain), syrinx formation or tethering (spinal cord), or neurogenic bladder or hydronephrosis (renal system). Early in life, most of these are more important than the orthopedic manifestations, and a team approach is needed to decide when and how best to coordinate management. The most pressing needs of the infant born with spina bifida are usually neural defect closure and ventricular shunting.

Orthopedic management depends on the deformities and the long-term mobility goals for the child. The level of paralysis often is helpful in determining whether the child will ultimately be able to walk (L5 or S1 function usually required) or will require a wheelchair (because of function only proximal to L4 or L5). Usually, foot deformities such as clubfoot or congenital vertical talus require surgery. If foot deformities recur or progress, tethered cord should be suspected.

Spina bifida is a static neurologic disease; progression of foot deformities, especially during growth spurts, suggests tethering (and therefore stretching) of the cord. Hip dislocations, although dramatic on radiograph, frequently require no treatment; they are painless and tend to occur in children with neurologic involvement at L2 to L4, which precludes long-term walking.

A young child with scoliosis may require bracing until the thorax is long enough for spinal fusion. Some scoliosis seen with spina bifida is congenital (see section on Scoliosis). If rapidly progressive scoliosis occurs, the physician should suspect a neurologic cause such as syrinx. Because of chronic exposure to latex materials in contact with mucous membranes and internal tissues (shunts, catheters), children with spina bifida are exceedingly susceptible to latex allergy, which can be fatal. Steps to limit latex exposure are essential in this population and must be observed by medical personnel working with them.

Bunch WH: Myelomeningocoele. Part I. General concepts. In: *American Academy of Orthopaedic Surgeons Instructional Course Lectures 25.* St. Louis: Mosby, 1976.

Mazur JM, Menelaus MB: Neurologic status of spina bifida patients and the orthopedic surgeon. Clin Orthop 1991;264:54.

3. Muscular Dystrophy

Duchenne's muscular dystrophy is an X-linked disorder that presents orthopedic features in 6–9-year-old boys. The disorder is one of progressive muscle weakness, usually first involving more proximal muscles of the limb girdles. Pseudohypertrophy caused by replacement of gastrocnemius muscles (or other muscles) with fat is a classic finding, as is Gower's sign (an inability to rise from the floor without using the hands to "walk up" the body and legs). As the muscles weaken, imbalance can cause fixed flexion contractures of the hip, knee, and ankle plantar flexors, which limits walking ability. Because weakness eventually forces patients into a wheelchair, a decision to brace or correct these contractures surgically depends on estimates of remaining strength and likely duration of ambulation after treatment. Most often, progressive foot deformities (usually equinovarus) require muscle release and correction (including bracing) because use of the wheelchair also requires relatively well-positioned feet.

As weakness progresses, the child requires an electric wheelchair for mobility. At this point, scoliosis begins to appear and is usually relentlessly progressive. Attempts to control the scoliosis of muscular dystrophy by wheelchair inserts and braces have been ineffective. Early surgery (before cardiorespiratory status deteriorates) is often the best answer. See Chapter 13 ("Rehabilitation") for more information.

4. Myotonic Dystrophy

Myotonic dystrophy is a genetic muscle disease whose name reflects the hallmark of the disease: myotonic EMG potentials. The disease is often associated with mild retardation, obesity, and foot deformities. Initial diagnosis is made by identifying the characteristic myotonic face (weak perioral muscles with a distinctive pyramidal mouth) and is confirmed by EMG. Myotonic dystrophy worsens with each succeeding generation; genetic markers are available for diagnosis.

The most frequent foot deformity is equinovarus, often with weakness of the anterior tibialis and overactivity of the posterior tibialis. Surgery is often required, and recurrence requiring additional surgery is common. Surgical treatment of myotonic dystrophy foot deformities includes joint release (for passive correction of the deformity) and muscle transfers (for rebalancing muscle forces).

5. Spinal Muscular Atrophy

This heterogeneous group of disorders includes static and degenerative lesions of the anterior horn cell population in the spinal cord. These disorders all involve muscle weakness caused by a lower motor neuron lesion, that is, flaccid paralysis. Sensation is intact, and the major goals are mobility (with electric wheelchair), adaptive devices to aid in daily living (eg, feeding devices), and control of scoliosis, which is similar to management of scoliosis in advanced muscular dystrophy (see section on Muscular Dystrophy).

Green NE: The orthopaedic care of children with muscular dystrophy. Instr Course Lect 1987;36:267.

6. Arthrogryposis (Arthrogryposis Multiplex Congenita)

Arthrogryposis is not a disease per se but rather a symptom complex that includes joint contractures or dislocations, rigid skeletal deformities (especially clubfoot), shiny skin with decreased wrinkling and subcutaneous tissue, weakness, and muscle wasting. Although many factors contribute to arthrogryposis, the common link among the symptoms appears to be decreased fetal movement during a critical period in limb development. This can be caused by neurologic lesions (congenital absence of anterior horn cells, Werdnig-Hoffman spinal muscular atrophy, myelomeningocele), myopathic lesions (myotonic dystrophy, congenital myopathies), various syndromes (Moebius syndrome), or physical restriction associated with oligohydramnios.

Arthrogrypotic infants frequently have extension or flexion contractures of knees and elbows, dislocated hips, and severe clubfeet. The contractures may partially resolve with passive range-of-motion therapy in the first 6–12 months of life; however, they must be released surgically after that if they interfere with walking or arm use. Hip dislocations may not limit function and often are not treated. Clubfeet require surgery, which is often of limited success; multiple operations are frequently necessary. Arthrogrypotic children are generally highly resourceful in learning to walk and care for themselves completely independently, despite seemingly overwhelming skeletal problems.

TUMORS

Skeletal neoplasms, particularly benign ones, are fairly common in children. Common benign bone lesions of childhood include osteochondroma, osteoid osteoma, unicameral (simple) bone cysts, chondroblastoma, hemangioma, histiocytosis X (eosinophilic granuloma), and fibrous dysplasia. Malignant tumors, which are usually seen after age 10, include Ewing's sarcoma and osteosarcoma. Certain systemic diseases can be manifested in childhood as apparent bone tumors (hyperparathyroidism, renal disease, leukemia). A detailed discussion of bone tumors can be found in Chapter 6.

AMPUTATIONS
Congenital Amputations & Absence of Segments

Congenital absence of limb segments at birth can occur sporadically, as part of a syndrome (Streeter's dysplasia), or as a result of mutagens (eg, thalidomide). Absence may be terminal (eg, congenital below-knee amputation) or intercalary (eg, congenital shortening or absence of the humerus).

Although congenital amputations can be dramatic in appearance, the missing limb is not part of the child's "body image." Thus, the child has a natural instinct to be mobile. Children with severe limb deficiencies at birth are almost always able to be completely independent and functional. They will accept prostheses quite readily but only if the device truly improves their efficiency. For example, nearly all congenital above-elbow amputees reject artificial limbs, opting for function over appearance. Parents may harbor strong feelings of guilt over the child's condition, so the psychologic issues associated with the condition are more those of the adults than the child.

It is not unusual for congenital amputations to require conversion to a level more easily fitted with a prosthesis. For example, fibular hemimelia (severe shortening of the tibia with absent fibula and foot deformity) sometimes can be most effectively treated by removing the foot and converting the limb to an ankle disarticulation level. This facilitates prosthetic fitting and simplifies management of the leg-length discrepancy, thus permitting normal function.

Aitken GT, Frantz CH: Management of the child amputee. In Reynolds FC (editor): *American Academy of Orthopaedic Surgeons Instructional Course Lectures 17.* St. Louis: Mosby, 1960.

Frantz CH, O'Rahilly R: Congenital skeletal limb deficiencies. J Bone Joint Surg Am 1961;43:1202.

Krebs DE, Fishman S: Characteristics of the child amputee population. J Pediatr Orthop 1984;4:8.

Traumatic Amputation

In contrast to the congenital amputee, the child with a traumatic amputation is particularly likely to be male, adolescent, rebellious, and troubled. Although pediatric traumatic amputations are often caused by inadvertent incidents, many result from high-risk behavior. These factors must be taken into account when dealing with the psychologic issues of the patient and family; social, as well as medical, intervention is often appropriate.

The orthopedic management of traumatic amputees is modified in children by the presence of growth plates and the remarkable healing and rehabilitation powers of children. This must be considered during surgical completion of amputations because injury to the physis may cause severe shortening or angulation of a stump, rendering the amputation far less satisfactory than a similar amputation in the adult. The child amputee rarely has vascular problems, however, and the use of split-thickness skin grafting may allow preservation of length that would be impossible in most adults.

Overgrowth of Amputation Stump

Amputations through the long bones of children exhibit the unique phenomenon of terminal overgrowth.

Eventually, the distal end of the stump may develop a long, thin, sometimes painful bony prominence. Overgrowth is not physeal in origin (ie, closure of the physis by epiphysiodesis does not eliminate its formation), and it appears to be related to aggressive bone formation associated with the periosteal membrane.

Although overgrowth can occur in any bone, it is most troublesome in the tibia, fibula, and humerus. When symptomatic, overgrowth is treated by resecting the spike of bone (revision of the amputation), but the process will continue, and recurrence is common. Some pediatric amputees require two or more surgical revisions during growth. Overgrowth ceases at skeletal maturity.

FRACTURES

Common Pediatric Fracture Patterns

Many fractures in children are similar to their counterparts in adults. However, the added factor of growth contributes to the unique issues of fracture care in children. Pediatric bone is "softer" and more easily broken than adult cortical bone. Thus, the amount of energy required to produce a fracture is less in the child, even as soft-tissue injury is frequently less severe in the child than in the adult. In addition, the periosteal membrane in children is far thicker and more osteogenic than in adults. The periosteum is so leathery in immature humans that it frequently holds bone ends together, contributing greatly to stability and ease of manipulative reduction. The excellent osteogenic potential of pediatric periosteum permits rapid, aggressive fracture healing, so that nonunions are extremely rare in children.

Less brittle pediatric bone is subject to fracture patterns unique to children (Figure 11–39): A greenstick fracture is a transverse crack that retains its continuity, just as a small moist twig would break without actually snapping apart.

A torus fracture is a small buckle or impaction of one cortex with a slight bend on the opposite cortex. Plastic deformation is a change in the natural shape of a bone without a detectable fracture line.

Remodeling (gradual correction in alignment or size of a fractured bone back to normal) is generally far more rapid in children than in adults. Remodeling of angular deformities is particularly rapid when the deformity is in the same plane of motion as the nearest joint (Figure 11–40) or when the deformity is near a rapidly growing physis. Remodeling of rotational deformities is less reliable. Overgrowth is a singular feature of remodeling that occurs in certain fractures of the long bones, particularly the femur. It is a product of physeal stimulation by the hyperemic response to fracture and heal-

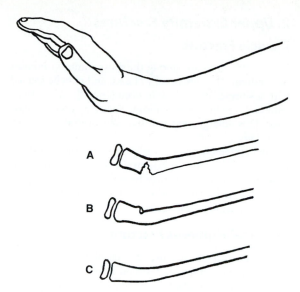

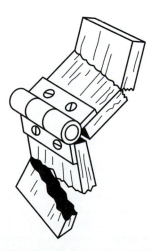

Figure 11–39. Softer bone in children can lead to unique fracture behavior (in addition to the fracture patterns seen in adults). **A:** Greenstick fracture; **B:** torus fracture; **C:** plastic deformation.

Figure 11–40. Remodeling of bone after fracture is most rapid when it is in the plane of a nearby joint. Schematically, if the joint is thought of as a hinge, the fracture above (in the plane of the hinge) is likely to remodel faster than the fracture below the hinge (out of plane).

ing and may increase the length of a bone by 2 cm or more over the course of a year.

The combination of low-energy injury, rapid bone healing, and dependable remodeling of angular deformity makes it possible to treat many pediatric fractures by simple closed reduction (often incomplete) and casting. Surgical management of children's fractures is rarely required. The surgeon may accept a less-than-perfect reduction if the fracture is known to remodel into satisfactory alignment.

1. Epiphyseal Fracture

The cartilage physeal plates are a region of low strength relative to the surrounding bone and are susceptible to fracture in the child. They are analogous to a scratch on a pane of glass, in which concentrated force facilitates damage. Once injury has occurred, the physis usually is able to recover and resume growth. But if an offset occurs in the physeal substance, bone may grow across it (from epiphyseal bone to metaphyseal bone), forming a bridge that anchors further growth and leads to either progressive shortening or a worsening angulation (Figure 11–41).

Because physes are near joints and physeal fractures are common, children may suffer injuries to joint surfaces that require careful surgical repair and realignment. Thus, open reduction is more likely in fractures involving physes and joints than in other pediatric fractures.

Most physeal fractures propagate through the weakest region of the cartilage. Physeal cartilage begins in a dense resting zone on the epiphyseal side, and chondrocytes gradually multiply, elongate, and arrange into longitudinal columns that produce longitudinal growth. Hypertrophic, balloonlike chondrocyte columns then undergo cell death, and the remaining cell walls are calcified and eventually ossify to form metaphyseal bone.

The weakest spot is usually the interface between hypertrophic dying columns of cells and the stiff calci-

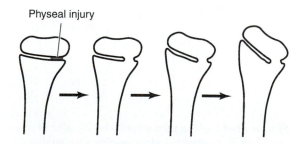

Figure 11–41. Progressive angular deformity can occur if there is asymmetric closure of the physis after fracture.

fied cell walls beneath them; this area is highly susceptible to shearing forces. Fortunately, the region also represents the boundary between the process of epiphyseal elongation (supported by the epiphyseal blood supply) and metaphyseal ossification (supported by the metaphyseal blood supply). Thus, physeal fractures do not often damage the growth potential of the physis, because they do not interrupt its critical blood supply.

Although physeal fractures can occur in a wide variety of configurations, certain patterns are seen frequently enough that a descriptive classification aids in understanding physeal injury (Figure 11–42). Fractures that either cross the joint or result in spatial malalignment of portions of the physis have the worst prognosis.

Physeal fractures heal rapidly, usually within 4 weeks. Careful monitoring is required to detect early posttraumatic closure of the growth plate. Occasionally, an epiphyseal-metaphyseal bony bridge will form and tether growth. If this growth is minor, surgical removal of the bridge (epiphyseal bar resection) may successfully restore physeal growth. Otherwise, the procedures for evaluation and treatment of limb-length inequality should be followed (see 1. Limb-length inequality).

Salter RB, Harris WR: Injuries involving the growth plate. J Bone Joint Surg Am 1963;45:587.

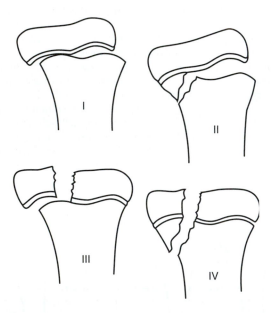

Figure 11–42. The Salter-Harris classification of physeal fractures is widely used to describe such injuries. With some exceptions, the potential for problems with growth arrest is greater in the higher numbered patterns.

2. Upper Extremity Fractures

Clavicle Fracture

Clavicle fractures are among the most common injuries in children. They are usually closed, and may be treated with a simple sling. Healing occurs rapidly with abundant callus, which leaves a lump that may concern parents. This enlargement will remodel over several years of growth.

An extremely rare condition, congenital pseudarthrosis of the clavicle, can mimic the radiographic appearance of fracture. It may be right-sided or bilateral, with little or no pain and no history of trauma. Treatment is generally unnecessary.

Proximal Humerus Fracture

Proximal humerus fractures are usually epiphyseal injuries (usually Salter-Harris type II injuries) that may progress into significant varus angulation (medial deviation). Fortunately, the proximal humerus is a rapidly growing physis and shoulder motion is full in all planes, so remodeling is rapid. These fractures generally require only a sling or shoulder immobilization for 3–4 weeks, without reduction. Rarely, fractures with extreme angulation (> 90 degrees) may require surgical reduction and fixation.

Elbow Region Fracture

Most elbow region fractures are indirect injuries caused by a fall on the outstretched hand. Both diagnosis and treatment can be difficult in this serious group of injuries. Epiphyseal ossification is incomplete in the age group that is susceptible to falls (2–10 years), making radiographs difficult to interpret (Figure 11–43). Swelling, if severe, can block venous or arterial structures and lead to forearm compartment syndromes. Reductions are often unstable, and operative intervention may be required. Most surgeons immobilize pediatric elbow fractures for 4 weeks after treatment. The most important fractures are listed as follows.

A. SUPRACONDYLAR FRACTURE OF HUMERUS

Supracondylar fracture of the humerus occurs at the metaphyseal bone, proximal to the elbow joint, and does not involve the growth plate (Figure 11–44). Displacement may be severe, and nerve injury, usually caused by stretching, is common. If swelling is marked, there may be interruption of the blood supply; it is not uncommon for such a distal extremity to lack a pulse.

The most appropriate treatment is rapid anatomic reduction under general anesthesia. Because the reduction is highly unstable, many surgeons prefer to fix the fracture after reduction with percutaneous wires. Once the fracture is reduced, the swelling recedes rapidly and

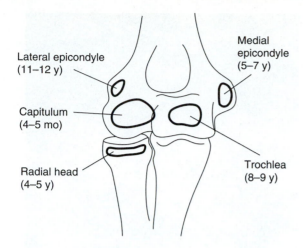

Medial epicondyle (5–7 y)

Lateral epicondyle (11–12 y)

Capitulum (4–5 mo)

Radial head (4–5 y)

Trochlea (8–9 y)

Figure 11–43. Ages of appearance of ossification centers. The ossification centers of the elbow region emerge at different ages as indicated and can complicate the interpretation of radiographs. It is often advisable to obtain comparison radiographs of the opposite elbow if injury is suspected.

the pulse returns. On rare occasions, the surgeon must perform vascular or nerve exploration or repair.

Some displaced supracondylar humerus fractures are incompletely reduced or lose position because of fracture instability after apparently adequate initial reduction. These progress to a characteristic malunion with an apex-lateral angular deformity of the elbow (known as cubitus varus). Although cosmetically unsightly, cubitus varus rarely has any significant functional consequences. If desired, it may be corrected by valgus osteotomy at the old fracture site.

B. LATERAL CONDYLE FRACTURE

The lateral condyle fracture is an oblique shearing fracture of the lateral portion of the joint surface that occurs when the radial head drives into the capitulum of the humerus during a fall. The lack of significant ossification may obscure the fracture or give the false appearance of a benign Salter-Harris II fracture pattern, but most lateral condyle fractures are highly unstable Salter-Harris IV fractures (Figure 11–45). Because both the joint surface and the physis are displaced, they usually require open reduction and fixation using pins.

C. RADIAL NECK FRACTURE

Fracture of the radial neck is similar to a lateral condyle fracture. The radial neck just distal to the joint may angulate up to 70–80 degrees, although lesser angulation is more common (Figure 11–46). It is important to de-

termine the location of the radial head despite traumatic angulation of the radial neck. Surprisingly, angulation of 45 degrees or less usually remodels spontaneously and requires only symptomatic treatment that permits early return to activity. Larger degrees of angulation can often respond to closed manipulation.

D. FOREARM FRACTURE

Forearm fractures are a common result of falls. If they involve both bones, one bone may be completely displaced while the other only bends or suffers a greenstick fracture. In children, most forearm fractures that involve both bones can be successfully treated by closed reduction and casting; minor angular malalignment can easily be tolerated if rotational alignment of the bone ends is accurate. In addition, the ends of fractured bones often overlap. This is not necessarily of concern if alignment is satisfactory, because side-to-side bone healing and remodeling are rapid in children.

E. MONTEGGIA FRACTURE

Monteggia fracture is fracture of the ulna only, with the radius remaining intact. Because two-bone systems generally must fail in two spots if they break at all, the radial head dislocates from the capitulum. In such cases, reduction must include the elbow component. As with other pediatric forearm fractures, closed reduction is usually successful, although some Monteggia fractures require open reduction. The physician should be alert to the possibility of Monteggia fracture because the fracture can lead to chronic loss of elbow motion if it is not properly reduced.

In children, Galeazzi fracture of the radius, in which the distal radioulnar joint is dislocated, is far less common than the analogous Monteggia fracture.

F. TORUS FRACTURE OF RADIUS

Torus fracture of the radius is a minor buckle of the dorsal cortex of the distal radius, usually 1–2 cm proximal to the distal radial physis. It occurs after a minor fall on the hand. Many torus fractures are mistaken for wrist sprains because they are stable and are not as painful as unstable fractures. They heal uneventfully in 3–4 weeks, with excellent long-term results.

Mintzer CM et al: Percutaneous pinning in the treatment of displaced lateral condyle fractures. J Pediatric Orthop 1994;14: 462.

Mirsky EC et al: Lateral condyle fractures in children: Evaluation of classification and treatment. J Orthop Trauma 1997;11: 117.

Metacarpal & Phalangeal Fractures

Fractures of the metacarpals and phalanges commonly occur from crush injuries in children (eg, catching a

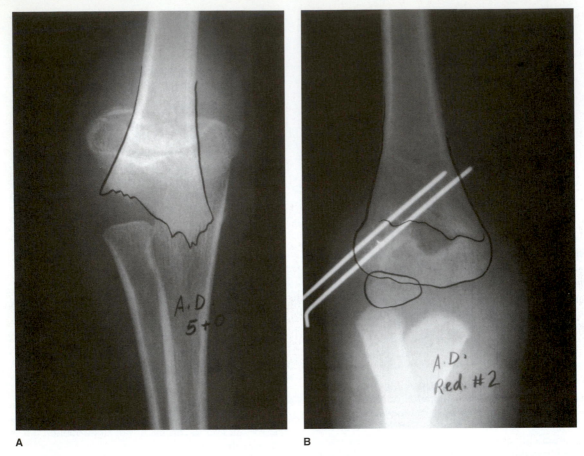

A   **B**

Figure 11–44.   Displaced supracondylar fracture of the humerus. Injury film (**A**); after closed reduction and internal fixation using percutaneous pins (**B**).

hand or finger in a door) and are generally quite stable because the periosteum remains intact. They are rarely severely angulated or rotationally malaligned, and usually can be managed by immobilization for 2–3 weeks.

3. Lower Extremity Fractures

Pelvic Fracture

Pelvic fractures in children are usually seen in conjunction with major blunt trauma. Gross displacement is fairly uncommon and usually can be treated symptomatically because the intact periosteum stabilizes the large flat bones. The patient should be carefully evaluated for intra-abdominal and other injuries. Properly treated pelvic fractures in an immature skeleton resolve satisfactorily.

Adolescents exhibit a special type of avulsion fracture of apophyses because aggressive pulling of mus-

cles during sports can detach an apophysis from its parent bone. These avulsion fractures are sometimes called transitional fractures because the physes are in transition within 2 years of skeletal maturity. During this time, relatively weak cartilage physes may not be strong enough to withstand the pull of growing muscles suddenly grown powerful under the influence of hormones. Transitional avulsion fractures may occur at the iliac crest (abdominal muscles), lesser trochanter of the femur (iliopsoas muscle), or ischial tuberosity (hamstring muscle). Transitional fractures of the pelvis and femur are treated symptomatically. Although these fractures do not require reduction, they may heal with a significant "bump" that requires excision later.

Hamsa WR: Epiphyseal injuries about the hip joint. Clin Orthop 1957;10:119.

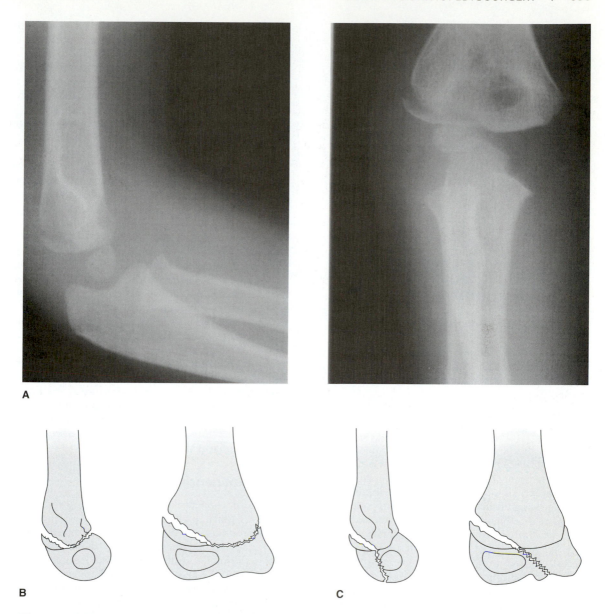

Figure 11–45. Lateral condyle fracture of the humerus (**A**) can easily be mistaken for a "simple" Salter-Harris type II injury, which carries a good prognosis (**B**). In reality, however, it is almost always a Salter-Harris type IV injury, with a fracture pattern crossing both the joint surface and the physis (**C**); unless it is not displaced, it requires open reduction.

Hip Fracture

Pediatric hip fractures are rare but may be serious, as trauma to this area may produce significant injury. As in the adult, the fracture pattern may disrupt the blood supply of the proximal femoral head and lead to avascu-

lar necrosis of the proximal femoral epiphysis, femoral neck, or both. In older children, this can be a devastating complication; it is treated like LCP but may result in such severe collapse that hip fusion is required.

Femoral neck fractures in children are highly unstable and are treated by reduction and internal fixation.

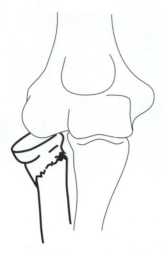

Figure 11–46. Fracture of the radial neck may angulate greatly yet still remodel spontaneously in the younger child.

The mechanical fixation may be imperfect because the surgeon must avoid injury to the proximal femoral physis. For this reason, a spica cast (body and legs) is generally used as well.

Femoral Shaft Fracture

Fractures of the femoral shaft are common injuries caused by falls as well as bicycle and motor vehicle accidents. In young children, they may be the result of child abuse. Although most are closed injuries, blood loss can be significant because of bleeding into the soft tissues of the thigh. Nerve injury is rare, and the fact that the fracture is surrounded by richly nourished muscle ensures rapid solid union (usually within 6 weeks).

Longitudinal muscle pull and spasm cause femoral shaft fractures to shorten and angulate. Initial treatment requires longitudinal traction (skin traction in younger children, skeletal traction in older children) to restore length and alignment. At this point, treatment largely depends on the patient's age.

Femur fractures in children age 2–10 years have a strong tendency to exhibit overgrowth of 1–2.5 cm because of fracture hyperemia. Therefore, in this age group, it may be desirable to use a cast and allow some shortening to occur. Rapid remodeling of the bone makes perfect reduction unnecessary. Most surgeons apply a spica cast immediately or within the first week.

Femoral overgrowth following fracture becomes unlikely in children older than 10 years of age. In these older children, the bone either must be kept to anatomic length by traction for 3–4 weeks (until sufficient callus has formed to stabilize length) or treated by intramedullary nails or other operative measures, as in the adult. Currently, flexible intramedullary nails are popular because they do not require reaming prior to insertion, and they are less likely to disrupt the precarious blood supply of the proximal femur.

After healing or cast removal, the child may begin walking. Limping is common in the first month after fracture because the hip girdle musculature regains its strength only slowly. No physical therapy is required, however, because normal walking permits spontaneous recovery, and long-term results of pediatric femur fractures are excellent.

Epiphyseal Separation

Epiphyseal separations (fracture) of the distal femoral physis are usually Salter-Harris type I or II injuries. All are caused by significant trauma, and injury to the growth mechanism of the plate is common. As many as 50% of cases exhibit subsequent growth arrest. Major neurovascular injury can occur, as with knee dislocations. Displaced epiphyseal separations require gentle reduction under general anesthesia. Some are so unstable, however, that they require percutaneous pin fixation for several weeks until the fracture is "sticky," or healed enough so that displacement does not occur. If physeal closure occurs, the treatment depends on age and remaining growth potential. (See discussion of limb-length inequality.)

Tibial Eminence Injury

The tibial eminence (spine), located entirely on the proximal tibial epiphysis, is the site of attachment of the anterior cruciate ligament. Twisting injuries of the knee can shear off the eminence and may displace it within the joint. Usually, the fragment reduces with full extension of the knee, but open reduction can be performed if necessary. Casting in extension is used for 6 weeks, until the bone has healed (Figure 11–47). Unlike many other pediatric fractures, tibial eminence injuries often lead to mild long-term knee symptoms, especially during athletic activities.

Tibial Tubercle Avulsion Fracture

Tibial tubercle avulsion fractures are most often seen in adolescent males (age 13–14) who suffer sports-related injuries. The anterior tongue of the proximal tibial epiphysis is the site of attachment of the patellar tendon. During strenuous jumping, as in basketball, the tongue may avulse and displace. Sometimes the fracture extends into the joint and across the tibial joint surface.

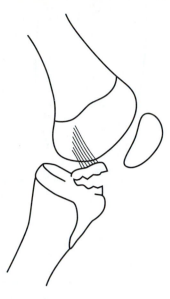

Figure 11–47. Tibial eminence fracture usually includes an anterior cruciate avulsion component. It can be treated nonoperatively if the fragment reduces with extension of the knee.

Tibial tubercle avulsions are transitional fractures in that they occur immediately before physeal closure and are not seen in younger children. Nearly all these fractures require open reduction and internal fixation, although the surgeon need not take the usual precautions when operating near the physis, because maturity follows too rapidly to permit deformity.

Proximal Tibial Metaphyseal Fracture

Proximal tibial metaphyseal fractures are usually undisplaced or minimally displaced. In the absence of fibular overgrowth (Figure 11–48) they can exhibit troublesome late angular deformity (valgus) caused by tibial overgrowth after fracture. The phenomenon is most pronounced at the age of maximum physiologic valgus (3–6 years). Over a number of years, the valgus has a tendency to remodel, so the best approach is observation.

Tibial Shaft Fracture

Tibial shaft fractures, which are usually accompanied by fibula fractures, generally result from major trauma. An exception is the nondisplaced, isolated spiral tibial fracture often seen after minor trauma in children just learning to walk (toddler's fracture). In the pediatric population, open tibia fractures are fairly common. As in the adult, injury to neurovascular structures and

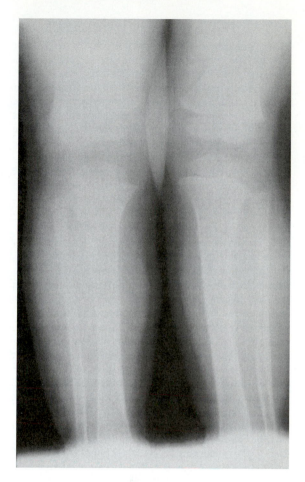

Figure 11–48. Even when not displaced, fracture of the proximal tibial metaphysis can stimulate the tibial physis and cause progressive valgus deformity, especially in patients younger than 6 years. Long-term observation indicates that slow remodeling eventually occurs.

compartment syndromes are major risks (see Chapter 3, "Musculoskeletal Trauma Surgery"). Open fractures of the tibia and fibula require surgical debridement, but because skin loss is less likely than in the adult, they can often be managed the same way as closed fractures, following lavage.

Most tibial fractures in children can be adequately aligned and immobilized in above-knee casts. Rare, unstable cases, some open fractures, or fractures in older children also may require external fixation or other devices to maintain reduction and alignment. As in the adult, pediatric tibia fractures are relatively slow to heal, frequently requiring 10–12 weeks; nonunion is rare, however.

Ankle Fracture & Distal Tibial Fracture

Ankle fractures and distal tibial fractures in younger children are often either metaphyseal or Salter-Harris type II distal tibial physeal injuries that heal rapidly. These fractures have very little tendency to suffer growth arrest or other serious consequences (Figure 11–49). In children age 8–11 years, inversion injuries can push off the medial malleolus, causing an oblique Salter-Harris type IV fracture that disrupts both the joint and the growth plate. These fractures generally require open reduction for accurate realignment of the physis and articular surface. Subsequent growth arrest can cause a medial physeal bridge and produce a progressive varus deformity of the distal tibial articular surface as the lateral physis continues untethered elongation. If this occurs, either epiphyseal bar resection or corrective tibial osteotomy should be considered.

The distal tibia is the site of several distinct transitional fracture patterns. These physeal injuries occur only at the end of growth, shortly before complete distal tibial physeal closure at maturity. The distal physis begins early closure medially, with gradual lateral closure over the next year. The exact fracture pattern depends on how much of the plate is still open and on the force applied (ie, mechanism of injury). When just the medial physis is closed, a triplane fracture (ie, sagittal, transverse, and frontal) of the distal tibia occurs (Figure 11–50). This fracture contains a complex of fracture lines and crosses the growth plate. Triplane fractures usually require open reduction, although minimally displaced injuries can be managed nonoperatively. CT scans may be necessary to define the exact fracture configuration for accurate treatment.

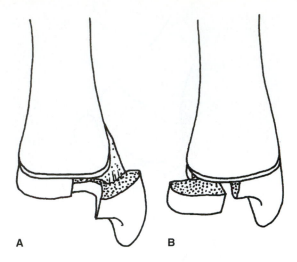

Figure 11–50. The triplane (**A**) and juvenile Tillaux (**B**) fractures are variations of ankle fracture that occur in the adolescent shortly before physeal closure. Because they involve the joint surface, such fractures may require open reduction.

In slightly older patients, when only a small anterolateral segment of the physis remains open, this anterolateral fragment can be avulsed by fibers of the distal tibiofibular syndesmosis (juvenile Tillaux fracture). This is a Salter-Harris type III fracture involving the articular surface and frequently requires open reduction to restore perfect joint anatomy.

Spiegel PG et al: Epiphyseal fractures of the distal ends of the tibia and fibula: A retrospective study of two hundred and thirty-seven cases in children. J Bone Joint Surg Am 1978;60:1046.

INJURIES RELATED TO CHILD ABUSE

Child abuse crosses all socioeconomic boundaries and takes many forms. The musculoskeletal system is frequently the site of abuse-related injuries, but findings may be subtle or misleading. The most critical issue to consider in suspected abuse is whether the injury can be adequately and believably explained by the history.

The classic radiographic picture of abuse is the presence of multiple healing fractures of various ages; in the absence of a bone fragility syndrome, the diagnosis may thus be obvious (Figure 11–51). Recent soft-tissue injuries have been found in 92% of children suspected of having been physically abused, with ecchymosis as the most common finding, increasing in incidence with age. Long bones (femur or humerus) are the bones most commonly fractured during child abuse. These fractures are transverse or oblique shaft injuries, a common pattern that is not by itself diagnostic. The history

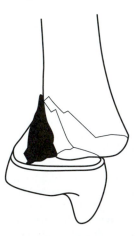

Figure 11–49. Simple fracture of the distal tibia (and fibula) at the ankle is usually a Salter-Harris type II pattern in patients younger than 10 years.

is often one of a minor fall or a limb "catching" in the side of the crib. It is important to realize that studies of fractures in young children have disclosed that injury mechanisms of this type are almost never the cause of serious skeletal injury, and the dichotomy between story and findings is highly suggestive of abuse. A good rule of thumb is to consider any long bone fracture in a child under age 3 years as abuse until proved otherwise.

The orthopedic management of abuse fractures is rarely complex, and simple closed methods usually suffice. Nearly all such fractures carry an excellent prognosis and heal or remodel rapidly. It is the detection of the abuse, and its subsequent social management, that are the main determinant of outcome.

Akbarnia BA, Akbarnia NO: The role of the orthopedist in child abuse and neglect. Orthop Clin North Am 1976;7:733.

King J et al: Analysis of 429 fractures in 189 battered children. J Pediatr Orthop 1988;8:585.

McMahon P et al: Soft-tissue injury as an indication of child abuse. J Bone Joint Surg 1995;77A:1179.

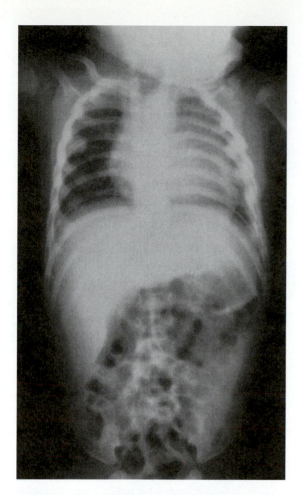

Figure 11–51. The presence of multiple fractures of various ages as well as unexplained long-bone fracture in a young child should suggest the diagnosis of child abuse.

Amputations

Douglas G. Smith, MD

Amputations are performed to remove extremities that are severely diseased, injured, or no longer functional. Although medical advances in antibiotics, trauma care, vascular surgery, and the treatment of neoplasms have improved the prospects for limb salvage, in many cases prolonged attempts to save a limb that should be amputated lead to excessive morbidity or even death. To adequately counsel a patient regarding amputation versus limb salvage, the physician must provide adequate information about the surgical and rehabilitative steps involved with each procedure and must also realistically appraise the probable outcome for function with each alternative. Attempting to salvage a limb is not always in the best interest of the patient.

The decision to amputate is an emotional process for the patient, the patient's family, and the surgeon. The value of taking a positive approach to amputation cannot be overemphasized. It is not a failure and should never be viewed as such. The amputation is a reconstructive procedure designed to help the patient create a new interface with the world and to resume his or her life. The residual limb must be surgically constructed with care to maintain muscle balance, appropriately transfer weight loads, and assume its new role of replacing the original limb.

For patients to achieve maximal function of the residual limb, they will also need a clear understanding of what to expect for an early postoperative prosthetic fitting, a rehabilitation program, and for long-term medical and prosthetic needs. For these discussions, the team approach to meeting the patients' needs can be especially rewarding. Nurses, prosthetists, physical and occupational therapists, and amputee support groups can be invaluable in providing the physical, psychologic, emotional, and educational support needed in returning patients to a full and active life. Many new amputees have stated that a peer visitor program was one of the most helpful events during their hospitalization and rehabilitation. The Amputee Coalition of America, a not-for-profit organization, supports this peer visitor training and can help locate programs that are available throughout the country.

SPECIAL CONSIDERATIONS IN THE TREATMENT OF PEDIATRIC PATIENTS

In infants and children, amputations are frequently associated with congenital limb deficiencies, trauma, and tumors.

Congenital limb deficiencies are commonly described using the Burtch revision of the Frantz and O'Rahilly classification system. Amelia is the complete absence of a limb; hemimelia is the absence of a major portion of a limb; and phocomelia is the attachment of the terminal limb at or near the trunk. Hemimelias can be further classified as terminal or intercalary. A terminal hemimelia is a complete transverse deficit at the end of the limb. An intercalary hemimelia is an internal segmental deficit with variable distal formation. In discussions of limb deficiencies, preaxial refers to the radial or tibial side of a limb, and postaxial refers to the ulnar or fibular side.

Reamputation of a congenital upper limb deficiency is rarely indicated, and even rudimentary appendages can often be functionally useful. In the lower limb, however, the ability to bear weight and the relative equality of leg lengths are mandatory for maximal function. Reamputation may be indicated in proximal femoral focal deficiency and congenital absence of the fibula or tibia, to produce a more functional residual limb and improve prosthetic placement.

In the growing child, proportional change occurs in residual limb length from childhood to adulthood—an important concept to keep in mind when determining the surgical approach. A diaphyseal amputation in an infant or young child removes one of the epiphyseal growth centers, and the involved bone therefore does not keep proportional growth with the rest of the body. What initially appears to be a long transfemoral amputation in a small child can turn out to be a short and troublesome residual limb when the child reaches skeletal maturity. All attempts should be made to save the distal-most epiphysis by disarticulation. If this is not technically possible, the greatest amount of bone length should be saved.

Terminal overgrowth occurs in 8–12% of pediatric patients who have had a surgical amputation. The growth of appositional bone at the transected end of a long bone exceeds the growth of the surrounding soft tissues. If left untreated, the appositional bone can penetrate through the skin (Figure 12–1). Terminal overgrowth of the transected bone does not occur as a result of the normal growth from the proximal physis pushing the distal end of the bone through the soft tissues, nor does it occur in limb disarticulations. Terminal overgrowth occurs most commonly in the humerus, fibula, tibia, and femur, in that order. Although numerous surgical procedures have been used to manage this problem, the best approach consists of stump revision with adequate bone resection or consists of autogenous osteochondral stump capping as originally described by Marquardt (Figure 12–2). If the stump-capping procedure is done at the time of original amputation, the graft material can be obtained from part of the amputated limb, such as the distal tibia, talus, or calcaneus. If a procedure is done later, the graft material can be obtained from the posterior iliac crest. Although techniques with nonautologous material have been used, significant complications have been reported. A recent report of using a modified Ertl osteomyoplasty to prevent terminal overgrowth in childhood limb deficiencies was not successful.

In a growing child, the fitting of a prosthesis can be challenging and requires frequent adjustments. Specialty pediatric amputee clinics can ease this process, provide family support, and make care more cost-effective. The timing of prosthetic fitting should be initiated

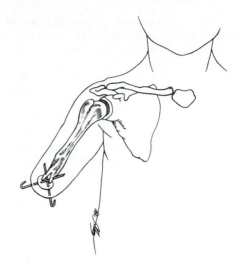

Figure 12–2. Stump-capping procedure. The bone end has been split longitudinally, and the osteochondral graft has been temporarily fixed with K wires.

to closely coincide with normal motor skill development.

Prosthetic fitting for the upper limb should begin near the time the child gains sitting balance, usually around 4–6 months of age. A passive terminal device with blunt rounded edges is used initially. Active cable control and a voluntary opening terminal device are added when the child exhibits initiative in placing objects in the terminal device, usually in the second year of life. Myoelectric devices are usually not prescribed until the child has mastered traditional body-powered devices. The physical demand placed on prosthetic devices by children can often exceed the durability of current myoelectric designs, so maintenance and repair costs must be considered. The decision to prescribe a myoelectric device for a child is individual and depends on many factors, including the physical characteristics of the residual limb, the desires of the child, the training available, the proximity of prosthetic facilities for fitting and maintenance, and issues about funding.

Prosthetic fitting for the lower limb commonly begins when the child develops the ability to crawl and pull to a standing position, which is usually at 8–12 months. A child with Syme's amputation or a transtibial amputation generally adapts to a prosthesis with surprising ease, and although formal gait training is not required, educational efforts are focused on teaching the parents about the prosthesis. For a child with a transfemoral amputation, control of a knee unit should not be expected immediately. The knee unit should be eliminated or locked in extension until the child is am-

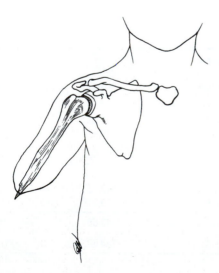

Figure 12–1. Terminal overgrowth of the transected bone in a pediatric amputee.

bulating well and demonstrates proficient use of the prosthesis. The initial gait pattern used by a child with a transfemoral amputation is not a normal heel-strike, midstance, toe-off gait pattern but is instead a more circumducted gait pattern with a prolonged foot flat phase. Formal gait training is seldom warranted until the child reaches 5 or 6 years of age. Attempts to force gait training too early can be frustrating for all involved. When pediatric patients are allowed to develop their own gait patterns as they grow and gain improved motor coordination, they are surprisingly adept at discovering the most efficient gait pattern without formal training.

Bernd L et al: The autologous stump plasty: Treatment for bony overgrowth in juvenile amputees. J Bone Joint Surg Br 1991; 73:203.

Birch JG et al: Syme amputation for the treatment of fibular deficiency. An evaluation of long-term physical and psychological functional status. J Bone Joint Surg Am. 1999;81(11):1511. [PMID: 10565642]

Davids JR et al: Operative treatment of bone overgrowth in children who have an acquired or congenital amputation. J Bone Joint Surg Am 1995;77:1490. [PMID: 7593057].

Greene WG, Cary JM: Partial foot amputation in children: A comparison of the several types with the Syme's amputation. J Bone Joint Surg Am 1982;64:438. [PMID: 7061561]

Pfeil J et al: The stump-capping procedure to prevent or treat terminal osseous overgrowth. Prosthet Orthot Int 1991;15:96.

Drvaric DM, Kruger LM: Modified Ertl oteomyoplasty for terminal overgrowth in childhood limb deficiencies. J Pediatr Orthop 2001;21(3):392. [PMID 1137827]

GENERAL PRINCIPLES OF AMPUTATION

Epidemiology

The most recent, accurate epidemiologic data on the incidence of amputation is from 1997 which shows an estimated 134,687 amputations were performed in the United States. This figure comes from totaling the National Hospital Discharge Survey and the Department of Veterans Affairs Hospitals' data. An unknown, but lesser number of amputations also occur in the military, private charitable, and Indian Health Services hospitals. Although persons with diabetes represent only approximately 3% of the total US population, 68% of the discharge diagnoses for amputation also list a diagnosis of diabetes. These data indicate that approximately 92,000 individuals with diabetes undergo lower extremity amputations every year.

Table 12–1 shows the estimated breakdown based on the National Hospital Discharge Survey and Veterans Administration data of the percent of lower extremity amputations performed by the surgical amputation level for persons with and without diabetes.

Preoperative Evaluation & Decision Making

The decision to amputate a limb and the choice of amputation level can be difficult and are often subject to differences in opinion. Advances in the treatment of in-

Table 12–1. Number and percent of U.S. amputation discharges by diabetes status and amputation level, 1997.

	Nationwide Inpatient Survey	Veterans Affairs Hospitals	Total	Percent
Diabetes				
Minor amputations[a]	46,680	1,987	48,667	53
Major amputations[b]	41,661	1,678	43,339	47
Subtotal	88,341	3,665	92,006	68
No Diabetes				
Minor amputations[a]	12,128	574	12,702	30
Major amputations[b]	28,574	1,405	29,979	70
Subtotal	40,702	1,997	42,681	32
Total	129,043	5,644	134,687	100

[a]Toe, ray, metatarsal or Syme's amputation.
[b]Transtibial or transfermoral amputation.

Reproduced, with permission, from Mayfield JA et al: *US Nationwide Inpatient Sample* (AHRQ 2000), Veterans Health Administration Patient Treatment File.

fection, peripheral vascular disease, replantation, and limb salvage complicate the decision-making process. The goals are to optimize a patient's function and reduce the level of morbidity.

A. Vascular Disease and Diabetes

Ischemia resulting from peripheral vascular disease remains the most frequent reason for amputation in the United States. More than half of patients with ischemia also have diabetes. The preoperative assessment of these patients includes a physical examination and an evaluation of perfusion, nutrition, and immunocompetence. Preoperative screening tests can be helpful, but no single test is 100% accurate in predicting successful healing. Clinical judgment based on experience in examining and following many patients with vascular disease and diabetes is still the most important factor in preoperative assessment.

1. Doppler ultrasound studies—The most readily available objective measurement of limb blood flow and perfusion is by Doppler ultrasound. Arterial wall calcification increases the pressure needed to compress the vessels of patients with vascular disease, and this often gives an artificially elevated reading. Low-pressure levels are indicative of poor perfusion, but normal and high levels can be confusing because of vessel wall calcification and are not predictive of normal perfusion or of wound healing. Digital vessels are not usually calcified, and blood pressure levels in the toes appear to be more predictive of healing than do those in the ankles.

2. Transcutaneous oxygen tension measurements—Tests to measure transcutaneous PO_2 are noninvasive and becoming more readily available in many vascular laboratories. These tests use a special temperature-controlled oxygen electrode to measure the partial pressure of oxygen diffusing through the skin. The ultimate reading is based on several factors: the delivery of oxygen to the tissue, the utilization of oxygen by the tissue, and the diffusion of oxygen through the tissue and skin. Caution in interpreting the transcutaneous PO_2 measurements during acute cellulitis or edema is warranted, because the presence of either of these disorders can increase oxygen utilization and decrease oxygen diffusion, thereby resulting in lower measurements of PO_2. Paradoxical measurements have also been reported on the plantar skin of the foot. In spite of these limitations, transcutaneous PO_2 and transcutaneous PCO_2 have both been shown to be statistically accurate in predicting amputation healing, but this does not rule out false-negative results.

3. Xenon (^{133}Xe) studies—Xenon-133 skin clearance studies have been used successfully to predict healing of amputations, but the preparation of the mixture containing xenon-133 gas and saline solution and the administration of the test are time-consuming, highly technician-dependent, and expensive. A small amount of the xenon and saline solution is injected intradermally at various sites, and the rate of washout is monitored by gamma camera. Xenon-133 is almost never used, and is primarily of historical interest.

4. Fluorescence studies—Skin fluorescence studies use intravenous injection of fluorescein dye and subjective observation or digital fluorometers to assess skin blood flow and correlate this with the likelihood of successful wound healing. The technique is not commonly used, and studies to assess its accuracy have yielded conflicting results.

5. Arteriography—Arteriography has not been helpful in predicting successful healing of amputations, and this invasive test is probably not indicated solely for the purpose of selecting the proper level of amputation. Arteriography is indicated if the patient is truly a candidate for arterial reconstruction or angioplasty.

6. Nutrition and immunocompetence studies—Both nutrition and immunocompetence have been shown to correlate directly with amputation wound healing. Many laboratory tests are available to assess nutrition and immunocompetence, but some are quite expensive. Screening tests for albumin level and total lymphocyte count are readily available and inexpensive. Several studies have shown increased healing of amputations in patients who have vascular disorders but have a serum albumin level of at least 3 g/dL and a total lymphocyte count exceeding 1500/mL. Nutritional screening is recommended to allow for nutritional improvement preoperatively and to help determine whether a higher level of amputation is needed.

7. Other issues—Activity level, ambulatory potential, cognitive skills, and overall medical condition must be evaluated to determine if the distal-most level of amputation is really appropriate for the patient.

For patients who are likely to remain ambulatory, the goals are to achieve healing at the distal-most level that can be fit with a prosthesis and to make successful rehabilitation possible. Recent studies of patients with vascular insufficiency and diabetes have demonstrated that successful wound healing can be achieved in 70–80% of these patients at the transtibial or more distal amputation level. This is in sharp contrast to 25 years ago, when because of a fear of wound failure, surgeons elected to perform 80% of all lower extremity amputations at the transfemoral level.

For nonambulatory patients, the goals are not simply to obtain wound healing but also to minimize complications, improve sitting balance, and facilitate position transfers. Occasionally, a more proximal amputation will more successfully meet these goals. For example, a bedridden patient with a knee flexion contracture might be better served with a knee disarticulation than a transtibial amputation, even if the biologic factors are present to heal the more distal amputation. Preoperative assessment of the patient's potential ability to use a prosthesis, the patient's specific needs for maintaining independent transfers, and the best weight distribution for seating can help in making wise decisions concerning the appropriate level of amputation and the most successful type of postoperative rehabilitation program.

Some nonambulatory patients do benefit from a partial foot amputation, or even transtibial amputation with prosthetic fitting, not with the goal of walking but to use that leg as a standing pivot for independent transfers. In these cases, prosthetic fitting is justified.

B. TRAUMA

As vascular reconstruction techniques improved, more attempts to salvage limbs were initially made, often with the result that multiple surgical procedures were subsequently required. In many cases, amputation was ultimately performed after a substantial investment of time, money, and emotional energy. Recent studies have offered guidelines for immediate or early amputation and shown the value of amputation not only in saving lives but also in preventing the emotional, marital, and financial disasters that can follow unwise and desperate limb salvage attempts. Although several scoring systems for mangled limbs have been published, none can perfectly predict when an amputation should be performed. These scores can help in the decision-making process, but good clinical experience and judgment are still required.

The absolute indication for amputation in trauma remains an ischemic limb with unreconstructible vascular injury. Massively crushed muscle and ischemic tissue release myoglobin and cell toxins, which can lead to renal failure, adult respiratory distress syndrome, and even death. In two groups of high-risk patients (multiply injured patients and elderly patients with a mangled extremity) limb salvage, even though technically possible, can become life-threatening and generally should be avoided. In all patients, the decision about whether to undertake immediate or early amputation of a mangled limb must also depend on whether it is an upper extremity or lower extremity.

An upper extremity can function with minimal or protective sensation, and even a severely compromised arm can serve as an assistive limb. An assistive upper extremity often functions better than the currently available prosthetic replacements. The decision of salvage versus amputation in the upper limb should be based on the chance of maintaining some useful function, even if that function is limited.

In the lower extremity, weight bearing is mandatory. A lower limb functions poorly without sensation, and an assistive limb is not useful. A salvaged lower limb often functions worse than a modern prosthetic replacement unless the limb can tolerate full weight bearing, is relatively pain free, has enough sensation to provide protective feedback, and has durable skin and soft-tissue coverage that does not break down whenever walking is attempted. The decision to salvage a mangled lower extremity should be based on providing a limb that can tolerate the demands of walking.

C. FROSTBITE

Exposure to cold temperatures can directly damage the tissue and cause a related vascular impairment from endothelial vessel injury and increased sympathetic tone. If the foot or hand is wet or directly exposed to the wind, cold injury can result even in temperatures above freezing. The immediate treatment involves restoring the core body temperature and then rewarming the injured body part in a water bath at a temperature of 40–44 °C for 20–30 min. Rewarming can be painful, and the patient often requires opiate analgesia. After rewarming, the involved part should be kept dry, blisters left intact, and dry gauze dressings used. The goals are to keep the injured extremity clean and dry and to prevent maceration, especially between the digits.

The temptation to perform early amputation should be avoided because the amount of recovery can be dramatic. As the extremity recovers from frostbite, a zone of mummification (dry gangrene) develops distally, and a zone of intermediate tissue injury forms just proximal to this. Even at the time of clear demarcation, the tissue just proximal to the zone of mummification continues to heal from the cold insult, and although the outward appearance is often pink and healthy, this tissue is not totally normal. Delaying amputation can improve the chance of primary wound healing. It is not unusual to wait 2–6 months for definitive surgery. In spite of having mummified tissue, infection is rare if the tissue is kept clean and dry.

D. TUMORS

Patients with musculoskeletal neoplasms face new choices in treatment with the development of limb salvage techniques and adjuvant chemotherapy and radiation therapy. If an amputation is chosen, the amputation incisions must be carefully planned to achieve the appropriate surgical margin.

Surgical margins (Figure 12–3) are characterized by the relationship of the surgical incision to the lesion, to the inflammatory zone surrounding the lesion, and to the anatomic compartment in which the lesion is located. The four types of margins are: the intralesional

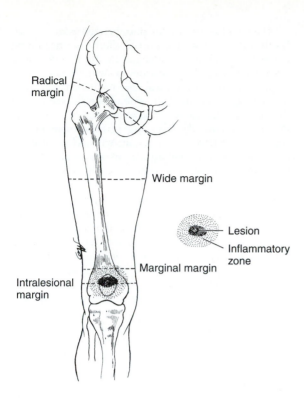

Radical margin

Wide margin

Intralesional margin

Marginal margin

Lesion

Inflammatory zone

Figure 12–3. Surgical margins in tumors of the extremity.

margin, in which the surgical incision enters the lesion; the marginal margin, in which the incision enters the inflammatory zone but not the lesion; the wide margin, in which the incision enters the same anatomic compartment as the lesion but is outside of the inflammatory zone; and the radical margin, in which the incision remains outside of the involved anatomic compartment. Biopsy incisions and amputation incisions must be planned with careful consideration as to the tumor margin required.

Recent studies continue to evaluate the complex issues and outcomes of amputation versus limb-sparing procedures for patients with extremity sarcomas. Studies continue to suggest that functional outcomes in terms of kinesiologic parameters are comparable with either limb salvage or amputation. Both treatment groups report quality of life problems involving employment, health insurance, social isolation, and poor self-esteem. Overall survival remains comparable with either treatment. In some tumors, amputation may achieve better local disease control. These results confirm that the decision about treatment must be made on an individual basis, according to the specific lifestyle and needs of the patient.

Surgical Definitions & Techniques

Terminology for amputation level has recently been changed to the accepted international nomenclature. Transtibial should be used instead of below-knee, and transfemoral instead of above-knee. In the upper extremity, the terms transradial and transhumeral have replaced the older terms below-elbow and above-elbow.

Careful surgical techniques, especially in soft-tissue handling, are more critical to wound healing and functional outcome in amputation procedures than in many other surgical procedures. The tissues are often traumatized or poorly vascularized, and the risk of wound failure is high, particularly if close attention is not paid to soft-tissue technique. Flaps should be kept thick, avoiding unnecessary dissection between the skin and subcutaneous, fascial, and muscle planes. In adults, periosteum should not be stripped proximal to the level of transection. In children, however, removing 0.5 cm of the distal periosteum may help prevent terminal overgrowth. The rounding of all bone edges and the beveling of prominences are necessary for optimal prosthetic use.

Muscle loses its contractile function when the skeletal attachments are divided during amputation. Stabilizing the distal insertion of muscle can improve residual limb function by preventing muscle atrophy, providing counterbalance to the deforming forces resulting from amputation, and providing stable padding over the end of the bone. Myodesis is the direct suturing of muscle or tendon to bone. Myodesis techniques are most effective in stabilizing strong muscles needed to counteract strong antagonistic muscle forces, such as in cases involving transfemoral or transhumeral amputation and in cases involving knee or elbow disarticulation. Myoplasty involves the suturing of muscle to periosteum or the suturing of muscle to muscle over the end of the bone. The distal stabilization of the muscle is more secure with myodesis than with myoplasty. Care must be taken to prevent a mobile sling of muscle over the distal end of the bone, which usually results in a painful bursa.

The transection of nerves always results in neuroma formation, but all neuromas are not symptomatic. Historical attempts to diminish symptomatic neuromas include clean transection, ligation, crushing, cauterization, capping, perineural closure, and end-loop anastomosis. No technique has proved more effective than careful and meticulous isolation, retraction, and clean transection of the nerve. This allows the cut end to retract into the soft tissues, away from the scar, pulsating vessels, and prosthetic pressure points. Ligation of a nerve is still indicated to control bleeding from the blood vessels contained within larger nerves, such as the sciatic.

Split-thickness skin grafts are generally discouraged except as a means to save a knee or elbow joint that has a stable bone and good muscle coverage. Skin grafts do best with adequate soft-tissue support and are least durable when closely adherent to bone. New prosthetic interfaces, such as silicone-based liners, can help reduce the shear at the interface and improve durability in skin-grafted residual limbs.

An open amputation is occasionally necessary to control a severe ascending infection. The term *guillotine amputation* should be avoided, as it gives the impression that the limb is transected at one level through skin, muscle, and bone. Open amputations need to be performed with careful planning and forethought as to how the amputation will eventually be closed. The surgical plan must obviously consider adequate debridement of tissue necrosis and drainage of infection but must also consider the surgical flaps and tissue needed for a functional closure of the amputation to allow prosthetic fitting.

The problem of ascending infection is seen, for example, in a diabetic patient with a severe infection of the foot and cellulitis extending upward to the calf. The open amputation removes the source of infection, provides adequate drainage, and allows the acute cellulitis to resolve. After resolution, a definitive amputation and closure can be done safely. In the case of a diabetic foot infection, an open ankle disarticulation is simple, relatively bloodless, and preserves the posterior calf flap for a definitive transtibial amputation. Occasionally, it is necessary to make a longitudinal incision to drain the posterior tibial, anterior tibial, or peroneal tendon sheaths, in which case care should be taken not to violate the posterior flap of the definitive amputation. This approach often prevents having open, transected muscle bellies that can retract and become edematous—a problem that commonly occurs if an open calf-level amputation was initially performed and one that can make the definitive amputation difficult. In more severe infections or in cases in which the level of the definitive amputation will clearly be transfemoral, an open knee disarticulation has the same advantages as the open ankle disarticulation.

Postoperative Care

A. POSTOPERATIVE CARE AND PLANNING

The terminal amputation allows the unique opportunity to manipulate the physical environment of the wound during healing. A variety of methods have been described, including rigid dressings, soft dressings, controlled environment chambers, air splints, and skin traction. The use of a rigid dressing controls edema, protects the limb from trauma, decreases postoperative pain, and allows early mobilization and rehabilitation.

The use of an immediate postoperative prosthesis, or IPOP (Figure 12–4), has proved effective in decreasing the time to limb maturation and the time to definitive prosthetic fitting. In most cases involving a lower limb amputation, the surgeon will have the patient start with partial weight bearing if the wound appears stable after the first cast change, which usually takes place between the fifth and tenth day after surgery. Immediate postoperative weight bearing can be initiated safely in selected patients, usually young patients in whom an amputation was performed following a traumatic injury and above the zone of injury. Rigid dressings and the IPOP need to be applied carefully, but their application is easily learned and well within the scope of interested physicians. For upper extremity amputations, an IPOP can be applied immediately. Early training with an IPOP is believed to increase the long-term acceptance and use of a prosthesis. See Chapter 13 for a detailed discussion of rehabilitation.

To adequately counsel patients, some insight into the typical surgical and postoperative course can be helpful. Many patients require inpatient hospital care for 6–8 days after a transtibial amputation. Epidural or patient-controlled analgesia is usually required for pain control. Assistance with basic mobility and emotional support are also necessary. Antibiotics can minimize the risk of infection. The cast that was applied at the end of the surgical procedure is changed about postoperative

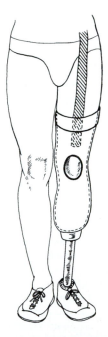

Figure 12–4. Immediate postoperative prosthetic cast for transtibial amputation.

day 5. If the wound healing is adequate, a new cast with a foot attachment is applied, and the patient can begin ambulating with approximately 30 lb of weight on the amputated extremity. Transtibial amputees are discharged to home or a nursing facility typically 6 or 8 days after surgery. Outpatient visits are scheduled weekly to change the cast, which frequently becomes loose as edema lessens, and to monitor wound healing and allow suture removal. Active and active-assisted knee range of motion is performed between each cast. On average, about six casts are applied on a weekly basis until the wound is healed, edema has resolved, wrinkles have returned to the skin, and the patient is ready for prosthetic fitting. The cast and the prosthetic foot attachment are applied and aligned by either the surgeon or the prosthetist. New, prefabricated, removable postoperative prosthetic systems are alternatives to the traditional casting techniques. Unfortunately, comparison trails versus traditional techniques have not been done.

Close interaction between the patient, the physical therapist, and the prosthetist is required in the first 12–18 months. The socket made for the first prosthesis must allow modifications as the residual limb continues to change shape during this time. Volume changes and mismatch between the shape of the socket and the evolving shape of the residual limb are treated with amputation socks and by adding pads to the socket or socket liner. Pads are usually needed in the region that contacts the anteromedial and anterolateral tibial flares, and posteriorly, in the popliteal region. Even with careful modifications, the prosthetic socket must be changed two or three times in the first 18 months. Because of these frequent prosthetic modifications, encouraging the patient to work with a prosthetic provider who is geographically close to the patient's residence can help tremendously in this rehabilitation phase. Many patients have an immediate desire to have the most advanced and high-tech components in their first prosthesis. But often these components are designed for higher activity levels than are typically achieved in the rehabilitation phase and are too rigid. Discussing how the prosthesis will evolve and be upgraded as the patient's activity increases can ease this process. A new prosthesis is typically required around month 18; often, the old components can be turned into a shower leg.

B. Prevention and Treatment of Complications

1. Failure of the wound to heal properly—Problems with wound healing, especially in diabetic and ischemic limbs, occur as the result of insufficient blood supply, infection, or errors in surgical technique. Healing failure rates are difficult to interpret because they are so dependent on the level of amputation selected.

Low failure rates can be achieved by doing amputations at an extremely proximal level in the majority of cases, but this sacrifices the rehabilitation potential of many patients because the ability to ambulate decreases dramatically with a transfemoral amputation. Wound healing failure that necessitates reamputation at a more proximal level occurs in approximately 5–10% of cases at centers specializing in amputee treatment.

Most surgeons prefer open wound care if the wound gap is less than 1 cm wide and prefer revision surgery if the gap is wider. If the surgical edema has resolved and some atrophy has already occurred, then a wedge excision of all nonviable tissue can be performed and still allow primary closure without any tension at the original level. If it is not possible to oppose the viable tissue gently without tension, then bone shortening or reamputation at a more proximal level should be performed.

In patients with small local areas of wound-healing failure, successful treatment with rigid dressings and an IPOP has been reported. The wounds are debrided weekly and packed open, and the IPOP is applied to allow some weight bearing. The stimulation of weight bearing can increase local circulation, decrease edema, and promote wound healing.

2. Infection—Infection without widespread tissue necrosis or flap failure may be seen after surgery, especially if active distal infection was present at the time of the definitive amputation or if the amputation was done near the zone of a traumatic injury. Hematomas can also predispose a wound to infection. In cases involving infection or hematomas, the wound must be opened, drained, and debrided. If the wound is allowed to remain open for an extended time, the flaps will retract and become edematous, which makes delayed closure difficult or impossible without shortening the bone. One solution, which can be instituted after thorough debridement and irrigation, is to close only the central one third to one half of the amputation wound and to use open packing for the medial and lateral corners (Figure 12–5). This method provides coverage of the bone but also allows adequate drainage and open wound management for the edges. If the original problem was truly infection and not tissue failure, the open portions of the wound will heal secondarily, and the result will still be a residual limb suitable for prosthetic fitting.

3. Phantom sensation—Phantom sensation is the feeling that all or a part of the amputated limb is still present. This sensation is felt by nearly everyone who undergoes surgical amputation, but it is not always bothersome. Phantom sensation usually diminishes over time, and telescoping (the sensation that the phantom foot or hand has moved proximally toward the stump) commonly occurs.

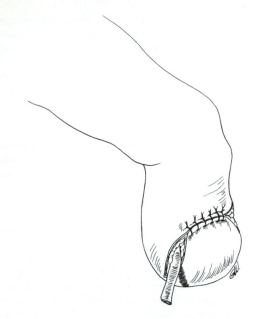

Figure 12–5. Partial closure of the infected transtibial amputation.

4. Pain and phantom pain—Phantom pain is defined as a bothersome, painful, or burning sensation in the part of the limb that is missing. Although from 60 to 70% of patients with acquired amputation experience some episodes of phantom pain, the episodes are often infrequent and brief. The dreaded problem of unrelenting phantom pain fortunately occurs only in a much smaller minority of patients. Surgical intervention for this problem has not been very successful.

Local physical measures including massage, cold packs, exercise, neuromuscular stimulation by external electrical currents, acupuncture, and regional sympathectomy may under given circumstances have a place in therapy when the pain is intractable. A technique that has gained some acceptance and success is the use of transcutaneous electrical nerve stimulators (TENS), incorporated either into a prosthesis or used as an isolated unit. The TENS system can be worn by the amputee at night and even during the day with the battery pack attached to the belt or inside a pocket. We have used this TENS system with moderate short-term success, but it is rare to see a patient who has continued to use a TENS system for more than a year.

Pharmacologic treatment has shown some success with several oral agents including amitriptyline, carbamazepine, phenytoin, gabapentin, and mexiletine. Medications can decrease the frequency of phantom pain episodes and decrease the intensity of these episodes. The appropriate use of an intravenous lidocaine challenge has been shown to be predictive of a favorable response to oral mexiletine. Unfortunately, no indicators are good at predicting who will respond to treatment with amitriptyline, carbamazepine, phenytoin, or gabapentin. Psychologic support can be beneficial, particularly when personality problems seem to accentuate the occurrence of pain. The individual needs patience and reassurance that the discomfort will improve with time, especially when a supportive social environment is present.

The sensations described by patients with phantom pain may be similar to the symptoms of reflex sympathetic dystrophy after an injury. Reflex sympathetic dystrophy can occur in amputated limbs and should be treated aggressively if present. Although rare, pain unrelated to the amputation can easily be overlooked. The differential diagnosis includes radicular nerve pain from proximal entrapment or disk herniation, arthritis of proximal joints, ischemic pain, and referred visceral pain.

Research has progressed in the prevention of phantom limb pain. Several authors have documented that the use of perioperative epidural anesthesia or intraneural anesthesia can block the acute pain associated with amputation surgery and decrease the opiate requirements in the immediate postoperative period. They have also suggested that perioperative analgesia can prevent or decrease the later incidence of phantom pain, although this is difficult to document. The literature is unfortunately not conclusive on whether preemptive measures can truly reduce the frequency or severity of phantom limb pain. Some reports dispute the claims that preemptive analgesia reduces the frequency of phantom limb problems. A recent randomized trial by Lambert and colleagues found that perioperative epidural block started 24 h before amputation is not superior to infusion of local anesthetic via a perineural catheter in preventing phantom pain but does give better relief in the immediate postoperative period.

5. Edema—Postoperative edema is common in patients who have undergone amputation. Rigid dressings can help reduce this problem. If soft dressings are used, they should be combined with stump wrapping to control edema, especially if the patient is a prosthetic candidate. The ideal shape of a residual limb is cylindrical, not conical. One common mistake is wrapping the stump too tightly at the proximal end. This can lead to congestion and worsening edema and can also cause the residual limb to become shaped like a dumbbell. Another common mistake is not wrapping transfemoral amputations in a waist-high soft spica cast that includes the groin. If wrapped incorrectly, the limb will have a narrow, conical shape, and a large adductor roll will develop. Because of the difficulty in wrapping the transfemoral amputation with elastic bandages, shrinker socks with a waist belt are frequently used as a safer alternative for the transfemoral level.

Stump edema syndrome is a condition commonly caused by proximal constriction and characterized by edema, pain, blood in the skin, and increased pigmentation. The syndrome usually responds to temporary removal of the prosthesis, elevation of the residual limb, and compression.

6. Joint contractures—Joint contractures usually develop between the time of amputation and prosthetic fitting. Contractures that exist preoperatively can seldom be corrected postoperatively.

In transfemoral amputees, the deforming forces are flexion and abduction. Adductor and hamstring stabilization can oppose the deforming forces. During the postoperative period, patients should avoid propping up the residual limb on a pillow and should begin active and passive motion exercises early, including lying prone to stretch the hip.

In transtibial amputees, knee flexion contractures greater than 15 degrees can cause major prosthetic problems and failure. Long leg rigid dressings, early postoperative prosthetic fitting, quadriceps-strengthening exercises, and hamstring stretching can prevent this complication. Because contractures in below-knee amputees can seldom be corrected, their prevention is paramount.

In the upper extremity amputee, shoulder and elbow flexion contractures often follow amputation, especially with short residual limbs. Efforts should be directed at prevention, with aggressive physical therapy beginning soon after surgery.

7. Dermatologic problems—Good general hygiene includes keeping the residual limb and prosthetic socket clean, rinsed well to remove all soap residual, and thoroughly dry. Patients should avoid the application of foreign materials and be encouraged not to shave a residual lower limb. Shaving seems to increase the problems with ingrown hairs and folliculitis.

Reactive hyperemia is the early onset of redness and tenderness after amputation. It is usually related to pressure and resolves spontaneously.

Epidermoid cysts commonly occur at the prosthetic socket brim, especially posteriorly. These cysts are difficult to treat and commonly recur, even after excision. The best initial approach is to modify the socket and relieve pressure over the cyst. Warm heat, often with a warm tea bag, topical agents, and oral antibiotics can be required as local treatment.

Verrucous hyperplasia is a wartlike overgrowth of skin that can occur on the distal end of the residual limb. It is caused by a lack of distal contact and failure to remove normal keratin. The disorder is characterized by a thick mass of keratin, sometimes accompanied by fissuring, oozing, and infection. The infection should be addressed first, and then the limb should be soaked and treated with salicylic acid paste to soften the keratin. Topical hydrocortisone is occasionally helpful in resistant cases. Prosthetic modifications to improve distal contact must be made to prevent recurrences. Because the distal limb is often tender and prosthetic modifications are uncomfortable, an aggressive preventive approach is warranted.

Contact dermatitis sometimes occurs in amputees and can be confused with infection. The primary irritation type of dermatitis is caused by contact with acids, bases, or caustics and frequently results from failure to rinse detergents and soaps from prosthetic socks. Patients should be instructed to use mild soap and to rinse extremely well. Allergic contact dermatitis is commonly caused by the nickel and chrome in metal, antioxidants in rubber, carbon in neoprene, chromium salts used to treat leather, and unpolymerized epoxy and polyester resins in plastic laminated sockets. After infection is ruled out and contact dermatitis is confirmed, treatment is begun and consists of removal of the irritant and use of soaks, corticosteroid creams, and compression with elastic wraps or shrinkers.

Superficial skin infections are common in amputees. Folliculitis occurs in hairy areas, often soon after the patient starts to wear a prosthesis. Pustules develop in the eccrine sweat glands surrounding the hair follicles, and this problem is often worse if the patient shaves. Hidradenitis, which occurs in apocrine glands in the groin and axilla, tends to be chronic and responds poorly to treatment. Socket modification to relieve any pressure in these areas can be helpful. Candidiasis and other dermatophytoses present with scaly, itchy skin, often with vesicles at the border and clearing centrally. Dermatophytoses are diagnosed with a potassium hydroxide preparation and treated with topical antifungal agents.

C. LENGTHENING OF RESIDUAL LIMBS

The ultimate function of an amputation depends on both the length of the bone and the quality of the soft-tissue envelope for the residual limb. Ilizarov techniques of distraction osteogenesis have been applied to lengthen the tibia or ulna in amputees. Bone lengthening can be successful, but often issues of soft-tissue coverage remain. Although great success has been described in recent small series of congenital short transradial amputations, another author describes the pending necrosis of the skin over the tip of the lengthened ulna. Nonadherent, mobile soft tissue that can pad the distal end of the bone is vitally important to successful prosthetic fitting. Microsurgical techniques have also been applied to use free tissue transfer to supply this type of coverage over bone in select patients, most often in trauma or tumor surgery. By using these techniques, the gracilis or latissimus dorsi muscle can be transferred to the end of the residual limb and covered with skin graft. The transposed tissues do not have sensation, and the bulk of the flap can lead to tremendous volume changes over the first two years. Lack of sensation and volume issues do complicate prosthetic fitting and function. These extraordinary techniques are probably best reserved for very select and unique circumstances.

D. PRESCRIPTION OF PROSTHETIC LIMBS

For lower limb prostheses, the major advances include the development of new lightweight structural materials (see Chapter 1), the incorporation of elastic response ("energy-storing") designs, the use of computer-assisted design and computer-assisted manufacturing technology in sockets, and microprocessor control of the prosthetic knee joint. For upper limb use, new electronic technology has increased the success and durability of myoelectric prostheses. The surgeon who prescribes prosthetic limbs should have a basic understanding of the general features available to optimally match the components with the patient's specific needs.

A good prosthetic prescription specifies the socket type, suspension, shank construction, specific joints, and terminal device. The socket can be a hard socket with no or minimal interface, or it can incorporate a liner. For the transfemoral amputee, a wide variety of socket shapes are available and range from the traditional quadrilateral design to the newer narrow mediolateral design. The prosthesis is suspended from the body by straps, belts, socket contour, suction, friction, or physiologic muscle control.

Shank construction can be either exoskeletal or endoskeletal. The older exoskeletal type has a rigid outer shell that is hollow in the center. The endoskeletal type has a central pylon or pipe that is surrounded by a soft and lightweight cosmetic foam cover. In the past, exoskeletal systems were more durable; however, as materials technology has improved, so has the durability and cosmetic appearance of endoskeletal systems. The endoskeletal systems also allow more adjustment and fine-tuning of alignment and are now considered structurally as durable as the older exoskeletal designs. However, the cosmetic and foam covers for the endoskeletal systems are not as durable as an exoskeletal shell. Exoskeletal systems are rarely prescribed, except for very active patients without easy access to prosthetic services, or for those involved in activities that would stain, tear, or destroy the endoskeletal cover. As the public's impression of disability has evolved, many active patients now decide not to cover the prosthesis and often take pride in the high-tech look of the titanium or carbon fiber components incorporated in an endoskeletal prosthesis.

A large variety of elbow, wrist, knee, and ankle joints are now available, as well as numerous terminal devices, including hands, hooks, feet, and special adaptive equipment for sports and work. The choice of an appropriate terminal device is extremely important. For an upper extremity amputee, there is no sensation in the prosthesis, and the critical feedback of touch and proprioception is missing. Initially, a hook may be a better choice than a prosthetic hand. This is because vision must substitute for upper extremity proprioception and a prosthetic hand will block vision and make dexterous use of the terminal device difficult and clumsy. In each case, the prosthetic prescription must be individualized to ensure the most efficient system for a particular patient.

Nearly all prosthetic sockets are fabricated by forming a thermoplastic or laminate socket over a plaster mold. It is important to note that an exact mold of the residual limb does not make a good socket for a prosthesis. The original mold must be modified to relieve the socket over areas that cannot tolerate pressure and to indent the socket over areas that can. Test sockets of clear plastic are commonly made to visualize the blanching of the skin at troublesome areas. Automated fabrication of mobility aids (AFMA) technology uses computer-assisted design and manufacturing to aid the prosthetist by digitizing the residual limb, adding the standard modifications usually applied to a mold, and allowing additional fine manipulation of the shape on the computer screen. The computer can direct the carving of the mold or fabrication of the socket. AFMA technology can decrease the time needed for the fabrication of prostheses and increase the time available for the evaluation and training of patients. The best use of AFMA is to allow fabrication of multiple sockets for one patient during the fitting process. By using computer modifications, refinements are added in each iteration to ultimately optimize the fit and comfort of the final socket. Before AFMA this technique was not cost-effective.

Myoelectric components are exciting but should generally not be prescribed for patients until they have mastered traditional body-powered devices and their residual limb volume is stable. Myoelectric devices have been most successfully used by patients with a mid-length transradial amputation. Although a long below-elbow limb has better rotation, it is less able to contain the electronics. The need for myoelectric devices is greater in patients with a more proximal upper extremity amputation, but the weight and slow speed of the myoelectric components has been a deterrent for their use. Hybrid devices utilizing body power and myoelectric components can be effective. Muscles that were stabilized by myodesis or myoplasty techniques seem to generate a better signal for myoelectric use.

Microprocessor control systems have been applied to the knee units for transfemoral amputees. The microprocessor control alters the resistance of the knee unit to flexion or extension appropriately by sensing the position and velocity of the shank relative to the thigh. The current microprocessor-controlled knee units still do not provide power for active knee extension that would assist in rising from the sitting position or in providing power to the amputee's gait and rise up stairs. The new microprocessor controlled, "intelligent" knee units do offer superior control when walking at varied speeds, descending ramps and stairs, and walking on uneven surfaces. Patients report improved confidence and a decrease in the tendency for the knee unit to buckle. One transfemoral amputee credits this new technology for his survival by allowing him to descend 70 stores in the World Trade center at a normal pace during the terrorist attacks.

Alekberov C et al: Lengthening of congenital below-elbow amputation stumps by the Ilizarov technique. J Bone Joint Surg Br 2000;82(2):239. [PMID: 10755433]

Bosse MJ et al: A prospective evaluation of the clinical utility of the lower-extremity injury-severity scores. J Bone Joint Surg Am 2001;83-A(1):3-14. [PMID: 11205855]

Boulas HJ: Amputations of the finger and hand: Indications for replantation. J Am Acad Orthop Surg 1998;6:104. [PMID: 9682072]

Boyko EJ et al: A prospective study of risk factors for diabetic foot ulcer. The Seattle Diabetic Foot Study. Diabetes Care 1999;22(7):1036. [PMID: 10388963]

Brooks B et al: TBI or not TBI: That is the question. Is it better to measure toe pressure than ankle pressure in diabetic patients? Diabet Med 2001;18(7):528. [PMID: 11553180]

Burgess EM et al: The Management of Lower-Extremity Amputations. Publication TR 10-6, US Government Printing Office, 1969.

Carter SA, Tate RB: The value of toe pulse waves in determination of risks for limb amputation and death in patients with peripheral arterial disease and skin ulcers or gangrene. J Vasc Surg 2001;33(4):708. [PMID: 11296321]

Davis RW: Successful treatment for phantom pain. Orthopedics 1993;16:691. [PMID: 8321759]

Ehde DM et al: Chronic phantom sensations, phantom pain, residual limb pain, and other regional pain after lower limb amputation. Arch Phys Med Rehabil 2000;81(8):1039. [PMID: 10943752]

Galer BS et al: Response to intravenous lidocaine predicts subsequent response to oral mexiletine: A prospective study. J Pain Symptom Manage 1996;12:161.

Lambert AW et al: Randomized prospective study comparing preoperative epidural and intraoperative perineural analgesia for the prevention of postoperative stump and phantom limb pain following major amputation. Reg Anesth Pain Med 2001;26(4):316. [PMID: 11464349]

Lane JM et al: Rehabilitation for limb salvage patients: Kinesiological parameters and psychological assessment. Cancer 2001; 92(4 Suppl):1013. [PMID: 11519028]

Marks LJ, Michael JW: Science, medicine, and the future: Artificial limbs. BMJ 2001;323(7315):732. [PMID: 11576982]

Martin C, Gonzalez del Pino J: Controversies in the treatment of fingertip amputations. Conservative versus surgical reconstruction. Clin Orthop 1998;(353):63. [PMID: 9728160]

Mayfield JA et al: Trends in lower limb amputation in the Veterans Health Administration, 1989-1998. J Rehabil Res Dev 2000; 37(1):23. [PMID: 10847569]

Melzack R: Phantom limbs. Sci Am 1992;266:120. [PMID: 1566028]

Mertens P, Lammens J: Short amputation stump lengthening with the Ilizarov method: Risks versus benefits. Acta Orthop Belg 2001;67(3):274. [PMID: 11486691]

Misuri A et al: Predictive value of transcutaneous oximetry for selection of the amputation level. J Cardiovasc Surg (Torino) 2000;41(1):83. [PMID: 10836229]

Nikolajsen L et al: Randomized trial of epidural bupivacaine and morphine in prevention of stump and phantom pain in lower limb amputation. Lancet 1997;350:1353.

Nikolajsen L et al: Phantom limb pain. Curr Rev Pain 2000;4 (2):166. [PMID: 10998730]Peabody TD et al: Evaluation and staging of musculoskeletal neoplasms. J Bone Joint Surg Am 1998;80(8):1204. [PMID: 9730132]

Reiber GE, Ledoux W: Epidemiology of foot ulcers and amputations in the diabetic foot: Evidence for prevention. In Williams R et al: The Evidence Base for Diabetes Care. New York: John Wiley & Sons, 2002.

Rosenberg JM et al: The effect of gabapentin on neuropathic pain. Clin J Pain 1997;13:251. [PMID: 9303258]

Smith DG, Burgess EM: The use of CAD/CAM technology in prosthetics and orthotics—Current clinical models and a view to the future. J Rehabil Res Dev 2001;38(3):327. [PMID: 11440264]

Stojadinovic A et al: Amputation for recurrent soft tissue sarcoma of the extremity: Indications and outcome. Ann Surg Oncol 2001;8(6):509. [PMID: 11456050]

Waters RL et al: The energy cost of walking of amputees: Influence of level of amputation. J Bone Joint Surg 1976;58A:42. [PMID: 1249111]

■ TYPES OF AMPUTATION

UPPER EXTREMITY AMPUTATIONS & DISARTICULATIONS

Hand Amputation

Although microsurgical replantation techniques have reduced the incidence of hand amputations, for many patients replantation is still not feasible or results in failure. There is considerable controversy about the best treatment for any given hand injury, and the optimal treatment takes into consideration the injured patient's occupation, hobbies, skills, and hand of dominance. The hand is a highly visible and important part of the body image. Many patients with partial hand amputations can benefit tremendously from using a cosmetic partial hand prosthesis.

A. FINGERTIP AMPUTATION

Fingertip injuries occur frequently, and fingertip amputation is the most common type of amputation. The treatment of choice usually depends on the geometry of the defect and whether or not bone is exposed. Although a large variety of local flap procedures have been used to cover defects of different shapes and sizes, there is also a growing understanding that allowing secondary healing of fingertip injuries is the treatment that is least prone to complications in adults as well as in children. Even if bone is exposed, simply rongeuring back the exposed bone proximal to the soft-tissue defect and allowing secondary healing can give excellent results. The amount of the bone that can be removed is limited because at least one third of the distal phalanx must be left intact to prevent a hook deformity of the nail.

Two problems frequently result from fingertip amputations: cold intolerance and hypersensitivity. Overall, regardless of which treatment is chosen, approximately 30-50% of patients will experience these problems. One criticism of the many local flap procedures used to obtain coverage and primary wound healing is that all of them involve incising and advancing uninjured tissue, which extends the area of scarring and damages the fine branches of the digital nerves. Recent studies suggest that the incidence of cold intolerance and hypersensitivity may be lower with secondary healing than with skin grafts or local flaps.

B. THUMB AMPUTATION

The thumb, with its unique range of motion, plays the major role in all three prehensile activities of the hand: palmar grip, side-to-side pinch, and tip-to-tip pinch. Amputation of the thumb can result in the loss of virtually all hand function. Thumb amputations can involve (1) the distal third of the thumb (ie, distal to the interphalangeal joint), (2) the middle third of the thumb (ie, from the metacarpophalangeal joint to the interphalangeal joint), or (3) the proximal third of the thumb.

Thumb amputation of the distal third allows the patient to retain a tremendous amount of thumb function. Cold intolerance and hypersensitivity are frequent problems, as noted in the previous discussion of fingertip amputations. Treatment of distal third injuries should allow secondary healing of the thumb or should use relatively uncomplicated techniques for coverage.

Thumb amputation in the middle third is more complicated. The issues here are length, stability, and sensate skin coverage. More aggressive procedures may well be warranted and may consist of crossfinger flaps, volar advancement flaps, neurovascular island flaps from the dorsal index finger (radial nerve) or volar mid-

dle finger (median nerve), bone lengthening, or web space deepening.

Thumb amputation in the proximal third has a devastating impact on hand function. Local reconstruction for this degree of loss is not generally successful. Pollicization of another digit, a toe-to-hand transfer, or other complicated surgical techniques may be indicated to restore function.

C. DIGIT AMPUTATION

Isolated amputation of a lesser digit can cause a variety of functional and cosmetic problems. Digit amputations distal to the insertion of the sublimis flexor tendon retain active flexor tendon activity and maintain useful metacarpophalangeal joint flexion. The long flexor tendon should not be sewn to the extensor tendon, because this will limit the excursion of both tendons and will definitely limit the function of the remaining digits.

Amputations proximal to the sublimis tendon insertion will retain approximately 45 degrees of proximal phalanx flexion at the metacarpophalangeal joint through the action of the intrinsic muscles. This is usually enough to keep small objects from falling through the defect and to allow the residual finger to participate to some degree in grip. If the patient uses a cosmetic finger prosthesis and wears a ring to cover the proximal edge of the prosthesis, the amputation is almost unnoticeable.

The index finger participates principally in side-to-side and tip-to-tip pinch with the thumb. After an amputation of the index finger at the metacarpophalangeal joint, the middle finger assumes this important role. The residual second metacarpal can interfere with side-to-side pinch between the thumb and the middle finger, however. Often, converting this amputation to a ray amputation can improve function and cosmesis, but the drawback is that it also narrows the width of the palm and can decrease grip and torque strength significantly. Surgical decisions must be individualized, but the second metacarpal should probably be retained if the patient uses hand tools extensively, as does a carpenter or machinist.

Amputation of the middle or ring finger at the metacarpophalangeal joint can make it difficult for the patient to hold small objects because they tend to fall through the defect. Full ray resection can narrow the central defect and occasionally improve function, but narrowing the palm can decrease grip and torque strength.

Amputation of the small finger at the metacarpophalangeal joint is often cosmetically unacceptable, because of the abrupt and noticeable change in contour of the hand. Although converting a fifth digital amputation to a ray amputation by including the metacarpal can improve cosmesis, it also narrows the width of the palm and can decrease grip and torque strength. Surgical decisions must be based on individual factors and concerns.

D. CARPUS AMPUTATION

Amputations through the carpus are generally discouraged. Most surgeons believe the result to have no real advantages over a wrist disarticulation or transradial amputation. There are isolated reports of patients valuing the little bit of wrist flexion and extension that allows them to hold objects against their body and to stabilize objects for two-handed grasp. The flexor and extensor carpi radialis and ulnaris tendons must be reattached to provide this limited motion. The prosthetic options are less standard and are generally considered to be less functional than the traditional transradial designs.

Carpus amputations should probably be considered in bilateral cases. Although rare, more patients sustaining tissue loss from ischemia are seen in the intensive care unit after prolonged resuscitations and the use of vasopressors. Without the vasopressors, these patients would die. Unfortunately, part of the body's response to these lifesaving medications can be to shunt blood flow from the distal extremities, resulting in demarcation and dry gangrene in the hands and feet. Just as in frostbite, if infection is not present, it is worthwhile to delay any surgical intervention and allow adequate time for tissue demarcation and recovery. Partial hand amputation is occasionally necessary, and if required, the carpus level should be considered.

Wrist Disarticulation

Wrist disarticulation continues to be controversial. Proponents frequently argue that it has two advantages over the shorter transradial amputation: it retains the distal radioulnar joint, which preserves more forearm rotation, and it retains the distal radial flare, which dramatically improves prosthetic suspension. Volar and dorsal fish-mouth incisions are usually best, and removal of the radial and ulnar styloids can prevent painful pressure points. Tenodesis of the major forearm motors stabilizes the muscle units and thereby improves physiologic and myoelectric performance.

Opponents of wrist disarticulation argue that prosthetic substitution after this procedure is slightly more complicated than it is after a standard transradial amputation. The prosthetic socket is more difficult to fabricate because of the bone contours. Conventional wrist units add too much length to the prosthetic arm after wrist disarticulation and therefore cannot be used. The terminal device for a wrist disarticulation also needs to be modified because of length. Myoelectric prostheses

are difficult to fit because there is less space to conceal the electronics and power supply.

In spite of these prosthetic concerns, wrist disarticulation patients are often excellent upper extremity prosthetic users. Some patients with an unsatisfactory hand can gain improved function by undergoing a wrist disarticulation and utilizing a standard prosthesis. This decision must be individualized and based on contributory factors such as severity of tissue loss, pain, functional requirements, and the patient's body image.

Transradial Amputation

The transradial amputation is extremely functional, and successful prosthetic rehabilitation and sustained use are achieved in 70–80% of patients who undergo amputation at this level. Forearm rotation and strength are proportional to the length retained. Surgical incisions are best with equal volar and dorsal flaps. A myodesis should be performed to prevent a painful bursa, facilitate physiologic muscular suspension, and allow for myoelectric prosthetic use. An extremely short transradial residual limb requires the use of a Muenster type socket, which molds up around the humeral condyles for added suspension. Occasionally, side hinges and a humeral cuff are required to achieve suspension of the prosthesis. Both of these types of suspension preserve elbow flexion and extension but limit rotation.

The value of preserving the elbow joint cannot be overemphasized. Skin grafts and even composite grafts should be considered to retain the tremendous functional benefit of an elbow with some active motion. Even a limited range of elbow motion can be useful, and an ingeniously designed, geared step-up elbow hinge can convert a limited active range of elbow motion to an improved prosthetic range of motion. Although body-powered prostheses are extremely functional at the transradial level of amputation, this level has also been the most successful level at which to use myoelectric devices.

Krukenberg's Amputation

Krukenberg's kineplastic operation transforms the transradial amputation stump into radial and ulnar digits that are capable of strong prehension and have excellent manipulative ability because of retained sensation on the "fingers" of the forearm. The operation should not be performed as a primary amputation.

Krukenberg's amputation can be performed as a secondary procedure in a transradial amputee who has a residual limb of at least 10 cm from the tip of the olecranon, an elbow flexion contracture of less than 70 degrees, and good psychologic preparation and acceptance. In this case, the amputee can become completely independent in daily activities owing to the retained sensory ability of the pincers as well as the quality of the grasping mechanism (Figure 12–6). Krukenberg's amputation has traditionally been indicated for blind patients with bilateral below-elbow amputations, but it also may be indicated at least unilaterally in bilateral below-elbow amputees who are able to see and in those who have limited access to prosthetic facilities.

A conventional prosthesis can be worn over the Krukenberg forearm, and myoelectric devices can be adapted to use the forearm motion. The major disadvantage is the appearance of the arm, which many people consider grotesque and will not accept. As society continues to become more understanding and accepting of disabled and handicapped individuals, concerns about appearance may diminish. Intensive preoperative preparation and counseling are mandatory.

Elbow Disarticulation

Elbow disarticulation can be a satisfactory amputation level and has the advantage of retaining the condylar flare to improve prosthetic suspension and allow for the transfer of humeral rotation to the prosthesis. The longer lever arm improves strength. The disadvantage is in the design of the prosthetic elbow hinge. An outside hinge is bulky and hard on clothing, while the conventional elbow unit provides a disproportionately long

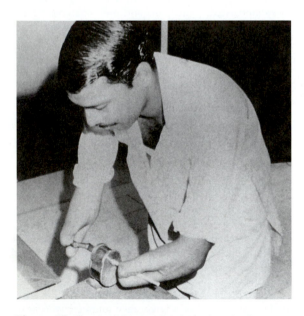

Figure 12–6. A patient with bilateral Krukenberg hands demonstrates bimanual dexterity in sharpening a pencil. (Reproduced, with permission, from Garst RJ: The Krukenberg hand. J Bone Joint Surg Br 1991;73:385.)

upper arm and short forearm. Whether the advantages of the elbow disarticulation outweigh the disadvantages remains controversial. Surgically, volar and dorsal flaps work best, and myodesis of the biceps and triceps tendons are needed to preserve the distal muscle attachments.

Transhumeral Amputation

When transhumeral amputation is performed, efforts should be made to retain as much as possible of the bone length that has suitable soft-tissue coverage. Even if only the humeral head remains and no functional length is salvageable, an improved shoulder contour and cosmetic appearance results. Myodesis helps preserve biceps and triceps strength, prosthetic control, and myoelectric signals. In most cases of transhumeral amputation, an immediate postoperative prosthesis and rigid dressings can be used successfully. Physical therapy should focus on proximal joint and muscle function. Because the terminal prosthetic device is usually controlled by active shoulder girdle motion, early prosthetic use and therapy can prevent contracture and maintain strength.

Prosthetic suspension has traditionally been incorporated in the body-powered harness, although this can be somewhat uncomfortable. Among the alternative techniques are humeral angulation osteotomy (which is rarely used), socket-suction suspension, and the newer elastomeric roll on locking liners. Many prosthetic options are available for the transhumeral amputee. One option is a prosthesis that is totally body-powered. Another is a hybrid prosthesis that uses myoelectric control of one component (either the terminal device or the elbow device) and body-powered control of the other. The transhumeral prosthesis is heavy, often considered slow, and requires much mental concentration to use effectively. These issues lead many unilateral transhumeral amputees to choose not to wear a prosthesis at all or to wear only a lightweight cosmetic prosthesis for special occasions.

Transhumeral amputation is sometimes elected to manage a dysfunctional arm following a severe brachial plexus injury. The advantages of amputation are that it unloads the weight from the shoulder and scapulothoracic joints and eliminates the problem of having a paralyzed arm that gets in the way and hinders body function. The decision to undertake shoulder arthrodesis in combination with transhumeral amputation is controversial and should be made on an individualized basis. Investigators who compared two groups of patients with transhumeral amputation because of brachial plexus injury—one group without shoulder arthrodesis and one group with it—found a somewhat better return-to-work rate in the group without shoulder arthrodesis. Prosthetic expectations in these patients should be limited because prosthetic fitting adds weight to a dysfunctional shoulder girdle, often defeating one of the original goals of the amputation.

Shoulder Disarticulation & Scapulothoracic (Forequarter) Amputation

The performance of shoulder disarticulation (Figure 12–7) or scapulothoracic amputation (Figure 12–8) is rare. When either operation is performed, it is usually in cases of cancer or severe trauma. Either operation results in a loss of the normal shoulder contour and causes the patient difficulty because clothing does not fit well. If it is possible to save the humeral head, this can improve the contour of a shoulder disarticulation tremendously. The scapulothoracic amputation, usually performed for proximal tumors, removes the arm, scapula, and clavicle. Dissection often extends into the neck and into the thorax.

Elaborate myoelectric prostheses are available for patients but are expensive, heavy, and require intensive maintenance. Body-powered prostheses are also heavy, hard to suspend comfortably, and are difficult to use. Most patients request prosthetic help for improved cos-

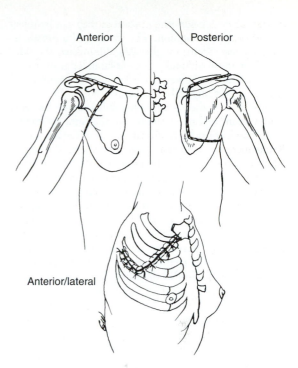

Figure 12–8. Forequarter amputation.

mesis and fitting of clothes. Often a simple soft mold to fill out the shoulder meets these expectations and is an alternative to a full-arm cosmetic prosthesis.

Postural Abnormalities After High Upper Extremity Amputation

Normally, the weight of the arm and the muscle activity associated with shoulder and arm function keep the shoulders appropriately level. Unilateral hypertrophy of an upper limb, including the shoulder girdle, occurs in certain occupations and is also seen in some sports. Some people are born with a degree of asymmetry of their shoulders. This is a relatively minor postural abnormality and does not require special clothing.

When the arm is removed and the clavicle and scapula remain, the muscles elevating the shoulder girdle are unopposed by both the weight of the arm and those muscles that pass across the shoulder and tend to depress the shoulder and arm. The consequence of this imbalance is an upward elevation described as "hiking" of the shoulder girdle. This "high shoulder" tends to accentuate the cosmetic loss, even when the individual is wearing a cosmetic shoulder filler or a cosmetic limb. Abnormal shoulder elevation can be countered by cor-

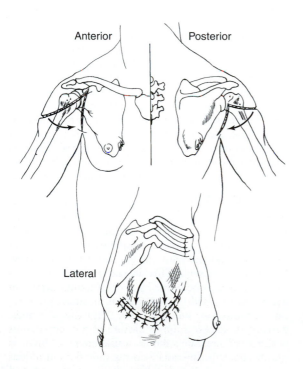

Figure 12–7. Shoulder disarticulation.

rective exercises beginning as soon as they can be tolerated after the amputation. The wearing of a prosthesis with its dependent weight also diminishes shoulder "hike." In most circumstances the shoulder girdle elevation is inevitable; however, its degree can be minimized by appropriate physical measures.

Removal of the entire upper limb in the growing skeleton can result in a scoliosis of the spine. Muscular imbalance is considered to be the cause of the deformity. It may be seen to a slighter degree in the adult but is primarily confined to the growing skeleton. The combined postural deformity of upper dorsal spine scoliosis and elevation of the shoulder girdle produces asymmetry of the head and neck on the trunk, with the head appearing to be placed asymmetrically as the person stands.

In general, no corrective splinting or orthotic device can successfully counteract the postural changes associated with shoulder-level amputation. Neck and shoulder-girdle exercises offer the most effective prophylaxis and treatment. The postural deficits are particularly evident with forequarter amputation. Soft, light polyurethane cosmetic restoration, either as part of a cosmetic prosthesis or separately used with the empty sleeve, will counter to some degree the unsightly upper body contour.

Hand Transplantation

Hand transplantation and the suppression of rejections is now technically possible. There have been approximately 10 documented cases of hand transplantation performed with varying degrees of success. The potential benefits for the amputee are certainly many, but must be balanced against the real risks. In general, skin, muscle and bone marrow appear to reject earlier and more aggressively than bone, cartilage or tendon. Preventing this rejection is a ongoing and lasting issue, with real consequences for the individual's health and life expectancy. The current immunosuppressive drugs needed to prevent rejection of a composite hand transplant include toxic side effects, opportunistic infections, and increase in malignancies.

Also, real psychologic impact following hand and other organ transplantation exists, and should not be underestimated. One study examining the issues 5 years following heart transplant showed a significant increase in emotional issues such as irritability, depression, and low self-esteem. Even for a patient with no pre-existing psychologic issues, living with a hand transplantation, which remains constantly in view, may not be easy.

Garst RJ: The Krukenberg hand. J Bone Joint Surg Br 1991;73: 385. [PMID: 1670433]

Goel A et al: Replantation and amputation of digits: User analysis. Am J Phys Med Rehabil 1995;74(2):134. [PMID: 7710728]

Hatrick NC, Tonkin MA: Hand transplantation: A current perspective. ANZ J Surg. 2001;71(4):245. [PMID: 11354126]

Martin C, Gonzalez del Pino J: Controversies in the treatment of fingertip amputations. Conservative versus surgical reconstruction. Clin Orthop 1998;(353):63. [PMID: 9728160]

Neusel E et al: Results of humeral stump angulation osteotomy. Arch Orthop Trauma Surg 1997;116:263. [PMID: 9177800]

Peimer CA et al: Hand function following single ray amputation. J Hand Surg [Am] 1999;24(6):1245. [PMID: 10584948]

Wilkinson MC et al: Brachial plexus injury: When to amputate? Injury. 1993;24(9):603. [PMID: 8288380]

Wright TW et al: Prosthetic usage in major upper extremity amputations. J Hand Surg [Am] 1995;20(4):619. [PMID: 7594289]

LOWER EXTREMITY AMPUTATIONS & DISARTICULATIONS

Foot Amputation

A. TOE AMPUTATION

Toe amputations can be performed with side-to-side or plantar-to-dorsal flaps to use the best available soft tissue. The bone should be shortened to a level that allows adequate soft-tissue closure without tension.

In great toe amputations, if the entire proximal phalanx is removed, the sesamoids can retract and expose the keel-shaped plantar surface of the first metatarsal to weight bearing. This often leads to high local pressure, callous formation, or ulceration. The sesamoids can be stabilized in position for weight bearing by leaving the base of the proximal phalanx intact or by performing tenodesis of the flexor hallucis brevis tendon.

An isolated amputation of the second toe commonly results in severe hallux valgus deformity of first toe (Figure 12–9). This may be prevented by amputation of the second ray or by fusion of the first metatarsal and phalanx. In the shorter toe amputations at the metatarsophalangeal joint level, transferring the extensor tendon to the capsule may help elevate the metatarsal head and maintain an even distribution for weight bearing. Prosthetic replacement is not required after toe amputations.

B. RAY AMPUTATION

A ray amputation removes the toe and all or some of the corresponding metatarsal. Isolated ray amputations can be durable. Multiple ray amputations, however, especially in patients with vascular disease, can narrow the foot excessively. This increases the amount of weight that must be borne by the remaining metatarsal heads and can lead to new areas of increased pressure, callous formation, and ulceration. Surgically, it is often difficult to achieve primary closure of ray amputation wounds because more skin is usually required than is readily apparent. Instead of closing these wounds under tension, it is usually advisable to leave them open and allow for secondary healing.

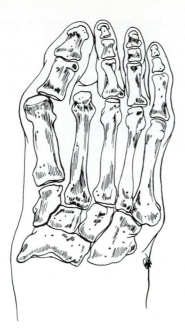

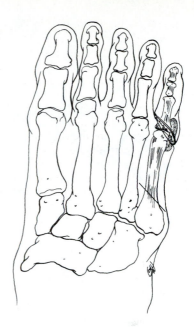

Figure 12–9. Severe hallux valgus deformity occurring after isolated second toe amputation.

Figure 12–10. Fifth ray amputation for fifth metatarsal head ulcer.

The fifth ray amputation has been the most useful of all the ray amputations. Plantar and lateral ulcers around the fifth metatarsal head often lead to exposed bone and osteomyelitis. A fifth ray amputation allows the entire ulcer to be excised and the wound to be closed primarily (Figure 12–10). In general, for more extensive involvement of the foot, a transverse amputation at the transmetatarsal level will be more durable. Prosthetic requirements after ray amputations include extra-depth shoes with custom-molded insoles. The insole should include a metatarsal pad that loads the shafts of the metatarsal and unloads some of the pressure at the metatarsal heads.

C. Midfoot Amputation

The transmetatarsal and Lisfranc amputations are reliable and durable. The Lisfranc amputation is actually a disarticulation just proximal to the metatarsals where the cuneiform and cuboid bones are retained. Surgically, a healthy, durable soft-tissue envelope is more important than a specific anatomic level of amputation, so the length of bone to be removed should be based on the ability to perform soft-tissue closure without tension. A long plantar flap is preferable, but equal dorsal and plantar flaps work well, especially for transmetatarsal amputation in the treatment of metatarsal head ulcers (Figure 12–11).

Muscle balance around the foot should be carefully evaluated preoperatively, with specific attention to tightness of the heel cord and strength of the anterior tibial, posterior tibial, and peroneal muscles. Midfoot amputations significantly shorten the lever arm of the foot, so lengthening of the Achilles tendon should be done if necessary. Tibial or peroneal muscle insertions should be reattached if they are released during bone resection. For example, if the base of the fifth metatarsal is resected, the peroneus brevis tendon should be reinserted into the cuboid bone. In patients with vascular disease, this can be performed with a minimal amount of dissection to prevent further compromise of the tissues.

Postoperative casting prevents deformities, controls edema, and speeds rehabilitation. Prosthetic requirements can vary widely. During the first year following amputation, many patients benefit from the use of an ankle-foot orthosis with a long footplate and a toe filler. To prevent an equinus deformity from developing, patients should be advised to wear the orthosis except when taking a bath or shower. Later, the use of a simple toe filler combined with a stiff-soled shoe may be adequate. Cosmetic partial foot prostheses are also available.

D. Hindfoot Amputation

A Chopart amputation removes the forefoot and midfoot and saves only the talus and calcaneus. Rebalancing procedures are required to prevent equinus and

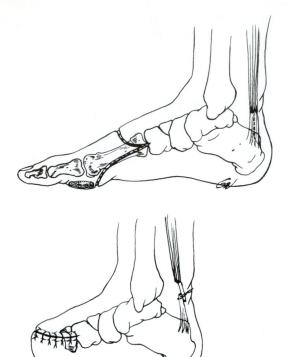

Figure 12–11. Transmetatarsal amputation with Achilles tendon lengthening.

varus deformities. Achilles tenotomy, transfer of the anterior tibial or extensor digitorum tendons, and postoperative casting are all usually necessary. Although tendon transfer to the talus has previously been recommended, transfer to the calcaneus is now done to minimize varus positioning. Beveling the inferior, anterior surface of the calcaneus can remove a potential bone pressure point.

Two other types of hindfoot amputations are the Boyd and the Pirogoff amputations. The Boyd procedure consists of a talectomy and calcaneal-tibial arthrodesis after forward translation of the calcaneus. The Pirogoff procedure consists of a talectomy with calcaneal-tibial arthrodesis after the vertical transection of the calcaneus through the midbody and a forward rotation of the posterior process of the calcaneus under the tibia. These two types of hindfoot amputations are done mostly in children to preserve length and growth centers, prevent heel pad migration, and improve socket suspension.

Studies in which various procedures in children have been compared showed that a hindfoot amputation results in better function than does a Syme's amputation (see section on Syme's amputation) in cases in which

the hindfoot is balanced and no equinus deformity has developed.

The hindfoot prosthesis requires more secure stabilization than a midfoot prosthesis to keep the heel from pistoning during gait. An anterior shell can be added to an ankle-foot prosthesis, or a posterior opening socket prosthesis can be used.

E. PARTIAL CALCANECTOMY

Partial calcanectomy, which consists of excising the posterior process of the calcaneus (Figure 12–12), should be considered an amputation of the back of the foot. In selected patients with large heel ulcerations or calcaneal osteomyelitis, partial calcanectomy can be a functional alternative to transtibial amputation. The removal of the entire posterior process of the calcaneus allows for fairly large soft-tissue defects to be closed primarily. Patients must have adequate vascular perfusion and nutritional competence for wound healing to occur. As with other amputations, partial calcanectomy creates a functional and cosmetic deformity. Use of an ankle-foot prosthesis with a cushion heel is usually required to replace the missing heel and prevent further skin ulceration.

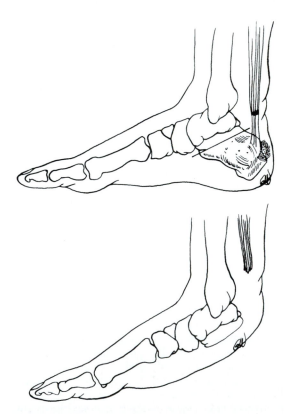

Figure 12–12. Partial calcanectomy.

Syme's Amputation

In Syme's amputation, the surgeon removes the calcaneus and talus while carefully dissecting on bone to preserve the heel skin and fat pad to cover the distal tibia (Figure 12–13). The surgeon must also remove and contour the malleoli, but there is controversy about whether this should be done during the initial operation or 6–8 weeks later. Proponents of the two-stage procedure argue that it can improve healing in patients with vascular disease. Opponents point out that it delays rehabilitation because the patient cannot bear weight until after the second stage of operation. A recent series supports the use of the one-stage procedure, even in the presence of vascular disease or diabetes. A late complication of Syme's amputation is the posterior and medial migration of the fat pad. One of the following surgical procedures can be done to stabilize the fat pad: tenodesis of the Achilles tendon to the posterior margin of the tibia through drill holes; transfer of the anterior tibial and extensor digitorum tendons to the anterior aspect of the fat pad; or removal of the cartilage and subchondral bone to allow scarring of the fat pad to bone, with or without pin fixation. Careful postoperative casting can also help keep the fat pad centered

under the tibia during healing. Syme's amputation is one of the most difficult amputations to perform in terms of surgical technique and achievement of primary healing and heel pad stability.

Syme's amputation should be designed to allow end-bearing. Retaining the smooth, broad surface of the distal tibia and the heel pad allows direct transfer of weight from the end of the residual limb to the prosthesis. A transtibial or transfemoral amputation does not allow this direct transfer of weight. Because of the ability to end-bear, the amputee can occasionally ambulate without a prosthesis in emergency situations or for bathroom activities.

Syme's prosthesis is wider at the ankle level than is a transtibial prosthesis, and this cosmetic problem can be bothersome to some patients. The surgical narrowing of the malleolar flare and the use of new materials in the prosthesis, however, can improve the appearance of the final prosthesis. Moreover, patients can now benefit from energy-storing technology provided by the newly designed lower profile elastic response feet. Sockets do not need the high contour of a patellar-tendon bearing design because of the end-bearing quality of the residual limb. The socket can be windowed either posteriorly or medially if the limb is bulbous, or a flexible socket within a rigid frame design can be used if the limb is less bulbous. Because of the tibial flare, the socket used following Syme's amputation is usually self-suspending.

Transtibial Amputation

Transtibial amputation is the most commonly performed major limb amputation. The long posterior flap technique (Figure 12–14) has become standard, and good results can be expected even in the majority of patients with vascular disease. Anterior and posterior flaps, sagittal flaps, and skewed flaps have been used and can be helpful in specific patients.

Efforts should be made to preserve as much bone length as possible between the tibial tubercle and the junction of the middle and distal thirds of the tibia, based on the available healthy soft tissues. Amputations in the distal third of the tibia should be avoided because they result in poor soft-tissue padding and are more difficult to comfortably fit with a prosthesis. The goal is a cylindrically shaped residual limb with muscle stabilization, distal tibial padding, and a nontender and nonadherent scar (Figure 12–15). The transtibial amputation is especially well suited to rigid dressings and immediate postoperative prosthetic management.

Distal tibiofibular synostosis (Ertl procedure) should be considered for the treatment of a wide trauma-induced diastasis to improve stabilization of the bone and soft tissue. The procedure is less often indicated in

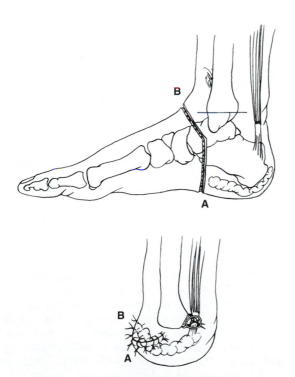

Figure 12–13. Syme's amputation with tenodesis of the Achilles tendon to the distal tibia.

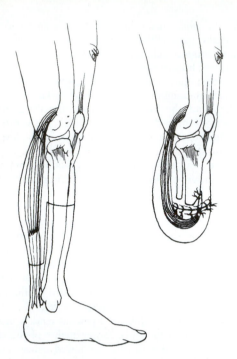

Figure 12–14. Transtibial amputation with long posterior flap technique.

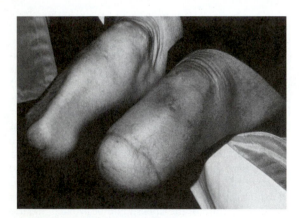

Figure 12–15. Bilateral transtibial amputations that emphasize the benefits of the long posterior flap technique. The right limb, amputated by using equal anterior and posterior flaps, is conically shaped and atrophic. The left limb, amputated by using the long posterior flap technique, is cylindrical and well padded. (Reproduced, with permission, from Smith DG et al: Fitting and Training the Bilateral Lower-Limb Amputee, *Atlas of Amputations and Prosthetics,* American Academy of Orthopaedic Surgeons, In press.)

the treatment of patients with vascular disease. The synostosis is developed to create a broad bone mass terminally to improve the distal end-bearing property of the limb and minimize motion between the tibia and fibula. Although there is renewed interest in these techniques, true comparison of patients with osteomyoplastic techniques versus standard techniques has not been done.

A wide variety of prosthetic designs are available for the transtibial amputee. Sockets can be designed to incorporate a liner, which offers the advantages of increased comfort and accommodation of minor changes in residual limb volume. Disadvantages include increased perspiration and a less sanitary, less comfortable feeling in hot humid weather. Hard sockets are designed to have cotton or wool stump socks of an appropriate ply or thickness as the interface between the leg and the socket. Hard sockets are easier to clean and are more durable than the liners are.

The Icelandic-Sweden-New York (ISNY) socket refers to the use of a more flexible socket material that is supported by a rigid frame. The flexible socket changes shape to accommodate underlying muscle contraction. This socket style can also be useful for limbs that are scarred or difficult to fit. Open-ended sockets with side joints and a thigh corset are not used much today except by patients who have worn them successfully in the past and by patients with limited access to prosthetic care. The patellar tendon-bearing shape is most commonly used for the transtibial amputee. In spite of its name, the majority of the weight is borne on the medial tibial flare and laterally on the interosseus space, whereas the rest of the weight is borne on the patellar tendon area. Even the new "total contact" transtibial socket, which is designed to have increased contact on all areas of the residual limb, preferentially loads the tibial flare and patellar tendon regions.

Numerous types of suspension devices are available for the transtibial prosthesis. The simplest and most common is a suprapatellar strap, which wraps above the femoral condyles and patella. Sockets can be designed to incorporate a supracondylar mold or wedge to grip above the femoral condyles, but this higher profile is bulkier and less cosmetic when the patient is sitting. A waist belt and fork strap are helpful for the patient who has a very short transtibial residual limb because these devices decrease pistoning in the socket; they are also helpful for the patient whose activities require extremely secure suspension. If the patient has a limb with poor soft tissue or has intrinsic knee pain, side hinges and a thigh corset can help unload the lower leg and transfer some of the weight to the thigh.

External suspension sleeves made of latex or neoprene are still used quite frequently . Latex is more cosmetic but less durable and can be constricting. Neoprene is more durable and not as constricting but sometimes causes contact dermatitis. The newest suspension uses an elastomeric or silicone-based liner that is rolled on over the residual leg and offers an intimate friction fit. A small metal post on the distal end of the liner then locks into a catch in the prosthetic socket to securely suspend the socket to the liner. Many patients who use these elastomeric locking liners like the secure suspension and feeling of improved control of the prosthesis. The liners have the disadvantages of being less durable and requiring frequent replacement. These elastomeric locking liners can be expensive. Although elastomeric locking liners were originally touted as preventing skin problems; rashes, skin irritation, and skin breakdown remain a frequent complaint even with this new technology. A recent presentation suggests that many amputees might actually walk less in these new liners than in a traditional system.

Many different designs for prosthetic feet are now available, ranging from the original solid ankle cushion heel (SACH) foot to the newer elastic response technology with a variety of keel, ankle, and pylon designs. Cost and function can vary widely, and care should be used in prescribing an appropriate prosthetic foot for an individual patient. A common error is to prescribe a foot that is either too stiff, or does not get to feel flat quickly enough for an individual patient, especially in the first 12–18 months after an amputation.

Knee Disarticulation

Disarticulation through the knee joint (Figure 12–16) is indicated in ambulatory patients when a below-knee amputation is not possible but suitable soft tissue is present for a knee disarticulation. These circumstances are most commonly found in cases involving traumatic injuries. In patients with vascular disease, the blood supply is such that if a knee disarticulation would heal, a short transtibial amputation would usually heal as well. The knee disarticulation is indicated in patients who have vascular problems and are nonambulatory, especially if knee flexion contractures or spasticity are present. Although sagittal flaps or the traditional long posterior flap can be used to take advantage of the best available soft-tissue coverage, recent literature supports use of the posterior flap technique when possible. The patella is retained and the patellar tendon sutured to the cruciate stumps to stabilize the quadriceps muscle complex. The biceps tendons can also be stabilized to the patellar tendon. A short section of gastrocnemius muscle can be sutured to the anterior capsule to pad the distal end. Although many techniques have been described to trim the condyles of the femur, trimming is rarely necessary and radical trimming can decrease some of the advantages of the knee disarticulation.

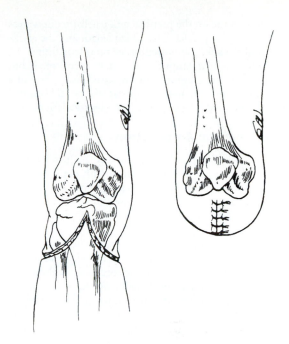

Figure 12–16. Knee disarticulation.

For ambulatory patients, the advantages that a knee disarticulation has over a transfemoral amputation include improved socket suspension by contouring above the femoral condyles, the added strength of a longer lever arm, the retained muscle balance of the thigh, and, most important, the end-bearing potential to directly transfer weight to the prosthesis. In the past, the objections to a bulky prosthesis and asymmetric knee-joint level led many surgeons to abandon the practice of performing knee disarticulations. New materials allow a less bulky prosthesis to be fabricated, and the four-bar linkage knee unit, which can fold under the socket, improves the appearance of the prosthesis when the patient is sitting. The four-bar linkage knee remains the prosthetic knee of choice for a knee disarticulation. It is low profile, has excellent stability, and can incorporate a hydraulic unit for control during the swing phase of gait in patients who can walk at different cadences.

For nonambulatory patients, a knee disarticulation will eliminate the problem of knee flexion contractures, provides a balanced thigh to decrease hip contractures, and provides a long lever arm for good sitting support and transfers.

The Gritti-Stokes amputation is not recommended. In this operation, the patella is advanced distally and fused by arthrodesis to the distal femur to theoretically allow direct weight bearing. The concept behind this operation is flawed because even in normal kneeling, the weight is borne on the pretibial and patellar tendon areas and not on the patella. The added length and the asymmetry of the knee joints complicate prosthetic fitting.

Transcondylar amputation can be performed, but the end-bearing comfort and improved suspension of a transcondylar amputation appear to be diminished when compared with the true knee disarticulation.

Transfemoral Amputation

Transfemoral amputation is usually performed with equal anterior and posterior fish-mouth flaps. Atypical flaps can and should be used to save all possible femoral length in cases of trauma because the amount of function is directly proportional to the length of the residual limb.

Muscle stabilization is more important in the transfemoral amputation than in any other major limb amputation. The major deforming force is into abduction and flexion. Myodesis of the adductor muscles through drill holes in the femur can counteract the abductors, prevent a difficult adductor tissue roll in the groin, and improve prosthetic control (Figure 12–17). Without muscle stabilization, the femur commonly migrates lat-

erally through the soft-tissue envelope to a subcutaneous location. Newer transfemoral socket designs attempt to better control the position of the femur, but they are not as effective as muscle stabilization. Even in nonambulatory patients, muscle stabilization is helpful in creating a more durable, padded residual limb by preventing migration of the femur.

An IPOP and rigid dressings are more difficult to apply and keep positioned after a transfemoral amputation than after more distal amputations. IPOP techniques do offer the advantages of early rehabilitation and control of edema and pain, and these techniques are preferred if the expertise to use them is available. The major complaints of patients with the transfemoral IPOP are the weight of the cast and the discomfort when sitting with this system. In many cases, only a soft compressive dressing alone is used, and in these patients, the dressing should be carried proximally around the waist as a spica to better suspend the dressing and to include the medial thigh to prevent the development of an adductor roll of tissue. Proper postoperative positioning and therapy are essential to prevent hip flexion contractures. The limb should be positioned flat on the bed, rather than elevated on a pillow, and hip extension exercises and prone positioning should be started early.

Suspension of the prosthesis is more complicated in transfemoral amputations than in more distal amputations because of the short residual limb, the lack of bony contours, and the increased weight of the prosthesis. The transfemoral amputation prosthesis can be suspended by suction, Silesian bandage, hip-joint and pelvic band, or by the newer elastomeric locking liners.

Traditional socket-suction suspension works when the skin forms an airtight seal against the socket. Air is forced distally through a small one-way valve when the prosthesis is donned and with each step during gait, thus maintaining negative pressure distally in the socket. No prosthetic sock or other liner is used between the hard socket and the limb because air leaks out around the sock and prevents suction from developing. Donning a socket-suction prosthesis requires skill and exertion, and patients must have good coordination, upper extremity function, and balance to perform this task. Socket-suction systems works well for average-to-long transfemoral residual limbs that have adequate soft tissues and stable shape and volume. It is usually comfortable and is the most cosmetically acceptable method of socket suspension.

A Silesian bandage is a flexible strap that attaches laterally to the prosthesis, wraps back around the waist and over the contralateral iliac crest, and then comes forward to attach to the anterior proximal socket (Figure 12–18). It provides good suspension and added rotational control of the prosthesis. A Silesian bandage is commonly used to augment suction suspension for pa-

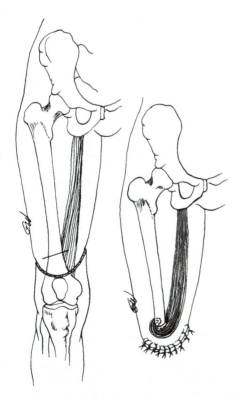

Figure 12–17. Transfemoral amputation with adductor myodesis.

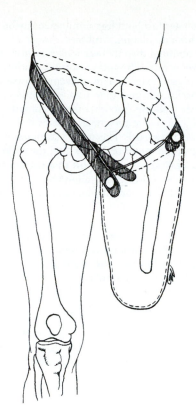

Figure 12-18. Silesian band suspension of a transfemoral prosthesis.

tients who have shorter-length limbs or for patients whose activities require more secure suspension than suction alone can offer.

As with the transtibial prosthesis, the newer elastomeric locking liners can provide excellent suspension and control. An elastomeric or silicone-based liner is rolled onto the leg similar to the manner in which a condom is applied. This liner has an intimate fit with the residual limb and avoids "pistoning" and rotational forces. A small metal post at the distal end of the liner locks down into a catch at the bottom of the prosthetic socket to create a secure mechanical suspension. A small button must be pushed to disengage the lock and release the prosthesis. Many amputees have expressed an improved sense of security and improved proprioception with these systems. The disadvantages continue to be the added cost, the need to replace the liners as they tear, and rarely, developing a contact dermatitis.

The hip joint and pelvic band provides extremely secure suspension and control, but the band is bulky, is the least cosmetically acceptable method of suspension, and is the least comfortable, especially when the patient

is sitting. The pelvic band is made of metal or plastic and is thicker than a Silesian bandage. The pelvic band runs from the hip hinge, around the waist, between the contralateral iliac crest and trochanter, and back to the hip hinge. The hinge is located laterally, just anterior to the trochanter, over the anatomic axis of the hip joint. Hip joint and pelvic band suspension is indicated for very short transfemoral limbs, geriatric patients who cannot don a suction suspension, and obese patients who cannot get adequate control with suction, silicone suspension sleeves, or Silesian band suspension.

Socket design for the transfemoral amputation has undergone recent changes. The traditional quadrilateral socket has a narrow anteroposterior diameter to keep the ischium positioned back and up on top of the posterior brim of the socket for weight bearing. The anterior wall of the socket is 5–7 cm higher than the posterior wall to hold the leg back on the ischial seat. Anterior pain is a frequent complaint and should be addressed by modification of the prosthetic socket in a small local area such as over the anterior superior iliac spine. If the entire anterior wall is lowered or relieved, the ischium will slip inside the socket and totally alter the load transfer and pressure areas. Even though the lateral wall is contoured to hold the femur in adduction, the overall dimensions of the quadrilateral socket are not anatomic and provide poor femoral stability in the coronal plane.

Narrow mediolateral transfemoral socket designs attempt to solve the problems of a traditional quadrilateral socket by contouring the posterior wall to set the ischium down inside the socket, not up on the brim. Weight is transferred through the gluteal muscle mass and lateral thigh instead of the ischium. This eliminates the need for anterior pressure from a high anterior wall. Attention is then focused on a narrow mediolateral contour to better hold the femur in adduction and minimize the relative motion between the limb and the socket. The normal shape and normal alignment (NSNA) socket and the contoured adducted trochanteric-controlled alignment method (CAT-CAM) socket are two of the narrow mediolateral designs available.

A socket made of flexible material with a rigid frame can also be used. The flexible material allows socket wall expansion with underlying muscle contraction. A flexible socket can be made in either the traditional quadrilateral or narrow mediolateral shapes. Advantages of this type of socket include improved comfort in walking and sitting and possibly improved muscular efficiency. One drawback is that the flexible material is less durable, and cracks can result in the loss of suction suspension and skin irritation.

Prosthetic knee joints are available in many designs to address specific patient needs. The traditional standard has been the single-axis constant-friction knee. The constant-friction knee is simple, durable, lightweight, and inexpensive. The friction can be set at only one level to optimize function at one cadence, and patients have difficulty when walking at different speeds.

Outside hinges were the old standard for the knee disarticulation patient, to better approximate the center of motion of the knee. Outside hinges are cosmetically poor but are still available for patients who have used them successfully in the past and remain satisfied with them. For new patients, other types of knee units are used.

The term *safety knee* has been replaced with the term *stance control knee*. It refers to a knee unit that has weight-activated friction to increase stability and resistance to buckling as more of the amputee's body weight is applied. This unit is particularly useful for patients who are older, feel less secure, have a very short residual limb, weak hip extensors, or hip flexion contractures.

A polycentric knee provides a changing center of rotation that is located more posterior than other knee joints. The posterior center of rotation offers more stability during stance and the first few degrees of flexion than other knee units do. The four-bar knee is one of many polycentric knee units available.

A hydraulic or pneumatic unit can be added to most knee joints to provide superior control of the prosthesis in swing phase by using fluid hydraulics to vary the resistance according to the speed of gait. This option is useful in active amputees who walk and run at different speeds.

The variable-friction knee unit can be a less expensive way to accommodate patients who walk at different speeds. This knee changes the friction according to the degree of flexion in the knee unit, and leads to an improvement in the swing phase of walking. Although a variable-friction knee is less costly and requires less maintenance than a hydraulic unit, it is not as effective in allowing the amputee to walk at different cadences.

A manual locking option can also be added to most knee units to lock the knee in full extension. Locking is helpful if the patient is blind, feels less secure, has a very short residual limb, or is a bilateral amputee.

As mentioned previously, microprocessor-controlled, "intelligent" knee units incorporate the latest technology to provide superior control of the swing and stance characteristics or the knee and respond to the amputees speed, cadence, and accelerations. Technology has not yet advanced enough for knee units to replace the tremendous motor power lost when an amputation is done above the knee.

The use of specifically designed prostheses known as **stubbies** are initially recommended for bilateral knee disarticulation or transfemoral amputees, regardless of age, who have lost both legs simultaneously but are candidates for ambulation. Stubbies consist of prosthetic sockets mounted directly over rocker-bottom platforms that serve as feet. The rocker-bottom platforms have a long posterior extension to prevent the patient from falling backward, and they have a shortened anterior process that allows smooth rollover into the push-off phase of gait. These prostheses look as if the foot were positioned backward. The use of stubbies results in a lowering of the center of gravity, and the rocker bottom provides a broad base of support that teaches trunk balance, provides stability, and allows the patient to build confidence during standing and ambulation. As the patient's confidence and skills improve, periodic lengthening of the stubbies is permitted until the height becomes nearly compatible with full-length prostheses, at which time the transition is attempted. Many patients reject full-length prostheses and prefer the stability and balance afforded by the stubbies.

Hip Disarticulation

Hip disarticulation (Figure 12–19) is rarely performed. Surgically, the traditional racket-shaped incision with an anterior apex is used in patients with vascular prob-

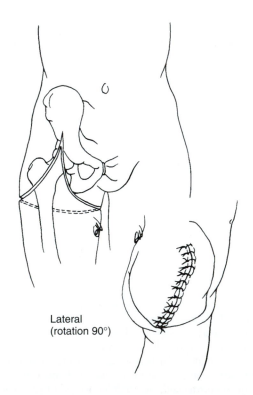

Lateral
(rotation 90°)

Figure 12-19. Hip disarticulation.

lems and in trauma-injured patients when possible. In tumor surgery, creative flaps based on the uninvolved anatomic compartments must be designed.

Prosthetic replacement can be successful in healthy young patients who required hip disarticulation because of trauma or cancer but is generally not indicated for patients with vascular disease. The standard prosthesis is the Canadian hip disarticulation prosthesis. The socket contains the involved hemipelvis and suspends over the iliac crests. Although the hip joint and other endoskeletal components are made of lightweight materials in an effort to keep the weight to a minimum, the prosthesis is still heavy and difficult to manipulate. Ambulation with the prosthesis usually requires more energy than it would take to ambulate with crutches and a swing-through gait. For this reason, many ambulatory patients will use crutches and no prosthesis. The advantage of the prosthesis is that it does allow freer use of the upper extremities.

Hemipelvectomy

Although a hemipelvectomy (Figure 12–20) is even less frequently required than a hip disarticulation, it is sometimes indicated for trauma injuries or cancer in-

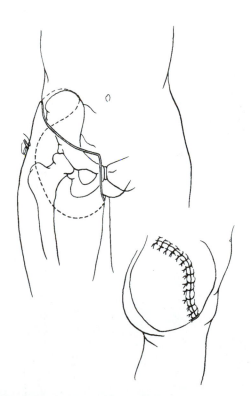

Figure 12-20. Hemipelvectomy.

volving the pelvis. Use of a prosthesis after this procedure is extremely rare because the body weight must be transferred onto the sacrum and thorax. Special considerations for seating are usually required after hemipelvectomy.

Prosthetic Prescription Following Amputation at or Above the Knee

To be considered a candidate for a high anatomic level prosthesis (knee disarticulation and higher), a patient must be able to transfer independently, rise from sitting to standing independently, and ambulate using one leg and a swing-through gait over a distance of 100 ft on the parallel bars or with a walker. Although these requirements seem extreme, they are necessary for the successful use of this heavy and complicated prosthesis. The use of a transtibial prosthesis can make it easier to transfer and to ambulate. But, a current transfemoral prosthesis can make it much more difficult to rise from sitting to standing because the powerful motor force required to extend the knee is not present. High-level prosthetic devices can actually increase the energy required for walking compared with one-leg swing-through gait. Unfortunately, without the ability to meet the activity demands unassisted, a prosthesis will act as an anchor to decrease overall independence. We use these same activity requirements as a functional test before prescribing a prosthesis for all transfemoral, hip disarticulation, and hemipelvectomy amputees.

Percutaneous Direct Skeletal Attachment of Artificial Limbs

The benefits of attaching prosthetic limbs through the skin, directly to the skeleton has been envisioned for nearly a hundred years. Documentation of temporary external fixation for fractures dates to Malgaigne in 1845. During and just after World War II independent attempts were made in Germany and the United States to directly attach a transtibial prosthesis to the tibia. Four humans were fit in May of 1946 by Drummer, a general surgeon in Pinneberg, Germany. The two major hurdles continue to be the bone-implant interface, and the skin-implant interface. Breakthrough work by PI Branemark in Gothenburg, Sweden, advance the use of titanium and improved design implants that have lead to over 30 years of successful dental and maxillofacial reconstruction with prosthetic devices directly connected to the bone of the mouth and face.

The skin of the extremities has posed a larger challenge to the cutaneous-implant interface. Recent improvement in implant design and surgical technique, however, have made it possible to successfully implant and fit thumb, forearm, and transfemoral amputees. Amputees have undergone surgical implantation and prosthetic fitting in Sweden, the United Kingdom, and Australia.

The early results confirm the potential promise of major improvements in attachment, proprioception, and function of osseointegrated prosthetic limbs compared with socket-style prostheses. Much work remains to be accomplished, however, especially in the skin-implant interface. A tremendous improvement in the bone-implant interface has lead to results that far outdistance historical attempts at directly attaching artificial limbs to the skeleton. Without true cutaneous-implant integration that provides a durable and biologic barrier, however, the risk of bacterial migration causing infection and loosening will continue. It is fantastic to see this dream continue and advance.

Bowker JH, Michael JW: *Atlas of Limb Prosthetics: Surgical, Prosthetic, and Rehabilitation Principles,* 2nd ed. St. Louis: Mosby, 1992.

Bowker JH et al: North American experience with knee disarticulation with use of a posterior myofasciocutaneous flap. Healing rate and functional results in seventy-seven patients. J Bone Joint Surg Am 2000;82-A(11):1571. [PMID: 11097446]

Branemark R et al: Osseointegration in skeletal reconstruction and rehabilitation: A review. J Rehabil Res Dev 2001;38(2):175. Review. No abstract available. [PMID: 11392650]

Gaine WJ, McCreath SW: Syme's amputation revisited: A review of 46 cases. J Bone Joint Surg Br 1996;78:461.

Gottschalk F et al: Does socket configuration influence the position of the femur in above-knee amputation? J Prosthet Orthot 1989;2:94.

Pinzur MS, Bowker JH, Smith DG, Gottschalk F: Amputation surgery in peripheral vascular disease. Instr Course Lect. 1999;48:687-91. [PMID: 10098097]

Unruh T et al: Hip disarticulation: An eleven-year experience. Arch Surg 1990;125:791.

Rehabilitation

13

Mary Ann E. Keenan, MD, & Robert L. Waters, MD

GENERAL PRINCIPLES OF REHABILITATION

In the past, rehabilitation was regarded as aftercare. Today, however, rehabilitation is recognized as an important part of the acute care program. Physicians, therapists, and other health care workers in the field of orthopedics are involved in rehabilitation programs for a variety of patients, including those with congenital or acquired musculoskeletal problems (eg, bone deformities, arthritis, or fractures) as well as those with neurologic trauma or diseases that affect limb function (eg, spinal cord injury, stroke, or poliomyelitis). Rehabilitation in these patients frequently involves correcting limb deformities, increasing muscle strength, maximizing motor control, training individuals to make the most effective use of residual function, and providing adaptive equipment.

The most successful model for rehabilitation addresses the physical, emotional, and other needs of the patient and is based on a team approach. Among those frequently included in the team are physicians and nurses from various medical specialties, physical and occupational therapists, speech therapists, psychologists, orthotists, and social workers as well as the patient and members of the patient's family. The shared goal of team members is to prevent barriers to rehabilitation by (1) accurately diagnosing all current problems in the patient, (2) adequately treating the problems, (3) establishing adequate nutrition, (4) monitoring the patient for any complications that might impede progress in recovery, (5) mobilizing the patient as soon as possible, and (6) restoring function or helping the patient adjust to an altered life-style.

Management of Common Problems in Rehabilitation

Inadequate nutrition, decubitus ulcers, urinary tract infections, impaired bladder control, spasticity, contractures, acquired musculoskeletal deformities, muscle weakness, and physiologic deconditioning are common complications that can obstruct rehabilitation efforts obstruct rehabilitation efforts and cause further loss of function in an already compromised patient. Because these problems are costly in both human and financial terms, every effort should be made to prevent them.

A. INADEQUATE NUTRITION

Good nutritional status is the basis for avoiding many of the previously listed complications. In trauma patients, the nutritional requirements are markedly increased from the normal maintenance requirement of 30 kcal/kg/d. Most trauma patients have been receiving intravenous fluids with minimal nutritional benefit and so arrive at the rehabilitation center in various degrees of malnutrition. Patients with chronic illnesses commonly have poor appetites. Physically handicapped people expend much of their energy performing simple activities of daily living and may also have difficulty in obtaining and preparing adequate amounts of food. Yet another form of poor nutrition that should be noted is obesity. Inactivity leads to diminished calorie need, but boredom may result in increased consumption.

B. DECUBITUS ULCERS (PRESSURE SORES)

The combination of poor nutritional status, lack of sensation at pressure points of the body, and decreased ability to move can cause decubitus ulcers (Figure 13–1) and will greatly add to the length and cost of the patient's hospital stay. The ulcer is a potential source of sepsis in an already compromised individual and often requires that a flap graft be rotated to cover the defect. After a sacral flap has been rotated, the patient must remain in a prone position until the graft has healed. This will significantly hamper the patient's participation in a rehabilitation program because mobility and ability to interact with others are hindered. Prevention is the best treatment. The clinical rule of protecting the patient's skin is to change position every 2 h. No cushion can completely prevent decubitus ulcers.

C. URINARY TRACT INFECTIONS AND IMPAIRED BLADDER CONTROL

Urinary tract infections are a common source of sepsis and prolonged illness. An indwelling catheter is the most frequent source of contamination. In an acutely ill or multiply injured patient, an indwelling catheter may be necessary for medical reasons but should be removed as soon as possible. Urinary incontinence is not sufficient reason for continued use of an indwelling catheter. In male patients, incontinence can be managed with a carefully applied condom catheter. Care must be taken to inspect the penis frequently for signs of skin

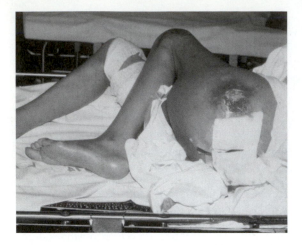

Figure 13–1. Patient with contractures and a decubitus ulcer over the greater trochanter of the femur.

maceration or pressure. In female patients, diapering and frequent linen changes are necessary.

Restoring bladder function to achieve adequate reflex voiding or a balanced bladder may require the use of an intermittent catheterization program. In a balanced bladder, the volume of residual urine should not exceed a third of the volume of voided urine. In general, an intermittent catheterization program is initiated if the residual volume is greater than 100 mL or if the voided volume exceeds 400 mL. The patient is catheterized every 4 h initially and then every 6 h for 24 h. After this, the patient is reassessed. Good records are necessary throughout the program.

D. MUSCLE WEAKNESS AND PHYSIOLOGIC DECONDITIONING

During sustained exercise, the metabolism is mainly aerobic. The principal fuels for aerobic metabolism are carbohydrates and fats. In aerobic oxidation, the substrates are oxidized through a series of enzymatic reactions that lead to the production of adenosine triphosphate (ATP) for muscular contraction. A physical conditioning program can increase the aerobic capacity by improving cardiac output, increasing hemoglobin levels, enhancing the capacity of cells to extract oxygen from the blood, and increasing the muscle mass by hypertrophy.

Prolonged immobilization of extremities, bed rest, and inactivity lead to pronounced muscle wasting and physiologic deconditioning in a short period of time. Because disabled patients generally expend more energy than normal individuals in performing the routine activities of daily living, it is important that they be mobilized as quickly as possible to prevent unnecessary phys-

iologic decline. They should also be placed on a daily exercise program to maximize muscle strength and aerobic capacity.

E. SPASTICITY

Patients with spasticity exhibit an excessive response to the quick stretch of a muscle. This leads to hyperactive deep tendon reflexes and clonus. Spasticity must be managed aggressively to prevent permanent deformities and joint contractures.

1. Spasmolytic drugs—Drugs can be of some assistance in controlling spasticity associated with upper motor neuron diseases. Drugs are used when spasticity affects multiple large muscle groups in the body and when the spasticity is not severe.

Baclofen (Lioresal) can inhibit both polysynaptic and monosynaptic reflexes at the spinal cord level. It does, however, depress general central nervous system function. Use of oral baclofen is avoided in traumatic brain-injured patients when possible, because it may cause sedation and impede cognitive recovery. Patients with attention deficits or memory disorders may be compromised by antispastic agents, such as baclofen, diazepam, and clonidine, that have sedating properties. The drug tizanidine (Zanaflex) has been reported to affect the central nervous system less than other agents and may be useful. Even a drug such as dantrolene sodium, which acts peripherally, may also cause drowsiness.

Baclofen pump technology has an advantage over oral drug therapy because of the small concentrations it introduces intrathecally. The small intrathecal doses control spasticity effectively while minimizing central side effects. The pump is placed in a subcutaneous pocket in the abdominal wall. A catheter is routed subcutaneously from the intrathecal space to the pump. The pump can be refilled by injection into the reservoir chamber. The dosage and rate of administration can be easily adjusted by using a laptop computer that sends radio signals to the pump.

Dantrolene (Dantrium) is another drug that can be used to control spasticity. Dantrolene is the drug of choice for treating clonus. Dantrolene produces relaxation by directly affecting the contractile response of skeletal muscle at a site beyond the myoneural junction. It causes dissociation of the excitation-contraction coupling probably by interfering with the release of calcium from the sarcoplasmic reticulum. Although it does not affect the central nervous system directly, it does cause drowsiness, dizziness, and generalized weakness, which may interfere with the patient's overall function. Use of dantrolene for the control of spasticity is indicated in upper motor neuron diseases, such as spinal cord injury, cerebral palsy, stroke, or multiple sclerosis. The most serious problem encountered with the use of dantrolene is hepatotoxicity. The risk appears greatest in females, in patients older than 35 years, and in patients taking other medications. When using dantrolene, the lowest effective dose should be used, and liver enzyme functions should be monitored closely. If no effect is noted after 45 days of use, the drug should be stopped.

2. Casts—Casting has been shown to temporarily reduce muscle tone and is frequently used to correct a contracture. The cast is changed weekly until the problem has been corrected. If a cast must be used for a prolonged period, the patient should be placed on anticoagulant therapy to prevent deep venous thrombosis.

3. Splints—Anterior and posterior clam-shell splints can be used to control joint position and still allow for active and passive range of motion of the joints in therapy. A splint applied to only one side of an extremity is not sufficient to control excessive spasticity and may result in skin breakdown from motion of the extremity against the splint. A splint can also obscure an early contracture.

4. Nerve-blocking agents—Anesthetic and phenol nerve blocks are often combined with a casting or splinting program.

Anesthetic nerve blocks are commonly used to temporarily eliminate muscle tone. They can be used diagnostically to evaluate what portion of a deformity is dynamic (occurring because of muscle spasticity) and what portion is secondary to myostatic contracture. The block can give an advanced indication of the likely results of surgical neurectomy or tendon lengthening. Repeated blocks of local anesthetics give a carryover effect to decrease muscle tone.

When muscle spasticity requires control for an extended period of time but the patient still has potential for spontaneous improvement, a phenol nerve block may be indicated. Phenol exerts two actions on the nerves. The first is a short-term effect, which is similar to the effect produced by a local anesthetic and is directly proportional to the thickness of the nerve fibers. The second is a long-term effect that results from protein denaturation. Although this leads to wallerian degeneration of the axons, experimental studies in animals have shown that the nerves will regenerate with time. In patients, the direct injection of a nerve with a 3–5% solution of phenol after surgical exposure gives relief of spasticity for up to 6 months. Mixed nerves containing sensory fibers should not be injected, because this could cause unwanted sensory loss or painful dysesthesia. Reduction of spasticity for up to 3 months can also be achieved by the percutaneous injection of muscle motor points with an aqueous solution of phenol after localization using a needle and nerve stimulator (Figure 13–2).

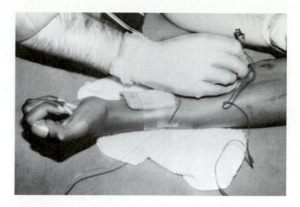

Figure 13–2. Use of a Teflon-coated needle and nerve stimulator to locate the motor points of spastic forearm muscles for phenol injection.

a. Botulinum toxin—Ordinarily, an action potential propagating down to a motor nerve to the neuromuscular junction triggers the release of acetylcholine (ACh) into the synaptic space. The released ACh causes depolarization of muscle membrane. Botulinum toxin type A is a protein produced by *Clostridium botulinum* that attaches to the presynaptic nerve terminal and inhibits the release of ACh at the neuromuscular junction. Botulinum toxin is injected directly into a spastic muscle. Clinical benefit lasts 3–5 months. Current practice is not to administer a total of more than 400 U in a single treatment session to avoid excessive weakness or paralysis. This upper limit of 400 U may be reached rather quickly when injecting a few large muscles. A delay of 3–7 days between injection of botulinum toxin A and the onset of clinical effect is typical. The patient will not see effects immediately, and usually a follow-up visit is arranged to check the result. Because botulinum toxin is the most potent biologic toxin known, and the cost is relatively high, the smallest possible dose should be used to achieve results.

5. Surgical procedures—If muscle spasticity is permanent and no change in muscle tone is anticipated, then definitive procedures such as dorsal rhizotomy, peripheral neurectomy, tendon lengthening or release, and tendon transfer should be considered.

F. Joint Contractures

Inactivity and uncontrolled spasticity often lead to joint contractures (Figure 13–3), which are difficult to correct and will greatly extend the needed rehabilitation program. Contractures may cause difficulties in positioning an individual in a bed or chair or problems in using orthotic devices. They can also cause difficulties with hygiene and skin care and increase the risk of de-

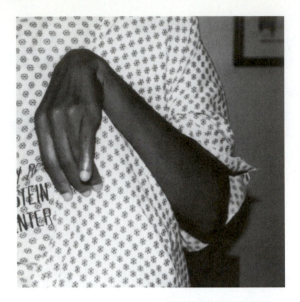

Figure 13–3. Upper extremity contractures in a patient with untreated spasticity.

cubitus ulcers. Shoe wear may be rendered impossible secondary to foot deformities.

Muscle weakness is accentuated by contractures and malalignment, which cause the muscle to function at a mechanical disadvantage. Sitting and standing balance are compromised when contractural deformities displace the location of the center of gravity relative to the base of support. Functional use of the extremities is severely limited by lack of adequate joint motion. Joint contractures may require surgical release, and this could further decrease function in an already compromised individual. Moreover, in children, joint contractures can lead to structural changes in the skeleton. Muscle growth lags behind skeletal growth, and this discrepancy in growth rates can cause increasing deformity with time.

To prevent contractures, exercises to maintain range of motion must be performed several times daily. The patient, family members, therapists, and nursing personnel should all participate in this task.

Splinting can help maintain joints in a functional position when motor control is lacking. Splints should be removed on a regular basis to inspect the skin condition and reassess their efficacy in maintaining the desired position.

Treatment of established contractures can be time-consuming and expensive. In general, if a contracture has been present for less than 3 months, it may be amenable to nonsurgical methods of correction such as serial casting or electrical stimulation of the antagonist muscles. Excessive muscle tone must be aggressively

treated if present because this will only accentuate the tendency to form contractures. An anesthetic nerve block can be given to temporarily eliminate excessive tone and provide analgesia prior to manipulation of the joint and application of a cast. Each week, the cast is removed, a nerve block is given, and a new cast is applied. When the desired limb position is obtained, a holding cast is used to maintain the position for an additional week. The cast can then be bivalved and made into anterior and posterior clam-shell splints, which can be removed for range-of-motion or other activities. Another useful technique is the application of a drop-out cast (Figure 13–4), which allows for further correction of the contracture while preventing the original deformity from recurring.

When contractural deformities are long-standing and fixed, surgical release is indicated. Tendons, ligaments, and joint capsules are all involved. If the deformity is severe, complete correction at the time of surgery may be impossible. Neurovascular structures must be protected from excessive traction. Serial casts or drop-out casts may be necessary following surgery to gain the desired limb position.

G. Other Acquired Musculoskeletal Deformities

Paralysis or weakness of trunk muscles can lead to scoliotic deformities of the spine. These deformities can impair respiratory function and tend to cause balance problems when the patient walks and sits. External support in the form of bracing or seating modifications can eliminate or minimize this tendency.

Disuse and lack of muscle tone lead to osteoporosis, which in turn predisposes patients to fractures. The fractures should be treated aggressively and in a manner that maximizes function rather than prolonging immobilization.

Peripheral nerve palsy can result from pressure secondary to decreased mobility in patients confined to a bed or chair. Pressure can also result from braces, splints, and casts, and these require careful monitoring. In those patients who form heterotopic ossification, the new bone formation and the accompanying inflamma-

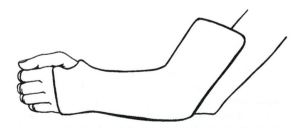

Figure 13–4. An elbow drop-out cast used to increase elbow extension while preventing flexion.

tion may impinge on peripheral nerves, thereby causing nerve palsy.

Evaluation of Impairment

A. NERVES

Many disabilities requiring rehabilitation result from diseases affecting the nervous system. The location and the extent of the primary lesion determine not only the degree of paralysis but also the extent to which motor control is impaired and spasticity is present. In injuries or diseases of the peripheral nerves, the damage is confined to the lower motor neurons. Normal motor control is preserved, spasticity is absent, and the magnitude of disability depends on the extent of paralysis and weakness (paresis). In pathologic conditions of the brain or spinal cord, the upper motor neurons are affected, and this not only causes muscular weakness but also impairs motor control.

Motor activity can be considered as a hierarchic system of voluntary and involuntary neurologic mechanisms.

1. Voluntary muscle activity—Two types of voluntary muscle activity are clinically identifiable: selective and patterned movements. The highest level of motor activity, selective movement, depends on the integrity of the cerebral cortex. Selective movement is the ability to preferentially flex or extend one joint without initiating a mass flexor or extensor motion at other joints of the limb. Patterned movement (synergy) at a joint refers to the ability to move one joint by invoking a mass flexion or extension synergy involving movement at other joints of the limb. Patients with central nervous system disorders may have voluntary patterned movement but lack selective movement. Because most patients have mixtures of selective and patterned movement at different joints, however, the strength of each type of activity must be assessed at each joint. Patterned flexion and extension movements of the lower limb can provide sufficient motor control for ambulation, but patterned motion does not provide sufficient fine control for upper extremity function.

2. Involuntary muscle activity—Spasticity relates to two types of involuntary muscle activity: clonic and tonic responses. Each type depends on the sensitivity of the muscle spindle to the rate of stretch. If a muscle is quickly extended above the threshold of the velocity-sensitive receptors of the spindle, a phasic response may be elicited. If spasticity is severe, sudden stretch may trigger clonus, which consists of repeated bursts of phasic activity at 6–8 cycles per second. The phasic stretch response has practical clinical significance. For example, if an ankle equinus deformity is present and spasticity is severe, clonus of the triceps surae may be triggered in

the stance phase each time the patient takes a step. A rigid ankle-foot orthosis (AFO) that blocks ankle motion and prevents the triceps surae from stretching may inhibit clonus, enabling the foot to be held in a neutral position. An articulated or flexible AFO that allows the ankle to move and the triceps surae to stretch may not prevent clonus from being elicited and may be less effective.

If the muscle is stretched slowly below the threshold of the velocity components of the spindle, a phasic response is not triggered, but the spindle is still capable of detecting changes in length that may generate a tonic response consisting of continuous muscle hypertonus. The tonic muscle activity during slow stretch is called **clasp-knife resistance.** This tonic activity is also of practical significance. Even if the ankle is slowly dorsiflexed for a prolonged time, hypertonus may persist in the triceps surae and restrict normal motion. Consequently, it may be necessary to differentiate spasticity from myostatic contracture by performing peripheral nerve blocks.

Patients with injury involving the brain stem may exhibit severe hypertonus that is continuously present and is called either **decorticate rigidity** or **decerebrate rigidity,** depending on the posture of the limbs. In decerebrate posturing, the patient's arms are held tightly flexed while the legs are held in extension. In decorticate posturing, both the upper and lower extremities are in rigid extension. Patients with severe muscular rigidity are at extreme risk of developing contractural deformities.

When a spastic patient is sitting or standing, labyrinthine activation increases tone in the extensor muscles of the lower extremity and also increases upper limb flexion. Consequently, patients who are examined for spasticity should be evaluated in the upright rather than supine position, to elicit the maximal stretch response. Conversely, patients who are examined for maximal range of motion should be evaluated in the supine position, to minimize muscle tone and enable maximal joint range. The limb posture of patients will also influence the intensity of reflex and voluntary activity.

3. Sensory perception—The final steps of sensory integration occur in the cerebral cortex, where basic sensory data are integrated into the more complex sensory phenomena. When central nervous system injury involves the cerebral cortex, the patient responds to basic modalities of touch and pain. Responses to tests of more complex aspects of sensation (such as shape, texture, and proprioception) and two-point discrimination may be impaired, however. These simple tests quickly determine the patient's ability to interpret basic sensory information. Patients with absent proprioception across the major lower joints have balance abnormalities or are unable to walk. Most patients do not routinely use an affected hand unless proprioception is intact. Patients without lesions of the cerebral cortex can generally discriminate between two points less than 10 mm apart applied simultaneously to the fingers.

B. MUSCLES

Manual muscle testing is often useful for evaluating an individual's ability to perform functional tasks and will also document progress made in the rehabilitation program. Several systems are currently used, but all are based on the grading system introduced by Robert Lovett in 1932. The evaluation is subjective, but the use of gravity resistance provides a measure of objective standardization (Table 13–1). A normal muscle grade as determined by manual testing does not always imply normal strength. A significant amount of weakness (a 25–30% loss of strength) must be present to be detected by this method.

C. GAIT

1. Normal gait—Normal gait is the combination of postures and muscle activities that produce forward motion with minimal energy expenditure (Figure 13–5).

a. Swing phase—The swing phase (Figures 13–5 and 13–6) is divided into three equal periods: initial swing, midswing, and terminal swing. During the three-part phase, the pelvis rotates from backward to forward and the hip flexes 20–30 degrees. The knee flexes to 60 degrees initially and then extends in preparation for contact with the ground. The knee flexion is largely responsible for the foot clearing the ground during swing. Knee flexion occurs as the result of the forward momentum of the limb swinging and not as a result of hamstring contraction. The ankle joint initially plantarflexes 10 degrees and then assumes a neutral po-

Table 13–1. Muscle strength.

Grade	Strength	Description
0	Absent	Muscle does not contract.
1	Trace	Muscle contracts, but no motion is generated.
2	Poor	Muscle contraction produces movement, but muscle cannot function against gravity.
3	Fair	Muscle functions against gravity.
4	Good	Muscle can overcome some outside resistance as well as gravity.
5	Normal	Muscle can overcome resistance to motion.

sition during terminal swing so that the heel normally contacts the floor first.

The hip flexor muscles provide the power for advancing the limb and are active during the initial two thirds of the swing phase. The ankle dorsiflexors become active during the latter two thirds of the phase to ensure foot clearance as the knee begins to extend. The hamstring muscles decelerate the forward motion of the thigh during the terminal period of the swing phase.

b. Stance phase—The stance phase (Figures 13–5 and 13–7) accounts for 60% of the gait cycle and can be divided into five distinct activities: initial contact, the loading response, midstance, terminal stance, and preswing. At initial ground contact, the ankle is in neutral position, the knee is extended, and the hip is flexed. The hip extensor muscles contract to stabilize the hip because the body's mass is behind the hip joint. During the loading response, the knee flexes to 15 degrees, and the ankle plantarflexes to absorb the downward force and conserve energy by minimizing the up-and-down movement of the body's center of gravity. As the knee flexes and the stance leg accepts the weight of the body, the quadriceps muscle becomes active to stabilize the knee. In midstance, the knee is extended, and the ankle is in a neutral position. As the body's mass moves forward of the ankle joint, the calf muscles become active to stabilize the ankle and allow the heel to rise from the floor. In terminal stance, the heel leaves the floor, and the knee begins to flex as momentum carries the body forward. In the final portion of terminal stance, as the body rolls forward over the forefoot, the toes dorsiflex at the metatarsophalangeal joints. During preswing, the knee is flexed to 35 degrees and the ankle plantarflexes to 20 degrees. Because the opposite extremity is also in contact with the floor, the preswing is called the time of double-limb support.

Throughout the stance phase, the hip gradually extends and the pelvis rotates backward. During the first portion of the stance phase, the ankle dorsiflexors and hamstring muscles remain active. During the loading response and early midstance, the gluteus and quadriceps muscles become active to provide hip and knee stability. In midstance, the gastrocnemius and soleus muscles become active to stabilize the ankle joint and control the forward advancement of the tibia. This allows the heel to rise from the floor and the body weight to roll forward over the forefoot.

2. Abnormal gait—The study of movement (kinesiology) has provided many important tools for evaluating patients with gait abnormalities. Among the areas of study are stride analysis, motion analysis (kinematics), force analysis (kinetics), and muscle activity analysis.

Three of the many specialized tools used in these studies are dynamic electromyography, force plate stud-

	SWING 40%			STANCE 60%				
	Initial swing	Mid-swing	Terminal swing	Initial contact	Loading response	Mid-stance	Terminal stance	Pre-swing
TRUNK	Erect neutral	Erect neutral	Erect neutral	Erect neutral	Erect neutral	Erect neutral	Erect neutral	Erect neutral
PELVIS	Level: backward rotation 5°	Level: neutral rotation	Level: forward rotation 5°	Level: maintains forward rotation	Level: less forward rotation	Level: neutral rotation	Level: backward rotation 5°	Level: backward rotation 5°
HIP	Flexion 20° Neutral rotation abduction adduction	Flexion 20°–30° Neutral rotation abduction adduction	Flexion 30° Neutral rotation abduction adduction	Flexion 30° Neutral rotation abduction adduction	Flexion 30° Neutral rotation abduction adduction	Extending to neutral Neutral rotation abduction adduction	Apparent hyperext 10° Neutral rotation abduction adduction	Neutral extension Neutral rotation abduction adduction
KNEE	Flexion 60°	Flexion 60°–30°	Extension to 0°	Full extension	Flexion 15°	Extending to neutral	Full extension	Flexion 35°
ANKLE	Plantar flexion 10°	Neutral	Neutral	Neutral heel first	Plantar flexion 15°	From plantar flexion to 10° dorsiflexion	Neutral with tibia stable and heel off prior to initial contact opposite foot	Plantar flexion 20°
TOES	Neutral	Neutral	Neutral	Neutral	Neutral	Neutral	Neutral IP extended MP	Neutral IP extended MP

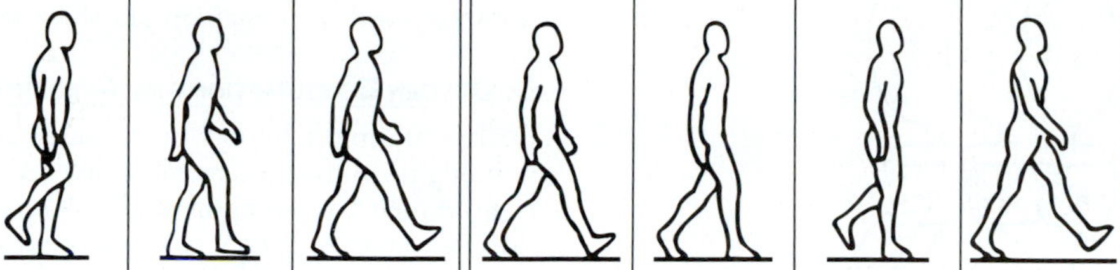

Figure 13–5. The normal gait cycle. (Reproduced, with permission, from American Academy of Orthopaedic Surgeons: Home study syllabus. In: *Orthopaedic Knowledge Update,* I. American Academy of Orthopaedic Surgeons, 1984.)

ies, and motion analysis. Dynamic electromyography, which records the electrical activity in multiple muscles simultaneously during functional activities, has elucidated the patterns of motor control in both the upper and the lower extremities and has helped in the management of spasticity and gait abnormalities. Force plate studies, which measure ground reaction forces and the fluctuations of the center of pressure, can be used to analyze gait problems and quantify balance reactions in impaired patients. Motion analysis uses multiple cameras located at different positions around the room. The cameras detect sensors placed on the patient and create a three-dimensional model of the patient moving through space.

Muscle strength can be accurately measured using torque, and this can be correlated with joint position. Joint stiffness can also be assessed by measuring torque while moving the joint through a passive arc of motion. Joint powers can be calculated by multiplying joint moment times angular velocity.

Measurement of velocity, stride length, cadence, and single- and double-limb support times can be combined

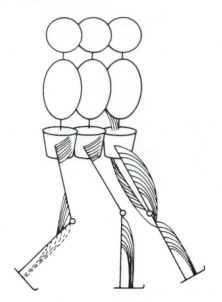

Figure 13–6. Swing phase of gait. (Reproduced, with permission, from American Academy of Orthopaedic Surgeons: Home study syllabus. In: *Orthopaedic Knowledge Update,* I. American Academy of Orthopaedic Surgeons, 1984.)

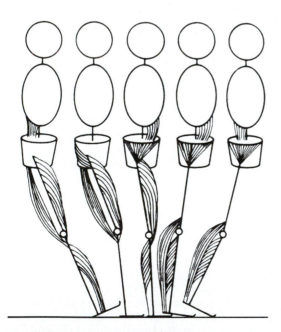

Figure 13–7. Stance phase of gait. (Reproduced, with permission, from American Academy of Orthopaedic Surgeons: Home study syllabus. In: *Orthopaedic Knowledge Update,* I. American Academy of Orthopaedic Surgeons, 1984.)

with dynamic electromyography, force plate studies, and joint goniometric recordings to present a complete analysis of gait dysfunction. These studies can also be used to assess the influence of surgery, orthotic corrections, or prosthetic design on gait characteristics.

D. Oxygen Consumption and Aerobic Capacity

Perhaps the most important measurement for understanding the difficulties faced by disabled people comes from oxygen consumption studies. Oxygen consumption indicates the energy required to perform an activity. Measuring an individual's maximal aerobic capacity is the single best indicator of the level of physical fitness.

1. Effects of disease and aging on energy expenditure—Cardiorespiratory disease, anemia, muscle atrophy, and any other condition that restricts oxygen uptake will cause a decrease in the maximal aerobic capacity. Even in a healthy person, 3 weeks of bed rest will decrease maximal aerobic capacity by up to 30%.

During normal walking, the rate of energy expenditure by adults varies from approximately 30 to 45% of the maximal aerobic capacity, with the higher percentage used in older people. Because of the decline in maximal aerobic capacity with age, an older person is more susceptible than a younger one to the penalties of a gait disability.

2. Effects of exercise on energy expenditure—When exercise is performed at less than 50% of an individual's maximal aerobic capacity, the exercise can be continued for prolonged periods because the adenosine triphosphate (ATP) needed for muscle contraction is provided by aerobic pathways. Anaerobic pathways of ATP production, which do not use oxygen, increasingly come into play when exercise is performed at work rates exceeding about 50% of maximal aerobic capacity. The amount of energy that can be delivered by anaerobic metabolism is limited, and fatigue ensues because of the accumulation of lactate in the muscle. Consequently, the normal activities of daily living and working that must be performed throughout an 8-h day, including walking, are performed below anaerobic threshold.

3. Effects of musculoskeletal impairment on energy expenditure—Gait abnormalities that interfere with efficient, coordinated limb movement can increase energy demand. Some affected patients respond to this increased demand by working harder, which increases the output of physiologic energy and is reflected in the higher-than-normal heart rate and oxygen consumption rate. Rather than increasing the rate of energy expenditure, however, most patients slow their gait velocity in an effort to keep the power requirement from exceeding normal limits.

Among amputees, patients progressively walk slower at increasingly more proximal amputation levels. Younger patients with traumatic or congenital amputations walk faster than older dysvascular amputees because of their greater maximal aerobic capacity. Patients with limited joint movement or with arthritis and painful joints also reduce their gait velocity. The heart rate and energy expenditure rate do not exceed normal in any of these groups of patients if crutches are not required.

Patients requiring crutches and exerting considerable force to support the body often have high heart rates and energy expenditure rates. A swing-through, crutch-assisted gait in a paraplegic or a patient who has a fracture and is unable to bear weight on one leg requires strenuous physical exertion, and this accounts for why few paraplegics use swing-through gait and why older patients with fractures can ambulate for only short distances. Even patients who use a reciprocal gait pattern, such as patients with low lumbar paraplegia resulting from spinal cord injury or myelodysplasia, use their arms for considerable exertion. Consequently, these types of patients may also be restricted ambulators in the community.

Patients with hip and knee flexion deformities caused by fixed or dynamic contractures require increasing muscle effort not only to walk but also to maintain an upright posture because the center of gravity during stance passes farther away from the axis of rotation of the joint. The fact that knee flexion greater than 30 degrees significantly increases the energy expenditure rate even in otherwise normal persons points to the importance of preventing and correcting contractures.

Children who have cerebral palsy and diplegia and who walk in a crouch gait may have energy expenditure rates that are above the anaerobic threshold. This accounts for why these children are restricted ambulators who frequently discontinue walking when they mature and their maximal aerobic capacities decrease.

Use of Orthoses

Orthotic (brace) prescription plays a vital role in rehabilitation. It is important for the physician to understand the functional needs of the patient and to provide the orthotist with an exact prescription that specifies the materials, type of joints, joint position, and range of motion. Brace prescriptions should not be left to the discretion of the patient and orthotist.

A temporary orthosis may be used in an early stage of illness until a definitive, custom-fitted orthosis is fabricated. Definitive orthoses for the lower extremity are the below-knee, ankle-foot orthosis (AFO) and the above-knee, knee-ankle-foot orthosis (KAFO).

The bichannel adjustable ankle-locking type of AFO is commonly applied as the first orthosis following stroke, head trauma, spinal injury, or other condition that causes extensive muscle imbalance about the foot and ankle (Figure 13–8). A rigid ankle is useful in controlling plantarflexion spasticity, stabilizing the ankle in a flaccid limb, and correcting a dynamic varus deformity (inversion of the foot). The adjustable ankle joint mechanism enables the clinician to determine the optimal ankle position in the acute period following onset of illness when the neurologic picture and orthotic requirement are changing. Once neurologic recovery has stabilized, a plastic (polypropylene) orthosis often becomes the treatment of choice (Figure 13–9).

The use of plastic materials in lower extremity orthotics has become widespread in recent years. Orthoses fabricated from plastics are lighter, more comfortable, and more attractive. A plastic AFO can be rigid or can be flexible, allowing motion at the ankle. Polypropylene is presently the most practical plastic material. Skillful fitting is critical because of the close skin and bone contact.

A. ANKLE-FOOT ORTHOSIS

1. Types—Of several currently available orthoses classified as limited-motion ankle joint orthoses, two are

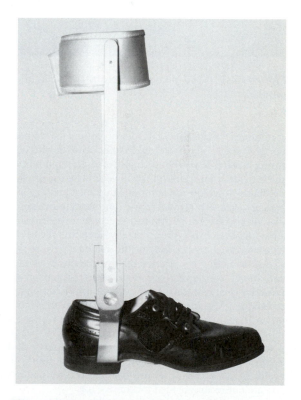

Figure 13–8. The bichannel adjustable ankle-locking (BiCAAL) type of ankle-foot orthosis.

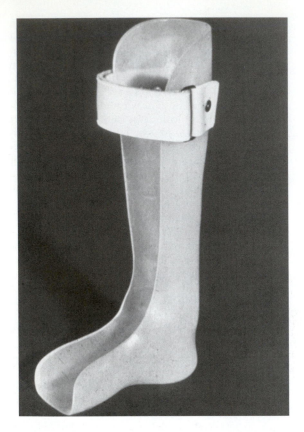

Figure 13–9. The molded polypropylene ankle-foot orthosis.

commonly used: the conventional metal, double-upright, single-adjustable ankle joint with dorsiflexion spring assist (Klenzak) and the molded plastic posterior shells made from ¹⁄₁₆-in. polypropylene. The use of plastic materials makes the latter design preferable for most patients. When a greater restriction of ankle motion is desired, rigidity can be attained in several ways: by using a thicker sheet of polypropylene, by extending the lateral trim lines farther anteriorly at the ankle to serve as side struts, by adding an anterior shell to the posterior shell and totally enveloping the ankle, or by stiffening the posterior shell with the use of carbon fiber or lamination techniques. The trim lines may be reinforced with metal or additional layers of plastic. The foot plate of the orthosis extends just proximal to the metatarsal heads. Total circumferential orthoses combining anterior and posterior shells require exceptionally careful fitting to avoid excessive skin pressure over bony prominences and are not recommended for routine use.

Insertion of a polypropylene orthosis inside a shoe generally requires a shoe size that is one-half size larger and wider than that previously worn by the patient. To eliminate the need to purchase two pairs of shoes of different sizes, an inlay can be inserted in the shoe of the sound limb to prevent excessive looseness once a shoe is fitted on the polypropylene side. The ankle position of the polypropylene orthosis should be assessed with the patient wearing his or her shoe with the normal heel height.

2. Indications—The primary requirement for orthotic support is that all joints must be passively capable of being positioned in adequate alignment. An orthosis will not correct a fixed bony deformity or fixed joint contracture.

a. Inadequate dorsiflexion for foot clearance during swing—An AFO is indicated for inadequate toe clearance (footdrop) during the midswing phase of gait. This problem may result from inadequate ankle dorsiflexion caused by weakness of the dorsiflexors or by the inability of dorsiflexors to overcome spasticity of the triceps surae. A lightweight, flexible polypropylene orthosis is indicated if inadequate dorsiflexion is the only problem at the ankle. A flexible orthosis can also be used for a mild swing-phase varus deformity (foot inversion). A rigid orthosis is needed in patients who have excessive plantarflexion resulting from severe spasticity and in patients who initiate a strong extensor pattern activity prior to heel strike.

b. Inadequate dorsiflexion for initial contact—A patient with inadequate dorsiflexion from any cause will contact the ground with the forefoot or with the foot flat and the tibia extended backward. This problem is commonly combined with varus deformity, and weight bearing is on the lateral edge of the foot. The results are a backward thrust to the limb, which decreases forward momentum and produces excessive hyperextension forces on the knee, which leads to knee instability in the patient who is a functional walker. A rigid AFO in the neutral position provides heel strike for the patient who has full-knee extension and allows the tibia to rotate forward during stance.

c. Medial-lateral subtalar instability during stance—Varus deformity is more common than valgus deformity. The patient walks on the lateral border of the foot and is hesitant to accept weight on the leg. A rigid orthosis will correct the varus deformity unless spasticity is severe. To correct a mild varus deformity, a limited ankle orthosis may be used. No orthosis is effective in controlling the severe spastic varus deformity.

d. Inadequate tibial stability during stance—Some patients have inadequate strength or control of the plantarflexors for maintenance of normal tibial position and alignment during stance. Early after midstance, this problem is manifested by excessive dorsiflexion and accompanying knee flexion. Whether or not the limb collapses during weight bearing depends on the amount of quadriceps muscle control and strength. Patients with sufficient proprioception learn to compensate by locking the knee in hyperextension as the foot contacts the floor, and this keeps the knee from buckling. A rigid orthosis that prevents both dorsiflexion and plantarflexion is indicated to provide vertical tibial alignment during midstance. Its use prevents tibial collapse forward during terminal stance as a substitution for adequate calf control.

A knee extension thrust, caused by inadequate calf control as described earlier, may result also from severe plantarflexion tone or fixed equinus deformity resulting from contracture. At foot strike, the forefoot will strike the floor first, resulting in a knee extension or hyperextension thrust. A rigid AFO with a plantarflexion block will prevent the development of knee instability and pain.

A T-strap (a leather T-shaped strap attached to the brace at the ankle and applied around the ankle to hold the foot from either an inverted or everted position) is usually not desirable for correction of severe varus deformity in patients fitted with metal orthoses. If a T-strap is applied with sufficient force to provide significant control to prevent foot-twisting, it will usually cause excessive pressure over the lateral malleolus in the patient with severe spasticity. This problem can be treated better by the use of a split anterior tibial tendon transfer or by the addition of a lateral wedge and flare to the shoe of the nonsurgical candidate.

B. KNEE-ANKLE-FOOT ORTHOSIS

Orthoses of this type may be used if quadriceps muscle weakness or hamstring muscle spasticity is present. A knee immobilizer may be used as a training aid before having a KAFO fabricated. A KAFO is more difficult to don than a below-knee brace, and most patients with a central nervous system disease such as stroke or cerebral palsy have difficulty walking with a KAFO. Consequently, if hamstring spasticity rather than quadriceps spasticity necessitates external support to align the knee in extension, it is preferable to perform hamstring tenotomy or tendon lengthening, thereby eliminating the need for knee support.

Most patients with lower extremity quadriceps paresis resulting from spinal cord injury lack sufficient proprioception to walk with a free-knee mechanism (unlocked knee joint mechanism).

When a KAFO is prescribed for quadriceps paresis, it is necessary to determine if the knee will be locked while walking or if it will be freely movable to allow knee flexion in swing. When a KAFO is prescribed because of knee instability or because of varus or valgus instability, a polycentric joint (a joint in which the center of rotation moves following the anatomic instantaneous center of rotation) permits flexion extension movement but blocks medial and lateral angulation. A posterior stop added to the knee mechanism will prevent excessive hyperextension.

If proprioception is intact, as is the case with poliomyelitis, even patients with considerable quadriceps weakness may be able to walk with an unlocked knee using an offset knee joint. This is accomplished by careful orthotic alignment. The center of rotation of the orthosis is positioned anterior to the center of rotation of the knee. As long as the patient can fully extend the knee in the swing stage preparatory to limb loading, the resulting movement caused by vertical loading will act to extend the knee against the posterior stop, thereby locking the knee in extension. This requires at least fair (grade 3) hip flexor strength (see Table 13–1) to provide sufficient forward momentum of the leg to position the knee in full extension.

The substitution of plastic components, such as a pretibial shell, has led to significantly improved fit and reduced weight in KAFOs.

Davis JA: Anaerobic threshold: Review of the concept and directions for future research. Med Sci Sports Exerc 1985;17:6.

DeLisa JA, Gans BM: *Rehabilitation Medicine.* Lippincott: Baltimore; 1993.

Goldberg B, Hsu JD: *Atlas of Orthoses and Assistive Devices.* Mosby-YearBook: St. Louis; 1997.

Keenan MA: Principles of Neuro-Orthopaedic Rehabilitation. In Fitzgerald RH et al (editors): *Orthopaedics.* Mosby Publishers: St Louis; 2002:71–85.

Keenan MAE et al: *Manual of Orthopaedic Surgery for Spasticity.* New York: Raven; 1993.

Keenan MAE, McDaid PJ: Orthopaedic Management of Spasticity. In Gelber DA, Jeffrey DR, eds: *Clinical Evaluation and Management of Spasticity.* Humana Press: Totowa, NJ; 2002:197–255.

Kendall FP et al: *Muscles: Testing and Function.* Baltimore: Williams & Wilkins; 1993.

Kendall FPM et al: *Muscles: Testing and Function.* Baltimore: Williams & Wilkins; 1993.

Nickel VL, Botte MJ: *Orthopaedic Rehabilitation.* New York: Churchill Livingstone; 1992.

Perry J: *Gait Analysis: Normal and Pathological Function.* Thorofare, NJ: Slack; 1992.

Torburn L: Principles of rehabilitation. Prim Care 1996;23:335.

Waters RL, Mulroy S: The energy expenditure of normal and pathologic gait. Gait Posture 1999;9:207.

Young J: Rehabilitation and older people. BMJ 1996;313:677.

SPINAL CORD INJURY

Trauma to the spinal cord causes dysfunction of the cord, with nonprogressive loss of sensory and motor function distal to the point of injury. Approximately

400,000 people have spinal cord damage in the United States, and the incidence rate is estimated to be 10,000 per year. The leading causes of spinal cord injury are motor vehicle accidents, gunshot wounds, falls, sports (especially diving) injuries, and water injuries.

Patients are generally categorized into three groups. The first consists predominately of younger individuals who sustained their injury from a motor vehicle collision or other high-energy traumatic accident. The second consists of older individuals with cervical spinal stenosis caused by congenital narrowing or spondylosis. Patients in this second group often sustained their injury from minor trauma and commonly have no vertebral fracture. The third group consists of people with gunshot wounds, which are now the leading cause of spinal injury in many urban centers in the United States. With the benefits of an organized program of medical care, the life expectancy of survivors of spinal cord injury is now approaching the normal level.

Terminology

A. TETRAPLEGIA

This term (preferred to *quadriplegia*) refers to loss or impairment of motor or sensory function (or both) in the cervical segments of the spinal cord with resulting impairment of function in the arms, trunk, legs, and pelvic organs.

B. PARAPLEGIA

Paraplegia refers to loss or impairment of motor or sensory function (or both) in the thoracic, lumbar, or sacral segments of the spinal cord. Arm function is intact but, depending on the level of the cord injured, impairment in the trunk, legs, and pelvic organs may be present.

C. COMPLETE INJURY

This term refers to an injury with no spared motor or sensory function in the lowest sacral segments.

D. INCOMPLETE INJURY

Incomplete injury refers to an injury with partial preservation of sensory or motor function (or both) below the neurologic level and includes the lowest sacral segments.

Neurologic Impairment & Recovery

A. NEUROLOGIC EXAMINATION

The neurologic examination is critical to the classification and treatment of spinal injuries because it determines the patient's potential level of recovery. The neurologic level of the lesion refers to the highest neural segment having normal motor and sensory function.

Patients are further subdivided according to whether they have complete or incomplete spinal cord function. This is determined by the absence or presence of motor or sensory function in the most distal part of the spinal cord innervating the sacral nerves. The presence of sacral nerve function is critical because patients with incomplete injuries have the potential to recover normal neurologic function over a time span of up to 2 years even if paralysis is initially complete.

1. Spinal shock—The diagnosis of complete spinal cord injury cannot be made until the period of spinal shock is over, as evidenced by the return of the bulbocavernosus reflex. To elicit this reflex, the clinician digitally examines the patient's rectum, feeling for contraction of the anal sphincter while squeezing the glans penis or clitoris. The concept of spinal shock is important and can be understood on the basis of the monosynaptic stretch reflex. At a given neural segment of the spinal cord, afferent sensory fibers enter the spinal cord and anastomose with the anterior motor neurons at the same level. If trauma to the spinal cord causes complete injury, reflex activity at the site of injury will not return because the reflex arc is permanently interrupted. When spinal shock disappears, however, reflex activity does return in the distal segments below the level of injury. In a patient with complete spinal cord injury, spinal shock may last for as little as several hours or as long as several months. Patients with complete spinal cord injury who have recovered from spinal shock have a negligible chance for any useful motor return.

2. Sacral reflexes—The presence or absence of sacral function determines the completeness of the injury. Sacral motor function is assessed by testing contraction of the external anal sphincter (graded as present or absent). Sacral sensation is tested at the anal mucocutaneous junction. Additionally, testing of the external anal sphincter is performed by assessing perceived deep sensation as present or absent when the examiner's finger is inserted.

B. SPINAL CORD SYNDROMES

1. Anterior cord syndrome—Anterior cord syndrome commonly results from direct contusion to the anterior cord by bone fragments or from damage to the anterior spinal artery. Depending on the extent of cord involvement, only posterior column function (proprioception and light touch) may be present. The ability to respond to pain (tested by sharp-dull discrimination) and to light touch (tested with a wisp of cotton) signifies that the entire posterior half of the cord has some intact function and thus offers a better prognosis for motor recovery. If there is no recovery of motor function and pain sensation 4 weeks after injury, the prognosis for significant motor return is poor.

2. Central cord syndrome—Central cord syndrome can be understood on the basis of the spinal cord anatomy. The gray matter in the spinal cord contains nerve cell bodies and is surrounded by white matter consisting primarily of ascending and descending myelinated tracts. The central gray matter has a higher metabolic requirement and is therefore more susceptible to the effects of trauma and ischemia. Central cord syndrome often results from a minor injury such as a fall in an older patient with cervical spinal canal stenosis. The overall prognosis for patients with central cord syndrome is variable. Most patients are able to walk despite severe paralysis of the upper extremity.

3. Brown-Séquard syndrome—Brown-Séquard syndrome is caused by a complete hemisection of the spinal cord, resulting in a greater ipsilateral proprioceptive motor loss and a greater contralateral loss of pain and temperature sensation. Affected patients have an excellent prognosis and will usually ambulate.

4. Mixed syndrome—Mixed syndrome is characterized by a diffuse involvement of the entire spinal cord. Affected patients have a good prognosis for recovery. As with all incomplete spinal cord injury syndromes, early motor recovery is the best prognostic indicator.

Management

A. LOWER EXTREMITIES

Prevention of contractures and maintenance of range of motion are important in all patients with spinal cord injury and should begin immediately following the injury. Teaching the patient to sleep in the prone position is the most effective means of preventing hip and knee flexion contractures. Passive stretching of the hamstring muscles with the knee extended is initiated to prevent shortening of these muscles secondary to spasticity. For patients to be able to dress the lower parts of their body independently, they must be able to flex the lumbar spine and hip 120 degrees with the knee extended.

Patients with extensive paralysis of the lower extremity need strength in both arms to manipulate crutches and bring the body to a standing position. Patients who lack at least fair (grade 3) strength in their quadriceps muscles (see Table 13–1) will require KAFOs to stabilize the knee and will also require the knee to be locked in extension while walking. Patients who have bilateral KAFOs commonly use a swing-through, crutch-assisted gait rather than a reciprocal gait. Because strenuous upper extremity exertion is required and the rate of energy expenditure is extremely high when crutches are used, nearly all patients prefer to use a wheelchair. In contrast, patients who have fair (grade 3) or greater strength in their hip flexors and knee extensors are able to walk with unlocked (free) knees and only require ankle-foot orthoses (AFOs) to stabilize their feet and ankles. These patients will also usually require crutches because of absent or impaired hip extensor and adductor muscles, but they are able to achieve a reciprocal gait pattern and can walk for a limited duration outside the home. Most of them prefer a wheelchair when ambulation over long distances is required.

Because most ambulatory patients with spinal cord injury have impaired hip extensor support, they learn to hyperextend the lumbar spine so that the center of gravity of the trunk is posterior to the hip joint in the stance phase of gait. This prevents forward collapse and decreases the demand on the arms during crutch use. Spine stabilization procedures that decrease the flexibility of the lower lumbar spine or reduce the amount of lordosis deprive the patient of an important gait maneuver.

B. UPPER BODY AND EXTREMITIES

1. C4 level function—Patients with cervical lesions above C4 may have impairment of respiratory function, depending on the extent of injury, and may require a tracheostomy and mechanical ventilatory assistance.

Phrenic nerve stimulation via implanted surgical electrodes will enable patients to use their own diaphragm and ventilate without mechanical assistance if the cause of their diaphragm paralysis was upper motor neuron injury. With training, these patients should be able to achieve a vital capacity that is 50–60% of normal using only the diaphragm.

Patients with high tetraplegia can use chin or tongue controls to operate an electric wheelchair with attached respiratory equipment. Mouth sticks that are lightweight rods attached to a dental bite plate enable patients to perform desktop skills, operate push-button equipment, and pursue vocational and recreational activities.

2. C5 level function—At the C5 level, the key muscles are the deltoid and biceps muscles, which are used for shoulder abduction and elbow flexion. If these muscles are weak, the patient will benefit from mobile arm supports attached to a wheelchair. Mobile arm supports are balanced to exert a vertical force to counteract gravity. This enables the patient with poor muscle strength to feed independently and perform other functional tasks with the hands. A ratchet wrist-hand orthosis (WHO) with a fixed wrist joint and a passively closing mechanism attached to the thumb and fingers enables the patient to grasp objects between the thumb and fingers.

Surgery can further enhance upper extremity function. The goals of surgery are to provide active elbow and wrist extension and to restore the ability to pinch the thumb against the index finger (key pinch or lateral pinch). Transferring the posterior deltoid to the triceps muscle will provide active elbow extension. Transferring the brachioradialis to the extensor carpi radialis brevis will provide active wrist extension. Attaching the flexor pollicis longus tendon to the distal radius and fusing the interphalangeal joint of the thumb will provide for key pinch by tenodesis when the wrist is extended.

3. C6 level function—At the C6 level, the key muscles are the wrist extensors, which enable the patient to manually propel a wheelchair, transfer from one position to another, and even live independently.

If wrist extensor strength is poor, an orthosis is indicated. A WHO with a free wrist joint and a rubber-band extensor-assist mechanism will enable the patient to complete wrist extension. A wrist-driven WHO with a flexor hinge mechanism that causes the metacarpophalangeal joint to flex when the wrist is extended will enable the patient to actively grasp between the fingers and thumb. Some patients will develop a natural tenodesis of their thumb and finger flexor muscles owing to myostatic contracture or spasticity, and this tenodesis enables them to grasp without the need of an orthosis.

Most patients with good wrist extensor strength are able to operate a manual wheelchair but may require an electric wheelchair for long distances. These patients may also be able to transfer independently if they have no elbow flexion contractures and they can passively lock their elbows in extension while transferring.

The goals of surgery in the C6 patient are the restoration of lateral pinch and active grasp. Lateral pinch can be restored either by tenodesis of the thumb flexor or by transfer of the brachioradialis to the flexor pollicis longus. Active grasp can be restored by transfer of the pronator teres to the flexor digitorum profundus.

4. C7 level function—At the C7 level, the key muscle is the triceps. All patients with intact triceps function should be able to transfer and live independently if no other complications are present. Despite their ability to extend the fingers, these patients may also require a WHO with a flexor hinge mechanism.

The goals of surgery in the C7 tetraplegic patient are active thumb flexion for pinch, active finger flexion for grasp, and hand opening by extensor tenodesis. Transfer of the brachioradialis to the flexor pollicis longus will provide active pinch. Transfer of the pronator teres to the flexor digitorum profundus allows for active finger flexion and grasp. If the finger extensors are weak, tenodesis of these tendons to the radius will provide hand opening with wrist flexion.

5. C8 level function—At the C8 level, the key muscles are the finger and thumb flexors, which enable a gross grasp. The functioning flexor pollicis longus enables patients to obtain lateral pinch between the thumb and the side of the index finger. Intrinsic muscle function is lacking, and clawing of the fingers is usually present. A capsulodesis of the metacarpophalangeal joints will correct the clawing and improve hand function. Active intrinsic function can be gained by splitting the superficial finger flexor tendon of the ring finger into four slips and transferring these tendons to the lumbrical insertions of each finger.

C. Skin

Maintaining skin integrity is crucial to spinal injury care. From the moment the patient enters the emergency room, preventive measures are instituted to avoid skin breakdown even while critical diagnostic procedures and lifesaving measures are performed. Only 4 h of continuous pressure on the sacrum is sufficient to cause full-thickness skin necrosis. Turning the patient from side to back to side every 2 h will avoid skin ulceration, a problem that greatly prolongs the cost and length of rehabilitation. Following the simple procedures outlined here will usually obviate the need for flotation devices, Stryker frames, cyclically rotating beds, and similar equipment.

Once the patient is allowed to sit, a progressive program to increase the time of sitting tolerance is undertaken. Paraplegics with normal upper extremity function are taught to automatically perform raises in the wheelchair and decompress the skin for approximately 15 s every 15 min. Tetraplegics who are unable to perform raises can lean to either side or lean forward for 1-min intervals on an hourly basis to achieve decompression. Those patients unable to perform decompressive maneuvers will require assistance from another person or may use an electric wheelchair with a powered recliner that enables them to assume a supine posture every hour.

All patients must be taught to inspect their skin at least twice a day, when dressing and undressing. Mirrors attached to a rod enable paraplegics to independently examine skin over the sacrum and ischia. Tetraplegics usually require assistance with skin inspection.

If there is evidence of chronic skin inflammation over bony prominences or if redness persists 30 min after removal of pressure, action must be taken to avoid incipient pressure necrosis. Pressure transducers placed under the bony prominences will determine if pressure exceeds acceptable levels. Up to 40 mm Hg is well tolerated by most patients. If pressures exceed this amount, then a custom-fitted foam cushion with appropriate cutouts is prescribed.

Development of any open areas in the skin over the ischia or sacrum, even superficial areas, is an indication to temporarily discontinue sitting. The patient must remain in a prone or side-lying position to avoid pressure until the lesion is healed. Failure to take aggressive steps to eliminate pressure and allow healing will lead to chronic inflammation, scarring, and a loss of elasticity, creating a vicious cycle that further increases susceptibility to pressure necrosis.

Excessive hip and knee flexor spasticity that prevents patients from assuming the prone position or lying supine and requires them to constantly assume a side-lying posture when in bed can lead to excessive pressure over the greater trochanters. Flexor spasticity or contracture that prevents continuous turning should be corrected medically prior to development of pressure sores and must be performed prior to skin flap placement. Failure to correct flexion deformities inevitably decreases the likelihood of successful skin closure. Surgical tenotomy and myotomy of hip and knee flexors is the most effective surgical method for correcting the problem when nonoperative measures fail. Neurosurgical procedures such as myelotomy or rhizotomy are usually less effective and run the risk of interfering with reflex bladder emptying and penile erections.

In the neglected patient with a full-thickness pressure sore, surgery will be necessary. The initial phase consists of debridement of all infected soft tissue and bone as well as treatment of spasticity and contractures that may have predisposed the patient to pressure sores. Once all wounds have a clean granulating base and the patient is able to remain prone 24 h a day, he or she becomes a candidate for a rotational flap. In recent years, the gluteus maximus, the tensor fasciae latae, and other types of musculocutaneous flaps have given the surgeon a superior and reliable method of providing skin coverage. Sitting tolerance must be carefully reestablished following flap surgery. Because most pressure sores in patients with chronic spinal cord injury are the result of failure to relieve pressure by appropriate measures, patient education is the key element of a successful rehabilitation outcome.

Ischial or trochanteric pressure sores commonly lead to septic arthritis of the hip. In such cases, femoral head and neck resection is required. In the paraplegic with an intact hip joint, the passive weight of the limbs cantilevered about the posterior thigh exerts an upward force on the pelvis, and this decompresses the ischia. Consequently, about 30% of the body weight is supported on the thigh. Femoral head and neck resection disrupts the bony leg of the femur to the pelvis and results in a greater concentration of pressure on the ischia, thereby increasing the chance of recurrence even after successful flap closure.

Pressure sores affecting the ankle commonly occur over the heel or malleolus. After initial debridement, wound healing can nearly always be obtained by placing the patient in a short leg cast that protects the wound from any external pressure. The cast is changed every 1 or 2 weeks until healing occurs. Rotational flaps are rarely needed.

D. Bladder Function

Intermittent catheterization has been the factor most responsible for the nearly normal life span of patients with spinal cord injuries. In this group, urinary tract infection is no longer the leading cause of death. Most patients who have intact sacral reflex activity following complete injury will be able to obtain reflex bladder emptying. Some patients with complete spinal cord injury will be able to trigger reflex bladder emptying by tapping the suprapubic area, stroking the thighs, or using Credé's method (applying external pressure on the bladder to induce emptying) or Valsalva's maneuver (forcibly exhaling against the closed glottis). These patients will require an external condom catheter for men or diapering for women. Patients with nonreflex bladders will void by the application of pressure on the bladder by Valsalva's maneuver or Credé's method. Not all so-called reflex bladders will empty reflexively, and some, despite reflex emptying, will have an excessive amount of residual urine. Anticholinergic medications to decrease bladder neck spasm of the smooth muscle of the internal sphincter or spasmolytic medications to decrease tone in the striated muscle of the external sphincter may improve bladder emptying. Some patients will require surgical sphincterotomy.

Bladder diversion using an ileal conduit as a primary means of achieving bladder drainage is contraindicated. This procedure leads to a chronic acid-base imbalance, osteoporosis, and, ultimately, renal failure from secondary infection. The suprapubic catheter also is to be avoided as a means of primary treatment for the same reasons that permanent indwelling catheters are contraindicated. The constant presence of an indwelling catheter leads to bladder constriction and increases the risks of renal calculi, infection, and death from renal failure. For male patients, the external condom catheter is the treatment of choice. For female patients, padding or diapering is the preferred treatment, although some women prefer an indwelling catheter despite the risks of a shortened life span.

E. Sexual Function

Women with or without intact reflex activity can perform coitus and deliver normal children. Approximately 90% of men with complete spinal cord injury and sacral reflex activity can be expected to have reflex erections. Most of these men will be able to perform coitus; however, fewer than half will be able to ejaculate. Sacral sparing plays a great role in prognosticating sexual potential in the male patient. Those able to distinguish pain (sharp-dull discrimination) will usually be able to achieve psychogenic erections.

F. AUTONOMIC DYSREFLEXIA

Splanchnic outflow conveying sympathetic fibers to the lower body exits at the T8 region. Patients with lesions above T8 are prone to autonomic dysreflexia. They are subject to bouts of hypertension that may be heralded by dizziness, sweating, and headaches. A plugged catheter is the most common precipitating cause of dysreflexia. The catheter should be carefully checked and the bladder irrigated. Other frequent causes of dysreflexia include calculi or infections in any portion of the urinary system, fecal impaction, and pressure sores. If the patient's blood pressure does not lower in response to treatment of the causative agent, management with antihypertensive medication is begun.

Recovery

The International Standards for Neurological and Functional classification of Spinal Cord Injury, published by the American Spinal Injury Association (ASIA) and the International Medical Society of Paraplegia (IMSOP) represent the most reliable instrument for assessing neurologic status in spinal cord injury. These standards provide a quantitative measure of sensory and motor function.

Neurologic recovery is assessed by determining the change in ASIA Motor Score (AMS) between successive neurologic examinations. The AMS is the sum of strength grades for each of the 10 key muscles tested bilaterally that represent neurologic segments from C5 to T1 and L2 to S1. In a neurologically intact individual, the total possible AMS is 100 points.

The most important prognostic indicator of recovery is completeness of injury using the sacral-sparing definition. Using completeness and level of injury (tetraplegia or paraplegia), patients are divided into four groups: complete tetraplegia, incomplete tetraplegia, complete paraplegia, and incomplete paraplegia. The rate of motor recovery in all groups declines rapidly in the first 6 months following injury with minimal further changes after this time (Figure 13–10).

A. COMPLETE PARAPLEGIA

Patients with paraplegia that remains complete 1 month after injury have a 96% chance of remaining complete. Thirty-eight percent of those with injuries at or below T9 will recover some lower extremity function. No patients with a neurologic level above T9 regained volitional lower extremity motor function. Only 5% of muscles with a strength of 0/5 at 1 month will recover to 3/5 or greater strength 1 year after injury. Furthermore, only 5% of individuals will become independent community ambulators at 1 year.

B. INCOMPLETE PARAPLEGIA

Motor recovery is better in individuals with incomplete injuries. Between 1 month and 1 year after injury, the AMS increases by an average of 12 points regardless of the level of injury. Additionally, these patients have a 76% chance of becoming community ambulators.

C. COMPLETE TETRAPLEGIA

Ninety percent of individuals with complete tetraplegia 1 month after injury will remain complete. Among the 10% who undergo late conversion to incomplete status, lower extremity motor recovery is minimal and inadequate for ambulation. Recovery of AMS points is independent of neurologic level. Waters and colleagues reported that with the exception of the triceps muscle, all upper extremity muscles with grade of at least 1/5

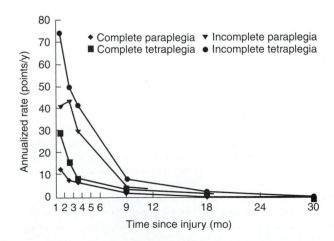

Figure 13–10. Recovery rates of ASIA Motor Score for persons with incomplete and complete paraplegia and tetraplegia. (Reproduced from Waters RL et al: Functional and neurological recovery following acute SCI. J Spinal Cord Med 1998;21:195.)

1 month after injury would recover to at least 3/5 1 year following injury.

D. INCOMPLETE TETRAPLEGIA

In patients with incomplete tetraplegia, motor recovery of upper and lower extremity muscles occurs concurrently. Nearly all muscles with at least 1/5 strength 1 month after injury recover to at least 3/5 1 year post injury. Forty-six percent of the patients examined by Waters and colleagues attained independent community ambulation status 1 year after injury. The number of individuals with incomplete tetraplegia who can attain independent community ambulation is less than for individuals with incomplete paraplegia and comparable lower extremity function. This is because upper extremity function may be insufficient to allow crutch-assisted ambulation in the former group, whereas those with incomplete paraplegia have normal upper extremity strength.

Taken as a whole, a minority of individuals with spinal cord injury can ambulate independently after injury. The proportion of patients who can ambulate does, however, vary with the level and completeness of the injury. The lower extremity motor scores (LEMS) which are the sum of the strength grades of the bilateral key lower extremity muscles, can be used to predict successful ambulation (Table 13–2). The motor groups are as follows: L2-hip flexors (iliopsoas), L3-knee extensors (quadriceps), L4-ankle dorsiflexors (tibialis anterior), L5-long toe extensors (extensor hallucis longus), and S1-ankle plantarflexors (gastrocnemius, soleus). In an individual with no deficit, the total possible LEMS is 50 points. The LEMS at 30 days is used to predict the chance of successful ambulation in incomplete tetraplegics, incomplete paraplegics, and complete paraplegics. All individuals with a LEMS of at least 20 and an incomplete injury are expected to be community ambulators 1 year after injury.

American Spinal Injury Association, International Medical Society of Paraplegia: *International Standards for Neurological and Functional Classification of Spinal Cord Injury,* Revised 1996. American Spinal Injury Association, Chicago, IL; 1996.

American Spinal Injury Association, International Medical Society of Paraplegia: *International Standards for Neurological Classification of Spinal Cord Injury,* Revised 2000. American Spinal Injury Association. Chicago, IL; 2000.

Banovac K et al: Prevention of heterotopic ossification after spinal cord injury with indomethacin. Spinal Cord 2001;39:370.

Bergman SB et al: Spinal cord injury rehabilitation. 2. Medical complications. Arch Phys Med Rehabil 1997;78(3 Suppl):S53.

Bracken MB: Methylprednisolone and acute spinal cord injury: An update of the randomized evidence. Spine 2001;26(24 Suppl):S47.

Burns AS, Ditunno JF: Establishing prognosis and maximizing functional outcomes after spinal cord injury: A review of current and future directions in rehabilitation management. Spine 2001;26:S137.

Delamarter RB, Coyle J: Acute management of spinal cord injury. J Am Acad Orthop Surg 1999;7(3):166.

Ditunno JF Jr et al: Neurological assessment in spinal cord injury. Adv Neurol 1997;72:325.

Keith MW: Neuroprosthesis for the upper extremity. Microsurgery 2001;21:256.

Kirshblum SC, O'Connor KC: Levels of spinal cord injury and predictors of neurologic recovery. Phys Med Rehabil Clin North Am 2000;11(1):1, vii.

Little JW et al: Neurologic recovery and neurologic decline after spinal cord injury. Phys Med Rehabil Clin North Am 2000;11(1):73.

Marino RJ et al: Neurologic recovery after traumatic spinal cord injury: Data from the Model Spinal Cord Injury Systems. Arch Phys Med Rehabil 1999;80(11):1391.

Nockels RP: Nonoperative management of acute spinal cord injury. Spine 2001;26(24 Suppl):S31.

Van der Putten JJ et al: Factors affecting functional outcome in patients with nontraumatic spinal cord lesions after inpatient rehabilitation. Neurorehabil Neural Repair 2001;15:99.

Table 13–2. Community ambulators at 1 year postinjury.

ASIA Lower Extremity Motor Score[a] (at 30 days postinjury)	Complete Paraplegia (%)	Incomplete Paraplegia (%)	Incomplete Tetraplegia (%)
0	< 1	33	0
1–9	45	70	2
10–19		100	63
20 or greater		100	100
Total	5	76	46

[a]Score based upon five key muscles.
Total possible 50 points for both lower extremities for normals.

Reprinted, with permission, from Waters RL et al: Functional and neurological recovery following acute SCI. J Spinal Cord Med 1998, 21:195.

Water RL, et al: Effect of surgery on motor recovery following traumatic spinal cord injury. Spinal Cord 1996;34:188.

Waters RL et al: Donal Munro Lecture: Functional and neurologic recovery following acute SCI. J Spinal Cord Med 1998;21(3): 195.

Waters RL et al: Prediction of ambulatory performance based on motor scores derived from Standards of the American Spinal Injury Association. Arch Phys Med Rehabil 1994;75:756.

Waters RL et al: Postrehabilitation outcomes after spinal cord injury caused by firearms and motor vehicle crash among ethnically diverse groups. Arch Phys Med Rehabil 1998;79:1237.

Waters RL et al: Motor and sensory recovery following complete tetraplegia. Arch Phys Med Rehabil 1993;74:242.

Waters RL et al: Emergency, acute and surgical management of spine trauma. Arch Phys Med Rehabil 1999;80:1383.

Waters RL et al: Rehabilitation of the patient with a spinal cord injury. Orthop Clin North Am 1995;26:117.

Waters RL et al: Injury pattern effect on motor recovery after traumatic spinal cord injury. Arch Phys Med Rehabil 1995;76: 440.

Waters RL et al: Motor recovery following spinal cord injury caused by stab wounds: A multicenter study. Paraplegia 1995; 33:98.

Waters RL et al: Functional hand surgery following tetraplegia. Arch Phys Med Rehabil 1996;77:86.

Waters RL et al: Gait performance after spinal cord injury. Clin Orthop 1993;288:87.

Waters RL, Adkins RH: Firearm versus motor vehicle related spinal cord injury: Preinjury factors, injury characteristics, and initial outcome comparisons among ethnically diverse groups. Arch Phys Med Rehabil 1997;78:150.

Waters RL et al: Motor recovery following spinal cord injury associated with cervical spondylosis: A collaborative study. Spinal Cord 1996;34:711.

Weiss DJ et al: Spinal cord injury and bladder recovery. Arch Phys Med Rehabil 1996;77(11):1133.

Yarkony GM et al: Spinal cord injury rehabilitation. 1. Assessment and management during acute care. Arch Phys Med Rehabil 1997;78(3 Suppl):S48.

Yoshida GM et al: Gunshot wounds to the spine. Orthop Clin North Am 1995;26:109.

STROKE

Stroke (cerebrovascular accident or brain attack) occurs when thrombosis, embolism, or hemorrhage interrupts cerebral oxygenation and causes the death of neurons in the brain. This leads to deficits in cognition and in motor and sensory function.

In the United States, where cerebrovascular accidents are the leading cause of hemiplegia in adults and the third leading cause of death, 2 million people have permanent neurologic deficits from stroke. The annual incidence of stroke is 1 in 1000, with cerebral thrombosis causing nearly three fourths of the cases. More than half of stroke victims survive and have an average life expectancy of about 6 years. Most survivors have the potential for significant function and useful lives if they receive the benefits of rehabilitation.

Neurologic Impairment & Recovery

Infarction of the cerebral cortex in the region of the brain supplied by the middle cerebral artery or one of its branches is most commonly responsible for stroke. Although the middle cerebral artery supplies the area of the cerebral cortex responsible for hand function, the anterior cerebral artery supplies the area responsible for lower extremity motion (Figure 13–11). The typical clinical picture following middle cerebral artery stroke is contralateral hemianesthesia (decreased sensation), homonymous hemianopia (visual field deficit), and spastic hemiplegia with more paralysis in the upper extremity than in the lower extremity. Because hand function requires relatively precise motor control, even for activities with assistive equipment, the prognosis for the functional use of the hand and arm is considerably worse than for the leg. Return of even gross motor control in the lower extremity may be sufficient for walking.

Infarction in the region of the anterior cerebral artery causes paralysis and sensory loss of the opposite

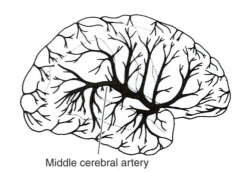

Middle cerebral artery

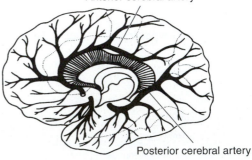

Anterior cerebral artery

Posterior cerebral artery

Figure 13–11. Cerebral artery circulation.

lower limb and to a lesser degree the arm. Patients who have cerebral arteriosclerosis and suffer repeated bilateral infarctions are likely to have severe cognitive impairment that limits their general ability to function even when motor function is good.

After stroke, motor recovery follows a fairly typical pattern. The size of the lesion and the amount of collateral circulation determine the amount of permanent damage. Most recovery occurs within 6 months, although functional improvement may continue as the patient receives further sensorimotor reeducation and learns to cope with disability.

Initially after a stroke, the limbs are completely flaccid. Over the next few weeks, muscle tone and spasticity gradually increase in the adductor muscles of the shoulder and in the flexor muscles of the elbow, wrist, and fingers. Spasticity also develops in the lower extremity muscles. Most commonly, there is an extensor pattern of spasticity in the leg, characterized by hip adduction, knee extension, and equinovarus deformities of the foot and ankle (Figure 13–12). In some cases, however, a flexion pattern of spasticity occurs, characterized by hip and knee flexion.

Whether the patient recovers the ability to move one joint independently of the others (selective movement) depends on the extent of the cerebral cortical damage. Dependence on the more neurologically primitive patterned movement (synergy) decreases as selective control improves. The extent to which motor impairment restricts function varies in the upper and lower extremities. Patterned movement is not functional in the upper extremity, but it may be useful in

the lower extremity, where the patient uses the flexion synergy to advance the limb forward and the mass extension synergy for limb stability during standing.

The final processes in sensory perception occur in the cerebral cortex, where basic sensory information is integrated to complex sensory phenomena such as vision, proprioception, and perception of spatial relationships, shape, and texture. Patients with severe parietal dysfunction and sensory loss may lack sufficient perception of space and awareness of the involved segment of their body to ambulate. Patients with severe perceptual loss may lack balance to sit, stand, or walk. A visual field deficit further interferes with limb use and may cause patients to be unaware of their own limbs.

Management

A. LOWER EXTREMITIES

1. Hemiplegia—To walk independently, the hemiplegic patient requires intact balance reactions, hip flexion to advance the limb, and stability of the limb for standing. If a patient meets these criteria and has acceptable cognition, the orthopedic surgeon can restore ambulation in most cases by prescribing an appropriate lower extremity orthosis and an upper extremity assistive device such as a cane. Surgery to rebalance the muscle forces in the leg can greatly enhance ambulation.

Except for the correction of severe contractures in nonambulatory patients, surgical procedures should be delayed for at least 6 months to allow spontaneous neurologic recovery to occur and the patient to learn how to cope with the disability. After this time, surgery may safely be performed to improve usage in the functional limb.

In the nonfunctional limb, surgery may be performed to relieve pain or correct severe hip and knee flexion contractures caused by spasticity. Most severe contractural deformities in the nonfunctional limb, however, are the result of an ineffective program of daily passive range of motion, splinting, and limb positioning.

Most hemiplegics with motor impairment have hip abductor and extensor weakness. A quad cane (cane with four feet to provide more stability) or a hemiwalker is prescribed to provide better balance. Because of paralysis in the upper extremity, the hemiplegic patient is unable to use a conventional walker.

2. Limb scissoring—Scissoring of the legs caused by overactive hip adductor muscles is a common problem. This gives the patient an extremely narrow base of support while standing and causes balance problems. When no fixed contracture of the hip adductor muscles

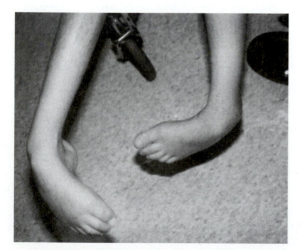

Figure 13–12. Equinovarus deformities of the feet in a patient with spasticity.

is present, transection of the anterior branches of the obturator nerve will denervate the adductors and allow the patient to stand with a broader base of support. If a contracture of the adductors has occurred, surgical release of the adductor longus, adductor brevis, and gracilis muscles should be performed (Figure 13–13).

3. Stiff-knee gait—Patients with a stiff-knee gait are unable to flex the knee during the swing phase of gait. The deformity is a dynamic one meaning that it only occurs during walking. Passive knee motion is not restricted, and the patient does not have difficulty sitting. Usually the knee is maintained in extension throughout the gait cycle. Toe drag, which is likely in the early swing phase may cause the patient to trip: thus balance and stability are also affected. The limb appears to be functionally longer. Circumduction of the involved limb, hiking of the pelvis, or contralateral limb vaulting may occur as compensatory maneuvers.

A gait study with dynamic electromyography (EMG) should be done preoperatively to document the activity of the individual muscles of the quadriceps. Dyssynergic activity is commonly seen in the rectus femoris from preswing through terminal swing throughout the gait cycle. Abnormal activity is also common in the vastus intermedius, vastus medialis, and vastus lateralis muscles. If knee flexion is improved with a block of the femoral nerve or with botulinum toxin injection of the quadriceps, the rationale for surgical intervention is strengthened. Any equinus deformity of the foot should be corrected prior to evaluation of a stiff-knee gait be-

cause equinus causes a knee extension force during stance. Because the amount of knee flexion during swing is directly related to the speed of walking, the patient should be able to ambulate with a reasonable velocity in order to benefit from surgery. Hip flexion strength is also needed for a good result because the forward momentum of the leg normally provides the inertial force to flex the knee. In the past a selective release of the rectus femoris or rectus and vastus intermedius was done to remove their inhibition of knee flexion. On average a 15 degree improvement in peak knee flexion was seen after surgery. Transfer of the rectus femoris to a hamstring tendon not only removes it as a deforming muscle force; it also converts the rectus into a corrective flexion force. This procedure provides improved knee flexion over selective release. When any of the vasti muscles are involved they can be selectively lengthened at their myotendinous junction (Figure 13–14) and knee flexion will improve.

4. Knee flexion deformity—A knee flexion deformity increases the physical demand on the quadriceps muscle, which must continually fire to hold the patient upright. Knee flexion often leads to knee instability and causes falls. It is most often caused by spasticity of the hamstring muscles. A KAFO can be used to hold the knee in extension on a temporary basis as a training aid in physical therapy. Such an orthosis, however, is difficult for the stroke patient to don and wear for permanent usage.

Surgical correction of the knee flexion deformity is the most desirable treatment. Hamstring tenotomy (Figure 13–15) eliminates the dynamic component of the deformity and generally results in a 50% correction of the contracture at the time of surgery. The residual joint contracture is then corrected by serial casting done weekly after surgery. Hamstring function posterior to the knee joint is not necessary for ambulation. In fact, ambulation may only be feasible in patients with knee flexion deformities of greater than 30 degrees if a hamstring release is done.

5. Equinus or equinovarus foot deformity—Surgical correction of an equinus deformity is indicated when the foot cannot be maintained in the neutral position with the heel in firm contact with the sole of the shoe in a well-fitted, rigid AFO. Despite a wide variety of surgical methods designed to decrease the triceps surae spasticity, none has proved more effective than Achilles tendon lengthening. In this procedure, triple hemisection tenotomy is performed via three stab incisions, with the most distal cut based medially to alleviate varus pull of the soleus muscle (Figure 13–16).

An anesthetic block of the posterior tibial nerve can be a valuable tool in preoperative assessment of the patient with equinus deformity because it will demon-

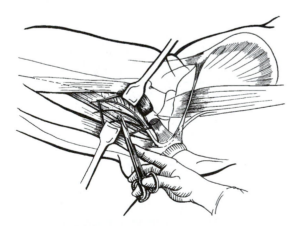

Figure 13–13. Release of the hip adductor tendons and neurectomy of the anterior branches of the obturator nerve to correct the problem of limb scissoring. (Illustration by Anthony C Berlet. Reproduced, with permission, from Keenan MAE et al: *Manual of Orthopaedic Surgery for Spasticity.* New York: Raven, 1993.)

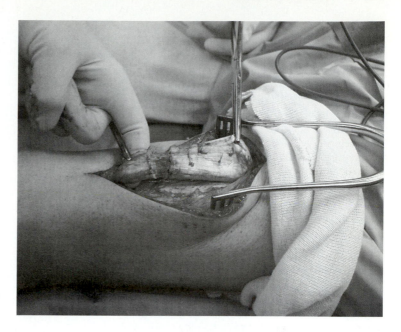

Figure 13–14. Selective lengthening of the rectus femoris tendon to correct a stiff-knee gait abnormality.

strate the potential benefits of Achilles tendon lengthening if the deformity is a result of increased muscle tone.

Surgical release of the flexor digitorum longus and brevis tendons at the base of each toe (Figure 13–17) is done prophylactically at the time of Achilles tendon lengthening, because increased ankle dorsiflexion following heel cord tenotomy increases tension on the long toe flexor and commonly leads to excessive toe flexion (toe

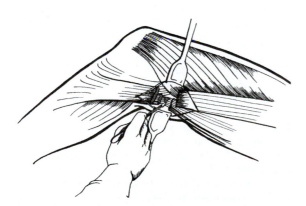

Figure 13–15. Distal release of the hamstring tendons to correct a knee flexion contracture. (Illustration by Anthony C Berlet. Reproduced, with permission, from Keenan MAE et al: *Manual of Orthopaedic Surgery for Spasticity*. New York: Raven, 1993.)

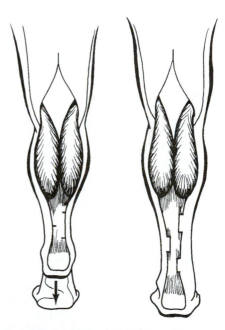

Figure 13–16. Hoke triple hemisection Achilles tendon lengthening to correct an equinus foot deformity. (Illustration by Anthony C Berlet. Reproduced, with permission, from Keenan MAE et al: *Manual of Orthopaedic Surgery for Spasticity*. New York: Raven, 1993.)

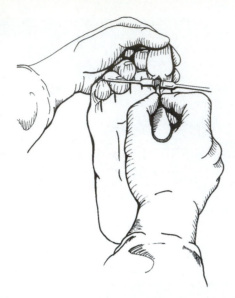

Figure 13–17. Release of the flexor digitorum longus and brevis tendons to correct the problem of toe curling. (Illustration by Anthony C Berlet. Reproduced, with permission, from Keenan MAE et al: *Manual of Orthopaedic Surgery for Spasticity*. New York: Raven, 1993.)

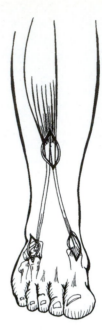

Figure 13–18. Split anterior tibial tendon transfer to correct a spastic varus foot deformity. (Illustration by Anthony C Berlet. Reproduced, with permission, from Keenan MAE et al: *Manual of Orthopaedic Surgery for Spasticity*. New York: Raven, 1993.)

curling). The flexor hallucis longus and flexor digitorum longus tendons can be transferred to the os calcis to provide additional support to the weakened calf muscles.

Surgical correction of varus deformity is indicated when the problem is not corrected by a well-fitted orthosis. It is also indicated to enable the patient to walk without an orthosis when varus deformity is the only significant problem. The tibialis anterior, tibialis posterior, extensor hallucis longus, flexor hallucis longus, flexor digitorum, and soleus pass medial to the axis of the subtalar joint and are potentially responsible for varus deformity. Electromyographic studies demonstrate that the peroneus longus and peroneus brevis are generally inactive, and the tibialis posterior is also usually inactive or minimally active.

The tibialis anterior is the key muscle responsible for varus deformity, and in most patients, this can be confirmed by visual examination or palpation while the patient walks. A procedure known as the split anterior tibial tendon transfer (Figure 13–18) diverts the inverting deforming force of the tibialis anterior to a corrective force. In this procedure, one half of the tendon is transferred laterally to the os cuboideum. When the extensor hallucis longus muscle is overactive, it can be transferred to the middorsum of the foot as well.

Treatment of equinovarus deformity consists of simultaneously performing the Achilles tendon lengthen-

ing procedure and the split anterior tibial tendon transfer. At surgery, the tibialis anterior is secured and held sufficiently taut to maintain the foot in a neutral position. After healing, 70% of patients are able to walk without an orthosis.

B. UPPER EXTREMITIES

1. Spasticity—The first objective in treating the spastic upper extremity is to prevent contracture. Severe deformities at the shoulder, elbow, and wrist are seen in the neglected or noncompliant patient. Assistive equipment can be used to position the upper extremity, to aid in prevention of contractures, and to support the shoulder. Positioning extends spastic muscles but does not subject them to sudden postural changes that trigger the stretch reflex and aggravate spasticity. Brief periods should be scheduled when the upper extremity is not suspended and time can be devoted to range-of-motion therapy and hygiene.

Most hemiplegics will not use their hand unless some selective motion is present at the fingers or thumb. Thumb opposition begins with opposition of the thumb to the side of the index finger (lateral or key pinch) and proceeds by circumduction to oppose each fingertip. In most stroke patients with selective thumb-finger extension, proximal muscle function is comparatively intact. Hence, orthotic stabilization of proximal joints is rarely necessary in the patient with a functional hand.

An overhead suspension sling attached to the wheelchair is used for patients with adductor or internal rotator spasticity of the shoulder. An alternative is an arm trough attached to the wheelchair.

It is usually not possible to maintain the wrist in neutral position with a WHO when wrist flexion spasticity is severe or when the wrist is flaccid. With minimal to moderate spasticity, either a volar or dorsal splint can be used. The splint should not extend to the fingers if the finger flexor spasticity is severe, because slight motion and sensory contact of the fingers or palm may elicit the stretch reflex or grasp response, causing the fingers to jackknife out of the splint.

2. Shoulder or arm pain—The hemiplegic shoulder deserves special attention because it is a common source of pain. A variety of different factors contribute to the painful shoulder: reflex sympathetic dystrophy, inferior subluxation, spasticity with internal rotation contracture, adhesive capsulitis, and degenerative changes about the shoulder. If early range-of-motion exercises are performed and the extremity is properly positioned with a sling to reduce subluxation, severe or chronic pain at the shoulder can usually be prevented or minimized.

The classic clinical signs of reflex sympathetic dystrophy (swelling and skin changes) may not be apparent in the hemiplegic patient. If the patient complains that the arm is painful and no cause is apparent, a technetium bone scan will assist in establishing the diagnosis (Figure 13–19). Treatment should be instituted immediately, and the patient should be given positive psychologic reinforcement. The use of narcotics must

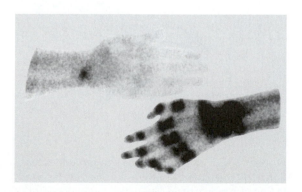

Figure 13–19. Technetium bone scan showing the periarticular increase in activity characteristic of reflex sympathetic dystrophy.

be avoided. Treatment options include the use of medications such as corticosteroids, amitriptyline, or gabapentin (Neurontin), physical therapy, or nerve blocks (stellate ganglion blocks, brachial plexus blocks, or Bier IV regional blocks). Each of these techniques is successful with some patients; however, none is reliable for all patients.

3. Shoulder contracture—Contracture of the shoulder can cause pain, hygiene problems in the axilla, and difficulty in dressing and positioning. Shoulder adduction and internal rotation are caused by spasticity and myostatic contracture of four muscles: the pectoralis major, the subscapularis, the latissimus dorsi, and the teres major.

When the deformity is not fixed, then lengthening of the pectoralis major, latissimus and teres major at their myotendinous junction provides satisfactory correction of the deformity. In a nonfunctional extremity, surgical release of all four muscles (Figure 13–20) is usually necessary to resolve the deformity. Release of the subscapularis muscle is performed without violating the glenohumeral joint capsule. The joint capsule should not be opened because instability or intra-articular adhesions may result. A Z-plasty of the axilla may be needed if the skin is contracted. After the wound has healed, an aggressive mobilization program is instituted. Gentle range-of-motion exercises are employed to correct any remaining contracture. Careful positioning of the limb in abduction and external rotation is necessary for several months to prevent recurrence.

4. Elbow flexion contracture—Persistent spasticity of the elbow flexors causes a myostatic contracture and flexion deformity of the elbow. Frequent accompanying problems include skin maceration, breakdown of the antecubital space, and compression neuropathy of the ulnar nerve.

Surgical release of the contracted muscles and gradual extension of the elbow will correct the deformity and decrease the ulnar nerve compression. The brachioradialis muscle and biceps tendon are transected. The brachialis muscle is fractionally lengthened at its myotendinous junction by transecting the tendinous fibers on the anterior surface of the muscle while leaving the underlying muscle intact (Figure 13–21). Complete release of the brachialis muscle is not performed unless a severe contracture has been present for several years. An anterior capsulectomy is not needed and should be avoided because of the associated increased stiffness and intra-articular adhesions that occur postoperatively. Anterior transposition of the ulnar nerve may be necessary to further improve ulnar nerve function.

Approximately 50% correction of the deformity can be expected at surgery without causing excessive tension on the contracted neurovascular structures. Serial casts

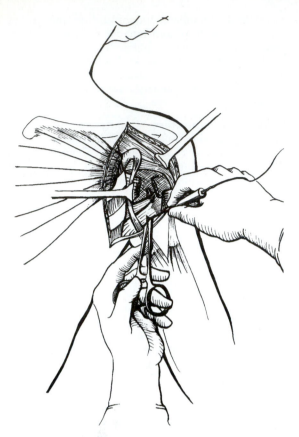

Figure 13–20. Release of the pectoralis major, subscapularis, latissimus dorsi, and teres major to correct an internal rotation and adduction contracture of the shoulder. (Illustration by Anthony C Berlet. Reproduced, with permission, from Keenan MAE et al: *Manual of Orthopaedic Surgery for Spasticity*. New York: Raven, 1993.)

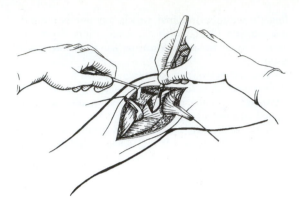

Figure 13–21. Surgery of the brachioradialis muscle, biceps tendon, and brachialis muscle to correct an elbow flexion contracture in a nonfunctional arm. (Illustration by Anthony C Berlet. Reproduced, with permission, from Keenan MAE et al: *Manual of Orthopaedic Surgery for Spasticity*. New York: Raven, 1993.)

of a passive tether to prevent a hyperextension deformity. The wrist deformity is corrected by release of the wrist flexors. A wrist arthrodesis is done to maintain the hand in a neutral position and to eliminate the need for a permanent splint. Because intrinsic muscle spasticity is always present in conjunction with severe spasticity of the extrinsic flexors, a neurectomy of the motor branches of the ulnar nerve in Guyon's canal should be routinely performed along with the superficialis-to-pro-

or drop-out casts can be used to obtain further correction over the ensuing weeks.

5. Clenched fist deformity—A spastic clenched fist deformity in a nonfunctional hand causes palmar skin breakdown and hygiene problems. Recurrent infections of the fingernail beds are also common.

Adequate flexor tendon lengthening to correct the deformity cannot be attained by fractional or myotendinous lengthening without causing discontinuity at the musculotendinous junction. Transection of the flexor tendons is not recommended because any remaining extensor muscle tone may result in an unopposed hyperextension deformity of the wrist and digits. The recommended procedure is a superficialis-to-profundus tendon transfer (Figure 13–22), which provides sufficient flexor tendon lengthening with preservation

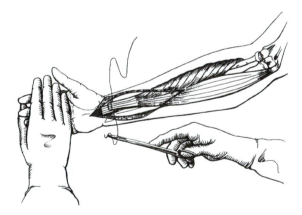

Figure 13–22. The superficialis-to-profundus tendon transfer to correct a severe clenched fist deformity in a nonfunctional hand. (Illustration by Anthony C Berlet. Reproduced, with permission, from Keenan MAE et al: *Manual of Orthopaedic Surgery for Spasticity*. New York: Raven, 1993.)

fundus tendon transfer to prevent the postsurgical development of an "intrinsic plus" deformity.

After surgery, the wrist and digits are immobilized for 4 weeks in a short arm cast extended to the fingertips.

Dorsey MK, Vaca KJ: The stroke patient and assessment of caregiver needs and patients. J Vasc Nurs 1998;16:62.

Hale LA, Eales CJ: Recovery of walking function in stroke patients after minimal rehabilitation. Physiother Res Int 1998;3:194.

Harvey RL et al: Stroke rehabilitation: Clinical predictors of resource utilization. Arch Phys Med Rehabil 1998;79:1349.

Hisey MS, Keenan MAE: Orthopaedic management of upper extremity dysfunction following stroke or brain injury. In Green DP et al (editors): *Operative Hand Surgery.* New York: Churchill Livingstone, 1998.

Jones F: The accuracy of predicting functional recovery in patients following a stroke, by physiotherapists and patients. Physiother Res Int 1998;3:244.

Keenan MAE et al: Improving calf muscle strength in patients with spastic equinovarus deformity by transfer of the long toe flexors to the os calcis. J Head Trauma Rehabil 1999;14:163.

Kwakkel G et al: Predicting disability in stroke: A critical review of the literature. Age Ageing 1996;25:479.

Lee GA, Keenan MA: Management of Lower Extremity Deformities Following Stroke and Brain Injury. In Chapman MW (editor): *Chapman's Orthopaedic Surgery,* Philadelphia: Lippincott Williams & Wilkins Publishers, 2001, pp 3201–3243.

Lincoln NB et al: Rehabilitation needs of community stroke patients. Disabil Rehabil 1998;20:457.

McDaid P, Keenan MA: Management of Upper Extremity Dysfunction Following Stroke and Brain Injury. In Chapman MW (editor): *Chapman's Orthopaedic Surgery,* Philadelphia: Lippincott Williams & Wilkins Publishers, 2001, pp 1809–1854.

Pomerance JF, Keenan MAE: Correction of severe spastic flexion contractures in the non-functional hand. J Hand Surg 1996; 21A:828.

Wressle E et al: The rehabilitation process for the geriatric stroke patient: An exploratory study of goal setting and interventions. Disabil Rehabil 1999;21:80.

GERIATRIC ORTHOPEDICS

General Principles

A major challenge facing society is the aging of the population. By the year 2020 there will be 52 million Americans over the age of 65. By 2040, 68 million people will be over the age of 65. Both the absolute numbers and proportion of elderly people is increasing dramatically. People are living longer and have higher expectations for a good quality of life. Despite this trend proportionally less disability occurs among the elderly now than in the past.

Although the passage of time, chronological age, is the convenient measure used, it is not necessarily the most precise marker of aging. A more sensitive marker would be to consider the person's functional age but this is often difficult to define and measure. Age 65 is generally considered the beginning of old age.

The young elderly are those individuals 65 to 75 years old. These people are usually functionally intact. They have isolated orthopaedic problems, such as mild osteoporosis, osteoarthrosis, overuse injuries (sports), and occasionally cancer.

The frail, very elderly are those persons who are greater than 80 years. These people tend to have multiple musculoskeletal impairments such as advanced osteoporosis, generalized muscle weakness, multiple organ diseases, and dementia.

1. Disability

The leading causes of death in the elderly are heart disease, malignant neoplasms, and cerebrovascular disease. The overall leading causes of disability in the elderly are cancer, heart disease, dementia, and musculoskeletal disorders. The leading causes of disease related disability before death are arthritis, hypertension, hearing impairment, heart disease, and orthopaedic conditions. Despite the increasing incidence of disability with aging, only 5% of Americans live in nursing homes.

When evaluating the elderly, five functional domains of disability need to be considered:

(1) *Physical activities of daily living* include activities such as bathing, dressing, eating, and walking.

(2) *Instrumental activities of daily living* are home management tasks such as shopping, meal preparation, money management, using the telephone, and performing light housework.

(3) *Cognitive functioning* is particularly important in the elderly. Dementia is one of the four leading causes of disability in the elderly and a principle reason for institutionalization.

(4) *Affective function* is important. Secondary depressions are common in the elderly and suicide is a more frequent cause of death in the elderly than in the young.

(5) *Social functioning* is less of a problem. Only one percent of the elderly rate their social interactions as inadequate.

2. Challenges for the Orthopaedic Surgeon

When working with the elderly the orthopaedic surgeon becomes a member of a multidisciplinary team. The people making up this team include internists, geriatricians, rehabilitation specialists, psychiatrists, psychologists, social workers, nutritionists, skin care specialists, physical and occupational therapists, and the "young elderly" children of the patient. Osteoporosis, fractures, arthritis, foot disorders, stroke, amputations are the most frequent causes of musculoskeletal impairment.

3. Osteoporosis

Osteoporosis is an age-related disorder characterized by decreased bone mass and increased fracture risk in the absence of other recognizable causes of bone loss. Osteoporosis can occur either as a primary disorder or secondary to other diseases.

A. PRIMARY OSTEOPOROSIS

Primary osteoporosis, the most common form of the disease, occurs in people from 51 to 65 years old with a female/male of ratio 6:1. Primary osteoporosis can be further subdivided into two types. Type I, postmenopausal osteoporosis, results from decreased circulating levels of estrogen. It is seen in postmenopausal women and affects the majority of persons older than 70 years. Bone loss is rapid. There is swift trabecular bone loss up to 8%/year. Type I osteoporosis causes primarily trabecular bone loss with only 0.5% cortical bone loss per year. Fractures occur in locations of trabecular bone loss such as the distal radius and vertebrae. The cause of primary osteoporosis is a changing hormonal milieu.

Type II, senile osteoporosis, is a consequence of aging. It causes a more global bone loss affecting cortical and cancellous bone such as in the femoral neck. Type II osteoporosis is seen in persons older than 70 years of age. The female/male ratio is 2:1. The bone loss occurs in both the trabecular and cortical bone and averages 0.3–0.5%/year. Fractures occurring as the result of type II osteoporosis typically involve the hip, pelvis, humerus, tibia, and vertebral bodies. The causes of senile osteoporosis are those seen with aging and include calcium deficiency, decreased vitamin D, and increased parathormone activity.

B. SECONDARY OSTEOPOROSIS

Secondary osteoporosis results from a variety of causes. The most common are chronic or prolonged corticosteroid use and endocrine disorders. The endocrine disorders associated with osteoporosis are hyperthyroidism; hyperparathyroidism; diabetes, Cushing's disease, and euplastic disorders.

Prevention Strategies

Restoration of bone is difficult. It is therefore imperative to maximize peak bone mass during skeletal growth and then to maintain it during maturity. This requires adequate dietary calcium and vitamin D intake. The recommended amounts for adults are 1200 mg/day of calcium and 400 mg of vitamin D. For postmenopausal women 1500 mg/day of calcium is recommended. Impact exercise has been shown effective in maintaining bone mass. It is also important to avoid those things that promote osteoporosis such as the use of tobacco products and excessive alcohol consumption.

Diagnosis

Osteoporosis is a clinical diagnosis often made following a fracture. Radiographic findings include osteopenia (seen with > 30% mineral loss), loss of horizontal trabeculae in vertebral bodies, thoracic wedge fractures; lumbar spine end-plate fractures, stress fractures of pelvis; and fractures of humerus, wrist, hip, supracondylar femur, tibial plateau. Quantification of bone mass is done for confirmation and follow-up. Dual energy x-ray absorption (DEXA) is used to quantify bone mass. The following criteria for diagnosis are based on the DEXA scan:

Normal—within 1 SD of young adult reference
Osteopenia—between 1.0–2.4 SD below reference
Osteoporosis—2.5 or more SD below reference
Severe osteoporosis—2.5 plus one or more fragility fractures

Treatment

Calcium alone will not prevent bone loss during the early postmenopausal period but adequate daily calcium replacement is helpful. In late menopause (> 6 years) calcium replacement does reduce bone loss. Weight-bearing exercise has also been shown useful in maintaining bone mass.

Newer treatments using bisphosphonates have recently shown promise in treating osteoporosis. The bisphosphonates are a class of compounds similar to pyrophosphate that are readily adsorbed by bone mineral surfaces. Once bound, they inhibit the bone absorption activity of osteoclasts. Currently two bisphosphonates are available for clinical use: alendronate sodium (Fosamax) and risedronate sodium (Actonel).

Only about one third of women in the United States diagnosed with osteoporosis during the 1990s were offered treatment for the condition. Fewer than 2% of the women age 60 and older were diagnosed with osteoporosis, but the rate increased from 1.2% in 1993 to 2.7% in 1997. Overall, 36% of women diagnosed with osteoporosis were prescribed calcium, vitamin D, or drugs to treat the disease, but this also increased, from 20% in 1993 to 55% in 1997.

Exercise

The ability to walk safely is vital for independent living. Both strength and endurance determine the capacity for independent movement. Muscle strength is associated with the capacity to perform activities of daily living. A reduction in strength with age is attributed to:

(1) a loss of muscle mass due to smaller and fewer fibers

(2) a loss of motor neurons (anterior horn cells)

(3) changes in muscle architecture

(4) a defect in the excitation-contraction mechanism

(5) psychosocial changes leading to reduced capacity to activate motor units.

Strength training can lead to major functional improvements in the elderly. The plasticity of the motor system to adapt to a training load appears to be maintained into the tenth decade of life. Strength training has no effect on the central determinants of aerobic capacity such as maximum heart rate, blood pressure hemoglobin concentration, and blood volume.

Aerobic exercise does lead to increased endurance and functional capacity. Endurance is the time a person can maintain either a static force or a power level involving a combination of concentric or eccentric muscular contractions. The stress that exercise imposes on a person and the tolerance or endurance for that exercise intensity depends on how much energy is needed to perform the task in relation to the person's maximal capacity. With training, activities become easier to perform. The person has increased endurance for submaximal exercise. Improvements in movement can lower the energy cost of an activity.

4. Arthritis

Osteoarthritis is very prevalent in the elderly. Total joint arthroplasty has dramatically improved the mobility and quality of life for the elderly. A variety of studies have confirmed the appropriateness and effectiveness of both total hip and total knee arthroplasty in the elderly with low complication rates. The elderly patient is more likely to require the use of an upper extremity assistive device for ambulation following joint replacement.

5. Fractures

A. General Considerations

In the elderly fractures result from low-energy injuries. Falls in the home most frequently result in fractures of the hip, distal radius, pelvis, proximal humerus, and ribs. Approximately 90% of fractures of the pelvis, hip, and forearm result from a fall. Only 3–5% of falls result in fractures.

Many of the risk factors for fracture are also risk factors for falls. Risk factors can be divided into categories. Risk factors associated with aspects of aging include primary osteoporosis, impaired vision or balance; gait abnormalities; and loss of muscle and fat padding the bones. Environmental risk factors consist of uneven surfaces; slippery surfaces; obstacles such as throw rugs, pets, and steps; poor lighting; and lack of railings or other supports for balance. Fall prevention programs include home safety measures such as the installation of safety bars in the bathtub and shower, elimination of heavily waxed floors and slippery rugs, and the use of rubber sole shoes with low wide heels that provide more stability.

Genetic factors are seen in both gender and race. Women sustain more fractures than men. Caucasians have more fractures than African Americans. Illnesses that are commonly associated with fractures include stroke, syncope, hypotension, secondary osteoporosis, Parkinson's disease, dementia, and paraparesis. The use of medications such as benzodiazepines, tricyclic antidepressants, antipsychotics, corticosteroids, and barbiturates are connected with fractures. Lifestyle factors include exercise, nutrition, alcohol or other substance abuse, immobilization, and shoe style.

Other factors contribute to the risk of traumatic fractures occurring in falls. The first is the orientation of the fall. A fall that happens while standing still or walking very slowly imparts little or no forward momentum so the point of impact will be near the hip. Gait velocity slows with aging putting the hip more at risk of injury in a fall. Protective responses during a fall decrease with age. Local shock absorbers, muscle and fat, that surround the bone decrease with age. Bone strength is less secondary to the osteoporosis associated with aging.

B. Hip Fractures

Fractures of the hip are classified by location and severity. The basic considerations are whether the fracture occurs in the intracapsular or extracapsular area and the stability of the fracture pattern. Intracapsular fractures occur along the neck of the femur. When they are displaced, the blood supply to the femoral head is likely to have been disrupted. This increases the possibility of osteonecrosis.

Treatment of hip fractures is operative whenever possible. The nonoperative treatment of hip fractures is very occasionally chosen for patients at high medical risk. It is sometimes recommended for demented, nonambulatory patients. The nonoperative treatment of a hip fracture involves months of bed rest and sometimes traction. It requires excellent nursing care to avoid decubitus ulcers and respiratory dysfunction. Fracture malunion, limb length inequality, pain, and higher mortality rates are common with nonoperative care. The chances for eventual ambulation are only 55% compared with 76% for patients treated operatively.

The basic principles of treatment of hip fractures have been well established. Nondisplaced fractures of the femoral neck are usually treated with multiple pins or screws. Displaced fractures of the femoral neck are usually treated with a hemiarthroplasty because of the high incidence of avascular necrosis. Stable intertrochanteric fractures are generally treated with a sliding screw and side plate system. Unstable intertrochanteric fractures may require additional measures to gain adequate medial support. In very osteoporotic bone, it may be necessary to add methyl methacrylate bone cement to gain sufficient fixation and stability. When a patient is known to have severe arthritis, a primary total hip arthroplasty may be performed.

The postoperative rehabilitation of the elderly patient is critical to a successful outcome. Non-weight–bearing ambulation is extremely difficult and more often impossible for elderly patients. Every effort should be made in the operative treatment to gain enough stability of the fracture to allow weight bearing as tolerated. The patient should be mobilized on the first or second day after surgery to prevent the many complications of immobility. Pain management is important to allow mobilization but over sedation of the elderly patient needs to be avoided. When a prosthesis has been inserted, dislocation must be avoided. The elderly patient may not remember the precautions. Use of elevated chairs and toilet seats will help to avoid the excessive hip flexion associated with posterior dislocation. A knee immobilizer splint while in bed will prevent knee flexion that in turn results in flexion of the hip. Occasionally it is prudent to place the patient in a hip brace which limits flexion and adduction while soft-tissue healing occurs.

C. Fractures of the Pelvis

A common pelvic classification is based on whether or not the ring of the pelvis is disrupted because this indicates the amount of energy involved with the initial trauma. A fracture which does not disrupt the pelvic ring such as a pubic ramus fracture is a low-energy injury. Formerly pelvic fractures were associated with high-energy trauma, were displaced, and occurred in young individuals. With the aging of America now more than 50% of fractures occur in those over 60 years of age, with a preponderance occurring in women. The majority of pelvis fractures in the elderly are low-energy injuries and can be treated nonoperatively with analgesia and bed rest. Early mobilization is desirable to prevent the complications of immobility. Full weight bearing is allowed. A walker or other assistive device is useful to decrease pain and increase stability during walking. Stool softeners are often helpful. Fractures of the coccyx and sacrum are treated in a similar manner.

D. Fractures of the Distal Femur

The management of distal femur fractures in the elderly patients must be individualized. Advanced age in itself is not a contraindication to surgery. The objects of surgical treatment of the distal femur are anatomic reduction and stable fixation. In the presence of severe osteopenia, stable fixation is difficult. The addition of methyl methacrylate or long-stem knee replacement can help with stability. Occasionally a postoperative cast brace is needed to supplement the internal fixation.

E. Fractures of the Forearm

Most fractures of the distal radius (Colles' fracture) can be treated by closed reduction and casting. Significant loss of radial height and dorsal comminution can occur in osteoporotic bone even after lower energy injuries. In this situation, most surgeons would agree that external fixation and bone grafting of the fracture are warranted to obtain and maintain a more anatomic reduction. Early range-of-motion exercises for both the shoulder and the fingers should be encouraged to avoid stiffness.

F. Fractures of the Proximal Humerus

Fractures of the proximal humerus account for 4–5% of all fractures and occur most commonly in the elderly. Humeral fractures in the elderly are minimally displaced 80% of the time. In these cases, sling immobilization is used to control pain. Pendulum exercises are begun early to prevent excessive stiffness in the shoulder. Limited external rotation of the shoulder predisposes to a future spiral fracture of the humerus during dressing. In unstable and markedly displaced fractures of the humeral head, a hemiarthroplasty can be considered. If coexisting severe osteoarthritis of the glenohumeral joint is present, a total shoulder arthroplasty can be considered.

6. Stroke

Stroke is a common cause of disability in the elderly. This topic is covered in detail elsewhere in this chapter.

7. Foot Disorders

The foot tends to widen with age as the transverse arch support weakens and abnormal bony alignments of the foot become common. Surgical reconstruction of foot deformities may be contraindicated in the frail elderly patient, particularly due to peripheral vascular disease. Nonoperative treatment consists of active and passive range-of-motion exercises of the foot to maximize flexibility. Strengthening exercises of the lower extremity can be useful to improve the overall gait pattern. The patient should try to optimize body weight to eliminate excessive forces on the foot. Functional orthoses of a semirigid material with little or no posting may improve the foot position and provide symptomatic relief. Accommodative orthoses of a soft material may also be used. These soft orthoses are designed to control foot posture and eliminate areas of pressure but are not intended to correct the foot position. Orthoses are used in combination with soft extra-depth shoes that provide more clearance for deformities of the toes. Flat shoes are helpful for forefoot deformities because they prevent the foot sliding forward in the shoe. A shoe with a low heel is desirable for patients with a severe pronation deformity because the Achilles tendon is commonly tight. Placing the heel cord on stretch only increases the pronation forces on the foot.

8. Amputation

The majority of amputations done in a civilian population are of the lower extremity. Most amputations are done in the sixth decade of life or later so this is largely a problem of the elderly. The issues associated with amputation are discussed in the chapter on amputation.

Esquenazi A, Thompson E: Management of foot disorders in the elderly. In Felsthal G et al (editors): *Rehabilitation of the Aging and Elderly Patient.* Baltimore: Williams and Wilkins, 1994, pp 153.

Frontera WR, Meredith CN: Exercise in the rehabilitation of the elderly. In Felsthal G et al (editors): *Rehabilitation of the Aging and Elderly Patient.* Baltimore: Williams and Wilkins, 1994, pp 35.

Garrison SJ: Geriatric stroke rehabilitation. In Felsthal G et al (editors): *Rehabilitation of the Aging and Elderly Patient.* Baltimore: Williams and Wilkins, 1994, p 175.

Gehlbach SH et al: Recognition of osteoporosis by primary care physicians. Am J Public Health 2002;92:271.

Karpman RR, Del Mar NB: Supracondylar femoral fractures in the frail elderly. Clin Orthop 1995; 316:21.

Karpman RR: Foot problems in the geriatric patient. Clin Orthop 1995;316:59.

Levy RN et al: Outcome and long-term results following total hip replacement in elderly patients. Clin Orthop 1995;316:25.

Lowner JH, Koval JK: Polytrauma in the elderly. Clin Orthop 1995;318:136.

Nicholas JJ, Rosenberg AN: Arthritis and arthroplasties. In Felsthal G et al (editors): *Rehabilitation of the Aging and Elderly Patient.* Baltimore: Williams and Wilkins, 1994, p. 97.

Pillar T et al: Operated vs non-operated hip fractures in a geriatric rehabilitation hospital. Disabil Studies 1989;10:104.

Silver JJ, Einhorn TA: Osteoporosis and aging. Current update. Clin Orthop 1995;316:10.

Stein BD, Felsenthal G: Rehabilitation of fractures in the geriatric population. In Felsthal G et al (editors): *Rehabilitation of the Aging and Elderly Patient.* Baltimore: Williams and Wilkins, 1994, p 123.

Tankersley WS, Hungerford DS: Total knee arthroplasty in the very aged. Clin Orthop 1995; 316:45.

Zimmerman SI et al: Demography and epidemiology of disabilities in the aged. In Felsthal G et al (editors): *Rehabilitation of the Aging and Elderly Patient.* Baltimore: Williams and Wilkins, 1994, p 11.

BRAIN INJURY

Brain injury resulting from trauma to the head is a leading cause of death and disability. Head injury is at least twice as common in males as in females and occurs most often in people age 15–24 years. About half of the injuries result from motor vehicle accidents. In the United States, 410,000 new cases of traumatic brain injury can be expected each year, with each case presenting a challenge to the team of health care providers involved in providing emergency treatment and long-term management.

Neurologic Impairment & Recovery

The Glasgow coma scale (Table 13–3) is frequently used to evaluate eye opening, motor response, and

Table 13–3. The Glasgow coma scale.

Response	Description	Numerical Value
Eye opening	Spontaneous response	4
	Response to speech	3
	Response to pain	2
	No response	1
Motor response	Obeying response	6
	Localized response	5
	Withdrawal	4
	Abnormal flexion	3
	Extension	2
	No response	1
Verbal response	Oriented conversation	5
	Confused conversation	4
	Inappropriate words	3
	Incomprehensible sounds	2
	No response	1

Adapted, with permission, from: Teasdale G, and Jennett B: Assessment of coma and impaired consciousness. A practical scale. Lancet 1974;2:81.

verbal response of patients with impaired consciousness. Analysis of scores from patients in several countries has shed light on the chances for survival and neurologic recovery. According to the data, about 50% of patients with impaired consciousness survived. Six months after injury, moderate or good neurologic recovery was seen in 82% of patients with initial (24-h) Glasgow scores of 11 or higher, 68% of patients with initial scores of 8 to 10, 34% with initial scores of 5 to 7, and 7% with initial scores of 3 or 4. Age was an important factor related to neurologic outcome, with 62% of patients under 20 years of age and 46% of patients between 20 and 29 years showing moderate or good recovery.

The incidence of good recovery declines not only with advancing age but also with advancing duration of coma. Patients recovering from coma within the first 2 weeks of injury have a 70% chance of good recovery. The recovery rate drops to 39% in the third week and to 17% in the fourth week. Decerebrate or decorticate posturing indicates a brain stem injury and is indicative of a poor prognosis.

Management

The rehabilitation process has three distinct phases: the acute injury period, the subacute period of neurologic recovery, and the residual period of functional adaptation. Health care workers from a variety of disciplines are involved in each phase.

A. PHASES OF PATIENT CARE AND REHABILITATION

1. Acute injury phase—The initial phase of rehabilitation begins as soon as the patient reaches the acute care hospital. Brain injury is frequently the result of a high-velocity accident. Diagnosis is problematic because multiple injuries are common, resuscitation and other lifesaving efforts make a complete examination difficult, and the patient who is comatose or disoriented cannot assist in the history or physical examination.

Under the circumstances, three important principles should be followed. The first is to make an accurate diagnosis based on a thorough examination. Fractures or dislocations are missed in 11% of patients, and peripheral nerve injuries are missed in 34%. The second is to assume that the patient will make a good neurologic recovery. Basic treatment principles should not be waived on the erroneous assumption that the patient will not survive. The third principle is to anticipate uncontrolled limb motion and lack of patient cooperation. The patient often goes through a period of agitation as neurologic recovery progresses. Traction and external fixation devices are best avoided for extremity injuries. Open reduction and internal fixation of fractures and dislocations will diminish complications, require less nursing care, allow for earlier mobilization, and result in fewer residual deformities.

2. Subacute phase of neurologic recovery—During the subacute phase, when the patient is generally in a rehabilitation facility, spontaneous neurologic recovery occurs. During this recovery period, which may last from 12 to 18 months, spasticity is frequently present and heterotopic ossification may develop. Management is aimed at preventing limb deformities, maintaining a functional arc of motion in the joints, and meeting both the physical and the psychologic needs of the patient.

3. Residual phase or period of functional adaptation—When neurologic recovery has reached a plateau, the third phase of rehabilitation begins. Medical and surgical management is aimed at correction of residual limb deformities and excision of heterotopic ossification, while specialists from various disciplines continue moving toward the goals planned for the individual patient.

B. THE TEAM APPROACH TO PATIENT CARE AND REHABILITATION

Members of the rehabilitation team are involved in setting short-term goals, which are meant to be accomplished by the time of discharge from the rehabilitation program, and long-term goals, which will take an extended period of time to achieve. The identification of needs and the setting of goals are performed independently by health care workers from each discipline. The team members then meet to discuss their goals and draw up a coordinated plan.

1. Medical management—General medical goals are usually straightforward. Because most patients with traumatic brain injuries are younger persons, chronic premorbid illnesses are uncommon. Prevention and treatment of infections are important goals, especially while shunts, tubes, and catheters are in place. If seizures are present, controlling them without causing sedation is vital.

In patients with decreased range of motion in a joint, the cause of the problem should be explored. Possible causes include increased muscle tone, pain, myostatic contracture, periarticular heterotopic ossification, an undetected fracture or dislocation, and lack of patient cooperation secondary to diminished cognition. Peripheral nerve blocks with local anesthetics are useful in distinguishing between severe spasticity and fixed contractures.

Phenol blocks or botulinum toxin injections are used to decrease spasticity only during the period of potential neurologic recovery. The rationale for phenol injection is that by the time the nerve has regenerated, the patient will have recovered more control of the affected muscle.

The technique for administering the phenol block will depend on the anatomic accessibility and composition of the nerve; the direct injection of a peripheral nerve gives the most complete and long-lasting block. If a peripheral nerve has a large sensory component, however, direct injection is not recommended, because loss of sensation is undesirable and some patients may develop painful hyperesthesia. In some cases, it is necessary to surgically dissect the individual motor branches of a nerve that runs to a muscle and inject each branch separately. In other cases, the motor points of the muscles can be localized using a needle electrode and nerve stimulator and then injected. Motor point injections do not completely relieve spasticity but can be helpful in reducing muscle tone. The duration of motor point blocks is approximately 2 months, and the blocks can be repeated as necessary.

Botulinum toxin is injected directly into the muscle belly. The onset of action is delayed but lasts for approximately 3 months. The injections can be repeated as needed and do not result in any scarring of the muscle. The limitation of botulinum toxin is the total dose tolerated at a given time and its high cost relative to phenol.

2. Nursing care—Nursing goals concentrate on basic bodily needs such as nutrition, hygiene, and handling of secretions. Removal of tubes at the earliest possible time is a desirable goal.

Tracheostomy tubes are commonly used in patients with brain injury. General principles of care include changing an uncuffed tube as soon as possible to prevent pressure necrosis of the trachea; adding mist if necessary to provide moisture to the artificial airway; establishing suctioning procedures to prevent trauma and infection; and eliminating the dressing once the tracheostomy incision is healed, because the dressing can be a source of infection. The size of the tube is gradually reduced, and the tube is then plugged to tolerance. When continual plugging is tolerated for 3 consecutive days, the tube can be removed.

Feeding tubes are also commonly used. If oral feeding is not anticipated in the near future, a percutaneous endoscopic gastrostomy tube is recommended. If oral feeding is anticipated soon, a nasogastric tube is inserted, cleaned daily, and changed once a week. Instituting and carrying out an oral feeding program will require the combined efforts of the nursing and physical therapy staffs. Head and trunk control are necessary to provide alignment of swallowing structures. The presence of a cough reflex indicates some measure of laryngeal control and the ability to clear the airway. The presence of a swallowing reflex indicates inherent coordination of swallowing structures. The gag reflex, although protective, is not necessary for functional swallowing. Oral feeding should be started with thickened liquids and pureed foods, which provide more oral stimulus and allow time to initiate swallowing. Thin liquids are more easily aspirated.

The ability to inhibit voiding is generally a cognitive function. Restoring continence in the brain-injured patient will require a consistent routine with repeated instructions and positive feedback. Bowel programs should be initiated as soon as the patient begins taking nourishment via the gastrointestinal tract. Again, a consistent routine is most successful.

3. Cognitive and neuropsychologic management—The return of cognitive abilities follows the same sequence of stages that normal cognitive development follows, with each new level of cognitive function stemming from the previous level. The eight levels are shown in Table 13–4. Cognitive and behavioral management focuses on providing stimulation for patients with a level II or III response; providing structure for patients with a level IV, V, or VI response; and encouraging community activities for patients with a level VII or VIII response.

Memory loss and diminished cognitive function are frequently the most pervasive limitations to overall function. Cognitive retraining is an essential part of the rehabilitation process at every stage. As cognition increases and the patient becomes more aware of the injury, he or she also becomes increasingly aware of the possible consequences of the injury and will require counseling and psychologic support.

4. Speech therapy—After traumatic brain injury, patients may have temporary or permanent physical handicaps that prevent them from communicating ef-

Table 13–4. Cognitive function.

Level	Description
I	No response
II	Generalized response
III	Localized response
IV	Confused, agitated response
V	Confused, inappropriate response
VI	Confused, appropriate response
VII	Automatic, appropriate response
VIII	Purposeful, appropriate response

Adapted, with permission, from: Malkmus D et al: Rehabilitation of the Head-Injured Adult. Comprehenisve Cognitive Management. Professional Staff Association of Rancho Los Amigos Hospital, Inc: Downey, CA. 1980.

fectively. In communicating with nonverbal patients, a variety of methods and devices can be used, ranging from yes-no signals to communication boards and electronic devices. Patients will need to acquire at least a minimal level of attentional, memory, and organizational skills to facilitate use of such communication devices. In verbal patients, language disorders may be present owing to an underlying cognitive disruption following head trauma. The most frequent residual language disorders are those seen in the areas of work retrieval and auditory processing. Language therapy in patients with these long-term disorders should be directed toward reorganization of the cognitive process.

5. Physical therapy—Areas of concern in physical therapy include patient positioning, mobility, and performance of daily activities. Making it possible for bedridden patients to sit can significantly improve the quality of life and greatly enhance the opportunities to interact with other people. In some patients, casts or orthotic devices may be required to maintain the desired limb positions. Aggressive joint range-of-motion exercises are necessary to prevent contractures.

Among the factors that influence whether a patient will be able to walk include limb stability, motor control, good balance reactions, and adequate proprioception. Equipment and devices to aid in movement (canes, walkers, wheelchairs, etc) should always be of the least complex design to accomplish the goal and should be chosen on the basis of the individual patient's cognitive and physical level of function.

In developing appropriate exercises and activities for a patient, the physical therapist should consider factors such as the joint range of motion, muscle tone, motor control, and cognitive functions of the patient. Even the confused and agitated patient may respond to simple, familiar functional activities such as washing the face and brushing the teeth. Patients with higher cognitive function should be encouraged to carry out hygiene, grooming, dressing, and feeding activities.

6. Surgical management of residual musculoskeletal problems—After neurologic recovery has stabilized, surgical procedures may be indicated to correct residual limb deformities and to excise heterotopic ossification.

a. Correction of limb deformities in the lower extremities—In functional lower limbs, surgery is most often directed at correcting the equinovarus deformity of the foot (see Figure 13–12). The procedures needed for correction of the deformity are determined by clinical evaluation combined with laboratory assessment using dynamic polyelectromyography. Commonly several procedures are done simultaneously: lengthening of the Achilles tendon (see Figure 13–16), release of the flexor digitorum longus, flexor hallucis longus and flexor brevis tendons (see Figure 13–17), a split anterior

tibial tendon transfer (see Figure 13–18), transfer of the flexor digitorum longus tendon to the heel. The object of surgery is to provide a plantigrade foot for standing and walking and the surgery is highly successful in this goal. Seventy percent of patients are able to ambulate without a brace after surgery.

A stiff-knee gait is a common deformity that causes the patient to hike the pelvis and circumduct the leg for clearance of the foot during the swing phase of walking. Inappropriate activity in the quadriceps muscle at this time prevents knee flexion. If the vasti muscles of the quadriceps muscle are firing out of phase, the affected head or heads can be surgically lengthened (see Figure 13–14) to allow knee flexion while retaining quadriceps function. Transfer of the rectus femoris muscle to the sartorius or gracilis muscle will provide active knee flexion during swing.

In nonfunctional lower limbs, surgery commonly consists of releasing contractures of the hips and knees.

b. Correction of limb deformities in the upper extremities—In functional upper limbs, surgery is frequently needed to correct problems of the wrist, fingers, and thumbs. If active hand opening is restricted by flexor spasticity, lengthening of the extrinsic finger flexors (Figure 13–23) will weaken the overactive flexors and improve hand function while preserving the ability of the patient to grasp objects. In cases in which spastic thenar muscles cause thumb-in-palm deformity, a procedure

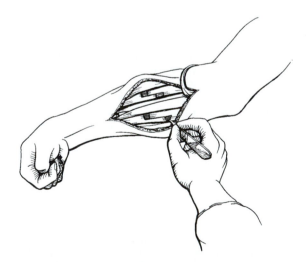

Figure 13–23. Lengthening of the extrinsic finger flexors to correct the problem of flexor spasticity and improve hand function while preserving the ability to grasp objects. (Illustration by Anthony C Berlet. Reproduced, with permission, from Keenan MAE et al: *Manual of Orthopaedic Surgery for Spasticity.* New York: Raven, 1993.)

consisting of proximal release of the thenar muscles (Figure 13–24) will correct the problem while preserving function of the thumb. In some patients, adequate placement of the hand for functional activities is impaired by elbow spasticity, although triceps function is generally normal. In these patients, lengthening the elbow flexors (Figure 13–25) will enhance the ability to extend the elbow smoothly while preserving active flexion.

In nonfunctional upper limbs, common procedures consist of releasing various contractures and performing neurectomies to eliminate muscle spasticity. The problems of shoulder contracture, elbow contracture, and clenched fist deformity are discussed in the section on stroke (see previous discussion), and the surgical procedures used in their treatment are shown in Figures 13–20, 13–21, and 13–22.

c. Excision of heterotopic ossification—Surgical measures for treatment of this problem are discussed in the next section of this chapter.

d. Occupational therapy and social services—Before patients are released from the hospital or rehabilitation facility, it is important to make sure that they and their families are informed about social service agencies, support groups, and special programs that can be of help. Social adjustment and the resumption of occupational pursuits and leisure activities are dependent on the recovery of mental factors first, personality status second, and physical factors third. Physical factors are more responsive to rehabilitation than are mental, personality, or social factors. Mental impairment, however,

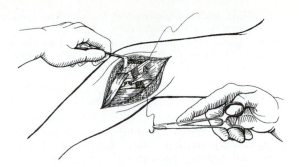

Figure 13–25. Lengthening of the elbow flexors to correct flexor spasticity and improve movement of the elbow. (Illustration by Anthony C Berlet. Reproduced, with permission, from Keenan MAE et al: *Manual of Orthopaedic Surgery for Spasticity.* New York: Raven, 1993.)

interferes the most with independence in activities of daily living.

Botte MJ et al: Heterotopic ossification in neuromuscular disorders. Orthopedics 1997;20:335.

Esquenazi A et al: Dynamic polyelectromyography, neurolysis, and chemodenervation with botulinum toxin A for assessment and treatment of gait dysfunction. Adv Neurol: Gait Disord 2001;87:321.

Hillier SL, Metzer J: Awareness and perceptions of outcomes after traumatic brain injury. Brain Inj 1997;11:525.

Hisey MS, Keenan MAE: Orthopaedic management of upper extremity dysfunction following stroke or brain injury. In Green DP et al (editors): *Operative Hand Surgery.* New York: Churchill Livingstone, 1998.

Keenan MAE, Haider T: The formation of heterotopic ossification after traumatic brain injury: A biopsy study with ultrastructural analysis. J Head Trauma Rehabil 1996;11:8.

Keenan MAE et al: Dynamic electromyography to assess elbow spasticity. J Hand Surg Am 1990;15:607.

Keenan MAE et al: Selective release of spastic elbow flexors in the patient with brain injury. J Head Trauma Rehabil 1996;11:8.

Keenan MA et al: A neuro-orthopaedic approach to the management of common patterns of upper motoneuron dysfunction after brain injury. J Neuro Rehabil 1999;12:119.

Kolessar DJ et al: Functional outcome following surgical resection of heterotopic ossification in patients with brain injury. J Head Trauma Rehabil 1996;11:78.

Lee GA, Keenan MA: Management of lower extremity deformities following stroke and brain injury. In Chapman MW (editor): *Chapman's Orthopaedic Surgery.* Philadelphia: Lippincott Williams & Wilkins Publishers, 2001, pp 3201–3243.

McDaid P, Keenan MA: Management of upper extremity dysfunction following stroke and brain injury. In Chapman MW (editor): *Chapman's Orthopaedic Surgery.* Philadelphia: Lippincott Williams & Wilkins Publishers, 2001, pp 1809–1854.

Mayer NH et al: Analysis and management of spasticity, contracture, and impaired motor control. In Horn ND, Zasler LJ

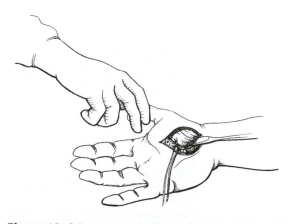

Figure 13–24. Proximal release of the thenar muscles to correct a thumb-in-palm deformity while preserving function of the thumb. (Illustration by Anthony C Berlet. Reproduced, with permission, from Keenan MAE et al: *Manual of Orthopaedic Surgery for Spasticity.* New York: Raven, 1993.)

(editors): *Medical Rehabilitation of Traumatic Brain Injury.* Hanley & Belfus, Philadelphia, 1996.

Young S, Keenan MAE: Extremity fractures in the brain-injured patient. In Nickel VL, Botte MJ (editors): *Orthopaedic Rehabilitation.* New York: Churchill Livingstone, 1992.

HETEROTOPIC OSSIFICATION

Heterotopic ossification is commonly detected 2 months after traumatic brain injury or spinal cord injury and is characterized by increasing pain and decreasing range of motion about a joint. The problem affects adults but is virtually unheard of in children. Although the cause of heterotopic ossification is unknown, a genetic predisposition is suspected. Unidentified humoral factors that enhance osteogenesis have been demonstrated in the sera of patients with brain injury. Other contributing factors include soft-tissue trauma and spasticity.

Clinical Findings

Clinically significant heterotopic ossification is seen in 20% of adults with traumatic brain injuries or spinal cord injuries and may affect one joint or multiple joints. The overall rate of joint ankylosis is 16%. In affected patients, the bone forms in association with spastic muscles, and the alkaline phosphatase level is elevated. Bone scans may aid in early diagnosis, and the diagnosis is most commonly confirmed by radiographs.

In 27% of patients with heterotopic ossification, shoulder involvement is found inferomedial to the glenohumeral joint. Although ankylosis of the joint in these cases is unusual, motion may be sufficiently restricted to require surgical resection. Elbow involvement is seen in 26% of patients with heterotopic ossification and in 89% of those who suffered a fracture or dislocation about the elbow. When ossification forms posterior to the elbow joint, pressure neuritis of the ulnar nerve is common. Anterior transposition of the ulnar nerve is frequently required to prevent entrapment, and this procedure also facilitates later bone resection. Joint ankylosis is a common complication in patients with elbow involvement. Hip involvement is seen in 44% of patients who form ectopic bone. Bilateral hip involvement and joint ankylosis are common in these patients. Heterotopic ossification in the knee joint is less common but significantly impedes both flexion and extension of the joint.

Management

A. Early Measures

Aggressive treatment of spasticity is necessary because this problem appears to play an etiologic role in mechanically stimulating bone formation. To eliminate spasticity in the muscle groups adjacent to the bone formation, phenol blocks are administered. To prevent the deposition of calcium crystals in the collagen matrix of the periarticular connective tissue, etidronate disodium (Didronel) is used. When the heterotopic bone is detected very early, the use of intravenous etidronate sodium 300 mg for 3 days followed by oral therapy has been shown to be very effective. The recommended dosage is 20 mg/kg/d orally in a single dose, and the drug should be taken on an empty stomach for proper absorption. Anti-inflammatory medications are also used to control the intense inflammatory reaction that occurs during the formation of heterotopic bone. The most commonly documented medication is indomethacin, 75–150 mg daily but in theory other medications are equally effective. Physical therapy is aimed at providing gentle range of motion to the joint to prevent ankylosis. Forceful joint manipulation is not advised because this can cause fractures or soft-tissue damage with contracture formation.

B. Definitive Treatment

Surgical excision is the definitive treatment for heterotopic ossification. To prevent recurrence of the problem, excision should be delayed until the heterotopic bone is fully mature. A true bone cortex should be visible radiographically. The serum alkaline phosphatase level does not need to be normal. If the patient has voluntary motion about the joint, surgical excision will predictably result in an increased range of motion. Following surgery a single dose of radiation therapy (800 rads) and oral etidronate therapy for 6 weeks is used to prevent recurrence. Physical therapy is continued after surgery.

Banovac K et al: Treatment of heterotopic ossification after spinal cord injury. *J Spinal Cord Med* 1997;20:60.

Botte MJ et al: Heterotopic ossification in neuromuscular disorders. Orthopedics 1997;20:335.

Burd TA et al: Indomethacin compared with localized irradiation for the prevention of heterotopic ossification following surgical treatment of acetabular fractures. J Bone Joint Surg Am 2001;83-A:1783.

Garland DE: A clinical perspective on common forms of acquired heterotopic ossification. Clin Orthop 1991;263:13.

Keenan MAE, Haider T: The formation of heterotopic ossification after traumatic brain injury: A biopsy study with ultrastructural analysis. J Head Trauma Rehabil 1996;11:8.

Kolessar DJ et al: Functional outcome following surgical resection of heterotopic ossification in patients with brain injury. J Head Trauma Rehabil 1996; 11:78.

Lazarus MD et al: Heterotopic ossification resection about the elbow. J Neuro Rehabil 1999;12:145.

Moore TJ: Functional outcome following surgical excision of heterotopic ossification in patients with traumatic brain injury. J Orthop Trauma 1993;7:11.

Schaeffer MA, Sosner J: Heterotopic ossification: Treatment of established bone with radiation therapy. Arch Phys Med Rehabil 1995;76:284.

Taly AB et al: Heterotopic ossification in non-traumatic myelopathies. Spinal Cord 1999;37:47.

Tsur A et al: Relationship between muscular tone, movement and periarticular new bone formation in postcoma-unaware (pcu) patients. Brain Inj 1996;10:259.

RHEUMATOID ARTHRITIS

Rheumatoid arthritis is a systemic disease that affects connective tissue and results in chronic inflammatory synovitis. The cause of the disease remains unknown. An infectious agent, perhaps viral, is suspected to be the initiating factor. A genetic predisposition may also be a factor.

Immune mechanisms are involved, as evidenced by the presence of large numbers of lymphocytes in the synovial tissue and by the presence of rheumatoid factor (IgM antibodies) in the serum and synovial fluid of 80% of patients. The antigen-antibody reactions activate the complement system and attract neutrophils to the joint fluid. The immune complexes are then phagocytized, and lysosomal enzymes are released into the synovial fluid. These enzymes and the inflammatory synovial pannus are in part responsible for the destruction of articular cartilage and periarticular structures. Tendons are also directly invaded by the inflammatory synovium and may attenuate and rupture. Ligaments and joint capsules become weakened by the chronic inflammatory process and may become stretched by repeated joint effusions (Figure 13–26).

The erosion of articular cartilage is greatly enhanced by the superimposition of mechanical derangements on a joint weakened by chronic inflammation and enzymatic deterioration. Osteoporosis results from the hyperemia of inflammation. Disuse of limbs secondary to pain, weakened muscle action, and mechanical derangements enhances the osteoporosis.

Clinical Findings

Rheumatoid arthritis affects synovial joints, bones, muscles, fasciae, ligaments, and tendons. Because it is a systemic disease, it can also affect internal organs. The diagnosis is made primarily on clinical grounds and supported by radiographic and laboratory data (Table 13–5). Rheumatoid arthritis is two or three times more common in women than men. The disease is seen in some children but has increasing prevalence with increasing age up to the seventh decade. Rheumatic complaints are responsible for the largest share of chronic disability in the United States.

The clinical course of rheumatoid arthritis is variable with respect to the extent and intensity of the disease. The time course of the disease is measured in months and years and is progressive. Several factors affect the course of disease and are associated with a poor prognosis. These factors include insidious onset, symmetric disease, presence of rheumatoid factor in the serum, and presence of rheumatoid nodules, which

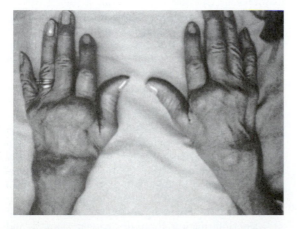

Figure 13–26. Chronic synovitis of the joints and extensor tendons in a patient with rheumatoid arthritis.

Table 13–5. American Rheumatism Association criteria for diagnosing and categorizing rheumatoid arthritis.

Category	Description
Classic rheumatoid arthritis	Presence of 7 of the following findings: (1) morning stiffness,[a] (2) pain on motion of 1 joint[a] (3) swelling of 1 joint[a] (4) swelling of an additional joint[a] (5) symmetric swelling of joints, (6) presence of subcutaneous nodules, (7) presence of rheumatoid factor in the serum, (8) poor results in the mucin clot test of synovial fluid, (9) characteristic roentgenographic changes, (10) characteristic histopathologic findings in the synovial fluid, and (11) characteristic histopathologic findings in nodule biopsies.
Definite rheumatoid arthritis	Presence of 5 of the above findings.
Probable rheumatoid arthritis	Presence of 3 of the above findings.

[a]Finding must be present for at least 6 weeks.

occur in patients with rheumatoid factor. In young adults with rheumatoid arthritis, females have a worse prognosis than males. Eosinophilia of 5% or greater is associated with an increased incidence of vasculitis, pleuropericarditis, pulmonary fibrosis, and subcutaneous nodules.

The multisystem nature of rheumatoid arthritis and its variable clinical pattern make it difficult to devise a precise system for describing the overall functional ability of the patient. The most commonly employed scale is the functional classification devised by the American Rheumatism Association (Table 13–6).

Management

A. THE TEAM APPROACH TO PATIENT CARE AND TREATMENT

Optimal management requires an interdisciplinary team approach involving many specialists, including a liaison nurse, rheumatologist, orthopedic surgeon, physical therapist, occupational therapist, psychologist, and social worker. The patient and members of his or her family are also important members of the team. Because the disease is an ongoing and progressive process, the goal of management is to prevent deformities and maintain function for the patient over a lifetime.

1. Nursing care and patient education—The liaison nurse functions as the coordinator of the team. The nurse provides the critical link between the inpatient medical and surgical management of the disease and the continuation of treatment in the outpatient environment.

Much of the responsibility for patient education in the daily care of the disease rests with the nurse, who explains the techniques for protecting joints; advises pa-

Table 13–6. American Rheumatism Association classification of function in patients with rheumatoid arthritis.

Class	Description
I	Complete function; able to perform usual duties without handicap.
II	Adequate function for normal activities, despite handicap of pain or limited range of motion in one or more joints.
III	Limited function; able to perform few or none of the duties of usual occupation or self-care.
IV	Largely or wholly incapacitated; bedridden or confined to a wheelchair; able to perform little or no self-care.

tients about the need to perform exercises for maintaining joint range of motion and optimizing failing muscle strength; cautions patients that exercising too vigorously can damage weakened joints and ligaments; and reminds patients that because the disease tends to decrease their physical activity, they will need regular periods of rest during the day and good nutrition to maximize their general health and to prevent obesity.

2. Medical and surgical management—The rheumatologist is commonly the team leader and is in charge of medical management, which is directed toward the control of synovitis, the relief of pain, and the prevention or treatment of other organ involvement by the disease. The medications used for treatment include aspirin, nonsteroidal anti-inflammatory drugs, corticosteroids, immunosuppressive drugs, and suppressive agents. A local injection of corticosteroids can be useful in controlling an acute inflammatory process in a specific joint. Corticosteroids can also be used systemically but are generally avoided because of undesirable side effects. Agents that produce suppression or remission of arthritis include gold salts, antimalarial drugs, and penicillamine. Immunosuppressive drugs or total lymphoid irradiation can also be used to suppress immune reactions.

The orthopedic surgeon should be involved early in the course of the patient's disease and not merely be called upon when medical management has failed to be effective. A knowledge of biomechanics, gait dynamics, and energy requirements can be useful in preserving function for the patient. The orthopedist can often recommend orthotic supports, walking aids, and shoe wear that will minimize unwanted stress on joints and maximize strength.

In selected situations, early surgical intervention may prevent excessive deterioration of joint structure and function. Synovectomy has been shown to be effective in preventing tendon rupture in the hand, whereas arthroscopic synovectomy of the knee and shoulder show promise for preventing joint destruction. Fusion of an unstable cervical spine can prevent the disastrous effect of a spinal cord injury.

Most surgical procedures are reconstructive. Because relief of pain is the most consistent result of reconstructive surgery, pain is the primary indication for surgery. Restoration of motion and function and the correction of deformity are additional indications for surgical intervention but are more difficult goals to achieve. Preoperative assessment is a painstaking process. In addition to performing a physical examination and reviewing radiographic findings, the surgeon must attempt to elicit sufficient information from the patient, family, and therapists to ascertain which deformities are causing the greatest functional losses. The patient can only tolerate a finite number of surgical procedures, and these must be carefully staged to obtain the maximal result.

For further discussion of medical and surgical treatment, see the section Management Approaches Based on the Area of Disease Involvement.

3. Physical therapy—The physical therapist uses modalities such as heat and ultrasound to decrease joint stiffness and relieve pain. An exercise program is essential for preserving the functional abilities of the patient. The exercise should gently put all joints through their full arc of motion to maintain this range.

Patients with joint effusions and synovitis will automatically assume positions that minimize intra-articular pressure and therefore minimize pain. These positions are usually not optimal for function and can result in flexion deformities. An abnormal position may be reversible if discovered early. Daily joint range-of-motion exercises are central to preventing unwanted contractures.

Muscles weakened by the concomitant myopathy need strengthening but are susceptible to damage from overuse or from an excessively vigorous exercise program. Orthotics may be indicated to support weakened ligaments and provide a means of joint protection and support for functional activities such as walking. Upper extremity walking aids may be useful to give the patients additional support. These aids often require modification to meet the specific needs of the individual. Forearm troughs will allow the patient to use the entire arm for support when the hands and wrists are weak or deformed. They are also useful for protecting the hands from excessive stress. A rolling walker, which does not require the patient to lift the walker for advancement, may be useful in patients with limited strength.

4. Occupational therapy—The occupational therapist evaluates and instructs the patient in modified techniques for performing activities of daily living, such as grooming, dressing, and meal preparation. Because of the weakness and deformities imposed by the arthritis, adaptive equipment and alternative methods are commonly needed. Modifications in clothing, such as larger fasteners for ease of manipulation, Velcro strips at seams or on shoes, and front openings, can all facilitate dressing. Upper extremity splints can be used to provide joint protection and stabilization and to prevent further deformity from occurring. The splints must be lightweight and easily donned by the patient.

5. Psychologic counseling—It is not uncommon for patients or their family members to have feelings of anxiety, denial, anger, or depression. The psychologist provides assistance in dealing with these feelings and coping with alterations in life-style and self-image. Comprehensive care involves an understanding of how patients respond to weakness, fatigue, altered physical appearance, progressive disability, diminished independence, and the financial burdens of chronic illness. Coping skills are needed to deal with these problems as well as with pain, which becomes an everyday occurrence and may interfere with both intellectual and emotional functioning.

6. Social services—A variety of modifications in lifestyle accompany chronic illness with rheumatoid arthritis. Occupational changes may be necessary, or the patient may no longer be able to work at all. Additional assistance may be needed in the home for housework and the preparation of meals. In more advanced stages, the patient may require help for personal care. Transportation needs become more complex, and the patient finds it increasingly difficult to leave the home. The social worker becomes an invaluable team member in helping families with the numerous practical arrangements required for everyday existence and for locating financial aid to help defray the mounting costs.

B. MANAGEMENT APPROACHES BASED ON THE AREA OF DISEASE INVOLVEMENT

Orthopedic surgery is frequently necessary for patients with rheumatoid arthritis affecting the cervical spine or extremities.

1. Cervical spine—Depending on the study and diagnostic criteria, involvement of the cervical spine is found in anywhere from 6.4 to 90% of patients with rheumatoid arthritis. Three forms of cervical spine involvement are seen.

The first and most common form is atlantoaxial instability (Figure 13–27), which results from erosion of

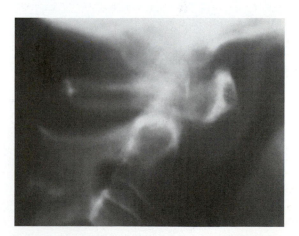

Figure 13–27. Tomogram of the upper cervical spine, showing atlantoaxial instability in a patient with rheumatoid arthritis.

the transverse and alar ligaments. These ligaments normally function to maintain the odontoid process of the axis within the anterior third of the atlas ring, where the two bones articulate with each other. Disruption of the transverse and alar ligaments results in excessive motion between C1 and C2. Forward flexion of the head causes anterior subluxation of the atlas on the axis and possible impingement of the spinal cord or occlusion of the vertebral arteries. This is best seen in lateral flexion and extension radiographs of the cervical spine.

The second form of cervical spine involvement is subaxial instability (Figure 13–28), which may lead to subluxation of two or more cervical vertebrae below the level of C2. If subluxation is severe or its appearance is sudden, it can exert sufficient pressure on the spinal cord to cause permanent quadriparesis. If subluxation occurs slowly over a long time, however, as commonly happens, the spinal cord is able to adapt to the pressure, so that a severe degree of deformity occurs before clinical symptoms appear.

The third and least common form of cervical spine involvement is superior migration of the odontoid process of C2 resulting from severe degrees of bone erosion (Figure 13–29). This form of involvement has been reported in from 3.8% to 15% of patients with rheumatoid arthritis. As the dens migrates proximally, radiographic detail is lost because of the overlapping of bony structures. Computed tomographic scanning is most useful in elucidating the exact nature of the involvement and can show rotational instability caused by asymmetric bone erosions (Figure 13–30).

Orthotic supports are useful in controlling the patient's symptoms. Posterior cervical fusion is indicated when the spinal cord is at risk of damage. The most common level of fusion is C1 to C2, supplemented by wire fixation. If the subluxation is irreducible or if severe osteoporosis is present, fusion to the occiput may be necessary. Occasionally, it is useful to supplement the bone graft with polymethyl methacrylate fixation.

In patients with severe erosive disease of the cervical spine and proximal migration of the odontoid process, a rotational deviation of the larynx may occur, making intubation impossible except with the use of a flexible fiberoptic scope (Figure 13–31). Because cervical spine disease often presents difficulties in endotracheal intubation at the time of surgery, the stability of the cervical

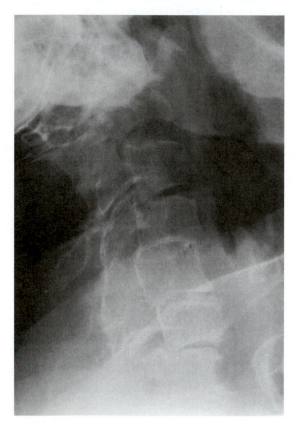

Figure 13–28. Radiograph of the cervical spine, showing multiple levels of subaxial instability in a patient with rheumatoid arthritis.

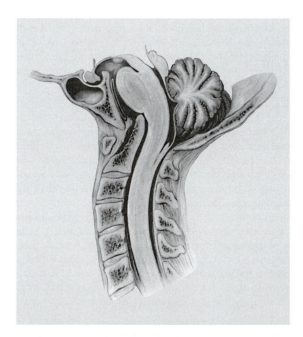

Figure 13–29. Diagram illustrating vertical penetration of the odontoid process into the foramen magnum following bone erosion in a patient with rheumatoid arthritis. (Illustration by Ted Bloodhart.)

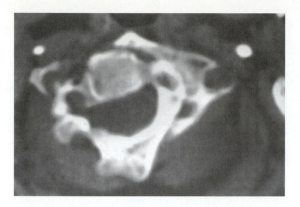

Figure 13–30. CT scan showing rotational instability of C1 on C2 in a patient with advanced psoriatic arthritis.

spine should be assessed preoperatively in all patients with rheumatoid arthritis. Lateral flexion-extension radiographs taken within 1 year of surgery are sufficient to detect significant instability problems. Use of the flexible fiberoptic bronchoscope for such problems has proved valuable. Among the indications for fiberoptic intubation in patients with arthritis are an unstable cervical spine on flexion and extension; limited mobility of the cervical spine; and impaired motion of the temporomandibular joints, with or without associated micrognathia.

2. Lower extremities

a. Hips—Total joint replacement has vastly improved the quality of life for patients with rheumatoid arthritis. Special problems exist in this group of patients, however, and must be considered before total hip arthroplasty is performed. Because osteoporosis is pronounced, fracture can occur easily during surgery. Protrusio acetabuli, another common problem, may require bone grafting. The risk of infection is increased in this population, and wound healing may also be delayed, especially if the patient has been taking systemic corticosteroids. In young patients, excess femoral anteversion may be present and distort the anatomy. Moreover, the small size of the bone may require a special prosthesis. Despite these problems, total joint arthroplasty remains the treatment of choice for the arthritic hip.

b. Knees—Knee pain is common and may be the result of a valgus deformity of the hindfoot, which places excessive stress on the knee proximally. Mild medial knee pain can be relieved with the use of an AFO to correct the valgus deformity. Knee pain may also be caused by the presence of a joint effusion, which increases the intra-articular pressure and thereby increases the pain. When patients attempt to minimize pain by placing the knee in 30 degrees of flexion, this encourages the formation of flexion contractures.

Arthroscopic evaluation of the rheumatoid knee has demonstrated the importance of the meniscus in the degeneration of the knee. The synovium directly invades the body of the meniscus and tears it. The mechanical derangement resulting from the torn meniscus then causes rapid deterioration of the articular surfaces, which have been rendered abnormal by the action of enzymes. Synovectomy of the joint line and partial meniscectomy are easily accomplished under arthroscopic control and may have a role in preventing articular damage in the rheumatoid knee.

Total knee arthroplasty has proved to be effective in restoring knee alignment and motion and relieving pain. When a valgus deformity is present, serial releases of the soft tissue should be performed to realign the limb prior to cutting the bone for insertion of the prosthetic components. The lateral retinaculum, popliteal tendon, proximal iliotibial band, posterolateral capsule, and lateral collateral ligament can be released in this sequence to provide soft-tissue balance. A flexion deformity is corrected at the time of arthroplasty by releasing the posterior capsule from the femur or by removing additional bone from the distal femur in severe cases.

c. Feet—Forefoot involvement is common in rheumatoid arthritis. Clawtoe deformities with plantar subluxation of the metatarsal heads result in painful callosities on the plantar surface of the forefoot. These problems are usually accompanied by a hallux valgus deformity. Skin ulcerations may form over bony prominences. Forefoot pain prevents the patient from transferring body weight over the foot during terminal stance, and this results in an awkward gait with a shortened step length. Extra-depth shoes with wide toe boxes and molded pressure-relieving inserts may be sufficient to relieve pain and improve gait. When the deformities are marked, resection of the metatarsal heads in conjunction with arthroplasty or fusion of the metatarsophalangeal joint of the great toe is indicated.

Hindfoot involvement is also common and results in a planovalgus or pronation deformity. A longitudinal arch support or similar shoe insert is not sufficient to hold the hindfoot in alignment. When the deformity is supple, an AFO with a well-molded arch support will control the position of the heel and subtalar joint during gait. This will also reduce the valgus thrust on the knee joint. If the deformity is fixed, a triple arthrodesis will align the hindfoot.

3. Upper extremities

a. Shoulders—In patients with rheumatoid arthritis, shoulder involvement is common but is generally insidious in onset or episodic in nature. Because the

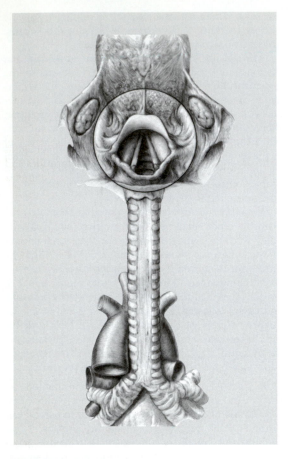 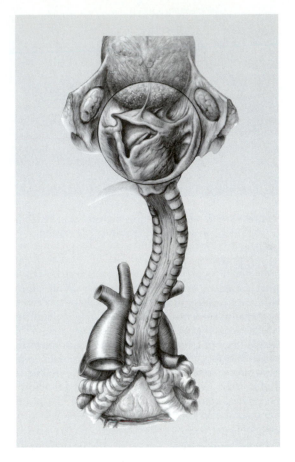

Figure 13–31. *Left*: Diagram showing the normal relationship of the trachea and larynx. The insert shows the view seen through the fiberoptic bronchoscope. *Right*: Diagram showing the triple-plane rotational deviation of the larynx noted secondary to cervical spine disease in inflammatory arthritis. (Illustrations by Ted Bloodhart. Reproduced, with permission, from Keenan MA et al: Acquired laryngeal deviation associated with cervical spine disease in erosive polyarticular arthritis. Anesthesiology 1983;58:441.)

pain is not constant early in the course of the disease, shoulder involvement is often not appreciated until a significant amount of destruction has occurred. It is important to examine the shoulders regularly so as to detect early loss of motion and function.

Arthroscopy provides a useful tool in examining the shoulder and assessing the integrity of the glenoid labrum, rotator cuff, and biceps tendon. Arthroscopy can also be used to perform synovectomy of the shoulder joint.

Normally, the glenohumeral joint has more motion than any other joint. This motion is rotation, and it is facilitated by the shallow shape of the glenoid labrum. The rotator cuff muscles, which are central to the normal functioning of the shoulder, provide stability to the humeral head and also provide rotation. If the rotator

cuff ruptures, the humeral head rides upward and is subjected to abnormal muscle forces as the patient attempts to compensate for the loss of motion. This results in the rapid deterioration of the glenohumeral joint. Normally, the anterior portion of the deltoid muscle provides forward elevation of the humerus. This is the position of function and the most common arc of motion for activities involving the upper extremity. The tendon of the long head of the biceps muscle serves to stabilize the humeral head against riding upward and also to reduce subacromial impingement. Whenever surgery of the shoulder is performed, it is important to preserve the deltoid muscle fibers and their attachments as well as the intra-articular portion of the biceps tendon.

The subacromial bursa is often involved with the inflammatory response of rheumatoid arthritis and may become thickened. The inflammatory process may cause a decrease in nutrition of the rotator cuff tendons and lead to attrition of the tendons with or without rupture of the rotator cuff. Subacromial bursitis can be treated by local injection of a corticosteroid preparation. When the inflammation has subsided, the patient is begun on a program of gentle range-of-motion exercises.

Repair of a ruptured rotator cuff is often possible and should be performed. If the rupture is detected early, excessive damage to the glenohumeral joint can be avoided. If extensive joint damage is already present, repair or reconstruction of the rotator cuff is done at the time of prosthetic arthroplasty of the glenohumeral joint. Preoperative radiographic evaluation should include axillary radiographs to assess the glenoid alignment. The glenoid labrum is often eroded asymmetrically, and the prosthetic component must be accurately aligned to ensure optimal function and to minimize the abnormal forces that might lead to prosthetic loosening. In patients with total shoulder replacement, pain is effectively alleviated. Shoulder function will depend on the integrity of the soft tissues and on muscle function. Resurfacing of the glenoid should be reserved for those patients with an intact rotator cuff. If the rotator cuff has been destroyed, humeral hemiarthroplasty is the preferred surgical treatment. A careful postoperative therapy program is essential for maximizing shoulder function.

b. Elbows—The elbow joint consists of three separate articulations: radiocapitellar, ulnotrochlear, and radioulnar. These articulations allow the hand to rotate 180 degrees around the longitudinal axis of the forearm. The function of the hand is dependent on being placed in space as necessary for use. The elbow is the most important joint for positioning the hand. Unlike the shoulder or wrist, if the elbow is fused, the functional loss is great. The goal of treatment is to maintain a painless arc of motion.

Olecranon bursitis is common in patients with rheumatoid arthritis. The usual treatment consists of aspirating the bursa and injecting a corticosteroid preparation. Rarely, chronic bursitis develops and requires surgical excision of the bursa.

Subcutaneous rheumatoid nodules are common along the extensor surface of the ulna. The nodules are often sensitive to pressure when the arm is resting on any surface, and they may interfere with the use of forearm troughs on walking aids. If they are bothersome, the nodules should be surgically excised. The patient should be advised, however, that nodules can recur.

Radiocapitellar arthritis is often the predominant feature of elbow involvement and can cause marked pain and a decrease in motion. The pain is most pronounced with pronation and supination of the forearm.

When the joint destruction is severe, prosthetic arthroplasty is indicated. Elbow prostheses fall into two basic categories: semiconstrained and unconstrained. An unconstrained design is less likely to loosen. The shoulder should be evaluated carefully prior to prosthetic elbow arthroplasty. A patient with limited shoulder motion will exert greater forces on the elbow in an effort to compensate for the decrease in shoulder function.

c. Wrists and hands—In patients with rheumatoid arthritis, evaluating the wrist and hand deformities and developing a rational treatment plan can be a complex task for the surgeon. Many joints, tendons, and ligaments are involved in a linked system of structure and function. Treatment can be divided into three categories: nonsurgical treatment, preventive surgery, and reconstructive or salvage surgery. Nonoperative treatment consists of resting inflamed joints; exercising joints for short periods of time but frequently and gently to maintain motion; using resting or dynamic splints to alleviate pain and prevent deformity; and judiciously using local corticosteroid injections for control of synovitis.

(1) Tendons—Dorsal tenosynovitis is common. It is of significance because it often results in rupture of the extensor tendons either from attrition or from direct invasion of the inflamed synovial tissue into the tendon substance. Tenosynovectomy should be performed in patients whose synovitis has persisted for 4–6 months despite medical treatment. Recurrence of the synovitis is rare following synovectomy, and the procedure has been shown to prevent extensor tendon rupture.

Rupture of an extensor tendon can result from attenuation of the tendon caused by chronic inflammation, friction against abnormal bony surfaces, ischemia secondary to interference with the normal circulation to the tendon, or direct invasion of the tendon by synovium. The most common tendons to rupture, listed in order of frequency, are the extensors of the fifth finger, the extensors of the ring finger, and the long extensor of the thumb (the extensor pollicis longus). Surgical repair by tendon transfer is more successful when fewer tendons are involved. Therefore, prompt diagnosis and treatment are essential for a successful outcome. For a single tendon rupture in the fifth and ring fingers, a side-to-side repair using the adjacent extensor tendon is advised. The tendon of the index finger extensor can be transferred to repair a rupture of the thumb extensor tendon or a rupture of two finger tendons. For more complex ruptures, tendon transfer from the wrist extensors or from the superficial flexor muscles of the fingers may restore function.

Synovitis in the flexor tendon sheaths is characterized by crepitation that is palpable in the palm during finger flexion and extension. Triggering of the fingers may result from the inflamed synovial tissue catching on the flexor pulleys with motion. Carpal tunnel syndrome may also occur as a result of swelling within the carpal canal, which causes pressure on the median nerve. Early treatment consists of local corticosteroid injection to reduce the inflammation, application of a splint, and medical management of the underlying synovitis. Persistent synovitis may require carpal tunnel release and synovectomy. Rupture of the flexor tendons is rare.

(2) Wrist joints—The wrist joint is a frequent site of synovitis and may begin to show radial deviation and volar subluxation. The radioulnar joint is commonly inflamed and painful. Early treatment consists of splinting for support and medical control of the synovitis. Dorsal synovectomy of the extensor compartments is indicated when medications do not adequately control the synovitis. Dorsal synovectomy will prevent rupture of the extensor tendons. Radial deviation of the carpus can be corrected by transfer of the extensor carpi radialis longus tendon to the extensor carpi ulnaris.

When the wrist becomes unstable, several choices of surgical treatment are available. If the deformity is mild, bone stock can be preserved and motion maintained by a limited carpal fusion. The lunate and scaphoid bones are fused to the distal radius to prevent further displacement of the carpus. The distal ulna can be fused to the distal radius to provide a platform to support the wrist. A segment of the ulna is removed just proximal to the fusion to allow for pronation and supination of the forearm. If the intercarpal joints are severely affected by the arthritis, the base of the capitate bone can be removed and a tendon spacer inserted to preserve motion at the intercarpal row.

Another option is to perform a prosthetic arthroplasty of the wrist. More bone stock is removed with this procedure, but revision is still possible in the event of fracture of the prosthesis. Several designs of total joint prosthesis have been developed for the wrist.

Fusion of the wrist joint provides a stable pain-free joint and remains a reasonable surgical choice for selected patients. Because fusion may interfere with personal hygiene tasks, it is advisable to avoid fusing both wrist joints.

(3) Metacarpophalangeal and carpometacarpal joints—Finger and wrist deformities commonly occur together in a collapsing zigzag pattern. The wrist deviates in a radial direction, and the fingers then drift ulnarward at the metacarpophalangeal joint level. When both deformities are present, it is important to realign the wrist prior to correcting the finger deformities, or the ulnar deviation of the fingers will recur.

Ulnar deviation and volar subluxation of the fingers at the metacarpophalangeal joint level are common. With ulnar deviation, the extensor tendons move into the valleys between the metacarpal heads. This condition can be confused with extensor tendon rupture. If the joint surfaces are preserved, function can be improved by a synovectomy, soft-tissue release of the volar capsule, and realignment of the extensor tendons. If the joint surfaces are destroyed, then a total wrist arthroplasty can be considered. If the joints are unstable because of ligament loss, it may be necessary to reconstruct the radial collateral ligament using a portion of the volar plate to provide a stable pinch. Tightness of the intrinsic tendons commonly occurs in conjunction with the subluxation of the metacarpophalangeal joints. To correct this problem, a release of the intrinsic tendons is performed along with the arthroplasty. Dynamic splinting of the fingers, which maintains alignment while allowing motion, is used continuously for 6 weeks following surgery and then for an additional 6 weeks at night.

Flexion of the metacarpophalangeal joint with extension of the interphalangeal joint in the thumb is the equivalent of a boutonnière deformity. The reverse deformity can also be seen, with extension of the metacarpophalangeal joint and flexion of the interphalangeal joint. An adduction deformity of the metacarpal bone places increased stress on the metacarpophalangeal joint and produces lateral instability and hyperextension. Adduction of the thumb occurs when the carpometacarpal joint has shifted radially. Derangements of the carpometacarpal joint can be treated by fusion or by arthroplasty. Interposition arthroplasty is desirable to maintain motion and can be performed using a Silastic spacer or soft tissue.

(4) Interphalangeal joints—Continued synovitis gradually attenuates the capsular and ligamentous structures and results in tendon imbalance. In the fingers, this will be seen as either a flexion or an extension deformity.

Flexion deformity results from rupture or attenuation of the central slip of the extensor mechanism, with gradual volar displacement of the lateral bands. As the lateral bands shift in the volar direction, a hyperextension deformity of the distal interphalangeal joint results. This flexion malalignment, which is called a **boutonnière,** or **buttonhole, deformity,** interferes with the ability to grasp large objects but does not usually impede the pinch function used for picking up small items. Interposition arthroplasty using a Silastic spacer has given unpredictable results. Fusion of the interphalangeal joints gives dependable results when the boutonnière deformity is fixed. In the index and long fingers, stability for pinch is required for good function and is more important than a large arc of motion. In the ring and small fingers, motion is more important for a functional grasp. When arthroplasty is considered, the ring and fifth fingers are usually selected.

Hyperextension deformities, or swan-neck deformities, can be either primary or secondary. Primary deformities are caused by stretching of the volar plate from synovitis or rupture of the flexor digitorum superficialis tendon. Secondary deformities are characterized by flexion of the metacarpophalangeal joints, with tightness of the intrinsic muscles proximally and presence of a mallet deformity distally. This hyperextension deformity interferes with picking up small objects but does not cause much difficulty with grasping larger objects. If the deformity is treated early and is secondary to intrinsic muscle tightness, a release of the intrinsic tendons will correct the imbalance. If the deformity is seen late and is rigid, joint fusion or arthroplasty is indicated.

Derangements of the distal interphalangeal joints are either mallet deformities secondary to rupture of the extensor tendon or lateral deformities from loss of capsular and ligamentous support. When the deformities interfere with function, fusion of the joint is indicated.

Anderson RJ: The orthopedic management of rheumatoid arthritis. Arthritis Care Res 1996;9:223.

Bellemans et al: Total knee arthroplasty in the young rheumatoid patient. Acta Orthop Belg 1997;63:189.

Belt EA et al: A 20-year follow-up study of subtalar changes in rheumatoid arthritis. Scand J Rheumatol 1997;26:266.

Belt EA et al: Destruction and arthroplasties of the metatarsophalangeal joints in seropositive rheumatoid arthritis. A 20-year follow-up study. Scand J Rheumatol 1998;27:194.

Belt EA et al: Destruction and reconstruction of hand joints in rheumatoid arthritis. A 20-year follow-up study. J Rheumatol 1998;25:459.

Belt EA et al: Outcome of ankle arthrodesis performed by dowel technique in patients with rheumatic disease. Foot Ankle Int 2001;22:666.

Bennett WF, Gerber C: Operative treatment of the rheumatoid shoulder [editorial]. Curr Opin Rheumatol 1994;6:177.

Berger RA et al: Long-term follow-up of the Miller-Galante total knee replacement. Clin Orthop 2001;388:56.

Bostrom C et al: Effects of static and dynamic shoulder rotator exercises in women with rheumatoid arthritis: A randomized comparison of impairment, disability, handicap, and health. Scand J Rheumatol 1998;27:281.

Burra G, Katchis SD: Rheumatoid arthritis of the forefoot. Rheum Dis Clin North Am 1998;24:173.

Creighton MG et al: Total hip arthroplasty with cement in patients who have rheumatoid arthritis. A minimum ten-year follow-up study. J Bone Joint Surg Am 1998; 80:1439.

Dionne RA et al: Analgesia and cox-2 inhibition. Clin Exp Rheumatol 2001;19:S63.

Dunbar RP, Alexiades MM: Decision making in rheumatoid arthritis. Determining surgical priorities. Rheum Dis Clin North Am 1998;24:35.

Gellman H et al: Total wrist arthroplasty in rheumatoid arthritis. A long-term clinical review. Clin Orthop 1997;342:71.

Gendi NS et al: Synovectomy of the elbow and radial head excision in rheumatoid arthritis. Predictive factors and long-term outcome. J Bone Joint Surg Br 1997;79:918.

Gill DR, Morrey BF: The Coonrad-Morrey total elbow arthroplasty in patients who have rheumatoid arthritis. A ten to fifteen-year follow-up study. J Bone Joint Surg Am 1998;80:1327.

Gordon P et al: A 10-year prospective followup of patients with rheumatoid arthritis 1986–96. J Rheumatol 2001;28:2409.

Johnstone BR: Proximal interphalangeal joint surface replacement arthroplasty. Hand Surg 2001;6:1.

Karbowski A et al: Arthroplasty of the forefoot in rheumatoid arthritis: Long-term results after Clayton procedure. Acta Orthop Belg 1998;64:401.

King JA, Tomaino MM: Surgical treatment of the rheumatoid thumb. Hand Clin 2001;17:275.

Lehtimaki MY et al: Hip involvement in seropositive rheumatoid arthritis. Survivorship analysis with a 15-year follow-up. Scand J Rheumatol 1998;27:406.

Madsen OR et al: Soft tissue composition, quadriceps strength, bone quality and bone mass in rheumatoid arthritis. Clin Exp Rheumatol 1998;16:27.

O'Connell PG et al: Forefoot deformity, pain, and mobility in rheumatoid and nonarthritic subjects. J Rheumatol 1998;25:1681.

Ramsey JL et al: Instability of the elbow treated with semiconstrained total elbow arthroplasty. J Bone Joint Surg Am 1999;81:38.

Ryu J et al: Risk factors and prophylactic tenosynovectomy for extensor tendon ruptures in the rheumatoid hand. J Hand Surg Br 1998;23:658.

Sculco TP: The knee joint in rheumatoid arthritis. Rheum Dis Clin North Am 1998;24:143.

Stein AB, Terrono AL: The rheumatoid thumb. Hand Clin 1996;12:541.

Toolan BC, Hansen ST Jr: Surgery of the rheumatoid foot and ankle. Curr Opin Rheumatol 1998;10:116.

Torchia ME et al: Total shoulder arthroplasty with the Neer prosthesis: Long-term results. J Shoulder Elbow Surg 1997;6:495.

van Den Ende CH et al: Assessment of shoulder function in rheumatoid arthritis. J Rheumatol 1996;23:2043.

Waldman BJ, Figgie MP: Indications, technique, and results of total shoulder arthroplasty in rheumatoid arthritis. Orthop Clin North Am 1998;29:435.

POLIOMYELITIS

Poliomyelitis is caused by an enterovirus that attacks the anterior horn cells of the spinal cord. Infection can lead to a variety of clinical findings, ranging from minor symptoms to paralysis. The last major epidemics in the United States occurred during the early 1950s. Because of effective immunization programs, acute poliomyelitis has now become rare in the United States and other developed nations of the world. Nevertheless, orthopedic surgeons today are frequently called upon to treat patients with postpoliomyelitis syndrome.

Classification

Four stages of poliomyelitis are recognized.

A. Acute Poliomyelitis

All of the anterior horn cells are attacked during the acute stage, and this accounts for the diffuse and severe paralysis seen with the initial infection. The anterior horn cells control the skeletal muscle cells of the trunk and limbs. Clinically, the infection is characterized by the sudden onset of paralysis and the presence of fever and acute muscle pain, often accompanied by stiff neck. Paralysis of the respiratory muscles is life-threatening in the acute stage. When the shoulder muscles are involved, respiratory compromise should be suspected because of the close proximity of the anterior horn cells controlling each in the spinal cord. Mechanical support of ventilation may be required.

A variable number of anterior horn cells survive the initial infection. The treatment in the acute stage of the disease consists of providing the needed respiratory support, decreasing muscle pain, and performing regular range of motion exercises to prevent the formation of joint contractures.

B. Subacute Poliomyelitis

Anterior horn cell survival, axon sprouting, and muscle hypertrophy occur in the subacute phase and provide three mechanisms for regaining strength. An average of 47% (range of 12–94%) of the anterior horn cells in the spinal cord survive the initial attack. Because cell survival occurs in a random fashion, the distribution of paralysis is variable and depends on which anterior horn cells have been destroyed. Each anterior horn cell innervates a group of muscle cells. When a group of muscle cells is "orphaned" by the death of the anterior horn cell that supports it, a nearby nerve cell can sprout additional axons and "adopt" some of the orphaned cells. By means of this process, a motor unit (defined as a nerve cell and the muscle cells it innervates) can expand greatly. Moreover, muscle cells in the unit will enlarge, and this hypertrophy will provide additional strength for the patient.

C. Residual Poliomyelitis

It is only after 16–24 months following onset that the ultimate extent of poliomyelitis can be determined and that procedures to restore lost function and provide structural stability can be instituted.

D. Postpoliomyelitis Syndrome

Patients who had acute poliomyelitis during childhood often complain of increased muscle weakness 30–40 years later. This weakness is not a result of infectious spread of the earlier disease but, rather, is caused by the overuse of muscles that were originally affected, whether or not they were known to have been affected at the onset of the disease. Studies have shown that a muscle must lose from 30 to 40% of its strength for weakness to be detected using manual muscle testing. Studies of gait have also demonstrated that the activities of daily living require more muscle strength and stamina than were previously appreciated. The traditional program, which encouraged patients to work harder to regain strength and which was based on the concept of "no pain, no gain," has proved detrimental because it has encouraged chronic overuse of muscles and resulted in further deterioration of function.

The diagnosis of postpoliomyelitis syndrome is based on a history of poliomyelitis; a pattern of increased muscle weakness that is random and does not follow any nerve root or peripheral nerve distribution; and the presence of additional symptoms such as muscle pain, severe fatigue, muscle cramping or fasciculations, joint pain or instability, sleep apnea, intolerance to cold, and depression. No pathognomonic tests for the syndrome are currently available. Electromyography can demonstrate the presence of large motor units resulting from the previous axon sprouting. This finding is supportive but not diagnostic of poliomyelitis.

Management

A. Acute Poliomyelitis

When the shoulder muscles are involved, respiratory compromise should be suspected, and mechanical support of ventilation should be instituted. Other measures are aimed at decreasing muscle pain and preventing complications. Regular range-of-motion exercises will prevent the formation of joint contractures.

B. Subacute Poliomyelitis

During the subacute stage, which may last as long as 24 months, the emphasis is on preventing deformities and preserving function. Splints and braces are often helpful for maintaining joint position and supplementing function.

C. Residual Poliomyelitis

Patients with compromised function of the diaphragm can be taught glossopharyngeal breathing. This method, in which air is swallowed into the lungs, provides sufficient air exchange for the patient to perform light activities in the sitting position. Mechanical support of ventilation may still need to be continued while the patient sleeps. It is during the residual stage that orthopedic surgery is commonly performed to restore lost function and provide structural stability. If the patient is still growing, it is important to prevent the formation of skeletal deformities that result from muscle imbalance. Before any surgery that requires general anesthesia or significant sedation is performed, the vital capacity should be assessed to determine the patient's need for respiratory support.

D. POSTPOLIOMYELITIS SYNDROME

Treatment is directed at preserving current muscle strength and preventing further weakness from occurring. Generally, strength cannot be restored in a muscle that has been weakened by poliomyelitis. Some gain in strength can be seen, however, when chronic overuse is corrected.

General management strategies consist of modifying the life-style to prevent chronic overuse of weak muscles; instituting a limited exercise program that incorporates frequent rest periods to prevent disuse atrophy and weakness; providing lightweight orthotic support of the limbs to protect joints and substitute for muscle function; and performing orthopedic surgery to correct limb or trunk deformities.

Specific management strategies will depend on the areas of disease involvement.

1. Spine—Back pain is a common complaint and usually results from postural strain caused by excessive lumbar extension in patients who have weak or paralyzed hip extensor muscles. Neck pain, like back pain, is a common complaint associated with slowly increasing weakness. Both complaints can be treated by the use of external supports. Patient education is imperative because many patients are reluctant to don braces again, after having passed decades without using them. Patients should be instructed in methods to relieve excess strain on the neck muscles and prevent further deterioration. Tilting the seat of a chair 10 degrees backward is often sufficient to relieve the fatigue of the posterior cervical muscles from supporting the head.

Paralysis of the cervical spine musculature can result in the inability to maintain the head erect and can interfere with the performance of a vast number of functions, including ambulation. Surgical fusion of the cervical spine will correct the problem.

Scoliosis is common in patients with muscle imbalance caused by paralysis. The condition is particularly pronounced in patients with leg-length discrepancies. External supports can be used to hold the spine in position, but these often interfere with respiration if the patient is dependent on the use of accessory muscles for breathing. Posterior spinal fusion may be needed to control the spine adequately. After fusion is performed, prolonged immobilization must be avoided. Segmental spine fixation may be helpful.

2. Lower extremities—Full range of motion of the hip and knee joints is needed for function. Contractures should be corrected when possible to permit more effective bracing. In iliotibial band contractures, which are common deformities, the hip assumes a position of flexion, external rotation, and abduction; the knee assumes a valgus alignment; and the tibia is externally ro-

tated on the femur. Release or lengthening of the iliotibial band will correct the deformity.

A patient with flailing lower extremities can stand using crutches and a KAFO with the knees locked in extension and the ankles in slight dorsiflexion by hyperextending the hips and using the strong anterior hip capsule for support. Flexion contractures of the hips or knees prevent this alignment. If trunk support and upper extremity strength are adequate, the patient could ambulate with a swing-through gait for short distances. This gait has high energy demands. With time, the posterior knee joint capsule becomes stretched, and the knee develops a recurvatum deformity that is painful and can lead to arthritic degeneration of the knee. A KAFO will protect the knee and provide improved stability for walking. If there is fair (grade 3) strength in the hip flexor muscles (see Table 13–1) and passive full-knee extension, then the knee joints can be left unlocked for walking. In this case, a posteriorly offset knee joint is used to stabilize the knee, and ankle dorsiflexion is limited to minus 3 degrees of neutral dorsiflexion to provide a hyperextension moment to the knee for stability. Thus, at stance phase, the net ankle plantarflexion locks the knee in hyperextension, restrained by posterior capsular static structures.

Quadriceps muscle strength is not essential for ambulation. A strong gluteus maximus and good calf strength can substitute by keeping the knee locked in extension. If the calf strength is inadequate to control the forward motion of the tibia in mid to late stance, an AFO is needed. It is not necessary to fix the ankle in mild plantarflexion to provide knee stability, and such a position could cause a recurvatum deformity in any case. An equinus position of the foot inhibits forward momentum and limits step length by preventing body weight from rolling over the forefoot prior to contact of the contralateral extremity with the ground. When good hamstring function is present, the biceps femoris and the semitendinosus can be transferred anteriorly to the quadriceps tendon to provide dynamic knee stability.

Muscle imbalances in the foot can lead to deformity. When muscle imbalances exist, tendon releases or transfers should be considered prior to the development of fixed deformities.

Equinus contracture of the ankle is a common problem and results in genu recurvatum. Accommodating the equinus posture by using an elevated heel places excessive stress on the calf muscles to control the leg. A surgical procedure to lengthen the Achilles tendon is frequently needed to correct the equinus contracture of the ankle and to permit adequate bracing.

A cavus foot deformity causes forefoot equinus, which also limits bracing. If no fixed bony abnormalities are present, then release of the plantar fascia will be sufficient to correct the deformity. If the cavus deformity is caused by bony abnormalities, then a closing wedge osteotomy is needed. A triple arthrodesis of the hindfoot can also be used to correct deformities and provide a stable base of support.

The long-standing muscle imbalances, patterns of muscle substitution, and resulting joint and ligament strains often lead to degenerative arthritis. Total joint replacement can be performed, but several special considerations are needed. In patients with postpoliomyelitis syndrome, osteoporosis is common because of prolonged lack of muscle action on the bone. Joint contractures must be corrected at the time of surgery to prevent excessive forces on the prosthetic components because these forces might lead to loosening of the prosthesis. Weak muscles must be supported with the appropriate orthoses after surgery. The rehabilitation program will be lengthy because it will take an extended period to regain joint motion and muscle function. Continuous passive motion devices and frequent joint range of motion must be used to gain joint mobility after surgery. Because the hip joint is difficult to brace, there must be at least fair (grade 3) strength (see Table 13–1) in the hip extensors, abductors, and flexors to provide stability to the hip after surgery. Surgery can be expected to weaken the surrounding muscles, and this must be taken into account before total hip arthroplasty is undertaken to prevent chronic dislocation.

3. Upper extremities

a. Shoulders—The shoulder is important for placing the hand in the desired position for use. The shoulder is totally dependent on muscle strength for active mobility. In patients who use a wheelchair, weak muscles about the shoulder can be made more functional with the use of mobile arm supports on the wheelchair. These supports allow the patient a greater arc of motion with less muscle strength. Shoulder stability is more important in the ambulatory patient who requires upper extremity aids. A glenohumeral fusion may be helpful if the patient has sufficient strength in the scapulothoracic muscles. When the shoulder is fused, scapulothoracic motion is maintained, allowing use of the extremity for tabletop activities. Glenohumeral fusion does restrict the ability of the patient to position the hand for bathroom hygiene, so it is undesirable to perform the procedure on both shoulders.

Preservation of shoulder strength should be a priority of treatment. Rotator cuff tears are a common problem in postpolio patients. Surgical repair of the torn rotator cuff should be done when possible. In large tears that cannot be repaired, arthroscopic debridement offers significant relief of pain. Shoulder weakness is found in 95% of patients with postpoliomyelitis syndrome and correlates closely with the amount of lower extremity weakness present. Patients with weak legs will use their arms to push up from a chair and pull themselves up stairs. They also lean heavily on upper extremity aids while walking. It is therefore important to remove as many unnecessary strains from the shoulders as possible. This can be done with the use of elevated seats, motorized lift chairs, elevators or motorized stair chair glides, and optimal lower extremity bracing. In minimally ambulatory or nonambulatory patients, an electric wheelchair or motorized scooter should be prescribed to prevent excessive strain on the shoulder muscles caused by propelling a manual wheelchair.

b. Elbows—The elbow requires sufficient flexor strength to lift an object against gravity for function. A mobile arm support can maximize the effectiveness of the muscle strength for the patient. Tendon transfers, such as those involving the deltoid and biceps muscles, may also be useful in restoring active flexion.

c. Wrists and hands—Opponens paralysis is common in the hand and results in a 50% loss of hand function. A splint used during the acute and recovery phases is useful in preventing an adduction contracture. Opponens function can be restored by tendon transfer. The most common muscle transferred is the flexor digitorum superficialis of the ring finger.

Paralysis of the intrinsic muscles of the hand interferes with function. A lumbrical bar orthosis will prevent hyperextension of the metacarpophalangeal joints and allow the long extensors to extend the fingers and open the hand. Surgical capsulodesis to limit metacarpophalangeal joint extension will accomplish the same result.

Paralysis of the finger flexors and extensors can be overcome with the use of a flexor hinge orthosis if wrist extensor function is present. Tendon transfers can provide the same result, allowing the tenodesis effect to provide grasp and pinch functions.

Agre JC: The role of exercise in the patient with post-polio syndrome. Ann N Y Acad Sci 1995;753:321.

Agre JC: Symposium on post-polio syndrome. Disabil Rehabil 1996;18:305.

Allen GM et al: Quantitative assessments of elbow flexor muscle performance using twitch interpolation in post-polio patients: No evidence for deterioration. Brain 1997;120:663.

Bartfeld H et al: Relevance of the post-polio syndrome to other motor neuron diseases: Relevance to viral (enteroviral) infections. Ann N Y Acad Sci 1995;753:237.

Bartfeld H, Ma D: Recognizing post-polio syndrome. Hosp Pract (Off Ed) 1996;31:95.

Halstead LS: Post-polio syndrome. Sci Am 1998;278:42.

Kidd D et al: Late functional deterioration following paralytic poliomyelitis. QJM 1997;90:189.

Kidd D et al: Poliomyelitis. Postgrad Med J 1996;72:641.

Klein MG et al: The relationship between lower extremity strength and shoulder overuse symptoms: A model based on polio survivors. Arch Phys Med Rehabil 2000;81:789.

Klein MG et al: Changes in strength over time among polio survivors. Arch Phys Med Rehabil 2000;81:1059.

LeCompte CM: Post-polio syndrome: An update for the primary health care provider. Nurse Pract 1997;22:133.

Nolan P, Beeston P: Post-polio syndrome. The late sequelae of poliomyelitis. Aust Fam Physician 1997;26:1055.

Perry J et al: Post-polio muscle function. Birth Defects Orig Artic Ser 1987;23:315.

Perry J et al: The relationship of lower-extremity strength and gait parameters in patients with post-polio syndrome. Arch Phys Med Rehabil 1993; 74:165.

Stanghelle JK, Festvag LV: Postpolio syndrome: A 5-year follow-up. Spinal Cord 1997;35:503.

CEREBRAL PALSY (STATIC ENCEPHALOPATHY)

Cerebral palsy is a nonprogressive and nonhereditary disorder of impaired motor function. The onset may be prenatal, perinatal, or postnatal. An exact cause is not always known, but the impairment is sometimes associated with prematurity, perinatal hypoxia, cerebral trauma, or neonatal jaundice. In the United States, over 500,000 people are affected by cerebral palsy. The degree of neurologic impairment is severe in one third of patients and mild in about one sixth.

Classification

Because of the diversity of neurologic findings seen in patients with cerebral palsy, a classification system is essential. The disease can be classified by the types of movement disorder and by the patterns of neurologic deficit.

A. TYPES OF MOVEMENT DISORDER

Three types of disorder are seen.

1. Spastic disorders—These are characterized by the presence of clonus and hyperactive deep tendon reflexes. Patients with spastic movement can be helped by orthopedic intervention.

2. Dyskinetic disorders—Among the conditions classified as dyskinetic disorders are athetosis, ballismus, chorea, dystonia, and ataxia. For practical purposes, these conditions are grouped together because they are not amenable to surgical correction.

3. Mixed disorders—These usually consist of a combination of spasticity and athetosis with total body involvement.

B. PATTERNS OF NEUROLOGIC INVOLVEMENT

1. Monoplegia—With single-limb involvement, the disorder is usually spastic in nature. Because monoplegia is rare, it is advisable to test the patient before making the diagnosis. The stress of performing an activity such as running at a fast pace will often uncover spasticity in another limb.

2. Hemiplegia—Spasticity affects the upper and lower extremities ipsilaterally. Equinovarus posturing is common in the lower extremity. The upper extremity is usually held with the elbow, wrist, and fingers flexed and the thumb adducted. The major problem interfering with upper extremity function, however, is a loss of proprioception and stereognosis. Surgery for the upper extremity is aimed at making the hand assistive and at improving cosmesis. An arm that is involuntarily held in severe flexion while the patient walks can present a major social disadvantage for the patient.

3. Paraplegia—In paraplegia, neurologic deficits involve only the lower extremities. Because paraplegia is rare in patients with spastic cerebral palsy, it is important to rule out the existence of a high spinal cord lesion that could also be responsible for the neurologic findings. Bladder problems coexist with spastic paralysis that affects the lower extremities and is secondary to spinal cord damage.

4. Diplegia—Spastic diplegia is seen in 50–60% of cerebral palsy patients in the United States and is the most common neurologic pattern. It is characterized by major involvement in both lower extremities with only minor incoordination in the upper extremities. Findings in the lower extremities include marked spasticity, particularly about the hips, hyperactive deep tendon reflexes, and a positive Babinski sign. The hips are commonly held in a position of flexion, adduction, and internal rotation secondary to the spasticity. The knees are in the valgus position and may have excessive external rotation of the tibia. The ankles are held in the equinus position, with a valgus attitude of the feet. Speech and intellectual functions are usually normal or only slightly impaired. Esotropia and visual perception problems are common.

5. Total body involvement—Sometimes referred to as quadriplegia, total body involvement is characterized by impairments affecting all four extremities, the head, and the trunk. Sensory deficits are typical, and speech and swallowing are commonly impaired. Often, the most serious deficit is the inability to communicate with others. Although mental retardation is found in approximately 45% of patients, intelligence is often masked by communication dysfunction. Ambulation is not usually a goal, because the equilibrium reactions of affected patients are severely impaired or absent. Sitting may require braces or adaptive supportive devices. Scoliosis, contractures, and dislocated hips are common orthopedic problems and may interfere with sitting.

Management

Because cerebral palsy in children is discussed elsewhere (see Chapter 11), the following discussion will concentrate on the needs of the adult with cerebral palsy.

A. SPECIAL CONSIDERATIONS IN ADULT PATIENTS

1. Musculoskeletal problems—Long-standing deformities may be rigid. Bony deformities are common and may preclude surgery for soft-tissue rebalancing unless concomitant osteotomies are done. In comparison with the young patient, the adult patient has a greater body mass to support and therefore has increased energy demands. Spastic muscles are weak and are frequently further compromised by the chronic overuse of muscles to compensate for contractural deformities.

2. Mobility—The patient who can sit independently has good balance and may propel a wheelchair. It may be easier to propel the wheelchair backward, using the feet to push. A self-propped sitter may require some external support to remain erect, whereas a propped sitter needs a straight spine and flexible hips to remain erect with support.

Ambulation can be divided into four categories: community ambulation, household ambulation, physiologic ambulation (exercise), and wheelchair ambulation. A patient categorized as a community ambulator is able to maneuver independently and safely around obstacles normally encountered in the community. Orthotics or upper extremity walking aids may be required. A household ambulator is able to walk independently for short distances but requires assistance to negotiate obstacles such as stairs or curbs and requires a wheelchair for long distances. A physiologic ambulator is someone who is capable of walking for short distances with assistance or walks as a means of exercise but finds it impractical to walk for normal activities. The energy requirements for walking determine the category to which a patient belongs and also determine the types of equipment that are recommended. It is unreasonable to expect patients to expend all their energy in merely transporting themselves from one location to another.

B. TREATMENT OF PATIENTS WITH LOWER EXTREMITY PROBLEMS

1. Hips—An adduction and internal rotation deformity of the hip is sometimes seen during ambulation. Release of the hip adductor tendons (see Figure 13–13) may be needed to correct this tendency.

A crouch gait and lumbar lordosis are evidence of hip flexion deformity. In patients with cerebral palsy, gait studies with dynamic polyelectromyography (poly-EMG) have demonstrated dysphasic activity of the iliopsoas, which is the main hip flexor muscle. Gait studies with poly-EMG should be undertaken to evaluate the activity of the iliopsoas and pectineus and to aid in surgical decision making. If release of the iliopsoas is indicated, the tendon is cut distally and allowed to retract proximally to the point where it reattaches to the anterior hip capsule (Figure 13–32). Release of the pectineus muscle is often also necessary.

2. Knees—Correction of a knee flexion deformity in a patient with a crouch gait may be necessary. Attention should first be paid to the hip deformity. Weakness of the gastrocnemius and soleus muscles and inability to maintain the position of the tibia may also contribute to a crouch posture and should be considered prior to performing any knee surgery. Gait electromyograms are useful in determining which muscles are responsible for the abnormal posture. Release of the offending hamstring tendons (see Figure 13–15) or hamstring lengthening may be useful.

3. Feet—Equinus posturing of the ankle is common. If no fixed contracture is present, an AFO will control the position of the foot. If the deformity is the result of an equinus contracture, Achilles tendon lengthening (see Figure 13–16) should be performed to bring the foot to a neutral position. The foot should be held in a short leg walking cast for 6 weeks following surgery. An AFO is then used to maintain the position of the foot and support the tibia during walking.

Equinovarus posturing of the ankle is also common. Although the anterior tibial muscle is the primary varus

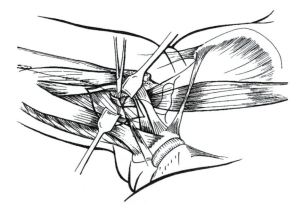

Figure 13–32. Release of the iliopsoas tendon from its insertion on the lesser trochanter of the femur to correct a hip flexion deformity. (Illustration by Anthony C Berlet. Reproduced, with permission, from Keenan MAE et al: *Manual of Orthopaedic Surgery for Spasticity*. New York: Raven, 1993.)

force in patients with stroke or traumatic brain injuries, it is equally likely that the posterior tibial muscle may be causing equinovarus posturing in patients with cerebral palsy. Therefore, in order to find the cause and make the correct decision concerning surgery, it is important to make dynamic EMG recordings while the patient walks.

If the anterior tibial muscle is overactive, Achilles tendon lengthening should be accompanied by a split anterior tibial tendon transfer (see Figure 13–18). If the posterior tibial muscle is overactive, it is advisable to lengthen the posterior tendon. If the EMG studies show that the posterior tibial muscle is active only during the swing phase of gait, then it may be more logical to transfer the posterior tendon through the interosseous membrane to the dorsum of the foot, rather than performing a split anterior tibial tendon transfer. After surgery is performed, a short leg cast that allows weight bearing is worn for 6 weeks, and the leg is then supported with an AFO. If hallux valgus subsequently develops, management consists of correcting the subtalar deformity and realigning the first digital ray.

A pes cavus deformity of the foot is occasionally seen in patients with spasticity of the intrinsic muscles. If the problem is detected early, it can be corrected by plantar fasciotomy and release of the flexor origins from the os calcis. If the problem has been detected late and a concomitant bony deformity is present, a wedge osteotomy of the midtarsal bones should be performed.

C. Treatment of Patients with Upper Extremity Problems

Function of the upper extremities is dependent on a variety of factors, including cognition, intact sensation, and the ability to place the hand in space. The amount of spasticity present will also affect the ability to control movement of the arm and hand. Surgery can influence hand placement and modify spasticity, but a successful outcome requires the ability to cooperate with postoperative therapy programs. Mental impairment, motion disorders, and poor sensation are relative contraindications to surgery in the functional arm and hand.

1. The functional upper extremity—In patients with problems involving the functional hand, treatment begins with careful clinical evaluation of motor and sensory deficits. Dynamic EMG is extremely useful in determining which muscles should be lengthened or transferred to improve function. The least severely involved hands exhibit a minor degree of spasticity in the flexor carpi ulnaris and a resulting mild flexion deformity of the wrist. In this case, all that is required to improve hand function and position is surgical lengthening of the flexor carpi ulnaris tendon.

In some patients, release of objects from the hand is a problem. In this case, the synergistic action of the finger extensors and wrist flexors causes difficulty with finger extension when the wrist is extended. This resembles the tenodesis effect seen in paralytic hands, but the mechanism is a dynamic one. Selective lengthening of the overactive finger flexors (see Figure 13–23) will improve hand function.

Transfer of a wrist flexor to a wrist extensor should be done with caution. Often a patient flexes the wrist to adjust the dynamic balance between the finger flexors and extensors. Holding the wrist in extension can rob the patient of this important method of compensation.

The thumb-in-palm deformity is treated by proximal release of the thenar muscles (see Figure 13–24) and lengthening of the flexor pollicis longus tendon. Distal release of the thenar muscles is not recommended because it may cause a hyperextension deformity of the metacarpophalangeal joint of the thumb.

2. The nonfunctional upper extremity—Surgery may be indicated in the nonfunctional upper extremity to prevent skin breakdown, to improve hygiene or cosmesis, or to make dressing easier. The problems of shoulder contracture and elbow contracture are discussed in the section on stroke, and the surgical procedures used in their treatment are shown in Figures 13–20 and 13–21. Patients who have a flexed wrist with flexed fingers and a thumb-in-palm deformity should be treated because severe wrist flexion can cause median nerve compression against the proximal edge of the transverse carpal ligament. An arthrodesis of the wrist in neutral position, combined with a superficialis-to-profundus tendon transfer (see Figure 13-22), will reliably correct the wrist deformity and also improve skin care. Management of the thumb deformity consists of lengthening the flexor pollicis longus tendon, fusing the interphalangeal joint, and performing a proximal release of the thenar muscles (see Figure 13–24).

D. Treatment of Patients with Total Body Involvement

These patients are rarely functional ambulators, although they may transfer from one position to another either independently or with assistance. They frequently have a combination of spasticity and motion disorders such as athetosis, and they spend most of their time in a chair. Flexible hips and a straight spine are needed for functional sitting.

Occasionally, knee flexion deformities require distal hamstring release or lengthening to allow for greater flexibility in positioning the patient. Rigid extension contractures of the knee are sometimes seen and will interfere with sitting tolerance. Lengthening of the quadriceps tendon (Figure 13–33) will allow the knee to flex.

Foot deformities in the spastic patient are extremely common and require treatment to allow shoe wear and to prevent skin breakdown. Sitting balance is improved when the feet can be positioned on the leg support of a wheelchair.

The spine is of major concern in patients with total body involvement because scoliosis is common. Adaptive seating or orthotics are useful in supporting the spine and helping the patient maintain an erect posture while seated. Spinal fusion with instrumentation is indicated for treatment of progressive scoliosis. Obliquity of the pelvis greatly interferes with sitting. When this problem is present, fusion should include the sacrum.

Buckon CE et al: Assessment of upper-extremity function in children with spastic diplegia before and after selective dorsal rhizotomy. Dev Med Child Neurol 1996;38:967.

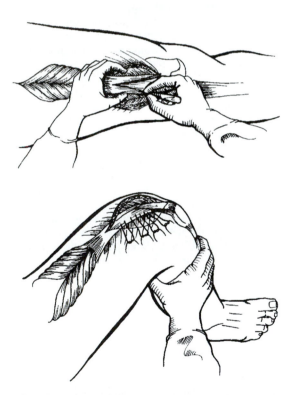

Figure 13–33. The dV-Y incision (*top*) and lengthening (*bottom*) of the quadriceps tendon to correct a rigid extension contracture of the knee and allow improved sitting. (Illustration by Anthony C Berlet. Reproduced, with permission, from Keenan MAE et al: *Manual of Orthopaedic Surgery for Spasticity*. New York: Raven, 1993.)

Chambers H et al: Prediction of outcome after rectus femoris surgery in cerebral palsy: The role of cocontraction of the rectus femoris and vastus lateralis. J Pediatr Orthop 1998; 18:703.

Dahlin LB et al: Surgery of the spastic hand in cerebral palsy. Improvement in stereognosis and hand function after surgery. J Hand Surg Br 1998;23:334.

O'Byrne JM et al: Split tibialis posterior tendon transfer in the treatment of spastic equinovarus foot. J Pediatr Orthop 1997; 17:481.

Rawlins P: Patient management of cerebral origin spasticity with intrathecal baclofen. J Neurosci Nurs 1998;30:32.

Roberts A, Evans GA: Orthopedic aspects of neuromuscular disorders in children. Curr Opin Pediatr 1993;5:379.

Vogt JC: Split anterior tibial transfer for spastic equinovarus foot deformity: Retrospective study of 73 operated feet. J Foot Ankle Surg 1998;37:2.

Waters PM, Van Heest A: Spastic hemiplegia of the upper extremity in children. Hand Clin 1998;14:119.

NEUROMUSCULAR DISORDERS

The neuromuscular disorders represent a diverse group of chronic diseases characterized by the progressive degeneration of skeletal musculature, which results in weakness, atrophy, joint contractures, and increasing disability. These disorders are best classified as motor unit diseases because the primary abnormality may involve the motor neuron, the neuromuscular junction, or the muscle fiber. Two broad categories are considered. Myopathies are diseases of the muscle fibers. Neuropathies are disorders in which muscle degeneration is seen secondary to lower motor neuron disease. Most of the neuromuscular disorders are hereditary (Table 13–7), although point mutations may result in spontaneous cases. Early diagnosis is important not only for initiation of appropriate therapy but also for genetic counseling. Treatment programs are aimed at symptomatic and supportive care. Appropriate orthopedic intervention can significantly increase the functional capacity of patients with neuromuscular disorders.

Diagnosis

A. History and Physical Examination

A careful genetic history is important. The clinical history and physical examination will delineate the onset and pattern of muscle involvement. Neuropathies generally present with distal involvement. Muscle fasciculation and spasticity are common, and muscle atrophy is in excess of the weakness. Myopathies usually display weakness of the proximal limb musculature initially. Fasciculations and spasticity are not seen. The weakness is more pronounced than the atrophy. Disorders of neuromuscular transmission, such as myasthenia gravis, present with fatigue and ptosis.

Table 13–7. Classification of the more commonly encountered neuromuscular disorders.

Disorder	Inherited	Creatine Phospho-kinase Level	Electromyo-graphic Pattern	Nerve Conduction	Biopsy Pattern
Muscular dystrophies					
Duchenne (pseudohypertrophic) type	Yes	Markedly elevated	Myopathic	Normal	Myopathic
Facioscapulohumeral type	Yes	Normal or elevated	Myopathic	Normal	Myopathic
Limb-girdle type	Yes	Elevated	Myopathic	Normal	Myopathic
Spinal muscular atrophy					
Werding-Hoffmann and Kugelberg-Welander types	Yes	Normal or slightly elevated	Neuropathic	Normal	Neuropathic
Hereditary motor and sensory neuropathies					
Type I (Charcot-Marie-Tooth disease)	Yes	Normal	Neuropathic	Markedly decreased	Neuropathic
Type II	Yes	Normal	Neuropathic	Decreased or normal	Neuropathic
Type III	Yes	Normal	Neuropathic	Decreased	Neuropathic
Type IV	Yes	Normal	Neuropathic		Neuropathic
Type V	Yes	Normal	Neuropathic	Normal	Neuropathic
Myopathies					
Central core, nemaline, minicore, mitochondrial, myotubular, and other types	Often	Often normal	Normal or mildly myopathic	Usually normal	Myopathic
Poliomyelitis	No		Neuropathic	Normal	Neuropathic
Guillain-Barré syndrome	No	Normal	Neuropathic	Slow in acute phase	Neuropathic
Polymyositis	No	Normal or elevated	Myopathic	Normal	Myopathic
Myotonic diseases	Usually	Usually normal	Diagnostic	Normal	
Myasthenia gravis	Sometimes		Diagnostic		

Data compiled by Irene Gilgoff, MD, Rancho Los Amigos Medical Center, Downey, CA.

B. MUSCLE ENZYME STUDIES

Serum levels of muscle enzymes are elevated in myopathies but normal in neuropathies. The enzymes studied include creatine phosphokinase (CPK), lactate dehydrogenase (LDH), aldolase, aspartate aminotransferase (AST, SGOT), and alanine aminotransferase (ALT, SGPT). CPK levels are the most elevated in the Duchenne type of muscular dystrophy and less elevated in the more slowly progressive disease forms. In Duchenne type muscular dystrophy, the highest enzyme levels are seen at birth and during the first few years of life, before the disease is clinically apparent. As the disease progresses and the muscle mass deteriorates, the enzyme levels will decrease.

C. ELECTROMYOGRAPHY AND NERVE CONDUCTION STUDIES

EMG and nerve conduction studies will differentiate between primary muscle diseases and neuropathies (see Table 13–7). EMG is useful in differentiating between muscle diseases, peripheral nerve disorders, and anterior horn cell abnormalities. A myopathic pattern on EMG is characterized by (1) increased frequency, (2) decreased duration, and (3) decreased amplitude of action potentials. In addition, increased insertional activity, short polyphasic potentials, and a retained interference pattern are evident. A neuropathic pattern on EMG is characterized by the opposite constellation of findings: (1) decreased frequency, (2) increased duration, and (3) increased amplitude of action potentials. In addition, frequent fibrillation potentials, a group polyphasic potential, and a decreased interference pattern can be seen. In myasthenia gravis and the myotonic diseases, the patterns on EMG are diagnostic. In myasthenia gravis, the fatigue phenomenon is exhibited. In myotonia, the EMG is characterized by positive waves and trains of potentials that fire at high frequency and then wax and wane until they slowly disappear.

D. MUSCLE BIOPSY

To gain the maximal amount of information from muscle biopsy, the clinician should choose a muscle that has mild to moderate involvement and has not been recently traumatized by electrodes during EMG. Muscle biopsy can be used to differentiate myopathy, neuropathy, and inflammatory myopathy. The biopsy, however, cannot be used to determine prognosis. Histochemical staining will further distinguish the congenital forms of myopathy.

Histologically, myopathies are characterized by muscle fiber necrosis, fatty degeneration, proliferation of the connective tissue, and an increased number of nuclei, some of which have migrated from their normal peripheral position to the center of the muscle fiber.

Neuropathies display small, angulated muscle fibers. Bundles of atrophic fibers are intermingled with bundles of normal fibers. There is no increase in the amount of connective tissue.

Biopsy findings in polymyositis include prominent collections of inflammatory cells, edema of the tissues, perivasculitis, and segmental necrosis with a mixed pattern of fiber degeneration and regeneration.

Dietz FR, Mathews KD: Update on the genetic bases of disorders with orthopaedic manifestations. J Bone Joint Surg 1996; 78:1583.

Esquenazi A et al: Dynamic polyelectromyography, neurolysis, and chemodenervation with Botulinum toxin A for assessment and treatment of gait dysfunction. In Ruzicka E et al, eds: *Advances in Neurology: Gait Disorders,* Vol 87 Lippincott Williams & Wilkins: Philadelphia;2001:321.

Roberts A, Evans GA: Orthopedic aspects of neuromuscular disorders in children. Curr Opin Pediatr 1993;5:379.

1. Duchenne-Type Muscular Dystrophy

Duchenne-type muscular dystrophy, which is also called **pseudohypertrophic muscular dystrophy,** is a progressive disease that affects males. It is inherited in an X-linked recessive manner and has its onset in early childhood. Generally, affected children have had a normal birth and developmental history. But by the time they reach 3–5 years of age, sufficient muscle mass has been lost to impair function.

Clinical Findings

Early signs of disease include pseudohypertrophy of the calf, which is the result of the increase in connective tissue; planovalgus deformity of the feet, which is secondary to heel cord contracture; and proximal muscle weakness. Muscle weakness in the hips may be exhibited by Gower's sign, in which the patient uses the arms to support the trunk while attempting to rise from the floor. Other signs are hesitance when climbing stairs, acceleration during the final stage of sitting, and shoulder weakness.

Weakness and contractures prevent independent ambulation in approximately 45% of patients by the age of 9 years and in the remainder by the age of 12 years. It is common for patients to have difficulty first in rising from the floor, next in ascending the stairs, and then in walking. Cardiac involvement is seen in 80% of patients. Findings generally include posterobasal fibrosis of the ventricle and electrocardiographic changes. In patients with a decreased level of activity, clinical evidence of cardiomyopathy may not be obvious. Pulmonary problems are common in the advanced stages of the disease and are found during periodic evaluations of pulmonary function. Mental retardation, which has been noted in 30–50% of patients, is present from birth and is not progressive.

Management

Efforts are made to keep patients ambulating for as many years as possible to prevent the complications of obesity, osteoporosis, and scoliosis. The hip flexors, tensor fasciae latae, and triceps surae develop ambulation-limiting contractures. With progressive weakness and contractures, the base of support decreases and the patient cannot use normal mechanisms to maintain upright balance. The patient walks with a wide-based gait, hips flexed and abducted, knees flexed, and the feet in equinus and varus position. Lumbar lordosis becomes exaggerated to compensate for the hip flexion contractures and weak hip extensor musculature.

Equinus contractures of the Achilles tendon occur early and are caused by the muscle imbalance between the calf and pretibial muscles. Initially, this problem can be managed by heel cord stretching exercises and night splints. A KAFO may be needed to control foot position and substitute for weak quadriceps muscles. Stretching exercises and pronation can be employed to treat early hip flexion contractures.

Surgical intervention is directed toward the release of ambulation-limiting contractures. Early postoperative mobilization is important to prevent further muscle weakness. Anesthetic risks are increased in these patients because of their limited pulmonary reserve and because the incidence of malignant hyperthermia is higher than normal in patients with muscle disease.

The triceps surae and tibialis posterior are the strongest muscles in the lower extremity of the patient with muscular dystrophy. These muscles are responsible for equinus and varus deformities. Management that consists of releasing the contracted tensor fasciae latae, lengthening the Achilles tendon, and transferring the tibialis posterior muscle anteriorly is indicated and will prolong walking for approximately 3 years. Postoperative bracing is required.

Scoliosis is common in nonambulatory patients confined to a wheelchair. Adaptive seating devices that hold the pelvis level and the spine erect are useful in preventing deformity. Alternatively, a rigid plastic spinal torso orthosis may be used for support. When external support is not effective, scoliosis develops rapidly. Spinal fusion is occasionally indicated. Blood loss during surgery is high, and the incidence of pseudarthrosis is increased. Postoperative immobilization is to be avoided; therefore, segmental spinal stabilization is often the preferred technique of internal stabilization.

Fractures in patients with myopathies occur secondary to osteoporosis from the inactivity and the loss of muscle tension. No abnormalities of bone mineralization are present. The incidence of fracture increases with the severity of the disease. Most fractures are metaphyseal in location, show little displacement, cause minimal pain, and heal in the expected time without complication.

Bach JR, McKeon J: Orthopedic surgery and rehabilitation for the prolongation of brace-free ambulation of patients with Duchenne muscular dystrophy. Am J Phys Med Rehabil 1991;70:323.

Bentley G et al: The treatment of scoliosis in muscular dystrophy using modified Luque and Harrington-Luque instrumentation. J Bone Joint Surg (Br) 2001;83:22.

Birch JG: Orthopedic management of neuromuscular disorders in children. Semin Pediatr Neurol 1998;5:78.

Botte MJ et al: Heterotopic ossification in neuromuscular disorders. Orthopedics 1997;20:335.

Brook PD et al: Spinal fusion in Duchenne's muscular dystrophy. J Pediatr Orthop 1996;16:324.

Dietz FR, Mathews KD: Update on the genetic bases of disorders with orthopaedic manifestations. J Bone Joint Surg Am 1996; 78:1583.

Forst R, Forst J: Importance of lower limb surgery in Duchenne muscular dystrophy. Arch Orthop Trauma Surg 1995; 114:106.

Fox HJ et al: Spinal instrumentation for Duchenne's muscular dystrophy: Experience of hypotensive anaesthesia to minimize blood loss [see comments]. J Pediatr Orthop 1997;17:750.

Goertzen M et al: Clinical results of early orthopaedic management in Duchenne muscular dystrophy. Neuropediatrics 1995; 26:257.

Hsu JD: Orthopedic approaches for the treatment of lower-extremity contractures in the Duchenne muscular dystrophy patient in the United States and Canada. Semin Neurol 1995;15:6.

Hsu JD, Furumasu J: Gait and posture changes in the Duchenne muscular dystrophy child. Clin Orthop 1993; 288:122.

Ramirez N et al: Complications after posterior spinal fusion in Duchenne's muscular dystrophy. J Pediatr Orthop 1997; 17:109.

Roberts A, Evans GA: Orthopedic aspects of neuromuscular disorders in children. Curr Opin Pediatr 1993;5:379.

Yamashita T et al: Prediction of progression of spinal deformity in Duchenne muscular dystrophy: a preliminary report. Spine 2001;26:E223.

2. Spinal Muscular Atrophy

Spinal muscular atrophy is a neuropathic disorder in which fewer anterior horn cells are present in the spinal cord congenitally. The severe infantile form of the disease is called **Werdnig-Hoffmann paralysis.** The disorder is inherited in an autosomal-recessive pattern.

About 20% of patients with spinal muscular atrophy are ambulatory, and 1% are totally dependent. Fractures are common in these patients and occur secondary to decreased mobility and function.

The goal of orthopedic intervention is to prevent collapse of the spine and contractures. Orthotic support is often needed to stabilize the spine. In the nonambulatory patient, adaptive seating devices or orthotics may be used. If collapse of the spine occurs, spinal fusion is indicated.

Bentley G et al: The treatment of scoliosis in muscular dystrophy using modified Luque and Harrington-Luque instrumentation. J Bone Joint Surg (Br) 2001;83:22.

Birch JG: Orthopedic management of neuromuscular disorders in children. Semin Pediatr Neurol 1998;5:78.

Biros I, Forrest S: Spinal muscular atrophy: Untangling the knot? J Med Genet 1999;36:1.

Noordeen MH et al: Blood loss in Duchenne muscular dystrophy: Vascular smooth muscle dysfunction? J Pediatr Orthop B 2001;8:212.

Stewart H et al: Molecular diagnosis of spinal muscular atrophy. Arch Dis Child 1998;78:531.

3. Charcot-Marie-Tooth Disease

Charcot-Marie-Tooth disease is the most common of the hereditary degenerative myopathies. It is generally inherited in an autosomal-dominant pattern. EMG studies show a neuropathic pattern, and the nerve conduction velocity of the involved nerves is markedly decreased. Muscle enzyme levels are normal. Clinical onset of the disease is between the ages of 5 and 15 years.

The peroneal muscles are affected early in the course of the disease. For this reason, Charcot-Marie-Tooth disease is sometimes referred to as **progressive peroneal muscular atrophy.** The intrinsic muscles of the feet and hands are affected later. Patients usually present with progressive clawtoe and cavus deformities of the feet. In the skeletally immature patient, release of the plantar fascia is done to correct the cavus deformity. This is often combined with transfer of the extensor digitorum longus tendon to the neck of the metatarsal and fusion of the proximal interphalangeal joints of the toes to correct the clawtoe deformities. If the tibialis posterior muscle is active during swing phase, then it can be transferred through the interosseous membrane to the lateral cuneiform bone. Triple arthrodesis is often necessary in the adult to correct the deformity.

The "intrinsic minus" hand deformity causes difficulty in grasping objects. An orthosis with a lumbrical bar to hold the metacarpophalangeal joints flexed will improve hand use. A capsulodesis of the volar portion of the metacarpophalangeal joints will accomplish the same objective. To restore active intrinsic muscle function in the hand, the flexor digitorum superficialis tendon of the ring finger can be divided into four slips and transferred through the lumbrical passages to the proximal phalanx.

Aktas S, Sussman MD: The radiological analysis of pes cavus deformity in Charcot Marie Tooth disease. J Pediatr Orthop B 2000;9:137.

Birch JG: Orthopedic management of neuromuscular disorders in children. Semin Pediatr Neurol 1998;5:78.

Borg K, Ericson-Gripenstedt U: Muscle biopsy abnormalities differ between Charcot-Marie-Tooth type 1 and 2: reflect different pathophysiology? Exerc Sport Sci Rev 2002;30:4.

Guyton GP, Mann RA: The pathogenesis and surgical management of foot deformity in Charcot-Marie-Tooth disease. Foot Ankle Clin 2000;5:317.

Holmes JR, Hansen ST Jr: Foot and ankle manifestations of Charcot-Marie-Tooth disease. Foot Ankle 1993;14:476.

Mann DC, Hsu JD: Triple arthrodesis in the treatment of fixed cavovarus deformity in adolescent patients with Charcot-Marie-Tooth disease. Foot Ankle 1992;13:1.

Martel J et al: Charcot-Marie-Tooth disease. J Manipulative Physiol Ther 1995;18:168.

Smith AG: Charcot-Marie-Tooth disease. Arch Neurol 2001;58:1014.

Sturtz F et al: Hereditary motor and sensory neuropathy of Charcot-Marie-Tooth disease. Arch Pediatr 1995;2:70.

Wood VE et al: Treatment of the upper limb in Charcot-Marie-Tooth disease. J Hand Surg Br 1995;20:511.

BURNS

More than 2 million people sustain burns of sufficient severity each year in the United States to require medical attention. Of these, 50,000 individuals remain hospitalized for more than 2 months, attesting to the serious nature of their injuries.

Thermal burns affect the skin most directly but can also involve the underlying muscles, tendons, joints, and bones. Scar contractures cause the greatest limitation to later function and the greatest deformity. Rehabilitation efforts ideally should begin when the patient first enters the hospital, immediately following acute resuscitation and continuing through the reconstruction process.

Classification

Burn wounds are traditionally classified as first-, second-, or third-degree, depending on the depth of the damage. Currently, it is thought to be more useful to simply divide burns into two categories: partial-thickness (involving part of the dermis) and full-thickness (involving the entire dermis).

First-degree burns damage only the epidermis. They cause erythema, minor edema, and pain. The skin surface remains intact, and healing occurs uneventfully in 5–10 days, without residual scar formation.

Second-degree burns involve the epidermis and a variable amount of the underlying corium. The depth of damage to the corium determines the outcome of healing. In the more superficial second-degree burns, blister formation is prominent and occurs secondary to the osmotic gradient formed by particles in the vesicle fluid. Superficial second-degree burns heal in 10–14 days, with minimal scarring. Deep dermal burns are characterized by either a reddish appearance or by the presence of a white tissue that is barely perceptible and adheres to the underlying viable dermis. These wounds may advance to a full-thickness loss if infection occurs. They heal with a fragile epithelial covering. Healing occurs over 25–30 days, and dense scar formation is common.

Third-degree burns are full-thickness injuries that damage the epidermis and the entire corium. Because of the loss of pain receptors, which are normally found within the corium, pain is absent. The burns have a thick leathery surface of dead tissue.

Management

A. TECHNIQUES FOR MAINTAINING FUNCTIONAL POSITION

Burn scars contract and become rigid, so it is critical to maintain the head, trunk, and extremities in a functional position. Contractures, if allowed to form, will severely limit later function. The location of the burns will determine which techniques are useful in preventing deformity.

To prevent deformities of the neck and jaw in patients with burns of the neck or upper torso, molded splints should be applied early to maintain the head and neck in a neutral position or in slight extension. Patients with burns in the shoulder region are at risk for contractures characterized by a protracted scapula with an adducted arm. Placing a roll between the scapulae and providing support with a firm mattress will help prevent scapula protraction. To keep the arms abducted 75–80 degrees and the shoulder flexed 20–30 degrees, axillary foam pads are used and can be held in position with a figure-of-eight wrapping. This will maintain the glenohumeral joint in a functional position. Untreated contractures not only limit limb motion but also can result in joint subluxation from extremes in positioning.

When the burns involve the torso, the goal is to maintain a straight spine in the face of contracting scar tissue. Burns involving only one side of the trunk sometimes result in scoliosis. This should be corrected by scar excision and splinting. If left uncorrected, the scoliosis will become structural, with resultant bony changes. Burns in the groin area tend to cause flexion and adduction contractures of the hip. To prevent this, the patient should be positioned with the hips extended and in 15–20 degrees of abduction. If the patient is lying on a soft mattress, mild flexion deformities of the hips may be masked. Daily pronation is useful in maintaining the extension range of the hips.

Regardless of the location of burn wounds on the extremities, the knees and elbows tend to develop flexion contractures. Custom-molded thermoplastic splints can be applied over dressings or skin grafts to maintain the extremities in extension. The splints should be removable to allow for daily wound care. Burns in the ankle area result in equinus contractures with inversion of the foot. Splints can be used here also to maintain the foot in a neutral position, but care must be taken to ensure that the splint is holding the foot adequately and not merely obscuring a deformity. Custom-molded splints applied to the anterior and posterior surfaces in a clamshell fashion are more effective in maintaining the desired position. They also will assist in the control of edema and can be removed for wound care and motion exercises. Burns on the dorsum of the foot cause hyperextension deformities of the toes. Early grafting and toe traction are useful.

Burns of the hands present special problems. Scar contracture results in a flexion deformity of the wrist and a clawhand position similar to that seen with loss of the intrinsic musculature. The hand should be splinted with the wrist in neutral or in a slightly extended position. The metacarpophalangeal joints should be flexed 60–75 degrees and the interphalangeal joints extended. The thumb should be held with the metacarpal in abduction and flexion, the metacarpophalangeal joint in mild flexion, and the interphalangeal joint in the extended position.

B. Skeletal Traction and External Suspension

In patients with circumferential burns on an extremity, the use of skeletal traction or external fixators and suspension is efficacious and has several advantages. It permits access to all surfaces, elevates the limb to decrease edema, and maintains the extremity in the desired position while allowing joint motion. Traction can be used to correct contractures. In addition, traction still allows for daily hydrotherapy. Generally, traction is only employed for a 2-week period because longer use may result in a pin tract infection with formation of sequestra.

Special splints have been fabricated for use in the hand. The traction frame is secured proximally with a pin inserted through the distal radius. Pins are also placed through the distal phalanges of the fingers and thumb by drilling through the nail bed from the dorsal to the volar surface. Traction is applied to the fingers in the desired direction by attaching rubber bands from the distal pins to the outrigger frame. The frame can be modified for use in the foot to apply traction to the toes. In this case, the traction frame is secured proximally with a pin inserted through the calcaneus.

C. Pressure Dressings

Consistent pressure of 25 torr applied evenly aids in the prevention of hypertrophic scar formation and contracture. Elastic wraps applied over splints are used early after the injury and following grafting because they can be adjusted for changes in the amount of edema present. Later, when the amount of swelling shows little fluctuation, custom elastic garments are employed. Pressure must be continued for as long as the scar tissue is biologically active. When the skin is soft and flat and has returned to normal color, the pressure can be discontinued. Pressure dressings should be employed for a minimum of 6 months and may be necessary for as long as a year. The daily application of lanolin will relieve dryness of grafted skin or will substitute for the loss of sebaceous gland secretions in deep burns.

D. Mobilization

Early motion is desirable for burned and uninvolved extremities. Splints should be removed frequently to allow for range-of-motion exercises. If the patient is being treated with skeletal traction, motion exercises can be performed on the extremities. If the patient is receiving hydrotherapy for the burn wounds, the motion exercises will be facilitated with the extremities supported in the fluid environment.

Patients with burns of the lower extremities can begin to stand or walk before skin grafts are performed, provided that the legs are wrapped with elastic supports to control edema. Ambulation should be resumed after skin grafting as soon as the grafts are stable. Early mobilization not only preserves joint motion but also decreases the incidence of sequelae such as osteoporosis, physiologic deconditioning, muscle atrophy, and heterotopic ossification.

E. TREATMENT OF SPECIAL PROBLEMS

1. Fractures—If fractures occurred at the time of the burn, they can be treated with the use of skeletal traction or external supports such as splints. Diagnosis may be delayed if the fractures have not resulted in any obvious deformity. If fractures occur secondary to disuse osteoporosis, they are usually minimally displaced and heal uneventfully. Pathologic fractures are less common with early mobilization.

2. Osteomyelitis—Osteomyelitis is not a common complication, despite the high incidence of sepsis associated with burns. Prolonged exposure of bone sometimes results in the formation of a tangential sequestrum in the devitalized cortex. Exposed bone surfaces can be drilled to promote the formation of a granulation tissue bed for skin grafting without an increased risk of infection. The prolonged use of pins for skeletal traction causes infection in 5% of patients who require traction. The use of threaded traction pins will minimize the motion of the pin in the bone. Pins should be removed as soon as possible.

3. Exposed joints—Children and adolescents with exposed joint surfaces may retain some function after healing, but adults often develop joint ankylosis or deformities that require arthrodesis at a later date. To maintain the joint in the desired position, traction can be used. The joint should be irrigated with hypochlorite solution daily and debrided as necessary. The exposed bone surfaces can be drilled to promote the formation of granulation tissue. When the bed of tissue covers the joint, skin grafting is performed.

4. Heterotopic ossification—Periarticular bone formation is seen in 2–3% of patients with severe burns. Although the cause is unknown, predisposing factors include full-thickness burns involving more than 30% of the body surface, prolonged immobilization, and superimposed trauma. The location of the heterotopic bone is not determined by the distribution of the burns. Ossification can occur in any of the major joints. In adults, the elbow is the joint most frequently affected, while the hip is rarely affected. In children, the hip and elbow are common sites, while the shoulder is an uncommon site.

Heterotopic bone can continue to form as long as open granulating wounds are present. If joint ankylosis does not occur, the ossification will gradually diminish after the burns have healed. In children, it may disappear completely. If joint ankylosis occurs, surgical resection is indicated and will usually restore a functional arc of motion, particularly when the heterotopic bone is in a single plane and the articular surface has not been violated. When the heterotopic bone is present in multiple planes, the problem may recur after resection. Early mobilization of patients with burns will decrease the incidence and severity of heterotopic ossification.

Goldberg DP et al: Reconstruction of the burned foot. Clin Plast Surg 2000;27:145.

James J: The treatment of severe burns of head, hands and feet. Trop Doct 2001;31:178.

Johnson CL, Cain VJ: Burn care. The rehab guide. Am J Nurs 1985;85:48.

Judkins K, Pike H: Prevention and rehabilitation: The community faces of burn care. Burns 1998;24:594.

Kane RL et al: Functional outcomes of posthospital care for stroke and hip fracture patients under Medicare. J Am Geriatr Soc 1998;46:1525.

Khorram-Sefat R et al: Long-term measurements of energy expenditure in severe burn injury. World J Surg 1999;23:115.

Luce EA: The acute and subacute management of the burned hand. Clin Plast Surg 2000;27:49.

Prakash V, Bajaj SP: A new concept for the treatment of postburn contracture of the elbow. Ann Plast Surg 2000;45:339.

Silverberg R et al: Gait variables of patients after lower extremity burn injuries. J Burn Care Rehabil 2000;21:259.

Smith MA et al: Burns of the hand upper limb-a review. Burns 1998;24:493.

Staley M et al: Return to school as an outcome measure after a burn injury. J Burn Care Rehabil 1999;20:91.

Tilley W et al: Rehabilitation of the burned upper extremity. Hand Clin 2000;16:303.

Torburn L: Principles of rehabilitation. Prim Care 1996;23:335.

Subject Index

NOTE: Page numbers in **boldface** type indicate a major discussion. A *t* following a page number indicates tabular material, and an *f* following a page number indicates a figure. Drugs are listed under their generic names. When a drug trade name is listed, the reader is referred to the generic name.